Inflammatory Bowel Disease:
From Bench to Bedside

2nd Edition

Inflammatory Bowel Disease: From Bench to Bedside
2nd Edition

Edited by

Stephan R. Targan
Cedars-Sinai IBD Center, Los Angeles, CA, USA

Fergus Shanahan
Cork University Hospital, Cork, Ireland

Loren C. Karp
Cedars-Sinai IBD Center, Los Angeles, CA, USA

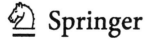 Springer

Library of Congress Cataloging-in-Publication Data

Inflammatory bowel disease : from bench to bedside / edited by Stephan R. Targan,
Fergus Shanahan, and Loren C. Karp-2nd ed.
    p. ; cm.
  Includes bibliographical references and index.

   1.Inflammatory bowel diseases. 1. Targan, Stephan R. II. Shanahan, Fergus. III. Karp, Loren C.
  [DNLM: 1. Inflammatory Bowel Diseases. WI 420 14237 2002]

ISBN 1-4020-0713-2 (HC)   ISBN – 10   0-387-25807-8 (SC)   E-ISBN 0-387-25808-6
                              ISBN – 13   978-0387-25807-2   E-ISBN 978-0387-25808-9

Printed on acid-free paper.

First softcover printing, 2005

9 8 7 6 5 4 3 2

springer.com

Preface

Why A Second Edition?

The pace of research in inflammatory bowel diseases has accelerated over the last decade, with a particularly rapid sprint occurring as we approached the new millennium. Advances in basic and technologic research have enabled scientists to examine the inflammatory process at the cellular and molecular levels. The powerful research tools of the current biotech and genotech era are now being applied successfully to inflammatory bowel disease research. Although there are many unanswered questions, today as before, the pathogenesis of inflammatory bowel disease can now be discussed at an increasingly fundamental level. Today, new therapeutic strategies are based on understanding of pathophysiology and are no longer introduced merely on an empiric basis. Many hitherto unexplained features of inflammatory bowel diseases can be accounted for because of improvements in understanding of the immune and inflammatory responses in the gut.

Like the first edition of *Inflammatory Bowel Diseases: From Bench to Bedside*, this book is intended to be more than a comprehensive compilation of reviews by individual authors on different aspects of these disorders. It is intended that the individual chapters be components of a coherent, albeit detailed, story of the local and systemic pathophysiology of intestinal inflammation, with a well-reasoned series of management strategies. Our goal was not only to produce a standard reference text, but also to present research advances and current concepts of etiopathogenesis in the context of what is already known of the clinicopathologic features of these disorders. Our vision was to have a book that would blend recent advances in the basic and clinical sciences as they relate to inflammatory bowel disease. It is our hope that that the book will illustrate the effectiveness of a team approach of basic scientists and clinician investigators in the field of inflammatory bowel disease. The book will give the reader a glimpse of where the field is moving and an idea of likely research directions in the future. Of course, it is our personal wish that this book will stimulate ideas for future research.

In early 1994, when the first edition of *Inflammatory Bowel Diseases: From Bench to Bedside*, was released, our introductory pages included predictions and considerations for the future of management of these disorders, as follows: (1) heterogeneity and the 'reagent grade' patient; (2) combination drug therapy rather than a stepwise progression; (3) emphasis on intestinal immunophysiology; (4) mucosa-specific rather than systemic immunomodulation; and (5) focus on factors promoting healing and remission rather than relapse. Each of these concepts has been validated and extended in the ensuing years, and are now the very foundation of current laboratory and clinical research on the inflammatory bowel diseases.

In addition, we posed three questions related to the predictions that we felt fundamental to research both at the bench and at the bedside. Perhaps the single most important technological advance toward answering these questions has been the application of molecular technology to the creation of a new society of colitic animal models, from which to learn about human disease. With the use of such models much progress has been made on first question, "Are Crohn's disease and ulcerative colitis different expressions of the same disease or are they discrete entities?" Based on numerous factors, including genetic associations, marker antibodies, and environmental agents, it has become increasingly clear that the varying clinical manifestations of inflammatory bowel disease reflect unique pathogenic processes in the mucosa. Indeed, there are numerous discrete entities that can be stratified by a variety of subclinical and clinical markers that may well identify which patients are likely to respond to any particular therapeutic intervention.

The second question, "Do infectious agents have a role in the etiology or pathogenesis of inflammatory

Stephan R. Targan, Fergus Shanahan and Loren C. Karp (eds.), *Inflammatory Bowel Disease: From Bench to Bedside, 2nd Edition*, v–vi.
© 2003 *Kluwer Academic Publishers. Printed in Great Britain*

bowel disease?" is a major focus for researchers at the present time. Mounting evidence, including the identification of specific bacterial products, implicate such agents in the pathogenic process. A key objective for investigators is to understand the interplay between bacteria and the altered immune response leading to mucosal inflammation. Evidence suggests that these immune responses are to normal commensal bacteria rather than any specific pathogen. In 2001, a Crohn's disease associated gene mutation was discovered in NOD2, a protein that is responsible for regulating appropriate responses between bacteria and host. This finding corroborates that an abnormality in this interaction is fundamental to the disease process in at least some forms of Crohn's disease, and further confirms that is unlikely that infectious agents will be directly correlated with the disease responses that are characteristic of the inflammatory bowel diseases. More likely, the process is indirect, requiring any number of combinations of genetics, immune responses, and environmental triggers, to manifest as disease. Specific manipulation of bacterial expression and the corresponding immune response may be the basis of very effective therapies in the near future.

Finally, we posed the questions, "Where is research taking us? How will it change the management of inflammatory bowel disease?" The effect of the research has already become apparent in the example of therapeutic anti-tumor necrosis factor-α monoclonal antibodies (anti-TNF-α). This treatment is targeted at a very specific point in the immune response, over-production of TNF-α, commonly found in patients with Crohn's disease. That this treatment is only effective in a portion of patients with Crohn's disease points to the fact that there are unique immune mechanisms that underly the intestinal inflammation in different subpopulations of patients. An even more recently developed therapeutic approach for those not responding to anti-TNF-α – or even those that do – involves using an antibody to α4 to prevent the recirculation of cells into the mucosa, a method which has been shown to decrease inflammation.

In the second edition, chapters across the spectrum of *Inflammatory Bowel Disease: From Bench to Bedside* will reflect the advances delineated above and lay the groundwork for ongoing research and treatment of these disorders. In the near future, the molecular basis of the interaction between host genetics and the environment will become more clear, and the linkage with the immune system will reveal not only more effective therapy but the ability to predict responders and non-responders to individual therapies.

We would like to express our gratitude to each of the authors for their carefully conceived contributions. In encouraging the authors to include their individual perspective and philosophical approaches, we likely made their job more difficult.

List of Authors

Maria T. Abreu
Director, Basic and Translational Research, IBD
   Center
Cedars-Sinai Medical Center
Los Angeles, CA
USA

David H. Alpers
William B. Kountz Professor of Medicine
Washington University School of Medicine
St Louis, MO
USA

Kristen O. Arseneau
Instructor of Research
Digestive Health Center of Excellence
University of Virginia Health System
Charlottesville, VA
USA

Filip Baert
Heilig Hartziekenhuis Roeselare Belgium
IBD Consultant
University Hospital Leuven
Belgium

Charles N. Bernstein
Professor of Medicine, Head Section of
   Gastroenterology and Director, University of
   Manitoba IBD Clinical and Research Center
University of Manitoba
Winnipeg, Manitoba
Canada

Scott W. Binder
Chief, Dermatopathology
Associate Professor of Pathology
UCLA Medical Center
Los Angeles, CA
USA

Richard S. Blumberg
Chief, Gastroenterology Division
Brigham and Women's Hospital
Harvard Medical School
Boston, MA
USA

Lawrence J. Brandt
Professor of Medicine and Surgery
Albert Einstein College of Medicine
Chief of Gastroenterology, Montefiore Medical
   Center and AECOM
Bronx, NY
USA

Jonathan Braun
Professor and Chair
Department of Pathology and Lab. Medicine
David Geffen School of Medicine at UCLA
Los Angeles, CA
USA

Arlene Caplan
Clinical Psychologist, Division of Gastroenterology,
   Hepatology, Hôpital Sainte Justine
Associated Professor, Department of Psychology
University of Montreal, Quebec
Canada

Roger Chapman
John Radcliffe Hospital
Oxford
UK

Gregg W. Van Citters
Research Fellow
Gonda Diabetes Research Center
City of Hope National Medical Center/Beckman
   Research Institute
Duarte, CA
USA

Offer Cohavy
Post-doctoral Fellow
Cedars-Sinai IBD Center
Los Angeles, CA
USA

Stephen M. Collins
Professor of Medicine, Chief of Gastroenterology
McMaster University
Hamilton, Ontario
Canada

Fabio Cominelli
David D. Stone Professor of Internal Medicine
Director, Digestive Health Center of Excellence
University of Virginia Health System
Charlottesville, VA
USA

William R. Connell
St Vincent's Hospital
Melbourne
Victoria
Australia

Galen Cortina
Assistant Professor Department of Pathology and
    Laboratory Medicine
University of California at Los Angeles
Los Angeles, CA
USA

Kenneth Croitoru
Associate Professor of Medicine, Division of
    Gastroenterology
McMaster University
Hamilton, Ontario
Canada

Cornelius C. Cronin
Consultant Physician/Gastroenterologist
Mallow General Hospital
University College Cork
Cork
Ireland

Sue Cullen
John Radcliffe Hospital
Oxford
UK

Themistocles Dassopoulos
Assistant Professor of Medicine
Department of Medicine, Division of
    Gastroenterology, Johns Hopkins University
Baltimore, MD
USA

Sander J.H. van Deventer
Professor of Gastroenterology
Academic Medical Center
Amsterdam
The Netherlands

Laurence J. Egan
Assistant Professor of Medicine
Mayo Medical School, Mayo Clinic
Rochester, MN
USA

Mark Eggena
Post-doctoral Fellow
Division of Infectious Diseases
University of California, San Francisco
San Francisco, CA
USA

Anders Ekbom
Professor, Department of Medicine at Karolinska
    Hospital, Karolinska Institutet
Stockholm
Sweden

Charles O. Elson
Basil I. Hirschowitz Chair inn Gastroenterology
Professor of Medicine and Microbiology
University of Alabama at Birmingham
Birmingham, AL
USA

Sue C. Eng
Senior Fellow in Gastroenterology
University of Washington School of Medicine
Seattle, WA
USA

Richard J. Farrell
Co-Director of the Center for IBD
Beth Israel Deaconess Medical Center
Assistant Professor of Medicine
Harvard Medical School
Boston, MA
USA

Michael J.G. Farthing
Professor of Medicine
Faculty of Medicine
University of Glasgow
Glasgow
Scotland, UK

Brian G. Feagan
Professor of Medicine, Epidemiology and
    Biostatistics
University of Western Ontario
London, Ontario
Canada

Claudio Fiocchi
Division of Gastroenterology
Professor of Medicine, Pathology and Pediatrics
Case Western Reserve University School of
    Medicine
Cleveland, OH
USA

Edward Fitzgerald
Consultant Radiologist
Mercy Hospital
Grenville Place
Cork
Ireland

Michael N. Göke
Priv.-Doz. Dr. med.
Gastroenterology, Hepatology and Endocrinology
Medizinische Hochschule Hannover
Hannover
Germany

D. Neil Granger
Professor
Department of Molecular and Cellular Physiology
LSU Health Sciences Center
Shreveport, LA
USA

Matthew B. Grisham
Professor
Department of Molecular and Cellular Physiology
LSU Health Sciences Center
Shreveport, LA
USA

Geert D'Haens
Gastroenterologist, Imelda General Hospital
Bonheiden and University Hospital Leuven
Leuven
Belgium

Rodger C. Haggitt (deceased)
Director of Hospital Pathology, University of Wa-
    shington Medical Center and Professor of
    Pathology and Adjunct Professor of Medicine
University of Washington
Seattle, WA
USA

Stephen B. Hanauer
Joseph B. Kirsner Professor of Medicine and
    Clinical Pharmacology
Chief, Section of Gastroenterology and Nutrition
University of Chicago
Chicago, IL
USA

Robert Hershberg
Corixa Corporation
Seattle, WA
USA

E. Jan Irvine
Professor of Medicine
McMaster University
Hamilton, Ontario
Canada

Derek P. Jewell
Professor of Gastroenterology
University of Oxford
Oxford
UK

Lori Kam
San Fernando Valley Gastroenterology Medical
    Group
Tarzana, CA
USA

Loren C. Karp
Researcher/Specialist, IBD Center
Cedars-Sinai Medical Center
Los Angeles, CA
USA

Ciarán P. Kelly
Chief, Blumgart Firm, and
Director Gastroenterology Fellowship Training
Beth Israel Deaconess Medical Center
Boston, MA
USA

Lorraine Kyne
Assistant Professor of Medicine
Harvard Medical School, and
Gerontology Division
Beth Israel Deaconess Medical Center
Boston, MA
USA

F. Stephen Laroux
Post-doctoral Fellow
Department of Molecular and Cellular Physiology
LSU Health Sciences Center
Shreveport, LA
USa

Klaus Lewin
Professor, Department of Pathology and
    Laboratory Medicine
University of California at Los Angeles
Los Angeles, CA
USA

Steven N. Lichtman
Professor of Pediatrics
University of North Carolina at Chapel Hill
Chapel Hill, NC
USA

Henry C. Lin
Director, GI Motility Program and Section of
    Nutrition
Cedars-Sinai Medical Center
Associate Professor of Medicine, UCLA
Los Angeles, CA
USA

Ian Lindsey
Consultant Colorectal Surgeon
John Radcliffe Hospital
Oxford
UK

Uma Mahadevan
Clinical Assistant Professor of Medicine
University of California at San Francisco
San Francisco, CA
USA

Phillipe Marteau
Professor, University of Paris (LHP)
Hepato-gastroenterology Unit
Laennec Hospital
Paris
France

Robin S. McLeod
Professor of Surgery and Health Policy, Manage-
    ment and Evaluation
University of Toronto
Head, Division of General Surgery
Mount Sinai Hospital
Toronto, Ontario
Canada

Stephen J. Meltzer
Professor of Medicine
University of Maryland School of Medicine
Baltimore, MD
USA

Neil J. McC. Mortensen
Professor of Colorectal Surgery
John Radcliffe Hospital
Oxford
UK

Diarmuid O'Donoghue
Gastroenterology Department
Centre for Colorectal Disease
St. Vincent's University Hospital
Dublin
Ireland

Timothy R. Orchard
Consultant Gastroenterology
St Mary's Hospital
Praed Street
London
UK

Remo Panaccione
Assistant Clinical Professor
University of Calgary
Calgary, Alberta
Canada

Konstantinos A. Papadakis
Assistant Professor of Medicine
UCLA School of Medicine, and
Research Staff Physician
Gastroenterology/IBD Center
Cedars-Sinai Medical Center
Los Angeles, CA
USA

Seth Persky
Gastroenterologist
Long Island Digestive Disease Consultants
Setauket, New York
Clinical Instructor of Medicine
SUNY-Stonybrook School of Medicine
Stonybrook, NY
USA

Theresa T. Pizarro
Assistant Professor of Internal Medicine
Digestive Health Center of Excellence
University of Virginia Health System
Charlottesville, VA
USA

Daniel K. Podolsky
Mallinckrodt Professor of Medicine
Harvard Medical School
Chief, Gastrointestinal Division
Massachusetts General Hospital
Boston, MA
USA

Robert H. Riddell
Pathologist, Mount Sinai Hospital and
Professor, Department of Laboratory Medicine and
    Pathobiology
University of Toronto
Canada

Gerhard Rogler
PD Dr. med. Dr. phil.
Department of Internal Medicine I
University Clinic of Regensburg
Regensburg
Germany

Jerome I Rotter
Director, Division of Medical Genetics and Board
    of Governors' Chair in Medical Genetics
Cedars-Sinai Medical Center
Professor of Medicine
Pediatrics and Human Genetics
UCLA School of Medicine
Los Angeles, CA
USA

Paul Rutgeerts
Professor of Medicine
Department of Gastroenterology
University Hospital of Gasthuisberg
3000 Leuven
Belgium

William J. Sandborn
Professor of Medicine
Mayo Medical School, Mayo Clinic
Rochester, MN
USA

R. Balfour Sartor
Professor of Medicine, Microbiology and
    Immunology
University of North Carolina at Chapel Hill
Chapel Hill, NC
USA

Ernest G. Seidman
Professor and Chief, Division of Gastroenterology,
    Hepatology and Nutrition
Sainte Justine Hospital
Department of Pediatrics
University of Montreal, Quebec
Canada

Fergus Shanahan
Professor of Medicine
Chairman, Department of Medicine
Cork University Hospital
University College Cork
Cork
Ireland

Kieran Sheahan
Consultant Histopathologist
Pathology Department
St Vincent's University Hospital
Dublin
Ireland

Konrad H. Soergel
Professor of Medicine and Physiology
Medical College of Wisconsin
Milwaukee, WI
USA

Catherine J. Streutker
Pathologist, St Michael's Hospital and Lecturer,
   Department of Laboratory Medicine and
   Pathobiology
University of Toronto, Ontario
Canada

Christina M. Surawicz
Professor of Medicine
Assistant Dean for Faculty Development
University of Washington School of Medicine
Seattle, WA
USA

Lloyd R. Sutherland
Professor of Medicine
University of Calgary
Calgary, Alberta
Canada

Stephan R. Targan
Director, Division of Gastroenterology, IBDCenter,
   and, Immunobiology Institute
Cedars-Sinai IBD Center
Los Angeles, CA
USA

Kent D. Taylor
Research Scientist
Medical Genetics and Birth Defects Center, and
   Inflammatory Bowel Disease Center
Cedars-Sinai Medical Center
Assistant Professor

Pediatrics, UCLA School of Medicine
Los Angeles, CA
USA

William J. Tremaine
Professor of Medicine
Director, IBD Clinic
Mayo Clinic
Rochester, MN
USA

Eric A. Vasiliauskas
Associate Clinical Director, IBD Center
Cedars-Sinai Medical Center
Assistant Professor of Medicine and Pediatrics
UCLA School of Medicine
Los Angeles, CA
USA

Huiying Yang
Director, Genetic Epidemiology Program
Medical Genetics Birth Defects Center
Cedars-Sinai Health System
Associate Professor of Pediatrics and Epidemiology
UCLA School Medicine and Public Health
Los Angeles, CA
USA

Casey T. Weaver
Professor of Pathology and Microbiology
University of Alabama at Birmingham
Birmingham, AL
USA

C. Mel Wilcox
Professor of Medicine
University of Alabama at Birmingham
Birmingham, AL
USA

Table of Contents

SECTION III: Back to the laboratory bench

Section I

THE LABORATORY BENCH

1 | Introduction: Inflammatory bowel disease: from bench to bedside

FERGUS SHANAHAN, LOREN C. KARP AND STEPHAN R. TARGAN

The adventurous physician goes on, and substitutes presumption for knowledge. From the scanty field of what is known, he launches into the boundless region of what is unknown
(Thomas Jefferson)

The introductory section of the first edition of this book closed with the following upbeat comments: 'inflammatory bowel disease is now an exciting field for the basic researcher, the clinician–investigator, and the clinical practitioner. Much work remains to be done ... Onward!'. In the same year the late Professor Anne Ferguson challenged the medical, political and research communities with a provocative editorial in which Crohn's disease and ulcerative colitis were referred to as 'important and disabling diseases, still under-researched.' Since then there have been remarkable improvements in our understanding of the pathophysiology of these disorders. The molecular mediators and major pathways of tissue injury have been identified. Improvements in molecular genetic technology have ensured that fundamental questions regarding mucosal inflammation can now be asked and answered. The new information promises to be translated into improvements in patient management. This is reflected in a progressive shift from therapeutic empiricism to evidence-based management.

Changes in research strategy have perhaps been even more important than technological progress in providing an integrated and coherent overview of disease mechanisms. Complex disorders require research input from a diversity of perspectives, including traditional disciplines, such as biochemistry, microbiology and immunology. It is at the interface of these seemingly disparate disciplines where incisive advances have been made; hence the emergence of hybrid disciplines such as microbial pathophysiology, immunophysiology and psycho-neuroimmunology. This is a recurring theme throughout this text with emphasis on trans-disciplinary topics such as intercellular crosstalk within the mucosa, lymphoepithelial dialog, neuroimmune interactions, and epithelial–microbe signalling (Chapters 3–11). This approach is also reflected in chapters explaining the fundamental basis of systemic symptoms and signs and extra-intestinal manifestations experienced by patients with Crohn's disease and ulcerative colitis (Chapters 11–13 and 16).

Understanding the role of endogenous outcome modifiers such as psychological stress, the brain–gut axis, and even the placebo response of the individual, requires the same transdisciplinary perspective. Perhaps the most intriguing convergence of research avenues is the interaction among the three major ingredients of the pathophysiology of inflammatory bowel disease (genetic predisposition, environmental bacteria and immune dysregulation). Indeed, the interface at the center of this triad appears to have become the basis of a unifying concept for the development of most autoimmune disorders. It is perhaps not surprising that one of the genes associated with increased susceptibility to Crohn's disease (*NOD2*) is linked to the mechanism of immune perception of the bacterial micro-environment (Chapter 2). One might predict that additional genes will be identified which regulate how the host immune system handles the microbial flora within the gut.

Unraveling the pathogenesis of inflammatory bowel disease is of more than passing interest to the clinician and has several immediate implications for patient management. Genetic studies have already come to the patient bedside with increasing emphasis on phamacogenomic prediction of drug efficacy and toxicity (Chapters 25 and 26). Immune mechanisms of tissue damage in inflammatory bowel disease have been successfully exploited for diagnostic and therapeutic purposes. Thus, immunologic alterations in patients with Crohn's disease and ulcerative colitis have utility as noninvasive diagnostic tools (Chapter

Stephan R. Targan, Fergus Shanahan and Loren C. Karp (eds.), Inflammatory Bowel Disease: From Bench to Bedside, 2nd Edition, 3–4.

20), and blockade of specific immune mediators has been one of the most elegant examples of bench to bedside medicine in recent years (Chapter 27). The challenge for clinicians now will be to establish the hierarchy of importance of site-specific therapeutics versus more traditional nonspecific modalities (Chapter 26) for different patients and the place of combination therapy.

What of the remaining contributors to the pathogenesis – the enteric bacteria? Here again there is already evidence for translation of research data to the clinical setting. Clinicians have been using the bacterial flora for decades to metabolize the prodrugs sulfasalazine or olsalazine to the active aminosalicylate moiety. The impact of enteral feeding in Crohn's disease is now thought to be mediated in part though effects on the flora and epithelial barrier function. Today, manipulation of the enteric flora with probiotics, prebiotics and synbiotics is an emerging therapeutic strategy as a safe adjunct to immunomodulation (Chapter 28). Tomorrow, perhaps one can predict that molecular fingerprinting of the enteric flora will help explain the timing of disease onset, the subset of bacteria driving the inflammatory response and the influence of the host on the composition of the indigenous flora. Because of the lesson of *Helicobacter pylori* and peptic disease, basic investigators and clinicians will be reluctant to dismiss the possibility of a specific infectious etiology in some or all patients with inflammatory bowel disease. Although this could account for the changing nature and prevalence of Crohn's disease and ulcerative colitis (Chapter 2), the information from animal models of disease suggests that more than one pathogenic pathway may be involved in leading to the same phenotypic outcome (Chapter 4). The animal models also indicate that a genetically determined defect in immune regulation can indeed lead to chronic inflammation in the presence of the normal bacterial flora, and this does not require a specific pathogenic infection in the traditional sense of a transmissible agent. Thus, these diseases are unlikely to represent a simple cause and effect relationship with a simple struggle between microbe and humans (Chapter 6).

Extrapolation of the diversity of animal models to the human condition has the obvious implication that clinicians need to contend with an extraordinary degree of patient heterogeneity. While this has not been particularly evident from conventional clinical criteria, improvements in genetic, immunologic and microbial molecular diagnostics are poised to facilitate categorization of patient subsets to improve the design and interpretation of clinical trials in the future (Chapter 23). Today the splitters appear to have the advantage over the lumpers. But the learning curve may have reached the point of inflexion, and with more research data the apparent complexity is likely to give way to commonalities and patterns of disease and therapeutic responsiveness.

Of course, the management of inflammatory bowel disease today must not only be evidence-based (Chapter 30), but must also be accountable in the context of modern concepts of disease management (Chapter 22) and outcome assessments (Chapter 23). In the midst of relentless scientific progress, clinicians will do well to uphold the traditional principles of caring for patients with chronic disease. Despite all the advances at the research bench, patients seem to have increasing expectations of health care and lower tolerance of illness. Dissatisfaction with modern medicine is reflected in greater litigation and expenditure on alternative medicine. Patient surveys consistently reflect the importance of the doctor–patient relationship. Compassion, time, and a commitment to long-term management are unlikely to become obsolete or superseded by any novel drug therapy.

In summary, inflammatory bowel disease is more exciting than ever; it remains a rewarding field for basic researchers and clinicians. Notwithstanding the extraordinary advances brought about by the genotech–biotech era, clinical clues at the bedside continue to pose the correct questions to be tackled in the research laboratory. Likewise, observations at the laboratory bench will continue to be translated into enhanced diagnostic and therapeutic strategies in the clinic. This bench-bedside interface shared by the clinician and the basic investigator needs to be nurtured, as it can pay handsome dividends for patient welfare. Therein lies the essence of what is intended with this book.

2 | The changing faces of Crohn's disease and ulcerative colitis

ANDERS EKBOM

Introduction

There are few diseases which have changed faces to such an extent as the inflammatory bowel diseases, i.e. ulcerative colitis (UC) and Crohn's disease (CD). At the beginning of the 20th century inflammatory bowel disease (IBD) was a rarity, and at the end of the same century these disease entities were something gastroenterologists in the Westernized world encounter not once, but repeatedly, on a daily basis. Fifty years ago high socioeconomic status and Jewish ethnicity were two commonly accepted risk factors, associations that today are either questioned or have been refuted in observational studies. Pancolitis, in the case of UC and CD confined to terminal ileum, were the most common clinical features during the first part of the 20th century as opposed to today. Nowadays ulcerative proctitis is the most common clinical presentation among UC patients and CD confined to the terminal ileum constitutes a minority of CD patients. Geographically there was a north–south gradient; a finding reproduced in different settings and continents that does not seem to exist today. Instead, we can see the emergence of an east–west gradient. A hypothesis of the origin of the diseases included *Mycobacterium paratuberculosis* as a potential agent, a hypothesis that was refuted early on, then reintroduced, and later refuted again.

These different faces of the two diseases are probably in part due to bad methodology or science, but this also illustrates that the two diseases have changed faces over time. It is a rather straightforward endeavor to describe the different faces over time, as we are fortunate to have clinicians and epidemiologists who, during the past 100 years, have taken a great interest in IBD. The difficult part is to interpret these findings and to make sense of them. The goal is to provide benchmarks for other scientists, which can be used to test the different hypotheses, which will emerge. This way we will eventually understand the etiology of IBD and primary prevention will become a possibility.

Occurrence

Temporal trends

Although historic figures such as Alfred the Great [1] and Bonnie Prince Charles [2] have been proposed to have suffered from CD and UC, respectively by clinicians turned historian, it is obvious that the two disease entities were rare until the 20th century. However, at the end of the 19th century there were quite a few case reports of patients with UC in Great Britain, and a symposium was held at the Royal Society of Medicine, London, as early as 1909, at which 317 patients from different hospitals in London were presented [3]. Similarly, in 1913 Kenneth Dalziel, a Scottish surgeon, reported nine patients with a new entity described as 'chronic intestinal enteritis and not tuberculosis' [4]. There is a consensus that those nine cases constitute the first case series of what later was called CD. Moreover, a retrospective study from Ireland has described 29 cases of CD treated during the latter half of the 19th century [5]. There are also reports outside the Anglo-Saxon world of early cases. For instance, the earliest bona-fide case of CD in Sweden is a 13-year-old boy operated on in 1918 due to suspected appendicitis. A bypass procedure was performed because of stenosis of the terminal ileum and, interestingly, the surgeon dismissed the diagnosis of tuberculosis as highly improbable. Nothing was heard from the patient until 1969 when he was admitted for perianal fistulas. As a subsequent barium enema was difficult to interpret, a laparotomy was performed and a resection including the bypassed segment of the ileum was done. The subsequent histopathologic examination revealed changes typical for CD of the terminal ileum. However, it was not until Dr Burrill B. Crohn,

Stephan R. Targan, Fergus Shanahan and Loren C. Karp (eds.), Inflammatory Bowel Disease: From Bench to Bedside, 2nd Edition, 5–20.
© 2003 *Kluwer Academic Publishers. Printed in Great Britain*

in 1932, introduced the term 'regional ileitis' for the disease that was later named after him, when CD became a distinct clinical entity [6].

There are no incidence figures available for either UC or CD until the 1930s. During this decade there are incidence rates from two retrospective studies in two defined populations. The first was done retrospectively in Rochester, Minnesota, where the authors were able to demonstrate an annual incidence of UC of 6.0 per 100 000 for the period 1934–1944 [7] and an annual incidence of CD of 1.9 per 100 000 for the period 1935–1954 [8]. In Europe there is only one estimate during the 1930s for CD, from Cardiff, United Kingdom, of 0.2 per 100 000 for the period 1935–1945 [9].

Thereafter, there have been an increasing number of incidence studies published either for both UC and CD, or for one of these conditions for different populations and different time periods. Besides cancer and cardiovascular diseases there are probably no other disease entities where so many incidence studies have been undertaken in so many different populations during the later part of the 20th century. However, most of these studies have generally dealt with small populations and/or short time periods; in most instances less than 10 years. Moreover, different case-finding methods have been used, and in many instances no age standardization has been done, making comparisons between different populations and time periods impossible to perform. In spite of these shortcomings there are remarkable similarities in the temporal trends for UC and CD in different populations in the Westernized world. There is a consistent finding from both western Europe and northern America of a substantial increase in incidence of both CD and UC since the Second World War.

There is also a strong correlation in the occurrence of the two diseases. Areas or populations with a high incidence or mortality attributed to UC also have a high incidence or mortality due to CD, and vice-versa [10]. Although misclassification of either disease could lead to a false correlation, the consistency of these findings in different settings argues convincingly against such a bias. Moreover, although this chapter will not deal with genetics, relatives of patients with UC are at higher risk for UC and also, to a lesser extent, for CD. Relatives of patients with CD are at higher risk for CD and, to a lesser extent, UC [11]. The temporal trends for both diseases and genetics consequently leave us with two different hypotheses: (1) UC and CD represent the opposite ends of a continuous spectrum of IBD, but with different clinical characteristics; or (2) there are some shared genetic and/or environmental risk factors for UC and CD.

Another common feature, with regard to the temporal trends for UC and CD, is that, in those instances where there are incidence figures for the shift from a low-incidence area to a high-incidence area, an increasing incidence of UC precedes an increase in CD with a time lag of around 15–20 years. The time lag is apparent in studies from Sweden [12–15], Iceland [16–18], Copenhagen [19–21], the Faroe Islands [22, 23], and the US [7, 8, 24–27]. In Fig. 1 the incidence figures for UC and CD are given for Uppsala County, Sweden, from 1945 to 1983. These figures are the result of four different studies performed in this population [12–15]. These studies are of additional interest as the different researchers have failed to identify more than a handful of prevalent cases, i.e. patients with symptoms or a diagnosis before 1945 for either disease. Different case-finding methods have been utilized in the different studies, but yielding the same results. These findings, like those from Cardiff [9, 28] and Minnesota [7, 8, 24–27], where a constant monitoring has been present, strongly suggest that the low incidence figures in the 1930s and 1940s are not due to flawed case-finding methods, but that this increase in incidence for both UC and CD is real.

Since the 1960s and 1970s the excess mortality compared to the background population is only marginal in patients with UC and CD. Thus, the presence of a shift, i.e. transition between low and high incidence of either UC or CD, makes prevalence figures less suitable to compare the occurrence of those diseases in different populations. The prevalence will then be a measure not only of the incidence but also of the duration since this change in incidence. Incidence figures should therefore be used in comparing populations and over time.

Another consistent finding in the descriptive epidemiology of IBD up to recently is that the incidence of UC is higher than for CD. In the case of CD there seems to be a leveling-off in most populations with an incidence of up to 6.0 per 100 000 and for UC an incidence between 15 and 20 per 100 000 although higher incidence figures have been reported for both diseases [9, 29]. This corresponds to a lifetime risk for either one of the two diseases in high-incidence areas between 0.5 and 1.0% which is close to the risk for a disease such as rheumatoid arthritis, which no one disputes constitutes a public health problem. How-

Incidence per 100,000

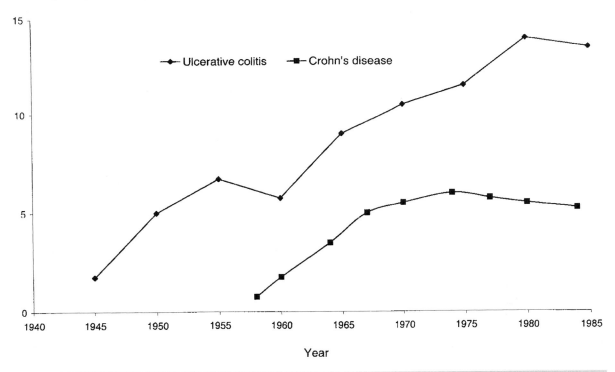

Figure 1. Annual incidence of ulcerative colitis and Crohn's disease in Uppsala County, Sweden, 1945–1983.

ever, as usual with IBD, there are different faces. Recent reports from both Belgium and France [30, 31] play havoc with the notion that UC is more common than CD as the opposite seems to be true in those two adjacent areas.

Age-specific incidence

The age-specific incidence rates for UC and CD vary substantially in different populations and over time. Populations with low annual incidence have an almost flat age-specific curve, and during periods of a rising annual incidence this increase will be most pronounced in the age group 20–40 years for both UC [27, 32] and CD [13, 26]. In Fig. 2 this is demonstrated by comparing the number of CD patients during the transient period in Uppsala County, Sweden, 1956–1961 versus 1962–1967.

To what extent there is a second peak in high incidence areas in the older age groups (60+) remains controversial. It has been argued that this peak represents a delayed diagnosis made when the disease relapses, as demonstrated in the first bona-

fide case of CD in Sweden and in the case of President Eisenhower [33]. However, in a study from the United Kingdom the authors demonstrated one of the highest incidence figures for CD ever reported, which was mainly due to a second peak [9]. The authors expressed concern that this would be the start of a new trend, but further data from the same population have to some extent challenged this [28].

Another area of recent interest is pediatric IBD. The incidence rates among juveniles have been stable for both diseases in different populations since the Second World War. However, during the 1980s there were reports of a substantial increase in juvenile onset of CD in Scotland [34]. An incidence of 1 per 100 000 inhabitants per year in 1968–1976 has changed to 3 per 100 000 in 1990–1992, with the largest increase in the age group 12–16 years. A similar finding was reported from Stockholm, Sweden, where an annual incidence of 1.1 per 100 000 during late 1980s has changed to an incidence of 5.4 during the late 1990s [35]. No such changes in the incidence of UC could be demonstrated. There was also a change in the pattern of the disease appearance, with a higher frequency of fistulating disease than could

No. of patients

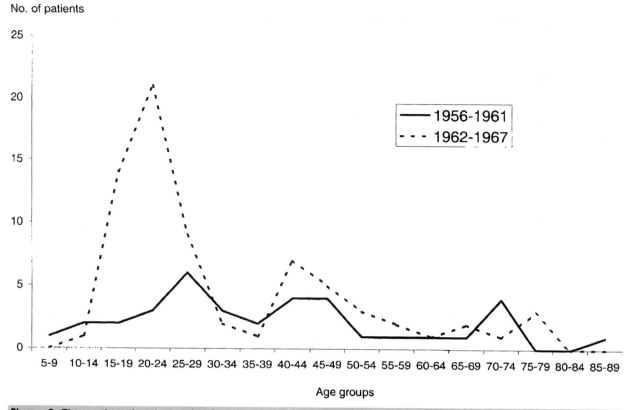

Figure 2. The number of patients with Crohn's disease in different age groups for the years 1956–1961 and 1962–1967 respectively according to the year of first diagnosis. (From Norlen BJ, Krause U, Bergman L. An epidemiological study of Crohn's disease. Scand J Gastroenterol 1970; 5: 385–90; permission to publish given by author BJ Norlen).

previously be demonstrated, as well as the presence of children with CD at very young age (below 5 years). This increase in incidence in juvenile CD seems to be confined to Stockholm, as other areas in Sweden have not been able to demonstrate any changes [36].

Gender

The sex distribution of UC and CD has also changed faces over time. In the case of UC there is a male predominance in high-incidence areas, most pronounced in patients with ulcerative proctitis or distal colitis [15]. Fig. 3 illustrates the change in sex distribution documented by 59 different descriptive studies over time [37]. In the case of CD there is an opposite trend compared to UC. Mortality from CD is higher among males in low-incidence areas but higher among females in high-incidence areas [10]. Temporal trends in incidence also show a similar

trend, from an even sex distribution to a female predominance in high-incidence areas [15].

Extent of disease

Extent of disease is probably the best example of the changing faces of IBD. In the case of UC, pancolitis constituted the majority of cases in some early epidemiologic studies [38] but not all [27]. In the 1960s and 1970s ulcerative proctitis or distal colitis started to emerge to an extent of disease as common as pancolitis. Patients with ulcerative proctitis have a more pronounced male predominance than patients with more extensive disease and also seem to have an older age at onset. It has therefore been discussed to what extent ulcerative proctitis should be a disease entity of its own [39], but it is quite common that patients with ulcerative proctitis will eventually experience a more extensive disease [40, 41], but very little is known about the long-term prognosis with regard to extent of disease in patients diagnosed with

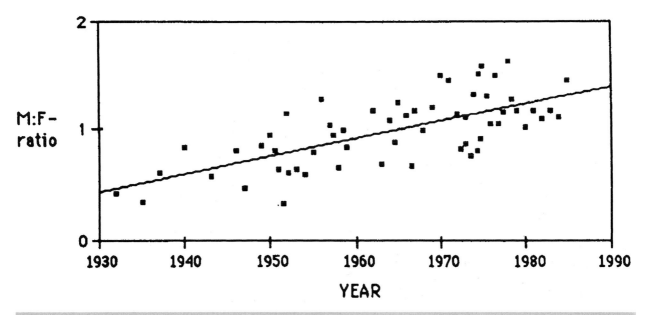

Figure 3. Male:female (M:F) ratio versus time period in 59 reported studies of uclerative colitis from 1930 to 1990. (From Tysk C, Jarnerot G. Has smoking changed the epidemiology of ulcerative colitis? Scand J Gastroenterol 1992; 27: 508–12; permission to publish given by author C Tysk).

ulcerative proctitis the past 20 years. This is a concern as patients with ulcerative proctitis or distal colitis presently constitute 50% of all patients with UC diagnosed in a defined catchment area [42].

Is this shift toward a less extensive disease only a sign of better ascertainment of cases? This might be, at least partly, the explanation in some studies, but it is not the underlying reason for the results in studies from Belgium and France. The proportions of ulcerative proctitis or distal colitis do not differ from those of other centers, arguing against the theory that the 'differences francaise and/or belgique' should be due to underascertainment.

In the case of CD, terminal ileitis was the original disease [6]. It is therefore of great interest to follow the patient's clinical characteristics at the original center over time even if a denominator is lacking [43]. Terminal ileitis was followed by ileocolitis and finally, during the 1960s, a new disease entity emerged – Crohn colitis. This shift can partly be explained by the understanding of Crohn colitis as an entity in the 1960s [44], but even thereafter there has been a decreased proportion of patients with terminal ileitis and an increased proportion of CD with colonic involvement at Mount Sinai as well as in most population-based studies.

Lately, a new entity has been introduced: indeterminate colitis [45]. Is this a new clinical entity or not? It has been argued that this is not the case. Classical CD of the colon is not always clear-cut in a clinical setting. The introduction of this entity could also be due to methodological problems. Most incidence studies published since the Second World War have been retrospective, i.e. data on cases have been assembled years or even decades after diagnosis. One major advantage of such a study design is that the evaluation process will include a long duration of follow-up of the clinical course. This additional information, compared with what is available at the time of diagnosis, will give an additional edge to retrospective studies compared to prospective ones. It has been shown repeatedly that in any cohort of patients with IBD there will be a continuous change in the diagnoses over time, and up to 10% will have a different final diagnosis to that originally assigned [15]. This is also shown by the frequent reports of patients with a definite UC being operated on with a pouch, who later will have a recurrence typical of that for CD [46]. Thus, the pressure to assign a definite diagnosis when a patient presents with a disease, which unequivocally can be classified as IBD, is probably one major reason for this disease entity.

In a prospective study from 20 European centers [47], 5% of all patients with IBD were classified as having indeterminate colitis, and there was a wide variation of that percentage in different populations. In Norway, for instance, there were 93 cases of indeterminate colitis compared to 525 cases of UC [29]. In a reevaluation of the Norwegian material 1 year after diagnosis [48], which included endoscopy and new histopathologic examination, 33% of the patients with indeterminate colitis were reclassified with UC and 17% with CD. There were also patients originally classified with UC or CD who were reclassified as indeterminate colitis. There are very few studies which have tried to assess the specific characteristics in patients with indeterminate colitis, but patients with indeterminate colitis seem to have a younger age at onset, a more extensive disease and a more severe clinical course than patients with UC [48, 49]. However, so far there are no compelling reasons to introduce a third clinical entity – indeterminate colitis.

Geographic differences

Observational studies during the 1960s and 1970s, both in Europe [50] and northern America [51], suggested a north–south gradient in IBD. As the existence of such a gradient could give new clues to the etiology of both diseases, a major study was undertaken in Europe to test this hypothesis [47]. Twenty European centers identified patients with either UC or CD prospectively during a 2-year period. There was a uniform diagnostic approach in all centers and close collaboration during the study period. Although there was a wide variation of the annual incidence in the different populations, there was no consistent pattern which would substantiate the presence of a north–south gradient. Even after adjusting for tobacco consumption as well as education no substantial gradient emerged.

Another interesting feature of IBD is the uniformity in incidence figures in different countries, and these features seem to follow not natural boundaries, but national borders. For instance, until 1 July 2000, there was 10 miles of water easily accessible by ferry between Copenhagen, Denmark, and Malmö, Sweden. In Fig. 4 the temporal trends for CD in these two adjacent cities are shown [20, 52], and it is obvious that the increase in incidence in CD occurred later in Copenhagen than in Malmö, and a similar time difference is present for UC [21, 49].

In contrast, the incidence of IBD in the northern part of Sweden [53] and the middle part of Sweden [14, 15, 32, 54–56] are similar to the one in Malmö, and likewise the temporal trends. A uniform incidence of IBD also seems to be present in Italy [57, 58]. Comparisons of the incidence of IBD made in Greece during the 1990s, on the other hand, revealed substantial differences, especially for CD which seems to be almost nonexistent in the northern part of Greece [59] as compared to Crete where the incidence does not differ from that of the rest of Europe [60, 61]. However, there are now strong indications of an east–west gradient evident from case reports [62, 63] and incidence figures [64] from Eastern Europe and the former Soviet Union.

Cohort effects

It is obvious from descriptive epidemiology that the increasing incidence in IBD occurred after the Second World War. However, this does not seem to be due exclusively to a period effect, but there are reports of a birth cohort phenomenon. This was first reported as early as the 1970s in a major incidence study of CD in Stockholm County, Sweden [54]. This finding was confirmed in an adjacent population in the Uppsala Health Care Region where a birth cohort phenomenon could be demonstrated both for UC and CD [15]. In the case of UC the birth a cohort phenomenon was more pronounced for extensive colitis than ulcerative proctitis. The existence of such a birth cohort phenomenon has, however, been questioned, and two studies [20, 55], one from Sweden and one from Denmark, failed to show any such effect. Both these studies, however, had problems with statistical power, and that could be the underlying reason for the inconsistent results.

In a slightly different approach, mortality data from England and Switzerland were used in order to analyze temporal trends in both UC and peptic ulcer disease [65]. The authors were able to demonstrate similar patterns for both diseases and the results were consistent with a birth cohort phenomenon. The major shortcoming with this study is that the authors have utilized mortality figures instead of incidence figures, and their finding of a peak in the incidence of UC among those born in the latter half of the 19th century is probably a result of this. However, the similarity in the temporal trends between duodenal ulcer disease and UC implicates early exposures, possibly of infectious origin. Moreover, a birth cohort phenomenon argues against genetic determi-

Incidence per 100,000

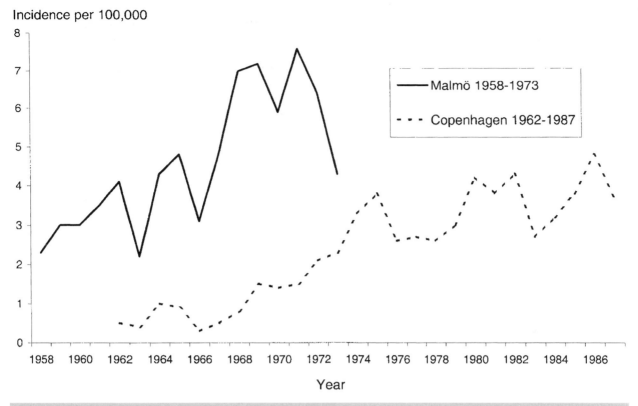

Figure 4. Annual incidences of Crohn's disease in Copenhagen County during the period 1962–1987 and Malmö during the period 1958–1973.

nants as the major cause, but strongly indicates environmental factors interacting with genetic susceptibility for the diseases.

Risk factors

There is no good hypothesis to explain and identify what sort of exposures are of importance for the emerging epidemic of IBD during the 20th century. This is probably the underlying reason for the abundance of different risk factors which have been proposed. With the exception of smoking, they all have in common that the results from different observational studies are not consistent, and quite often lack any biologic rationale. There has been an uniform pattern during the past 50 years: a hypothesis is proposed, followed by enthusiastic early reports of an association, and then a nullifying of the initial results in better-conducted epidemiologic studies. This includes different dietary habits, food items such as margarine and cornflakes, toothpaste,

chewing gum, etc. There are, however, some exposures which are worth discussing more in detail.

Ethnicity

In Crohn's original description all 14 patients were Jewish [6]. Ever since that time there has been a perceived association between Jewish ethnicity and an increased risk of IBD. This has been further substantiated by data from the US Army, where the risk of UC in 1944 was higher among those with a Jewish ethnicity compared to other groups [66]. Analytical studies from Sweden [52, 54], South Africa [67], the United Kingdom [68] and the US [69] have given further credence to such an association. However, there are reasons to question the methodology in most of these studies. In the two Swedish studies [52, 54] the nominator – that is the number of subjects with Jewish ethnicity – was assessed through the family name, but the denominator was assessed in a different manner, an approach that would yield an incidence rate which is bound to be inflated. The study from South Africa [67] has similar drawbacks as the denominator was unknown and therefore ascertained from old census data, probably too low, thus generating inflated incidence rates. It is also of interest that descriptive epidemiologic studies from Israel do not find any incidence or prevalence rates, which differs from other high-incidence areas such as the United Kingdom and Scandinavia [47]. The country of origin seems to be a strong predictor for the risk of IBD, and in subgroup analyses of data from Israel, Jews born either in North America or western Europe seemed to be at highest risk [70]. Similar findings have been reported from Los Angeles, US, where the authors could demonstrate that the Jews originating from Central Europe had a higher risk for CD compared to those originating for Poland or Russia [71]. The authors' conclusion that there is a subset of individuals of Jewish origin with an especially high predisposition for CD might be valid, but the suggestion that all individuals with a Jewish background show an increased risk of either UC or CD still remains to be proven.

In areas with high incidence of IBD, certain ethnic minorities, especially those with lower socio-economic status, often have a lower annual incidence. Such associations have been seen among blacks in Baltimore [69], Indian migrants in the United Kingdom [72], blacks in South Africa [67] and Bedouin Arabs in Israel [73]. However, these observations are not constant over time – changing faces – and there are examples of these differences being diminished over time [72, 74, 75]. In some instances, as in Great Britain, even opposite associations have been reported. In a study using data from the National Representative British Birth Cohort utilizing everyone born in Britain during one week in 1970, the authors could demonstrate a more than 6-fold increased risk for IBD among those with a parent from India, Pakistan or Bangladesh compared to the indigenous British population [76]. Similar results were found in a study from Leicester in the United Kingdom, where the mean incidence in the south Asian community was more than double that of those of European descent [77]. Thus, although ethnicity previously was a good predictor for the risk of IBD, this does not seem to be the case today.

Socioeconomic status

Another consistent finding in early observational studies of both UC and CD was the association between high socioeconomic status and an increased risk [78, 79]. This finding has been used by some authors to explain the lower incidence of IBD in minority groups. However, this accepted truth is another example of the changing faces of IBD, as recent studies in different populations have failed to find such an association [80, 81].

Socioeconomic status as such is of course not a biologically relevant marker. It stands for differences in diet, crowding, and hygiene, exposures that change over time in various ways in different populations. Thus, it is not surprising that the faces have changed, but the question which remains to be answered is: 'What is the underlying mechanism?'

Diet

Because both UC and CD mainly affect the gastro-intestinal tract, it is natural that different dietary exposures have been proposed as the main etiologic factor for the increase in incidence. As early as 1925 it was proposed that UC was due to food allergy [82]. Further credence to this has been lent by the fact that an elimination diet has a beneficial effect on quite a substantial number of patients with UC, where avoidance to cow milk was recognized early to have an effect [2, 83].

Exposure to dairy products therefore seems to be of importance for a clinical course of the disease, and it has been shown that patients with more severe UC have decreased levels of lactase compared to other patients with UC [84]. It is, however, highly unlikely that milk or milk products are of any etiologic relevance for either UC or CD, as there is no consistent finding of such an association in different etiologic studies [85].

Besides milk and milk products, an abundance of other dietary compounds have been implicated in different studies. However, in a review of all such studies conducted up to the mid-1980s for both UC and CD [86], the authors were highly critical of those studies and concluded that both the study design and data analysis made it impossible to infer anything from the results presented that far. Studies since then have not improved our understanding, as they face substantial methodologic problems as in most instances they rely on retrospective assembled data. Any researcher dealing with diet and IBD has to face one major issue: the insidious onset of the disease, i.e. symptoms might have changed the dietary habits, and this is probably one of the reasons why exposure to refined sugar, as well as an inverse association with diet rich in fiber, have been implicated repeatedly, especially for CD [86]. One should also refrain from infering a causal association through ecologic data such as the rise in incidence in IBD and the introduction of margarine in the Westernized world [87], a hypothesis which could be refuted by a well-conducted correlation study [88]. Cornflakes [89], fast food [85], and cola drinks [90] are examples of other food items which have been proposed to be casually linked with IBD, but here also the underlying biologic mechanisms remain elusive [85]. In conclusion, although some interactions with diet cannot be ruled out, it is at present highly unlikely that the increase in incidence of IBD is due to any of those dietary compounds mentioned above.

Smoking

During the 1950s an Austrian physician made the observation that smoking was less prevalent among patients with UC than among other patient groups [91]. Unfortunately, he used as a comparison group patients with duodenal ulcer disease, where smoking is an accepted risk factor. A report from Sweden during the 1970s, published only in Swedish, reported the same association [92]. It was not until the 1980s that this observation spread to the Anglo-Saxon medical literature [93]. Since then there has been an abundance of studies which have shown that smoking is protective against UC, and non-smoking or former smoking is associated with an increased risk [94]. This finding is present in both sexes, all age groups and all extents of disease. It has, however, been argued to what extent smoking cessation is an even stronger risk factor than lifelong non-smoking status [56]. The consistency of these results has even led to the initiation of pharmacologic therapy by nicotine, mostly as patches, which in most instances have shown beneficial effects [95].

In contrast to UC, smoking is a risk factor for CD in almost all analytical studies with a more than doubled risk [74], but even higher risk estimates have been reported [96]. There are clear signs of a dose–response gradient, which further strengthens the hypothesis of a causal association. However, the risk of former smoking does not differ from the risk of never smoking [97], indicating that smoking is perhaps not an initiator but rather a promoting

factor. Further credence to this theory comes from the fact that the clinical course in CD seems to differ among smokers compared to non-smokers where smokers seem to have a more severe clinical course [98].

The contradictory findings in UC and CD have led to speculations that smoking may determine the type of IBD that develops in a predisposed individual. This speculation, as mentioned previously, assumes an otherwise common etiology for the two diseases, which is at least partly contradicted both by the genetics and the temporal trends.

In the case of CD there is a reasonable biologic model for such an association if one assumes that part of the disease process is a multifocal gastrointestinal infarction which would be potentiated by cigarette smoke [99], similar to what has been proposed in the process of arteriosclerosis. This is also in line with smoking as a promoting factor more than initiating. In the case of UC, so far no biologic model exists, but there are quite a few speculations [100].

To what extent can smoking and changes in smoking habits explain the time trends in IBD? In the case of UC we should keep in mind that the majority of patients are never smokers, thus the introduction of cigarette smoking as a common feature in a population during the 20th century could not explain the emergence of this disease. It has been proposed that the change in sex ratios over time in UC can be explained by a higher frequency of former smokers in the male section of the population compared to the female population over time [37]. The authors speculate that this male predominance will eventually disappear when the same frequency of ex-smokers is present among females. So far, however, there are no signs of such a trend.

There are exceptions to the reported associations between IBD and smoking in studies from Israel [101, 102]. It has been proposed that this could be due to a genetic interaction, i.e. higher genetic predisposition to IBD, especially CD, among Jews. The incidence figures for Israel, as mentioned previously, do not substantiate such a predisposition, and even if that were the case, it is rare that a known risk factor will not show up among the genetically predisposed. It is, however, not unlikely that the results from these two studies illustrate the problem with a reported control group in case–control studies.

Oral contraceptives

The introduction of oral contraceptives in the 1960s among women in the Westernized world and the emerging epidemics of IBD have led some authors to infer a casual association, especially for CD [103]. It was therefore not surprising that in the early 1980s there were quite a few case reports describing an association between the use of oral contraceptives and the occurrence of CD [104]. Since then there have been many analytic studies dealing with the subject but, in contrast to smoking, the results have not been consistent [105]. The underlying biologic mechanism which has been proposed is similar to that for smoking, i.e. multifocal gastrointestinal infarction mediated by chronic mesenteric vasculitis which is aggravated by oral contraceptives [99]. Oral contraceptives would then, similar to smoking, be a promoter and not an initiator. However, in contrast to smoking, the use of oral contraceptives does not seem to affect the recurrence rate or severity of the disease [106].

There is also an absence of a consistent interaction between smoking and oral contraceptive use, and opposite findings showing the presence of such an interaction [107] and the non-presence [108] have been reported. However, oral contraceptives are still the focus of interest, and in a study from the US [109], the relative risk of 5.5 was presented following oral contraceptive use for more than 6 years. The authors also calculated the attributable fraction and concluded that almost 16% of all CD patients in the American population was due to oral contraceptives. There are, however, reasons to be very skeptic of such numbers, especially as the incidence of CD in some populations such as Sweden [15] and Great Britain [28] have not increased since the introduction of oral contraceptives.

Clusters

There have been reports of clusters both in time and space for CD [110–112]. This includes CD occurring in spouses [113–115] and affected families in France [116]. These findings have been interpreted as an indication for a transmittable agent. However, in the case of spouses it has so far not been shown that the number of affected pairs differs from that expected. There are always inherent problems in the analyses of clusters. Any researcher has to be aware of the potential presence of a Texan sharpshooter, i.e. the target is decided after the use of the gun. Some of the clusters that have been described can possibly be explained by such a bias, but especially from France the report indicates that some transmittable agent is operating. However, so far the search for this agent has failed [116], but it would be premature to rule out an infectious cause, keeping in mind the history of duodenal ulcer disease. There are also quite a few reports of seasonality of both onset and exacerbation in IBD, especially UC, indicating the existence of an infectious agent triggering the disease [117–121]. To what extent this is of etiologic importance remains unanswered, and the less frequent reports of seasonality for CD could be due to this disease having a more insidious onset, which makes it difficult to establish the start of the symptoms.

Transmittable agents

Chronic mycobacterial infection was proposed by Dalziel as early as 1913 [4] to be the cause for what would later be CD. The similarities between Johne's disease in cattle, sheep, and goats [122] and CD have been used as one of the major arguments. Johne's disease is due to an early infection by *Mycobacterium paratuberculosis* and clusters of patients in England [110] and Wales [123] have been attributed to exposure to this agent [124]. It has been proposed that *M. paratuberculosis* is spread by clinically or subclinically infected animals around the implicated areas, and this could be the underlying explanation for the higher incidence described in urban compared to rural areas.

However, it was pointed out in a recent review [125] that morphologic similarities between Johne's disease and CD are superficial and more suggestive of differing etiopathogenesis. Bacteriologic cultures for *M. paratuberculosis*, immunocytochemistry, use of polymerase chain reaction and trials to transmit CD to animals have all been negative or inconclusive [125]. Moreover, trials with antibiotics directed against *M. paratuberculosis* has also been inconclusive or negative [126, 127]. One should also be aware that in areas such as Iceland, where *M. paratuberculosis* is a problem, especially in sheep, is not characterized by any remarkably high incidence of CD. On the contrary, the increase in incidence of CD emerged later in Iceland compared with other Scandinavian countries [16–18]. Thus, it presently seems very unlikely that *M. paratuberculosis* is an etiologic factor for CD, although one cannot rule out that its presence in patients with IBD can have a clinical impact. Other transmittable agents which could lead to a persistent infection, such as *Listeria* [128], *Mycoplasma* [129] and viruses, especially measles [130], have also been suggested. There are, however, no consistent results so far, and the search for a transmittable agent will continue. As the story of *H. pylori* demonstrates, one should be cautious before ruling out a persistent infection as a cause.

Psychological factors

An association between stressful events and both UC and CD has been proposed repeatedly. It is, however, highly unlikely that psychological stress should be the underlying reason for the emerging epidemic of IBD. An extensive review published 1990 of 138 studies of psychiatric factors and their relation to UC, and to some extent to CD also, seemingly refutes such an association [131]. The authors were able to demonstrate that those studies where a positive association was found were particularly likely to be flawed, and those reporting solely systematic investigations failed to find any association. However, stressful events as an aggravating or even initiating factor cannot be ruled out, especially with the emerging understanding of a brain–gut interaction [132].

Appendectomy

As early as the 1980s the first report was published which showed that patients with UC were less likely to have been subjected to appendectomy compared to controls [80]. Further research in this area has shown that this protective effect seems to be most pronounced if the appendectomy was done before the age of 20 [133, 134]. There are two mutually exclusive interpretations of these findings. One is that the removal of the appendix is causally linked to a decreased risk of UC, and animal models have given some credence to this [135]. There have even been trials to utilize appendectomy in a clinical setting as an alternative therapy. The other is that there is an association between appendicitis and UC, i.e. patients who will get appendicitis are less likely to succumb to UC [136]. Data from a Swedish study seem to support this latter alternative, as the authors could find no protective effect against UC following the removal of a non-diseased appendix [137].

In Sweden there has been a dramatic decline in appendectomies. For instance, during the past 10 years the decrease was close to 20%, from 13 000 to 10 000, and this decline has been most pronounced in the younger age groups [138]. There are reasons to believe that this decline is not due to better diagnostic procedures, but actually reflects a decrease in the incidence of appendicitis. Appendicitis is another disease where the underlying etiology remains an enigma. There was a rise in appendicitis in the late 19th century, which seemed to peak in the 1950s followed by a decline in the Westernized world. It has been hypothesized that the rise in appendicitis could be due to improvements in sewage disposal and water supplies, leading to an enteric infection in childhood at an older age [139]. It is therefore not unlikely that appendicitis, UC and CD are part of the same disease spectrum, perhaps similar to other disease where hygiene in childhood is of importance for the future risk for disorders such as allergy and asthma [140].

Early exposures

The hypothesis of early exposures as of major importance for the risk of IBD was introduced in the 1970s by Whorwell *et al.* [141]. In two subsequent studies from Canada [142, 143] the authors were able to demonstrate that both early gastroenteritis and bottle feeding was associated with an increased risk for both UC and CD. Early weaning has also been reported as a risk factor [144], but the results have not been consistent [80]. Hygiene in early childhood with access to hot tap water has been implicated as a risk factor for CD [133, 134], as has being a single child or a first-born [146], which indicates later exposure to infectious events. As mentioned previously, similar associations have been proposed for the increasing incidence of appendicitis during the early 20th century.

There has also been a dramatic decrease in perinatal mortality during this century, and this has been proposed to be the underlying reason for the emergence of IBD [147]. Ecologic data (Fig. 5), where perinatal mortality 20–30 years before and incidence figures for CD are compared, are seductive. The underlying hypothesis is that children who previously should have been most vulnerable due to infectious events or an impaired immunologic defense are those who will succumb in a population with high perinatal mortality, and those survivors will be individuals who today will cause the rising incidence. The reasons for the decrease in perinatal

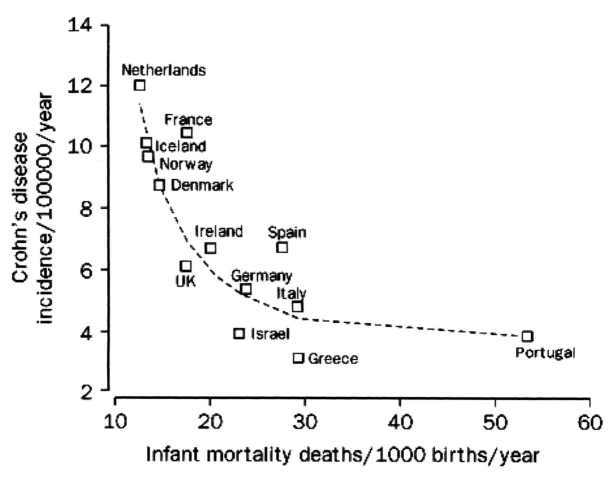

Figure 5. Incidence of Crohn's disease for ages 15–44 in 1991–1993 by infant mortality rate for 1960–1980, when the majority of patients with Crohn's disease were infants. (From Montgomery SM, Pounder RE, Wakefield AJ. Infant mortality and the incidence of inflammatory bowel disease. Lancet 1997; 349: 472–3; permission to publish given by author SM Montgomery).

mortality are better hygiene, better nutrition, and improved maternal and pediatric care, and this could therefore explain the changing faces of IBD from that of a disease much more common in higher socioeconomic classes than lower, during the emerging epidemic until now, when no such difference exists.

Clustering at time and place of birth has been reported for IBD [148], also indicating the importance of early exposures to infectious events. Besides gastroenteritis, different viral infections have been implicated, such as measles, varicella, herpes zoster, influenza and mumps [81]. Although a persistent viral infection has been proposed to be an underlying cause [149] this hypothesis remains unproven. Another hypothesis is that early viral infectious events would affect the immune response, especially if there is a history of repeated infections early in life [150].

The disappearance of a north–south gradient in Europe might be an illustration of what will happen when a society gains affluence. It will therefore be of extreme interest to follow the temporal trends for IBD in Eastern Europe and the former Soviet Union. They have already encountered a substantial increase in childhood disorders such as allergies and asthma since 1989 [140]. One of the more promising hypotheses to explain this phenomenon is that this is due to an altered microflora of the gastrointestinal tract. There have been substantial changes in the diet which will affect the bacterial flora in the intestines. There are strong indications that colonization in early life will determine the subsequent microflora. Early infectious events can therefore be of importance by interaction with this colonization. If this hypothesis is true, we will see the emergence of an epidemic of IBD during the next decade affecting the younger age groups in countries such as the Baltic States, Poland, Hungary, etc. Japan [151] and Korea [152] are other countries with a low incidence of IBD, which have had substantial changes in their dietary habits during the past decade. We should therefore, in my opinion, focus our interest on these populations in order to learn more about the changes in the microflora of the gastrointestinal tract and the subsequent risk for IBD.

Conclusion

During the past 50 years IBD has become one of the major gastroenterologic problems in the Westernized world. It is disheartening that we have so far been unsuccessful in identifying the underlying reason for this. What we presently know for certain is that there is a genetic component, that smoking is protective against UC, but seemingly a risk factor for CD, and that a history of appendicitis under the age of 20 is protective against UC. All other faces of these two diseases have not been consistent over time. We are not even sure that there is a common factor for the two disease entities, although the uniformity in temporal trends over time in different populations indicates that this is the case. There are also strong reasons to believe that exposures early in life are of major determinance for the risk. However, what exposures, and the underlying mechanisms for them, still remain elusive.

On the other hand, it is very likely that for the next 10 years we will have a unique opportunity to learn more of the underlying mechanisms for IBD by conducting good epidemiologic studies in those populations where we might expect a change in incidence. We should also broaden our understanding of the underlying mechanism for appendicitis in younger age groups as that would probably give us some insights on what factors are operating early in life, determining the two different outcomes, appendicitis or UC. We should therefore not be too pessimistic; we have gained some insights during the past 50 years, but in order to proceed we must accept that both UC and CD change faces at different places and times, and adapt ourselves to this paradigm in both our clinical work and our research.

References

1. Craig G. Alfred the Great: a diagnosis. J R Soc Med 1991; 84: 303–5.
2. Wilson PJE. The young pretender. (Correspondence) Br Med J 1961; 1: 1226.
3. Hawkins HP. Natural history of ulcerative colitis and its bearing on treatment. Br Med J 1909; 1: 765–70.
4. Dalziel TK. Chronic interstitial enteritis. Br J Med 1913; 2: 1068–70.
5. Walker JF, Fielding JF. Crohn's disease in Dublin in the latter half of the nineteenth century. Ir J Med Sci 1988; 157: 235–7.
6. Crohn BB, Ginzburg L, Oppenheimer GD. Regional ileitis. A pathological and clinical entity. J Am Med Assoc 1932; 99: 1323–9.
7. Stonnington CM, Phillips SF, Melton III LJ, Zinsmeister AR. Chronic ulcerative colitis: incidence and prevalence in a community. Gut 1987; 28: 402–9.
8. Sedlack RE, Nobrega FT, Kurland LT, Sauer WG. Inflammatory colon disease in Rochester, Minnesota, 1935–1964. Gastroenterology 1972; 62: 935–41.
9. Rose JDR, Roberts GM, Williams, Mayberry JF, Rhodes J. Cardiff Crohn's disease jubilee: the incidence over 50 years. Gut 1988; 29: 346–51.
10. Sonnenberg A. Geographic variation in the incidence of and mortality from inflammatory bowel disease. Dis Colon Rectum 1986; 29: 854–61.
11. Orholm M, Munkholm P, Langholz E, Haagen Nielsen O, Sörensen TIA, Binder V. Familial occurrence of inflammatory bowel disease. N Engl J Med 1991; 324: 84–8.
12. Samuelsson SM. Ulcerös colit och proctit. Uppsala: Department of Social Medicine. University of Uppsala: thesis, 1976.
13. Norlén BJ, Krause U, Bergman L. An epidemiologic study of Crohn's disease. Scand J Gastroenterol 1970; 5: 385–90.
14. Bergman L, Krause U. The incidence of Crohn's disease in central Sweden. Scand J Gastroenterol 1975; 10: 725–9.
15. Ekbom A, Helmick C, Zack M, Adami HO. The epidemiology of inflammatory bowel disease: a large, population-based study in Sweden. Gastroenterology 1991; 100: 350–8.
16. Björnsson S. Inflammatory bowel disease in Iceland during a 30-year period, 1950–1979. Scand J Gastroenterol 1989; 24(Suppl. 170): 47–9.
17. Bjornsson S, Johannsson JH, Oddsson E. Inflammatory bowel disease in Iceland, 1980–89. A retrospective nationwide epidemiologic study. Scand J Gastroenterol 1998; 33: 71–7.
18. Bjornsson S, Johannsson JH. Inflammatory bowel disease in Iceland, 1990–1994: a prospective, nationwide, epidemiological study. Eur J Gastroenterol Hepatol 2000; 12: 31–8.
19. Binder V, Both H, Hansen PK, Hendriksen C, Kreiner S, Torp-Pedersen K. Incidence and prevalence of ulcerative colitis and Crohn's disease in the County of Copenhagen 1962–1978. Gastroenterology 1982; 83: 563–8.
20. Munkholm P, Langholtz E, Haagen Nielsen O, Kreiner S, Binder V. Incidence and prevalence of Crohn's disease in the County of Copenhagen, 1962–87: a sixfold increase in incidence. Scand J Gastroenterol 1992; 27: 609–14.
21. Langholz E, Munkholm P, Nielsen OH, Kreiner S, Binder V. Incidence and prevalence of ulcerative colitis in Copenhagen county from 1962 to 1987. Scand J Gastroenterol 1991; 26: 1247–56.
22. Berner J, Kiaer T. Ulcerative colitis and Crohn's disease on the Faroe Islands 1964–1983. Scand J Gastroenterol 1986; 21: 188–92.
23. Roin F, Roin J. Inflammatory bowel disease of the Faroe Islands, 1981–1988. Scand J Gastroenterol 1989; 24(Suppl. 170): 44–6.

24. Sedlack RE, Whisnant J, Elveback LR, Kurland LT. Incidence of Crohn's disease in Olmstead County, Minnesota, 1935–1975. Am J Epidemiol 1980; 112: 759–63.
25. Gollop JH, Phillips SF, Melton LJD, Zinsmeister AR. Epidemiologic aspects of Crohn's disease: a population based study in Olmsted County, Minnesota, 1943–1982. Gut 1988; 29: 49–56.
26. Loftus EV, Jr, Silverstein MD, Sandborn WJ, Tremaine WJ, Harmsen WS, Zinsmeister AR. Crohn's disease in Olmsted County, Minnesota, 1940–1993: incidence, prevalence, and survival. Gastroenterology 1998; 114: 1161–8.
27. Loftus EV, Jr, Silverstein MD, Sandborn WJ, Tremaine WJ, Harmsen WS, Zinsmeister AR. Ulcerative colitis in Olmsted County, Minnesota, 1940–1993: incidence, prevalence, and survival. Gut 2000; 46: 336–43.
28. Thomas GA, Millar-Jones D, Rhodes J, Roberts GM, Williams GT, Mayberry JF. Incidence of Crohn's disease in Cardiff over 60 years: 1986–1990; an update. Eur J Gastroenterol Hepatol 1995; 7: 401–5.
29. Moum B, Vatn MH, Ekbom A et al. Incidence of ulcerative colitis and indeterminate colitis in four counties in southeastern Norway, 1990–1993. Scand J Gastroenterol 1996; 31: 362–6.
30. Gower-Rousseau C, Salomez JL, Dupas JL et al. Incidence of inflammatory bowel disease in northern France (1988–1990). Gut 1994; 35: 1433–8.
31. Latour P, Louis E, Belaiche J. Incidence of inflammatory bowel disease in the area of Liege: a 3 years prospective study (1993–1996). Acta Gastroenterol Belg 1998; 61: 410–13.
32. Nordenvall B, Brostrom O, Berglund M, et al. Incidence of ulcerative colitis in Stockholm County 1955–1979. Scand J Gastroenterol 1985; 20: 783–90.
33. Hughes CW, Baugh JH, Mologne LA, Heaton LD. A review of the late General Eisenhower's operations: epilog to a footnote to history. Ann Surg 1971; 173: 793–9.
34. Armitage E, Drummond H, Ghosh S, Ferguson A. Incidence of juvenile-onset Crohn's disease in Scotland. Lancet 1999; 353: 1496–7.
35. Askling J, Grahnquist L, Ekbom A, Finkel Y. Incidence of paediatric Crohn's disease in Stockholm, Sweden. Lancet 1999; 354: 1179.
36. Lindberg E, Lindquist B, Holmquist L, Hildebrand H. Inflammatory bowel disease in children and adolescents in Sweden, 1984–1995. J Pediatr Gastroenterol Nutr 2000; 30: 259–64.
37. Tysk C, Jarnerot G. Has smoking changed the epidemiology of ulcerative colitis? Scand J Gastroenterol 1992; 27: 508–12.
38. Evans JG, Acheson ED. An epidemiological study of ulcerative colitis and regional enteritis in the Oxford area. Gut 1965; 6: 311–24.
39. Ekbom A, Helmick C, Zack M, Adami HO. Ulcerative proctitis in central Sweden 1965–1983. A population-based epidemiological study. Dig Dis Sci 1991; 36: 97–102.
40. Farmer RG, Brown CH. Course and prognosis of ulcerative proctosigmoiditis. Am J Gastroenterol 1971; 56: 227–34.
41. Powell-Tuck J, Ritchie JK, Lennard-Jones JE. The prognosis of idiopathic proctitis. Scand J Gastroenterol 1977; 12: 727–32.
42. Ghosh S, Shand A, Ferguson A. Ulcerative colitis. Br Med J 2000; 320: 1119–23.
43. Korelitz BI. From Crohn to Crohn's disease: 1979; an epidemiologic study in New York City. Mt Sinai J Med 1979; 46: 533–40.
44. Lockhart-Mummery HE, Morson BC. Crohn's disease (regional enteritis) of the large intestine and its distribution from ulcerative colitis. Gut 1960; 1: 87–105.
45. Price AB. Overlap in the spectrum of non-spectrum inflammatory bowel disease – 'colitis-indeterminate'. J Clin Pathol 1978; 31: 567–77.
46. Leijonmarck CE, Lofberg R, Ost A, Hellers G. Long-term results of ileorectal anastomosis in ulcerative colitis in Stockholm County. Dis Colon Rectum 1990; 33: 195–200.
47. Shivananda S, Lennard-Jones J, Logan R et al. Incidence of inflammatory bowel disease across Europe: is there a difference between north and south? Results of the European Collaborative Study on Inflammatory Bowel Disease (EC-IBD). Gut. 1996; 39(5): 690–7.
48. Moum B, Ekbom A, Vatn MH et al. Inflammatory bowel disease: re-evaluation of the diagnosis in a prospective population based study in south eastern Norway. Gut 1997; 40: 328–32.
49. Stewenius J, Adnerhill I, Ekelund G et al. Ulcerative colitis and indeterminate colitis in the city of Malmo, Sweden. A 25-year incidence study. Scand J Gastroenterol 1995; 30: 38–43.
50. Kyle J. Crohn's disease in the northeastern and northern Isles of Scotland: an epidemiological review. Gastroenterology 1992; 103: 392–9.
51. Sonnenberg A, McCarty DJ, Jacobsen SJ. Geographic variation in inflammatory bowel disease within the United States. Gastroenterology 1991; 100: 143–9.
52. Brahme F, Lindstrom C, Wenckert A. Crohn's disease in a defined population. An epidemiological study of incidence, prevalence, mortality, and secular trends in the city of Malmo, Sweden. Gastroenterology 1975; 69: 342–51.
53. Nyhlin H, Danielsson Å. Incidence of Crohn's disease in a defined population in Northern Sweden. Scand J Gastroenterol 1986; 21: 1185–92.
54. Hellers G. Crohn's disease in Stockholm County, 1955–1974. Acta Chir Scand 1979; 490(Suppl. 1): 1–84.
55. Lindberg E, Järnerot G. The incidence of Crohn's disease is not decreasing in Sweden. Scand J Gastroenterol 1991; 26: 495–500.
56. Tysk C, Jarnerot G. Ulcerative proctocolitis in Orebro, Sweden. A retrospective epidemiologic study, 1963–1987. Scand J Gastroenterol 1992; 27: 945–50.
57. Trallori G, d'Albasio G, Palli D et al. Epidemiology of inflammatory bowel disease over a 10-year period in Florence (1978–1987). Ital J Gastroenterol 1991; 23: 559–63.
58. Cottone M, Cipolla C, Orlando A, Olivia L, Salerno G, Pagliaro L. Hospital incidence of Crohn's disease in the province of Palermo. Scand J Gastroenterol 1989; 24(Suppl. 170): 27–8.
59. Tsianos EV, Masalas CN, Merkouropoulos M, Dalekos GN, Logan RF. Incidence of inflammatory bowel disease in northwest Greece: rarity of Crohn's disease in an area where ulcerative colitis is common. Gut 1994; 35: 369–72.
60. Manousos ON, Koutroubakis I, Potamianos S, Roussomoustakaki M, Gourtsoyiannis N, Vlachonikolis IG. A prospective epidemiologic study of Crohn's disease in Heraklion, Crete. Incidence over a 5-year period. Scand J Gastroenterol 1996; 31: 599–603.
61. Manousos ON, Giannadaki E, Mouzas IA et al. Ulcerative colitis is as common in Crete as in northern Europe: a 5-year prospective study. Eur J Gastroenterol Hepatol 1996; 8: 893–8.
62. Kull K, Salupere R, Uibo R, Ots M, Salupere V. Antineutrophil cytoplasmic antibodies in Estonian patients with inflammatory bowel disease. Prevalence and diagnostic role. Hepatogastroenterology 1998; 45: 2132–7.
63. Ihasz M, Batorfi J, Balint A et al. Surgical relations of Crohn's disease and the frequency of recurrence. Acta Chir Hung 1995; 35: 63–75.

64. Vucelic B, Korac B, Sentic M, *et al*. Ulcerative colitis in Zagreb, Yugoslavia: incidence and prevalence 1980–1989. Int J Epidemiol 1991; 20: 1043–7.

65. Delco F, Sonnenberg A. Exposure to risk factors for ulcerative colitis occurs during an early period of life. Am J Gastroenterol 1999; 94: 679–84.

66. Acheson ED. The distribution of ulcerative colitis and regional enteritis in United States veterans with particular reference to the Jewish religion. Gut 1960; 1: 291–3.

67. Wright JP, Froggatt J, O'Keefe EA *et al*. The epidemiology of inflammatory bowel disease in Cape Town 1980–1984. S Afr Med J 1986; 70: 10–15.

68. Mayberry JF, Judd D, Smart H, Rhodes J, Calcraft B, Morris JS. Crohn's disease in Jewish people – an epidemiological study in south-east Wales. Digestion 1986; 35: 237–40.

69. Monk M, Mendeloff AI, Siegel CI, Lilienfeld A. An epidemiological study of ulcerative colitis and regional enteritis among adults in Baltimore. I. Hospital incidence and prevalence, 1960 to 1963. Gastroenterology 1968; 54:(Suppl.): 822–4.

70. Odes HS, Locker C, Neumann L *et al*. Epidemiology of Crohn's disease in southern Israel. Am J Gastroenterol 1994; 89: 1859–62.

71. Roth MP, Petersen GM, McElree C, Feldman E, Rotter JI. Geographic origins of Jewish patients with inflammatory bowel disease. Gastroenterology 1989; 97: 900–4.

72. Jayanthi V, Probert CSJ, Pinder D, Wicks ACB, Mayberry JF. Epidemiology of Crohn's disease in Indian migrants and the indigenous population in Leicestershire. Q J Med 1992; 298: 125–38.

73. Odes HS, Fraser D, Krugliak P, Fenyves D, Fraser GM, Sperber AD. Inflammatory bowel disease in the Bedouin Arabs of southern Israel: rarity of diagnosis and clinical features. Gut 1991; 32: 1024–6.

74. Calkins BM, Lilienfeld AM, Garland CF, Mendeloff AI. Trends in incidence rates of ulcerative colitis and Crohn's disease. Dig Dis Sci 1984; 29: 913–20.

75. Kurata JH, Kantor-Fish S, Frankl H, Godby P, Vadheim CM. Crohn's disease among ethnic groups in a large health maintenance organization. Gastroenterology 1992; 102: 1940–8.

76. Thompson NP, Montgomery SM, Wadsworth ME, Pounder RE, Wakefield AJ. Early determinants of inflammatory bowel disease: use of two national longitudinal birth cohorts. Eur J Gastroenterol Hepatol 2000; 12: 25–30.

77. Carr I, Mayberry JF. The effects of migration on ulcerative colitis: a three-year prospective study among Europeans and first- and second-generation South Asians in Leicester (1991–1994). Am J Gastroenterol 1999; 94: 2918–22.

78. Acheson ED, Nefzger MD. Ulcerative colitis in the United States Army in 1944. Epidemiology: comparisons between patients and controls. Gastroenterology 1963; 44: 7–19.

79. Sonnenberg A. Disability from inflammatory bowel disease among employees in West Germany. Gut 1989; 30: 367–70.

80. Gilat T, Hacohen D, Lilos P, Langman MJS. Childhood factors in ulcerative colitis and Crohn's disease. Scand J Gastroenterol 1987; 22: 1009–24.

81. Ekbom A, Adami HO, Helmick CG, Jonzon A, Zack MM. Perinatal risk factors for inflammatory bowel disease: a case–control study. Am J Epidemiol 1990; 132: 1111–19.

82. Andresen AFR. Gastrointestinal manifestations of food allergy. Med J Rec 1925; 122(Suppl.): 271–5.

83. Truelove SC. Ulcerative colitis provoked by milk. Br Med J 1961; 1: 154–60.

84. Pena AS, Truelove SC. Hypolactasia and ulcerative colitis. Gastroenterology 1973; 64: 400–4.

85. Persson PG, Ahlbom A, Hellers G. Diet and inflammatory bowel disease: a case–control study. Epidemiology 1992; 3: 47–52.

86. Persson PG, Ahlbom A, Hellers G. Crohn's disease and ulcerative colitis. A review of dietary studies with emphasis on methodologic aspects. Scand J Gastroenterol 1987; 22: 385–9.

87. Guthy E. Morbus Crohn and Nahrungsfette – Hypothese zur Ätiologie der Enteritis regionalis. Dt Med Wochenschr 1982; 107: 71–3.

88. Sonnenberg A. Geographic and temporal variations of sugar and margarine consumption in relation to Crohn's disease. Digestion 1988; 41: 161–71.

89. James AH. Breakfast and Crohn's disease. Br Med J 1977; 1: 943–5.

90. Russel MG, Engels LG, Muris JW *et al*. 'Modern life' in the epidemiology of inflammatory bowel disease: a case–control study with special emphasis on nutritional factors. Eur J Gastroenterol Hepatol 1998; 10: 243–9.

91. Boller R. Erfahrungen an 89 Colitis-ulcerosa-Fällen der Abteilung Boller im allgemeinen Krankenhaus Wien. Gastroenterologia 1956; 86: 693–6.

92. Samuelsson SM, Ekbom A, Zack M, Helmick CG, Adami HO. Risk factors for extensive ulcerative colitis and ulcerative proctitis: a population based case–control study. Gut 1991; 32: 1526–30.

93. Harries AD, Baird A, Rhodes J. Non-smoking: a feature of ulcerative colitis. Br Med J (Clin Res Ed) 1982; 284: 706.

94. Calkins BM. A meta-analysis of the role of smoking in inflammatory bowel disease. Dig Dis Sci 1989; 34: 1841–54.

95. Pullan RD, Rhodes J, Ganesh S *et al*. Transdermal nicotine for active ulcerative colitis. N Engl J Med 1994; 330: 811–5.

96. Franceschi S, Panza E, La Vecchia C, Parazzini F, Decarli A, Bianchi Porro G. Nonspecific inflammatory bowel disease and smoking. Am J Epidemiol 1987; 125: 445–52.

97. Benoni C, Nilsson Å. Smoking habits in patients with inflammatory bowel disease. Scand J Gastroenterol 1987; 22: 1130–6.

98. Cottone M, Rosselli M, Orlando A *et al*. Smoking habits and recurrence in Crohn's disease. Gastroenterology 1994; 106: 643–8.

99. Wakefield AD, Sawyerr AM, Hudson M, Dhillon AP, Pounder RE. Smoking, the oral contraceptive pill, and Crohn's disease. Dig Dis Sci 1991; 36: 1147–50.

100. Rachmilewitz D. On smoking, rats, and inflammatory bowel disease. Gastroenterology. 1999; 117: 1008–11.

101. Reif S, Klein I, Arber N, Gilat T. Lack of association between smoking and inflammatory bowel disease in Jewish patients in Israel. Gastroenterology 1995; 108: 1683–7.

102. Reif S, Lavy A, Keter D *et al*. Lack of association between smoking and Crohn's disease but the usual association with ulcerative colitis in Jewish patients in Israel: a multicenter study. Am J Gastroenterol 2000; 95: 474–8.

103. Lesko SM, Kaufman DW, Rosenberg L *et al*. Evidence for an increased risk of Crohn's disease in oral contraceptive users. Gastroenterology 1985; 89: 1046–9.

104. Rhodes JM, Cockel R, Allan RN, Hawker PC, Dawson J, Elias E. Colonic Crohn's disease and use of oral contraception. Br Med J 1984; 1: 595–96.

105. Lashner BA, Kane SV, Hanauer SB. Lack of association between oral contraceptive use and Crohn's disease colitis. Gastroenterology 1989; 97: 1442–7.

106. Sutherland LR, Ramcharan S, Bryant H, Fick G. Effect of oral contraceptive use on reoperation following surgery for Crohn's disease. Dig Dis Sci 1992; 37: 1377–82.

107. Sandler RS, Wurzelmann JI, Lyles CM. Oral contraceptive use and the risk of inflammatory bowel disease. Epidemiology 1992; 3: 374–8.

108. Katschinski B, Fingerle D, Scherbaum B, Goebell H. Oral contraceptive use and cigarette smoking in Crohn's disease. Dig Dis Sci 1993; 38: 1596–600.

109. Boyko EJ, Theis MK, Vaughan TL, Nicol-Blades B. Increased risk of inflammatory bowel disease associated with oral contraceptive use. Am J Epidemiol 1994; 140: 268–78.

110. Allan R, Pease P, Ibbotson JP. Clustering of Crohn's disease in a Cotswold village. Q J Med 1986; 229: 473–8.

111. Reilly RP, Robinson TJ. Crohn's disease – is there a long latent period? Postgrad Med J 1986; 62: 353–4.

112. Aisenberg J, Janowitz HD. Cluster of inflammatory bowel disease in three close college friends? J Clin Gastroenterol 1993; 17: 18–20.

113. Rhodes JM, Marshall T, Hamer JD, Allan RN. Crohn's disease in two married couples. Gut 1985; 26: 1086–7.

114. Lobo AJ, Foster PN, Sobala GM, Axon ATR. Crohn's disease in married couples. Lancet 1988; i: 704–5.

115. Comes MC, Gower-Rousseau C, Colombel JF *et al*. Inflammatory bowel disease in married couples: 10 cases in Nord Pas de Calais region of France and Liege county of Belgium. Gut 1994; 35: 1316–18.

116. van Kruiningen HJ, Colombel JF, Cartun RW *et al*. An in-depth study of Crohn's disease in two French families. Gastroenterology 1993; 104: 351–60.

117. Cave DR, Freedman LS. Seasonal variations in the clinical presentation of Crohn's disease and ulcerative colitis. Int J Epidemiol 1975; 4: 317–20.

118. Myszor M, Calam J. Seasonality of ulcerative colitis. Lancet 1984; 2: 522–3.

119. Sellu DR. Seasonal variation in onset of exacerbations of ulcerative proctocolitis. J R Coll Surg Edinb 1986; 31: 158–60.

120. Tysk C, Jarnerot G. Seasonal variation in exacerbations of ulcerative colitis. Scand J Gastroenterol. 1993; 28: 95–6.

121. Moum B, Aadland E, Ekbom A, Vatn MH. Seasonal variations in the onset of ulcerative colitis. Gut 1996; 38: 376–8.

122. Morgan KL. Johne's and Crohn's. Chronic inflammatory bowel disease of infectious aetiology? Lancet 1987;1i: 1017–19.

123. Mayberry JF, Hitchens RAN. Distribution of Crohn's disease in Cardiff. Soc Sci Med 1978; 12: 137–8.

124. Hermon-Taylor J. Causation of Crohn's disease: the impact of clusters. Gastroenterology 1993; 104: 643–6.

125. Van Kruiningen HJ. Lack of support for a common etiology in Johne's disease of animals and Crohn's disease in humans. Inflam Bowel Dis 1999; 5: 183–91.

126. Afdhal NH, Long A, Lennon J, Crowe J, O'Donoghue DP. Controlled trial of antimycobacterial therapy in Crohn's disease. Clofazimine versus placebo. Dig Dis Sci 1991; 36: 449–53.

127. Rutgeerts P, Geboes K, Vantrappen G *et al*. Rifabutin and ethambutol do not help recurrent Crohn's disease in the neoterminal ileum. J Clin Gastroenterol 1992; 15: 24–8.

128. Liu Y, van Kruiningen HJ, West AB, Cartun RW, Cortot A, Colombel JF. Immunocytochemical evidence of *Listeria*, *Escherichia coli*, and *Streptococcus* antigens in Crohn's disease. Gastroenterology 1995; 108: 1396–404.

129. Kangro HO, Chong SK, Hardiman A, Heath RB, Walker-Smith JA. A prospective study of viral and *Mycoplasma* infections in chronic inflammatory bowel disease. Gastroenterology 1990; 98: 549–53.

130. Ekbom A, Daszak P, Kraaz W, Wakefield AJ. Crohn's disease after *in-utero* measles virus exposure. Lancet 1996; 348: 515–17.

131. North CS, Clouse RE, Spitznagel EL, Alpers DH. The relation of ulcerative colitis to psychiatric factors: a review of findings and methods. Am J Psychiatry 1990; 147: 974–81.

132. Peck OC, Wood JD. Brain–gut interactions in ulcerative colitis. Gastroenterology 2000; 118: 807–8.

133. Rutgeerts P, D'Haens G, Hiele M, Geboes K, Vantrappen G. Appendectomy protects against ulcerative colitis. Gastroenterology 1994; 106: 1251–3.

134. Duggan AE, Usmani I, Neal KR, Logan RF. Appendicectomy, childhood hygiene, *Helicobacter pylori* status, and risk of inflammatory bowel disease: a case control study. Gut 1998; 43: 494–8.

135. Mizoguchi A, Mizoguchi E, Chiba C, Bhan AK. Role of appendix in the development of inflammatory bowel disease in TCR-α mutant mice. J Exp Med 1996; 184: 707–15.

136. Ekbom A. Appendicectomy and childhood hygiene: different sides of the same coin? Gut 1998; 43: 451.

137. Andersson RE, Olaison G, Tysk C, Ekbom A. Appendectomy and protection against ulcerative colitis. N Engl J Med 2001; 344: 808–14.

138. Blomqvist P, Ljung H, Nyrén O, Ekbom A. Appendectomy in Sweden 1989–1993 assessed by the Inpatient Register. J Clin Epidemiol 1998; 51: 859–65.

139. Barker DJP, Morris JA. Acute appendicitis, bathrooms, and diet in Britain and Ireland. Br Med J 1988; 296: 953–8.

140. Bjorksten B. Environment and infant immunity. Proc Nutr Soc 1999; 58: 729–32.

141. Whorwell PJ, Holdstock G, Whorwell GM, Wright R. Bottle feeding, early gastroenteritis and inflammatory bowel disease. Br Med J 1979; 1: 382.

142. Koletzko S, Griffiths A, Corey M, Smith C, Sherman P. Infant feeding practices and ulcerative colitis in childhood. Br Med J 1991; 302: 1580–1.

143. Koletzko S, Sherman P, Corey M, Griffiths A, Smith C. Role of infant feeding practices in development of Crohn's disease in childhood. Br Med J 1989; 298: 1617–18.

144. Bergstrand O, Hellers G. Breast-feeding during infancy in patients who later develop Crohn's disease. Scand J Gastroenterol 1983; 18: 903–6.

145. Gent AE, Hellier MD, Grace RH, Swarbick ET, Coggon D. Inflammatory bowel disease and domestic hygiene in infancy. Lancet 1994; 343: 766–7.

146. Persson PG, Leijonmarck CE, Bernell O, Hellers G, Ahlbom A. Risk indicators for inflammatory bowel disease. Int J Epidemiol 1993; 22: 268–72.

147. Montgomery SM, Pounder RE, Wakefield AJ. Infant mortality and the incidence of inflammatory bowel disease. Lancet 1997; 349: 472–3.

148. Ekbom A, Zack M, Adami HO, Helmick C. Is there clustering of inflammatory bowel disease at birth? Am J Epidemiol 1991; 134: 876–86.

149. Wakefield AJ, Ekbom A, Dhillon AP, Pittilo RM, Pounder RE. Crohn's disease: pathogenesis and persistent measles virus infection. Gastroenterology 1995; 108: 911–16.

150. Montgomery SM, Morris DL, Pounder RE, Wakefield AJ. Paramyxovirus infections in childhood and subsequent inflammatory bowel disease. Gastroenterology 1999; 116: 796–803.

151. Morita N, Toki S, Hirohashi T *et al*. Incidence and prevalence of inflammatory bowel disease in Japan: nationwide epidemiological survey during the year 1991. J Gastroenterol 1995; 30(Suppl. 8): 1–4.

152. Yoon CM, Kim SB, Park IJ *et al*. Clinical features of Crohn's disease in Korea. Gastroenterol Jpn 1988; 23: 576–81.

3 | Genetics of inflammatory bowel disease

KENT D. TAYLOR, JEROME I. ROTTER AND HUIYING YANG

Introduction

There is ample evidence that the inflammatory bowel diseases (IBD) – Crohn's disease (CD) and ulcerative colitis (UC) – are in large part determined by genetic predispositions. The supporting lines of evidence reviewed in this chapter include ethnic differences in disease frequency, familial aggregation, an increased monozygotic twin concordance rate compared with that in dizygotic twins, the existence of genetic syndromes that feature IBD, associations between various forms of IBD and specific genetic markers, and most recent linkage between specific chromosomal regions and IBD in families. It is the principal thesis of this chapter that the IBD are fundamentally genetic diseases with complex non-Mendelian patterns of inheritance. The support for this proposition will occupy the majority of this chapter. However, before we turn to this evidence it is important to note two important implications of such a conclusion. First, since the various forms of IBD are caused by specific genetic susceptibilities, we must identify those genes and understand how they act, since it is at that fundamental step that the disease process is presumably initiated. This is essential if we are ever to develop methods of disease prevention or fundamentally different therapies. Second, the individual genetic susceptibility will vary tremendously in the population; thus we will need genetic methods to identify those who are susceptible, to initiate prevention strategies.

Thus the existence of a genetic predisposition or predispositions to IBD means that etiologic studies must include a consideration of the genetic components. Genetic studies are essential for the delineation of the basic etiologies of the various forms of IBD. It is only through understanding of these etiologies that we can develop radically new and specific therapies for these disorders. Such knowledge will eventually provide the means to identify those at high risk as well as means for prevention.

General genetic and epidemiologic evidence

Epidemiology and ethnic differences

Because the etiology of IBD is unknown, descriptive epidemiologic studies could play an important role in

Glossary

ANCA	anti-neutrophil cytoplasmic antibody	MHC	major histocompatibility complex
AS	ankylosing spondylitis	MLS	multipoint LOD score
ASCA	anti-*Saccharomyces cerevisiae* antibody	MTHFR	methylene tetrahydrofolate reductase
CD	Crohn's disease	MUC3	mucin 3
cM	centimorgan	NPL	non-parametric LOD score
HLA	human leukocyte antigen	NRAMP1	natural resistance-associated macrophage protein 1
HPS	Hermansky–Pudlak syndrome	pANCA	ANCA with perinuclear staining on indirect immunofluorescence
IBD	inflammatory bowel disease	PSC	primary sclerosing cholangitis
ICAM1	intracellular adhesion molecule 1	SCID	severe combined immunodeficincy
IFN-γ	interferon gamma	TCR	T-cell receptor
IL	interleukin	TGF	transforming growth factor
IL-1RA	interleukin 1 receptor antagonist	TNF	tumor necrosis factor
IPAA	ileal pouch–anal anastomosis	TNR	trinucleotide repeat
LTA	lymphotoxin alpha	UC	ulcerative colitis
LTB	lymphotoxin beta	VNTR	variable number of tandem repeats

Stephan R. Targan, Fergus Shanahan and Loren C. Karp (eds.), Inflammatory Bowel Disease: From Bench to Bedside, 2nd Edition 21–65.
© 2003 *Kluwer Academic Publishers. Printed in Great Britain*

indicating the potential importance of genetic and environmental factors. However, due to the difficulty of conducting population-based epidemiologic studies for these diseases, insufficient studies have been done to estimate incidence and prevalence fully, especially in non-Caucasian populations. With the available data the following can be generalized. Caucasians have a higher risk than non-Caucasian populations [1–3]. There seems to be a north to south gradient [2, 4, 5] and IBD appears to be less common in developing countries, but accurate data are lacking and the rate may increase with industrialization. In the Western world the most rapid increase of IBD occurred during the period 1960–1980 and reached a plateau in most countries [6, 7]. For the Caucasian population in North America the annual incidence rate of IBD (per 100 000) during 1989–1994 in the central Canadian province of Manitoba was 14.6 for CD and 14.3 for UC. The prevalence (per 100 000) in 1994 was 198.5 for CD and 169.7 for UC [8]. For a similar period (1983–1993) a lower incidence and prevalence was observed in Olmsted County, Minnesota (incidence: 6.9 and 8.3 per 100 000 for

CD and UC, respectively [7, 9]. European countries have a similar population risk as reported in the North American population [4, 6, 10–12]. In the United States the Caucasian population has the highest risk among all racial groups, followed by Blacks and Hispanics; the Asian population has the lowest risk [2, 3].

Although the differences in IBD frequency between various ethnic groups can have both environmental and genetic explanations, an important finding is the repeated observation that the Ashkenazi Jewish population has a consistently increased incidence/prevalence compared with other ethnic groups in the same geographic location. The fact that the Jewish and non-Jewish differences occur across different time periods as well as different geographic areas [13–15], strongly suggests the existence of a genetic predisposition as the most parsimonious explanation (see Table 1). Further support for such a hypothesis comes from studies of historical origins of Jewish subgroups and their relation to IBD frequency [14, 16, 17].

Table 1. Inflammatory bowel disease incidence/prevalence rates (per 100 000) among Jewish and non-Jewish populations by area and time period

Area (ref. no)	Disease	Period	Jews	Non-Jews	Ratio[a]
Incidence comparisons					
North America					
Baltimore, MD [18]	IBD	1960–1963	16.7	5.4	3.1
	UC	1960–1963	13.3	3.4	3.9
New York City [19]	CD	1960–1963	3.4	1.7	2.0
	CD	?	12.6[b]	5.4	2.3
Scandinavia					
Malmo, Sweden [20]	CD	1965–1973	24.0[b]	6.0	4.0
Stockholm, Sweden [21]	CD	1960–1974	10.0	3.0	3.3
South Africa					
Western Cape [22]	CD	1970–1974	2.8	0.8	3.5
Prevalence comparisons					
Edmonton, Canada [23]	CD		309	143	2.2
	UC		143	76	1.9
Southern Israel [24]	CD	30 June 1990	30	3.2[c]	9.4
	UC		89	9.8[c]	9.1

[a]Ratio-Jewish/non-Jewish.

[b]As estimated in ref. 25.

[c]Israeli Arab.

Table 2. Positive family history of inflammatory bowel disease in ulcerative colitis (UC) and Crohn's disease probands[a]: an example

Disease in proband[b]	Number of probands	Disease in relatives			
		UC (%)	CD (%)	Mixed[c] (%)	Total (%)
UC	269	37 (13.8)	6 (2.2)	4 (1.5)	47 (17.5)
CD	258	19 (7.4)	32 (12.4)	9 (3.5)	60 (23.3)
Total	527	56 (10.6)	38 (7.2)	13 (2.5)	107 (20.3)

[a]Adapted from ref. 33.

[b]Both Jews and non-Jews have the same trend.

[c]With several affected relatives, some affected with UC and some with CD.

Family epidemiology

Family studies

More than a dozen studies have demonstrated that familial aggregation is clearly increased in IBD, although the data fit no simple Mendelian pattern of inheritance [13, 26, 27]. Several studies have shown there is an approximate 10–30-fold increase in disease prevalence among siblings compared to the community-wide prevalence [28–32]. UC is increased among the relatives of UC patients and CD is increased among the relatives of CD patients. However, the two diseases do exist in the same family with an increased frequency higher than just the co-occurrence by chance alone, suggesting an etiologic relationship between UC and CD [33, 34] (see Table 2). This may even identify a specific subset of IBD (mixed IBD), which currently would be defined by family history [33]. It has been observed that a positive family history is somewhat greater among CD patients than among UC patients [33–35], and that the relatives of CD patients have a higher risk for IBD than those of UC patients [33, 36]. This suggests that CD is to some degree more often familial than UC, and may indicate a more important role for genetic predisposition in this form of IBD. (As will be seen below, this is supported by the twin data.) The authors' family data well represent the observations regarding familiality (Table 2) [33]. In that study the age of relatives was also taken into account to estimate the lifetime risks for disease. The lifetime risks for the relatives of non-Jewish patients were consistently lower than the corresponding risks for relatives of Jewish patients from the same geographic area [33] (Table 3). This has implications for the mode of inheritance of genetic susceptibility (see below).

Genetic contributions supported by twin and spouse studies

Furthermore, while familial aggregation can be due to environmental factors alone, the increased monozygotic twin concordance rates, the rarity of IBD concordance in spouses, and the numerous instances of affected relatives whose disease onset is completely separated geographically and temporally from other affected family members [37], all provide support for a major genetic component to disease susceptibility.

A number of reports on twin data showed increased concordance rate of both CD and UC in monozygotic (MZ) twins as compared with dizygotic (DZ) twins [38, 39]. However, potential selection bias should be considered in reviewing these data since concordant pairs are more likely than discordant pairs to be reported. Nevertheless, in a population-based twin study the same higher concordance rate for MZ twins than that for DZ twins, in both CD and UC (shown in Table 4) was also observed [40]. In addition, it seems that there is a greater concordance rate for CD than that for UC. The higher concordance rate in MZ twins than in DZ twins supports the argument that genetic factors are an important component in the development of IBD and that such genetic factors account for much of the familial aggregation. The observation that less than 100% of MZ twins are concordant indicates that there is reduced penetrance for the IBD genotype, presumably due to non-genetic factors. These non-genetic factors may be environmental, or they may be due to random stochastic variation such as occurs in development of B cells and T cells of the immune system [41]. The observation that the risk to DZ twins is not

Table 3. Empiric risks for inflammatory bowel disease in first-degree relatives of patients with inflammatory bowel disease (percentages)[a]

	Sibling	Parents	Offspring	Total
1. *Uncorrected empiric risks for relatives of IBD probands*				
Jewish probands affected with				
CD	8.0	3.0	1.8	4.5
UC	2.4	3.2	1.9	2.6
Non-Jewish probands affected with				
CD	3.0	3.7	0	2.7
UC.	0.4	0.9	2.3	0.9
2. *Corrected empiric lifetime risk for relatives of IBD probands*[b]				
Jewish probands affected with				
CD	16.8	3.8	7.4	7.8
UC	4.6	4.1	7.4	4.5
Non-Jewish probands affected with				
CD	7.0	4.8	0	5.2
UC.	0.9	1.2	11.0	1.6

[a]Adapted from [33]

[b]Corrected for age of at-risk relatives, using age-specific incidence data

Table 4. Ulcerative colitis and Crohn's disease in monozygotic and dizygotic twins from unselected twin registry[a]

	Monozygotic twins		Dizygotic twins	
	Concordant	Discordant	Concordant	Discordant
CD	8 (44%)	10 (56%)	1 (4%)	25 (96%)
UC	1 (6%)	15 (94%)	0 (0%)	20 (100%)

[a]Adapted from Ref. 40.

higher than the risk to siblings argues that environmental factors are population-wide in their effect.

From the limited number of family studies investigating the risk in spouses, it seems that the incidence of reported spouse concordance does not appear to be increased over population risks, and is dramatically less than the risk to siblings [26, 28, 38]. This would argue against any rapid-acting environmental agents, though there are case reports of husband–wife couples who both developed IBD after marriage [42] (also see below, Gene–environmental interaction).

Rare genetic syndromes which include IBD

IBD is clearly associated with three well-defined genetic syndromes [43]: Turner syndrome, also characterized by its association with autoimmunity [44], the autosomal recessive Hermansky–Pudlak syndrome (HPS, oculocutaneous albinism with a defect in the second phase of platelet aggregation leading to a bleeding diathesis and a ceroid-like pigment accumulation) [45–48], and glycogen storage disease type Ib in which there is neutropenia and abnormal neutrophil function [49, 50]. The gene for HPS, located on the long arm of chromosome 10 has recently been cloned [51–53]. Mutations, as well as locus heterogeneity, have been identified [54, 55]. Different mutations at the HPS locus have been shown to be associated with IBD [56]. As regards glycogen storage disease, it seems likely that the neutropenia or the neutrophil dysfunction that occurs in this latter syndrome is the predisposing factor for the development of the Crohn's-like lesions in the bowel. Further circumstantial evidence implicating the neutrophil defect is the recognized occurrence of Crohn's-like lesions in other neutrophil or bone marrow stem-cell disorders such as chronic granulomatous disease [57–59], congenital neutropenia [60], autoimmune neutropenia [61], leukocyte adhesion deficiency [62], and myelodysplastic syndromes [63–65]. In addition, IBD has been less dramatically associated with several rare syndromes associated with immunodeficiency [43]. These studies of rare syndrome associations with IBD suggest that a variety of immunodeficiency states, autoimmune diseases, as well as miscellaneous genetic syndromes [66, 67], appear to increase the risk for IBD. These associations had suggested that studies of elements of the immune pathways may be useful in understanding the etiologies of at least some forms of IBD, a hypothesis subsequently supported by HLA and cytokine gene marker studies (see Genetic marker studies below).

Inferences regarding mode of inheritance

Although there is strong familial aggregation of IBD, and genetic susceptibility contributes to such familiality, there is no one simple genetic model that can explain the mode of inheritance of this disorder. The following observations should be kept in mind when one attempts to explore potential genetic models.

1. From the MZ twin data these are diseases with reduced penetrance, i.e. genetic susceptibility does not appear to be the only determinant of disease.

2. The fact that DZ twins have a similar risk as that of siblings suggest that it is macro-, not micro-environmental factors that determine the risk to IBD.

3. CD and UC are clearly genetically related, since they are found together with increased frequency in families; they are both increased in the Jewish population compared to the surrounding Caucasian population; and the distinct distribution of countries of origin of US Ashkenazi Jewish patients with IBD is true for both CD and UC [68].

4. Based on the stronger family history of IBD and greater MZ twin concordance for CD, genetic determinants appear to play a more deterministic role in CD than in UC. This does not mean that UC is any less genetic, but may be more influenced by stochastic variation, such as occurs in the development of the immune system.

5. There is now evidence for involvement of specific loci and genes (see below, Gene identification).

6. Genetically modified animal models suggest that different genes can cause the same clinical phenotype.

7. Animal models also indicate the importance of gene and environmental interactions.

Simple Mendelian model

It seems clear that the susceptibility to IBD as a whole is not inherited in any simple Mendelian mode of inheritance [43, 69]. One approach is to ask whether the aggregation of disease within families is consistent with a specific mode of inheritance, an approach termed segregation analysis. Utilizing a computerized genetic analytic technique termed complex segregation analysis, a recessive gene with incomplete penetrance was suggested for CD [70, 71], while an additive major gene or a dominant major gene was proposed for UC [71, 72]. It is important to realize that the major gene effect concluded from complex segregation analysis is not equivalent to a major gene with simple Mendelian inheritance. While these analyses argue strongly against the multifactorial/polygenic model (discussed below), they cannot distinguish between simple Mendelian models and models with several major genes interacting (also known as a multilocus or oligogenic model, see below), or models of genetic heterogeneity (i.e. several genetically distinct diseases with a similar phenotype). Nevertheless, keeping the genetic heterogeneity of IBD in mind (see below), the possibility of simple Mendelian susceptibility may be true for a subset of IBD.

Multifactorial/polygenic models

A common explanation that used to be invoked frequently for diseases that demonstrate familial aggregation, but whose aggregation does not follow a Mendelian pattern of inheritance, is that they are due to multiple genes each of small effect (hence the term polygenic), acting together to provide the susceptibility to disease. Only when one has a sufficient number of these genes would an individual pass beyond a threshold and clinical disease result. If environmental factors were also required, then the term multifactorial is applied. Since IBD does not fit a Mendelian pattern, the polygenic model was suggested.

McConnell had proposed a polygenic model as an explanation of the association between CD and UC: that there is one genotype, with perhaps 10 or 15 genes, which makes people liable to develop inflammatory bowel disease [35, 73] . Under this model, if a person has only a few of these genes, he/she is liable to develop UC; if such a person has many of these genes (a more complete genotype), the clinical and pathological picture that develops would more likely be CD. This would explain why the relatives of people with CD are much more likely to have IBD than relatives of people with UC. If a patient has a large number of these genes (and has CD), his or her relatives would be more likely to have a larger number of the genes compared to relatives of a patient with only a moderate number of the risk genes (i.e. a UC patient). Thus, CD patients would be more likely to have relatives with UC, and most of the relatives of UC patients would be likely to have too few of the high-risk genes to have any form of IBD.

However, the formal mathematical genetic analyses of large family data sets of both UC [71, 72] and CD [70, 71] have allowed rejection of the simple polygenic model. Basically what these formal genetic analyses have concluded is that the risk to relatives is too great to be explained by the polygenic model. In addition, genetically modified animal models (including knockouts) suggest that if one gene in the immunoregulatory pathway is sufficiently altered, it can lead to clinical disease; thus it may not require multiple genes with equal small effect to lead to disease.

Multilocus (oligogenic) models

There is increasing evidence that the genetic predisposition to a number of diseases is due to the interaction of two or more major genes, a form of inheritance termed two-locus (if two major genes are involved), multilocus or oligogenic (if more than two are involved) [74–78]. This concept is important for IBD for several reasons. First it is an etiologically attractive hypothesis that could explain more than one pathophysiologic defect being found in IBD patients. For example, in order to develop clinical Crohn's disease, one may need both a permeability defect that leads to increased exposure of the body's immune system to antigenic substances that ordinarily do not cross the gut mucosal barrier and a particular genetically determined immune response. An analogous hypothesis might include abnormal mucins and certain autoantibodies as the etiologic

factors in UC. Second, the recurrence risks for multilocus disorders are very different from Mendelian disorders [76–78]. Third, a multilocus model could explain the relationship of UC and CD in families, i.e. one gene may be insufficient by itself to lead to clinical disease yet predisposes to both diseases, but clinical disease occurs only when a second more specific gene, or genes, interacts with the first, thus leading to the specific disease, CD or UC. Finally, if such a model for these diseases is indeed confirmed, it has important implications for genetic counseling and risk identification in relatives, since if even one locus is identified, family-based genetic marker risk assessment begins to become feasible, as has been demonstrated for other autoimmune diseases [78].

There has been one intriguing study (as opposed to anecdotal case reports) of the risks to offspring for IBD when both parents themselves have IBD [79]. The results suggested that the risk was substantially greater than that of twice the empiric risk to offspring of couples when one parent has IBD, and was starting to approach the identical-twin risks. This suggests another high-risk group, albeit somewhat rare. It also appears that there is a proclivity toward CD in these offspring, especially when the parents are concordant for CD. When the children were further divided into three groups according to whether both parents, one parent, or neither parent had yet developed symptoms of IBD at the time of the children's conception, the risks for IBD were similar among these three groups. In addition, the concordance rate for the type of IBD (UC or CD) in those couples in whom both had onset of IBD after marriage, was not greater than those in whom both or one was affected before marriage. These data argue for the position that some intrinsic (e.g. genetic) and not acquired factors are essential in the development of IBD and in the determination of the type of IBD. While strong environmental determinants limited to certain families could be an explanation, these data more likely argue for a limited number of genetically determined forms of IBD. In other words, such data are consistent with the assumption of a limited number of IBD-predisposing genes. The logic for such a conclusion is that if many different genes were required, i.e. if there were many different genetic forms of IBD, then the occurrence of genetic complementation would reduce the risks to offspring. But if instead there are a limited number of such genes, then the offspring of two affected parents are more likely to be homozygous at the loci for such genes and consequently affected. These data suggest that the actual number of genes predisposing is limited, and thus more consistent with the multi-locus/oligogenic models, rather than polygenic, encouraging the search for the major genes that predispose to these diseases. The success of the genome scan efforts (reviewed below) also supports the multilocus model.

Genetic heterogeneity models

The concept of genetic heterogeneity is that IBD is not a single disease, but rather is several etiologically and genetically distinct diseases presenting a similar clinical picture. Each of the individual component diseases could conceivably be inherited in a Mendelian, polygenic, or multilocus mode of inheritance. Increasing evidence, from clinical differences, to subclinical markers, to genetic markers, supports this concept. The apparent physiologic and immunologic complexity of IBD argues that a heterogeneity model, while at first glance apparently more complex, may in the end be the most parsimonious. The etiology of specific subtypes of IBD may be more easily understood once these subgroups can be identified. Indeed, certain of these etiologically distinct IBD 'diseases' may even be inherited in a Mendelian manner. The existence of the several genetic syndromes that feature IBD and several IBD knockout mice models is an immediate proof of at least some degree of genetic heterogeneity. In this context the interrelationship of CD and UC may mean that there is a form (or forms) of disease that result in UC alone, others that result in CD alone, and some that can present either as CD or UC. The different relative frequency of mixed disease (CD and UC) in the same family in Jewish versus non-Jewish families argue that the mixed form may be a distinct subgroup [33]. A major advantage of the heterogeneity model is that it can lead to directly testable etiologic hypotheses. For example, one possible corollary of such a model is that genetically determined physiologic abnormalities in the affected case are likely to be shared with their relatives, and these can differ in different groups of patients. Thus, clinically unaffected relatives of cases with a particular defect can be tested to see: (1) if the defect is familial; (2) whether it is present prior to disease. Along these lines, several different potential defects (reviewed below, Disease Pathophysiology) have been found in families with IBD (see Table 5). The available data on the familiality of antineutrophil cytoplasmic antibodies argue for genetic heterogeneity within UC; similarly the data on ASCA argue for heterogeneity

of CD. In addition, the genetic marker associations also suggest heterogeneity within CD and within UC (see below). If the heterogeneity model is indeed the appropriate model, an understanding of the etiologies will only be possible by the subdivision of IBD on the basis of both physiologic defects and genetic marker associations into more etiologically homogeneous groups.

As will be seen below, the available evidence argues that IBD is a heterogeneous group of disorders, with each subform an oligogenic disorder due primarily to the interaction of a limited number of genes, though there may be more minor contributions from modifying genes.

Genetic anticipation

Anticipation refers to the progressive increase in severity of an illness as it manifests in its transmission from parent to child, occurring in a more severe form and at an earlier age with succeeding generations. For a long time the cause of anticipation had been attributed to artifact, due to ascertainment bias [80]. It was thought that, when a more severe case of a disease presented clinically, milder clinical forms were identified among the parents and this gave the appearance of anticipation. However, a prospective study of one paradigmatic disorder, myotonic dystrophy, clearly demonstrated the clinical phenomenon of anticipation [81]. Subsequently, the molecular basis of myotonic dystrophy, expansion of a trinucleotide (CTG) repeat (TNRs) at the 3' end of a transcript encoding a protein kinase family member, was identified [82]. Expansion of TNRs over subsequent generations is now known to be associated with a number of disorders, especially in the neuropsychiatric diseases. The significance and cause of anticipation is clear in those diseases that demonstrate both clinical anticipation and association with expansions in TNRs, e.g. Huntington disease [83], myotonic dystrophy, fragile X syndrome [84], and spinocerebellar ataxia type 1 [85]. If the phenomenon of anticipation can be established for a disorder, then expansion of TNRs should be searched for, because at the moment that is the only biologic mechanism established for the etiology of anticipation. However, our understanding of the molecular events related to anticipation is far from complete [80].

A number of studies have examined the possibility of anticipation in IBD. A lower age at diagnosis and a greater extent of disease in the younger member of two-generation pairs affected with CD was observed in a retrospective study [86]. In another study it was shown that, while children were younger than their parents at diagnosis, in most, but not all, parent–offspring pairs, the children did not have more severe disease than their parents [87]. In contrast, two large studies have found no evidence for genetic anticipation and have attributed the younger age of onset in the children to ascertainment bias [88, 89].

Anticipation is clearly an interesting hypothesis worth further pursuing in IBD. To date the data have been inconclusive. It should be kept in mind that the expanding trinucleotide repeats are not the only cause of apparent anticipation [90]. Other molecular mechanisms, termed epigenetic factors, may also be involved in events similar to genetic anticipation, such as DNA methylation and chromatin conformation [91]. Furthermore, rapid changes in the environment could also mimic the phenomenon of anticipation.

Associations with other diseases

It has been observed for many years that IBD is associated with several other disorders whose etiologies are unknown, but which appear to involve the immune system. The best-documented disease associations are with ankylosing spondylitis, primary sclerosing cholangitis, and psoriasis. All of these diseases occur more often than expected in IBD cases and in also their unaffected family members as well.

Ankylosing spondylitis (AS)

Most disease association studies have shown that the frequency of UC patients with AS ranges from 1% to 6%, and the frequency of arthritis in UC patient series ranges from 2% to 15% [92]. Among case series of CD patients the frequency of peripheral arthropathies ranges from 5% to 10% [92, 93]. Approximately 90% of all AS patients are HLA-B27 positive, compared to a frequency of less than 10% in the general population. While the frequency of HLA-B27 in IBD patients reflects that of the general population, about 60–80% of IBD patients with spondylitis are HLA-B27 positive [94–97]. There are also reports that the individuals with the phenotype B27, B44 are especially at high risk (estimated relative risk = 69) for the concurrent manifestation of CD and AS [93, 98, 99]. This strongly suggests that IBD is a potent initiating or potentiating factor in the development of AS. It is still not certain whether AS should be considered a complication of IBD, or an associated disease. The accumulated data suggest that bowel disease may be present even when it is not manifested clinically [100–103], and that patients with non-AS spondyloarthropathy and inflammatory gut lesions have greater risk of developing AS than patients without gut inflammation [104, 105]. Of note is the increased risk for ankylosing spondylitis seen in the relatives of IBD patients even when the patients themselves have no evidence of AS [106]. These data suggest that the intestinal inflammation may lead to joint disease in individuals who are genetically predisposed to these diseases, perhaps by allowing passage of potential antigens through the gut mucosa, or by other mechanisms yet to be defined. It also suggests that there may well be subclinical, yet active, bowel disease in those patients in whom AS appears to develop prior to the bowel disease. Based on these data, the hypothesis should be actively considered that, etiologically, AS may often be secondary to a form of the idiopathic IBD with the bowel disease being subclinical. It is conceivable that this spectrum of disease could occur in relatives of IBD patients, in whom clinical bowel disease is not apparent but in whom subclinical bowel disease leads to spondylitis. Thus, IBD is associated with factors that increase the risk for AS in persons genetically predisposed to this disease, and particularly in those with HLA-B27. The link between gut inflammation and arthropathy has also been demonstrated in animal models, notably the human leukocyte antigen B27 transgenic rats (see below, Animal models) [107].

Psoriasis

The frequency of psoriasis, an inflammatory autoimmune disease of the skin, is increased in CD patients (7–11%) as compared to that of the general population (1.1–1.6%) [108, 109]. It is of interest that the increased occurrence of psoriasis was also observed in the relatives of CD patients [109, 110]. As with other IBD-associated diseases, the concurrence of psoriasis and CD at both the individual level and family level suggests the possibility of a genetic link between the two disorders. In genome-wide scans for psoriasis susceptibility loci the HLA region, along with several other novel loci, including loci on 16q (the long arm of chromosome 16), 20q, and 17q, were identified [111–114]. The chromosome 16q region overlaps with a susceptibility locus of CD-*IBD1* [115] (see Genome-wide linkage studies, below). These data are consistent with the hypothesis that some genetic determinants are common for both disorders. Thus attention should be paid in the IBD community as regard any advances in the 16q region with psoriasis (and vice-versa).

Primary sclerosing cholangitis (PSC)

In the case of PSC the association is almost exclusively with UC [116, 117]. This association between PSC and UC has been recognized for several decades, and the most recent surveys of UC series have found the prevalence of PSC among UC patients to be approximately 5% overall and a 10–15% prevalence among UC patients with hepatic abnormalities [118–120]. The converse association is much stronger. Approximately 50–70% of all PSC cases are affected with UC. This may be an underestimate, since IBD onset may have a substantial subclinical phase of IBD far longer than previously appreciated [121].

The significance of such association of PSC with UC has at least two aspects. The first is its obvious clinical importance. The second implication of the PSC–IBD association is pathogenetic, and pertains to the possible immunologic mechanisms linking colitis and cholangitis. Although the pathogenesis of such association is still unknown, the following studies demonstrated the similarities between the two disorders in the immune response: (1) a higher proportion of patients with PSC and UC have anticolon antibodies (63%) and antibodies to portal tract antigens of the liver (compared to 17% of patients with UC alone) [122]; (2) a 40 000 molecular weight colonic epithelial protein has been identified with a unique epitope or epitopes that is shared by the skin and biliary tract epithelial cells [123]; (3) antineutrophil cytoplasmic antibodies have been found in high frequency in both UC and PSC [124–127]. If in fact there is a common antigenic target for immune-mediated attack on both colonic and biliary epithelial cells, identification of this antigen may facilitate understanding of not only the links between IBD and PSC, but also the basic immunoregulatory disorder underlying both diseases, and also allow development of an improved assay(s) for a disease marker or markers in UC and PSC.

Many diseases with a suspected autoimmune etiology or pathogenesis, or both, have been found to be associated with genes of the HLA class II region (discussed in more detail in Gene identification, candidate genes, below). PSC is associated with the HLA antigens B8 and DR3 [117, 128]. Although one study reported that, of 29 patients with PSC, 100%

had the HLA-DRw52a antigen, compared with 35% in the general population [129], such results could not be confirmed in Swedish patients with PSC [130, 131]. A dual association of both HLA-DR2 and HLA-DR3 with PSC has been described [132]. After all the DR3-positive individuals were removed, a significant secondary association with DR2 was noted (69% in PSC vs. 34% in controls). These data suggest that both DR2 and the HLA haplotype A1-B8-DR3 are independent factors that influence the development of PSC. This observation is particularly of interest because most HLA class II association studies with IBD observed a DR2–UC association [133–135] (see below for details) and this was substituted by a DR3–UC association in a population in which the HLA-DRB1*1502 (serologically DR2) is rare [136].

Although it is preliminary, it is worth noting that the degree of association between PSC and UC seems to vary with race and sex. Turkish patients with IBD do not have an increased risk for PSC [137] while Africans and Afro-Caribbeans, especially women, may be at increased risk for PSC [138]. Such a difference suggests a different pathogenesis between PSC and IBD, though some aspects may be common for both diseases.

Pouchitis

Restorative proctocolectomy with ileal reservoir is a widely accepted procedure in the surgical treatment of UC. However, the most frequent long-term complication after ileal pouch–anal anastomosis (IPAA) for UC is a non-specific inflammation of the ileal reservoir known as pouchitis. This complication seems to be disease-related and not operation-related since the occurrence of pouchitis in patients after IPAA for familial adenomatous polyposis is significantly lower than those due to UC [139]. The cumulative risk of developing pouchitis varies between 15% and 46%, depending on the duration of follow-up [140].

The etiology and pathophysiology of pouchitis are not well understood. Many of the risk factors are similar to those for UC. Pouchitis has been found to be associated not only with UC, but with the presence of extraintestinal manifestations of the disease [141, 142], with the presence of pANCA [143, 144] and with the protective effect of smoking [145]. Therefore, it appears that pouchitis reflects the same underlying etiology and pathophysiology of UC, indicating the importance of host factors, such as genetic susceptibility and immunologic functions.

Other immunologic diseases

Multiple sclerosis (MS) is another disorder associated with IBD. Such an association has been demonstrated by the concurrence of MS and IBD both within families [146, 147] and within individuals [148–150]. It is of interest that a study of intestinal permeability in MS patients found that a fourth of patients with MS also had increased intestinal permeability [151]. An explanation, which could also be the explanation for several of the IBD-associated diseases, is that what is inherited is a generalized defect of the immune system which can predispose to several different autoimmune diseases. In support of this hypothesis for at least one form of IBD are studies of large series of IBD patients in which an increased frequency of a series of classic organ-specific autoimmune disorders are observed (e.g. autoimmune thyroid disease, insulin-dependent diabetes, and systemic lupus erythematosus) in UC patients, but not in those with Crohn's [152–154]. An increased co-occurrence of UC and celiac disease has also been reported [155, 156]. In addition, in this genome scan era, multiple putative susceptibility loci have been identified for a number of autoimmune disorders. Importantly, some of these loci are shared among many of the autoimmune diseases [157].

It is interesting to speculate whether other complications of IBD, whose etiology is currently unknown, and which affect only a portion of IBD patients, may have a similar etiologic relationship as the above-mentioned organ-specific autoimmune disorders and UC (i.e. an example of genetic pleiotropy). Complications which might be included in this etiologic model might include uveitis, erythema nodosum, pyoderma gangrenosum, hepatitis, pancreatitis, and cirrhosis. In a large family with members affected with different autoimmune disorders, including rheumatoid arthritis, systemic lupus erythematosus, psoriasis, and IBD, it appears that family members with the same disease tend to share the same HLA haplotypes [158]. If this holds true it may raise a possibility that one set of genes, such as HLA, determine an individual's general auto-immunity, and phenotypic specificity is governed by other genes.

Gene and environmental interaction

The family and twin studies discussed above, and the genetic linkage and association studies reviewed below, are evidence that genetic factors play an essential role in the development of IBD. However, the following observations also argue for an environmental contribution to human IBD: (1) disease incidence has exhibited temporal trends and is correlated with industrialization, (2) there is a much less than a 100% concordance rate in MZ twins, and (3) different disease risks have been observed for the same ethnic group residing in different geographic locations. Therefore, it is likely that both gene and environmental factors determine the risk of developing IBD. Epidemiologic studies have identified several environmental factors, including smoking, appendectomy, oral contraceptive use, and infection. However, the relationships of these environmental factors with IBD seem to be quite complex. For instance, smoking shows a protective effect for UC [159] while it has a deleterious effect for CD [160]. There is a negative correlation between infant mortality or household hygiene and incidence of CD [161–163] while childhood viral infection (e.g. measles and mumps) may increase risk for both UC and CD [164].

The importance of gene and environmental interactions in the development of IBD is clearly demonstrated in animal models [165]. For example, using recombinant DNA technology, transgenic rats expressing the human HLA-B27 and β_2-microglobulin genes have been produced. Certain transgenic rat lines developed a multiorgan disease manifested by colitis, arthritis, orchitis, and psoriasiform changes of the skin and nails [166], features that resemble the human spondyloarthropathies. However, colitis and arthritis do not occur when B27 transgenic rats are raised under germfree conditions, implicating the normal enteric bacterial flora as the source of the antigens driving these diseases [167]. Another model is that mice homozygous for the SCID mutation develop IBD with adoptive transfer of CD4$^+$ T cells expressing high levels of CD45RB (see below, Animal models). However, these mice do not develop IBD in germfree conditions. Other studies have demonstrated that an abnormal immune response in the presence of a single murine pathogen, *Helicobacter hepaticus*, resulted in IBD [168]. Similarly, IL-2 knockout mice do not develop colitis when raised in germfree conditions [165]. Although what genetic and environmental factors interact to cause human IBD is still unknown, such a model may explain at least some forms of IBD, and direct research efforts are necessary to study not only genes, but also environmental factors, simultaneously in the etiologic studies of IBD.

In human studies, environmental factors, such as sanitation, measles virus infection, and other perinatal or childhood infections, *Mycobacterium* infection, appendectomy, oral contraceptive agents, and smoking, etc. have been investigated, but none of these environmental studies has been evaluated taking genetic interactions into account.

If both environmental and genetic factors play an important role in the development of a disease, which factor will be identified as a predominant risk factor will depend on the relative distribution of these factors. For example, in Western societies a common environment may have brought the majority of people to an equal footing in terms of good hygiene, better nutrition, and improved maternal and pediatric care. Those with susceptibility genes will be more likely to develop the disease as compared with those who do not have such genes, given the same environment. In such cases it will be difficult to evaluate environmental factors. In contrast, the increasing incidence in developing countries may provide a window of opportunity for researchers to study gene–environmental interactions since the changing environmental factors (modernization) in a society from a progressive process, and those who develop the disease will be those who are both genetically susceptible and environmentally vulnerable. Therefore, well-designed genetic epidemiologic studies in developing countries are warranted.

An evolutionary perspective

One question that should be raised in the context of this broad discussion of the genetic susceptibility to IBD is why these genes are so frequent. One theoretical possibility is that this could be just due to new mutations. However, these genes clearly cause clinical disease – with major morbidity and even mortality. The mortality was certainly greater until modern supportive management became available. Thus, if new mutations were the explanation, the mutation rate would have to equal both the mortality rate and the decreased reproduction due to the disease. For mutation to explain the IBD disease frequency in the modern world the mutation rate clearly would have to be much greater than the estimated range of 1 in 100 000 to 1 in 1 million per gene locus that appears to be the mutation rate in humans.

If new mutations are an inadequate explanation, there remain two other possible explanations – founder effect and genetic selection. Founder effect refers to the concept that a given gene appeared (presumably by mutation) in a small ancestral population (i.e. in a founder) and by random chance was transmitted to a large number of that founder's offspring. This would establish the gene in relatively high frequency in the original small population and its subsequent ancestors [169]. Although this founder effect is a reasonable explanation for the high frequency of certain genes in certain ethnic groups, it is inadequate explanation for a disease (or diseases) with as wide a distribution and as high a frequency as IBD.

This means we must turn to the consideration of selective advantage [170]. This suggests that the reason these genes are so relatively frequent, even though they are deleterious, i.e. cause disease, is that they also provide some compensating advantage to those individuals who have them [170]. That is, these IBD-predisposing genes presumably provide some advantage in certain environments to which humans have been exposed. This advantage allows those humans with the gene (or genes) to survive better under these conditions, and thus the genes increase in frequency. A balance is achieved when the advantageous effect of the genes is matched by the frequency and severity of the diseases for which they predispose.

There are two reasons why it would be useful to understand how these IBD genes provide their selective advantage. One is that it would contribute to our understanding of human evolution and history. But there is an even more important reason. Understanding of the actual mechanism of the selective advantage (or advantages) will provide an understanding of the underlying physiologic process at a very fundamental level; such understanding may allow us to identify the actual predisposing genes, provide a new understanding of disease pathogenesis, and thus suggest entirely new therapeutic approaches.

Is there any information that would allow us to speculate on the selective advantage provided by the IBD susceptibility genes? There are several basic observations that would underlie any such speculation. First, from the discussion throughout this chapter, it is apparent that IBD is indeed genetic, is clearly common, and occurs in many different ethnic groups throughout the world. Hence a selective advantage is likely necessary to account for its high frequency. Second, it is also apparent that IBD is genetically complex and is likely several different diseases. This means that there are likely several steps in the etiologic pathway that can contribute to any proposed selective advantage. Third, IBD appears to have increased dramatically in the developed world over the past century and is now appearing (or being recognized) with increasing frequency in the developing world. This indicates that some environmental factor or factors, still operating in historical times, provides the advantage in the developing world. It also raises the possibility that the disease is occurring because the selective advantage is no longer acting against the environmental factors that provided the selective advantage. Fourth, given the data reviewed above – that the DZ twin rate is no larger than the sibling recurrence risk – it seems whatever environmental factors are responsible are likely to affect the entire population. That is, the environmental factors are probably ubiquitous, rather than varying dramatically in frequency between families within a population or over a short time period (the few years of childhood). Fifth, IBD is an inflammatory and likely immunologic disease of the gut, so it is likely that environmental factors that provided the selective advantage also operated at the level of the gut.

Putting this information together, the authors have proposed the following hypothesis: that the genes that predispose to the various forms of IBD provided a selective advantage in the form of mucosal immunoprotection in an unsanitary world [162]. Truly effective public sanitation is a development of modern civilization. The development of such sanitation then removes the selective advantage. But the mucosal immunoprotection is still primed genetically in those with the IBD genes, armed, if you will, to defend the organism. Thus, the authors have proposed that, when the IBD predisposing genes are not adequately used in mucosal defense, as they would not be in the developed world, one of two events could occur: (1) later exposure to an infectious agent could result in hyperstimulation of the immune response and subsequent chronic inflammation (analogous to paralytic polio, which occurs when infection occurs after early infancy); or (2) even more likely, failure of exposure to a potentially injurious agent conceivably leaves the gut immunologic system in a continually primed state and thus sets up the system for subsequent dysregulation, i.e. an autoimmune reaction that eventuates in the diseases we recognize as UC and CD [162].

This hypothesis could provide a possible explanation for the relatively high frequency of IBD in the Jewish population [162]. It appears that IBD is highest in frequency in Ashkenazi Jews (i.e. those whose origin is middle and eastern Europe), suggesting that the selective factor or factors had their greatest influence after the Ashkenazi/Sephardic division [14]. This would correspond to the historical division of Europe and the Mediterranean between the Christian and Islamic kingdoms. However, the greatest frequency of IBD appears to arise in those Ashkenazi Jews whose origin is in middle Europe [16, 17] and is similar to the distribution of Tay-Sachs gene carriers [171]. These are the countries that imposed the greatest ghetto urbanization on the Jews and presumably greatest overcrowding and the consequent greatest defects in sanitation. This situation eased when the Ashkenazi Jews were invited to settle in eastern Europe, that is, Poland, Ukraine, and Russia. The origin of both Tay-Sachs heterozygotes and IBD patients is highest in individuals from middle as opposed to eastern Europe [17, 171]. The lower frequency of IBD in Israel compared to western Europe or the United States would then be a possible consequence of the more developing nature of that society. Regardless, if the specific details of this hypothesis are correct, it will be important to determine if indeed a genetically hyperresponding mucosal immune system is responsible for the susceptibility to IBD.

Pathophysiology: biologic basis of genetic susceptibility

Recent, parallel progress in the genetic and immunologic studies of human and rodent models has contributed much detail to our understanding of the pathophysiology of IBD. Several genetic abnormalities have now been shown to affect the balance of T cell responses to the antigens of bacteria commensal to the gut. Susceptibility to disease arises from an unfavorable genetic profile that creates an imbalance between antigen-specific effector and regulatory cells (e.g. Th-1, Th-2, TR-1/IL-10, or Th-3 /TGF-β cells). Disorders in T cell responses have been associated with the presence of marker serum antibodies, each with a particular antigen specificity, as well as with distinct patterns of mucosal damage that together result in the broad spectrum of clinical manifestations of UC and CD. A clinical implication of this working hypothesis is that each distinct pattern will respond best to that therapy that addresses the specific imbalance at the foundation of that pattern. Future therapies may address these imbalances by altering cytokine profiles, by augmenting regulatory

T cell functions, or by changing the bacterial micro-environment in the gut.

Phenotypic heterogeneity

Current evidence strongly supports the concepts that: (1) IBD is not a single or even two diseases (e.g. CD and UC), but rather is likely to be several distinct diseases presenting within the broad clinical picture of CD or UC; (2) these distinct diseases may have distinct etiologies and may require distinct therapies for successful treatment; and (3) close attention to clinical phenotype, to marker antibodies, and ultimately to polymorphisms of specific genes may identify these subgroups of CD and UC. These concepts are further supported by the fact that manipulation of many different genes in numerous rodent models of IBD (reviewed below) produces a wide spectrum of intestinal inflammation, broadly classifiable as CD-like or UC-like, yet each also with specific characteristics unique to each model. Indeed, the wide spectrum of human intestinal inflammation seen in the clinic is mimicked by the wide spectrum of intestinal inflammation seen in the animal models.

The numerous rodent models further suggest that genetic heterogeneity, wherein defects in different genes or different combinations of genes lead to similar clinical manifestations, poses a major problem in elucidating the pathophysiology of IBD. Studies of the association of genetic variation with more homogeneous subgroups of disease, defined either by close attention to clinical detail or by subclinical markers, will therefore play an important role in sorting out the etiology of the different forms of IBD and ultimately lead to the specific therapies needed for each subgroup.

Patients with UC or CD show great variability in their disease phenotype for such characteristics as age of onset; rate of relapse; fibrostenosis; perforating/fistulizing; internal or perianal 'penetrating disease' (fistulas, abscesses, or perforations); presence of diarrhea bleeding or mucus discharge; duration of disease; location of disease (small bowel only, ileocolonic, colon only); number and types of surgery; development of chronic pouchitis after colectomy; and response to classes of medications such as corticosteroids, sulfasalazine or oral mesalamine, immunomodulatory agents (e.g. 6-mercaptopurine/azathioprine, methotrexate, cyclosporine), antibiotics, and topical therapies for distal colonic disease [172–174]. Some patients can be clearly classified as having CD based on histologic criteria yet have the 'UC-like' features of left-sided colitis, more continuous and more shallow inflammation on endoscopy, and response to topical therapy [173]. As discussed above, some patients present with intermediate inflammation and cannot be classified as either CD or UC ('indeterminate colitis').

Several lines of evidence suggest these phenotypic differences reflect underlying differences in immunologic processes. IL-1β and IL-1 receptor antagonist mRNAs are increased in resected intestinal tissue from patients with non-perforating CD (the more benign form of CD) when compared with perforating CD [175]. CD patients from families with multiple cases tend to have an early age at onset and more extensive disease as compared with those from families with no other cases [176]. Within families with multiply-affected cases of CD, common familial patterns have been observed in the disease aggressi [176, 178]. Such familial distribution of clinical features suggests that certain genetic or environmental factors shared by family members may determine the clinical course of the disease. Thus, it may be beneficial to study a clinically homogeneous group in order to understand the role of certain genetic or environmental factors.

Genetic studies of pathophysiology

Subclinical markers – ANCA and ASCA

As commonly used, subclinical markers can be considered as 'intermediate phenotypes' or parameters which occur in the process of a disease's development, and are hopefully highly specific for that disease, e.g. abnormal glucose tolerance and islet cell antibodies in diabetes, serum cholesterol in coronary artery disease, and adenomatous polyps in colon cancer [179]. The study of subclinical markers promises to be a great aid to unravel the phenotypic heterogeneity of IBD. Markers with the greatest value in IBD research will be those that are closely related to the various underlying immunologic processes that lead to the broad categories of intestinal inflammation.

As discussed above, the use of anti-neutrophil cytoplasmic antibodies with perinuclear immunofluorescent binding pattern (pANCA) in combination with antibodies to the cell-wall mannan of *Saccharomyces cerevisiae* (ASCA) distinguish UC and CD. Several lines of evidence support the concept that the *serum* expression of these antibodies reflects *mucosal* processes. For pANCA, B cell clones taken from the mucosa of UC patients express pANCA [180], directly demonstrating pANCA in the intestinal mucosa. Further, pANCA is present in the sera of a high proportion of IL-10 knockout mice [181]. This reaction is eliminated by prior absorption of the pANCA+ mouse sera with homogenized mouse cecal bacteria, suggesting that pANCA cross-reacts with enteric bacterial antigens. For ASCA the specificity of the expression of anti-mannan antibodies, rather than anti-gliadin or anti-ovalbumin in CD patients [182], of antibodies to *Saccharomyces* and not to *Candida* [183] and of the expression of ASCA in patients with CD, rather than with UC or other colitides, suggests that ASCA expression manifests a CD-related immune response rather than reflecting a non-specific intestinal insult resulting from the inflammation.

The expression of pANCA or ASCA has also been shown to extend the observed variability in IBD phenotype and provides further evidence for distinct subgroups within UC and CD. Within UC the presence of pANCA has been associated with more severe forms of UC (treatment-resistant and left-sided UC [184]), and the development of pouchitis following an ileal pouch–anal anastomosis procedure [144]. Within CD the presence of pANCA is associated with a more 'UC-like' disease (more left-sided colitis, more distal, continuous, or shallow endoscopic appearance, more superficial histopathology [173]). Utilizing pANCA as a phenotype the authors have also provided evidence for heterogeneity within UC with family data [185] and this heterogeneity appears to have a genetic basis as demonstrated by the use of HLA class II [186] and the intercellular adhesion molecule-1 molecular polymorphisms [187] (see below, Candidate genes). High titers of ASCA in CD are associated with early age of disease onset as well as both fibrostenosing and internal penetrating disease; in contrast, high ANCA levels are associated with a later age of onset and different disease location [174].

Recent studies support the hypothesis that genetic factors determine ANCA and ASCA expression, at least in part. First, ANCA and ASCA have been observed to be familial traits. For ANCA an increased frequency of positive ANCAs has been observed in the clinically healthy relatives of UC patients compared with environmental controls [185]. Second-degree relatives, who did not share the same household with the probands, had an increased prevalence of ANCAs and the household controls

were not at increased risk for ANCA. These results were further confirmed by an independent study [188], but not observed in another study [189]. In a small twin study, 64% (9/14) of identical twins with UC had a positive ANCA, while of their 10 healthy monozygotic twins, two had ANCA (20%), which was greater than the frequency in healthy controls (5.8%) [190]. These important epidemiologic observations suggest that the familial aggregation of ANCAs is due to shared genetic factors among the family members, and not due to shared environmental factors. Further, in these family studies there was a significant difference in the frequency of ANCAs in the relatives of probands whose sera were ANCA(+) compared with the relatives of probands whose sera were ANCA(–) [185, 188]. This concordant familial distribution indicates heterogeneity within UC. Thus, ANCAs may be used as a marker of an underlying immunologic disturbance that is genetically determined [191].

For ASCA the level of ASCA expression as a quantitative trait has been shown to be familial in both affected and unaffected relatives of CD patients using intraclass correlation analysis [192]. A high percentage of CD patients (approximately half) and affected family members (also approximately half but with a lower level of expression) were seropositive for anti-mannan Ig, compared to the normal control population (3.7%). Seropositivity or seronegativity was correlated among all affected relatives, and this association was stronger in affected first-degree relatives. Intraclass correlations revealed less variation in ASCA levels within, rather than between, families, and a significant familial aggregation was observed. There was no significant correlation among marital pairs. These findings demonstrated that ASCA in family members affected and unaffected with CD is a familial trait for both affected and unaffected relatives. The lack of correlation in marital pairs suggested that this familial aggregation is due in part to a genetic factor or childhood environmental exposure.

Second, preliminary observations suggest that genetic loci are associated with ANCA and ASCA expression. For ANCA the intracellular adhesion molecule-1 *ICAM1* G241R allele has been associated with ANCA expression [187] (see below, Candidate gene studies, *ICAM1*). For ANCA and ASCA an allele in the MHC *Notch4* gene has been associated with high ASCA expression combined with absence of pANCA expression (see below) [193]. For ASCA the TNF microsatellite 'a' (see

Candidate gene studies – TNF, below) has been associated with ASCA seropositivity, irregardless of whether the patient has CD or UC [194]. In addition, ASCA expression appears to be linked to markers near the MHC on chromosome 6 (IBD3) but not with the IBD1 locus on chromosome 16 [195].

When taken together, these observations suggest that ASCA and pANCA are serum markers for different mucosal inflammatory mechanisms that underlie distinct disease expression, and that genetic variation may underlie these mechanisms. Use of clinical (fistulizing, perforating, fibrostenotic) and subclinical (ANCA, ASCA) characteristics may be useful in subdividing patient populations into more etiologically homogeneous groups for genetic studies, and may thus be the means for unraveling the genetic heterogeneity of these diseases in the future.

Other subclinical markers

Other potential subclinical markers are summarized in Table 5. Some of these, if confirmed, may lead to the understanding of host and environmental interactions, such as obligate anerobic fecal flora.

The complement system plays a major role in the immune response and in the inflammatory process, thus making it a potential candidate in the etiology of IBD. Subnormal release of chemotactic activity for neutrophils (elicited by C5a2 from complement), increased *in-vivo* C3 catabolism, increased levels of circulating C3c split products, and positive immunoconglutinin titers have all been reported in CD patients, and suggest that complement may play a role in this disease [198, 209–213]. Complement levels are also known to vary with disease activity, supporting the possibility that the complement system could play a role in IBD etiology or pathophysiology [214–216]. Evidence supporting this concept includes the observation of enhanced local production of complement components in the small intestine of patients with CD [216–218]. Furthermore, the proposal that the pathogenesis of CD is mediated by multifocal gastrointestinal infarction is also consistent with a complement-mediated process [219–221]. A study of the protein polymorphism of the third component of complement (C3) was reported in a series of Danish patients with CD [222]. In this series, the 'F' and 'FS' phenotypes occurred significantly more often in the CD patients than in either UC patients or normal controls. The gene frequency of the 'F' allele was 0.33 in CD with small bowel involvement only, 0.23 in all CD patients, 0.18 in UC patients and 0.17 in healthy volunteers. These

data suggest that there may be etiologic differences not only between UC and CD, but also between CD with and without colonic involvement. The molecular basis of polymorphisms between C3S and C3F has been suggested to be due to a single nucleotide change [223]. The complement *C3* gene is located within the peak linkage reported for IBD on chromosome 19 (see below).

One trait that has been investigated a number of times is that of intestinal permeability. Since the initial family study of intestinal permeability in CD [224], there have been a number of several additional family studies. On first inspection the results may appear somewhat inconsistent. It seems that a number of related factors may affect the results of an intestinal permeability study. These may include the type of probes, the method of administration of the probe, e.g. fasting/non-fasting, with meals/without meals [199], day urine collection/overnight urine collection, length of urine collection, and use of aspirin as a challenge [225]. It is important for this area of investigation to identify a sensitive and reproducible protocol for permeability testing that reliably separates Crohn's patients (or a subgroup of CD) from controls. In addition, it has been proposed that some of the statistical methods used to illustrate the increased permeability in the relatives of patients with CD may give misleading results [199]. Rather than comparing the means of permeability between the two groups – relatives and controls – one can examine the proportion of the asymptomatic relatives of patients with CD who have permeability values above the upper limits of the range of values in normal controls. The logic of this latter approach is that presumably only a proportion of CD relatives is genetically susceptible. Where this was done the investigators found that approximately 10% of these relatives had a significant increase in intestinal permeability [226]. When re-examining the published studies by this same approach (i.e. defining an increased level as greater than two standard deviations above the mean in controls), the majority of such studies showed a significant increase in intestinal permeability in a fraction of the asymptomatic relatives of patients with CD [199]. Although there may be familiality of increased intestinal permeability, some family and twin studies do not support the hypothesis of a genetically determined intestinal leakiness in CD [201, 202]. In addition, a variety of other disorders have shown increased permeability, such as celiac disease, relatives of celiac disease patients [227] and even AIDS patients [228].

Table 5. Subclinical markers for inflammatory bowel disease

Specific disease	Marker	Type of relatives studied	Observations	Reference
Combined IBD	Autoantibodies to epithelial cell-associated components (ECAC) antigens	Family members	ECAC-C observed in 69.7% CD patients, 55.7% relatives, and only 8.0% control subjects	196
	Antinuclear autoantibodies (ANA)	Family members	ANA observed in 18% CD patients, 43% UC patients, 13% relatives of CD, 24% relatives of UC, 2% control subjects	197
	Goblet cell autoantibodies (GABs)	Family members	Positive GABs in 39% UC, 30% CD, 21% first-degree relatives of UC, 19% first-degree relatives of CD, 3% infectious enterocolitis, 2% healthy control subjects	197
CD	C3 dysfunction	Family members	Greater C3 dysfunction in CD (38%) and relatives (18%) than in control subjects	198
	Intestinal permeability	Family members and twins	Increased in CD patients, conflicting results regarding relatives	Review in 1999 200–202
	Obligate anaerobic fecal flora	Family members	The flora of CD patients contained more anerobic Gram-positive coccoid rods and more Gram-negative rods than that of healthy subjects; during 5–7 years follow-up, three of nine children with CD with a CD floral pattern showed CD symptoms and one such child was diagnosed as CD. None of 17 children with a normal flora showed CD symptoms	203
	Anti-*Saccharomyces cerevisiae* antibodies (ASCA)	Family members and twins	ASCA increased in CD patients as compared with control subjects ASCA positive in 50% CD, increased in healthy relatives	182, 204, 192; also see text
	Pancreatic autoantibodies	Family members	Positive pancreatic autoantibodies in 27% CD (144% type I, 13% type II), subtype showed familial cluster, 0.5% in first-degree relatives	205
UC	Antineutrophil cytoplasmic antibodies	Family members and twins	Specific for UC, increased in healthy relatives of UC patients, occur in a subset of CD patients	185, 188, 189, 206; also see text
	Colonic mucins	Twins	HCM species IV (mucin subtype) reduced in both UC and healthy co-twins as compared with control subjects	207
	Mucosal production of gG subclass	Twins	UC patients and their healthy MZ co-twins showed a raised proportion of IgG1 (78%) as compared with control subjects (56%)	208
	IgA against gliadin	Twins	High IgA titers against gliadin in both UC patients and their healthy co-twins	182

These cumulative data would argue that these permeability abnormalities are likely not a fundamental inborn defect which predispose an individual to develop IBD, but indicate early intestinal damage (preclinical expression). Natural history studies will be useful to resolve this 'chicken and egg' issue and clarify the interpretation from cross-sectional family studies. Genetic marker studies may also shed some light on this issue, especially those genes coding for structures in the permeability channels of the gut.

The potential importance of T cell receptor γ/δ genes in IBD has been suggested by a phenotypic study of γ/δ T lymphocytes in the intestinal mucosa of UC and CD [229]. The different characterization and distribution of γ/δ lymphocytes was found not only between patients with IBD and normal controls, but also between patients with UC and those with CD. The T cell receptor α/δ complex lies in the chromosomal 14 linkage region (see below).

Immunoglobulin levels and subtypes have been investigated between IBD patients and controls, and also between CD and UC patients. One report observed a difference in immunoglobulin G (Gm allotype) markers in CD patients versus controls, with a significant increase in frequency of the Gm (a,x,f;b,g) phenotype and Gm (a,x;g) haplotypes [230]. However, these results could not be replicated in later studies [231–234]. No evidence for association or linkage with any specific immunoglobulin allotype was found in these latter studies. Given the studies of IgG subclass distribution in patients with UC or CD [235] and their family members [208] (see section on Subclinical markers above for details), immunoglobulin genes still remain as potential candidate genes for IBD genetic studies.

Animal models

Recognition and development of animal models of IBD has progressed rapidly in recent years [165, 236] (see Table 6). Chronic intestinal inflammation has been observed to occur in animals: (1) spontaneously (e.g. the rainforest cottontop tamarin grown in the temperate climate of North America, or the C3H/HeJBir mouse strain); (2) after application or ingestion of chemicals (e.g. acetic acid instilled into the rectum or dextran sulfate sodium given in drinking water); (3) after genetic manipulation (e.g. rats expressing the human HLA-B27 molecule or various 'knockout' strains of mice); and (4) after tissue transfer from one strain to another (e.g. transplantation of T cell-depleted wild-type bone marrow into T

cell-deficient (tgε 26) mice or transfer of CD4$^+$ CD45RB^{hi} T cells into B and T cell-deficient SCID mice). No single model completely reproduces the spectrum of human IBD, but each model is useful depending on the question being asked. Indeed, the wide spectrum of intestinal inflammation manifested by the sum total of these animal models is further evidence for the likely heterogeneity of human IBD.

The basic lessons for IBD pathophysiology learned from these models are:

1. *There are multiple paths to chronic intestinal inflammation.* Chronic inflammation can be produced by creating transgenic animals in different genes: (1) targeted disruption ('knockout') of various genes in the mouse, interleukin-2 or its receptor, interleukin-10 (IL-10$^{-/-}$), T-cell receptor α or β, transforming growth factor β, or G protein-α_{i2}; (2) enhancing expression of the tumor necrosis factor gene (TNF$^{\Delta ARE}$ 'knockin'); or (3) adding of the human HLA-B27 and β_2-microglobulin genes to the rat (HLA-B27/β2m). The involvement of different paths in these models is further supported by differences in cytokine profiles, for example, inflammation in the TNF$^{\Delta ARE}$ model is characterized by high levels of TNF [240], inflammation in the IL-10$^{-/-}$ knockout model is characterized by high levels of IFN-γ [251], and the inflammation in the T-cell receptor $\alpha^{-/-}$ knockout model is characterized by high levels of IL-1α,β, and IL-4, but not IFN-γ [257, 258].

2. *Intestinal inflammation is determined by multiple genes.* In addition to the observations that several human genomic regions show linkage to IBD (see below) and that disruption of several different genes can lead to chronic intestinal inflammation (see previous section), breeding studies with mouse models also support the idea that many genes acting in concert predispose to IBD. For example, with the dextran sulfate sodium (DSS) mouse model, observed major differences in genetic susceptibility to DSS-induced colitis were observed [237]: strains C3H/HeJ and NOD/LtJ were particularly susceptible, strain C57BL/6J(B6) was partially resistant, and NON/LtJ was fully resistant to induction of inflammation. By crossing the susceptible C3H/HeJ strain to the partially resistant C57BL/6 strain and analyzing the colitis as a quantitative trait, these authors identified two loci with significant link-

Table 6. Genetically mediated rodent models of IBD

Model	Symbols	Inflammation	Bacteria required	Comments	References
Induced by agents					
Dextran sulfate sodium	DSS	Entire colon		Identification of linkage to 5 genomic regions – multiple genes are required; this colitis is not T cell-dependent	237, 238
Transgenic					
HLA-B27/β_2-microglobulin rat	HLAB27/β_2m	Entire colon, small bowel, stomach	Yes	Increased colitis with *Bacteroides* spp.	107, 167, 239
TNF knockin mouse, increased TNP production	TNF$^{\Delta ARE}$	Chronic ileitis	Unknown	No colitis in TNF$^{\Delta ARE}$ + TNF receptor 1 double mutants	240, 241
Targeted disruption (knockouts)					
IL-2 knockout mouse	IL-2$^{-/-}$	Entire colon	Colitis decreased, but not eliminated in germfree environment	Increased transforming growth factor β, CD14, inducible nitric oxide synthase; IL-12 induces thymocytes to become colitis-inducing	242–246
IL-2 knockout mouse, raised pathogen-free, with colitis induced by keyhole limpet hemocyanin	IL-2$^{-/-}$ with TNP-KLH induction	Entire colon	Mild colitis increased by induction with TNP-KLH in germ-free environment	Colitis reduced by anti-integrin $\alpha E\beta 7$	247, 248
IL-10 knockout mouse	IL-10$^{-/-}$	Colon, duodenum, jejunum	Yes; colitis can also be induced by *Helicobacter hepaticus* alone	Overproduction of Th1 cytokines; mediated by CD4^{+} Th1 cells	243, 249–252
Tumor necrosis factor knockout mouse	TNF$^{-/-}$	None	No	Defective antibacterial response; formation of B lymphocyte follicles; TNF receptor 1 also deficient in antibacterial response	253–255
T-cell receptor α knockout mouse	TCR$\alpha^{-/-}$	Entire colon		No colitis in TCR$\alpha^{-/-}$ and IL-4$^{-/-}$ double mutants (suggests Th2 pathway), but colitis in TCR$\alpha^{-/-}$ and IFN-$\gamma^{-/-}$ double mutants; B cells suppress colitis development but not required for initiation; initiation may require overproduction of IL-1α and IL-1β	256–258
				IL-4 but not IFN-γ required	258
Transplantation					
CD45RB^{hi} cells to SCID mouse or to RAG minus mouse		Entire colon	Yes	STAT-4/IL-12 pathway involved; CD45RB^{lo} cells from IL-10$^{-/-}$ mouse no longer protect; TGF-β is required for suppression of colitis by CD45RB^{lo}; accelerated disease if T cells are depleted of natural killer cells	259–263
				Role of natural killer (NK) cells in down-regulation of Th1-mediated colitis	263

age to colitis, *D5Mit216* and *D2Mit94*, and a further three loci with suggestive evidence for linkage, *D18Mit119*, *D1Mit386*, and *D11Mit140* [238]. The linkage of DSS-induced colitis to the region on mouse chromosome 2 was confirmed using a NOD/LtJ X NON/LtJ cross. The *D5Mit216* locus is syntenic with human linkage results on chromosome 5 [264]. These results demonstrated that, similar to the human colitis, the rodent colitis in this model had more than one determining locus, and further work may lead to the identification of the specific genes determining colitis in this model.

3. *Intestinal inflammation may require the presence of bacteria in the gut.* When raised in bacteria-free conditions, inflammation does not occur with the *IL-10* and *TCRα* knockouts [243, 256]. Using the HLA-B27/β2m rat, it was observed that animals raised under germfree conditions developed colitis only after gut colonization by bacterial mixtures containing *Bacteroides* species [107]. When directly compared, inflammation induced by *Bacteroides vulgatus* was significantly more severe than that induced by *Escherichia coli* [239]. This latter model raises the possibility that the HLA-B molecule may interact with bacterial antigens to produce IBD in humans. In contrast, inflammation is greatly reduced, but not eliminated, when the IL-2 knockout is raised in germfree, compared with specific pathogen-free, conditions [243]. When taken together, these results suggest that live gut bacteria increase colonic inflammation in IBD and may be necessary for initiation of inflammation in some, but not all, models of disease.

4. *Both pathogenic and protective CD4+ cells are present in the normal animal.* Intestinal inflammation occurs when a subpopulation of T cells from spleen or lymph node, CD4+ CD45RB^{hi}, are transferred into isogenic mice with severe combined immunodeficiency (SCID) or with a disruption of the recombination activating gene (RAG$^{-/-}$). In contrast, transfer of the entire CD4+ population, or of the CD4+ CD45RB^{lo} subpopulation, does not induce inflammation. The CD4+ CD45RB^{lo} subset inhibits the CD4+ CD45RB^{hi} subset from inducing inflammation [265]. These observations suggested that normal mice have subsets of T cells that are capable of causing gut

inflammation and that these subsets are kept in check by other subsets of T cells that protect the animal from inflammation. The induction by CD4+ CD45RB^{hi} cells can also be significantly reduced by treating the animal with anti-IFN-γ, anti-IL-12, and IL-10, suggesting that pathogenesis in this model follows the Th1 pathway [259, 260, 266]. The suppression of inflammation by the CD4+ CD45RB^{lo} subset was inhibited by treatment with anti-transforming growth factor beta (anti-TGB-β) but not anti-IL-4, suggesting a role for TGF-β in this suppression and that the inhibitory cells in the CD4+ CD45RB^{lo} subset may not be simply Th2 cells [261].

IBD pathogenesis in this model can be dissected further by isolating the CD4+ CD45RB^{hi} cells from transgenics with alterations in various genes. Inflammation was greatly reduced, but not eliminated, when the CD4+ CD45RB^{hi} cells were isolated from knockouts in the signal transducer and activator of transcription-4 (STAT-4$^{-/-}$) [260], demonstrating that the IL-12/STAT-4 pathway plays the major role in the development of inflammation in this model. While this pathway controls IFN-γ production and anti-IFN-γ does reduce inflammation, conflicting results have been reported with CD4+ CD45RB^{hi} cells from IFN-γ knockouts [260, 267]. These conflicts, and the fact that some disease occurs with CD4+ CD45RB^{hi} cells from STAT-4 knockouts, further reiterates the observations that there are multiple pathways to intestinal inflammation.

Gene mapping approaches

Analytic approaches to gene identification

Before we turn to strategies of gene-finding based on prior hypotheses (e.g. candidate genes) or chromosomal locations (e.g. systematic genome scans), it is worthwhile to briefly review the analytic approaches and molecular tools that are utilized in all such studies.

The goal of gene-finding efforts is to identify the specific gene(s), and the specific molecular variation(s) in that gene (known as alleles), that predispose to one or more forms of IBD. Classically, this problem was approached by finding a physiologic abnormality in a disease, then the responsible biochemical abnormality, and then the abnormal protein responsible for the biochemical abnormality. One could then sequence the protein and infer the responsible DNA variation leading to the variant protein. Limitations to this approach included lack of understanding of the biochemical processes involved, thereby limiting the ability to examine for abnormal enzyme activity. Furthermore, the abnormal protein may not be abnormal *per se*, but only be abnormal in the amount expressed. In addition, with modern molecular techniques it is considerably easier to sequence DNA than it is to sequence a protein. Thus the more expeditious approach is to study some level of phenotype (e.g. disease, antibody) together with variation defined at the DNA level. Gene-finding efforts take advantage of the fact that DNA is a linear structure, i.e. that a gene is a linear sequence of DNA base pairs, and that individual genes are arranged linearly along a chromosome.

Polymorphic markers

All gene-finding studies require variation in a gene, or along the DNA of a chromosome. This variation is known as a gene marker. While historically any trait that varied (the formal term is that the trait is polymorphic) was used as a genetic marker (examples include red blood cell antigens, HLA antigens, serum protein polymorphisms), by far the greatest variation occurs at the DNA level itself. The most common is variation in the sequence of the four DNA bases, i.e. one base replacing another, known as single-nucleotide polymorphisms (SNPs). There can also be deletion or addition of one or more base pairs. When either of these variations affects a sequence of base pairs that is recognized by a specific DNA endonuclease (which in digesting the DNA will result in fragments of different sizes), then one has a restriction enzyme fragment length polymorphism (RFLP). A different class of polymorphism is due to variation in the length of a sequence, e.g. an individual might have a sequence of CACA on one chromosome, and CACACACA on the other. When the unit (repeated sequence) of DNA base pairs being repeated is small, they are termed microsatellites, or simple sequence repeats (SSRs), or alternatively simple tandem repeats (STRs). When the unit is large they are termed variable number of tandem repeats (VNTRs). There are a whole host of molecular methods to assess these variations, including Southern blotting, oligonucleotide hybridization, restriction enzyme digestion, and direct sequencing (to name a few), all of which have been greatly expedited by the discovery of the polymerase chain reaction (PCR), which allows the *in vitro* amplification of virtually any sequence of DNA in any quantities desired.

Linkage and association

Using these molecular tools the two basic study approaches are family-based linkage studies and population (usually case–control) association studies (see Table 7). Linkage studies ask the question: does the trait of interest (e.g. the presence of CD) travel together in families with a particular chromosomal segment, identified by one or more genetic markers? Linkage studies take advantage of the fact that genes are arranged linearly along the 23 pairs (i.e. 46 total) of human chromosomes. During meiosis, the cellular division that produces the gametes, each chromosome pairs with its partner (known as the homologous chromosome, hence 22 autosomal pairs, and a pair of sex chromosomes), and exchanges genetic material. This exchange, termed recombination, is the basis of linkage. If two genes are close together on a chromosome, then the chance that they would recombine is small. If they are far apart on the chromosome, then the chance that they would recombine is large. The frequency of recombination is reported in units termed centimorgans (cM), with one centimorgan equivalent to a frequency of 1% recombination. The genetic distance of all the human chromosomes combined is somewhat greater than 3000 cM. Since the 23 pairs of chromosomes are approximately 3 billion DNA base pairs long, the genetic distance of 1 cM is, on average, equivalent to a physical distance of 1 million base pairs.

Within one or two generations there are only a few recombinant events per chromosome, so large chromosomal segments are shared between parents and offspring and between siblings. Linkage asks whether a certain allele of a genetic marker is transmitted within a family (also referred to as cosegregation) with the disease or trait of interest. Because large chromosomal segments are shared in families, if the actual disease predisposing gene is within 10–20 cM (equivalent to 10–20 million base pairs) of the genetic marker, then linkage will usually be observed. In performing a linkage analysis one can have a prior hypothesis that a specific gene is involved. In that case, existence of linkage with a genetic marker at or near the gene of interest indicates that this is indeed the gene causing the disease, or that the disease gene is located in close physical proximity to that gene. Alternatively, one can perform a linkage analysis of the entire genome (the entire complement of human chromosomes), known as systematic mapping (also known as a genome scan). Here there is no prior hypothesis regarding the disease gene's location.

Table 7. Contrasting linkage and association

	Linkage	Association
Theoretical basis	Predisposing gene is located on a chromosomal segment which contains tested polymorphic genetic markers. Depends on the fact that family members share chromosome segments that are transmitted as a unit	Testing specific predisposing variant allele of a predisposing gene; or testing a marker that is extremely close to the gene
Type of sample	Pedigrees, sibpairs, relative pairs	Case-control, nuclear families
Role to identify contribution of specific gene	Major genes easily identified Genes of modest effect: difficult to identify, requires large number of families	Major genes, moderate genes, minor genes can be identified
Polymorphic marker locations relative to specific gene	Can be some genetic distance away, i.e. 5–20 cM (centimorgans), approximately 5–20 million base pairs For a genome-wide search, ~ 400 markers with ~ 10 cM map density is generally sufficient	Must be extremely close, either within the gene, or within several hundred kilobases of the gene (less than 1 cM). For a genome-wide search, it is stimated that 50 000–500 000 markers are required
Advantages	If linkage is observed, it is likely that a major gene is identified. Can see the effect some distance from the disease gene. Can identify an effect even there is allelic heterogeneity (i.e. multiple alleles contribute to the disease susceptibility). A powerful approach for genome-wide search	Can identify genes of minor effect. Can identify specific genetic variants that contribute to the disease susceptibility. Can easily incorporate gene–gene and gene–environmental interactions in data analysis. A preferred approach for candidate gene studies

Instead one is taking advantage of the fact that 300–400 evenly spaced DNA markers will likely identify most linkages, because such a number of markers will on average be 10 cM apart, and linkage usually extends over that distance. It is important to note that, in conducting a linkage analysis, the form of the genetic marker, the allele, can differ between one family and another. The important question is whether the alleles travel together with the disease in families, but the measure is not allele-specific.

In contrast to linkage, which asks whether chromosomal segments are shared between two family members with a disease, association tests whether a specific allele of a genetic marker is found with increased frequency in individuals with the disease compared to the frequency of that marker in individuals without the disease. If a disorder is found to be associated with a particular allele, this may suggest a causal relationship (i.e. the association may be due to one of the effects of the gene in which the marker allele lies), or may be due to very nearby genes, a phenomenon known as linkage disequilibrium (see further discussion of linkage disequilibrium, below). Just as linkage takes advantage of recombination within current families, linkage disequilibrium takes advantage of the many more recombinant events that have occurred historically in a population. Thus, in contrast to linkage which covers a chromosomal region of 10–20 cM (10–20 million base pairs), association due to linkage disequilibrium will usually occur over less than 1 cM (say 0.1–0.2 cM), therefore over a distance of only a few hundred thousand base pairs.

Linkage and association approaches each have their advantages and disadvantages (see Table 7). The most information is gained when they are used in a complementary fashion. Thus, for example, if one has no prior hypothesis, then one starts first with a systematic linkage genome scan to identify potential chromosomal regions, and then one can study the positive regions in more detail with association approaches. If one starts out with a candidate gene, it may be easier to first conduct an association study. Such studies have the advantage that, even if the responsible gene has a minor effect (often referred to as a polygene), such effects can be identified. However, regardless of the association result, it is still important to conduct a linkage study. One, linkage can be observed even when an association does not exist, or the associated marker has not been identified. Two, if linkage is found along with an association for a particular gene locus (the address of the gene), then this suggests that the association has identified a major gene for the disease. That is, interestingly, linkage studies, at the sample sizes currently being conducted, can usually only identify major gene effects. Such, for example, has been the case for the chromosome 6 HLA class II locus associations with type 1 insulin-dependent diabetes [268]. Thus linkage can help prioritize the order in which associations should be further explored. Studies of type 1 diabetes well illustrate these concepts. Associations were seen in the mid-1970s with HLA class I alleles on chromosome 6, but these were of only modest magnitude. Similar magnitude associations were seen with the insulin gene on chromosome 11 in the mid-1980s. However, the importance of the HLA gene region was recognized very quickly in the 1970s, because strong evidence for linkage was seen with family studies of modest size (tens of families), indicating that the actual responsible genetic variation was nearby. In contrast, it was not until the 1990s that family studies had attained the sample size (many hundreds) to help confirm the role of polymorphic variation in the insulin gene. Indeed, the nearby HLA class II genes are major genes for type 1 diabetes, while the insulin gene is comparatively a minor gene.

Advantages and challenges of a systematic linkage mapping approach

Due to the complexity and incomplete understanding of the pathophysiology of IBD, the number of potential candidates for these abnormalities could easily extend to well over a hundred, and at the same time it may not be possible to identify all possible candidates. As the number of biologically relevant candidate genes in IBD becomes more numerous, a candidate gene strategy becomes more cumbersome and resource-expensive, because in many cases one has to identify new polymorphic markers for each gene and optimize the genotyping condition individually for these markers. Fortunately, the systematic linkage mapping approach gives us a solution to this dilemma. That is, we can now test for linkage between a disease and evenly spaced, highly polymorphic markers along the whole genome. Then one can follow those results by testing candidate genes in the regions showing evidence for linkage – the positional candidate approach – or alternatively, identify novel susceptibility genes to the disease.

In the systematic mapping approach, no *a-priori* hypothesis is made as to the nature or location of the specific genetic susceptibility genes for the disease or trait of interest. Instead, the genetic determinants of these phenotypes are tested with a large number of highly polymorphic DNA markers scattered at equal intervals throughout the estimated 3300 cM comprising the human genome. One is simply asking if there is cosegregation between the disease (or related phenotype) and one or more of the tested markers. This approach has been successfully applied in Mendelian disorders, such as cystic fibrosis, Huntington's disease, and diastrophic dysplasia, with investigations proceeding from positive linkage results, to linkage disequilibrium mapping, to gene identification, and then to functional studies both *in vitro* and in genetically manipulated animal models.

Genome scans in complex diseases

It is a much greater challenge to apply this approach to genetically complex disorders, since the strict one-to-one relationship between genotypes and phenotypes observed in monogenic disorders breaks down for complex diseases. For most complex diseases it is likely that multiple genes influence the expression of the disease which, in turn, makes it difficult to isolate and characterize the effects of each and every individual locus determining the disease. Such multiple genes may interact (epistasis) or induce susceptibility independently (locus heterogeneity). In addition, most complex diseases such as IBD are also influenced by environmental factors. As a consequence, genetic mapping in a complex disorder is considerably more difficult than for a Mendelian disorder. However, success is now being achieved, due to advances in rapid molecular genotyping, development of non-parametric linkage methods, studies of adequate sample size, and better definition of phenotypes.

Experience has now shown us that it has become possible to determine the approximate location of genes with only a moderate effect on complex disease expression. In this regard, work in diabetes, especially type 1 insulin-dependent diabetes mellitus IDDM) has served as a leading model. Since the initial recognition of the HLA region contribution to type 1 diabetes (reviewed in ref. 268), several other chromosome regions that may contain loci leading to susceptibility to IDDM have been detected by genome-wide linkage studies [269–273], although none of these loci appears to make a contribution to familial risk that is as strong as that of HLA. For example, the estimated sibling relative risks (ls) of *IDDM2*, the insulin gene (*INS*) minisatellite on chromosome 11p15, is only 1.3 as compared to 2.6 for HLA [274]. The effect of the non-HLA loci became more pronounced after stratified analysis on HLA [270, 275]. Once linkage has been established, it is possible to obtain additional evidence for the location of a putative susceptibility locus by linkage disequilibrium or association studies. The presence of association and linkage at *INS* demonstrated unambiguously its involvement in type 1 diabetes susceptibility [276, 277].

In the past few years it has become clear that highly polymorphic sequences, such as microsatellites, offer important advantages and are present at a sufficiently high density to allow construction of detailed linkage maps in both humans and animal models [278, 279]. The high degree of microsatellite polymorphism, combined with the relative ease of analysis by PCR, makes whole genome scanning an attractive method for genetic studies [280]. Rapid genotyping of the human genome is now feasible and, indeed, becoming routine in many laboratories.

The primary advantage of whole genome mapping is that it can use PCR markers that can be typed by semi-automated, high-throughput methods. In particular, groups of markers can be simultaneously amplified from a single template (multiplex PCR) and combined on a single gel lane where each marker is resolved from the others on the basis of size or fluorescent tag (multiplex electrophoresis). Moreover, analysis of the genotypes is now largely automated. A computer image of the fluorescent bands is transferred to disk by laser scanning the gel during electrophoresis. Imaging software identifies bands and computes their sizes from fluorescent size standards included with the samples. Database software can then associate the allele sizes with each individual's DNA on the basis of standardized lane positions. Although the computer-generated allele sizes need to be checked visually on the computer screen, most of the arduous lane-identification and allele-calling work is rapid and automatic.

The technical developments described above are obviously of major importance in our ability to address the genetics of IBD. Additionally, however, it is also necessary to have the ability to appropriately perform the complex mathematical linkage analyses of the data produced in the laboratory.

Statistical and study design issues

Linkage analysis is a statistical method to test whether a disease gene and a marker locus are located in the same chromosomal region. The LOD score method, also known as a model-based method, involves calculating the likelihood of obtaining the observed phenotypes in a sample of pedigrees, given that the recombination fraction between the relevant loci is a value theta (θ). This likelihood is compared to the likelihood of observing the same data assuming no linkage between the two loci (recombination fraction = 0.5). The resulting value provides an estimate proportional to the odds in favor of linkage at recombination fraction θ compared to no linkage. In general, such linkage analyses have been applied primarily to disorders with 'simple' inheritance patterns (that is, inheritance patterns due to a single, completely penetrant, Mendelian gene where the mode of inheritance and the allele frequencies are known). Misspecifying any of these parameters may lead to incorrect results which miss the real linkage or find false linkage when it does not exist.

However, optimally, statistical tools for gene mapping involving complex traits should be model-free, since one does not know *a priori* how many genes are involved in the disease, the mode of inheritance of each gene, or the penetrance or gene frequencies. Hence, model-free or non-parametric methods are the primary methods used in linkage analysis of complex traits, such as type 1 diabetes and IBD. In the model-free approach the concept is that, if the disease gene is located very close to a marker locus, the sibs (or other relatives) who have similar phenotype (i.e. affection status is concordant) will likely share the same marker alleles (i.e. identity-by-descent). Thus, it is important to determine whether the two sibs are truly sharing identical alleles from a common ancestor by studying not only affected sibs, but also parents and/or unaffected sibs from a nuclear family.

The power to detect linkage in complex traits depends on many factors, for some of which the relative effects are still unknown. The more a gene contributes to a disorder, the easier it will be identified. A commonly used measurement for a genetic determination of a discrete trait is λ_s as defined by Risch [281] – the risk to a relative of an affected individual given that they share a particular allele compared to the general population. For a quantitative trait, heritability can be used as a substitute. As discussed above, in the IBD and type 1 diabetes studies, some loci with λ_s as low as 1.3 were identified (*INS* in type 1 diabetes).

As reviewed above, the single greatest risk factor for IBD is a positive family history [26]. The observed empirical risks of IBD in siblings of IBD patients ranges from 0.4% to 8% and depends on the type of the disease in probands and ethnicity [33]. Familial risk in CD is greater than that in UC and it is greater in Jewish individuals than in non-Jewish cases. If we take 5% as the average risk to sibs of CD probands and 1.5% as the risk to sibs of UC probands, and prevalence data summarized by Calkins and Mendeloff for North America [282], i.e. 0.04–0.1% for CD and 0.04–0.15% for UC, estimated relative risk to sibs (λs) are approximately 50–100 for CD and 10–30 for UC.

It is almost certain that there is genetic heterogeneity within IBD, e.g. CD vs. UC, pANCA-positive UC/CD vs. pANCA-negative UC/CD. That is, these different forms of the disease may result from the expression of different genes. One way of reducing the analytic problem of heterogeneity is to divide the clinical phenotype into 'subphenotypes'. Thus, the families can be subdivided into families exhibiting only certain phenotypes such as CD only, UC only, pANCA-positive only, or some combinations of these traits to obtain more genetically homogeneous groups. Another way of obtaining etiologically homogeneous families is to divide families by ethnicity. That is because different ethnic groups may have different evolutionary histories so that they may have different distributions of predisposing genes, different relative proportions of forms of the diseases, and different levels of linkage disequilibrium, all of which will affect the efficiency of a linkage study. While such phenotypic subdivision does not automatically translate into complete genetic homogeneity, it does tend to reduce the extent of genetic heterogeneity. The trade-off for obtaining homogeneous families is a decrease in the available sample size. Thus far, all available systematic linkage studies either analyzed CD alone, and UC alone (with or without mixed families), or IBD all together.

Gene identification

Genome-wide linkage studies

An intensive search for the susceptibility loci for IBD using the systematic mapping approach is currently under way in numerous laboratories worldwide. In this approach no prior hypothesis is made as to the nature or location of the genetic susceptibility to disease. A *linkage panel*, or set of genetic markers equally spaced along the human genome, is systematically tested for linkage to the trait of interest using the appropriate statistical methods. A panel of 400 markers is necessary to give the 8–10 cM spacing over the entire human genome needed to detect a genetic effect in a complex trait. One of the problems with this approach is that it may be difficult to distinguish a genetic effect in a complex trait from a random effect that occurs because so many markers are tested in a sample of IBD patients from a given locale. This problem can be potentially overcome whenever more than one laboratory observes linkage; thus the confirmation of linkage of a particular chromosomal region to IBD gives greater confidence that a susceptibility locus has in fact been detected.

Several genome scans have now been completed; these have examined linkage to CD, UC, or IBD combined. The putative regions identified by these scans have been further confirmed by yet more laboratories. This international effort is noteworthy within the study of the genetics of complex diseases in that several susceptibility loci for IBD have been identified by more than one laboratory. These results are summarized in Tables 8 and 9.

Table 8 shows the major IBD loci identified thus far. Consensus has been reached by an international consortium on IBD genetics (IBD Genetics Consortium) that the genome-wide approach provides evidence for susceptibility loci for IBD on chromosome 16 (IBD1) and on chromosome 12 (IBD2). Further agreement has been reached by some of the members of this consortium that this approach has also provided evidence for a third locus at or near the major histocompatibility complex (MHC) on chromosome 6 (IBD3), a fourth locus on chromosome 14, and a likely fifth locus on chromosome 5. More loci likely exist; some have probably already been detected by this effort. If a 'cut-of' is arbitrarily set at LOD·2 or at $p < 0.001$ or at replication in two studies, then additional tentative loci may have also been identified on chromosomes 1, 3, 4, 5, 7 and 19.

Even though some of these results will represent 'false-positives' incurred during the analysis of the genome screen data, clearly these results already support the following ideas: (1) there are multiple susceptibility loci for IBD, (2) CD and UC share some loci in common and do not share other loci, (3) some of these loci interact, and (4) different loci play different roles in the IBD susceptibility of different populations.

Table 8. Susceptibility loci for IBD

Locus	Location	Initial report and replications	Reference
IBD1	16q12	Hugot *et al.* 1996	115
		Ohmen *et al.* 1996	283
		Parkes *et al.* 1996	284
		Mirza *et al.* 1998	285
		Cho *et al.* 1998	286
		Cavanaugh *et al.* 1998	287
		Curran *et al.* 1998	288
		Brant *et al.* 1998	289
		Hugot *et al.* 1998	290
IBD2	12q13	Satsangi *et al.* 1996	291
		Duerr *et al.* 1998	292
		Curran *et al.* 1998	288
		Yang *et al.* 1999	293
IBD3	6p21 (MHC)	Yang *et al.* 1999	294
		Hampe *et al.* 1999	295
		Rioux *et al.* 2000	296
IBD4	14q11	Ma *et al.* 1999	264
		Duerr *et al.* 2000	297
IBD5	19p13	Cho *et al.* 1998	286
		Rioux *et al.* 2000	296
		Duerr *et al.* 1998	292
IBD6	5q31-q33	Ma *et al.* 1999	264
		Rioux *et al.* 2000	296

Chromosome 16 (IBD1)

The chromosome 16 locus was the first to be identified by a whole genome approach [115], was quickly confirmed [283], and currently has the strongest experimental support worldwide (Table 9a). A two-point LOD score of 2.04 and an increased sharing of 0.67 between affected sibpairs was observed for marker D16S409 in an initial family panel with 25 sibling pairs affected with CD with no known cases of UC (CD-only families) [115]. Significant linkage to this region was also observed in a second panel of 53 families. By further genotyping and multipoint analysis methods, linkage was localized to the region D16S409 and D16S419 with a significance of $p < 1.5 \times 10^{-5}$. This result was confirmed in an independent sample the same year [283]. Subsequent genotyping to a 1 cM resolution has resulted in a multipoint LOD score (MLS) of $Z = 2.81$ ($p = 0.0003$) at D16S416 to D16S3117 [290]. Linkage of this region was also observed in families with UC only (NPL = 2.02, $p = 0.02$ at D16S3120) but, surprisingly, not in families with both CD and UC subjects (mixed families) [285].

A peak MLS of 2.1 at D16S411 was observed using two-point and multipoint analysis to replicate this finding [283]. After stratifying based on non-Jewish or Jewish ethnicity, the MLS increased to 2.4 for the non-Jewish families and decreased to lack of evidence for linkage in the Jewish families. This suggested that the chromosome 16 region contained a susceptibility locus for CD important for the non-Jewish population. In this latter study no linkage was observed in UC only or in mixed families. Linkage of either CD or UC to this region of chromosome 16 has subsequently been observed by many, but not all, laboratories (summarized in Table 9a).

In one study, linkage of IBD1 was strongest in families with an earlier age of onset of disease [309]. Since an earlier age of disease onset is also associated with severity of CD, this observation suggests that IBD1 may play a role in determining the natural history of CD.

In an effort to combine the observations of the various laboratories worldwide in a single non-parametric analysis, members of the International IBD Genetics Consortium have combined genotype data for the same six markers broadly spanning the IBD1 region [310]. A total of 581 families (382 CD only, 91 UC only, 108 mixed) had data available for both parents and at least two affected sibpairs. A multipoint LOD score of 5.2 for this locus was observed in CD but not UC [310]. This is among the highest LOD score observed in any complex trait and demonstrates the importance of the study of a large number of families in order to detect modest genetic effects by linkage. Approximately 10–15% of the susceptibility to CD was estimated to be accounted for by this locus. The interval containing multipoint evidence within 1 LOD of the peak spans a less than 10 cM region between D16S753 and the interval between the markers D16S411 and D16S419.

After 5 years of intensive research, recently, the IBD1 gene (*NOD2*) has been identified by Hugot *et al.* [392] using a positional cloning strategy – linkage followed by linkage disequilibrium mapping. They identified three independent associations for CD: a frameshift variant and two missense variants in the *NOD2* gene, which encodes a member of the Apaf-1/Ced-4 superfamily of apoptosis regulators that is expressed in monocytes. These associated NOD2 variants alter the structure of either the leucine-rich repeat domain of the protein or the adjacent region.

Table 9a. Linkage studies on chromosome 16 (IBD1)

Type of families	Multipoint linkage LOD scores	Two-point linkage p-value	Association	Population	Comments	Reference
CD only	3.2	0.0004	–	France	Did not examine UC or mixed families	115
CD only	2.4	0.02	–	North American	No linkage in UC and mixed families. Linkage was observed in non-Jewish families only	283
CD only	2.4	0.21	–	North American	No linkage in UC or mixed families and no Jewish and non-Jewish difference. Interaction with locus on chromosome 1	298
CD only	6.3	0.000002	+	Australia	No linkage in mixed families	287
IBD		CD, 0.045; IBD-0.058		UK	A marker 40cM distal to this region , D16S407 gave a LOD 1.5 (p = 0.004) in CD families, zero in UC families	291
IBD	CD, 1.5; UC, 2; IBD, 2.4			North central European		288
UC	2.2			France	Did not report CD results	285
CD	2.8	0.003		France	Families for this study different from the families used in Hugot *et al.* 1996	299
CD	2.8			North American	This linkage was conducted in a large pedigree containing seven relatives affected with CD	289
IBD		0.5	–	Belgian		300
IBD				Canadian	Exclusion of λ_s 2.0	301

The leucine-rich repeat domain plays a critical role in activating nuclear factor NF-κB. The potential etiologic role of NF-κB dysregulation or its pathway in CD has been indicated by the efficacy of antibiotic therapy in some patients [393] and the use of sulfasalazine and glucocorticoids – two known NF-κB inhibitors, for CD treatment [394, 395]. The relative risks for simple heterozygotes, homozygotes, and compound heterozygotes as compared with those individuals with no variants are 3, 38, and 44, respectively. The frequencies of the three variant alleles are 7%, 5%, and 29% in controls, UC, and CD patients, respectively. It is of interest that: (1) there are three different, independent predisposing variations in the same gene; and (2) these three variants seem to have arisen independently from the same ancestral haplotype. These data argue strongly for the hypothesis of genetic selection as an explanation for the frequency of these predisposing variants in this gene (see discussion of selection above and in Chapter 4 of this volume). Simultaneously, by a candidate gene approach, an independent group also demonstrated association between the *NOD2* and CD [396], thus supporting the findings of Hugot *et al.* [392]. Clearly, *NOD2* is a susceptibility gene to CD, that is, it increases an individual's risk for CD, but it is neither sufficient nor necessary for the development of CD. As reviewed below, there are other loci to be identified. The identification of the *NOD2* will shed light on the etiologic pathways of IBD and accelerate the discovery of additional susceptibility genes for IBD. The identification of the IBD1 gene is one of few successes to date in genetic studies of complex diseases, but this success validates this approach and thus presents a promising future for genetic research of complex diseases.

Chromosome 12 (IBD2)

The chromosome 12 locus (IBD2) was the second region to be identified by a whole genome approach [291]. A two-point LOD score of 5.47 ($p = 2.66 \times 10^{-7}$) was observed in their complete set of 186 sib pairs from CD only, UC only, and mixed families at the marker D12S83. An association between a '4-1-3' haplotype constructed with markers D12S83, D12S1662, and D12S1655 and UC was observed in further work using the transmission disequilibrium test [302]. Both the linkage and association findings have been replicated in North American studies: one observing an association to the same marker D12S83 in both CD and UC families using the transmission disequilibrium test [292], and one to a marker 14 cM away at D12S85 in CD families [293]. Other linkage studies of this region are summarized in Table 9b. The differences in the results for this interval have raised the possibility that there may be two loci in this region, one for CD and one for UC.

Thus far, a few candidate genes have been tested based for association to either IBD, CD, or UC based on their location within the IBD2 region, and negative results have been reported for IFN-γ [303] and the natural resistance-associated macrophage protein (NRAMP2) [311].

Major histocompatibility complex (MHC; Chromosome 6p21.3; IBD3)

Based on the hypothesis that IBD pathogenesis may involve immunoregulatory factors, candidate genes within the MHC on chromosome 6p21.3 have long been tested for IBD susceptibility with conflicting results (see Candidate gene studies, below). In a recent study of the sharing of MHC haplotypes, which allowed the delineation of identity by descent of all markers [294], linkage to the MHC was observed using several non-parametric methods: (1) an increased *number* of sib pairs sharing one or more haplotypes ($p = 0.004$); (2) an increased *mean proportion* of sharing between concordant affected ($p = 0.002$) and concordant unaffected ($p = 0.031$) pairs along with a decreased proportion in discordant pairs ($p = 0.007$); (3) a significant linear relation

Table 9b. Linkage and association studies on chromosome 12 (IBD2)

Region	Type of families	Multipoint linkage LOD scores	Two-point linkage *p*-value	Association	Population	Comments	Reference
~80 cM[a]	IBD		CD, 0.0073; UC, 0.0025; IBD, 2.7×10^{-7}	+	UK	Linkage and association were reported in different papers	291, 302
	IBD	CD, 1.8; UC, 1.8;		+	North American		292
	CD	2.0	0.0004	+	North American	This peak is at D12S85 and is approximately 10–15 cM away from the peak observed in English families. No linkage was observed in UC and mixed families	293
	IBD	CD, 1.8; UC, 0.8					288
	IBD		0.24	−	Belgian		300
IFN-γ				−	European		303
VDR gene	Case–control			CD+, UC−	UK	VDR gene maps to the region on chromosome 12 linked to IBD	304

cM[a] distance from p telomere.

between the similarity of phenotype between members of a sibpair and the proportion of their shared haplotypes by regression analysis ($p = 0.00003$); and (4) an increased sharing between pairs more distantly related than sibpairs ($p = 0.001$). Linkage was also observed in this region in a genome scan by the same investigators [264]. Further support for linkage of the MHC region to IBD has been observed by two additional laboratories following the systematic mapping approach (summarized in Table 9c): (1) a multipoint LOD score of 4.2 for D6S461 [312] and (2) a peak non-parametric LOD score of 2.3 ($p = 0.0026$) for D6S1017 with other NPL scores over 2 for nearby markers [296]. These observations suggest that the MHC is a third susceptibility region for IBD and could be referred to as IBD3.

Chromosome 14 (IBD4)

Evidence for linkage between CD and the marker D14S261 has been observed in two studies [264, 297] and to the general region of this marker in a third [313]. This confirmation argues that this region constitutes the fourth IBD susceptibility locus, IBD4. Candidate genes in this region include the T-cell receptor α/δ complex.

Chromosome 19

Significant linkage of IBD to the marker D19S591 with a multipoint LOD of 4.6 has been observed in Canadian sib pair families [296]. Some evidence for linkage to this same marker has also been reported by a second group [297] (two-point LOD score 1.6, $p = 0.0067$) and to a neighboring region by a third group [286] (multipoint $p = 0.0059$). This region contains the genes for ICAM-1, complement component 3, thromboxane A_2 receptor, leukotriene B_4 hydroxylase, and the janus protein tyrosine kinases TYK2 and JAK3.

Chromosome 5

Evidence for linkage to the region D5S393–D5S673 has been observed in Jewish CD-only families [264] and in CD families with early-onset disease (multipoint LOD 3.9) [296]. This region contains the genes for the cytokines interleukin 3, 4, 5, 13 and colony stimulating factor 2, and is syntenic to a mouse region implicated in the dextran sulfate-induced colitis model [238]. While this volume was in press, a specific 250 kb haplotype that confers susceptibility to CD was identified within a cluster of cytokine genes [397]. However, due to the complex genomic structure of this cluster, the specific causal mutation within this region was not identifiable using genetic methods alone.

Other loci

The published genome scans have also proposed that other regions contain suscepibility loci for IBD. The following evidence for linkage is worthy of note:

Table 9c. Linkage studies on chromosome 6 (MHC)

Type of families	Multipoint linkage LOD score	Two-point linkage *p*-value	Association	Population	Comments	Reference
CD only		0.002	+	North American	Linkage observed using several non-parametric methods	294
IBD, UC	4.2		+	North American	D6S461 and D6S426 fine mapping peak outside of MHC, but nearby	295
	2.3		+	Canadian		305
UC		0.032			D6S276. HLA-DRB1 $p = 0.017$	306
CD				European	Exclusion of MHC with parametric and non parametric methods	307
IBD				UK	Exclusion of MHC with parametric methods	308
CD, UC, IBD					Evidence that MHC plays a minor role, if any	298

Chromosomes 3 and 7

A suggestion of linkage to the regions D3S1076–D3S1573 (mostly contributed by CD-only families) and D7S484–D7S527 (contributed by both CD and UC families, depending on the marker in the region) was observed in the same study that reported the initial linkage to chromosome 12 [291]. With further fine mapping, a peak single-point linkage to CD has been observed by this group at marker D3S3521 (LOD = 3.5, p = 0.00003) with the support region (LOD within 1 of the peak) spanning D3S11–D3S3559 [314]. Evidence for linkage to these two regions has been observed in another study, with a multipoint p = 0.014 for CD-only families to the chromosome 3 region, and a multipoint p = 0.01 for all IBD families to the chromosome 7 region [286]. A mouse chromosome region containing a susceptibility locus for dextran sulfate-induced colitis, *Dssc-1* [238], is syntenic with this human chromosome 7 region.

For the chromosome 3 region, negative results have been reported for the G protein G-alpha-i-2 gene (GNAI2) [315]. A modest association between markers near the mutL homologue 1 gene (colon cancer, non-polyposis type I; MLH1) and has been observed in a small sample of 45 CD, 36 UC and 45 controls [316].

For chromosome 7 the mucin-3 (MUC3) gene has been tested for association to IBD; alleles of a 51 bp VNTR polymorphism are increased in UC patients from both Great Britain and Japan [317]. This observation of an association from two populations combined with the observation of a reduction of altered mucin species IV in UC patients [318] make this an attractive finding.

Chromosome 1

Two studies have observed evidence for linkage to the D1S2670–D1S2682 region [286, 295]. Families with linkage to this region also show greater linkage to IBD1, suggesting that this susceptibility locus interacts with IBD1 [286]. Further narrowing of this region to 130 kb near D1S2697 and D1S3669 has been accomplished by homozygosity mapping in a collection of American Iraqi Chaldean families with IBD [319]. Since both CD and UC are observed in these families, these authors have proposed that this locus determines a generic susceptibility to IBD, with the concomitant inheritance of IBD1 then determining CD [319].

Candidate gene studies

In the candidate gene approach, genetic variants are tested based on a prior hypothesis regarding the role of that gene or gene product in the pathophysiology of the disease. Such a hypothesis may be based on evidence from clinical observation or physiologic studies of affected individuals (*in-vivo* studies), from studies of known disease-related processes (*in-vitro* studies), from animal models of disease (transgenic construction or targeted disruption), and from the effects of drugs or chemicals on disease in either humans or animals (pharmacogenetic studies). For IBD, possible candidates could be selected from genes involved in the regulation of the balance between Th1 and Th2 cells, the response of humans to gut flora, and the release of cytokines during the immunologic destruction and healing of the intestinal mucosa.

The major histocompatibility complex (MHC)

The MHC on chromosome 6p21.3 is the most gene-dense region of the human genome sequenced thus far, with 224 genes identified within 3.6 megabases (Mb) [320]. Since many of the genes in this cluster function in the regulation of the immune system and in antigen processing and presentation, the MHC is a candidate region for most, if not all, diseases with dysregulation of the immune system as the possible underlying pathophysiology. The MHC has therefore long been considered a candidate region for IBD. However, also among these genes are the most polymorphic human proteins known, the class I and class II molecules; and some of these proteins have over 100 allelic variants. This great variation and the high gene density of the MHC have contributed to the difficulty of assigning the specific role of a specific gene to the pathophysiology of IBD.

The MHC class II region

In general, the class II molecules are dimeric, with an α-chain and a β-chain that form a groove for presenting an extracellular antigenic peptide to CD4$^+$ T cells. The three class II molecules are HLA-DP, HLA-DQ, and HLA-DR. In each case the α- and β-chains are encoded by A and B genes, respectively. For HLA-DR there is an invariant HLA-DRA gene and up to three distinct and highly polymorphic HLA-DRB genes. One of these HLA-DRB genes, HLA-DRB1, is present in all individuals and is the most polymorphic. The study of HLA-DRB1 genes has been an important tool in the study of the role of

Table 10. Associations of Crohn's disease and ulcerative colitis with HLA class II alleles

Serologic	Genetic allele		OR	p	Reference
DR					
DR1	DRB1*01	15% CD, 9% controls not	1.75	0.003 (corr)	322
	DRB1*03	found in ANCA neg UC			135
	DRB1*07	17% CD, 11% controls	1.58	0.008 (corr)	322
	DRB1*07	18% CD, 10% controls	1.9 RR	0.0001	323
	DRB1*0103	8.6% UC, 3.2% controls	2.9	0.0074	306
		14% UC (16% extensive UC),		< 0.0001	324
		23% extraintestinal manifestations			
		6% UC, 0.2% control increased	27.6	0.0002	325
		with extensive UC, colectomy	33, 84	< 0.0001	325
		7.9% CD, 2.2% controls	3.9	0.004	326
		8.9% UC, 2.2% controls	4.4	0.001	326
		meta-analysis, association with UC	3.42		321
DR2		70% UC, 31% controls	5.1 RR	‹0.001	327
		41% UC, 21% control	2.6	0.008	133
		44% ANCA+UC, 21% ANCA- UC		0.01	186
		meta-analysis, association with UC	2.0		321
	DRB1*15	42% UC, 26% controls	2.1	0.006	325
		35% ANCA positive UC, 15% controls	2.9	0.004	135
		meta-analysis, association with UC	1.65		321
	DRB1*1501 and DRB1*1502	increased in ANCA pos UC			135
	DRB1*1502	49% UC, 18% controls	2.8 RR	< 0.0001	328
		12% UC, 5% controls	2.7	0.005	326
		meta-analysis, association with UC	3.74		321
		negative for DR2 alleles			329
		negative for DRB1*1502			330
DR4	DRB1*0410	13% CD, 3% controls	5.02 RR	0.001 (corr)	331
	DRB1*0410/DQA1*03/ DQB1*0402 haplotype	13% CD, 2.7% controls	5.6 RR	0.00011 (corr)	331
DR13	DRB1*1302/DRB3*030 1 haplotype	21% CD, 5.4% controls	4.6 RR	0.0066	330, 332
	DRB3*0301	meta-analysis, associated with CD	1.18		321
DP					
	DPB1*0401	74% CD, 71% controls, stratified on Jew/non-Jew	1.6	0.015	326
DQ					
	DQA1*03	88% CD, 68% control	3.36 RR	0.03 (corr)	331
	DQA1*0201	19% CD, 11% control	1.9 RR	0.0001	323
	DQB1*0402	19% CD, 6% control	3.89 RR	0.001 (corr)	331
	DQB1*0501	16% CD, 10% control	10.6	0.01 (corr)	322

RR, relative risk; (corr), *p* value corrected for the multiple comparisons performed.

class II genes in IBD. Serologic methods identify several HLA-DR types and subtypes and were used in the older studies, while molecular methods reveal even more subtypes at the nucleotide level and are the preferred techniques today. A meta-analysis of 29 studies reporting HLA-DR or HLA-DQ frequencies in CD and UC patients and in controls has recently been published [321]. The results of this analysis and of recent association studies using molecular methods are summarized in Table 10.

The authors have identified an association between the combination of HLA-DR1/HLA-DQ w5 alleles and CD in Caucasians in the United States and HLA-DR2 and UC [133]. The association

Table 11. Summary of class II associations with Crohn's disease, ulcerative colitis, or both (inflammatory bowel disease)

Disease	Class II allele or haplotype	% affected	% control	p	OR
IBD	DRB1*0103	8.3	2.2	0.001	4.6
CD		7.9	2.2	0.002	4.4
UC		8.9	2.2	0.001	4.9
IBD	DRB1*0103-DQA1*0501-DQB1*0303	2.8	0.4	0.034	6.9
IBD	DRB1*0103-DQA1*0101-DQB1*0501	6.4	2.2	0.007	3.5
UC	DRB1*1502	11.9	4.7	0.006	2.6
CD	DPB1*0401	74.1	64.7	0.014	1.6

Total subjects: 232 control, 304 for CD, 270 for UC [326].

between HLA-DR1 and CD has also been observed in France [322] and in the Netherlands [333]. Further molecular typing revealed that, of all the DR1 alleles, only the HLA-DRB1*0103 allele, and not other DR1 subtypes, was associated with CD as well as UC (see Table 11) [326]. This finding pointed to the importance of molecular typing over serologic typing as the means to clarify the associations between class II alleles and IBD; an example of the associations between IBD and HLA alleles typed using molecular methods in one of the largest studies to date is given in Table 11.

An association between HLA-DRB1*0103 and UC has also been reported in the Japanese population [306] and in Britain [324]. This latter report observed that this allele is associated with extensive UC, extraintestinal manifestations of UC, or with some complications of UC (mouth ulcers, arthritis, or uveitis). In Britain, HLA-DRB1*0103 has also been associated with the extraintestinal manifestation of peripheral arthropathy in IBD patients when compared with controls [334]. The authors have further observed that the association of DR2 with UC was due to the HLA-DRB1*1502 allele [326]. In addition, a rare HLA-DRB1*0103–DQA1*0501–DQB1*0301 haplotype was dramatically associated with IBD with an odds ratio of 6.6, and a more common DR1 haplotype, HLA-DRB1*0103–DQA1*0101–DQB1*0501, was also associated with IBD. This result suggested that an interaction between HLA-DR and HLA-DQ may determine the extent of disease risk.

A new association at another MHC class II locus, HLA-DP, has been recently observed; the common HLA-DPB1*0401 allele and CD confers a modest risk [326].

The results summarized in Tables 10 and 11 clearly point to a role for the MHC class II genes in the pathogenesis of IBD. HLA-DRB1*0103 differs from other HLA-DRB1 alleles by an LLEQR to ILEDE change at positions 67–71 in exon 2 [326]. This change alters the peptide binding groove and may be involved in the binding of an IBD-related peptide to this antigen-presenting molecule. However, these results also suggest there are interactions between multiple class II genes in the MHC, and that further studies with larger sample sizes will be necessary in order to unravel the complex role of this region in the pathogenesis of IBD. Further, although great progress has been made in further defining the association between IBD and MHC class II genes, three lines of evidence suggest that the contribution of the MHC to IBD is likely to consist of more than that provided by the class II region:

1. While some investigators have confirmed associations to the same class II alleles, others have observed associations to other class II alleles, particularly when studying other populations. This suggests that at least some MHC class II alleles are not the IBD susceptibility alleles but are in linkage disequilibrium with susceptibility alleles.

2. The results of two genome scans [264, 312] suggest that the peak linkage to IBD in this region may be several centimorgans telomeric from the MHC and the result of a third [296] suggests that the peak may be centromeric.

3. The magnitude of the linkage effect revealed above is not explained by the relatively modest associations of the MHC class II alleles heretofore observed. This evidence suggests that further fine linkage disequilibrium mapping of the MHC and IBD is also warranted. Strategies

to unravel the role of the potentially multiple MHC genes involved in the susceptibility to IBD are: (a) to carry out this fine mapping using both case–control and family-based association tests (the TDT) and to follow leads that are positive with both methods, and (b) to examine the contribution of each locus in isolation from the others by methods that stratify the genotyping data at one locus with respect to another locus.

Notch4

A preliminary example of such a fine-mapping effort has revealed further susceptibility loci in the MHC class III region around *Notch4*. The *Notch4* gene is located in the MHC class III region close to the border with the class II region. The function of the human *Notch4* gene is not currently known, but the family of Notch proteins are involved in the control of cell fate decisions during development [335] including hematopoiesis [336] and gut epithelium [337]. Notch receptors and ligands are also expressed in the thymus, and the overexpression of Notch1 in a mouse transgenic strain directs $CD4^+$ $CD8^+$ precursors to the CD8 lineage [338]. The authors have observed that an allele of *Notch4* is associated with CD in Ashkenazi Jews in both a case–control study and a family-based study by TDT [339]. This genetic association was independent of the HLA-DRB1 associations discussed above, suggesting that multiple genes in the MHC may be determining IBD. In a study of well-characterized CD patients this same allele was also associated with a subset of CD patients characterized by an earlier age of onset of CD and no expression of pANCA combined with a high expression of ASCA [193]. These observations suggest that either the *Notch4* gene itself or a gene close by may also determine one of the subtypes of CD.

Tumor necrosis factor (TNF)

TNF is involved in the regulation of inflammation at many levels; of particular interest for IBD is the role of TNF in the recruitment of circulating inflammatory cells to local tissue sites and in granuloma formation. An important role for TNF as a pro-inflammatory cytokine in CD has emerged in recent years [340], and this pivotal role is prominent in the mouse models of intestinal inflammation that are the result of the alteration of the regulation of the TNF gene (reviewed above) and in the success of the use of anti-TNF antibody in the treatment of moderate to severe CD [341].

The genes for three members of the TNF superfamily, TNF, lymphotoxin alpha (LTA) and lymphotoxin beta (LTB) are located adjacent to each other at the border between the class III and class I region of the MHC [320, 342]. Several studies have observed an association between polymorphisms in this region and (1) changes in TNF expression [343, 344], (2) altered immune response to infectious diseases [345–349], and (3) increased joint damage in rheumatoid arthritis [350]. Five microsatellite markers, denoted as TNFa–e, broadly encompass this region [350–353]. The authors have observed an association between a haplotype of these microsatellite markers and CD [354]. TNF promoter polymorphisms have also been associated with CD [355, 356]. Two of the authors' recent observations suggest that genetic variation in the TNF region may determine the course of disease in subsets of IBD: (1) a haplotype in the LTA region may be associated with a lack of response to anti-TNF therapy in a group of patients with moderate to severe CD [357]; and (2) TNF microsatellite a is associated with the level of expression of ASCA antibody [194].

Other observed associations

Interleukin 1-beta (IL-1β) and interleukin 1 receptor antagonist (IL-1RA)

The interleukin 1 (IL-1) family consists of three related proteins: interleukin-1α (IL-1α), IL-1β and IL-1RA. The genes for all three proteins are located together on chromosome 2q14 but not within a region of linkage observed in a genome scan (see Table 11). IL-1A and IL-1B are cytokines with a wide spectrum of pro-inflammatory actions in many cell types, and IL-1RA inhibits the action of IL-1α and IL-1β by blocking the IL-1 receptor [358]. When these cytokines were measured in freshly isolated intestinal mucosal cells from IBD patients and controls, an imbalance in the ratio of IL-1 to IL-1RA was observed in both CD and UC patients, with the ratio correlating closely with the clinical severity of disease [359]. This observation was confirmed using biopsies from the inflamed mucosa of IBD patients [360]. Further, removal of IL-1RA by treating animals with anti-IL-1RA or by gene knockout increases susceptibility to experimentally induced colitis [361]. These observations support the hypothesis that an imbalance between IL-1 and IL-1RA is important in the etiology of IBD [362, 363].

The authors and others have observed an association between the *IL-1RA* gene and UC, with an increased frequency of allele 2 of an 86 bp variable number of tandem repeats (VNTR) polymorphism in intron 2 of the *IL-1RA* gene in UC [362, 364]. This increased frequency was observed in patients from the Los Angeles area, particularly in a subset of UC patients from the Ashkenazi Jewish population, but not in patients from Milan. Biopsies from IBD patients with this genotype have a slight reduction of IL-1RA [360]. These results suggest that genetic variation in the *IL-1RA* gene may alter the ratio between IL-1 and its receptor antagonist and thus contribute to susceptibility to IBD. An association between polymorphisms in the *IL-1RA* gene has been observed in some but not all subsequent studies [365–369]. Furthermore, some evidence supports the concept that *IL-1RA* polymorphisms may also participate in determining the course and severity of IBD: (1) a significant association has been observed between two polymorphisms in the *IL-1β* gene (IL-1β; variants at –511 in the promoter and in exon 5) and non-perforating CD but not with perforating–fistulizing disease [369]; and (2) the *IL-1RA* allele 2 has a higher frequency in surgically treated UC patients compared with non-surgically treated patients or controls [366]. When taken together, the evidence supports an association between polymorphisms in the *IL-1RA* gene and both CD and UC; the differences in these reports may be due to sample size problems and differences between the ethnic groups studied in these reports.

Intercellular adhesion molecule 1 (ICAM1)

ICAM1 is involved in one of the several steps of the normal capture and migration of leukocytes from the blood stream to the site of inflammation [370, 371]. Several observations suggest that ICAM1 plays a direct role in IBD: (1) in mucosa taken from IBD patients and controls, a massive infiltration of ICAM1-positive cells has been correlated with the amount of inflammation in IBD [372] and the concentration of ICAM1 is significantly elevated in CD and UC patients and is also higher in active UC compared with inactive UC [373]; (2) plasma soluble ICAM1 is also higher in patients with active UC, pouchitis, and CD [374]; and (3) anti-ICAM treatment of rats reduces intestinal inflammation in the acetic-acid-induced model of colitis [375]. The *ICAM1* G241R polymorphism has been tested for association to IBD and the frequency of the mutant allele was higher for the ANCA-negative UC and for ANCA-positive CD subsets of disease but not CD or UC as a whole when compared with controls [187]. This polymorphism may therefore play a role in determining the disease course of subsets of IBD. A negative result was reported for ANCA-positive UC [135], but it should also be noted that the method of ANCA determination is not uniform on both sides of the Atlantic. As discussed above, *ICAM1* is located within the chromosome 19 linkage peak (see Table 8).

Interferon gamma receptor subunit 1

Mutations in the IFN-γ receptor subunit 1 gene (*IFNGR1*) have been associated with impaired response to IFN-γ [376, 377] and susceptibility to mycobacterial infection [378–380]. The authors have observed an association between a polymorphism in this gene and the development of chronic pouchitis in UC patients who have undergone ileal pouch–anal anastomosis surgery [381]. This observation raises the intriguing possibility that this receptor plays a role in determining the course of severe forms of UC. This gene is located in a peak of linkage to IBD [264].

Prothrombotic gene variants

Since IBD patients are also at a greater risk for thrombosis, the most frequent hereditary prothrombotic mutations have been tested for association with IBD. Currently the results are contradictory, probably due to the small sample sizes of some of the studies and geographic/ethnic differences. As in other diseases, the factor V Leiden mutation seems to confer a higher relative risk for venous thrombosis in IBD patients. The thermolabile variant of the methylene tetrahydrofolate reductase gene (*MTHFR* C677T) was associated with IBD and probably accounts for a higher plasma homocysteine concentration in IBD patients when compared with controls [382]. Negative results have been reported for the following genetic variants: Factor V Leiden [383, 384], the thermolabile variant of the methylene tetrahydrofolate reductase gene (*MTHFR* C677T), and prothrombin [384].

Natural resistance-associated macrophage protein 1 (NRAMP1)

The *NRAMP1* gene may be an important gene controlling response to infection by pathogens, particularly to *Mycobacteria* spp. [385–387]. An association has been observed between CD and a haplotype composed of two markers that flank *NRAMP1*, D2S434 and D2S1323 [388]. A negative result has also been reported [311].

In summary, the linkage data clearly identify specific genetic loci as contributing to the etiology of IBD. At least four, and likely more, loci can be identified from the current data. In moving from linkage to positional candidates the best available data are for genes in both the MHC class II and in the border between the MHC class II and class III regions. Other candidate genes have been studied from functional hypotheses (as has the MHC class II and TNF), and the best-established of these is the interleukin receptor 1 family cluster.

Clinical application of genetic information

In general, the genetic information described here is not yet used in clinical practice. Typing for ANCA and ASCA is on the verge of utility in diagnosing CD versus UC and in clarifying the cases of 'indeterminate colitis'. At the current time genetic markers are not used diagnostically. As for the serum antibody markers pANCA and ASCA, they can be used in diagnosis. Even though they are found at increased risk in relatives, screening relatives clinically is not recommended as there is no recognized intervention. Counseling is based on empiric risk, which was reviewed in family epidemiology, and are for the most part modest.

In the long term, genotyping patients for CD- and UC-associated genes will enable the determination of risk to relatives of IBD patients and of the optimal therapy for each individual, and identifying the genes that predispose to each pathogenetic mechanism of IBD will point research into new directions to develop therapies, and will enable the construction of mouse models for the testing of those therapies before starting clinical trials. The use of this genetic information in the nearest term is perhaps suggested by several preliminary IBD pharmacogenetic studies.

Since glucocorticoids are known substrates for a drug efflux pump protein (P-glycoprotein 170) expressed by the multidrug resistance gene (MDR), Farrell and co-workers compared the expression of this pump on the surface of lymphocytes obtained from IBD patients and controls, and observed that MDR expression was significantly elevated in CD and UC patients who required surgery because they failed medical therapy [389]. This observation suggests that a genetic variation that affects the pharmacology of steroids may lead to the ineffectiveness of these drugs in some IBD patients. Inflammation of the large intestine has been observed in a mouse knockout of this gene, and this observation

raises the possibility that MDR also plays a more direct role in intestinal inflammation as well [390].

Clinical response to 6-mercaptopurine (6-MP) depends on its conversion to 6-thioguanine (6-TG) and reaching a TG level greater than 235 (pmol/ 8×10^{-8} erythrocytes) [391]. Patients heterozygous for mutations that reduce the level of the enzyme thiopurine methyltransferase (TPMT) are able to attain this therapeutic level more readily on a given dose of 6-MP, because the drug is not converted into inactive nucleotides by this enzyme (e.g. 6-methylmercaptopurine or 6-MMP). These results suggest that TPMT genotyping may assist the clinician in optimizing the therapeutic response to 6-MP and in identifying individuals at increased risk for drug-induced toxicity.

Patients in the original clinical trial of the anti-TNF antibody were also typed for ANCA status and genotyped in the TNF region of the MHC. The response of pANCA patients was the lowest and not significantly different from placebo, and the response of sANCA patients (a different type of staining from pANCA) was the highest in this study. Homozygotes for the LTA NcoI-TNFc-aa13L-aa26 haplotype '1-1-1-1' did not respond to treatment. While these results must be interpreted with a great deal of caution, because of the many comparisons made in this small study, they raise the intriguing possibility that sANCA may identify a CD subgroup with a better response to infliximab and that pANCA and homozygosity for the LTA '1-1-1-1' haplotype may identify CD subgroups with a poorer response.

While these studies are all recent, they each raise the possibility that the use of specific genetic markers, involved in either metabolism of the therapeutic agent or in the susceptibility to a form of IBD, may well guide therapy in the not-too-distant future.

References

1. Probert CS, Jayanthi V, Hughes AO, Thompson JR, Wicks AC, Mayberry JF. Prevalence and family risk of ulcerative colitis and Crohn's disease: an epidemiological study among Europeans and south Asians in Leicestershire. Gut 1993; 34: 1547-51.
2. Sonnenberg A, Wasserman IH. Epidemiology of inflammatory bowel disease among U.S. military veterans. Gastroenterology 1991; 101: 122–30.
3. Kurata JH, Kantor-Fish S, Frankl H, Godby P, Vadheim CM. Crohn's disease among ethnic groups in a large health maintenance organization. Gastroenterology 1992; 102: 1940–8.
4. Shivananda S, Lennard-Jones J, Logan R *et al*. Incidence of inflammatory bowel disease across Europe: is there a difference between north and south? Results of the Eur-

opean Collaborative Study on Inflammatory Bowel Disease (EC-IBD). Gut 1996; 39: 690–7.

5. Sonnenberg A, McCarty DJ, Jacobsen SJ. Geographic variation of inflammatory bowel disease within the United States. Gastroenterology 1991; 100: 143–9.

6. Trallori G, Palli D, Saieva C *et al.* A population-based study of inflammatory bowel disease in Florence over 15 years (1978 92). Scand J Gastroenterol 1996; 31: 892–9.

7. Loftus EV Jr, Silverstein MD, Sandborn WJ, Tremaine WJ, Harmsen WS, Zinsmeister AR. Crohn's disease in Olmsted County, Minnesota, 1940–1993: incidence, prevalence, and survival. Gastroenterology 1998; 114: 1161–8.

8. Bernstein CN, Blanchard JF, Rawsthorne P, Wajda A. Epidemiology of Crohn's disease and ulcerative colitis in a central Canadian province: a population-based study. Am J Epidemiol 1999; 149: 916–24.

9. Loftus EV Jr, Silverstein MD, Sandborn WJ, Tremaine WJ, Harmsen WS, Zinsmeister AR. Ulcerative colitis in Olmsted County, Minnesota, 1940–1993: incidence, prevalence, and survival. Gut 2000; 46: 336 43.

10. Palli D, Masala G, Trallori G, Bardazzi G, Saieva C. A capture–recapture estimate of inflammatory bowel disease prevalence: the Florence population-based study. Ital J Gastroenterol Hepatol 1998; 30: 50–3.

11. Russel MG, Dorant E, Volovics A *et al.* High incidence of inflammatory bowel disease in The Netherlands: results of a prospective study. The South Limburg IBD Study Group. Dis Colon Rectum 1998; 41: 33–40.

12. Russel MG, Stockbrugger RW. Epidemiology of inflammatory bowel disease: an update. Scand J Gastroenterol 1996; 31: 417–27.

13. Yang H, Rotter JI. The genetics of inflammatory bowel disease. In: Targan SR, Shanahan F, eds. Inflammatory Bowel Disease: From Bench to Bedside. Baltimore: Williams & Wilkins, 1994: 32–64.

14. Rotter JI, Yang H, Shohat T. Genetic complexities of inflammatory bowel disease and its distribution among the Jewish people. In: Bonne-Tamir B, Adam A, eds. Genetic Diversity Among Jews: Diseases and Markers at the DNA Level. New York: Oxford University Press, 1992: 395–411.

15. Gilat T, Grossman A, Fireman Z, Rozen P. Inflammatory bowel disease in Jews. In: McConnell R, Rozen P, Langman M, Gilat T, eds. The Genetics and Epidemiology of Inflammatory Bowel Disease. New York: Krager, 1986: 135–40.

16. Roth M-P, Petersen GM, McElree C, Feldman E, Rotter JI. Geographic origins of Jewish patientis with inflammatory bowel disease. Gastroenterology 1989; 97: 900–4.

17. Zlotogora J, Zimmerman J, Rachmilewitz D. Crohn's disease in Ashkenazi Jews. Gastroenterology 1990; 99: 286–90.

18. Monk M, Mendeloff AI, Siegel CI, Lilienfeld A. An epidemiological study of ulcerative colitis and regional enteritis among adults in Baltimore. I. Hospital incidence and prevalence, 1960–1963. Gastroenterology 1967; 53: 198–210.

19. Korelitz BI. From Crohn to Crohn's disease – 1979: an epidemiologic study in New York city. Mt Sinai J Med 1979; 46: 533–40.

20. Brahme F, Lindstrom G, Wenckert A. Crohn's disease in a defined population. Gastroenterology 1975; 69: 342–51.

21. Hellers G. Crohn's disease in Stockholm county, 1955–1974: a study of epidemiology, results of surgical treatment and long term prognosis. Acta Chir Scand 1979; Suppl 490: 1–84.

22. Novis BH, Marks IN, Louw JH, Bank S. Incidence of Crohn's disease at Groote Schuur Hospital during 1970–1974. S Afr Med J 1975; 49: 693–7.

23. Pinchbeck BR, Kirdeikis J, Thomson ABR. Effect of religious affiliation and education status on the prevalence of inflammatory bowel disease in northern Alberta. Can J Gastroenterol 1988; 2(Suppl. A): 95–100.

24. Odes HS, Fraser D, Krugliak P, Fenyves D, Fraser GM, Sperber AD. Inflammatory bowel disease in the Bedouin Arabs of southern Israel: rarity of diagnosis and clinical features. Gut 1991; 32: 1024–6.

25. Krawiec J, Odes HSL, Krugliak P, Weitzman S. Aspects of the epidemiology of Crohn's disease in the Jewish population in Beer Sheva, Israel. Israel J Med Sci 1984; 20: 16–21.

26. Yang H, Rotter JI. Genetic aspects of idiopathic inflammatory bowel disease. In: Kirsner JB, Shorter RG, eds. Inflammatory Bowel Disease, 4th edn. Baltimore: Williams & Wilkins, 1995: 301–31.

27. Russel MGVM, Pastoor CJ, Janssen KMW *et al.* Familial aggregation of inflammatory bowel disease: a population-based study in South Limburg, the Netherlands. Scand J Gastroenterol 1997; 32: 88–91.

28. Mayberry JF, Rhodes J, Newcombe RG. Familial prevalence of inflammatory bowel disease in relatives of patients with Crohn's disease. Br Med J 1980; 280: 84.

29. Fielding JF. The relative risk of inflammatory bowel disease among parents and siblings of Crohn's disease patients. J Clin Gastroenterol 1986; 8: 655–7.

30. Orholm M, Munkholm P, Langholz E, Nielsen OH, Sorensen IA, Binder V. Familial occurrence of inflammatory bowel disease. N Engl J Med 1991; 324: 84–8.

31. Binder V. Genetic epidemiology in inflammatory bowel disease. Dig Dis 1998; 16: 351–5.

32. Orholm M, Fonager K, Sorensen HT. Risk of ulcerative colitis and Crohn's disease among offspring of patients with chronic inflammatory bowel disease. Am J Gastroenterol 1999; 94: 3236–8.

33. Yang H, McElree C, Roth M-P, Shanahan F, Targan SR, Rotter JI. Familial empiric risks for inflammatory bowel disease: differences between Jews and non-Jews. Gut 1993; 34: 517–24.

34. Kirsner JB, Spencer JA. Family occurrences of ulcerative colitis, regional enteritis and ileocolitis. Ann Intern Med 1963; 59: 539–46.

35. McConnell RB, Vadheim CM. Inflammatory bowel disease. In: King RA, Rotter JI, Motulsky AG, eds. The Genetic Basis of Common Diseases. New York: Oxford University Press, 1992: 326–48.

36. Roth MP, Petersen GM, McElree C, Vadheim CM, Panish JF, Rotter JI. Familial empiric risk estimates of inflammatory bowel disease in Ashkenazi Jews. Gastroenterology 1989; 96: 1016–20.

37. Kirsner JB. Genetic aspects of inflammatory bowel disease. Clin Gastroenterol 1973; 2: 557–76.

38. Weterman IT, Pena AS. Familial incidence of Crohn's disease in the Netherlands and a review of the literature. Gastroenterology 1984; 86: 449–52.

39. McConnell RB. Ulcerative colitis – genetic features. Scand J Gastroenterol Supplement 1983; 88: 14–16.

40. Tysk C, Lindberg E, Jarnerot G, Floderus-Myrhed B. Ulcerative colitis and Crohn's disease in an unselected population of monozygotic and dizygotic twins: a study of heritability and the influence of smoking. Gut 1988; 29: 990–6.

41. Hayward AR. Lymphoid cell development. In: Litwin SD, Scott DW, Reisfeld RA, Flaherty L, Marcus DM, eds. Human Immunogenetics. New York: Marcel Dekker, 1989: 145–62.

42. Comes MC, Gower-Rousseau C, Colombel JF *et al.* Inflammatory bowel disease in married couples: 10 cases in Nord Pas de Calais region of France and Liege county of Belgium. Gut 1994; 35: 1316–18.

43. Yang H, Rotter JI. Inflammatory bowel disease. In: Rimoin DL, Connor JM, Pyeritz RE, Emery AEH, eds. Principles

and Practice of Medical Genetics, 3rd edn. London: Churchill Livingstone, 1997: 1533–53.

44. Hall JG. Turner syndrome. In: King RA, Rotter JI, Motulsky AG, eds. The Genetic Basis of Common Diseases. New York: Oxford University Press, 1992: 895–914.

45. Witkop CJ, Quevedo WC, Fitzpatrick TB, King RA. Albinism. In: Scriver C, Beaudet AL, Sly WS, Valle D, eds. The Metabolic Basic of Inherited Disease, 6th edn. New York: McGraw-Hill, 1989: 2905–48.

46. Schinella RA, Grego A, Cobert BT, Denmark LW, Cox RP. Hermansky–Pudlak syndrome with granulomatous colitis. Ann Intern Med 1980; 92: 20–3.

47. Mahadero R, Markowitz J, Fisher S, Daum F. Hermansky–Pudlak syndrome with granulomatous colitis in children. J Pediatr 1991; 118: 904–6.

48. Shanahan F, Randolph LM, King R et al. The Hermansky–Pudlak syndrome: an immunological assessment of 15 cases. Am J Med 1989; 85: 823–8.

49. Couper R, Kapelushnik J, Griffiths AM. Neutrophil dysfunction in glycogen storage disease IB: association with Crohn's-like colitis. Gastroenterology 1991; 100: 549–54.

50. Roe TF, Coates TD, Thomas DW, Miller JH, Gilsanz V. Brief report: treatment of chronic inflammatory bowel disease in glycogen storage disease type Ib with colony-stimulating factors. N Engl J Med 1992; 326: 1666–9.

51. Wildenberg SC, Oetting WS, Almodovar C, Krumwiede M, White JG, King RA. A gene causing Hermansky–Pudlak syndrome in a Puerto Rican population maps to chromosome 10q2. Am J Hum Genet 1995; 57: 755–65.

52. Oh J, Bailin T, Fukai K et al. Positional cloning of a gene for Hermansky–Pudlak syndrome, a disorder of cytoplasmic organelles. Nat Genet 1996; 14: 300–6.

53. Gardner JM, Wildenberg SC, Keiper NM et al. The mouse pale ear (ep) mutation is the homologue of human Hermansky–Pudlak syndrome. Proc Natl Acad Sci USA 1997; 94: 9238–43.

54. Hazelwood S, Shotelersuk V, Wildenberg SC et al. Evidence for locus heterogeneity in Puerto Ricans with Hermansky–Pudlak syndrome. Am J Hum Genet 1997; 61: 1088–94.

55. Oh J, Ho L, Ala-Mello S et al. Mutation analysis of patients with Hermansky–Pudlak syndrome: a frameshift hot spot in the HPS gene and apparent locus heterogeneity. Am J Hum Genet 1998; 62: 593–8.

56. Gahl WA, Brantly M, Kaiser-Kupfer MI et al. Genetic defects and clinical characteristics of patients with a form of oculocutaneous albinism (Hermansky–Pudlak syndrome). N Engl J Med 1998; 338: 1258–64.

57. Ament ME, Ochs HD. Gastrointestinal manifestations of chronic granulomatous disease. N Engl J Med 1973; 288: 382–7.

58. Werlin SL, Chusid MJ, Caya J, Oechler HW. Colitis in chronic granulomatous disease. Gastroenterology 1982; 82: 328–31.

59. Sloan JM, Cameron CHS, Maxwell RJ, McClusky DR, Collins JSA. Colitis complicating chronic granulomatous disease. A clinicopathological case report. Gut 1996; 38: 619–22.

60. Vannier JP, Arnaud-Battandier F, Ricour C et al. Chronic neutropenia and Crohn's disease in childhood. Report of 2 cases. Arch Fr Pediatr 1982; 39: 367–70.

61. Stevens C, Peppercorn MA, Grand RJ. Crohn's disease associated with autoimmune neutropenia. J Clin Gastroenterol 1991; 13: 328–30.

62. D'Agata ID, Paradis K, Chad Z, Bonny Y, Seidman E. Leucocyte adhesion deficiency presenting as a chronic ileocolitis. Gut 1996; 39: 5–8.

63. Eng C, Farraye FA, Shulman LN et al. The association between the myelodysplastic syndromes and Crohn disease. Ann Intern Med 1992; 117: 661–2.

64. Seymour JF. Association between myelodysplastic syndromes and inflammatory bowel diseases. Report of seven new cases and review of the literature. Leukemia 1998; 12: 1331–2.

65. Hebbar M, Kozlowski D, Wattel E et al. Association between myelodysplastic syndromes and inflammatory bowel diseases. Report of seven new cases and review of the literature. Leukemia 1997; 11: 2188–91.

66. Compton RF, Sandborn WJ, Yang H et al. A new syndrome of Crohn's disease and pachydermoperiostosis in a family. Gastroenterology 1997; 112: 241–9.

67. Caruso ML, Cristofaro G, Lynch HT. HNPCC-Lynch syndrome and idiopathic inflammatory bowel disease. A hypothesis on sharing of genes. Anticancer Res 1997; 17: 2647–9.

68. Yang H, Shohat T, Rotter JI. The genetics of inflammatory bowel disease. In: McDermott RP, Stenson WF, eds. Inflammatory Bowel Disease. New York: Elsevier, 1992: 17–51.

69. Kirsner JB. Inflammatory bowel disease – clinical, etiological and genetic aspects. In: Rotter JI, Samloff IM, Rimoin DL, eds. Genetics and Heterogeneity of Common Gastrointestinal Disorders. New York: Academic Press, 1980: 261–80.

70. Kuster W, Pascoe L, Purrmann J, Funk S, Majewski F. The genetics of Crohn disease: complex segregation analysis of a family study with 265 patients with Crohn disease and 5,387 relatives. Am J Med Genet 1989; 32: 105–8.

71. Orholm M, Iselius L, Sorensen TIA, Munkholm P, Langholz E, Binder V. Investigation of inheritance of chronic inflammatory bowel disease by complex segregation anslysis. Br Med J 1993; 306: 20–4.

72. Monsen U, Iselius L, Johansson C, Hellers G. Evidence for a major additive gene in ulcerative colitis. Clin Genet 1989; 36: 411–14.

73. McConnell RB. Inflammatory bowel disease: newer views of genetic influences. In: Berk JE, eds. Developments in Digestive Disease, Vol 3, 3rd edn. Philadelphia: Lea and Febiger, 1980: 129–37.

74. Rotter JI. The genetics of peptic ulcer disease – more than one gene,more than one disease. Prog Med Genet 1980; 4: 1–58.

75. Rotter JI. Genetics in gastroenterology. In: Gitnick G, Hollander D, Kaplowitz N, Samloff IM, Schoenfield LJ, eds. Principles and Practices of Gastroenterology. New York: Elsevier, 1988: 1501–25.

76. Greenberg DA, Rotter JI. Two locus models for gluten sensitive eneropathy: population genetic considerations. Am J Med Genet 1981; 8: 205–14.

77. Rotter JI, Landaw EM. Measuring the genetic contribution of a single locus to a multilocus disease. Clin Genet 1984; 26: 529–42.

78. Lin HJ, Rotter JI, Conte WJ. Use of HLA marker associations and HLA haplotype linkage to estimate disease risks in families with gluten-sensitive enteropathy. Clin Genet 1985; 28: 185–98.

79. Bennett RA, Rubin PH, Present DH. Frequency of inflammatory bowel disease in offspring of couples both presenting with inflammatory bowel disease. Gastroenterology 1991; 100: 1638–43.

80. McInnis MG. Anticipation: an old idea in new genes. Am J Hum Genet 1996; 59: 973–9.

81. Howeler CJ, Busch HFM, Geraedts JPM, Niermeijer MF, Staal A. Anticipation in myotonic dystrophy: fact or fiction? Brain 1989; 112: 779–97.

82. Brook JD, McCurrach ME, Harley HG et al. Molecular basis of myotonic dystrophy: expansion of a trinucleotide (CTG) repeat at the 3′ end of a transcript encoding a protein kinase family member. Cell 1992; 68: 799–808.

83. Huntington's Disease Collaborative Research Group. A novel gene containing a trinucleotide repeat that is expanded and unstable on Huntington's disease chromosomes. Cell 1993; 72: 971–83.

84. Verkerk AJ, Pieretti M, Sutcliffe JS *et al.* Identification of a gene (FMR-1) containing a CGG repeat coincident with a breakpoint cluster region exhibiting length variation in fragile X syndrome. Cell 1991; 65: 905–14.

85. Orr HT, Chung MY, Banfi S *et al.* Expansion of an unstable trinucleotide CAG repeat in spinocerebellar ataxia type 1. Nat Genet 1993; 4: 221–6.

86. Polito JM, Rees RC, Childs B, Mendeloff AI, Harris ML, Bayless TM. Preliminary evidence for genetic anticipation in Crohn's disease. Lancet 1996; 347: 798–800.

87. Grandbastien B, Peeters M, Franchimont D *et al.* Anticipation in familial Crohn's disease. Gut 1998; 42: 170–4.

88. Lee JC, Bridger S, McGregor C, Macpherson AJ, Jones JE. Why children with inflammatory bowel disease are diagnosed at a younger age than their affected parent. Gut 1999; 44: 808–11.

89. Hampe J, Heymann K, Kruis W, Raedler A, Folsch UR, Schreiber S. Anticipation in inflammatory bowel disease: a phenomenon caused by an accumulation of confounders. Am J Med Genet 2000; 92: 178–83.

90. Fraser FC. Trinucleotide repeats are not the only cause of genetic anticipation. Am J Med Genet 1997; 75: 337.

91. Petronis A, Kennedy JL, Paterson AD. Genetic anticipation: fact or artifact, genetics or epigenetics? Lancet 1997; 350: 1403–4.

92. Moll JMH. Inflammatory bowel disease. Clin Rheum Dis 1985; 11: 87–111.

93. Purrmann J, Zeidler H, Bertrams J *et al.* HLA antigens in ankylosing spondylitis associated with Crohn's disease. Increased frequency of the HLA phenotype B27,B44. J Rheumatol 1988; 15: 1658–61.

94. Mallas EG, Mackintosh P, Asquith P, Cooke WT. Histocompatibility antigens in inflammatory bowel disease. Their clinical significance and their association with arthropathy with special reference to HLA-B27 (w27). Gut 1976; 17: 906–10.

95. Russell AS. Transplantation antigens in Crohn's disease: linkage of associated ankylosing spondylistis with HLAw27. Am J Dig Dis 1975; 20: 359–61.

96. Dekker-Saeys BJ, Meuwissen SG, Van Den Berg-Loonen EM, De Haas WH, Meijers KA, Tytgat GN. Ankylosing spondylitis and inflammatory bowel disease. III. Clinical characteristics and results of histocompatibility typing (HLA B27) in 50 patients with both ankylosing spondylitis and inflammatory bowel disease. Ann Rheum Dis 1978; 37: 36–41.

97. Huaux JP, Fiasse R, de Bruyere M, Nigant de Deuxchaisnes C. HLA-B27 in sacroilitis. J Rheumatol 1977; 3: 60–3.

98. Khan MA. HLA-B27 and B12 (B44) in Crohn's disease with ankylosing spondylitis. J Rheumatol 1989; 16: 851–2.

99. Gilvarry J, Keeling F, Fielding JF. Sibship Crohn's disease and ankylosing spondylitis. J Clin Gastroenterol 1990; 12: 711–12.

100. Jayson MIV, Salmon PR, Harrison WJ. Inflammatory bowel disease in ankylosing spondylitis. Gut 1970; 11: 506–11.

101. Mielants H, Veys EM. Ileal inflammation in B27-positive reactive arthritis. Lancet 1984; 1: 1072.

102. Mielants H, Veys EM. Inflammation of the ileum in patients with B27-positive reactive arthritis. Lancet 1984; 1: 288.

103. De Keyser F, Elewaut D, De Vos M *et al.* Bowel inflammation and the spondyloarthropathies. Rheum Dis Clin N Am 1998; 24: 785–813, ix–x.

104. Mielants H, Veys EM, Cuvelier C *et al.* The evolution of spondyloarthropathies in relation to gut histology. II. Histological aspects. J Rheumatol 1995; 22: 2273–8.

105. De Vos M, Mielants H, Cuvelier C, Elewaut A, Veys E. Long-term evolution of gut inflammation in patients with spondyloarthropathy. Gastroenterology 1996; 110: 1696–703.

106. Russell AS. Arthritis, inflammatory bowel disease, and histocompatibility antigens. Ann Intern Med 1977; 86: 820–1.

107. Rath HC, Herfarth HH, Ikeda JS *et al.* Normal luminal bacteria, especially *Bacteroides* species, mediate chronic colitis, gastritis, and arthritis in HLA-B27/human beta2 microglobulin transgenic rats. J Clin Invest 1996; 98: 945–53.

108. Yates VM, Watkinson G, Kelman A. Further evidence for an association between psoriasis, Crohn's disease and ulcerative colitis. Br J Dermatol 1982; 106: 323–30.

109. Lee FI, Bellary SV, Francis C. Increased occurrence of psoriasis in patients with Crohn's disease and their relatives. Am J Gastroenterol 1990; 85: 962–3.

110. Hammer B, Ashurst P, Naish J. Diseases associated with ulcerative colitis and Crohn's disease. Gut 1968; 9: 17–21.

111. Trembath RC, Clough RL, Rosbotham JL *et al.* Identification of a major susceptibility locus on chromosome 6p and evidence for further disease loci revealed by a two stage genome-wide search in psoriasis. Hum Mol Genet 1997; 6: 813–20.

112. Matthews D, Fry L, Powles A *et al.* Evidence that a locus for familial psoriasis maps to chromosome 4q. Nat Genet 1996; 14: 231–3.

113. Nair RP, Henseler T, Jenisch S *et al.* Evidence for two psoriasis susceptibility loci (HLA and 17q) and two novel candidate regions (16q and 20p) by genome-wide scan. Hum Mol Genet 1997; 6: 1349–56.

114. Bhalerao J, Bowcock AM. The genetics of psoriasis: a complex disorder of the skin and immune system. Hum Mol Genet 1998; 7: 1537–45.

115. Hugot JP, Laurent-Puig P, Gower-Rousseau C *et al.* Mapping of a susceptibility locus for Crohn's disease on chromosome 16 by a genome-wide nonparametric linkage analysis. Nature 1996; 379: 821–3.

116. Weisner RH, LaRusso NF. Clinicopathologic features of the syndrome of primary sclerosing cholangitis. Gastroenterology 1980; 79: 200–6.

117. Chapman RW, Arborgh BA, Rhodes JM *et al.* Primary sclerosing cholangitis: a review of its clinical features, cholangiography, and hepatic histology. Gut 1980; 21: 870–7.

118. Wewer V, Gluud C, Schlichting P, Burcharth F, Binder V. Prevalence of hepatobiliary dysfunction in a regional group of patients with chronic inflammatory bowel disease. Scand J Gastroenterol 1991; 26: 97–102.

119. Olsson R, Danielsson A, Jarnerot G *et al.* Prevalence of primary sclerosing cholangitis in patients with ulcerative colitis. Gastroenterology 1991; 100: 1319–23.

120. Rasmussen HH, Fallingborg J, Mortensen PB *et al.* Primary sclerosing cholangitis in patients with ulcerative colitis. Scand J Gastroenterol 1992; 27: 732–6.

121. Broome U, Lofberg R, Lundqvist K, Veress B. Subclinical time span of inflammatory bowel disease in patients with primary sclerosing cholangitis. Dis Colon Rectum 1995; 38: 1301–5.

122. Chapman RW, Cottone M, Selby WS, Shepherd HA, Sherlock S, Jewell DP. Serum autoantibodies, ulcerative colitis and primary sclerosing cholangitis. Gut 1986; 27: 86–91.

123. Das KM, Vecchi M, Sakamaki S. A shared and unique epitope(s) on human colon, skin, and biliary epithelium detected by a monoclonal antibody. Gastroenterology 1990; 98: 464–9.

124. Duerr RH, Targan SR, Landers CJ, Sutherland LR, Shanahan F. Anti-neutrophil cytoplasmic antibodies in ulcerative colitis. Comparison with other colitides/diarrheal illnesses. Gastroenterology 1991; 100: 1590–6.

125. Zauli D, Baffoni L, Cassani F. Antineutrophil cytoplasmic antibodies in primary sclerosing cholangitis, ulcerative colitis, and autoimmune diseases. Gastroenterology 1992; 102: 1088–95.

126. Lo SK, Fleming KA, Chapman RW. Prevalence of anti-neutrophil antibody in primary sclerosing cholangitis and ulcerative colitis using an alkaline phosphatase technique. Gut 1992; 33: 1370–5.

127. Seibold F, Weber P, Klein R, Berg PA, Wiedmann KH. Clinical significance of antibodies against neutrophils in patients with inflammatory bowel disease and primary sclerosing cholangitis. Gut 1992; 33: 657–62.

128. Shepherd HA. Ulcerative colitis and persistent liver dysfunction. Q J Med 1983; 52: 503–13.

129. Prochazka EJ, Terasaki PI, Park MS, Goldstein LI, Busuttil RW. Association of primary sclerosing cholangitis with HLA-DRw52a. N Engl J Med 1990; 322: 1842–4.

130. Zetterquist H, Broome U, Einarsson K, Olerup O. HLA class II genes in primary sclerosing cholangitis and chronic inflammatory bowel disease: no HLA-DRw52a association in Swedish patients with sclerosing cholangitis. Gut 1992; 33: 942–6.

131. Olerup O, Broome U, Einarsson K, Zetterquist H. Inability to attribute susceptibility to primary sclerosing cholangitis to specific amino acid positions of the HLA-DRw52 allele. N Engl J Med 1991; 325: 1251–2.

132. Donaldson PT. Dual association of HLA DR2 and DR3 with primary sclerosing cholangitis. Hepatology 1991; 13: 129–33.

133. Toyoda H, Wang SJ, Yang HY et al. Distinct associations of HLA class II genes with inflammatory bowel disease. Gastroenterology 1993; 104: 741–8.

134. Sugimura K, Asakura H, Mizuki N et al. Analysis of genes within the HLA region affecting susceptibility to ulcerative colitis. Hum Immunol 1993; 36: 112–18.

135. Hirv K, Seyfarth M, Uibo R et al. Polymorphisms in tumour necrosis factor and adhesion molecule genes in patients with inflammatory bowel disease: associations with HLA-DR and -DQ alleles and subclinical markers. Scand J Gastroenterol 1999; 34: 1025–32.

136. Satsangi J, Landers CJ, Welsh KI, Koss K, Targan S, Jewell DP. The presence of anti-neutrophil antibodies reflects clinical and genetic heterogeneity within inflammatory bowel disease. Inflam Bowel Dis 1998; 4: 18–26.

137. Bayraktar Y, Arslan S, Saglam F, Uzunalimoglu B, Kayhan B. What is the association of primary sclerosing cholangitis with sex and inflammatory bowel disease in Turkish patients? Hepato-Gastroenterology 1998; 45: 2064–72.

138. Kelly P, Patchett S, McCloskey D, Alstead E, Farthing M, Fairclough P. Sclerosing cholangitis, race and sex. Gut 1997; 41: 688–9.

139. Dozois RR, Kelly KA, Welling DR et al. Ileal pouch-anal anastomosis: comparison of results in familial adenomatous polyposis and chronic ulcerative colitis. Ann Surg 1989; 210: 268–71.

140. Sandborn WJ. Pouchitis following ileal pouch-anal anastomosis: definition, pathogenesis, and treatment. Gastroenterology 1994; 107: 1856–60.

141. Lohmuller JL, Pemberton JH, Dozois RR, Ilstrup D, van Heerden J. Pouchitis and extraintestinal manifestations of inflammatory bowel disease after ileal pouch–anal anastomosis. Ann Surg 1990; 211: 622–67.

142. Penna C, Dozois R, Tremaine W et al. Pouchitis after ileal pouch–anal anastomosis for ulcerative colitis occurs with increased frequency in patients with associated primary sclerosing cholangitis. Gut 1996; 38: 234–9.

143. Yang P, Oresland T, Jarnerot G, Hulten L, Danielsson D. Perinuclear antineutrophil cytoplasmic antibody in pouchitis after proctocolectomy with ileal pouch–anal anastomosis for ulcerative colitis. Scand J Gastroenterol 1996; 31: 594–8.

144. Sandborn WJ, Landers CJ, Tremaine WJ, Targan SR. Anti-neutrophil cytoplasmic antibody correlates with chronic pouchitis after ileal pouch–anal anastomosis. Am J Gastroenterol 1995; 90: 740–7.

145. Merrett MN, Mortensen N, Kettlewell M, Jewell DO. Smoking may prevent pouchitis in patients with restorative proctocolectomy for ulcerative colitis. Gut 1996; 38: 362–4.

146. Sadovnick AD, Paty DW, Yannakoulias G. Concurrence of multiple sclerosis and inflammatory bowel disease. N Engl J Med 1989; 321: 762–3.

147. Minuk GY, Lewkonia RM. Possible familial association of multiple sclerosis and inflammatory bowel disease. N Engl J Med 1986; 314: 580–6.

148. Rang EH, Brooke BN, Hermon-Taylor J. Association of ulcerative colitis and multiple sclerosis. Lancet 1982; 2: 555.

149. Kitchin LI, Knobler RL, Friedman LS. Crohn's disease in a patient with multiple sclerosis. J Clin Gastroenterol 1991; 13: 331–4.

150. Purrmannn J, Arendt G, Cleveland S et al. Association of Crohn's disease and multiple sclerosis. Is there a common background? J Clin Gastroenterol 1992; 14: 43–6.

151. Yacyshyn B, Meddings J, Sadowski D, Bowen-Yachyshyn MB. Multiple sclerosis patients have peripheral blood CD45RO+ B cells and increased intestinal permeability. Dig Dis Sci 1996; 41: 2493–8.

152. Jarnerot G, Azad Khan AK, Truelove SC. The thyroid in ulcerative colitis and Crohn's disease. II. Thyroid enlargement and hyperthyroidism in ulcerative colitis. Acta Med Scand 1975; 197: 83–7.

153. Snook JA, de Silva HJ, Jewell DP. The association of autoimmune disorders with inflammatory bowel disease. Q J Med 1989; 72: 835–40.

154. Snook J. Are the inflammatory bowel diseases autoimmune disorders? Gut 1990; 31: 961–3.

155. Cottone M, Cappello M, Puleo A, Cipolla C, Filippazzo MG. Familial association of Crohn's and coeliac diseases. Lancet 1989; 2: 338.

156. Breen EG, Coughlan G, Connolly CE, Stevens FM. Coeliac proctitis. Scand J Gastroenterol 1987; 22: 471–7.

157. Becker KG, Simon RM, Biddison WE, Bailey-Wilson JE, McFarland HF, Trent JM. Clustering of non-MHC susceptibility candidate loci in human autoimmune diseases. Am J Hum Genet 1997; 61: A267.

158. Sels F, Westhovens R, Emonds MP, Vandermeulen E, Dequeker J. HLA typing in a large family with multiple cases of different autoimmune diseases. J Rheumatol 1997; 24: 856–9.

159. Jick H, Walker AM. Cigarette smoking and ulcerative colitis. N Engl J Med 1983; 308: 261–3.

160. Calkins BM. A meta-analysis of the role of smoking in inflammatory bowel disease. Dig Dis Sci 1989; 34: 1841–54.

161. Gent AE, Hellier MD, Grace RH, Swarbrick ET, Coggon D. Inflammatory bowel disease and domestic hygiene in infancy. Lancet 1994; 343: 766–7.

162. Rotter JI. Inflammatory bowel disease. Lancet 1994; 343: 1360.

163. Montgomery SM, Pounder RE, Wakefield AJ. Infant mortality and the incidence of inflammatory bowel disease. Lancet 1997; 349: 472–3.

164. Montgomery SM, Morris DL, Pounder RE, Wakefield AJ. Paramyxovirus infections in childhood and subsequent inflammatory bowel disease. Gastroenterology 1999; 116: 796–803.

165. Elson CO, Sartor RB, Tennyson GS, Riddell RH. Experimental models of inflammatory bowel disease. Gastroenterology 1995; 109: 1344–67.

166. Hammer RE, Maika SD, Richardson JA, Tang JP, Taurog JD. Spontaneous inflammatory disease in transgenic rats expressing HLA-B27 and human beta 2m: an animal model of HLA-B27-associated human disorders. Cell 1990; 63: 1099–112.

167. Taurog JD, Richardson JA, Croft JT et al. The germfree state prevents development of gut and joint inflammatory disease in HLA-B27 transgenic rats. J Exp Med 1994; 180: 2359–64.

168. Cahill RJ, Foltz CJ, Fox JG, Dangler CA, Powrie F, Schauer DB. Inflammatory bowel disease: an immunity-mediated condition triggered by bacterial infection with Helicobacter hepaticus. Infect Immun 1997; 65: 3126–31.

169. Diamond JM, Rotter JI. Observing the founder effect in human evolution. Nature 1987; 329: 105–6.

170. Rotter JI, Diamond JM. What maintains the frequencies of human genetic diseases? Nature 1987; 329: 289–90.

171. Petersen GM, Rotter JI, Cantor RM et al. The Tay-Sachs disease gene in North American Jewish populations: geographic variations and origin. Am J Hum Genet 1983; 35: 1258–69.

172. Targan SR, Murphy LK. Clarifying the causes of Crohn's. Nat Med 1995; 1: 1241–3.

173. Vasiliauskas EA, Plevy SE, Landers CJ et al. Perinuclear antineutrophil cytoplasmic antibodies in patients with Crohn's disease define a clinical subgroup. Gastroenterology 1996; 110: 1810–9.

174. Vasiliauskas EA, Kam LY, Karp LC, Gaiennie J, Yang H, Targan SR. Marker antibody expression stratifies Crohn's disease into immunologically homogeneous subgroups with clinical characteristics. Gut 2000; 47: 487–96.

175. Gilberts EC, Greenstein AJ, Katsel P, Harpaz N, Greenstein RJ. Molecular evidence for two forms of Crohn disease. Proc Natl Acad Sci USA 1994; 91: 12721–4.

176. Colombel JF, Grandbastien B, Gower-Rousseau B et al. Clinical characteristics of Crohn's disease in 72 families. Gastroenterology 1996; 111: 604–7.

177. Bayless TM, Tokayer AZ, Polito JM, Quaskey SA, Mellits ED, Harris ML. Crohn's disease: concordance for site and clinical type in affected family members – potential hereditary influences. Gastroenterology 1996; 111: 573–9.

178. Cottone M, Brignola C, Rosselli M et al. Relationship between site of disease and familial occurrence in Crohn's disease. Dig Dis Sci 1997; 42: 129–32.

179. King RA, Rotter JI, Motulsky AG. The Genetic Basis of Common Diseases. New York: Oxford University Press, 1992.

180. Targan SR, Deem RL, Liu M, Wang S, Nel A. Definition of a lamina propria T cell responsive state. Enhanced cytokine responsiveness of T cells stimulated through the CD2 pathway. J Immunol 1995; 154: 664–75.

181. Seibold F, Brandwein S, Simpson S, Terhorst C, Elson CO. pANCA represents a cross-reactivity to enteric bacterial antigens. J Clin Immunol 1998; 18: 153–60.

182. Lindberg E, Magnusson K-E, Tysk C, Jarnerot G. Antibody (IgG,IgA,and IgM) to baker's yeast (*Saccharomyces cerevisiae*), yeast mannan, gliadin, ovalbumin and betalactoglobulin in monozygotic twins with inflammatory bowel disease. Gut 1992; 33: 909–13.

183. McKenzie H, Main J, Pennington CR, Parratt D. Antibody to selected strains of *Saccharomyces cerevisiae* (baker's and brewer's yeast) and *Candida albicans* in Crohn's disease. Gut 1990; 31: 536–8.

184. Vecchi M, Gionchetti P, Bianchi MB et al. p-ANCA and development of pouchitis in ulcerative colitis patients after proctocolectomy and ileoanal pouch anastomosis. Lancet 1994; 344: 886–7.

185. Shanahan F, Duerr RH, Rotter JI et al. Neutrophil autoantibodies in ulcerative colitis: familial aggregation and genetic heterogeneity. Gastroenterology 1992; 103: 456–61.

186. Yang H, Rotter JI, Toyoda H et al. Ulcerative colitis: a genetically heterogeneous disorder defined by genetic (HLA class II) and subclinical (anti-neutrophil cytoplasmic antibodies) markers. J Clin Invest 1993; 92: 1080–4.

187. Yang H, Vora DK, Targan SR, Toyoda H, Beaudet AL, Rotter JI. Intercellular adhesion molecule 1 gene associations with immunologic subsets of inflammatory bowel disease. Gastroenterology 1995; 109: 440–8.

188. Seibold F, Slametschka D, Gregor M, Weber P. Neutrophil autoantibodies: a genetic marker in primary sclerosing cholangitis and ulcerative colitis. Gastroenterology 1994; 107: 532–6.

189. Lee JCW, Lennard-Jones JE, Cambridge G. Antineutrophil antibodies in familial inflammatory bowel disease. Gastroenterology 1995; 108: 428–33.

190. Yang P, Jarnerot G, Danielsson D, Tysk C, Lindberg E. P ANCA in monozygotic twins with inflammatory bowel disease. Gut 1995; 36: 887–90.

191. Shanahan F. Neutrophil autoantibodies in inflammatory bowel disease: are they important? Gastroenterology 1994; 107: 586–9.

192. Sutton CL, Yang H, Li Z, Rotter JI, Targan SR, Braun J. Familial expression of anti-*Saccharomyces cerevisiae* mannan antibodies in affected and unaffected relatives of patients with Crohn's disease. Gut 2000; 46: 58–63.

193. Taylor KD, Vasiliauskas EA, Kam LY et al. Specific clinical and immunological features in Crohn's disease patients are associated with the MHC class III marker Notch4. Gastroenterology 2000; 118: A869.

194. Taylor KD, Li Z, Barry M et al. Tumor necrosis factor microsatellite haplotype A11B4C1D3E3 is associated with anti-*Saccharomyces cerevisiae* antibody (ASCA) across clinical forms of inflammatory bowel disease. Gastroenterology 1998; 114: A1098.

195. Yang H, Taylor KD, Lin YC, Targan SR, Rotter JI. Magnitude of anti-*Saccharomyces cerevisiae* antibody (ASCA) expression is linked in Crohn's disease families to the major histocompatibility complex (MHC) region. Gastroenterology 2000; 118: A339.

196. Fiocchi C, Roche JK, Michener WM. High prevalence of antibodies to intestinal epithelial antigens in patients with inflammatory bowel disease and their relatives. Ann Intern Med 1989; 110: 786–94.

197. Folwaczny C, Noehl N, Endres SP, Heldwein W, Loeschke K, Fricke H. Antinuclear autoantibodies in patients with inflammatory bowel disease. High prevalence in first-degree relatives. Dig Dis Sci 1997; 42: 1593–7.

198. Elmgreen J, Both H, Binder V. Familial occurrence of complement dysfunction in Crohn's disease: correlation with intestinal symptoms and hypercatabolism of complement. Gut 1985; 26: 151–7.

199. Hollander D. Permeability in Crohn's disease: altered barrier functions in healthy relatives? Gastroenterology 1993; 104: 1848–51.

200. Munkholm P, Langholz E, Hollander D et al. Intestinal permeability in patients with Crohn's disease and ulcerative colitis and their first degree relatives. Gut 1994; 35: 68–72.

201. Lindberg E, Soderholm JD, Olaison G, Tysk C, Jarnerot G. Intestinal permeability to polyethylene glycols in monozygotic twins with Crohn's disease. Scand J Gastroenterol 1995; 30: 780–3.

202. Peeters M, Geypens B, Claus D et al. Clustering of increased small intestinal permeability in families with Crohn's disease. Gastroenterology 1997; 113: 802–7.

203. Van de Merwe JP, Schroder AM, Wensinck F, Hazenberg MP. The obligate anaerobic faecal flora of patients with Crohn's disease and their first-degree relatives. Scand J Gastroenterol 1988; 23: 1125–31.

204. Sendid B, Quinton JF, Charrier G et al. Anti *Saccharomyces cerevisiae* mannan antibodies (ASCA) in healthy relatives of patients with Crohn's disease. Gut 1997; 41: A177.

205. Seibold F, Mork H, Tanza S et al. Pancreatic autoantibodies in Crohn's disease: a family study. Gut 1997; 40: 481–4.

206. Yang H, Rotter JI. Subclinical markers of human inflammatory bowel disease. Can J Gastroenterol 1995; 9: 161–7.

207. Tysk C, Riedesel H, Lindberg E, Panzini B, Podolsky D, Jarnerot G. Colonic glycoproteins in monozygotic twins with inflammatory bowel disease. Gastroenterology 1991; 100: 419–23.

208. Helgeland L, Tysk C, Jarnerot G. IgG subclass distribution in serum and rectal mucosa of monozygotic twins with or without inflammatory bowel disease. Gut 1992; 33: 1358–64.

209. Amelio RD, Rossi P, Moli SLE, Ricci R, Montano S, Pallone F. *In vitro* studies on cellular and humoral chemotaxis in Crohn's disease using the under agarose gel technique. Gut 1981; 22: 566–70.

210. Elmgreen J, Berkowicz A, Sorensen H. Hypercatabolism of complement in Crohn's disease. Acta Med Scand 1983; 214: 403–7.

211. Lake AM, Stitzel AE, Urmson RJ, Walker WA, Spitzer RE. Complement alterations in inflammatory bowel disease. Gastroenterology 1979; 76: 374–9.

212. Hodgson HJF, Potter BJ, Jewell DP. C3 metabolism in ulcerative colitis and Crohn's disease. Clin Exp Immunol 1977; 28: 490–5.

213. Potter BJ, Brown DJC, Watson A, Jewell DP. Complement inhibitors and immunoconglutinins in ulcerative colitis and Crohn's disease. Gut 1980; 2: 1030–4.

214. Halstensen TS, Mollnes TE, Brandzaeg P. Persistent complement activation in submucosal blood vessels of active inflammatory bowel disease: Immunohistochemical evidence. Gastroenterology 1989; 97: 10–19.

215. Halstensen TS, Mollnes TE, Garred P, Fausa O, Brandtzaeg P. Epithelial deposition of immunoglobulin G1 and activated complement (C3b and terminal complement complex) in ulcerative colitis. Gastroenterology 1990; 98: 1264–71.

216. Ahrenstedt O, Knutson L, Nisson B, Nilsson-Ekdahl K, Odlind B, Hallgren R. Enhanced local production of complement components in the small intestines of patients with Crohn's disease. N Engl J Med 1990; 322: 1345–9.

217. Ueki T, Mizuno M, Uesu T et al. Distribution of activated complement, C3b, and its degraded fragments, iC3b/C3dg, in the colonic mucosa of ulcerative colitis (UC). Clin Exp Immunol 1996; 104: 286–92.

218. Laufer J, Oren R, Goldberg I et al. Cellular localization of complement C3 and C4 transcripts in intestinal specimens from patients with Crohn's disease. Clin Exp Immunol 2000; 120: 30–7.

219. Wakefield AJ, Sawyer AM, Dhillon AP et al. Pathogenesis of Crohn's disease: multifocal gastrointestinal infarction. Lancet 1989; 2: 1057–62.

220. Wakefield AJ, Sankey EA, Dhillon AP et al. Granulomatous vasculitis in Crohn's disease. Gastroenterology 1991; 100: 1279–87.

221. Hudson M, Piasecki C, Sankey EA et al. A ferret model of acute multifocal gastrointestinal infarction. Gastroenterology 1992; 102: 1591–6.

222. Elmgreen J, Sorensen H, Berkowicz A. Polymorphism of complement C3 in chronic inflammatory bowel disease. Predominance of the C3F gene in Crohn's disease. Acta Med Scand 1984; 215: 375–8.

223. Botto M, Fong KY, So AK, Koch C, Walport MJ. Molecular basis of polymorphisms of human complement component C3. J Exp Med 1990; 172: 1011–17.

224. Hollander D, Vadheim CM, Brettholtz E, Petersen GM, Delahunty T, Rotter JI. Increased intestinal permeability in Crohn's patients and their relatives: an etiological factor? Ann Intern Med 1986; 105: 883–95.

225. Bjarnason I, Smethurst P, Levi AJ, Menzies IS, Peters TJ. The effect of polyacrylic acid polymers on small-intestinal function and permeability changes caused by indomethacin. Scand J Gastroenterol 1991; 26: 685–8.

226. May GR, Sutherland LR, Meddings JB. Is small intestinal permeability really increased in relatives of patients with Crohn's disease? Gastroenterology 1993; 104: 1627–32.

227. van Elburg RM, Uil JJ, Mulder CJ, Heymans HS. Intestinal permeability in patients with coeliac disease and relatives of patients with coeliac disease. Gut 1993; 34: 354–7.

228. Lim SG, Menzies IS, Lee CA, Johnson MA, Pounder RE. Intestinal permeability and function in patients infected with human immunodeficiency virus. A comparison with coeliac disease. Scand J Gastroenterol 1993; 28: 573–80.

229. Fukushima K. Immunohistochemical characterization, distribution, and ultrastructure of lymphocytes bearing T-cell receptors in inflammatory bowel disease. Gastroenterology 1991; 101: 670–8.

230. Kagnoff MF, Brown RJ, Schanfield MS. Association between Crohn's disease and immunoglobulin heavy chain (Gm) allotypes. Gastroenterology 1983; 85: 1044–7.

231. Biemond I, Delange GG, Weterman IT, Pena AS. Immunoglobulin allotypes in Crohn's disease in the Netherlands. Gut 1987; 28: 610–12.

232. Ockhuizen T, Westra H, Bijzet J, Post J, van Leeuwen M, van Rijswijk M. Immunoglobulin allotypes are not involved in systemic amyloidosis. J Rheumatol 1985; 12: 742–6.

233. Gudjonsson H, Schanfield MS, Albertini RJ, McAuliffe TL, Beeken WL, Krawitt EL. Association and linkage studies of immunoglobulin heavy chain allotypes in inflammatory bowel disease. Tissue Antigens 1988; 31: 243–9.

234. Field LL, Boyd N, Bowen TJ, Kelly JK, Sutherland LR. Genetic markers and inflammatory bowel disease: immunoglobulin allotypes (GM, KM) and protease inhibitor. Am J Gastroenterol 1989; 84: 753–5.

235. Kett K, Rognum TO, Brandtzaeg P. Mucosal subclass distribution of immunoglobulin G-producing cells is different in ulcerative colitis and Crohn's disease of the colon. Gastroenterology 1987; 93: 919–24.

236. Elson CO, Cong Y, Brandwein S et al. Experimental models to study molecular mechanisms underlying intestinal inflammation. Ann NY Acad Sci 1998; 859: 85–95.

237. Mahler M, Bristol IJ, Leiter EH et al. Differential susceptibility of inbred mouse strains to dextran sulfate sodium-induced colitis. Am J Physiol 1998; 274: G544–51.

238. Mahler M, Bristol IJ, Sundberg JP et al. Genetic analysis of susceptibility to dextran sulfate sodium-induced colitis in mice. Genomics 1999; 55: 147–56.

239. Rath HC, Wilson KH, Sartor RB. Differential induction of colitis and gastritis in HLA-B27 transgenic rats selectively colonized with *Bacteroides vulgatus* or *Escherichia coli*. Infect Immun 1999; 67: 2969–74.

240. Kontoyiannis D, Pasparakis M, Pizarro TT, Cominelli F, Kollias G. Impaired on/off regulation of TNF biosynthesis in mice lacking TNF AU-rich elements: implications for joint and gut-associated immunopathologies. Immunity 1999; 10: 387–98.

241. Cominelli F, Kontoyiannis D, Pizarro T, Kollias G. Contribution of TNF receptor (TNFR) types and T lymphocyte population to the pathogenesis of experimental Crohn's disease (CD) in TNF^{DARE} mutant mice. Gastroenterology 1999; 116: A690.

242. Sadlack B, Merz H, Schorle H, Schimpl A, Feller AC, Horak I. Ulcerative colitis-like disease in mice with a disrupted interleukin-2 gene. Cell 1993; 75: 253–61.

243. Schultz M, Tonkonogy SL, Sellon RK *et al.* IL-2-deficient mice raised under germfree conditions develop delayed mild focal intestinal inflammation. Am J Physiol 1999; 276: G1461–72.

244. Meijssen MA, Brandwein SL, Reinecker HC, Bhan AK, Podolsky DK. Alteration of gene expression by intestinal epithelial cells precedes colitis in interleukin-2-deficient mice. Am J Physiol 1998; 274: G472–9.

245. Harren M, Schonfelder G, Paul M *et al.* High expression of inducible nitric oxide synthase correlates with intestinal inflammation of interleukin-2-deficient mice. Ann NY Acad Sci 1998; 859: 210–15.

246. Ludviksson BR, Gray B, Strober W, Ehrhardt RO. Dysregulated intrathymic development in the IL-2-deficient mouse leads to colitis-inducing thymocytes. J Immunol 1997; 158: 104–11.

247. Ehrhardt RO, Ludviksson BR, Gray B, Neurath M, Strober W. Induction and prevention of colonic inflammation in IL-2-deficient mice. J Immunol 1997; 158: 566–73.

248. Ludviksson BR, Strober W, Nishikomori R, Hasan SK, Ehrhardt RO. Administration of mAb against alpha E beta 7 prevents and ameliorates immunization-induced colitis in IL-2-/- mice. J Immunol 1999; 162: 4975–82.

249. Kuhn R, Lohler J, Rennick D, Rajewsky K, Muller W. Interleukin-10-deficient mice develop chronic enterocolitis. Cell 1993; 75: 263–74.

250. Davidson NJ, Leach MW, Fort MM *et al.* T helper cell 1-type CD4$^+$ T cells, but not B cells, mediate colitis in interleukin 10-deficient mice. J Exp Med 1996; 184: 241–51.

251. Berg DJ, Davidson N, Kuhn R *et al.* Enterocolitis and colon cancer in interleukin-10-deficient mice are associated with aberrant cytokine production and CD4(+) Th1-like responses. J Clin Invest 1996; 98: 1010–20.

252. Kullberg MC, Ward JM, Gorelick PL *et al. Helicobacter hepaticus* triggers colitis in specific-pathogen-free interleukin-10 (IL-10)-deficient mice through an IL-12- and gamma interferon-dependent mechanism. Infect Immun 1998; 66: 5157–66.

253. Pasparakis M, Alexopoulou L, Episkopou V, Kollias G. Immune and inflammatory responses in TNF alpha-deficient mice: a critical requirement for TNF alpha in the formation of primary B cell follicles, follicular dendritic cell networks and germinal centers, and in the maturation of the humoral immune response. J Exp Med 1996; 184: 1397–411.

254. Pasparakis M, Alexopoulou L, Grell M, Pfizenmaier K, Bluethmann H, Kollias G. Peyer's patch organogenesis is intact yet formation of B lymphocyte follicles is defective in peripheral lymphoid organs of mice deficient for tumor necrosis factor and its 55-kDa receptor. Proc Nat Acad Sci USA 1997; 94: 6319–23.

255. Kaneko H, Yamada H, Mizuno S *et al.* Role of tumor necrosis factor-alpha in *Mycobacterium*-induced granuloma formation in tumor necrosis factor-alpha-deficient mice. Lab Invest 1999; 79: 379–86.

256. Dianda L, Hanby AM, Wright NA, Sebesteny A, Hayday AC, Owen MJ. T cell receptor-alpha beta-deficient mice fail to develop colitis in the absence of a microbial environment. Am J Pathol 1997; 150: 91–7.

257. Mizoguchi E, Mizoguchi A, Bhan AK. Role of cytokines in the early stages of chronic colitis in TCR alpha-mutant mice. Lab Invest 1997; 76: 385–97.

258. Mizoguchi A, Mizoguchi E, Bhan AK. The critical role of interleukin 4 but not interferon gamma in the pathogenesis of colitis in T-cell receptor alpha mutant mice. Gastroenterology 1999; 116: 320–6.

259. De Winter H, Cheroutre H, Kronenberg M. Mucosal immunity and inflammation. II. The yin and yang of T cells in intestinal inflammation: pathogenic and protective roles in a mouse colitis model. Am J Physiol 1999; 276: G1317–21.

260. Simpson SJ, Shah S, Comiskey M *et al.* T cell-mediated pathology in two models of experimental colitis depends predominantly on the interleukin 12/Signal transducer and activator of transcription (Stat)-4 pathway, but is not conditional on interferon gamma expression by T cells. J Exp Med 1998; 187: 1225–34.

261. Powrie F, Carlino J, Leach MW, Mauze S, Coffman RL. A critical role for transforming growth factor-beta but not interleukin 4 in the suppression of T helper type 1-mediated colitis by CD45RB(low) CD4$^+$ T cells. J Exp Med 1996; 183: 2669–74.

262. Asseman C, Mauze S, Leach MW, Coffman RL, Powrie F. An essential role for interleukin 10 in the function of regulatory T cells that inhibit intestinal inflammation. J Exp Med 1999; 190: 995–1004.

263. Fort MM, Leach MW, Rennick DM. A role for NK cells as regulators of CD4$^+$ T cells in a transfer model of colitis. J Immunol 1998; 161: 3256–61.

264. Ma Y, Ohmen JD, Li Z *et al.* A genome-wide search identifies potential new susceptibility loci for Crohn's disease. Inflam Bowel Dis 1999; 5: 271–8.

265. Powrie F, Leach MW, Mauze S, Caddle LB, Coffman RL. Phenotypically distinct subsets of CD4$^+$ T cells induce or protect from chronic intestinal inflammation in C. B-17 scid mice. Int Immunol 1993; 5: 1461–71.

266. Powrie F, Leach MW, Mauze S, Menon S, Caddle LB, Coffman RL. Inhibition of Th1 responses prevents inflammatory bowel disease in scid mice reconstituted with CD45RBhi CD4$^+$ T cells. Immunity 1994; 1: 553–62.

267. Ito H, Fathman CG. CD45RBhigh CD4$^+$ T cells from IFN-gamma knockout mice do not induce wasting disease. J Autoimmunity 1997; 10: 455–9.

268. Rotter JI, Vadheim CM, Rimoin DL. Diabetes mellitus. In: King RA, Rotter JI, Motulsky AG, eds. The Genetic Basis of Common Diseases, 1st edn. New York: Oxford University Press, 1992: 413–81.

269. Hashimoto L, Habita C, Beressi JP *et al.* Genetic mapping of a susceptibility locus for insulin-dependent diabetes mellitus on chromosome 11q. Nature 1994; 371: 161–4.

270. Davies JL, Kawaguchi Y, Bennett S *et al.* A genome-wide search for human type 1 diabetes susceptibility genes. Nature 1994; 371: 130–6.

271. Field LL, Tobias R, Magnus T. A locus on chromosome 15q26 (IDDM3) produces susceptibility to insulin-dependent diabetes mellitus. Nature Genet 1994; 8: 189–94.

272. Luo DF, Bui MM, Muir A, Maclaren NK, Thomson G, She JX. Affected sib-pair mapping of a novel susceptibility gene to insulin-dependent diabetes mellitus (IDDM8) on chromosome 6q25-q27. Am J Hum Genet 1995; 57: 911–19.

273. Luo DF, Buzzetti R, Rotter JI *et al.* Confirmation of three susceptibility genes to insulin-dependent diabetes mellitus: IDDM4, IDDM5 and IDDM8. Hum Mol Genet 1996; 5: 693–8.

274. Todd JA, Farrall M. Panning for gold: genome-wide scanning for linkage in type 1 diabetes. Hum Mol Genet 1996; 5: 1443–8.

275. Delepine M, Pociot F, Habita C *et al.* Evidence of a non-MHC susceptibility locus in type I diabetes linked to HLA on chromosome 6. Am J Hum Genet 1997; 60: 174–87.

276. Julier C, Hyer RN, Davies J *et al.* Insulin–IGF2 region on chromosome 11p encodes a gene implicated in HLA-DR4-dependent diabetes susceptibility. Nature 1991; 354: 155–9.

277. Bennett ST, Lucassen AM, Gough SCL *et al.* Susceptibility to human type 1 diabetes at *IDDM2* is determined by

tandem repeat variation at the insulin gene minisatellite locus. Nature Genet 1995; 9: 284–92.

278. Lander ES. Mapping complex genetic traits in humans. In: Davies RE, editor. Genome Analysis. Oxford: IRL Press, 1988: 171–89.

279. Szpirer C, Riviere M, Szpirer J *et al*. Chromosomal assignment of human and rat hypertension candidate genes: Type 1 angiotensin II receptor genes and the SA gene. J Hypertens 1993; 11: 919–25.

280. Lander ES, Botstein D. Mapping complex genetic traits in humans: new methods using a complete RFLP linkage map. 1986; 51; 49–62.

281. Risch N. Assessing the role of HLA-linked and unlinked determinants of disease. Am J Hum Genet 1987; 40: 1–14.

282. Calkins BM, Mendeloff AI. The epidemiology of idiopathic inflammatory bowel disease. In: Kirsner JB, Shorter RG, eds. Inflammatory Bowel Disease, 4th edn. Baltimore: Williams & Wilkins, 1995: 31–68.

283. Ohmen JD, Yang HY, Yamamoto KK *et al*. Susceptibility locus for inflammatory bowel disease on chromosome 16 has a role in Crohn's disease, but not in ulcerative colitis. Hum Mol Genet 1996; 5: 1679–83.

284. Parkes M, Satsangi J, Lathrop GM, Bell JI, Jewell DP. Susceptibility loci in inflammatory bowel disease. Lancet 1996; 348: 1588.

285. Mirza MM, Lee J, Teare D *et al*. Evidence of linkage of the inflammatory bowel disease susceptibility locus on chromosome 16 (IBD1) to ulcerative colitis. J Med Genet 1998; 35: 218–21.

286. Cho JH, Nicolae DL, Gold LH *et al*. Identification of novel susceptibility loci for inflammatory bowel disease on chromosomes 1p, 3q, and 4q: evidence for epistasis between 1p and *IBD1*. Proc Natl Acad Sci USA 1998; 95: 7502–7.

287. Cavanaugh JA, Callen DF, Wilson SR *et al*. Analysis of Australian Crohn's disease pedigrees refines the localization for susceptibility to inflammatory bowel disease on chromosome 16. Ann Hum Genet 1998; 62 : 291–8.

288. Curran ME, Lau KF, Hampe J *et al*. Genetic analysis of inflammatory bowel disease in a large European cohort supports linkage to chromosomes 12 and 16. Gastroenterology 1998; 115: 1066–71.

289. Brant SR, Fu Y, Fields CT *et al*. American families with Crohn's disease have strong evidence for linkage to chromosome 16 but not chromosome 12. Gastroenterology 1998; 115: 1056–61.

290. Hugot JP, Zouali H, Colombel JF *et al*. Fine mapping of the inflammatory bowel disease susceptibility locus 1 (IBD1) in the pericentromeric region of chromosome 16. Gastroenterology 1998; 114: A999.

291. Satsangi J, Parkes M, Louis E *et al*. Two stage genome-wide search in inflammatory bowel disease provides evidence for susceptibility loci on chromosomes 3, 7 and 12. Nat Genet 1996; 14: 199–202.

292. Duerr RH, Barmada MM, Zhang L *et al*. Linkage and association between inflammatory bowel disease and a locus on chromosome 12. Am J Hum Genet 1998; 63: 95–100.

293. Yang H, Ohmen JD, Ma Y, Targan SR, Fischel-Ghodsian N, Rotter JI. Additional evidence of linkage between Crohn's disease and a putative locus on chromosome 12. Genet Med 1999; 1: 194–9.

294. Yang H, Plevy SE, Taylor K *et al*. Linkage of Crohn's disease to the major histocompatibility complex region is detected by multiple non-parametric analyses. Gut 1999; 44: 519–26.

295. Hampe J, Schreiber S, Shaw SH *et al*. A genomewide analysis provides evidence for novel linkages in inflammatory bowel disease in a large European cohort. Am J Hum Genet 1999; 64: 808–16.

296. Rioux JD, Silverberg MS, Daly MJ *et al*. Genomewide search in Canadian families with inflammatory bowel disease reveals two novel susceptibility loci. Am J Hum Genet 2000; 66: 1863–70.

297. Duerr RH, Barmada MM, Zhang L, Pfutzer R, Weeks DE. High-density genome scan in Crohn disease shows confirmed linkage to chromosme 14q11-12. Am J Hum Genet 2000; 66: 1857–62.

298. Cho JH, Fu Y, Kirschner BS, Hanauer SB. Confirmation of a susceptibility locus for Crohn's disease on chromosome 16. Inflam Bowel Dis 1997; 3: 186–90.

299. Hugot JP, Thomas G. Genome-wide scanning in inflammatory bowel diseases. Dig Dis 1998; 16: 364–9.

300. Vermeire S, Peeters M, Vlietinck R *et al*. No evidence for linkage on chromosomes 16-12-7 and 3 in the Belgian population may reflect genetic heterogeneity of inflammatory bowel disease. Gastroenterology 1998; 114: A1109.

301. Rioux JD, Daly MJ, Green T *et al*. Absence of linkage between inflammatory bowel disease and selected loci on chromosomes 3, 7, 12, and 16. Gastroenterology 1998; 115: 1062–5.

302. Parkes M, Satsangi J, Merriman A, Jewell DP. Precision mapping of chromosome 12 linkage in IBD: evidence for a haplotype association. Gastroenterology 1998; 114: A1058.

303. Hampe J, Hermann B, Bridger S, MacPherson AJ, Mathew CG, Schreiber S. The interferon-gamma gene as a positional and functional candidate gene for inflammatory bowel disease. Int J Colorect Dis 1998; 13: 260–3.

304. Simmons JD, Mullighan C, Welsh KI, Jewell DP. Vitamin D receptor gene polymorphism further evidence for an association with Crohn's disease. Gastroenterology 1998; 114: A1086.

305. Broman KW, Murray JC, Shefield VC, White RL, Weber JL. Comprehensive human genetic maps: individual and sex-specific variation in recombination. Am J Hum Genet 1998; 63: 861–9.

306. Satsangi J, Welsh KI, Bunce M *et al*. Contribution of genes of the major histocompatibility complex to susceptibility and disease phenotype in inflammatory bowel disease. Lancet 1996; 347: 1212–17.

307. Hugot JP, Laurent-Puig P, Gower-Rousseau C *et al*. Linkage analyses of chromosome 6 loci, including HLA, in familial aggregations of Crohn disease. Am J Med Genet 1994; 52: 207–13.

308. Naom I, Lee J, Ford D *et al*. Analysis of the contribution of HLA genes to genetic predisposition in inflammatory bowel disease. Am J Hum Genet 1996; 59: 226–33.

309. Brant SR, Panhuysen C, Bailey-Wilson J *et al*. Crohn's disease diagnosis before age 22 and with greater severity of disease identifies multiplex pedigrees at greater risk for locus IBD1. Gastroenterology 2000; 118: A708.

310. IBD Genetics Consortium. The international IBD consortium confirms linkage of Crohn's disease to a locus on chromosome 16 (IBD1). Gastroenterology 2000; 118: A463.

311. Stokkers PC, Huibregtse K Jr, Leegwater AC, Reitsma PH, Tytgat GN, van Deventer SJ. Analysis of a positional candidate gene for inflammatory bowel disease: NRAMP2. Inflam Bowel Dis 2000; 6: 92–8.

312. Hampe J, Shaw SH, Saiz R *et al*. Linkage of inflammatory bowel disease to human chromosome 6p. Am J Hum Genet 1999; 65: 1647–55.

313. Vermeire S, Vlietinck R, Groenen P, Peeters M, Rutgeerts P. Replication of linkage on 14q11-12 in inflammatory bowel disease. Gastroenterology 2000; 118: A338.

314. Parkes M, Vyas P, Satsangi J, Jewell DP. Fine mapping the IBD linkage on chromosome 3. Gastroenterology 1999; 116: A792.

315. Zhang WJ, Koltun WA, Tilberg AF, Page MJ, Chorney MJ. Absence of GNAI2 codon 179 oncogene mutations in

inflammatory bowel disease. Inflam Bowel Dis 2000; 6: 103–6.

316. Pokorny RM, Hofmeister A, Galandiuk S, Dietz AB, Cohen ND, Neibergs HL. Crohn's disease and ulcerative colitis are associated with the DNA repair gene MLH1. Ann Surg 1997; 225: 718–25.

317. Kyo K, Parkes M, Takei Y et al. Association of ulcerative colitis with rare VNTR alleles of the human intestinal mucin gene, MUC3. Hum Mol Genet 1999; 8: 307–11.

318. Podolsky DK, Fournier DA. Alterations in mucosal content of colonic glycoconjugates in inflammatory bowel disease defined by monoclonal antibodies. Gastroenterology 1988; 95: 379–87.

319. Cho JH, Nicolae DL, Ramos R et al. Linkage and linkage disequilibrium in chromosome band 1p36 in American Chaldeans with inflammatory bowel disease. Hum Mol Genet 2000; 9: 1425–32.

320. MHC Sequencing Consortium. Complete sequence and gene map of a human major histocompatibility complex. Nature 1999; 401: 921–3.

321. Stokkers PC, Reitsma PH, Tytgat GN, van Deventer SJ. HLA-DR and -DQ phenotypes in inflammatory bowel disease: a meta-analysis. Gut 1999; 45: 395–401.

322. Danze PM, Colombel JF, Jacquot S et al. Association of HLA class II genes with susceptibility to Crohn's disease. Gut 1996; 39: 69–72.

323. Reinshagen M, Loeliger C, Kuehnl P et al. HLA class II gene frequencies in Crohn's disease: a population based analysis in Germany. Gut 1996; 38: 538–42.

324. Roussomoustakaki M, Satsangi J, Welsh K et al. Genetic markers may predict disease behavior in patients with ulcerative colitis. Gastroenterology 1997; 112: 1845–53.

325. Bouma G, Crusius JB, Garcia-Gonzalez MA et al. Genetic markers in clinically well defined patients with ulcerative colitis (UC). Clin Exp Immunol 1999; 115: 294–300.

326. Trachtenberg EA, Yang H, Hayes E et al. HLA class II haplotype associations with inflammatory bowel disease in Jewish (Ashkenazi) and non-Jewish caucasian populations. Hum Immunol 2000; 61: 326–33.

327. Asakura H, Tsuchiya M, Aiso S et al. Association of the human lymphocyte-DR2 antigen with Japanese ulcerative colitis. Gastroenterology 1982; 82: 413–18.

328. Futami S, Aoyama N, Honsako Y et al. HLA-DRB1*1502 allele, subtype of DR15, is associated with susceptibility to ulcerative colitis and its progression. Dig Dis Sci 1995; 40: 814–18.

329. Duerr RH, Neigut DA. Molecularly defined HLA-DR2 alleles in ulcerative colitis and an antineutrophil cytoplasmic antibody-positive subgroup. Gastroenterology 1995; 108: 423–7.

330. Cariappa A, Sands B, Forcione D, Finkelstein D, Podolsky DK, Pillai S. Analysis of MHC class II DP, DQ and DR alleles in Crohn's disease. Gut 1998; 43: 210–15.

331. Nakajima A, Matsuhashi N, Kodama T, Yazaki Y, Takazoe M, Kimura A. HLA-linked susceptibility and resistance genes in Crohn's disease. Gastroenterology 1995; 109: 1462–7.

332. Forcione DG, Sands B, Isselbacher KJ, Rustgi A, Podolsky DK, Pillai S. An increased risk of Crohn's disease in individuals who inherit the HLA class II DRB3*0301 allele. Proc Natl Acad Sci USA 1996; 93: 5094–8.

333. Bouma G, Oudkerk Pool M, Crusius JB et al. Evidence for genetic heterogeneity in inflammatory bowel disease (IBD); HLA genes in the predisposition to suffer from ulcerative colitis (UC) and Crohn's disease (CD). Clin Exp Immunol 1997; 109: 175–9.

334. Orchard TR, Thiyagaraja S, Welsh KI, Wordsworth BP, Hill Gaston JS, Jewell DP. Clinical phenotype is related to HLA genotype in the peripheral arthropathies of inflammatory bowel disease. Gastroenterology 2000; 118: 274–8.

335. Artavanis-Tsakonas S, Rand MD, Lake RJ. Notch signaling: cell fate control and signal integration in development. Science 1999; 284: 770–6.

336. Milner LA, Bigas A. Notch as a mediator of cell fate determination in hematopoiesis: evidence and speculation. Blood 1999; 93: 2431–48.

337. Skipper M, Lewis J. Getting to the guts of enteroendocrine differentiation. Nat Genet 2000; 24: 3–4.

338. Robey E. Regulation of T cell fate by Notch. Annu Rev Immunol 1999; 17: 283–95.

339. Taylor KD, Yang H, Hang TD et al. Linkage disequilibrium mapping identifies a class III major histocompatibility complex (MHC) susceptibility haplotype to Crohn's disease in Ashkenazi Jews. Am J Hum Genet 1999; 65: A102.

340. Van Deventer SJ. Tumour necrosis factor and Crohn's disease. Gut 1997; 40: 443–8.

341. Targan SR, Hanauer SB, van Deventer SJ et al. A short-term study of chimeric monoclonal antibody cA2 to tumor necrosis factor alpha for Crohn's disease. Crohn's Disease cA2 Study Group. N Engl J Med 1997; 337: 1029–35.

342. Bazzoni F, Beutler B. The tumor necrosis factor ligand and receptor families. N Engl J Med 1996; 334: 1717–25.

343. Kroeger KM, Carville KS, Abraham LJ. The –308 tumor necrosis factor-alpha promoter polymorphism effects transcription. Mol Immunol 199; 34: 391–9.

344. Louis E, Franchimont D, Piron A et al. Tumour necrosis factor (TNF) gene polymorphism influences TNF-alpha production in lipopolysaccharide (LPS)-stimulated whole blood cell culture in healthy humans. Clin Exp Immunol 1998; 113: 401–6.

345. McGuire W, Hill AV, Allsopp CE, Greenwood BM, Kwiatkowski D. Variation in the TNF-alpha promoter region associated with susceptibility to cerebral malaria. Nature 1994; 371: 508–10.

346. McGuire W, Knight JC, Hill AV, Allsopp CE, Greenwood BM, Kwiatkowski D. Severe malarial anemia and cerebral malaria are associated with different tumor necrosis factor promoter alleles. J Infect Dis 1999; 179: 287–90.

347. Wilson AG, di Giovine FS, Duff GW. Genetics of tumour necrosis factor-alpha in autoimmune, infectious, and neoplastic diseases. J Inflammation 1995; 45: 1–12.

348. Nadel S, Newport MJ, Booy R, Levin M. Variation in the tumor necrosis factor-alpha gene promoter region may be associated with death from meningococcal disease. J Infect Dis 1996; 174: 878–80.

349. Hohler T, Kruger A, Gerken G, Schneider PM, Meyer zum Buschenfelde KH, Rittner C. Tumor necrosis factor alpha promoter polymorphism at position –238 is associated with chronic active hepatitis C infection. J Med Virol 1998; 54: 173–7.

350. Kaijzel EL, van Krugten MV, Brinkman BM et al. Functional analysis of a human tumor necrosis factor alpha (TNF-alpha) promoter polymorphism related to joint damage in rheumatoid arthritis. Mol Med 1998; 4: 724–33.

351. Nedospasov SA, Udalova IA, Kuprash DV, Turetskaya RL. DNA sequence polymorphism at the human tumor necrosis factor (TNF) locus. Numerous TNF/lymphotoxin alleles tagged by two closely linked microsatellites in the upstream region of the lymphotoxin (TNF-beta) gene. J Immunol 1991; 147: 1053–9.

352. Udalova IA, Nedospasov SA, Webb GC, Chaplin DD, Turetskaya RL. Highly informative typing of the human TNF locus using six adjacent polymorphic markers. Genomics 1993; 16: 180–6.

353. Iris FJ, Bougueleret L, Prieur S et al. Dense Alu clustering and a potential new member of the NF kappa B family

within a 90 kilobase HLA class III segment. Nat Genet 1993; 3: 137–45.

354. Plevy SE, Targan SR, Yang H, Fernandez D, Rotter JI, Toyoda H. Tumor necrosis factor microsatellites define a Crohn's disease-associated haplotype on chromosome 6. Gastroenterology 1996; 110: 1053–60.

355. Kinouchi Y, Simmon J, Van Heel D, Jewell DP. Polymorphism at position –1031 in the TNF gene confers susceptibility to Crohn's disease. Gastroenterology 2000; 118: A334.

356. Bonen DK, Ramos R, Lee S et al. Characterization of genomic and functional variation throughout the TNF gene in patients with IBD. Gastroenterology 2000; 118: A330–1.

357. Plevy SE, Taylor K, DeWoody KL, Schaible YF, Shealy D, Targan SR. Tumor necrosis factor (TNF) microsatellite haplotypes and perinuclear anti-neutrophil cytoplasmic antibody (pANCA) identify Crohn's disease (CD) patients with poor clinical responses to anti-TNF monoclonal antibody. Gastroenterology 1997; 112: A1062.

358. Dinarello CA, Wolff SM. The role of interleukin-1 in disease. N Engl J Med 1993; 328: 106–13.

359. Casini-Raggi V, Kam L, Chong YJ, Fiocchi C, Pizarro TT, Cominelli F. Mucosal imbalance of IL-1 and IL-1 receptor antagonist in inflammatory bowel disease. A novel mechanism of chronic intestinal inflammation. J Immunol 1995; 154: 2434–40.

360. Andus T, Daig R, Vogl D et al. Imbalance of the interleukin 1 system in colonic mucosa – association with intestinal inflammation and interleukin 1 receptor antagonist genotype 2. Gut 1997; 41: 651–7.

361. Ferretti M, Casini-Raggi V, Pizarro TT, Eisenberg SP, Nast CC, Cominelli F. Neutralization of endogenous IL-1 receptor antagonist exacerbates and prolongs inflammation in rabbit immune colitis. J Clin Invest 1994; 94: 449–53.

362. Tountas NA, Casini-Raggi V, Yang H et al. Functional and ethnic association of allele 2 of the interleukin-1 receptor antagonist gene in ulcerative colitis. Gastroenterology 1999; 117: 806–13.

363. Dinarello CA. The role of the interleukin-1-receptor antagonist in blocking inflammation mediated by interleukin-1. N Engl J Med 2000; 343: 732–4.

364. Mansfield JC, Holden H, Tarlow JK et al. Novel genetic association between ulcerative colitis and the anti-inflammatory cytokine interleukin-1 receptor antagonist. Gastroenterology 1994; 106: 637–42.

365. Louis E, Satsangi J, Roussomoustakaki M et al. Cytokine gene polymorphisms in inflammatory bowel disease. Gut 1996; 39: 705–10.

366. Heresbach D, Alizadeh M, Dabadie A et al. Significance of interleukin-1beta and interleukin-1 receptor antagonist genetic polymorphism in inflammatory bowel diseases. Am J Gastroenterol 1997; 92: 1164–9.

367. Stokkers PC, van Aken BE, Basoski N, Reitsma PH, Tytgat GN, van Deventer SJ. Five genetic markers in the interleukin 1 family in relation to inflammatory bowel disease. Gut 1998; 43: 33–9.

368. Nemetz A, Kope A, Molnar T et al. Significant differences in the interleukin-1beta and interleukin-1 receptor antagonist gene polymorphisms in a Hungarian population with inflammatory bowel disease. Scand J Gastroenterol 1999; 34: 175–9.

369. Nemetz A, Nosti-Escanilla MP, Molnar T et al. IL1B gene polymorphisms influence the course and severity of inflammatory bowel disease. Immunogenetics 1999; 49: 527–31.

370. Etzioni A. Adhesion molecules – their role in health and disease. Pediatr Res 1996; 39: 191–8.

371. Vainer B. Role of cell adhesion molecules in inflammatory bowel diseases. Scand J Gastroenterol 1997; 32: 401–10.

372. Nakamura S, Ohtani H, Watanabe Y et al. In situ expression of the cell adhesion molecules in inflammatory bowel

disease. Evidence of immunologic activation of vascular endothelial cells. Lab Invest 1993; 69: 77–85.

373. Vainer B, Nielsen OH. Changed colonic profile of P-selectin, platelet-endothelial cell adhesion molecule-1 (PECAM-1), intercellular adhesion molecule-1 (ICAM-1), ICAM-2, and ICAM-3 in inflammatory bowel disease. Clin Exp Immunol 2000; 121: 242–7.

374. Patel RT, Pall AA, Adu D, Keighley MR. Circulating soluble adhesion molecules in inflammatory bowel disease. Eur J Gastroenterol Hepatol 1995; 7: 1037–41.

375. Wong PY, Yue G, Yin K et al. Antibodies to intercellular adhesion molecule-1 ameliorate the inflammatory response in acetic acid-induced inflammatory bowel disease. J Pharmacol Exp Ther 1995; 274: 475–80.

376. Altare F, Jouanguy E, Lamhamedi-Cherradi S et al. A causative relationship between mutant IFNGR1 alleles and impaired cellular response to IFNG in a compound heterozygous child. Am J Hum Genet 1998; 62: 723–6.

377. Jouanguy E, Dupuis S, Pallier A et al. In a novel form of IFN-gamma receptor 1 deficiency, cell surface receptors fail to bind IFN-gamma. J Clin Invest 2000; 105: 1429–36.

378. Newport MJ, Huxley CM, Huston S et al. A mutation in the interferon-gamma-receptor gene and susceptibility to mycobacterial infection. N Engl J Med 1996; 335: 1941–9.

379. Jouanguy E, Lamhamedi-Cherradi S, Altare F et al. Partial interferon-gamma receptor 1 deficiency in a child with tuberculoid bacillus Calmette-Guerin infection and a sibling with clinical tuberculosis. J Clin Invest 1997; 100: 2658–64.

380. Jouanguy E, Lamhamedi-Cherradi S, Lammas D et al. A human IFNGR1 small deletion hotspot associated with dominant susceptibility to mycobacterial infection. Nat Genet 1999; 21: 370–8.

381. Fleshner PR, Taylor KD, Yang H et al. Chronic pouchitis after ileal pouch–anal anastomosis for ulcerative colitis (UC) is associated with the interferon gamma receptor alpha gene independent of perinuclear antineutrophil cytoplasmic antibody (pANCA) level. Gastroenterology 2000; 118: A338.

382. Mahmud N, Molloy A, McPartlin J et al. Increased prevalence of methylenetetrahydrofolate reductase C677T variant in patients with inflammatory bowel disease, and its clinical implications. Gut 1999; 45: 389–94.

383. Helio T, Wartiovaara U, Halme L et al. Arg506Gln factor V mutation and Val34Leu factor XIII polymorphism in Finnish patients with inflammatory bowel disease. Scand J Gastroenterol 1999; 34: 170–4.

384. Vecchi M, Sacchi E, Saibeni S et al. Inflammatory bowel diseases are not associated with major hereditary conditions predisposing to thrombosis. Dig Dis Sci 2000; 45: 1465–9.

385. Govoni G, Gros P. Macrophage NRAMP1 and its role in resistance to microbial infections. Inflam Res 1998; 47: 277–84.

386. Bellamy R. Identifying genetic susceptibility factors for tuberculosis in Africans: a combined approach using a candidate gene study and a genome-wide screen. Clin Sci 2000; 98: 245–50.

387. Bellamy R. The natural resistance-associated macrophage protein and susceptibility to intracellular pathogens. Microbes Infect 1999; 1: 23–7.

388. Hofmeister A, Neibergs HL, Pokorny RM, Galandiuk S. The natural resistance-associated macrophage protein gene is associated with Crohn's disease. Surgery 1997; 122: 173–9.

389. Farrell RJ, Murphy A, Long A et al. High multidrug resistance (P-glycoprotein 170) expression in inflammatory bowel disease patients who fail medical therapy. Gastroenterology 2000; 118: 279–88.

390. Panwala CM, Jones JC, Viney JL. A novel model of inflammatory bowel disease: mice deficient for the multiple

drug resistance gene, mdr1a, spontaneously develop colitis. J Immunol 1998; 161: 5733–44.

391. Dubinsky MC, Lamothe S, Yang HY *et al.* Pharmacogenomics and metabolite measurement for 6-mercaptopurine therapy in inflammatory bowel disease. Gastroenterology 2000; 118: 705–13.

392. Hugot JP, Chamaillard M, Zouali H *et al.* Association of NOD2 leucine-rich repeat variants with susceptibility to Crohn's disease. Nature 2001; 411: 599–603.

393. McKay DM. Intestinal inflammation and the gut microflora. Can J Gastroenterol 1999; 13: 509–16.

394. Auphan N, DiDonato JA, Rosette C, Helmberg A, Karin M. Immunosuppression by glucocorticoids: inhibition of

NF–kB activity through induction of 1kB synthesis. Science 1995; 270: 286–90.

395. Wahl C, Liptay S, Adler G, Schmid RM. Sulfasalazine: a potent and specific inhibitor of nuclear factor kB. J Clin Invest 1998; 101: 1163–74.

396. Ogura Y, Bonen DK, Inohara N *et al.* A frameshift mutation in NOD2 associated with susceptibility to Crohn's disease. Nature 2001; 411: 603–6.

397. Rioux JD, Daly MJ, Silverberg MS *et al.* Genetic variation in the 5q31 cytokine gene cluster confers susceptibility to Crohn disease. Nat Genet 2001; 29: 223–8.

4 Experimental mouse models of inflammatory bowel disease: new insights into pathogenic mechanisms

CHARLES O. ELSON AND CASEY T. WEAVER

Introduction

Inflammatory bowel disease (IBD) is a term that comprises two chronic inflammatory diseases of humans, namely ulcerative colitis and Crohn's disease. Despite many years of study the exact etiology and pathogenesis of these disorders have remained elusive. Various infections can mimic the tissue pathology seen in each of these diseases; however, no organism or infectious cause has yet been identified. As with chronic inflammatory disorders in other organs, these diseases appear to involve complex interactions among immunologic, environmental, and genetic components. The early inductive phases of these diseases are particularly difficult to study in humans because patients come to clinic only after their symptoms are established. Experimental models in animals have a number of advantages in this regard, in that the environmental conditions and genetics can be either controlled or defined. No animal model exactly reproduces human IBD, nor could it. There cannot be precise models of imprecise, ill-defined diseases. The value of the models, as is illustrated in this chapter, is the insight they allow into the complex, multifaceted processes and mechanisms that can result in chronic intestinal inflammation. In recent years quite a number of new experimental models of chronic intestinal inflammation have been described. The focus here will be mainly on these new models. The reader is referred to a previous review for others not discussed here [1]. Knowledge gained from these experimental models has already resulted in the development of new hypotheses and therapies that are being tested in patients with IBD.

The growth in this area is remarkable considering that the first such model of IBD was reported only as recently as 1994. Most of these new models involve some form of genetic manipulation, either insertion (transgenic) or selective deletion (knockout) of a gene. Mice resulting from such genetic manipulation are now collectively referred to as 'induced mutants' to distinguish them from mice with spontaneously occurring mutations. The induced mutants that develop IBD, usually in the absence of any further manipulation, represent a small subset of the total number of immune system genes that have been mutated. This argues that the mutations that have resulted in disease must represent genes involved in pathways critical to the maintenance of mucosal homeostasis. The results that have been obtained from these models to date provide strong support for the immunologic hypothesis that a dysregulated mucosal immune response, particularly a CD4+ T cell response, to antigens of the enteric bacteria in a genetically susceptible host result in chronic intestinal inflammation. This hypothesis has been advanced in various forms over the past several decades as knowledge of the immune system grew, as did the recognition that many microbial products are intensely stimulatory for immune cells. Given the large number and variety of microbes resident in the intestine, which outnumber the cells in the body by 10 to 1, the mystery has been why all of us do not have IBD. The answer to that mystery is now emerging through study of these new models. These studies have shown that the host interaction with the flora is complex, but that there are a select number of cells and molecules that are critical to this effort. When these key pathways are impaired, the host response to the bacterial flora results in IBD. That the bacterial flora can cause IBD under these circumstances has been demonstrated in multiple models in which animals rendered germfree do not contract IBD unless they are reconstituted with an enteric bacterial flora. There is clearly a genetic influence to this host response, in that certain strains are much more susceptible to develop colitis than others. This has been shown to be due to the presence of modifier genes that confer susceptibility in some strains.

Stephan R. Targan, Fergus Shanahan and Loren C. Karp (eds.), Inflammatory Bowel Disease: From Bench to Bedside, 2nd Edition, 67–99.
© 2003 *Kluwer Academic Publishers. Printed in Great Britain*

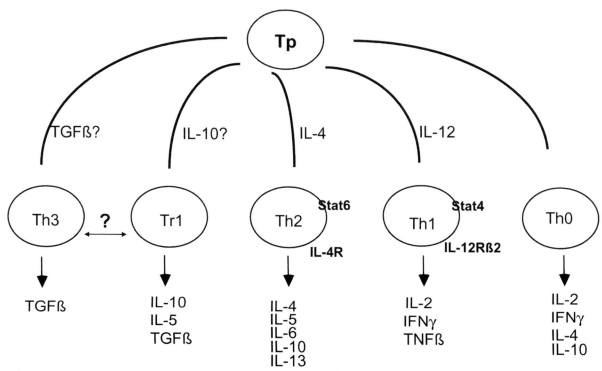

Th1, Th2 and more ...

Figure 1. CD4$^+$ T cell subsets. Precursor CD4$^+$ T cells can differentiate into one of a number of subsets, each of which has a different function and is marked by production of a distinct assortment of cytokines. The differentiation of Tp into Th1 or Th2 subsets is influenced by IL-12 and IL-4, respectively. The factors which determine regulatory T cell differentiation are largely unknown. Several regulatory T cell subsets have been defined and others are likely. Regulatory T cells control both effector subsets in the mucosa.

Another important finding from these models is that the key effector cell responsible for disease in most instances is the CD4$^+$ T cell. CD4 T cells can be placed into several functional subsets based on the types of cytokines that they produce (Fig. 1). Th1 cells produce IFN-γ, IL-2, and TNF-β, cytokines that are important in delayed hypersensitivity and cellular immunity. Th2 cells produce instead IL-4, IL-5, IL-6, IL-10, and IL-13, cytokines important in humoral immunity. The type of CD4$^+$ T cell response to a given pathogen can be critical for the host in that inbred mouse strains that respond to a microbial pathogen such as *Leishmania major* with a Th2 response succumb to the infection and die, whereas inbred strains that respond to the same infection with a predominant Th1 response recover and are resistant to reinfection [2]. Although there are data in some systems showing that Th1 and Th2 subsets can

reciprocally regulate one another via IFN-γ inhibition of Th2 responses and IL-10 inhibition of Th1 responses, each of these CD4 T cell effector CD4 T cell subsets has been found to mediate colitis in various mouse models. There are no data at present that demonstrate that Th2 cells regulate Th1 cells in the intestine or vice versa; thus, experimental colitis is not explained as an imbalance between Th1 and Th2 subsets. To the contrary, administration of exogenous IL-4 has been shown to exacerbate Th1-mediated colitis in one model [3]. At present, the data are compatible with the concept that excessive responses of either the Th1 or Th2 effector subsets are detrimental and can result in IBD. The tissue damage resulting from the CD4$^+$ T cell in either case is likely to be indirectly mediated through cytokines rather than by direct cytotoxicity, and a critical molecule in the Th1 pathway is likely to be TNF-α [4].

In regard to application of the Th1/Th2 paradigm to human disease, Crohn's disease (CD) does appear to be mediated by Th1 effector cells. Mucosal lesions in CD have increased numbers of IFN-γ-producing T cells, increased IL-12 mRNA levels, and increased levels of the STAT-4 transcription factor which is the intracellular messenger of IL-12 signaling. Ulcerative colitis has been called 'Th2-like' because of increased T cell production of IL-5 by cells isolated from the mucosa [5], but does not fit the Th2 pattern in that there is no increase in IL-4, the hallmark Th2 cytokine. Nevertheless, the data being generated in these models are highly germane to our understanding of IBD in humans.

Additional CD4$^+$ T cell subsets with regulatory activity for CD4$^+$ effector T cells have been identified in recent years. The effects of regulatory cells have been seen in various experimental systems for many years, but because they have been difficult to isolate and culture, their existence has been questioned. These cells are now being isolated and characterized. It is unclear how many distinct subsets of regulatory CD4 T cells there are, but three deserve special mention. T-regulatory-1 (Tr1) cells produce high levels of IL-10, variable levels of TGF-β_1, low levels of IFN and IL-4, and no IL-2. They are generated by chronic activation of CD4$^+$ T cells in the presence of IL-10. Tr1 cells were originally identified in humans [6] and subsequently in mice [7]. Tr1 cells have been shown to be capable of suppressing the induction of colitis in the CD45RB transfer model, which is discussed below. Another regulatory subset that has been found to be important in intestinal regulation are T-helper-3 cells (Th3) that produce high amounts of active TGF-β_1 when stimulated with specific antigen. Th3 cells have been identified in experiments examining mechanisms of oral tolerance induced by autoantigen feeding in mice [8, 9] and in the peripheral blood of humans with multiple sclerosis [10]. Th3 cells mediate protective oral tolerance in mice fed TNP-colon proteins prior to induction of TNBS-induced colitis [11]. Lastly, there is evidence that deficient mucosal TGF-β_1 production is associated with the development of TNP-KLH-induced colitis in IL-2-deficient mice [12], suggesting that this form of experimental colitis is due to lack of development of the Th3 subset. A third important T regulatory subset is the CD4$^+$, CD25$^+$ lineage that is generated in the thymus early in life. This subset comprises some 10% of peripheral CD4$^+$ T cells in adults. In mice this subset has been shown to maintain peripheral tolerance to autoantigens. It may play a similar role in regulating the mucosal immune response to commensal bacterial antigens but that is not yet established. It is also unknown whether this subset is the precursor for Tr1 and/or Th3 regulatory CD4$^+$ T cells.

Although the experimental data indicate that CD4$^+$ T cells are the key regulatory cells in the intestine, other cell types very likely also contribute to maintaining mucosal homeostasis. Data supporting such a role for CD8$^+$ T cells [13, 14], NK cells [15], NK-T cells [16], and B cells/antibody [17] have been generated in various experimental model systems.

In this chapter, experimental models have been clustered into certain categories for ease of discussion. These are somewhat arbitrary assignments and new findings may well shift these assignments. Most of the models in some way affect T cell function and these have been further subdivided based on the concept, discussed above, of disease resulting from an imbalance between regulatory and effector T cells (Fig. 2). Thus the first major category represents instances in which impaired regulatory T cell activity appears responsible for disease. A second category comprises models in which excessive effector T cell function overcomes normal regulatory function to cause disease. A third category clusters models in which perturbations of the epithelium appear to result in chronic intestinal inflammation. An important emerging concept is that the epithelium is an active participant in mucosal immune defense, communicating with both the bacterial flora and the mucosal lymphoid cells. Thus perturbations of the epithelial layer may lead to abnormal immune responses and inflammation. There are additional categories which do not quite fit into any of the above at present, i.e. models with spontaneous IBD, models involving chemical stressors or injury, and models as yet unclassified into any of these other categories. It is likely that, as more is learned about models in these latter categories, they could be reclassified into one of the first two or three. In the sections that follow, a short summary of the different models from each category is provided, and a table with major features of the models in each category is provided to facilitate comparisons among them.

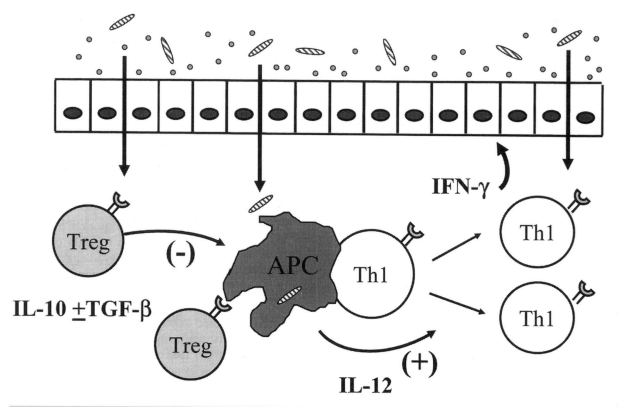

Figure 2. Mucosal immune homeostasis. The mucosal immune response to the enteric bacteria is composed of both regulatory T cells (T reg) and effector T cells, here shown as Th1 effector cells (Th1). In health the T reg population is dominant, and thus the intestine is in a state of controlled inflammation. Either deficient T reg function or excessive T effector cell function can result in chronic intestinal inflammation.

Models of impaired T cell regulation

As mentioned above, results obtained in experimental models of colitis do indicate that there are local mucosal regulatory mechanisms that limit the immune response to antigens of the bacterial flora. Disruption of these processes results in excessive responses to intestinal bacteria and chronic intestinal inflammation (Table 1). CD4[+] T regulatory cells appear to be predominant; however, there is likely to be more than one cell type involved in mucosal regulation. The occurrence of IBD in mice deficient of certain immune molecules but not of others is helping to identify the critical, nonredundant pathways of mucosal immune regulation.

CD4[+], CD45RB[hi] transfer model

Severe combined immunodeficient (SCID) mice have a spontaneous mutation in a DNA-dependent protein kinase catalytic subunit gene [18] which results in a deficiency of both B cells and T cells, but their innate immune system remains intact. The immune system of SCID mice can be partially reconstituted by adoptive transfer of normal B cells and T cells, and such transfers of selected subsets of lymphocytes allow definition of the function of that isolated subset *in vivo*. The adoptive transfer of normal CD4[+] T cells that express high levels of the surface molecule CD45RB (CD4[+], CD45RB[hi]), results in colitis and wasting over the following weeks to 2–3 months. Transfer of the whole CD4[+] T cell subset does not result in disease in this time frame, nor does transfer of the reciprocal CD4 subset expressing low levels of the CD45RB molecule (CD4[+], CD45RB[lo]) [19, 20].

Table 1. Models with deficient immune regulation

Model	Area involved	Effector cell	Key cytokines	Bacterial flora driven	Strain variation/ genetic modifiers	Reference
CD4+, CD45RB^{hi} transfer	Cecum, colon	CD4+ Th1	IFN-γ, TNF-α, IL-12, IL-1, IL-6	Yes	BALB > B6	20
IL-10-deficient	Cecum, colon	CD4+ Th1	IFN-γ, TNF-α, IL-12, IL-1, IL-6	Yes	C3H, BALB, 129 > (129 × B6)F1 > B6	37
CRF2-4-deficient	Cecum, colon	CD4+ Th1	IFN-γ, TNF-α, IL-12 probable	Probable	B6	48
Macrophage-PMN STAT3-deficient	Cecum, colon	CD4+ Th1	IFN-γ, TNF-α, IL-12 probable	Probable	Undefined	109
IL-2-deficient	Cecum, colon	CD4+ Th1	IFN-γ, IL-12	Yes	C3H, BALB > B6	163
IL-2 receptor alpha-deficient	Cecum, colon	CD4+ Th1	IFN-γ, IL-12	Probable	Undefined	164
Bone marrow transfer to Tgε26	Cecum, colon	CD4+ Th1	IFN-γ, TNF-α, IL-12	Yes	AKR	63
TCRα-deficient	Cecum, colon	CD4+ Th2	IL-4, IL-13	Yes	C3H, 129 > (129 × B6)F1 > B6	67
TGF-β_1-deficient*	Multiple organs	CD4+	Undefined	No	Undefined	165
TGF-βRII-deficient*	Multiple organs	Unknown	Undefined	Unknown	Undefined	86
SMAD3-deficient*	Multiple organs	Unknown	Undefined	Unknown	Undefined	88

*Multiorgan inflammation not limited to intestine.

SCID mice receiving CD4+, CD45RB^{hi} T cells develop weight loss and diarrhea within weeks of the transfer secondary to a colitis that is unremitting and eventuates in the death of the animal (Table 1). The colon is markedly thickened due to both hyperplasia of the epithelium and infiltration of the lamina propria and the submucosa by lymphocytes and macrophages. The small intestine is usually unaffected, aside from a variable, diffuse infiltration of mononuclear cells in the lamina propria. Disease can be prevented by treatment with anti-IFN-γ, anti-TNF-α or murine IL-10 but not by administration of IL-4 [21], indicating that the colitis is mediated by Th1 effector cells. Transfer of small numbers of whole CD4+ T cells into SCID mice has also been reported to induce colitis [22] under certain environmental conditions, if one extends the experimental period

to many months; this is due presumably to *in vivo* separation of the pathogenic from the protective CD4 subsets, perhaps by a more rapid expansion of the former. The disease in this latter variation of the CD4 transfer model has the same Th1 cytokine pattern in the mucosa as that seen after shorter-term transfers of the CD4, CD45RB^{hi} subset [23].

One of the most important findings in the CD45RB transfer model is that colitis is abrogated by co-transfer of the CD4+, CD45RB^{lo} T cell subset or of whole CD4 T cells along with the pathogenic CD4+ CD45RB^{hi} T cell subset [20]. Prevention of colitis by this subset can be abrogated by administration of either anti-TGF-β [24] or anti-IL-10R1 [25]. These results are consistent with the presence in this subset of regulatory population(s) producing IL-10 and TGF-β_1. It is unclear whether this is one or more than one regulatory subsets, i.e. the Tr1 and/or Th3 subsets discussed above. Recent data suggest this regulatory population may be derived from the $CD4^+$, $CD25^+$ subset that appears to be generated in the thymus and acts to maintain peripheral tolerance for autoantigens. $CD45RB^{lo}$ cells from germfree mice have been reported as capable of suppressing colitis induced by $CD45RB^{hi}$ T cells [26], suggesting the regulatory cells are not generated by bacterial antigens in intestine. $CD4^+$, $CD25^+$ cells constitutively express CTLA-4, and this molecule may play a role in their regulatory activity [27, 28]. Exogenously generated Tr1 cells have also been shown capable of inhibiting the induction of colitis in this model *in vivo*. Tr1 cells producing high levels of IL-10 in response to ovalbumin (OVA) were generated by culturing TCR transgenic T cells specific for OVA *in vitro* with OVA in the presence of IL-10. Such Tr1, OVA-specific T cells were administered to SCID mice along with pathogenic $CD4^+$, $CD45RB^{hi}$ cells from normal, histocompatible donors [7]. $CD4^+$, $CD45RB^{hi}$ cells induced colitis in the recipients when transferred alone or with Tr1 cells in the absence of OVA. However, colitis was prevented in the mice co-transferred with both subsets if they were fed OVA in order to trigger the Tr1 regulatory subset. Because the Tr1 cells were specific for a different antigen than the effector cells, this is an example of what has been termed 'bystander suppression'. This is due to release of inhibitory cytokines in the local microenvironment that act nonspecifically on all adjacent cells. Somewhat similar results were obtained with T cells from a mouse transgenic for IL-10 under the regulation of the IL-2 promoter [29]. Because this promoter is restricted to the T cell lineage, IL-10 is overproduced only when such transgenic T cells are activated. $CD4^+$, $CD45RB^{hi}$ T cells from these IL-10 transgenic mice did not induce disease in SCID recipients; moreover, they prevented colitis when cotransferred with control, non-transgenic pathogenic $CD4^+$, $CD45RB^{hi}$ T cells. Thus, T cell production of IL-10, either by the Tr1 subset or by a transgenic, IL-10-producing T cell subset, can prevent the induction of colitis in the $CD45RB^{hi}$ transfer model. Whether either T cell subset can treat established, active disease remains to be seen.

After transfer to SCID mice, both $CD4^+$, $CD45RB^{hi}$ and $CD4^+$, $CD45RB^{lo}$ T cells, traffic to the intestine and reconstitute both lamina propria and intraepithelial compartments [30]. The cell surface markers that they express are typical of mucosal lymphocytes, i.e. $\alpha E\beta_7^{hi}$, $CD69^{hi}$, L-selectin^{lo}, and $CD45RB^{lo}$. Inhibition of cell trafficking to the intestine with anti-β_7 integrin or anti-MAdCAM-1 attenuates disease [31], as does disruption of secondary lymphoid tissue organization by administration of lymphotoxin β-immunoglobulin fusion protein [32]. Although lymphocytes migrate to both colon and small intestine, lesions occur only in the colon. IL-12 is required for disease initiation and perpetuation. Antibody blockade of CD40L, which is required for sustained IL-12 production, prevents colitis and ameliorates established disease [33]. When $CD4^+$, $CD45RB^{hi}$ T cells are transferred to SCID recipients with a reduced flora [30], or to recipients treated with antibiotics [34], the colitis is ameliorated. These results strongly implicate the bacterial flora as driving the colitis; indeed, the T cells became oligoclonal after transfer [35] and demonstrate reactivity to antigens of the bacterial flora [36]. This model does illustrate two important concepts; namely that normal T cells can cause intestinal inflammation, and secondly, that such inflammation is prevented in normal mice by the effects of regulatory cells.

IL-10-deficient mice

IL-10 is an important cytokine produced by T cells, certain B cells, macrophages, thymocytes, and keratinocytes. IL-10 is a potent direct inhibitor of macrophage function and an indirect inhibitor of Th1 and NK cells. IL-10-deficient mice have normal lymphocyte development and antibody responses initially; however, with age the animals develop anemia, growth retardation, and chronic IBD [37]. The bowel lesions consist of focal ulcerations and focal epithelial hyperplasia. The lamina propria and submucosa of affected areas is heavily infiltrated with T cells, macrophages, neutrophils, B cells, plasma cells, and occasional multinucleated giant cells. Some animals develop perforating ulceration. There is an increased and aberrant expression of MHC class II on the epithelium of both small intestine and colon. More than 60% of mice surviving 6 months or more develop colon adenocarcinomas. The disease is progressive and does not remit. When IL-10-deficient mice are raised under germfree conditions, IBD does not occur unless they are reconstituted with a bacterial flora [38].

The earliest immunologic abnormalities in C57BL/6 IL-10-deficient mice occur as early as 3 weeks, even under specific pathogen-free (SPF) conditions, and consist mainly of focal infiltrations of mononuclear cells in the cecum and right colon; these develop into overt lesions by 3 months of age. $CD4^+$ and $CD4^+CD8^+$ T cells can be increased up to 50–200-fold, respectively, above background levels in the focal lesions. Because IL-10-deficient mice have exaggerated DTH responses in general [39], the supposition has been that the disease would likely be T cell-mediated. Indeed, double mutant mice deficient in both IL-10 and B cells still develop colitis, eliminating an obligatory role for B cells and antibody in the development of lesions [40].

The effector cell mediating colitis in the IL-10-deficient mouse is the $CD4^+$ T cell. Thus, transfer of $CD4^+$ or $CD4^+CD8^+$ T cells isolated from the lamina propria (LP) of IL-10 mice into syngeneic $RAG-2^{-/-}$ recipients results in colitis, whereas the transfer of $CD8^+$ LP T cells does not. The LP lymphocytes in the $RAG-2^{-/-}$ recipients are $CD4^+$ or $CD4^+CD8^+$, $CD45RB^{lo}$ and $CD44^+$ [36]. Moreover, the $CD4^+$ T cell that is mediating disease is the Th1 subset in that IFN-γ is the predominant cytokine produced by lamina propria (LP) cells isolated both from the $IL-10^{-/-}$ itself and from $RAG-2^{-/-}$ recipients of $CD4^+$ T cells from $IL-10^{-/-}$ mice [36, 37]. The central role played by the CD4 Th1 subset is confirmed by experiments showing that anti-IFN-γ therapy given to young IL-10-deficient mice attenuates their colitis [41], as does the administration of IL-10 [42] or anti-IL-12 [43]. Anti-IL-12 can also treat established disease in adult IL-10-deficient mice [43]. These data indicate that the pathogenic mechanism is an enhanced Th1 response in the mucosa due to a lack of inhibition by IL-10 (Fig. 3). This leads to macrophage activation and overproduction of inflammatory cytokines such as IL-1, IL-6 and TNF-α, all of which have been demonstrated in the lesions.

Although IL-10 deficiency in these mice is global, the lesions are confined to the colon and are focal. The presumption is that the disease is localized in the colon because of the large quantities of bacteria there. Certainly the environmental conditions in which the mice are housed can have a major effect on disease expression, i.e. mice held in SPF conditions do not have small bowel lesions [37] and mice raised under germfree conditions do not develop colitis at all [38]. The bacterial species that are involved, as well as whether disease is stimulated by antigens, superantigens, or mitogens, remains unclear but *Bacteroides* species do not appear to play a role [38, 39]. IL-10-deficient mice have circulating antibodies to a highly selective number of antigens of

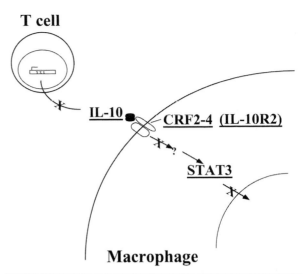

Figure 3. An IL-10 pathway to colitis. IL-10 exerts its effects by interacting with a receptor on the surface of target cells such as macrophages and neutrophils. The receptor is composed of two subunits, IL-10R1 and IL-10R2. The latter is encoded by the CRF2-4 gene. The binding of IL-10 to its receptor eventuates in phosphorylation of STAT-3 which enters the nucleus and alters the expression of multiple target genes. Disruption of the IL-10 gene itself, of the IL-10R2 gene (CRF2-4), or of STAT-3 in monocytes and neutrophils all result in a similar phenotype, i.e. colitis. Thus disease can result by abnormal function of any of a number of molecules along a regulatory pathway.

the enteric bacteria (unpublished data), a selective reactivity also identified in a C3H/HeJBir mouse [44]. At least one of the putative autoantibodies that develop in IL-10 knockout mice, anti-pANCA, is likely to be due to a cross-reactivity to conventional enteric bacterial antigens, in that this reactivity can be removed by absorption with homogenates of normal enteric bacteria [45].

In addition to environmental influences, the background genes of the inbred strains carrying the IL-10 null mutation strongly influence the age of onset and severity of disease. Thus, 129SvEv, BALB/c, and C3H/HeJBir strains have severe disease early in life, 129SvEv × C57BL/6 outbreed mice have intermediate disease, and C57BL/6 mice have disease onset after 3 months of age [41]. This pattern of susceptibility and resistance among inbred strains is quite similar to that identified in other models. The difference in susceptibility for colitis in IL-10-deficient C3H/HeJBir versus C57BL/6 strains has been shown to be a genetic trait [46]. Mapping studies in (C3H × B6) F2 mice have identified multiple different genes with a major locus on chromosome 3, derived from the highly susceptible C3H/HeJBir mouse [47].

An IL-10 pathway to colitis

IL-10 mediates its effects by binding to a specific IL-10 receptor on target cells such as macrophages and neutrophils. After binding its ligand the IL-10 receptor activates members of a family of cytoplasmic proteins named STATs (signal transducers and activators of transcription) by tyrosine phosphorylation via receptor-associated Janus kinases. The phosphorylated STAT proteins translocate to the nucleus and induce gene expression (Fig. 3). It follows that deficiency of key signaling molecules along this pathway could result in a disease phenotype similar to that found with a disrupted IL-10 gene. To date, two genes encoding proteins along this IL-10 pathway have been mutated and in both instances a disease similar to that seen in IL-10-deficient mice has resulted. In the first of these, an orphan receptor termed CRF2-4 of the class II cytokine receptor family was deleted by gene targeting. Cells from CRF2-4-deficient mice do not respond to IL-10 and the mice develop colitis by 12 weeks of age. These results are consistent with CRF2-4 encoding the β chain of the IL-10R [48]. In other studies, STAT-3 was selectively deleted in macrophages and neutrophils which rendered them unresponsive to the suppressive effects of IL-10 on the production of inflammatory cytokines such as TNF-α, IL-1, IL-6, and IFN-γ. Macrophage–neutrophil STAT-3-deficient mice developed chronic enterocolitis as they aged, similar to IL-10-deficient mice. These results indicate that STAT-3 is critical for transduction of IL-10–IL-10R signaling in macrophages and neutrophils. Taken together these experiments are defining an IL-10 pathway in which deficiency of any one of a number of molecules can result in disease (Fig. 3). This is important conceptually when considering genetic susceptibility to disease among different populations or among different species. Results that appear discordant may not be if different genes along the same pathway are involved.

IL-2-deficient mice

IL-2 is an important cytokine with multiple effects, including the growth, expansion and eventual activation-induced cell death of T cells, differentiation of B cells, and activation of macrophages, LAK and NK cells. Mice homozygous for a disrupted *IL-2* gene on a mixed genetic background (129/Ola, C57BL/6) develop normally for the first 4 weeks of life [49]. However, approximately half of the animals die between the fifth through ninth week of age with splenomegaly, lymphadenopathy, and a severe autoimmune hemolytic anemia. Mice surviving past 10 weeks of age uniformly develop a pancolitis with diarrhea, intermittent bleeding and frequent rectal prolapse [49]. There is a pronounced thickening of the colon due to hyperplasia of the epithelial layer, an extensive infiltration of the lamina propria with acute and chronic inflammatory cells, and ulceration. The small intestine is not affected. The colitis is unremitting and results in progressive weight loss and death. Immune abnormalities include a high number of activated T cells and B cells, elevated IgG$_1$ and IgE levels, anti-colon antibodies and increased expression of MHC class II antigens on colon epithelial cells.

Recent studies have shed light on the immunologic pathogenesis. As the mice age a polyclonal B cell and T cell activation occurs with lymphocytic infiltration of the gut and other organs and production of multiple autoantibodies. Several studies have shown that the crucial effector cell in the colitis of IL-2-deficient mice is a T cell [50–52]. Among T cells the CD4$^+$ Th1 subset is critical for disease development. Activated CD4$^+$ T cells are present in the colon early in the disease course [13, 52], and mice deficient in both IL-2 and β$_2$-microglobulin, in which the mice lack both IL-2 and CD8$^+$ T cells, still develop disease [13]. Moreover, depletion of CD4$^+$ T cells abrogates colitis [52, 53]. Both IFN-γ and IL-12 are increased in the colonic mucosa [53], indicating that the pathogenic CD4$^+$ T cells are of the Th1 subset. IL-12 produced by macrophages and dendritic cells enhances T cell production of IFN-γ and vice versa. This feedback loop appears important in disease perpetuation because administration of antibodies to IL-12 abrogates colitis. The Th1 effector cells may have to be continually replenished because antibody blockade of the α$_4$β$_7$ gut homing receptor on lymphocytes prevents and partially treats colitis in B6 IL-2-deficient mice [54]. Lastly, IL-2 is an important permissive cytokine for activation-induced programmed cell death; not surprisingly, IL-2-deficient mice have defective T cell apoptosis [55]. However, the role this defect plays in disease is unclear. IL-2-deficient mice have a marked decrease in CD8αα IEL of both TCRαβ and TCRαδ lineage [56]; whether this IEL depletion contributes to disease pathogenesis is unknown.

Why do CD4$^+$ Th1 cells develop sustained activation in IL-2-deficient mice? Several studies point to a defect of regulatory T cells. For example, *RAG-2*$^{-/-}$ mice reconstituted with IL-2-deficient bone marrow develop disease. However, if the *RAG-2*$^{-/-}$ mice are reconstituted with mixtures of both IL-2$^{-/-}$ and wild-type bone marrow, disease development is prevented if greater than 30% of the resulting T cells are wild-type [51]. More direct evidence is the observation that IL-2-deficient mice fail to generate the CD4$^+$, CD25$^+$ regulatory T cell subset which has been found to be important in maintaining peripheral tolerance to autoantigens [57]. Depletion of the CD4$^+$, CD25$^+$ T cell subset in mice results in activation and expansion of autoreactive T cells and a wide spectrum of organ-specific autoimmune disease [58]. The report that IL-2 receptor alpha chain-deficient mice also develop a disease very similar to that of *IL-2*$^{-/-}$ mice would be consistent with this idea, because they also lack this subset. Curiously, although gut inflammation in the form of autoimmune gastritis can occur after such CD4$^+$, CD25$^+$ T cell depletion, there are no reports that colitis occurs after depletion of this subset. This may reflect heterogeneity within the IL-2-dependent regulatory T cell population or a different time course of sensitivity to IL-2 or T cell perturbation.

The environment strongly influences whether and how the disease is expressed in IL-2-deficient mice. IL-2-deficient mice derived germfree do not develop colitis, although they still develop anemia, extra-intestinal lymphoid hyperplasia, and autoimmunity [59]. Indeed, C56BL/6.IL-2$^{-/-}$ mice that are housed under certain SPF conditions do not develop colitis [53]. Interestingly, parenteral immunization of such SPF C56BL/6.IL-2$^{-/-}$ mice with TNP-KLH induces a disease similar to that which occurs in IL-2-deficient mice housed in conventional conditions [53]. Whether such an immunization would trigger disease in germfree C56BL/6.IL-2$^{-/-}$ mice is unknown. The exact mechanism by which the enteric flora induces colitis in conventional IL-2-deficient mice remains unknown. The disease course and its mortality have been found to be strongly influenced by the genetic background of the mice. BALB/c.IL-2$^{-/-}$ mice develop a severe hemolytic anemia and die by 5 weeks of age [52]. C3H/HeJ.IL-2$^{-/-}$ mice also develop early and severe anemia whereas C57BL/6J.IL-2$^{-/-}$ mice develop it at 3–6 months of age. Although the time course to development of lesions differs among these strains, the histopathology is similar, namely mononuclear cell infiltration of most organs, with the intestine most severely affected [60].

Transgenic epsilon 26 (Tgε26) bone marrow transfer model

Mice transgenic for the human CD3ε chain gene (Tgε26) have a block at a very early stage of thymic T cell development, resulting in complete T cell and NK cell deficiency [61]. The thymus develops abnormally and becomes involuted in these mice unless they receive normal bone marrow cells early in life, which corrects the thymic abnormality, a result demonstrating that T cells participate in normal thymic development [62]. The transfer of normal T cell-depleted bone marrow into adult Tgε26 mice whose thymus is already abnormal does not restore a normal thymus, but instead results in marked weight loss and diarrhea some 5–8 weeks after transfer. Such bone marrow recipients have general lymphadenopathy, especially in the mesenteric lymph node, and a severe pancolitis with crypt hyperplasia and branching, mucin depletion, scattered crypt abscesses, and a substantial infiltration of lymphocytes, macrophages and neutrophils [63]. This disease does not occur in Tgε26 mice if a normal fetal thymus is transplanted into them at the same time that they receive the transfer of T cell-depleted normal bone marrow. These data are consistent with disease being due to either abnormal thymic selection of pathogenic T cells, or alternatively the lack of development of a critical regulatory T cell population that does develop in the normal thymus, such as the CD4$^+$, CD25$^+$ lineage discussed above. Because the T cell response is directed at environmental enteric bacterial antigens [64], it is difficult to postulate the former and thus the lack of development of a regulatory T cell population seems more likely.

The majority of the lymphocytes infiltrating the intestinal mucosa are CD3$^+$CD4$^+$ in both the lamina propria and epithelium. Most of the intraepithelial lymphocytes (IELs) are not only CD4$^+$, but also CD5$^+$, suggesting a thymic-dependent origin, and both IEL and LPL are activated (L-selectin^{lo}, CD69^{hi}, CD44^{hi}, and CD45RB^{lo}). Mucosal CD3$^+$ T cells show increased cytotoxic activity in redirected lysis assays but the significance of this is unclear because transfers of bone marrow from perforin or FAS ligand-deficient mice still results in colitis [65]. The effector cell mediating disease is an αβTCR cell as shown by the transfer of colitis into C57BL/6.RAG-2$^{-/-}$ mice by transfer of peripheral (PLN or MLN) $\alpha\beta$ T cells from bone marrow transplanted, colitic Tgϵ26 donors [66]. Transfer of similar cells from control animals does not cause colitis. The predominant cytokine phenotype in the colon is a Th1 response with increased production of IFN-γ and TNF-α by both CD4$^+$ and CD8$^+$ T cells [66]. Production of IL-12 is required for colitis to occur, in that antibody to IL-12 or antibody blockade of CD40L, which is required for sustained production of IL-12, prevents disease [33]. Response of effector cells to IL-12 is also required, in that transfer of STAT-4-deficient (IL-12-unresponsive) bone marrow results in only mild disease. Disruption of lymphotoxin α/β receptor signaling, which is important in development and maintenance of secondary lymphoid tissues, also attenuates development of colitis [32] to an extent equal to antibody treatment with anti-TNF.

Recent studies utilizing bone marrow transplanted germfree Tgϵ26 mice have demonstrated that colitis does not occur in the absence of the bacterial flora [64]. Interestingly, transfers of fully pathogenic T cells from colitic mice to germfree recipients did not result in colitis, even though these T cells migrated to the intestine and maintained their activation and memory markers. This result demonstrates that perpetuation of colitis in this model was completely dependent on the continual presence of enteric bacteria, and moreover that the T cell response to bacteria did not crossreact with any intestinal auto-antigens.

T cell receptor (TCR) α-chain-deficient mice

Mice with targeted mutations of each of the four T cell receptor chains have now been produced (α, β, γ, and δ). Of these, spontaneous development of colitis has been observed in both TCRα- and β-deficient mice, although only TCRα-deficient mice have consistently developed spontaneous colitis [67, 68]. TCRα-deficient mice develop normally for the first 3–4 months of life, but then develop unremitting chronic diarrhea, rectal prolapse and wasting [69]. The colon and cecum of diseased animals are thickened, shortened and dilated. Histologically, the colitis is characterized by marked epithelial hyperplasia and elongation of crypts with acute and chronic inflammation in the colonic lamina propria, mucin depletion, and occasional crypt abscesses. Mucosal ulceration is unusual. No inflammation is found in the small intestine or in extraintestinal tissues.

TCRα-deficient mice demonstrate a number of immunologic abnormalities such as a poor immune response to protein antigens such as OVA, and deficient rejection of skin grafts [70]. There is evidence of polyclonal expansion and activation of B cells with the production of multiple autoantibodies [69] including anti-colon and anti-tropomyosin, which have been previously reported in patients with ulcerative colitis [71]. Mice also develop antibodies to multiple enteric bacterial antigens. The immunologic defect in TCRα-deficient mice results from aberrant thymic selection and deficiency of circulating $\alpha\beta$ T cells. In developing thymocytes, gene rearrangement of the T cell receptor β chain locus precedes that of the TCRα locus resulting in 'β-selection' by association of TCRβ chains with the pre-TCRα (pTα) molecule. In TCRα-deficient mice, functional TCRβ rearrangement and pairing with the pTα chain occurs; however, the absence of subsequent α chain rearrangement results in defective TCR repertoire selection in the thymus. Nevertheless, these mice populate peripheral immune tissues with a unique population of T cells that express the TCRβ chain without TCRα chain [69, 70, 72]. This novel TCRβ^+ T cell subset responds to polyclonal activators, is enriched in Peyer's patches and in colon lymphoid follicles early in life, and is abundant in the colon lamina propria and draining mesenteric lymph nodes of mice with colitis. This TCRβ^+ subset produces IL-4 and is the effector cell mediating disease, in that treatment of mice with antibodies to the TCRβ chain abrogates colitis and polyclonal B cell activation [73]. Analysis of the TCR repertoire indicates that the pathogenic T cell utilizes a restricted Vb8.2$^+$ chain with a conserved motif in the CDR3 region, and that this TCR might cross-react with both epithelial and bacterial antigens [74].

Similar to several other colitis models, development of disease in TCRα-deficient mice requires the bacterial flora. Colitis fails to develop in TCRα-deficient mice that are maintained under germfree conditions [72, 75], suggesting that reactivity to antigens produced by commensal organisms, drives disease development. Removal of the distal cecum ('appendectomy') at 1 month of age, reduces colitis incidence later in life from 80% to 3%, suggesting that the dysregulated immune response may develop in the cecum [76]. Transition from a polyclonal to oligoclonal antibody response to enteric bacterial antigen has been described in TCRα mice and parallels the development of colitis [77]. The mechanism by which TCRα⁻β⁺ T cells are primed to recognize enteric bacterial antigens is unclear, but CD4 T cells expressing only the TCRβ chain are immunologically competent in these animals, and produce cytokines in response to stimulation with plate-bound anti-TCRβ and anti-CD3 monoclonal antibodies. Further, the development of antibody responses in these mice indicates that CD4⁺ TCRα⁻β⁺ cells can provide functional B cell help.

In contrast to most other models where IFN-γ is the critical effector cytokine, T cells in the lesions of TCRα-deficient mice produce IL-4 predominantly [69]. Double knockout mice deficient for both TCRα and IFN-γ demonstrate no significant attenuation of disease development [78], but IL-4-deficient TCRα knockout mice show markedly attenuated colitis development [72, 78]. More recent studies of TCRα-deficient mice that are both IL-4- and IL-13-deficient show complete absence of colitis, suggesting that both of these cytokines contribute to pathogenesis. Thus, TCRα-deficient colitis appears to be a Th2-mediated inflammatory disease.

An interesting facet of the TCRα model concerns the role of the B cell response in modifying disease. Studies using B cell-deficient, TCRα-deficient mice clearly demonstrate that B cells are not required for development of colitis [79]. In contrast, these mice develop colitis at an earlier age and of greater severity than B cell-competent TCRα-deficient mice. This finding suggests that B cells have a regulatory role in the colitis in TCRα-deficient mice. Indeed, B cells from TCRα-deficient mice inhibit colitis induction in RAG-1⁻/⁻ recipients given TCRα-deficient mesenteric lymph node cells. Moreover, administration of TCRα-deficient serum immunoglobulin or of a mixture of monoclonal anti-colon autoantibodies to mice deficient in both TCRα and B cells (Igμ⁻/⁻) ameliorates their colitis. The mechanism of this B cell/autoantibody regulatory effect is postulated to be rapid clearance of autoantigens released by apoptotic cells, thus reducing sensitization of autoreactive T cells [80]. In addition, there appears to be a direct regulatory effect of B cells on the pathogenic TCRβ⁺ cell mediated through surface CD40 and CD86 molecules [17]. To date, this is the only model that has shown such regulation by B cells and their antibodies.

TGF-β₁-deficient mice

TGF-β is a member of a family of cytokines involved in growth and differentiation. TGF-β has pleiotropic effects including inflammation, fibrosis, and immunosuppression. It is produced by most cells, including intestinal epithelial cells, as an inactive precursor and must be enzymatically activated to exert its effects. Mice deficient in TGF-β₁ develop a multi-organ inflammatory disease involving the heart, lungs, diaphragm, salivary glands and pancreas and die by 5 weeks of age [81, 82]. Gastritis, enteritis, and colitis can occur on certain genetic backgrounds but is mild. Germfree TGF-β-deficient mice develop the same lesions as conventionally reared mice [83]. TGF-β₁ mice crossed onto a SCID or MHC class II deficient background do not develop inflammation [84, 85], nor do TGF-β₁-deficient mice treated with monoclonal anti-CD4, indicating that CD4 T cells mediate the inflammation. The cytokines expressed in the lesions have not been characterized (see Table 1).

TGF-β₁ exerts its effects on target cells by binding to its specific receptor. The TGF-β receptor is a heterodimer consisting of an RI chain that binds TGF-β on the cell surface, and then associates with the RII chain which has an intracellular kinase domain that transmits the signal by causing the phosphorylation of SMAD2 and SMAD3. These SMADs translocate to the nucleus and mediate activation of target genes. Similar to the IL-10 pathway (Fig. 3), this TGF-β signaling pathway can be interrupted at multiple points. Two groups have blocked TGF-β signaling in T cells by expressing a dominant negative form of the TGF-β receptor II as a transgene under the control of a T lineage specific promoter. One line of such mice, on a mixed genetic background, and using a CD4 promoter, developed wasting and diarrhea and were found to have severe colitis [86]. There was also mononuclear infiltration of multiple other organs. Interestingly, another mouse line expressing this transgene on the C57BL/6 background using a CD2 promoter did not develop any inflammation, but did demonstrate a marked expansion of CD8⁺ T cells [87] for reasons that are not clear. Targeted disruption of the *Smad3* gene blocked T cell and neutrophil responses to TGF-β. SMAD3-deficient mice develop runting and wasting and most die between 1 and 3 months of age with multifocal pyogenic abscesses in the wall of the intestine and at other mucosal surfaces. Cultures of these abscesses grew commensal bacteria [88]. The small fraction of mice which lived more than 6

Table 2. Models with excessive effector cell function

Model	Area involved	Effector cell	Key cytokines	Bacterial flora driven	Strain variation/ genetic modifiers	Reference
STAT4 transgenic	Colon, ileum	CD4$^+$ T cell	IFN-γ	Probable	FVB/NHSD	161
IL-7 transgenic	Colon	CD4$^+$ T cell	IFN-γ, IL-2, IL-7	Unknown	B6	92
TNF$^{\Delta ARE}$ *	Terminal ileum > proximal colon	T cell	Undefined	Unknown	B6 × 129	94
A20-deficient*	Colon	T and B cell independent ? macrophage	Undefined	Unknown	Unknown	96
B7-related protein 1-Fc transgenic	Colon	T cell	Undefined	Unknown	Unknown	97
CD40L transgenic*	Colon, small bowel, other organs	T cell	IFN-γ, IL-12 probable	Unknown	B6	100

*Multiorgan inflammation not limited to intestine.

months had chronic IBD. The effector cell mediating this disease has not been identified, nor have the cytokines expressed in the lesions.

The phenotypes expressed due to deficiency of TGF-β_1, TGF-βRII, or SMAD3 are remarkably variable, although multiorgan inflammation is a common feature. Colitis occurred in some but not others, which is likely due to differences in the genetic backgrounds and possibly in the enteric bacterial flora. This variability illustrates the difficulty in studying and understanding this complex cytokine. A TGF-β_1-producing regulatory cell that prevents colitis has been implicated in a number of models including TNBS colitis [11] and IL-2-deficient mice [12]. Yet TGF-β_1 deficiency itself has resulted in only mild enteritis and colitis. Moreover, the TGF-β-producing regulatory cell does not protect IL-10-deficient mice from developing colitis. Clearly many questions remain to be answered about this cytokine and its role in IBD.

Models of excessive effector cell function

If normal mucosal homeostasis is maintained by a balance between regulatory and effector cells, then disease could result from impaired regulation, as discussed, or from excessive effector cell function that overcomes a normal regulatory tone. The net effect of either is the same. In this section we will consider some models where the latter appears to be occurring (Table 2).

STAT-4 transgenic mice

The clearest example of experimental models that involve excessive effector cell function is the STAT-4 transgenic mouse. STAT-4 is a transcription factor that is phosphorylated (along with STAT-3) following IL-12 binding to its receptor on the surface of CD4$^+$ T cells. The phosphorylated STAT-3/STAT-4 complex translocates into the nucleus of the cell and activates the expression of genes such as IFN-γ. As already mentioned, IL-12 is a cytokine produced by antigen-presenting cells that drives naïve CD4$^+$ T cells to differentiate down the Th1 pathway. Over-expression of STAT-4 in T cells should make them more sensitive to IL-12 signaling and thus should result in enhanced Th1 responses. To test this idea, mice transgenic for STAT-4 under control of the CMV promoter were generated in the FVB/NHSD strain (Table 2). Interestingly STAT-4 mRNA was not increased in cells from unperturbed transgenic mice. However, when the mice were immunized with DNP-KLH in CFA, transgene expression was increased in both spleen and colon. DNP-KLH immunization was performed because this antigen is thought to mimic antigens of the bacterial flora in some way. Some 7–14 days after DNP-KLH immunization, STAT-4 transgenic mice developed an unremitting colitis manifested by diarrhea, weight loss, and a grossly thickened colon. On histology the ileum and colon had severe transmural inflammation with dense infiltrates of $CD4^+$ T cells expressing nuclear STAT-4 and producing IFN-γ and TNF-α. Lymphocytes isolated from STAT-4 transgenic mice with colitis proliferated and produced large amounts of IFN-γ when stimulated with lysates of intestinal bacteria. Transfer of bacterial antigen-activated transgenic $CD4^+$ T cells from spleen or lymph nodes of colitic STAT-4 transgenic mice into SCID mice transferred colitis to the recipients. Transfer of similarly treated wild type, non-transgenic $CD4^+$ T cells did not cause disease.

STAT-4 transgenic mice would be expected to have a normal regulatory cell activity; thus this model is the clearest example of excessive effector cell activity overwhelming endogenous regulatory mechanisms to cause disease. An interesting feature in this model was the requirement of antigen-specific activation for colitis to occur. Colitis did not occur in STAT-4 transgenic mice given complete Freund's adjuvant intraperitoneally without the DNP-KLH incorporated into it. Thus, these genetically susceptible mice did not develop excessive $CD4^+$ T cell reactivity to the bacterial flora with subsequent colitis unless they sustained a triggering event that activated the pathogenic process. The exact relationship of DNP-KLH to the flora is unclear and other types of antigens were not tested. However, CFA contains mycobacterial antigens as an adjuvant and these mycobacterial antigens were not sufficient to trigger disease on their own, suggesting that some specificity was required for triggering of disease. Little is known about how colitis is triggered in genetically susceptible hosts, and this seems to be an excellent model to explore such questions further.

IL-7 transgenic mice

IL-7 is a pleiotrophic cytokine with growth-promoting activity for both immature and mature lymphocytes. IL-7 is produced by stromal cells in the bone marrow and thymus, as well as stroma in other organs. IL-7 mRNA and protein expression have been demonstrated in both mouse and human intestinal epithelium and the IL-7 receptor (IL-7R) is expressed by intestinal lymphocytes in both the IEL and lamina propria (LP) compartments [89, 90]. Indeed, $\gamma\delta$ IEL T cells are deficient in IL-7- and IL-7R-deficient mice [91], and IL-7 has been implicated as a growth factor for local, extrathymic T cell development in the intestine.

To examine the role of IL-7 in mucosal immune homeostasis, transgenic mice were generated that expressed IL-7 under control of the SV40/HTLV1 LTR viral promoter [92]. In at least one of the SRα/IL-7 transgenic founder lines, clinical evidence of colitis (diarrhea, weight loss, rectal prolapse, and perianal bleeding) was observed at 6–10 weeks of age, although significant variability in the penetrance and age of onset of colitis was found. Intestinal inflammation was most severe in the rectum, although involvement of the ileum and colon was also found. Histologically, the inflammatory lesions were characterized by dense infiltrates of $CD4^+$ T cells, with lesser numbers of monocytes/macrophages, $CD8^+$ T cells, and neutrophils. Focal erosions were noted, but there was no ulceration. Goblet cell depletion, crypt abscesses, and Paneth cell metaplasia were also described.

The composition of the infiltrating lymphocyte population was dominated by $CD4^+$ $\alpha\beta$ T cells. *Ex vivo* stimulation of $CD4^+$ T cells isolated from colitic lesions demonstrated increased production of IFN-γ and IL-2 but decreased production of IL-4 compared to those isolated from control mice [92]. Curiously, increased IL-7 production in the inflammatory lesions of transgenic mice was due to increased expression by infiltrating lymphocytes, not inflamed epithelial cells. Similarly, IL-7R expression was increased on colonic mucosal lymphocytes. Although the mechanism by which dysregulated IL-7 production generates colitis/proctitis in this model is unclear, variable expression of disease suggests that environmental cofactors, such as commensal bacteria, may be contributory.

TNF-α 'knockin' (TNF$^{\Delta ARE}$) mice

Evidence from a number of animal models of IBD supports a central role for tumor necrosis factor (TNF) in the pathogenesis of chronic intestinal inflammation. Human clinical trials have also implicated TNF, and agents that block TNF activity have recently been used with success in treating patients with Crohn's disease [93]. Mice with impaired regulation of TNF biosynthesis that develop chronic, unremitting inflammation in the intestines and joints were recently described [94]. In this model, deletion of a repeated octanucleotide AU-rich motif in the 3'-untranslated region of the *Tnfα* gene results in enhanced mRNA stability and increased TNF production by macrophages and other hemato-poietically derived cells. Mutant mice homozygous ($TNF^{\Delta ARE/\Delta ARE}$) or heterozygous ($TNF^{\Delta ARE/+}$) for the ARE deletion have elevated circulating levels of TNF-α. Homozygous animals fail to thrive and die between 5 and 12 weeks of age.

Both homozygous and heterozygous $TNF^{\Delta ARE}$ mice develop intestinal inflammation, although the tempo of disease development and progression is accelerated in homozygous mice. Disease is localized primarily to the terminal ileum and, less frequently, the proximal colon. Initial lesions consist of villus blunting and broadening that is associated with mucosal and submucosal infiltration of chronic and acute inflammatory cells, including mononuclear leukocytes, plasma cells, and scattered neutrophils. Severe intestinal inflammation is usually observed by 4 weeks of age in homozygous mice and 8 weeks of age in heterozygous mice, with an increased number of submucosal lymphoid aggregates and follicles becoming evident at this time. With disease progression there is transmural extension of inflammation, and in older heterozygous mice (4–7 months), complete loss of villus structure and poorly organized granulomas. Focal skin lesions and severe symmetrical joint disease develop concomitantly with the intestinal lesions.

The roles of the two TNF receptor family members in intestinal disease have been evaluated by crossing the $TNF^{\Delta ARE}$ mutation into the TNFRI- and TNFRII-gene backgrounds [94, 95]. $TNF^{\Delta ARE/\Delta ARE}$ mice show complete elimination of gut and joint pathology when backcrossed onto a TNFRI-deficient background. Similarly, backcross of the $TNF^{\Delta ARE/\Delta ARE}$ mice onto a TNFRII-deficient background results in significant attenuation in intestinal inflammation, although there is mild mucosal and submucosal inflammation in these mice. This is in contrast to joint disease in the TNFRII background, which is much more aggressive than in the control. Similarly, introduction of the $TNF^{\Delta ARE}$ mutation into a RAG-1-deficient background lacking both mature T and B lymphocytes results in marked attenuation of intestinal disease but retention of the severe arthritic phenotype, suggesting distinct chronic inflammatory mechanisms in the intestinal and joint tissues.

This model supports a central role for TNF in the pathogenesis of chronic intestinal inflammation. Interestingly, there is clearly a gene dosage effect of the mutated TNF allele because homozygous mice develop the clinical phenotype much more rapidly

than heterozygotes. Studies with this model suggest that excessive or dysregulated production of TNF-α in response to otherwise normal inflammatory stimuli in the gut results in disease development. This model further provides evidence that TNF-dependent IBD pathogenesis requires the adaptive immune response and is dependent on the presence of both TNF receptor family members (TNFRI and TNFRII). TNFRII is expressed primarily on hematopoietic cells, suggesting that TNF modulation of cells of hematopoietic origin is important in maintenance of mucosal immune homeostasis.

A20-deficient mice

Many of the inflammatory responses induced by TNF and IL-1 are mediated by activation of nuclear factor κB (NF-κB), which regulates the transcription of genes of multiple other proinflammatory cytokines. In its inactive form, NF-κB is sequestered in the cytoplasm, bound by members of the IκB family of inhibitory proteins, including IκBα. Stimuli that activate NF-κB, such as TNF-α or IL-1, result in the phosphorylation of IκB, which is followed by its ubiquitination and subsequent degradation. The release of NF-κB following IκB degradation results in its nuclear translocation where it binds to a consensus sequence present in a number of genes, thus activating their transcription. A20 is a cytoplasmic zinc finger protein that inhibits the TNF-α-stimulated activation of NF-κB at multiple points along the TNF-α receptor signaling cascade.

Mice deficient in the A20 protein were recently generated by gene targeting [96]. Mice heterozygous for the *A20* gene deficiency ($A20^{+/-}$) develop normally and show no evidence of pathology. In contrast, homozygous A20-deficient mice ($A20^{-/-}$) were runted as early as 1 week of age and died shortly thereafter. Gross and histological examination of 3–6-week-old $A20^{-/-}$ mice demonstrated severe, multiorgan inflammation, including severe intestinal inflammation. The inflammatory lesions were characterized by increased numbers of activated T cells, granulocytes, and macrophages. Interestingly, $A20^{-/-}$ mice bred into a RAG-1-deficient background demonstrated similar multiorgan inflammation, indicating that the adaptive immune response is not required for disease to develop in this model. Similar multiorgan inflammation has been described in IκBα-deficient mice, indicating that attenuation of TNF-α-mediated inflammatory effects by regulators of NFκB are essential for maintenance of gut homeostasis. The mechanism of A20-mediated attenuation of TNF-induced NFκB activation is not yet defined. The effector cell and cytokines mediating the inflammation are not known.

B7-related protein 1-Fc transgenic

B7-related protein-1 (B7RP-1) is a costimulatory molecule expressed on antigen-presenting cells, which is related to but distinct from B7 (CD80, CD86). This molecule interacts with its ligand ICOS (inducible co-stimulator) on the surface of activated T cells. Transgenic mice overexpressing B7RP-1 fused to a human IgG$_1$ Fc region have been generated [97]. Transgene expression was driven by the apolipoprotein E promoter in the liver. One-third of the transgenic mice developed intestinal inflammation between 5 and 12 months of age, with the most severe involvement in the proximal and distal colon and milder changes in the small intestine. In the colon there was transmural inflammation and fissuring ulceration. The effector cell and cytokines are not yet known, but increased levels of serum IgE were found, suggesting a Th2 pathway.

CD40 ligand transgenic mice

CD40 ligand (CD40L) is a member of the TNF family that is expressed primarily by activated T lymphocytes. Engagement of CD40L on activated T cells by its receptor, CD40, provides an important signal for naïve T cell activation and differentiation. Conversely, binding of CD40L expressed on the T cell surface by CD40 expressed on B cells during cognate B–T interactions provides a critical costimulatory signal for B cell proliferation, differentiation, and Ig class switching [98]. CD40 is also expressed on other cell lineages, including monocytes and dendritic cells, where it plays an important role in proinflammatory signaling. Engagement of CD40 on monocytes and dendritic cells during interactions with activated T cells induces expression of proinflammatory cytokines including TNF-α, IL-1, IL-8 and IL-12, as well as various cell surface molecules such as CD54 and CD86. CD40L–CD40 interactions are required for sustained release of IL-12 which is needed to initiate and sustain Th1 responses.

CD40- and CD40L-deficient mice generated by gene targeting demonstrate profound defects in both cellular and humoral immunity [99]. In contrast, transgenic mice that overexpress CD40L under control of the LCK proximal promoter, which directs transgene expression to T cells and some B cells, demonstrate multiorgan inflammation and morbid-

Table 3. Models with perturbations of the epithelium

Model	Area involved	Effector cell	Key cytokines	Bacterial flora driven	Strain variation/ genetic modifiers	Reference
Multi-drug resistance gene 1α-deficient	Colon	CD4$^+$ Th1	IFN-γ, IL-1, IL-6, TNF-α, IL-12	Probable: antibiotics prevent *and* treat	FVB	120
NCADΔ chimera	Small bowel, cecum	Unknown	Undefined	Unknown	Unknown	119
Gαi2-deficient	Entire colon	CD4$^+$ Th1	IFN-γ, IL-1, IL-6, TNF-α, IL-12	Unnown	129, C3H > (129 × B6)F1 > B6	122, 166
Intestinal trefoil factor-deficient (with DSS)	Colon	Unknown	Undefined	Unknown	BALB/c	124
Keratin 8-deficient	Cecum, colon	Unknown	Undefined	Unknown	FVB/N strain; embryonic lethal in 129, B6	125

Table 4. Models with spontaneous intestinal inflammation

Model	Area involved	Effector cell	Key cytokines	Bacterial flora driven	Strain variation/ genetic modifiers	Reference
C3H/HeJBir	Cecum > colon	CD4$^+$ Th1	IFN-γ, TNF-α, IL-1, IL-6, IL-12	Yes	Yes; multiple loci chromosome 3 > 8, 1	102, 105
SAMP1/Yit	Ileum > cecum, perianal	CD4$^+$ Th1	IFN-γ, TNF-α	Yes	AKR	110
Cotton-top tamarin	Colon	Unknown	Undefined	Unknown	NHo colitis in other tamarin strains	167

ity associated with IBD [100]. Different founder lines show a transgene dose-dependent alteration in thymic development, such that founders with higher transgene copy number demonstrate progressively profound depletion of thymocytes of all subsets, a loss of thymic cortical epithelium, increased thymic B cells in the medulla, and splenomegaly with myeloid hyperplasia. Mononuclear cell infiltrates are found in the lung, liver, pancreas, and intestinal tract. The degree of tissue inflammation, like the degree of disrupted thymic and peripheral lymphoid tissue organization, shows a direct correlation with transgene copy number. In the highest copy number lines there is severe IBD that is associated with early-onset wasting and diarrhea beginning at 3–6 weeks of age. Morbidity and mortality in high copy number mice appears to correlate with the severity of intestinal inflammation. Inflammation in the intestine was most marked in the colon but extended into the small bowel. In the colon there was multifocal ulceration, which could be transmural and granulomatous in areas. There were large numbers of CD40L$^+$ T cells in the inflamed intestine as well as large numbers of B cells and activated T cells in the mesenteric lymph node.

In light of studies in several mouse models of IBD, wherein blockade of CD40–CD40L interactions is associated with diminished IL-12 and IFN-γ production and inflammation [33, 52, 101], one can speculate that constitutive, high level expression of CD40L by peripheral T cells results in increased proinflammatory cytokine expression by cells of the innate immune system. As yet no characterization of the effector cell or cytokines in the inflammatory lesions of CD40L transgenic mice has been reported.

Similarly, it is unknown whether the bacterial flora plays a role in the inflammation seen in this model.

Models of spontaneous IBD

Colitis has been reported to occur spontaneously in animals, but this has been sporadic and uncommon. There are now several instances in which colitis has occurred in high frequency in a strain of animals: C3H/HeJBir mice, SAMP1/Yit mice, and the cotton-top tamarin (Table 4). The cottontop tamarin is an interesting model but little is known about the pathogenesis. The interested reader is referred to an earlier review [1].

C3H/HeJBir mice

C3H/HeJBir is a substrain of C3H/HeJ mice which was generated by a program of selective breeding at the Jackson Laboratory. These mice are highly susceptible to the development of colitis, and under certain housing conditions can develop colitis spontaneously. In the original studies, the spontaneous colitis was localized mainly to the cecum and right colon of young mice, with onset in the third to fourth week of life. Colitis was usually mild, resolving by 10–12 weeks of age. The lesions were focal, mainly in the cecum but sometimes extending into the right colon. There was acute and chronic inflammation, ulceration, crypt abscesses, and epithelial regeneration, but no thickening of the mucosal layer or granulomas [102].

A comparison of immunologic cell types and their functions between C3H/HeJBir and the C3H/HeJ strain reveals few differences in the systemic compartment. Both have the Lps[d] mutation, now known to be a mutation of toll-like receptor (TLR) 4, which renders them unresponsive to bacterial endotoxin. The differences that have been found are compatible with a potential defect in mucosal immune regulation including increased secretory IgA, high titer serum antibodies to commensal bacterial antigens, and increased T cell responses to orally delivered antigen in C3H/HeJBir mice [103]. IEL of C3H/HeJBir mice have been reported to have increased cytotoxicity and homotypic aggregation due to increased expression of β_7 integrins [104].

C3H/HeJBir mice have no significant B cell or T cell reactivity to food or intestinal epithelial cell antigens, but do have strong B cell and T cell responses to cecal bacterial antigens. Serum IgG antibodies, particularly IgG$_{2a}$, bind to a set of antigens on Western blots of electrophoresed homogenates of cecal bacteria. This antibody reactivity is highly selective, recognizing a limited but reproducible subset of antigens from the thousands of proteins present [44]. These antibodies probably do not play a major role in disease pathogenesis in that most mice develop them after colitis has resolved.

C3H/HeJBir CD4[+] T cells demonstrate strong proliferative and cytokine responses to cecal bacterial antigens which are detectable as early as 4 weeks of age. This T cell response is directed at protein antigens and is MHC class II restricted. The cytokines produced are mainly IFN-γ and IL-2, consistent with a predominantly Th1 response. Adoptive transfer of bacterial antigen-activated CD4[+] T cells from C3H/HeJBir but not from control C3H/HeJ mice into histocompatible C3H/HeSnJ *Scid/Scid* recipients induces focal ulcers and colitis mainly in the cecum, similar to what has been found in the C3H/HcJBir donors [105]. This formally demonstrates that CD4[+] T cells reactive with conventional antigens of the enteric bacterial flora can mediate chronic IBD. The number of antigens stimulating this T cell response also appears to be limited in that a restricted number of TCRβ chain gene families is expanded after antigen stimulation *in vitro* [101].

A number of CD4[+] T cell lines reactive with enteric bacterial antigens has been generated *in vitro*. Most of these are predominantly Th1 and cause colitis in all recipients after adoptive transfer into C3H SCID recipients. High levels of IFN-γ and IL-12 are found in colon explant cultures of colitic mice. The sustained IL-12 production in the mucosa that is required for disease to occur depends on CD40L–CD40 interactions, in that antibodies to CD40L

block IL-12 production *in vitro* and prevent colitis *in vivo* [101]. A bacterially reactive CD4[+] T cell line with properties similar to Tr1 cells has also been generated. This cell line is able to block the development of colitis by a pathogenic Th1 cell line when both are transferred together into SCID recipients [106].

Again, environmental factors appear to be important in disease expression, in that the expression of the phenotype of spontaneous colitis is reduced or eliminated when the mice are housed in SPF conditions. However, C3H/HeJBir (and C3H/HeJ) remain very susceptible to several forms of colitis, including both TNBS-induced and DSS-induced colitis [107]. In addition, C3H/HeJBir carrying the IL-10 null mutation contract severe disease in the first weeks of life [46]. Thus C3H/HeJBir mice have a high susceptibility for colitis, possibly due to defects in mucosal immune regulation, that can express spontaneous colitis when stressed by certain conventional housing conditions.

SAMP1/Yit mice

Another model of spontaneous intestinal inflammation is the recently described SAMP1/Yit mouse [108]. The SAMP1/Yit strain is a subline of the SAM (Senescence Accelerated Mice) P1 strain, which was derived by extended sibling mating of AKR/J mice. SAMP1 mice are so named because of their shortened life span (approximately 9 months) and propensity to develop early senescence associated with spontaneous amyloidosis, alopecia, and osteoporosis [109]. The SAMP1/Yit subline of the SAMP1 strain was derived by selective sibling breeding of SAMP1 mice with spontaneous skin ulcerations [108]. Unlike the parent SAMP1 strain, the SAMP1/Yit strain shows no shortened life span or features of early senescence, but does develop a spontaneous enteritis and cecitis under SPF conditions.

Unlike most of the IBD models described in this chapter, the intestinal inflammation in SAMP1/Yit mice is unusual in its preferential development in the small intestine; the absence of colonic involvement is characteristic. Extraintestinal manifestations of disease include focal lymphocytic infiltrates in the liver and inflammatory skin lesions on the dorsum and eyelids. Animals maintained under SPF conditions develop discontinuous inflammatory lesions of the distal small intestine as early as 10 weeks of age, and show 100% penetrance by 30 weeks of age [110].

Grossly, there is thickening of the distal ileum with focal stricture formation. Histologically, the disease is most severe in the terminal ileum with progressively diminished inflammation in the proximal ileum and variable, mild involvement of the cecum. There is no significant involvement of the jejunum, duodenum, stomach, colon, or rectum. Early lesions are characterized by neutrophilic infiltrates of the epithelium, particularly that over Peyer's patches or preexisting lymphoid follicles, an injury that resembles aphthous ulceration in human IBD. Mature lesions are characterized by villus atrophy and crypt hyperplasia with transmural inflammatory cell infiltrates. There is a mixed inflammatory cell infiltrate composed of mononuclear cells (lymphocytes, macrophages, and plasma cells) and neutrophils. Loose aggregates of macrophages consistent with granuloma formation and focal microabscess formation have been described in mature lesions. In more advanced disease there can be development of mucosal fibrosis with budding and branching of glands, as well as muscular and neural hyperplasia.

Phenotypic analyses of inflammatory cell infiltrates by immunohistochemistry and flow cytometric analysis have demonstrated increases in activated T cells [110]. There is an increase in the ratio of $CD8\alpha^+$ IEL T cells bearing $\alpha\beta$ versus $\gamma\delta$ TCRs. Disease can be transferred into MHC-matched SCID mice by unfractionated or $CD4^+$ T cell-enriched mesenteric lymph node (MLN) cells from 30-week-old SAMP1/ Yit mice in a dose- and time-dependent manner. The cytokine profile of MLN cells from SAMP1/Yit or adoptive transfer recipient mice is characterized by increased production of IFN-γ and TNF-α. Treatment of adoptive transfer recipients with neutralizing antibodies to either TNF-α or IL-12 suppressed disease incidence and severity. Thus, Th1-type cytokines play a pathogenic role in this model. Administration of antibodies to adhesion molecules that have been implicated in T cell homing and neutrophil trafficking (E- and P-selectin and α4-integrin) also attenuates disease development in SAMP1/Yit mice.

Development of terminal ileitis in SAMP1/Yit mice requires the endogenous flora. Germfree SAMP1/Yit mice fail to develop intestinal inflammation, whereas germfree SAMP1/Yit mice reconstituted by transfer of the flora from SPF SAMP1/ Yit mice developed disease as early as 15 weeks post-conventionalization [108]. These results suggest that T cell reactivity to bacterial antigens localized in the terminal ileum, presumably the commensal flora, may be responsible for disease pathogenesis. It is unknown whether disease progression represents continued reactivity to antigens provided by the commensal flora or rather represents cross-reactivity to self antigens expressed in the terminal ileum.

Models with perturbations of the epithelium

The intestinal epithelium is recognized increasingly as an active partner in the mucosal immune system. Epithelial (IEC) cells produce and respond to a wide variety of cytokines and express molecules able to interact with lymphoid cells. Epithelial cells signal the innate immune system by rapid release of chemokines upon bacterial invasion [111, 112]. The epithelial layer is exposed to and interacts also with luminal bacteria. IEC express a number of toll-like receptors (TLR), proteins which bind to and thus recognize certain classes of microbial products based on molecular patterns. There are some 9–10 TLR genes identified to date, and each appears to recognize a different assortment of microbial molecules, e.g. TLR2 binds CpG nucleotides, TLR4 binds lipopolysaccharides, and TLR5 binds flagellins. Epithelial cells alter the expression of some genes based on the composition of the bacterial flora, and so are able to detect changes in the flora, perhaps via TLR or other pattern-recognition receptors. Thus, one could more accurately view the dynamic interactions at the mucosal surface as a bacterial–epithelial–lymphoid circuit with each component communicating with the others (Fig. 4). It is of some interest that NOD2, the first gene identified as conferring susceptibility to Crohn's disease, appears to be a microbial pattern-recognition receptor [113, 114].

The epithelial hypothesis of the pathogenesis of IBD proposes that abnormal epithelial cell function can result in chronic intestinal inflammation even in a host with a normal immune system. The inflammation is viewed as secondary to the epithelial abnormality. Support for this hypothesis comes from the observations that some patients with Crohn's disease have increased intestinal permeability for small molecules [115] and that enterocytes from patients with IBD demonstrate abnormal stimulation of allogenic T cells due to deficient expression of a glycoprotein (gp 180) on their surface [116]. Further support for this hypothesis comes from experimental animal models in which the major abnormality appears to be epithelial. The best example of this is the *mdr1a*-deficient mouse, as

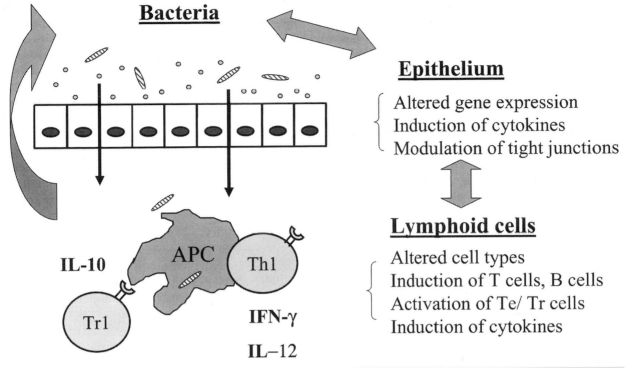

Figure 4. Bacterial–epithelial–lymphoid circuit. Enteric bacteria and their products can act on epithelial cells to alter epithelial gene expression and function. The epithelial cells in turn are interacting with lymphoid cells within the epithelial layer itself and in the lamina propria. Mucosal lymphoid cells can influence the bacterial flora through the production of cytokines and immunoglobulins such as IgA. Thus there is a very dynamic dialog or circuit occurring at the mucosal surface. From this viewpoint it is not difficult to see how abnormal epithelial function could perturb this dialog and skew the lymphoid response into an inflammatory one.

discussed below. However, this hypothesis is not incompatible with the immunological hypothesis discussed above, particularly when one views the epithelial layer as an active player in a dynamic bacterial–epithelial–lymphoid circuit at the mucosal surface.

From this perspective it is not surprising that mutations that affect or target epithelial cells can result in perturbation of the mucosal immune system and thus eventuate in chronic intestinal inflammation (Table 3). Providing a barrier is one important function of the epithelium, but only one of them [117]. Although increased permeability is generally assumed to equate to increased mucosal immune reactivity and thus chronic intestinal inflammation, direct proof that this is true is lacking. The chronicity of the altered barrier function is likely an important variable. For example, instillation of acetic acid into the colon of mice, which interrupts the mucosal barrier for days, results in inflammation and increased mRNA for IL-1, TNF, and IL-6 but no

up-regulation of T cell cytokine mRNA despite the presence of memory T cells in the lamina propria [118]. The best support for a role of increased permeability leading to IBD comes from the N-cadherin dominant negative mutant chimera, discussed below, and in this model the inflammation takes months to develop and remains histologically mild [119]. Given the advances in understanding of the many roles epithelial cells play in mucosal immune homeostasis, concepts of their potential role in intestinal inflammation need to be expanded beyond alterations in permeability.

Multi-drug resistance gene 1α (*mdr1a*)-deficient mice

The murine multiple drug resistance gene, *mdr1a* encodes a 170 kDa transmembrane transporter protein that is expressed by intestinal epithelial cells, as well as a subset of lymphoid cells and hematopoietic cells. *mdr1a* is one of a family of transporters known as ATP-binding transporters that are characterized by their ability to transport small amphiphilic and hydrophobic molecules across cell membranes in an ATP-dependent manner. Three *mdr* genes have been identified in rodents, each with a restricted pattern of tissue expression and presumably distinct functions. Two *mdr* genes have been identified in humans. Originally defined on the basis of their ability to confer resistance to chemotherapeutic agents in neoplasia, thus the name, the physiologic function of these transporters is not known.

Mice with a targeted deletion of the *mdr1a* gene were recently generated on a FVB background; 2-0-25% of *mdr1a*-deficient mice studied for a 1-year period developed clinical signs of intestinal inflammation (loose stools and anal mucous discharge) with an average age of disease onset of 20 weeks. Disease was primarily limited to the large intestine and characterized by mucosal thickening, a dense infiltration of the lamina propria by inflammatory cells, crypt hyperplasia with focal ulceration, and occasional crypt abscesses. The majority of the infiltrating cells were CD4$^+$ TCR$\alpha\beta^+$cells, plus granulocytes and clustered collections of B cells. Cytokine analysis of the colonic lesions revealed increased expression of IFN-γ, TNF-α, IL-12, IL-6 and IL-1 compared to controls. There was also increased expression of the chemokine receptors CCR2 and CCR5, as well as the chemokines MCP-1, MIP1α, and RANTES. These features are consistent with a Th1-type chronic inflammatory response.

Treatment of *mdr1a*$^{-/-}$ mice with broad-spectrum antibiotics both prevented disease development and treated active disease [120]. In mice with active disease who showed clinical improvement following 10 weeks of treatment with antibiotics, there was no evidence of persistent granulocytic infiltrates or B cell follicles, although increased numbers of CD3$^+$ T cells remained in the colon lamina propria. Characterization of the intestinal flora showed only commensal organisms, although there were differences in the relative frequency of species between experimental groups. Notably, analysis for *Helicobacter* spp. was negative.

Interestingly, T cells isolated from the mesenteric lymph node of *mdr1a*-deficient mice with clinical evidence of IBD demonstrated proliferative responses to bacterial antigens, whereas cells from non-colitic *mdr1a*$^{-/-}$ and control FVB mice did not. The absence of T cell or antibody reactivity to the intestinal flora in noncolitic *mdr1a*-deficient mice

suggests that antigenic reactivity to the intestinal flora followed rather than preceded disease development.

Because the *mdr1a* transporter is expressed in both intestinal epithelium and mucosal lymphocytes, irradiation bone marrow chimeras were generated to determine which cell populations might be responsible for disease. Bone marrow chimeras in which irradiated FVB animals were reconstituted with bone marrow from mdr1a$^{-/-}$ or FVB donors, or irradiated mdr1a$^{-/-}$ recipients were reconstituted with FVB or mdr1a$^{-/-}$ bone marrow were generated. Only mdr1a$^{-/-}$ recipients developed disease, whereas FVB recipients failed to develop disease irrespective of the origin of the bone marrow donor. Thus, defects in the *mdr1a* expression by the gut epithelium may be associated with development of colitis. Because no immune defects have been described in *mdr1a*$^{-/-}$ mice, these results suggest that spontaneous colitis can develop from an epithelial abnormality in animals with a normal immune system.

N-cadherin dominant negative mutant chimeric mice

This model provides support for the notion that primary abnormalities of epithelial barrier function may cause chronic intestinal inflammation. A dominant negative N-cadherin mutant (NCADΔ) transgene lacking an extracellular domain was transfected into 129/Sv embryonic stem cells which were then introduced into normal C57BL/6 blastocysts [119]. The chimeric mice that resulted had patches of mutant 129/Sv-derived epithelium dispersed in normal C57BL/6-derived intestinal epithelium. The two could be distinguished by differences in lectin binding. The 129/Sv epithelium, but not the C57BL/6 epithelium, had a defect in epithelial adhesion due to disruption of E-cadherin expression, a molecule critical to cell–cell and cell–matrix adhesion. Two types of chimeras were generated using different promoters, one of which caused expression of the NCADΔ in both the small intestinal crypt and villus cells and another that caused expression only in villus cells. Focal inflammation and adenomas occurred in the chimeras which expressed the epithelial defect in both crypt and villus cells, but neither occurred in mice expressing NCADΔ only in villus cells. The earliest changes in 129/Sv epithelium were an increase in the number and size of lymphoid follicles/aggregates, expansion of the lamina propria in the same areas, and increased 129/Sv epithelial cell MHC class II expression. By age 3 months the inflammation in the 129/Sv mucosal patches became transmural and was associated with numerous lymphoid aggregates, lymphangiectasia, cryptitis, and some small ulcerations. This inflammation appeared to be mild based on the histopathology presented. Small intestinal adenomas developed between 3 and 9 months of age, but did not progress to adenocarcinoma.

This model gives support to the idea that primary abnormalities of the epithelial barrier could result in significant secondary inflammation because there should be no direct effect of NCADΔ on the immune system. The authors postulated that antigen coming across the crypts induces an immune response different from that to antigen coming through villus epithelium. Because the initial phenotypic change is an expansion of the lymphoid follicles with later extension of inflammation from them, an alternative explanation of these results is that altered mucosal barrier function of the dome epithelium over the Peyer's patches is the critical factor. The crypts supply cells not only to the villus epithelium, but also to the dome epithelium covering lymphoid follicles. If this is the explanation, it implies that the dome epithelium not only samples antigen, but also serves a barrier function, regulating the quantity of antigen being delivered in a fashion that maintains mucosal homeostasis. All of these are very interesting hypotheses and this model could provide some important insights into both epithelial and mucosal immune cell homeostasis.

Gαi2-deficient mice

G proteins are important signal transductors that couple cell surface receptors to various effector pathways inside the cell. They are composed of alpha, beta, and gamma chains. The alpha subunit of *Gi2* is part of the heterotrimeric complex that regulates signal transduction through adenylate cyclase. Gi2 is widely distributed in most cell types, including gut epithelial cells and lymphocytes. In lymphocytes, *Gi2* is known to regulate certain events in thymogenesis, T cell recirculation, T cell activation and production of certain cytokines. Gαi2-deficient mice are normal at birth, but exhibit slow growth and increased mortality due to a pancolitis that begins at 8–12 weeks of age. The colitis is gradually progressive and more severe in the distal vs proximal colon [121] and rectal prolapse is common. The colon is grossly

irregular with a focally thickened wall. The histopathology is marked by acute and chronic inflammation, crypt abscesses, crypt distortion, focal fibrosis, and both superficial and deep, sometimes perforating, ulcerations. Other organs are not involved. The colonic mucosa has foci of intense regenerative proliferation bordering on dysplasia. Indeed, up to one-third of animals develop adenocarcinoma of the colon between 15 and 33 weeks of age [121].

Gαi2-deficient mice manifest a variety of immune abnormalities, particularly in lymphocytes isolated from the colon. There are increased numbers of activated/memory CD4$^+$ T cells (CD44^{hi}, CD44RB^{lo}, CD62^{lo}), and a marked increase in IFN-γ and IL-1β production and lesser increases of IL-6 and TNF-α in mice with colitis as compared to wild-type mice or Gαi2-deficient mice without colitis [122]. IL-12 p40 mRNA is detectable in the colon but not small bowel, but there is no increase in IL-2, IL-4, IL-5 or IL-10. B cells producing IgG in the colon, predominantly IgG$_{2a}$, are markedly increased, which is reflected by elevated levels of IgG and particularly IgG$_{2a}$ in colonic secretions [122]. Thus, the immunologic data are consistent with an unrestrained Th1 response in the colon. Activation of the mucosal immune system precedes development of the colitis by several weeks [123], but this would not exclude a major role for an abnormal epithelium in the process.

Mice housed under specific pathogen-free conditions continue to develop the disease at a similar frequency, including the development of adenocarcinoma. The mice are colonized with *Helicobacter hepaticus*, a potential opportunistic pathogen, but the role of this bacterium in the overall disease process is not defined. Genetic background has an important influence (Table 2): the Gαi2 knockout mutation on the 129/Sv background results in severe disease, but the same mutation on a mixed 129/Sv, C57BL/6 background has a much lower severity and incidence of colitis [122].

Intestinal trefoil factor-deficient mice

Intestinal trefoil factor (ITF) is a member of the trefoil family of proteins which are expressed by goblet cells in the intestinal mucosa. Members of this family share a distinctive three-loop secondary structure that confers upon them resistance to acid and proteases. ITF has been shown to enhance epithelial restitution *in vitro* in a wounded monolayer system. Its role *in vivo* was explored by the generation of an

ITF-deficient mouse [124]. These mice are born and develop normally, although they do have a relative defect of epithelial migration to the mucosal surface. However, ITF-deficient mice stressed by administration of dextran sulfate sodium in their drinking water develop more severe colitis than wild-type controls, and half of them die. Histologic sections revealed a marked defect in epithelial repair. ITF-deficient mice given acetic acid enemas also developed colitis with markedly impaired healing, but this was corrected by delivery of exogenous recombinant ITF to the colonic mucosa. Although these studies involved acute injury to the colonic mucosa, they do provide a proof of principle that impaired mucosal healing can contribute to the severity and progression of colitis. These data also provide support for the notion that agents that enhance healing of the inflamed mucosa will be useful in the therapy of IBD.

Keratin 8-deficient mice

Keratin filaments are present in all epithelial cells and are thought to provide strength to the cell. The keratin 8 gene encodes a type II keratin filament which pairs with type I filaments to form extended keratins within single-layered epithelia such as that in the intestine. Disruption of the keratin 8 gene is lethal in embryonic mice of a mixed B6, 129 genetic background. However, a proportion of keratin 8-deficient FVB/N strain mice do not die *in utero*

[125]. These mice develop colitis between 2 and 12 months of age while housed under SPF conditions. The colitis is heralded by rectal prolapse and involves the whole colon and the cecum, but not the small intestine. There is epithelial hyperplasia and inflammation of the colon lamina propria and submucosa, but no ulcerations, goblet cell depletion, or crypt distortion. The epithelial hyperplasia is thought to precede the inflammation. No anemia or leukocytosis occurs, nor are any other organs affected, aside from mild splenomegaly. The cytokines involved have not been identified. Curiously, deletion of keratin 18, the filament that pairs with keratin 8 in enterocytes, does not result in IBD [126].

Models involving chemical or environmental stressors

Models clustered together in this category are diverse although each involves a chemical stress or other injury to elicit disease (Table 5). Some are limited to acute tissue injury; in others, the tissue injury is part of a more complex immunologic reactivity. Three models have been reviewed previously [1] and will not be discussed further here.

Table 5. Models involving chemical stress or injury

Model	Area involved	Effector cell	Key cytokines	Bacterial flora driven	Strain variation/ genetic modifiers	Reference
Dextran sulfate sodium	Colon	Unknown	IL-1, IL-6, TNF-α	Possible; metronidazole prevents	C3H, NOD, BALB > B6 > NON; multiple genes [107]	127
TNBS/ethanol	Colon	CD4$^+$ Th1	IFN-γ, IL-12, TNF-α	Probable	SJL, C3H, BALB > B6 > DBA/2	168
Oxazalone	Colon	CD4$^+$ Th2	IL-4, IL-5, TGF-β	Unknown	SJL	169
Acetic acid	Colon	Unknown	IL-1, IL-6, TNF-α	No	BALB/c	118
Indomethacin (rat)	Small intestine	Unknown	Undefined	Yes	Lewis > Fischer	170, 171
Peptidoglycan– polysaccharide (rat)	Injection site: ileum, cecum	T cells	IL-1, IL-6, TNF-α	Yes	Lewis, S-W susceptible; Buffulo resistant	172

Dextran sulfate sodium (DSS)-induced colitis

Addition of 30–5 kDa DSS to the drinking water at 3–10% will induce colitis in hamsters, rats and mice [127], which is manifested by bloody diarrhea, weight loss, shortening of the colon, mucosal ulceration and neutrophilic infiltration. In Swiss-Webster mice a chronic colitis can be induced by feeding multiple cycles of DSS [128]. Such chronic lesions demonstrate increased lymphoid cells, prominent lymphoid aggregates in the lamina propria and serosa, a patchy distribution of inflammation and fissuring ulceration. Prolonged low-dose feeding of DSS has resulted in colitis, dysplasia and colon cancer in hamsters [129] and rats [130].

The earliest change of acute DSS-induced colitis is a progressive noninflammatory dropout of crypts [128], suggesting a primary effect on epithelial cells. Indeed, DSS inhibits proliferation of mouse epithelial cells *in vitro* [131]. Early lesions occur mainly in the left colon and over lymphoid aggregates. In established lesions multiple inflammatory mediators are increased, including thromboxane, leukotriene B_4, IL-2, IL-4 and IL-6. Colitis occurs in SCID mice fed DSS, indicating that the T cells and B cells are not required for acute colitis to develop [131]. Luminal bacteria may play a role in the pathogenesis of these lesions in that colonic concentrations of *Bacteroides* spp., especially *B. distasonis*, are increased in acute and chronic phases of inflammation [127]; concomitant metronidazole therapy prevents DSS colitis [129].

The DSS model has some advantages and some limitations. It is a fairly simple method of inducing damage in the colon of most strains of mice. The lesions are fairly reproducible and the clinical and histologic severity can be quantitated. Because of these features, DSS colitis has been used for screening of potential therapeutic agents, and a large number of them have shown benefit in this model, indicating it is a sensitive screening system. There are also limitations of this model, mainly that it represents a nonspecific injury model that does not require either T cells or B cells; thus, it is not well suited to address immunologic or therapeutic issues involving the acquired immune system.

The significant and substantial variations in DSS-induced colon lesions among inbred strains of mice have been shown to represent a quantitative genetic trait [107]. The reproducibility of lesions produced by DSS has allowed the identification and mapping of genes important in susceptibility to colitis, genes that are likely to be of general importance in maintaining mucosal homeostasis. The location of a number of candidate genes has been identified through quantitative trait locus mapping [132]. Interestingly, the same pattern of susceptibility and resistance among strains found with DSS is seen in a number of induced mutant mouse models (Tables 1–6), suggesting either that the same set of genes or different genes affecting similar pathways may be involved.

Trinitrobenzene sulfonic acid (TNBS)/ethanol enema-induced colitis

This model is a hybrid one involving both chemical damage and T cell immune reactivity. The administration of an enema containing the contact sensitizing agent TNBS in 50% ethanol induces colitis in rodents. The ethanol breaks the mucosal barrier and is a crucial component; no colitis ensues if TNBS alone is given [133]. Because TNBS is a covalently reactive compound, its administration results in acute necrosis of the wall of the distal colon due to oxidative damage. The occurrence of such necrosis appears to be an important factor for the development of colitis, which may explain why the effective dose of TNBS in mice is close to the lethal dose. In a few strains of rats and mice a single enema can result in prolonged chronic colitis [133, 134]. However, in most strains of mice multiple enemas are required to generate chronicity and the duration of colitis following administration is a matter of days.

Discrete foci of acute necrosis and inflammation shortly after the enema are followed by submucosal chronic inflammation that lasts a variable amount of time. In mice, TNBS colitis appears to be a classic delayed-type hypersensitivity response mediated by T cells responding to 'hapten-modified self antigen'. The latter is formed by the covalent attachment of the hapten, trinitrophenyl (TNP), to self peptides. Such reactions in mice are under complex regulation by T cells and B cells. The colitic mucosa is infiltrated with $CD4^+$ T cells [134] and increased IgG- and IgA-producing B cells [135], the latter being reminiscent of the changes in plasma cells that occur in the mucosa in human IBD [136]. There is a marked increase in B cells producing IgG anti-TNP in the inflamed colon, including the IgG_1, IgG_{2a}, and IgG_{2b} subclasses.

Mucosal $CD4^+$ T cells produce increased amounts of IFN-γ and IL-2, but not IL-4 [134], consistent with a Th1 effector response. Administration of monoclonal anti-IL-12 to mice with TNBS/ethanol colitis significantly prevents or treats the colitis [134], indicating that the interaction between antigen-presenting cells producing IL-12 and T cells producing IFN-γ contributes to both the induction and progression of colitis. Antibody blockade of interactions of CD40L (CD154) prevents induction of TNBS colitis by reducing IL-12 production [137]. Furthermore, other agents that can inhibit IL-12 production, such as IL-10 [138] or an anti-sense oligonucleotide to the transcription factor NFκB p65 [139], have similar beneficial effects.

A significant finding originating from the TNBS model is that regulatory cells able to inhibit colitis can be manipulated. Contact allergens are classic oral tolerogens and thus TNBS itself [135] or TNP-conjugated tissue homogenates [11] have been fed to mice to induce oral tolerance prior to the induction of colitis. The resulting colonic inflammation was less severe, the mucosal IgG anti-TNP cells were markedly reduced, and the cytokines produced by mucosal CD4$^+$ T cells were altered with production of less IFN-γ and more TGF-β$_1$, IL-10, and IL-4. Mucosal production of IL-12 was also reduced. Administration of antibodies to TGF-β reversed the protective effects of TNP-colon homogenate feeding in one study [11], suggesting that the regulatory cells induced by feeding were producing TGF-β.

Oxazolone/ethanol-induced colitis

Similar to the induction of colitis initiated by TNBS administration, administration of the contact sensitizing agent oxazolone in 50% ethanol as an enema also induces distal colitis in mice. In contrast to the colitis initiated by TNBS administration, however, colitis induced by high-dose oxazolone given in an ethanol enema has quite distinct clinical, histopathologic and immunologic features. Colonic instillation of 6 mg oxazolone in 50% ETOH as an enema results in rapid onset of distal colitis, diarrhea, and weight loss in SJL mice which peaks on day 2. Approximately 50% of the animals dosed died by day 4. Surviving animals showed progressive clinical improvement with apparent complete resolution by 10–12 days.

Histologically, oxazolone-induced lesions were confluent and characterized by superficial inflammation of the mucosa associated with severe epithelial loss, focal ulceration, and severe edema of the submucosal layers. The inflammatory infiltrate was mixed, composed predominantly of lymphocytes and neutrophils with a limited number of eosino-

phils. Severe goblet cell depletion and reduction of the density of tubular glands was noted. No crypt abscesses, crypt elongation, granulomatous inflammation, or fistulas were found.

Examination of the cytokine profiles of T cells isolated from the lamina propria of distal colon at day 2 demonstrated elevations of both IL-4 and IL-5 in CD3/CD28-stimulated T cell cultures, with no change in IFN-γ production. TGF-β was also markedly elevated in both spontaneous and stimulated cultures. Interestingly, levels of TGF-β were even higher in T cells isolated from uninvolved proximal segments of colon of diseased animals, as were IL-4 levels. A pathologic role for IL-4 in oxazolone/ ethanol colitis was demonstrated by neutralizing antibody studies. Animals that received a single neutralizing dose of IL-4 at the time of oxazolone/ ethanol administration displayed an abbreviated and attenuated transient weight loss and only minimal inflammation. In contrast, treatment of mice with neutralizing antibodies to TGF-β or IL-12 resulted in more severe disease and weight loss. Tissues from anti-TGF-β- and anti-IL-12-treated mice demonstrated a pancolitis instead of the distal colitis that was characteristic of control animals. Both anti-TGF-β and anti-IL-12 treatment resulted in sustained elevation of IL-4 production in diseased colons.

The oxazolone/ethanol colitis model represents an intriguing contrast to the TNBS model, and is unusual in its expression of a Th2 pattern of response. The mechanistic basis for the very different patterns of disease induced by oxazolone and TNBS is unknown, but promises to provide insights into antigenic features that may predispose to dysregulated Th1- or Th2-polarized intestinal responses. An important caveat regarding this model, however, is the role of antigen-induced Th2 cell responses in their development. The time course of disease development is very rapid compared to the inductive phase typically required for Th1 or Th2 development. It remains possible that this model represents a preferential recruitment of pre-committed Th2 cells, rather than induction of polarized effectors from naïve intestinal T cell precursors. Also, the basis for the resolution of lesions in the oxazolone/ethanol colitis model is unknown. Given the exacerbation of disease that accompanies neutralization of TGF-β, it is speculated that this pleiotropic cytokine may play a central role in rapid attenuation of the inflammatory response. Further studies will be needed to define the role of TGF-β in this model, and to

Table 6. Models as yet unclassified

Model	Area involved	Effector cell	Key cytokines	Bacterial flora driven	Strain variation/ genetic modifiers	Reference
HLA-B27 transgenic rat	Entire intestine, other organs	T cell CD4+/CD8+	IFNγ, IL-1, IL-6, TNF-α	Yes	Undefined	173
Wiskott-Aldrich syndrome protein deficient	Colon	? T cell	Undefined	Unknown	Undefined	144
Fucosyltransferase transgenic	Cecum, colon	Unknown	Undefined	Unknown	BALB/c	146
Pigeon cytochrome c T cell receptor transgenic	Cecum, colon	CD4+	Undefined	Probable	B10, B6	145

determine whether TGF-β may play a role in suppressing the Th2 response.

Models as yet unclassified

There remain a number of models that cannot be classified easily into the other categories as yet, mostly because there are insufficient data available (Table 6).

HLA-B27/β2M transgenic rat

Because the human HLA-B27 class I MHC molecule is strongly associated with ankylosing spondylitis and the spondyloarthropathies, transgenic rats expressing the human HLA-B27 and β2-microglobulin genes were generated. Certain of these transgenic rat lines develop a multiorgan disease manifested by colitis, arthritis, orchitis, and psoriasiform changes of the skin and nails in the absence of any further manipulation [140]. These features resemble the human spondyloarthropathies. Rats transgenic for other class I molecules such as HLA-A2 or HLA-B7, have not developed inflammatory disease. In the most susceptible 21-4H line, disease occurs in all animals surviving past 10 weeks of age and is manifest primarily by watery diarrhea (Table 6). A diffuse enteritis with mononuclear cell infiltrate is present that is variable in the stomach and small intestine, but prominent in the colon where it is associated with hyperplasia of crypts and mucin

depletion. Crypt abscesses or transmural inflammation are uncommon. The mechanisms by which the human B27 molecule induces this disease are unclear [140]. The HLA-B27 transgene is not expressed on gut epithelial cells but is present on antigen-presenting cells. CD4+ T cells are abundant in the intestinal lesions. Disease can be transferred with transgenic bone marrow and a critical role for T cells in disease is demonstrated by the observation that athymic (nude) rats bearing the transgene fail to develop disease, although bone marrow cells from these nude rats can transfer disease [141]. These results suggest disease requires B27 expression on antigen-presenting cells which then interact with host T cells. Interestingly, colitis and arthritis do not occur when B27 transgenic rats are raised under germfree conditions [142] but both develop when the flora, particularly *Bacteroides* spp., are restored [143].

Wiskott-Aldrich syndrome protein (WASP)-deficient mice

The Wiskott-Aldrich syndrome is an immunodeficiency disease due to mutations in a gene on the X chromosome encoding a cytoplasmic protein, WASP, that is expressed in lymphocytes and megakaryocytes. WASP appears to function in cell signaling and cytoskeletal interactions. WASP-deficient mice exhibit normal lymphocyte development in lymphoid tissues but have decreased numbers of lymphocytes and platelets in the blood. T cells from

WASP-deficient mice proliferate poorly after stimulation via the TCR which may be related to deficient receptor clustering or 'capping' which was also observed. Although colitis is not a feature in humans with WAS, most of the WASP-deficient mice developed acute and chronic colitis by 4 months of age. Large numbers of CD4$^+$ T cells infiltrated the mucosa of colitic mice. The effector cells mediating the colitis and cytokines involved remain unknown [144].

Lymphopenic T cell receptor transgenic mice

One report described an unusual form of spontaneous colitis that arose in a subset of T cell receptor transgenic mouse lines [145]. In this study two lines of mice with rearranged, transgenic α and β TCR chains specific for the antigen cytochrome C (5C.C7 and -D TCR transgenic lines). When these TCR transgenes were crossed onto a SCID or RAG background, colitis developed early in life and was characterized by marked mucosal hyperplasia, crypt elongation, and mixed inflammatory cell infiltrates with a predominance of mononuclear cells. Focal mucosal ulceration and crypt abscesses were also identified.

Lesions were more severe in the descending colon and rectum with progressively diminished disease in the cecum and ascending colon. The stomach, small intestine, and liver were uninvolved. Intestinal inflammation in each of these transgenic lines seemed to correlate with low numbers of circulating CD4$^+$ T cells, suggesting that lymphopenia played a role. Curiously, the dominant T cell population found in colon lesions expresses the transgenic β chain, but not the transgenic α chain (Tgα$^-$). Presumably the transgenic β chain is paired with nontransgenic, endogenous α chains. These cells have an activated phenotype (CD45RB^{lo}, CD44^{hi}, CD69^{hi}) and are expanded both in the intestine as well as in extraintestinal lymphoid tissues. The polyclonal nature of the pathogenic Tgα$^-$ cell population correlates with 'leakiness' of endogenous α chain rearrangement during thymic development in these mice, such that a small circulating population with potential cross-reactivity to intestinal antigens may be present. The ability of endogenous α chains to undergo rearrangement in the *scid* and *rag1*$^{-/-}$ background is unusual. The role of a relative lymphopenia in these mice and its association with development of colitis is unknown. It is speculated that crossreactivity with enteric bacterial antigens in mice with a 'brittle' T cell repertoire may predispose to colitis, perhaps due to the absence of sufficient regulatory T cells.

Fucosyltransferase transgenic mice

A primary abnormality in the glycosylation of colonic mucins resulting in a defective mucosal barrier function is hypothesized as a mechanism by which genetic factors may be involved in the etiology of ulcerative colitis. In a recent study, mice transgenic for α1,2-fucosyltransferase (H transferase, HTF) were observed to spontaneously develop colitis with a mixed acute and chronic inflammatory infiltrate and crypt abscesses, similar to human ulcerative colitis [146]. The inflammation was limited to the colon and cecum. Changes in mucin glycosylation were demonstrated; there is no evidence of impaired immunologic function in these transgenic mice. On lectin histochemistry there was increased peanut agglutinin staining in the colonic mucus layer of pre-colitic HTF mice compared with wild-type littermates. Further, monosaccharide analysis of purified colonic mucins demonstrated marked decreases in galactose and sialic acid in non-diseased HTF mice compared with wild-type littermates. The incidence of colitis was increased with successive backcrossing onto a BALB/c background. These studies suggest a novel model of ulcerative colitis based on genetic modification of colonic mucin glycosylation.

Discussion

The inflammatory bowel diseases represent a complex interplay among environmental, genetic, and immunologic components. New insight into each of these factors has been generated from experimental models. Some facets of what has been learned in each of these areas will be considered in turn.

Environmental factors

The major environmental factor revealed in the different experimental models is the enteric bacterial flora. On the luminal side of the epithelial layer there are a large number of bacterial species, estimated at 10^{14} organisms per gram of stool. On the other side of the epithelium are a large number of immune cells and molecules. The concept of a microbial–epithelial–lymphoid circuit with all components in communication with one another has already been presented, as have examples in which perturbations of either lymphocytes or epithelium can lead to chronic intestinal inflammation (Tables 1–3). It is unknown whether abnormalities of the flora alone can lead to disease in a similar manner, but this is possible. An altered or abnormal flora has been raised as a possible explanation for the rapid increase in immune-mediated diseases, including IBD, in the Western world. Sometimes called 'the hygiene hypothesis' this theory postulates that early childhood exposure to microbes primes the immune system to respond in certain ways later in life. In the Western world such priming either does not occur or is abnormal and results in a variety of immune diseases occurring later in life, including autoimmunity, atopy, asthma, and IBD. One factor that has changed substantially in the Western world is the bacterial flora, and a leading hypothesis is that this altered flora is responsible for the abnormal priming of the immune system early in life and thus later immune-mediated diseases. This theory is being tested by interventions to alter the bacterial flora early in life, and initial results indicate a 50% reduction in atopy in young children from atopic families who were given a probiotic flora as newborns [147].

The microbial flora is very complex and comprises hundreds of different organisms [148]. Many more have never been cultured but are being identified by new molecular methods that can identify novel organisms without having to culture them. The bacterial flora is the major stimulus to the development of the intestinal immune system. For example, germfree animals have little or no intestinal lymphoid tissue or IgA despite exposure to a variety of food antigens. When germfree animals are reconstituted with an intestinal flora they develop abundant mucosal lymphoid cells along the length of the intestine, and secretory IgA is produced in large amounts [149]. However, not all organisms among the flora are equally able to stimulate the mucosal immune system [150]. One example is segmented filamentous bacteria (SFB) which colonizes the intestine of a number of species including both mice and humans [151]. Colonization of germfree mice with SFB alone stimulates a large mucosal immune response, one which is greater in extent than colonization with a more complex bacterial flora not containing SFB [152, 153]. *Helicobacter* comprises another species that appears to be immunostimulatory in the intestine as a member of the flora, and some *Helicobacter* strains can contribute to colitis in selected immunodeficient strains. In most mice with an intact immune system, *Helicobacter* species are

commensals and do not cause disease. At the other end of the spectrum there may be organisms which are delivering inhibitory signals to the mucosal immune system [154, 155]. An interesting recent observation is that a non-pathogenic *Salmonella* species was able to inactivate NF-κB signaling in epithelial cells, by delivery of flagellin into them, thereby down-regulating inflammatory cytokine production [156]. If this result extends to commensal bacteria it suggests that some bacteria may be actively inhibiting mucosal immune responses. Indeed, certain bacterial strains have been classified as 'probiotics', i.e. bacteria that promote health. Probiotic bacteria are being tested in both experimental models and in humans with IBD with some promising early results [157, 158]. In the future, the probiotic approach may be taken one step further by genetically altering commensal bacteria to express cytokines. This has been done in a recent report in which *Lactococcus* were genetically altered to express IL-10 [159]. These organisms were able to treat colitis in two different experimental models. As we learn more about the bacterial flora, its manipulation may represent an effective treatment modality, particularly for maintaining remission of disease.

The variation in immune stimulating capability among organisms extends to their antigens. For example, in the colitic C3H/HeJBir mouse only a small fraction of the total enteric bacterial proteins present in the cecum are recognized by serum antibody, and this set of antigens is highly reproducible among individual members of this strain [44]. Similarly, a selective IgG reactivity has been found in other strains with colitis, although the bacterial antigens detected are different from those detected by serum from C3H/HeJBir mouse. The implication is that there are not only immunodominant organisms, but also a limited set of immunodominant antigens recognized by the host immune system which may vary from one strain to another. Such immunodominant antigens need to be defined in both mice and humans. This will be crucial to understanding the complex immune response to the flora, and particularly how this response is regulated. Availability of these dominant microbial antigens will allow us to test whether immunologic tolerance to enteric flora does indeed exist, as has been proposed [138, 160]. Identification of these microbial antigens may allow manipulation of the immune response to them, which would be a novel approach to the treatment of IBD.

Genetic factors

Disease expression can vary greatly when the same mutant gene is bred onto different inbred mouse strains. Each inbred strain carries a set of genes that are identical within that inbred strain but differs from other inbred strains. These 'background genes' can greatly influence or modify the expression of a disease resulting from a defined mutation. With regard to experimental IBD, many of the same strains appear to be susceptible or resistant regardless of how the disease was induced (Tables 1–6). This variation has been examined in detail in DSS-induced colitis where reproducible quantitative differences were found among the inbred strains. These differences were shown to be heritable and due to the effects of multiple genes [107]. Using quantitative trait locus mapping the location of a number of genes responsible for this variation has been identified [132]. A similar effort using IL-10 deficiency as the stimulus for colitis has also revealed the influence of multiple genes determining susceptibility [46, 47]. These results in mice mirror the results of similar efforts in patients with IBD in whom multiple genetic loci contributing to susceptibility have been identified. Similar approaches are under way in humans. The first gene conferring susceptibility to Crohn's disease has been identified on chromosome 16 [113, 114]. The NOD2 gene encodes an intracellular protein that recognizes microbial products such as endotoxin. The mechanism of NOD2 function, and how its deficiency can lead to Crohn's disease, will require the generation of a NOD2-deficient line of mice, an effort that is under way. This illustrates how the genetic studies in experimental models and in human patients complement one another.

Immunologic factors

The immunologic pathogenesis has been discussed in the introduction and sections on each experimental model. However, there are some overall themes that recur through multiple models that are worth considering. These include triggering factors, progression or perpetuation of disease, and immune regulation, i.e. the immunologic stages of IBD.

A number of models demonstrate that an animal that is genetically susceptible to IBD may not become ill unless the process is triggered by some event that perturbs the system. Initiating or 'triggering' factors seem to operate also in humans with IBD whose disease may initiate from a viral or bacterial infection, emotional shock, etc. Very little is known about these initiating factors but several examples of their requirement for disease to occur are demonstrated in the experimental models. One example is the specific pathogen-free C57Bl/6 IL-2-deficient mouse, which under strict SPF housing conditions can remain healthy. However, immunization with DNP-KLH in complete Freund's adjuvant triggers the typical disease associated with IL-2 deficiency, including a severe colitis [53]. Another is the STAT-4 transgenic mouse which remains healthy unless immunized with the same material [161]. The ITF-deficient mouse, which has a genetic defect in the epithelial healing, remains well as long as epithelium is not perturbed. Feeding of DSS to ITF-deficient mice injures the epithelium and results in a severe colitis [124]. Non-steroidal anti-inflammatory drugs have long been thought to activate human IBD, but data supporting this idea are lacking. Thus it is quite interesting that an NSAID, piroxicam, can accelerate the onset of colitis in C57Bl/IL-10-deficient mice [162]. Even from this short list it is clear that the triggering factors can be quite diverse and can involve either systemic or mucosal perturbations. Experimental models should allow further dissection and understanding of this aspect of IBD.

Initiating factors and those responsible for disease perpetuation or progression are likely to be different. With regard to Th1-mediated disease a key factor in disease perpetuation is sustained IL-12 production. The latter in turn requires interactions of CD40L on T cells and CD40 on antigen-presenting cells. Antibodies to IL-12 and to CD40L have been shown to be effective in multiple models and each of these agents is currently being tested in patients. Another factor required for perpetuation of the disease is the recruitment of new effector cells into the mucosa. Effector cells, including dendritic cells, macrophages, neutrophils, and activated lymphocytes, have fairly short life spans. Thus all these different cell types need to be renewed for chronic inflammation to persist, and this involves recruitment of such cells from the circulation. Supporting this idea are the findings that agents which block trafficking of cells into the intestine are able to prevent and treat colitis in a number of experimental models. In addition, a lymphotoxin β–Fc fusion protein, which perturbs secondary lymphoid structure, was able to treat active colitis in two different experimental models, probably by altering cell trafficking.

A third immunologic aspect important to pathogenesis of IBD is immune regulation. Deficiency of regulatory cells has been implicated in a significant number of models (Table 1). One of the most exciting developments in modern immunology is the identification of these regulatory cells. Their effects have long been seen, but identification of the cells responsible for those effects have been elusive. Many different types of regulatory cells are being defined and a great deal of information will be generated in coming years. Much of the basic immunology will come from experimental systems in the mouse and will need to be translated to humans. This area has great promise for novel therapeutic approaches to IBD therapies that could potentially alter the natural history of these diseases. Based on what has been learned from the models to date, the most rational therapy for IBD is to enhance regulatory cell function, to inhibit effector cell function, or to accomplish both. Such an approach is within sight at present, but will need to be validated in experimental models before it is translated to the treatment of human IBD.

References

1. Elson CO, Sartor RB, Tennyson GS, Riddell RH. Experimental models of inflammatory bowel disease. Gastroenterology 1995; 109: 1344–67.
2. Mosmann TR, Sad S. The expanding universe of T-cell subsets: Th1, Th2 and more. Immunol Today 1996; 17: 138–46.
3. Fort MM, Lesley R, Davidson NJ *et al.* IL-4 exacerbates disease in a Th1 cell transfer model of colitis. J Immunol 2001; 166: 2793–800.
4. Neurath MF, Fuss I, Pasparakis M *et al.* Predominant pathogenic role of tumor necrosis factor in experimental colitis in mice. Eur J Immunol 1997; 27: 1743–50.
5. Fuss IJ, Neurath M, Boirivant M *et al.* Disparate CD4$^+$ lamina propria (LP) lymphokine secretion profiles in inflammatory bowel disease. Crohn's disease LP cells manifest increased secretion of IFN-gamma, whereas ulcerative colitis LP cells manifest increased secretion of IL-5. J Immunol 1996; 157: 1261–70.
6. Bacchetta R, Bigler M, Touraine JL *et al.* High levels of interleukin 10 production *in vivo* are associated with tolerance in SCID patients transplanted with HLA mismatched hematopoietic stem cells. J Exp Med 1994; 179: 493–502.
7. Groux H, O'Garra A, Bigler M *et al.* A CD4$^+$ T cell subset inhibits antigen-specific T-cell responses and prevents colitis. Nature 1997; 389: 737–42.
8. Santos LM, al-Sabbagh A, Londono A, Weiner HL. Oral tolerance to myelin basic protein induces regulatory TGF-beta-secreting T cells in Peyer's patches of SJL mice. Cell Immunol 1994; 157: 439–47.
9. Chen Y, Kuchroo VK, Inobe J, Hafler DA, Weiner HL. Regulatory T cell clones induced by oral tolerance: suppression of autoimmune encephalomyelitis. Science 1994; 265: 1237–40.
10. Fukaura H, Kent SC, Pietrusewicz MJ, Khoury SJ, Weiner HL, Hafler DA. Induction of circulating myelin basic protein and proteolipid protein-specific transforming growth factor-beta1-secreting Th3 T cells by oral administration of myelin in multiple sclerosis patients. J Clin Invest 1996; 98: 70–7.
11. Neurath MF, Fuss I, Kelsall BL, Presky DH, Waegell W, Strober W. Experimental granulomatous colitis in mice is abrogated by induction of TGF-beta-mediated oral tolerance. J Exp Med 1996; 183: 2605–16.
12. Ludviksson BR, Ehrhardt RO, Strober W. TGF-beta production regulates the development of the 2,4,6-trinitrophenol-conjugated keyhole limpet hemocyanin-induced colonic inflammation in IL-2-deficient mice. J Immunol 1997; 159: 3622–8.
13. Simpson SJ, Mizoguchi E, Allen D, Bhan AK, Terhorst C. Evidence that CD4$^+$, but not CD8$^+$ T cells are responsible for murine interleukin-2-deficient colitis. Eur J Immunol 1995; 25: 2618–25.
14. Cong Y, Weaver CT, Nguyen H, Lazenby A, Sundberg JP, Elson CO. CD8+ T cells, but not B cells inhibit enteric bacterial antigen-specific CD4$^+$ T cell-induced colitis. Gastroenterology 1999; 116: A690.
15. Fort MM, Leach MW, Rennick DM. A role for NK cells as regulators of CD4$^+$ T cells in a transfer model of colitis. J Immunol 1998; 161: 3256–61.
16. Saubermann LJ, Beck P, De Jong YP *et al.* Activation of natural killer T cells by alpha-galactosylceramide in the presence of CD1d provides protection against colitis in mice. Gastroenterology 2000; 119: 119–28.
17. Mizoguchi E, Mizoguchi A, Preffer FI, Bhan AK. Regulatory role of mature B cells in a murine model of inflammatory bowel disease. Int Immunol 2000; 12: 597–605.
18. Blunt T, Gell D, Fox M *et al.* Identification of a nonsense mutation in the carboxyl-terminal region of DNA-dependent protein kinase catalytic subunit in the scid mouse. Proc Natl Acad Sci USA 1996; 93: 10285–90.
19. Morrissey PJ, Charrier K, Braddy S, Liggitt D, Watson JD. CD4$^+$ T cells that express high levels of CD45RB induce wasting disease when transferred into congenic severe combined immunodeficient mice. Disease development is prevented by cotransfer of purified CD4$^+$ T cells. J Exp Med 1993; 178: 237–44.
20. Powrie F, Leach MW, Mauze S, Caddle LB, Coffman RL. Phenotypically distinct subsets of CD4$^+$ T cells induce or protect from chronic intestinal inflammation in C. B-17 scid mice. Int Immunol 1993; 5: 1461–71.
21. Powrie F, Leach MW, Mauze S, Menon S, Caddle LB, Coffman RL. Inhibition of Th1 responses prevents inflammatory bowel disease in scid mice reconstituted with CD45RBhi CD4$^+$ T cells. Immunity 1994; 1: 553–62.
22. Rudolphi A, Bonhagen K, Reimann J. Polyclonal expansion of adoptively transferred CD4$^+$ alpha beta T cells in the colonic lamina propria of scid mice with colitis. Eur J Immunol 1996; 26: 1156–63.
23. Bregenholt S, Claesson MH. Splenic T helper cell type 1 cytokine profile and extramedullary haematopoiesis in severe combined immunodeficient (scid) mice with inflammatory bowel disease (IBD). Clin Exp Immunol 1998; 111: 166–72.
24. Powrie F, Carlino J, Leach MW, Mauze S, Coffman RL. A critical role for transforming growth factor-beta but not interleukin 4 in the suppression of T helper type 1-mediated colitis by CD45RB(low) CD4$^+$ T cells. J Exp Med 1996; 183: 2669–74.
25. Asseman C, Mauze S, Leach MW, Coffman RL, Powrie F. An essential role for interleukin 10 in the function of regulatory T cells that inhibit intestinal inflammation. J Exp Med 1999; 190: 995–1004.
26. Annacker O, Burlen-Defranoux O, Pimenta-Araujo R, Cumano A, Bandeira A. Regulatory CD4 T cells control

the size of the peripheral activated/memory CD4 T cell compartment. J Immunol 2000; 164: 3573–80.

27. Takahashi T, Tagami T, Yamazaki S *et al*. Immunologic self-tolerance maintained by CD25(+)CD4(+) regulatory T cells constitutively expressing cytotoxic T lymphocyte-associated antigen 4. J Exp Med 2000; 192: 303–10.

28. Read S, Malmstrom V, Powrie F. Cytotoxic T lymphocyte-associated antigen 4 plays an essential role in the function of CD25(+)CD4(+) regulatory cells that control intestinal inflammation. J Exp Med 2000; 192: 295–302.

29. Hagenbaugh A, Sharma S, Dubinett SM *et al*. Altered immune responses in interleukin 10 transgenic mice. J Exp Med 1997; 185: 2101–10.

30. Aranda R, Sydora BC, McAllister PL *et al*. Analysis of intestinal lymphocytes in mouse colitis mediated by transfer of CD4$^+$, CD45RBhigh T cells to SCID recipients. J Immunol 1997; 158: 3464–73.

31. Picarella D, Hurlbut P, Rottman J, Shi X, Butcher E, Ringler DJ. Monoclonal antibodies specific for beta 7 integrin and mucosal addressin cell adhesion molecule-1 (MAdCAM-1) reduce inflammation in the colon of scid mice reconstituted with CD45RBhigh CD4$^+$ T cells. J Immunol 1997; 158: 2099–106.

32. Mackay F, Browning JL, Lawton P *et al*. Both the lymphotoxin and tumor necrosis factor pathways are involved in experimental murine models of colitis. Gastroenterology 1998; 115: 1464–75.

33. De Jong YP, Comiskey M, Kalled SL *et al*. Chronic murine colitis is dependent on the CD154/CD40 pathway and can be attenuated by anti-CD154 administration. Gastroenterology 2000; 119: 715–23.

34. Morrissey PJ, Charrier K. Induction of wasting disease in SCID mice by the transfer of normal CD4$^+$/CD45RBhi T cells and the regulation of this autoreactivity by CD4$^+$/CD45RB^{lo} T cells. Res Immunol 1994; 145: 357–62.

35. Matsuda JL, Gapin L, Sydora BC, Systemic activation and antigen-driven oligoclonal expansion of T cells in a mouse model of colitis. J Immunol 2000; 164: 2797–806.

36. Brimnes J, Reimann J, Mogens MH, Claessen MH. Enteric bacterial antigens activate CD4$^+$ T cells from scid mice with inflammatory bowel disease. Eur J Immunol 2001; 31: 23–31.

37. Kuhn R, Lohler J, Rennick D, Rajewsky K, Muller W. Interleukin-10-deficient mice develop chronic enterocolitis. Cell 1993; 75: 263–74.

38. Sellon RK, Tonkonogy S, Schultz M *et al*. Resident enteric bacteria are necessary for development of spontaneous colitis and immune system activation in interleukin-10-deficient mice. Infect Immun 1998; 66: 5224–31.

39. Berg DJ, Kuhn R, Rajewsky K *et al*. Interleukin-10 is a central regulator of the response to LPS in murine models of endotoxic shock and the Shwartzman reaction but not endotoxin tolerance. J Clin Invest 1995; 96: 2339–47.

40. Davidson NJ, Leach MW, Fort MM *et al*. T helper cell 1-type CD4$^+$ T cells, but not B cells, mediate colitis in interleukin-10-deficient mice. J Exp Med 1996; 184: 241–51.

41. Berg D, Davidson N, Kuhn R *et al*. Enterocolitis and colon cancer interleukin-10-deficient mice are associated with aberrant cytokine production and CD4$^+$ Th1-like responses. J Clin Invest 1996; 98: 1010–20.

42. Rennick DM, Fort MM, Davidson NJ. Studies with IL-10–/– mice: an overview. J Leuk Biol 1997; 61: 389–96.

43. Davidson NJ, Hudak SA, Lesley RE, Menon S, Leach MW, Rennick DM. IL-12, but not IFN-gamma, plays a major role in sustaining the chronic phase of colitis in IL-10-deficient mice. J Immunol 1998; 161: 3143–9.

44. Brandwein SL, McCabe RP, Cong Y *et al*. Spontaneously colitic C3H/HeJBir mice demonstrate selective antibody reactivity to antigens of the enteric bacterial flora. J Immunol 1997; 159: 44–52.

45. Seibold F, Brandwein S, Simpson S, Terhorst C, Elson CO. pANCA represents a cross-reactivity to enteric bacterial antigens. J Clin Immunol 1998; 18: 153–60.

46. Bristol IJ, Farmer MA, Cong Y *et al*. Heritable susceptibility for colitis in mice induced by IL-10 deficiency. Inflam Bowel Dis 2000; 6: 290–302.

47. Farmer MA, Leiter EH, Churchill GA, Sundberg JP, Elson CO. Complex interactions among modifier genes controlling colitis severity in IL-10 deficient mice. Gastroenterology 2001; 120: A36.

48. Spencer SD, Di Marco F, Hooley J *et al*. The orphan receptor CRF2-4 is an essential subunit of the interleukin 10 receptor. J Exp Med 1998; 187: 571–8.

49. Kundig TM, Schorle H, Bachmann MF, Hengartner H, Zinkernagel RM, Horak I. Immune responses in interleukin-2-deficient mice. Science 1993; 262: 1059–61.

50. Ma A, Datta M, Margosian E, Chen J, Horak I. T cells, but not B cells, are required for bowel inflammation in interleukin 2-deficient mice. J Exp Med 1995; 182: 1567–72.

51. Kramer S, Schimpl A, Hunig T. Immunopathology of interleukin (IL) 2-deficient mice: thymus dependence and suppression by thymus-dependent cells with an intact IL-2 gene. J Exp Med 1995; 182: 1769–76.

52. Sadlack B, Lohler J, Schorle H *et al*. Generalized autoimmune disease in interleukin-2-deficient mice is triggered by an uncontrolled activation and proliferation of CD4$^+$ T cells. Eur J Immunol 1995; 25: 3053–9.

53. Ehrhardt RO, Ludviksson BR, Gray B, Neurath M, Strober W. Induction and prevention of colonic inflammation in IL-2-deficient mice. J Immunol 1997; 158: 566-73.

54. Ludviksson BR, Strober W, Nishikomori R, Hasan SK, Ehrhardt RO. Administration of mAb against alpha E beta 7 prevents and ameliorates immunization-induced colitis in IL-2–/– mice. J Immunol 1999; 162: 4975–82.

55. Kneitz B, Herrmann T, Yonehara S, Schimpl A. Normal clonal expansion but impaired Fas-mediated cell death and anergy induction in interleukin-2-deficient mice. Eur J Immunol 1995; 25: 2572-7.

56. Poussier P, Ning T, Chen J, Banerjee D, Julius M. Intestinal inflammation observed in IL-2R/IL-2 mutant mice is associated with impaired intestinal T lymphopoiesis. Gastroenterology 2000; 118: 880–91.

57. Papiernik M, de Moraes ML, Pontoux C, Vasseur F, Penit C. Regulatory CD4 T cells: expression of IL-2R alpha chain, resistance to clonal deletion and IL-2 dependency. Int Immunol 1998; 10: 371–8.

58. Sakaguchi S, Toda M, Asano M, Itoh M, Morse SS, Sakaguchi N. T cell-mediated maintenance of natural self-tolerance: its breakdown as a possible cause of various autoimmune diseases. J Autoimmun 1996; 9: 211–20.

59. Contractor NV, Bassiri H, Reya T *et al*. Lymphoid hyperplasia, autoimmunity, and compromised intestinal intraepithelial lymphocyte development in colitis-free gnotobiotic IL-2-deficient mice. J Immunol 1998; 160: 385–94.

60. Mähler M, Serreze D, Evans R, Linder CD, Leiter EH, Sundberg JP. IL-2^{tm1Hor}, an interleukin-2 gene targeted mutation: the Jackson Laboratory, Bar Harbor, ME; Fall 1996. Report No. 467.

61. Wang B, Biron C, She J *et al*. A block in both early T lymphocyte and natural killer cell development in transgenic mice with high-copy numbers of the human CD3E gene. Proc Natl Acad Sci USA 1994; 91: 9402–6.

62. Hollander GA, Wang B, Nichogiannopoulou A *et al*. Developmental control point in induction of thymic cortex regulated by a subpopulation of prothymocytes. Nature 1995; 373: 350–3.

63. Hollander GA, Simpson SJ, Mizoguchi E *et al.* Severe colitis in mice with aberrant thymic selection. Immunity 1995; 3: 27–38.

64. Velkamp C, Tonkonogy SL, De Jong YP *et al.* Continuous stimulation by normal luminal bacteria is essential for the development and perpetuation of colitis in Tg epsilon 26 mice. Gastroenterology 2001; 120: 900–13.

65. Simpson SJ, Dc Jong YP, Shah SA *et al.* Consequences of Fas-ligand and perforin expression by colon T cells in a mouse model of inflammatory bowel disease. Gastroenterology 1998; 115: 849–55.

66. Simpson SJ, Hollander GA, Mizoguchi E *et al.* Expression of pro-inflammatory cytokines by TCR alpha beta+ and TCR gamma delta+ T cells in an experimental model of colitis. Eur J Immunol 1997; 27: 17–25.

67. Mombaerts P, Mizoguchi E, Grusby MJ, Glimcher LH, Bhan AK, Tonegawa S. Spontaneous development of inflammatory bowel disease in T cell receptor mutant mice. Cell 1993; 75: 1–20.

68. Mizoguchi E, Mizoguchi A, Bhan AK. Role of cytokines in the early stages of chronic colitis in TCR alpha-mutant mice. Lab Invest 1997; 76: 385–97.

69. Mizoguchi A, Mizoguchi E, Chiba C *et al.* Cytokine imbalance and autoantibody production in T cell receptor-alpha mutant mice with inflammatory bowel disease. J Exp Med 1996; 183: 847–56.

70. Mombaerts P, Mizoguchi E, Ljunggren HG *et al.* Peripheral lymphoid development and function in TCR mutant mice. Int Immunol 1994; 6: 1061–70.

71. Das KM, Dasgupta A, Mandal A, Geng X. Autoimmunity to cytoskeletal protein tropomyosin. A clue to the pathogenetic mechanism for ulcerative colitis. J Immunol 1993; 150: 2487–93.

72. Bhan AK, Mizoguchi E, Smith RN, Mizoguchi A. Colitis in transgenic and knockout animals as models of human inflammatory bowel disease. Immunol Rev 1999; 169: 195–207.

73. Takahashi I, Kiyono H, Hamada S. A CD4$^+$ T-cell population mediates development of inflammatory bowel disease in T-cell receptor alpha-deficient mice. Gastroenterology 1997; 112: 1876–82.

74. Mizoguchi A, Mizoguchi E, Saubermann LJ, Higaki K, Blumberg RS, Bhan AK. Limited CD4 T-cell diversity associated with colitis in T-cell receptor alpha mutant mice requires a T helper 2 environment. Gastroenterology 2000; 119: 983–95.

75. Dianda L, Hanby AM, Wright NA, Sebesteny A, Hayday AC, Owen MJ. T cell receptor-alpha beta-deficient mice fail to dcvclop colitis in the absence of a microbial environment. Am J Pathol 1997; 150: 91–7.

76. Mizoguchi A, Mizoguchi E, Chiba C, Bhan AK. Role of appendix in the development of inflammatory bowel disease in TCR-alpha mutant mice. J Exp Med 1996; 184: 707–15.

77. Mizoguchi A, Mizoguchi E, Tonegawa S, Bhan AK. Alteration of a polyclonal to an oligoclonal immune response to cecal aerobic bacterial antigens in TCRα mutant mice with inflammatory bowel disease. Int Immunol 1996; 8: 1387–94.

78. Mizoguchi A, Mizoguchi E, Bhan AK. The critical role of interleukin 4 but not interferon gamma in the pathogenesis of colitis in T-cell receptor alpha mutant mice. Gastroenterology 1999; 116: 320–6.

79. Mizoguchi A, Mizoguchi E, Smith RN, Preffer FI, Bhan AK. Suppressive role of B cells in chronic colitis of T cell receptor alpha mutant mice. J Exp Med 1997; 186: 1749–56.

80. Mizoguchi A, Mizoguchi E, Smith RN, Preffer FI, Bhan AK. Suppressive role of B cells in chronic colitis of T cell receptor α mutant mice. J Exp Med 1997; 186: 1749–56.

81. Kulkarni AB, Ward JM, Yaswen L, Transforming growth factor-beta 1 null mice. An animal model for inflammatory disorders. Am J Pathol 1995; 146: 264–75.

82. Boivin GP, O'Toole BA, Orsmby IE *et al.* Onset and progression of pathological lesions in transforming growth factor-beta 1-deficient mice. Am J Pathol 1995; 146: 276–88.

83. Boivin GP, Ormsby I, Jones-Carson J, O'Toole BA, Doetschman T. Germ-free and barrier-raised TGF beta 1-deficient mice have similar inflammatory lesions. Transgenic Res 1997; 6: 197–202.

84. Letterio JJ, Geiser AG, Kulkarni AB *et al.* Autoimmunity associated with TGF-beta1-deficiency in mice is dependent on MHC class II antigen expression. J Clin Invest 1996; 98: 2109–19.

85. Diebold RJ, Eis MJ, Yin M *et al.* Early-onset multifocal inflammation in the transforming growth factor beta 1-null mouse is lymphocyte mediated. Proc Natl Acad Sci USA 1995; 92: 12215–19.

86. Gorelik L, Flavell RA. Abrogation of TGFbeta signaling in T cells leads to spontaneous T cell differentiation and autoimmune disease. Immunity 2000; 12: 171–81.

87. Lucas PJ, Kim SJ, Melby SJ, Gress RE. Disruption of T cell homeostasis in mice expressing a T cell-specific dominant negative transforming growth factor beta II receptor. J Exp Med 2000; 191: 1187–96.

88. Yang X, Letterio JJ, Lechleider RJ *et al.* Targeted disruption of SMAD3 results in impaired mucosal immunity and diminished T cell responsiveness to TGF-beta. EMBO J 1999; 18: 1280–91.

89. Watanabe M, Ueno Y, Yajima T *et al.* Interleukin 7 is produced by human intestinal epithelial cells and regulates the proliferation of intestinal mucosal lymphocytes. J Clin Invest 1995; 95: 2945–53.

90. Fujihashi K, Kawabata S, Hiroi T, Interleukin 2 (IL-2) and interleukin 7 (IL-7) reciprocally induce IL-7 and IL-2 receptors on gamma delta T-cell receptor-positive intraepithelial lymphocytes. Proc Natl Acad Sci USA 1996; 93: 3613–8.

91. Fujihashi K, McGhee JR, Yamamoto M, Peschon JJ, Kiyono H. An interleukin-7 internet for intestinal intraepithelial T cell development: knockout of ligand or receptor reveal differences in the immunodeficient state. Eur J Immunol 1997; 27: 2133–8.

92. Watanabe M, Ueno Y, Yajima T *et al.* Interleukin 7 transgenic mice develop chronic colitis with decreased interleukin 7 protein accumulation in the colonic mucosa. J Exp Med 1998; 187: 389–402.

93. Targan SR, Hanauer SB, van Deventer SJ *et al.* A short-term study of chimeric monoclonal antibody cA2 to tumor necrosis factor alpha for Crohn's disease. Crohn's Disease cA2 Study Group. N Engl J Med 1997; 337: 1029–35.

94. Kontoyiannis D, Pasparakis M, Pizarro TT, Cominelli F, Kollias G. Impaired on/off regulation of TNF biosynthesis in mice lacking TNF AU-rich elements: implications for joint and gut-associated immunopathologies. Immunity 1999; 10: 387–98.

95. Kollias G, Douni E, Kassiotis G, Kontoyiannis D. On the role of tumor necrosis factor and receptors in models of multiorgan failure, rheumatoid arthritis, multiple sclerosis and inflammatory bowel disease. Immunol Rev 1999; 169: 175–94.

96. Lee EG, Boone DL, Chai S *et al.* Failure to regulate TNF-induced NF-kappaB and cell death responses in A20-deficient mice. Science 2000; 289: 2350–4.

97. Byrne FR, Whoriskey JS, Sarmiento U *et al.* Transgenic mice over-expressing the B7 related protein-1 (B7RP-1) develop an intestinal pathology similar to human Crohn's disease. A new mouse model of inflammatory bowel disease. Gastroenterology 2001: A47.

98. Foy TM, Aruffo A, Bajorath J, Buhlmann JE, Noelle RJ. Immune regulation by CD40 and its ligand GP39. Annu Rev Immunol 1996; 14: 591–617.

99. Grewal IS, Flavell RA. CD40 and CD154 in cell-mediated immunity. Annu Rev Immunol 1998; 16: 111–35.

100. Clegg CH, Rulffes JT, Haugen HS *et al.* Thymus dysfunction and chronic inflammatory disease in gp39 transgenic mice. Int Immunol 1997; 9: 1111–22.

101. Cong Y, Weaver CT, Lazenby A, Elson CO. Colitis induced by enteric bacterial antigen-specific CD4+ T cells requires CD40–CD40 ligand interactions for a sustained increase in mucosal IL-12. J Immunol 2000; 165: 2173–82.

102. Sundberg JP, Elson CO, Bedigian H, Birkenmeier EH. Spontaneous, heritable colitis in a new substrain of C3H/HeJ mice. Gastroenterology 1994; 107: 1726–35.

103. McCabe RP, Sharmanov A, Birkenmeier E, Sundberg J, Elson CO. Mucosal immune abnormalities in C3H/HeJBir mice with susceptibility to colitis. Gastroenterology 1994; 106: A731.

104. Ni J, Chen SF, Hollander D. Immunological abnormality in C3H/HeJ mice with heritable inflammatory bowel disease. Cell Immunol 1996; 169: 7–15.

105. Cong Y, Brandwein SL, McCabe RP *et al.* CD4+ T cells reactive to enteric bacterial antigens in spontaneously colitic C3H/HeJBir mice: increased T helper cell type 1 response and ability to transfer disease. J Exp Med 1998; 187: 855–64.

106. Cong Y, Weaver CT, Lazenby A, Elson CO. T-regulatory-1 (Tr1) cells that prevent CD4+ T cell colitis inhibit the antigen-presenting function and IL-12 production of dendritic cells. Gastroenterology 2001; 120: A38.

107. Mahler M, Bristol IJ, Leiter EH *et al.* Differential susceptibility of inbred mouse strains to dextran sulfate sodium-induced colitis. Am J Physiol 1998; 274: G544–51.

108. Matsumoto S, Okabe Y, Setoyama H *et al.* Inflammatory bowel disease-like enteritis and caecitis in a senescence accelerated mouse P1/Yit strain. Gut 1998; 43: 71–8.

109. Takeda K, Clausen BE, Kaisho T *et al.* Enhanced Th1 activity and development of chronic enterocolitis in mice devoid of Stat3 in macrophages and neutrophils. Immunity 1999; 10: 39–49.

110. Kosiewicz MM, Nast CC, Krishnan A *et al.* Th1-type responses mediate spontaneous ileitis in a novel murine model of Crohn's disease. J Clin Invest 2001; 107: 695–702.

111. Eckmann L, Kagnoff MF, Fierer J. Epithelial cells secrete the chemokine interleukin-8 in response to bacterial entry. Infect Immun 1993; 61: 4569–74.

112. McCormick BA, Colgan SP, Delp-Archer C, Miller SI, Madara JL. *Salmonella typhimurium* attachment to human intestinal epithelial monolayers: transcellular signalling to subepithelial neutrophils. J Cell Biol 1993; 123: 895–907.

113. Hugot J-P, Chamaillard M, Zouali H *et al.* Association of NOD2 leucine-rich repeat variants with susceptibility to Crohn's disease. Nature 2001; 411: 599–603.

114. Ogura Y, Bonen DK, Inohara N *et al.* A frameshift mutation in NOD2 associated with susceptibility to Crohn's disease. Nature 2001; 411: 603–606.

115. Katz KD, Hollander D, Vadheim CM *et al.* Intestinal permeability in patients with Crohn's disease and their healthy relatives. Gastroenterology 1989; 97: 927–31.

116. Toy LS, Yio XY, Lin A, Honig S, Mayer L. Defective expression of gp180, a novel CD8 ligand on intestinal epithelial cells, in inflammatory bowel disease. J Clin Invest 1997; 100: 2062–71.

117. Madara J, Stafford J. Interferon-γamma directly affects barrier function of cultured intestinal epithelial monolayers. J Clin Invest 1989; 83: 724.

118. Dieleman LA, Elson CO, Tennyson GS, Beagley KW. Kinetics of cytokine expression during healing of acute colitis in mice. Am J Physiol 1996; 34: G 130–6.

119. Hermiston ML, Gordon JI. Inflammatory bowel disease and adenomas in mice expressing a dominant negative N-cadherin. Science 1995; 270: 1203–7.

120. Panwala CM, Jones JC, Viney JL. A novel model of inflammatory bowel disease: mice deficient for the multiple drug resistance gene, mdr1a, spontaneously develop colitis. J Immunol 1998; 161: 5733–44.

121. Rudolph U, Finegold MJ, Rich SS *et al.* Ulcerative colitis and adenocarcinoma of the colon in G alpha i2-deficient mice. Nat Genet 1995; 10: 143–50.

122. Hornquist CE, Lu X, Rogers-Fani PM *et al.* G(alpha)i2-deficient mice with colitis exhibit a local increase in memory CD4+ T cells and proinflammatory Th1-type cytokines. J Immunol 1997; 158: 1068–77.

123. Ohman L, Franzen L, Rudolph U, Harriman GR, Hultgren-Hornquist E. Immune activation in the intestinal mucosa before the onset of colitis in Galphai2-deficient mice. Scand J Immunol 2000; 52: 80–90.

124. Mashimo H, Wu DC, Podolsky DK, Fishman MC. Impaired defense of intestinal mucosa in mice lacking intestinal trefoil factor. Science 1996; 274: 262–5.

125. Baribault H, Penner J, Iozzo RV, Wilson-Heiner M. Colorectal hyperplasia and inflammation in keratin 8-deficient FVB/N mice. Genes Devel 1994; 8: 2964–73.

126. Magin TM, Schroder R, Leitgeb S *et al.* Lessons from keratin 18 knockout mice: formation of novel keratin filaments, secondary loss of keratin 7 and accumulation of liver-specific keratin 8-positive aggregates. J Cell Biol 1998; 140: 1441–51.

127. Okayasu I, Hatakeyama S, Yamada M, Ohkusa T, Inagaki Y, Nakaya R. A novel method in the induction of reliable experimental acute and chronic ulcerative colitis in mice. Gastroenterology 1990; 98: 694–702.

128. Cooper HS, Murthy SN, Shah RS, Sedergran DJ. Clinicopathologic study of dextran sulfate sodium experimental murine colitis. Lab Invest 1993; 69: 238–49.

129. Yamada M, Ohkusa T, Okayasu I. Occurrence of dysplasia and adenocarcinoma after experimental chronic ulcerative colitis in hamsters induced by dextran sulphate sodium. Gut 1992; 33: 1521–7.

130. Hirono I, Kuhara K, Hosaka S, Tomizawa S, Goldberg L. Induction of intestinal tumors in rats by dextran sulfate sodium. J Natl Cancer Inst 1981; 66: 579–83.

131. Dieleman LA, Ridwan BU, Tennyson GS, Beagley KW, Bucy RP, Elson CO. Dextran sulfate sodium-induced colitis occurs in severe combined immunodeficient mice. Gastroenterology 1994; 107: 1643–52.

132. Mahler M, Bristol IJ, Sundberg JP *et al.* Genetic analysis of susceptibility to dextran sulfate sodium-induced colitis in mice. Genomics 1999; 55: 147–56.

133. Morris GP, Beck PL, Herridge MS, Depew WT, Szewczuk MR, Wallace JL. Hapten-induced model of chronic inflammation and ulceration in the rat colon. Gastroenterology 1989; 96: 795–803.

134. Neurath MF, Fuss I, Kelsall BL, Stuber E, Strober W. Antibodies to interleukin 12 abrogate established experimental colitis in mice. J Exp Med 1995; 182: 1281–90.

135. Elson CO, Beagley KW, Sharmanov AT, Hapten-induced model of murine inflammatory bowel disease – mucosal immune responses and protection by tolerance. J Immunol 1996; 157: 2174–85.

136. Brandtzaeg P, Valnes K, Scott H, Rognum TO, Bjerke K, Baklien K. The human gastrointestinal secretory system in health and disease. Scand J Gastroenterol 1985; 20: 17–38.

137. Kelsall BL, Stuber E, Neurath M, Strober W. Interleukin-12 production by dendritic cells. The role of CD40–CD40L

interactions in Th1 T-cell responses. Ann NY Acad Sci 1996; 795: 116–26.

138. Duchmann R, Schmitt E, Knolle P, Meyer zum Buschenfelde KH, Neurath M. Tolerance towards resident intestinal flora in mice is abrogated in experimental colitis and restored by treatment with interleukin-10 or antibodies to interleukin-12. Eur J Immunol 1996; 26: 934–8.

139. Neurath MF, Pettersson S, Meyer Zum Buuschenfeld K-H, Strober W. Local administration of antisense phosphorothionate oligonucleotides to the p65 subunit of NFkB abrogates established experimental colitis in mice. Nature Med 1996; 2: 998–1004.

140. Hammer RE, Maika SD, Richardson JA, Tang JP, Taurog JD. Spontaneous inflammatory disease in transgenic rats expressing HLA-B27 and human beta 2m: an animal model of HLA-B27-associated human disorders. Cell 1990; 63: 1099–112.

141. Breban M, Hammer RE, Richardson JA, Taurog JD. Transfer of the inflammatory disease of HLA-B27 transgenic rats by bone marrow engraftment. J Exp Med 1993; 178: 1607–16.

142. Taurog JD, Richardson JA, Croft JT et al. The germfree state prevents development of gut and joint inflammatory disease in HLA-B27 transgenic rats. J Exp Med 1994; 180: 2359–64.

143. Rath HC, Herfarth HH, Ikeda JS et al. Normal luminal bacteria, especially *Bacteroides* species, mediate chronic colitis, gastritis, and arthritis in HLA-B27/human beta2 microglobulin transgenic rats. J Clin Invest 1996; 98: 945–53.

144. Snapper SB, Rosen FS, Mizoguchi E et al. Wiskott–Aldrich syndrome protein-deficient mice reveal a role for WASP in T but not B cell activation. Immunity 1998; 9: 81–91.

145. Koh WP, Chan E, Scott K, McCaughan G, France M, Fazekas de St Groth B. TCR-mediated involvement of CD4+ transgenic T cells in spontaneous inflammatory bowel disease in lymphopenic mice. J Immunol 1999; 162: 7208–16.

146. Miller AM, Elliot PR, Connell W, Desmond PV, d'Apice AJ. A novel model of ulcerative colitis based on genetic manipulation of the glycosylation of colonic mucins. Gastroenterology 2000; 118: A687.

147. Kalliomaki M, Salminen S, Arvilommi H, Kero P, Koskinen P, Isolauri E. Probiotics in primary prevention of atopic disease: a randomized placebo-controlled trial. Lancet 2001; 357: 1076–9.

148. Moore WEC, Holdeman LV. Human fecal flora: the normal flora of 20 Japanese-Hawaiians. Appl Microbiol 1974; 27: 961–79.

149. Crabbe PA, Bazin H, Eyssen H, Heremans JF. The normal microbial flora as a major stimulus for proliferation of plasma cells synthesizing IgA in the gut. The germ-free intestinal tract. Int Arch Allergy 1968; 34: 362–75.

150. Okada Y, Setoyama H, Matsumoto S et al. Effects of fecal microorganisms and their chloroform-resistant variants derived from mice, rats, and humans on immunological and physiological characteristics of the intestines of exγermfree mice. Infect Immun 1994; 62: 5442–6.

151. Klaasen HL, Koopman JP, Van den Brink ME, Bakker MH, Poelma FG, Beynen AC. Intestinal, segmented, filamentous bacteria in a wide range of vertebrate species. Lab Anim 1993; 27: 141–50.

152. Klaasen HL, Van der Heijden PJ, Stok W et al. Apathogenic, intestinal, segmented, filamentous bacteria stimulate the mucosal immune system of mice. Infect Immun 1993; 61: 303–6.

153. Umesaki Y, Okada Y, Matsumoto S, Imaoka A, Setoyama H. Segmented filamentous bacteria are indigenous intestinal bacteria that activate intraepithelial lymphocytes and in-

duce MHC class II molecules and fucosyl asialo GM1 glycolipids on the small intestinal epithelial cells in the exγerm-free mouse. Microb Immunol 1995; 39: 555–62.

154. Klapproth JM, Donnenberg MS, Abraham JM, James SP. Products of enteropathogenic *E. coli* inhibit lymphokine production by gastrointestinal lymphocytes. Am J Physiol 1996; 271: G841–8.

155. Klapproth JM, Donnenberg MS, Abraham JM, Mobley HL, James SP. Products of enteropathogenic *Escherichia coli* inhibit lymphocyte activation and lymphokine production. Infect Immun 1995; 63: 2248–54.

156. Neish AS, Gewirtz AT, Zeng H et al. Prokaryotic regulation of epithelial responses by inhibition of IkappaB-alpha ubiquitination. Science 2000; 289: 1560–3.

157. Madsen KL, Doyle JS, Jewell LD, Tavernini MM, Fedorak RN. *Lactobacillus* species prevents colitis in interleukin 10 gene-deficient mice. Gastroenterology 1999; 116: 1107–14.

158. Schultz M, Sartor RB. Probiotics and inflammatory bowel diseases. Am J Gastroenterol 2000; 95(Suppl. 1): S19–21.

159. Steidler L, Hans W, Schotte L et al. Treatment of murine colitis by *Lactococcus lactis* secreting interleukin-10. Science 2000; 289: 1352–5.

160. Duchmann R, Kaiser I, Hermann E, Mayet W, Ewe K, Meyer zum Buschenfelde KH. Tolerance exists towards resident intestinal flora but is broken in active inflammatory bowel disease (IBD). Clin Exp Immunol 1995; 102: 448–55.

161. Wirtz S, Finotto S, Kanzler S et al. Cutting edge: chronic intestinal inflammation in STAT-4 transgenic mice: characterization of disease and adoptive transfer by TNF- plus IFN-gamma-producing CD4(+) T cells that respond to bacterial antigens. J Immunol 1999; 162: 1884–8.

162. Berg DJ, Weinstock J, Lynch R. Rapid induction of inflammatory bowel disease in NSAID-treated IL-10 –/– mice. Gastroenterology 2001; 120: A685.

163. Sadlack B, Merz H, Schorle H, Schimpl A, Feller AC, Horak I. Ulcerative colitis-like disease in mice with a disrupted interleukin-2 gene. Cell 1993; 75: 253–61.

164. Willerford D, Chen J, Ferry J, Davidson L, Ma A, Alt F. Interleukin-2 receptor alpha chain regulates the size and content of the peripheral lymphoid compartment. Immunity 1995; 3: 521–30.

165. Shull MM, Ormsby I, Kier AB et al. Targeted disruption of the mouse transforming growth factor-beta 1 gene results in multifocal inflammatory disease. Nature 1992; 359: 693–9.

166. Rudolph U, Finegold MJ, Rich SS et al. G(i2)alpha protein deficiency: A model for inflammatory bowel disease. J Clin Immunol 1995; 15(Suppl 6.): S101–5.

167. Madara JL, Podolsky DK, King NW, Sehgal PK, Moore R, Winter HS. Characterization of spontaneous colitis in cotton-top tamarins (*Saguinus oedipus*) and its response to sulfasalazine. Gastroenterology 1985; 88: 13–9.

168. Neurath M, Fuss I, Strober W. TNBS-colitis. Int Rev Immunol 2000; 19: 51–62.

169. Boirivant M, Fuss IJ, Chu A, Strober W. Oxazolone colitis: a murine model of T helper cell type 2 colitis treatable with antibodies to interleukin 4. J Exp Med 1998; 188: 1929–39.

170. Sartor RB, Cromartie WJ, Powell DW, Schwab JH. Granulomatous enterocolitis induced in rats by purified bacterial cell wall fragments. Gastroenterology 1985; 89: 587–95.

171. Sartor RB, Bender DE, Allen JB et al. Chronic experimental enterocolitis and extraintestinal inflammation are T lymphocyte dependent. Gastroenterology 1993; 104: A775.

172. Sartor RB, Bender DE, Holt LC. Susceptibility of inbred rat strains to intestinal inflammation induced by indomethacin. Gastroenterology 1992; 102: A690.

173. Taurog JD, Maika SD, Simmons WA, Breban M, Hammer RE. Susceptibility to inflammatory disease in HLA-B27 transgenic rat lines correlates with the level of B27 expression. J Immunol 1993; 150: 4168–78.

5 | The normal intestinal mucosa: a state of 'controlled inflammation'

CLAUDIO FIOCCHI

Introduction

The focus of investigation in inflammatory bowel disease (IBD) is almost invariably centered on the various cellular and soluble components of the mucosal immune system whose abnormal number or functions presumably underlies the pathogenesis of chronic intestinal inflammation. Although this approach is obviously justified, it is easy to lose sight of the peculiar conditions that allow the normal intestinal immune system to exert a protective rather than an aggressive role. As a matter of fact the intestinal immune system is not only the largest of the body, but primarily a biological shield functioning in unique ways that distinguish it from all other defense mechanisms. Because it is constantly exposed to the external environment, and carries an extremely rich and varied endogenous flora, the gut mucosa is adapted to work under intense, yet physiological, conditions of permanent antigenic pressure. This pressure requires and brings into action an enormous amount of organized (Peyer's patches and lymphoid follicles) and diffuse (intraepithelial lymphocytes and lamina propria mononuclear cells) lymphoid cells that respectively form the gut-associated lymphoid tissue (GALT) and the mucosa-associated lymphoid tissue (MALT) [1]. The existence of this population of mature immunocytes all along the lining of the gastrointestinal tract is quantitatively and qualitatively unparalleled in other organs, including those with a mucosal surface such as the oral cavity, the lungs and airways, the genitourinary tract, and the mammary glands. For this reason the term 'controlled' or 'physiological intestinal inflammation' has been coined to reflect the fact that activated immunocytes are present in large numbers and, rather than causing injury, afford instead an essential protection to the gut and indirectly the rest of the body. Despite its importance this terminology is seldom used outside of the realm of mucosal immunology and it is difficult to find it even in comprehensive textbooks of mucosal immunology [2].

Interestingly, the majority of components and functions involved in physiological intestinal inflammation are the same responsible for pathological inflammation as found in IBD and other conditions. Thus, the question arises of what distinguishes one from the other, and the answer is the appropriateness or not of the local defense mechanisms. There is not enough information to clearly define what constitutes an inappropriate defense response in IBD and why it endures over time, but there is a reasonably good knowledge of the components responsible for physiological intestinal inflammation (Fig. 1). Since avoiding all dietary, microbial or self stimuli that are potentially harmful is practically impossible, the intestine has devised control mechanisms that allow it to limit the quantity and quality of the antigens presented to the mucosa and GALT. According to Fig. 1 an appropriate response resulting in physiological inflammation relies on two types of control mechanisms: physical and biological. The first depends on the intrinsic properties of the gut and epithelium, while the latter involves circulatory, humoral and immune mechanisms. Immune mechanisms rely on both innate and adaptive responses, and when specific immunity is required it can either incite a switch-on response by the induction of effector cells that eliminate the antigen (active immunity), or a switch-off response resulting in a lack or suppression of response to the antigen (tolerance). An elaborate discussion of each component and function listed in the diagram is beyond the scope of this review, and some of these topics will be covered more comprehensively in other chapters of this book. Instead, the goal of this review is to provide the reader with an integrated overview of the components that together are presumably

Stephan R. Targan, Fergus Shanahan and Loren C. Karp (eds.), Inflammatory Bowel Disease: From Bench to Bedside, 2nd Edition, 101–120.
© 2003 *Kluwer Academic Publishers. Printed in Great Britain*

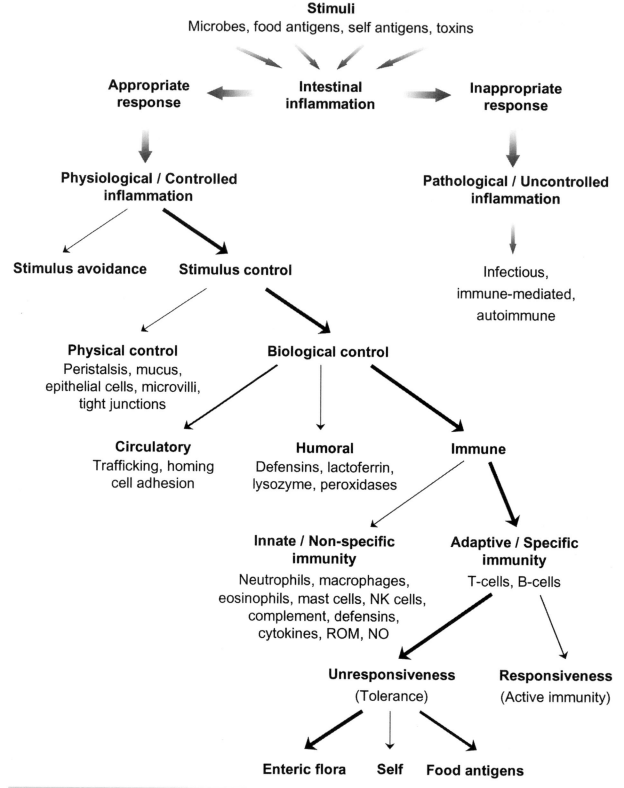

Figure 1. Diagram of the various components responsible for the induction and maintenance of physiological intestinal inflammation. The relative thickness of the solid arrows indicates the proportional contribution of single components to each defensive system.

responsible for the induction and maintenance of physiological inflammation in the human intestine.

Physical control mechanisms

Physical control mechanisms that contribute to physiological intestinal inflammation include primarily those that exclude, limit or select the amount and type of antigenic stimuli that can activate local lymphoid cells. This classification is arbitrary and somewhat artificial because even elements that exert an essentially pure mechanical function, such as peristalsis and the mucus coat, depend on and are integrated with other biological functions. These control mechanisms form what is commonly referred to as intestinal mucosal barrier.

Peristalsis

Peristalsis, the coordinated contraction of the bowel propelling its luminal content aborally, prevents the unnecessary accumulation of food-derived proteins, bacteria, parasites or toxins, and therefore decreases the possibility of absorbing an excessive antigenic load that may induce inflammation [3].

Mucus

The clinical observation that mucus production and release is enhanced during gut inflammation has long been associated with a protective function. Intestinal mucus is a viscoelastic gel composed of large mucin molecules made up by a small protein core and a complex array of oligosaccharide chains. The various mucin gene products are selectively expressed by different cells along the small and large bowel, suggesting that each mucin plays a distinctive role in mucosal protection [4]. Mucus prevents mechanical damage of the mucosa, enables shedding and renewal of mucosal surfaces, functions as a selective barrier for macromolecules and micro-organisms and a trap impeding the penetration of larger microbes, and retains defensive molecules on the luminal surface, such as secretory IgA (sIgA) [5]. Together, these integrated activities generate an important barrier that lowers the damaging and proinflammatory potential of the luminal contents.

Epithelial cells

Just underneath the mucus coat lies a single cell layer of intestinal epithelial cells that offer a variety of physical and functional protective mechanisms. Intestinal epithelial cells are heterogeneous and include columnar, goblet, Paneth, enteroendocrine and undifferentiated stem cells [6]. Each type has unique morphological features translating distinct physiological and defensive roles. In addition, there are specialized epithelial cells overlying lymphoid follicles called follicle-associated epithelium. Such cells are referred to as M cells; they have less developed microvilli and play a significant role in limiting and selecting antigen sampling [7]. Epithelial cells provide diverse protective systems that include the microvilli with their large surface and negative charge, the lipid bilayer of the plasma membrane, intracellular organelles containing degradative enzymes, and the junctions between adjacent cells. Prominent among the effector mechanisms mediated by these various systems are enhanced salt and water secretion, expression of antimicrobial proteins and peptides, and production of mucin [8]. Most of these systems are regulated by locally produced cytokines [9], and epithelial cells themselves are a source of proinflammatory cytokines, especially in response to bacterial invasion [10]. This paradoxical phenomenon has been proposed to actually represent an early protective defense mechanism of the mucosa by limiting bacterial invasion through a repertoire of regulatory molecules including cytokines, chemokines, adhesion molecules, prostanoids, nitric oxide and the induction of epithelial cell apoptosis [11, 12].

Antigens can penetrate the epithelium directly through individual epithelial cells (transcellular route) or the space between two cells (paracellular route). When antigens are absorbed transcellularly they are internally processed by individual cells, destroyed or degraded for exposure on the cell surface in the context of major histocompatibility complex (MHC) class II antigens for presentation to local T cells. Although this series of events could be construed as stimulatory and potentially proinflammatory, under normal circumstances the ultimate effect is a limitation in antigen presentation and the selective activation of T cell subsets [13]. First, intestinal epithelial cells are less efficient than professional antigen-presenting cells (APC) such as macrophages and dendritic cells. Second, they activate preferentially CD8[+] cytotoxic/suppressor T cells or CD4[+] T cells putatively involved in induction of tolerance [13, 14]. Thus, the overall response is actually one promoting containment of excessive immune reactivity at the mucosal level.

When antigens penetrate the epithelium paracellularly the pathway utilized consists of the tight junctions (zonulae occludentes) and the subjunctional space. The tight junction is a complex and dynamic structure that constitutes a considerable barrier to large molecules and regulates the frequency, quality and quantity of antigen presentation to the adjacent and underlying immunocytes [15]. Various probes used for clinical measurement of small bowel permeability, including L-rhamnose, PEG400, and [51Cr]EDTA, are believed to permeate the intestinal epithelial barrier through the paracellular tight junctions [16]. Their increased absorption in conditions such as Crohn's disease, celiac disease, infections, allergy and food intolerance indicates a loss of the protective function of the tight junctions under inflammatory conditions. The same apparently occurs in uninflamed ileal mucosa of Crohn's disease, and this could increase the antigen load in the mucosa and predispose to intestinal inflammation [17].

Biological control mechanisms
Circulatory control
GALT and MALT

The impressive size and diffusiveness of the normal MALT, which forms the anatomical basis for physiological intestinal inflammation, imply the existence of highly efficient mechanisms that direct the circulation of lymphoid cells to the intestine and allow their retention in the mucosa where they can mediate a protective effector function. Under physiological conditions lymphocytes circulate constantly throughout the body. This movement does not take place in a random fashion, but rather occurs under the control of a tightly regulated process coordinating the traffic of specific cell subsets to inductive (e.g. lymph nodes) and effector (e.g. mucosal surfaces) sites. In this regard there is a significant dichotomy in lymphocyte trafficking and distribution between naive (CD45A$^+$) and memory (antigen-primed CD45RO$^+$) cells: naive lymphocytes are programmed to circulate mainly among secondary lymphoid tissues (lymph nodes, tonsils, spleen and Peyer's patches) while memory cells preferentially access and recirculate to immune effector sites such as the intestinal lamina propria [18]. This distinction is of major importance to the intestinal immunity because the vast majority of lymphocytes populating the normal intestinal mucosa is composed of mature memory cells [19]. These derive primarily from naive cells which have been primed by antigens sampled by M cells in the Peyer's patches and other organized GALT and recirculate to finally home in the lamina propria [1]. The implementation of this complex distribution system requires a series of signals and receptors on circulating leukocytes as well as the microvasculature to which immunocytes must adhere in order to penetrate the interstitial tissue. This task is accomplished through a proposed multi-step paradigm in which leukocyte attachment to the vascular endothelium and the subsequent rolling, activation, arrest, spreading and transendothelial migration are mediated by specific cell adhesion and chemoattractant molecules [20]. Once in the interstitium the combined influence of local mesenchymal cells and the extracellular matrix provides a protective anti-apoptotic environment that prolongs the survival of immigrated lymphocytes [21] (Fig. 2).

Cell adhesion molecules

Cell adhesion molecules are a large number of structurally and functionally related and unrelated molecules forming four major families: the *selectin family* which is primarily responsible for leukocyte-endothelial cell interactions; the *integrin family* which mediates cell–cell and cell–extracellular matrix interactions, the *immunoglobulin superfamily* which mediates homophilic adhesion between an identical cell adhesion molecule and another cell, and the *cadherin family* which establishes molecular links between adjacent cells [22] (Table 1). The process of lymphocyte migration to and retention in the intestinal mucosa has two basic requirements. The first is the expression of a combination of adhesion molecules that impart tissue specificity to memory/effector cells, which for mucosal homing lymphocytes is represented by high levels of the integrin α4β7 and αLβ2 (LFA-1, leukocyte function-associated molecule) and low levels of L-selectin to avoid trapping in secondary lymphoid tissues. The second requirement is the coordinated participation of several cell adhesion molecules from different families, particularly those regulating the adhesion of leukocytes to the vascular endothelial cells (homing) and subsequent translocation into the interstitial space. These include L-, E-, and P-selectin of the selectin family, CD11/CD18, very late activation antigen (VLA) -4, and α4β7 of the integrin family, intercellular cell adhesion molecule (ICAM) 1,

Intestinal lumen

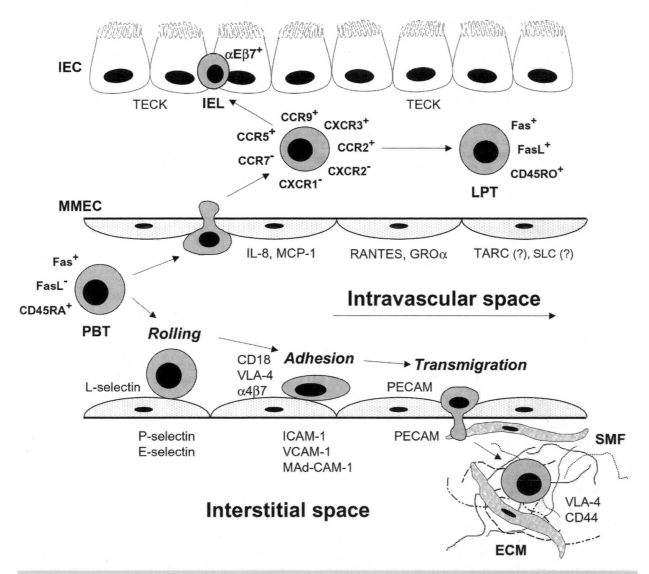

Figure 2. Major chemokines, chemokine receptors, and cell adhesion molecules involved in the multiple steps necessary to attract and translocate (rolling, adhesion and transmigration) T cells from the intravascular to the interstitial space, and to distribute and retain T cells in the intraepithelial and lamina propria compartments. In the upper part of the figure chemokines (TECK, IL-8, MCP-1, RANTES, GROα, TARC, and SLC) are shown below their respective cellular source: intestinal epithelial cells (IEC) and mucosal microvascular endothelial cells (MMEC). Receptors for CC and CXC chemokines (CCR2, CCR5, CCR7, CCR9, CXCR1, CXCR2, and CXCR3) are shown around the translocated T cells (+ indicates the expression and – indicates the absence of expression of each chemokine receptor). In the lower part of the figure cell adhesion molecules expressed by T cells are shown to their left and cell adhesion molecules expressed by MMEC are shown below them. ECM, extracellular matrix; GRO, growth-related oncogene; ICAM, intercellular adhesion molecule; IEL, intraepithelial lymphocyte; IL-8, interleukin-8; LPT, lamina propria T cell; PBT, peripheral blood T cell; PECAM, platelet–endothelial cell adhesion molecule; RANTES, regulated on activation, normal T cell expressed and secreted; SLC, secondary lymphoid organ chemokine; SMF, subepithelial myofibroblast; TARC, thymus and activation-regulated chemokine; TECK, thymus expressed chemokine; VCAM, vascular cell adhesion molecule; VLA, very late activation antigen.

Table 1. Cell adhesion molecules relevant to intestinal immunity

Cell adhesion molecule	Main cellular source	Main ligand	Main target
Selectin family			
E-selectin	Endothelial cells	L-selectin	Neutrophils, monocytes, T cells
L-selectin	Lymphocytes, neutrophils, monocytes	MAd-CAM1	Mucosal HEV, endothelial cells
P-selectin	Platelets, endothelial cells	L-selectin	Neutrophils, monocytes, platelets
Integrin family			
LFA-1 (CD11a/CD18)	All leukocytes	ICAM1, -2, -3	Lymphoid, non-lymphoid cells
LFA-3	All cells, some T cells	CD2	T cells, natural killer cells
Mac-1 (CD11b/CD18)	Neutrophils, monocytes	ICAM1, -3, fibrinogen	Lymphoid, non-lymphoid cells, ECM
VLA-1, -2, -3		Collagen, laminin	ECM
VLA-4	Lymphocytes, monocytes	VCAM1, fibronectin	Endothelial cells, fibroblasts, monocytes, ECM
VLA-5	Lymphocytes, monocytes	Fibronectin	ECM
VLA-6	Lymphocytes, monocytes	Laminin	ECM
$\alpha 4\beta 7$	Lymphocytes	MAd-CAM1, fibronectin	Mucosal HEV, ECM
Immunoglobulin superfamily			
ICAM1 (CD54)	Lymphoid, non-lymphoid cells	LFA-1, Mac-1	Neutrophils, lymphocytes, monocytes
VCAM1 (CD106)	Endothelial cells, fibroblasts, monocytes	VLA-4, $\alpha 4\beta 7$	Neutrophils, lymphocytes, monocytes
MAd-CAM1	Mucosal HEV	$\alpha 4\beta 7$, L-selectin	Lymphocytes, monocytes, neutrophils
PECAM1	Endothelial cells, neutrophils	PECAM1	Endothelial cells, neutrophils
Cadherin family			
Cadherin, α-, β-catenin	Adjacent cells	Cadherin	Same cell type
Other			
CD44 (Hermes)	Lymphoid, non-lymphoid cells	Hyaluronan, collagen	Endothelial cells, ECM

ECM, extracellular matrix; HEV, high endothelial venule; ICAM, intercellular cell adhesion molecule; LFA, leukocyte function-associated antigen; MAd-CAM, mucosal addressin cell adhesion molecule; PECAM, platelet–endothelial cell adhesion molecule; VCAM, vascular cell adhesion molecule; VLA, very late activation antigen vascular cell adhesion molecule (VCAM) 1, and mucosal addressin cell adhesion molecule (MAd-CAM) 1 of the Ig superfamily, and PECAM (platelet-endothelial cell adhesion molecule) 1 [23] (Fig. 2). Among these molecules, some play more dominant roles than others do in lymphocyte migration to the gut. Of pivotal importance is the mucosal vascular addressin MAdCAM1 which is expressed by high endothelial venules (HEV), specialized postcapillary microvessels that support high levels of lymphocyte extravasation from the blood in both GALT and MALT [24], and is the target of lymphocytes expressing the intestinal homing receptor α4β7. Another molecule specifically involved in intestinal lymphocyte–epithelial interaction is the integrin αEβ7 which determines the destination of intraepithelial lymphocytes through binding to E-cadherin present on intestinal epithelial cells [25].

Chemoattractants

In addition to classical adhesion molecules, a series of chemoattractant molecules also triggers the migration and controls the directional movement of leukocytes. They include complement factor C5a, the tripeptide f.Met-Leu-Phe, the leukotriene LTB$_4$ and a vast number of *chemokines*. Among these groups, considerable experimental evidence indicates that chemokines and their receptors play a previously unrecognized but fundamental role in the direction, selection, entry and retention of lymphocytes in the various tissues of the body under both physiological and pathological conditions [26, 27]. Chemokines are a large group of molecules with considerable amino acid sequence homology that function primarily as chemotactic cytokines but also mediate a variety of other biological activities [28]. They are divided into four families depending on the number of amino acids separating the first two cysteine residues, and they are discussed in greater detail in Chapter 7. Most cells produce chemokines, including human intestinal microvascular endothelial cells [29]. The response to chemokines is mediated through chemokine receptors, an equally large and complex series of cell surface molecules that can be specific, shared or promiscuous for individual chemokine molecules [30] (Table 2). Perhaps even more important than their chemokine ligands, chemokine receptors are essential in regulating the direction, selection, entry and retention of lymphocytes in distinct body compartments.

Table 2. Major human chemokines and their receptors

Chemokine ligand	Chemokine receptor
C chemokines	
Lymphotactin/SCM-1α	XCR1
SCM-1β	XCR1
CC chemokines	
I-309	CCR8
MCP-1/MCAF	CCR2
MIP-1α	CCR1, CCR5
MIP-1β	CCR5
RANTES	CCR1, CCR3, CCR5
MCP-3	CCR1, CCR2, CCR3
MCP-2	CCR3
Eotaxin	CCR3
MCP-4	CCR2, CCR3
HCC-1	CCR1
HCC-2/MIP-1δ	CCR1, CCR3
HCC-4/LEC	CCR1
TARC	CCR4
MIP-3β/ELC/exodus-3	CCR7
MIP-3α/LARC/exodus-1	CCR6
SLC/exodus-2	CCR7
MDC/STCP-1	CCR4
MPIF-1	CCR1
MPIF-2/eotaxin-2	CCR3
TECK	CCR9
Eotaxin-3	CCR3
CTACK/ILC	CCR10
CXC chemokines	
GROα	CXCR1, CXCR2
GROβ	CXCR2
GROγ	CXCR2
ENA-78	CXCR2
GCP-2	CXCR1, CXCR2
NAP-2	CXCR2
IL-8	CXCR1, CXCR2
MIG	CXCR3
IP-10	CXCR3
I-TAC	CXCR3
SDF-1α/β	CXCR4
BLC/BCA-1	CXCR5
CX3C chemokines	
Fractalkine	CX3CR1

BCA, B-cell attracting chemokine; BLC, B lymphocyte chemoattractant; ELC, EBI1-ligand chemokine; ENA-78, epithelial cell-derived neutrophil-activating peptide 78; GCP, granulocyte chemotactic protein; GRO, growth-related oncogene; HCC, hemofiltrate CC chemokine; IL-8, interleukin-8; IP-10, interferon-γ-inducible protein-10; I-TAC, interferon-inducible T cell α chemoattractant; LARC, liver and activation-regulated chemokine; MCP, monocyte chemotactic protein; MDC, macrophage-derived chemokine; MIG, monokine induced by interferon-γ; MIP, macrophage inflammatory protein; NAP, neutrophil-activating protein; RANTES, regulated on activation, normal T cell expressed and secreted; SDF, stromal cell-derived factor; SLC, secondary lymphoid organ chemokine; TARC, thymus- and activation-regulated chemokine; TECK, thymus-expressed chemokine.

Chemokine receptors

Knowledge in this area is still evolving, but it is clear that chemokines and their receptors have an impact on the overall biology of T cells. By virtue of their diversity, members of the four chemokine families can attract various subsets of T cells, and impart signals that cause them to traffic from the intravascular to extravascular compartments and within lymph nodes, as well as recirculate from tissues to lymphatics [31], all events directly relevant to homing to and retention of T cells in the MALT. The effect on a T cell responding to chemokines is strictly dependent on the types of chemokine receptors displayed on the cell surface, because this controls the relationship between the functional activity of lymphocytes and their migratory and functional properties. The net effect of this relationship includes: (a) distinct migratory patterns of naive and memory cells, (b) the final destination to distinct tissues and organs, and (c) the decision to prime a Th1- or a Th2-mediated response. For instance, the chemokine receptor CCR4 is expressed by memory T cells that migrate to the skin but not the intestine [32]. By the same token the chemokine receptor CCR7 discriminates between two subsets of CD45O$^+$ T cells, and its loss after antigen-induced differentiation generates effector cells homing to the intestinal mucosa [33]. Small intestinal epithelial cells produce selected chemokines such as TECK (thymus-expressed chemokine, also expressed in the thymus) whose receptor is the newly discovered GPR-9-6/CCR9 which is expressed by all intestinal lamina propria and intraepithelial lymphocytes [34]. TECK is also produced by small bowel but not colonic endothelial cells and a subset of cells in the intestinal crypts and lamina propria [35]. TECK is selectively chemotactic for small bowel but not colonic lamina propria mononuclear cells (LPMC), which display high and low CCR9 levels, respectively. This restricted expression of TECK and CCR9 implies the existence of unique chemokine–chemokine receptors pairs involved in the development and maintenance of physiological intestinal inflammation which is compartmentalized to the small or large bowel. There is also evidence that the differential expression of chemokine receptors is a strong determinant of Th1 vs Th2 responses. CXCR3 and CCR5 are preferentially expressed by human Th1 cells, whereas Th2 preferentially express the CCR4 and CCR3 receptors [36]. This has obvious implications not only in the physical positioning of T cells in the immune response, but also the composition and function of cell-mediated

immune responses in the gut. Supporting this notion is recent evidence showing that normal human lamina propria and intraepithelial lymphocytes express the CXCR2, CCR3 and CCR5 receptors which are associated with Th1/Th0 responses, but not the CCR1, CXCR2 and CXCR7 receptors that are associated with Th2 responses [37] (Fig. 2).

Under inflammatory conditions the normal traffic of mucosal lymphocytes is drastically disrupted by hemodynamic changes combined with the abnormal expression of adhesion molecules and receptors by both leukocytes and microvascular cells. Levels of MAdCAM1, ICAM1, E- and L-selectins are up-regulated, resulting in an aberrant and enhanced influx of activated and naive lymphocytes in the mucosa [23, 38]. Production of mucosal chemokines is markedly increased in the inflamed intestine and presumably the level of expression and the types of chemokine receptors are also altered [39]. A direct evaluation of all cell surface and secreted molecules in normal and inflamed gut mucosa will be needed to fully understand all migratory patterns and their implication in physiological intestinal inflammation.

Humoral control

Several organs, particularly those with mucosal surfaces, contain a variety of substances with intrinsic antimicrobial activity. In the intestinal tract the most prominent of these substances are the defensins, peptides similar to the ones found in granules of phagocytic leukocytes [40]. The two major classes of defensins are the α- and β-defensins; α-defensins are abundant constituents of Paneth cells, where they are stored in and released from granules in response to bacterial stimuli [41]. Paneth cell α-defensins exhibit selective activity against several Gram-positive and Gram-negative bacteria, but also against mycobacteria and spirochetes, fungi and certain viruses. There is also considerable evidence that defensins may play other safeguarding roles including immunomodulation, opsonization, and stimulation of wound repair [42]. Because of their multiple defensive functions and spontaneous presence in normal intestine defensins can also be considered components of innate intestinal immunity. In reality the protective functions of defensins probably extend beyond the natural ability to kill bacteria, in view of recent evidence that human defensins are chemotactic for dendritic cells and memory T cells [43], an observation that establishes a link between innate and adaptive immunity.

In addition to defensins a whole host of other substances exists with properties potentially relevant to mucosal protection. The best known is lactoferrin, a single-chain glycoprotein bound to one or two molecules of ferric iron [44]. Among other several functions, lactoferrin has antimicrobial activity against viruses, bacteria, fungi and parasites and can bind sIgA. Additional substances that can contribute to mucosal defenses are lysozyme, peroxidases, histatins, cystatins, calprotectin, and secretory phospholipase A2, all of which display different degrees of microbicidal activity [42].

Immune control

Although systemic and local immunity are often interrelated, the health of each organ depends fundamentally on regulatory events which have been developmentally adapted to optimize and maintain the unique physiological conditions of each specific tissue microenvironment. In view of the preponderance of the immune system in the gut, and its lifelong stimulation by dietary and microbial antigens, robust but finely tuned immunomodulatory mechanisms must be constantly at work to preserve the state of physiological intestinal inflammation. The response of the immune system against any aggression has been traditionally divided in two separate but complementary compartments, innate immunity and adaptive immunity [45]. Mechanisms of *innate immunity*, such as phagocytosis, microbial killing and complement-dependent lysis, are primarily employed against infectious agents, become active immediately, have a limited receptor repertoire, and are largely non-specific [46]. In contrast, *adaptive immunity*, organized around T cells and B cells, has an almost unlimited target and receptor repertoire, requires a delayed onset, is strictly dependent on clonal expansion, and displays exquisite specificity. This separation is somewhat arbitrary in view of the sharing of several mediator and effector molecules, and the mutual interplay between innate and adaptive immunity [47]. Knowledge of innate and adaptive immunity in the intestine is fairly uneven, more abundant information existing in regard to the latter than the former. The following two sections will review the basic elements of innate intestinal immunity and provide a more extended discussion on adaptive immunity, with particular emphasis on tolerance as a key controller of physiological intestinal inflammation.

Innate immunity

Components of innate immunity relevant to normal gut physiology include both cellular and soluble mediators. Macrophages, eosinophils, mast cells, natural killer (NK) cells and neutrophils are the cellular mediators. Soluble mediators include the complement system, mannose-binding lectin (collectin), C-reactive protein (pentraxin), coagulation actors, defensins, various cytokines and chemokines, and reactive oxygen (ROM) and nitrogen (nitric oxide, NO) metabolites. It should be noted that very few studies have investigated in detail the role of the above components in the normal human intestine, and existing knowledge is almost exclusively derived from control data in studies of inflammatory conditions such as IBD or celiac disease. The paucity of information in this area will be supplemented by more extensive discussion of several of the same mediators in Chapters 7, 8 and 9, dealing with their involvement in pathological intestinal inflammation.

Cellular mediators

Macrophages are important to innate immunity because of their role as phagocytic and scavenger cells, but they are also involved in adaptive immunity because of their essential role in antigen presentation. Macrophages are blood-derived monocytes that have differentiated into very efficient cells for recognition and elimination of invading microbes, processes mediated by specialized receptor systems. Products of Gram-negative bacteria such as lipopolysaccharide (LPS/endotoxin) bind to a receptor that stimulates microbicidal activity and cytokine secretion. This LPS-sensing system consists of a combination of a plasma LPS-binding protein, the cell surface receptor CD14, and a signal-transducing receptor subunit called Toll-like receptor protein 4 [48]. Additional receptors include seven α-helical transmembrane receptors for N-formylmethionyl peptides, lipid mediators and chemokines, as well as phagocytic receptors such as the mannose and Fc receptors for opsonized and non-opsonized microbes. In the normal small and large bowel mucosa macrophages form a heterogeneous HLA-DR+ cell population with different morphological and phenotypic features of interdigitating dendritic cells or scavenger cells with weak expression of the B7-1 or B7-2 costimulatory molecules [49–51]. *In vitro* they show a limited capacity for phagocytosis and generation of oxygen radicals [52, 53], but produce substantial levels of interleukin (IL)-1α, IL-1β, tumor necrosis factor (TNF)-α and IL-6 in response to mitogens, LPS or interferon (IFN)-γ [54]. Together, these characteristics suggest that mucosal macrophages are normally involved in baseline antimicrobial and antigen-presenting activities, though they have the capacity to up-regulate both activities under inflammatory conditions [50, 51, 53, 54].

NK cells are a subset of lymphocytes that spontaneously lyse virus-infected cells and tumor cells. They are rare in the normal human mucosa and their contribution to innate immunity is uncertain. After plasma cells, T cells and macrophages, eosinophils represent the next most common type of mucosal immune cells, followed by mast cells and rare basophils. Little is known about these cells in maintenance of physiological inflammation, but they are presumably in a readiness state to provide defense against allergic and parasitic insults. Neutrophils are notably absent in a healthy intestine and their presence, no matter how small, should be interpreted as an early sign of infection or pathological inflammation.

Soluble mediators

Knowledge of the various soluble mediators of intestinal innate immunity is heavily skewed towards cytokines, chemokines and reactive metabolites. Cytokines involved in innate immunity include IL-1α/β and TNF-α because of their role in inflammation, IFN-α, and IFN-β because they promote resistance against viral infections, IFN-γ for its macrophage-activating activity, IL-12 for stimulating IFN-γ production by NK and T cells, IL-15 because of its T cell proliferation inducing ability, and IL-10 and transforming growth factor (TGF)-β due to their anti-inflammatory activity [55]. A comprehensive discussion on cytokines in intestinal immunity and inflammation is found in another chapter entirely dedicated to them.

Reactive metabolites

Reactive metabolites are also discussed in Chapter 8 but they will be briefly mentioned here to point out that these toxic molecules are also produced in the healthy intestine where they contribute to defense against microorganisms and other physiological activities. Using chemiluminescence or histochemical techniques low levels of ROM can be detected in the normal colon [56, 57]. The intestine, on the other hand, also produces several antioxidant molecules such as urate, glutathione, α-tocopherol, and ubiquinol-10 [58], which help in maintaining a protective physiological balance between pro- and anti-oxidative activities. The role of NO in intestinal physiology is still somewhat unclear because it participates in both physiological and pathological phenomena. In the healthy mucosa the constitutive endothelial NO synthase (eNOS) is present while the inducible NOS (iNOS) is absent [59], although the latter markedly increases during inflammation [59, 60]. The paradox that NO may be beneficial in physiological inflammation but injurious in pathological inflammation may be explained by the ability of different concentrations of NO to produce completely opposite effects in the same tissue [61]. In small amounts NO generally exerts beneficial effects, whereas generation of NO in large amounts is usually detrimental. The beneficial effects of NO that contribute to mucosal defense include increased secretion of mucus, reduction in neutrophil adherence, acceleration of wound repair, inhibition of cytokine release and of mast cell degranulation [61].

Complement

The complement system consists of several plasma proteins linking recognition of microbes to microbicidal activity and development of inflammation [62]. Recognition of microbes can occur through the classical or alternative pathway, both of which result in sequential recruitment and assembly of additional proteins into protease complexes such as C5, followed by formation of a complex with C6, C7, C8 and C9 which ultimately cause lysis of cells where complement is activated. Low expression of complement proteins C3d, C5, C9, terminal complement complex and S-protein can be found in submucosal blood vessels of the normal small and large bowel [63], while other proteins such as C3, C4 and factor B can be detected in perfusates of healthy small bowel [64].

Other soluble molecules

Defensins have been previously discussed as part of humoral control mechanisms but they can also rightfully belong to innate immunity. The mannose-binding lectin is a plasma protein that functions as an opsonin. Like the mannose receptor found on macrophages, it binds carbohydrates with terminal mannose and fucose which are typically found in microbial cell walls. C-reactive protein is another plasma protein that also functions as a bacterial opsonin. Finally, coagulation factors contribute to healing by protecting vessel integrity and limit bacterial spreading by walling off microvasculature.

Adaptive immunity

The central feature of adaptive immunity is the ability to generate defense mechanisms that respond specifically to the antigen inciting the immune response. Since adaptive immunity is centered around B cells and T cells, often the response elicited by a single antigen results in antibody production accompanied by a concomitant cell-mediated response. However, one type of reactivity may predominate over the other, depending on the nature of the antigen as well as the conditions and site of stimulation, since the characteristics of the lymphoid tissue in each organ influence the quality and quantity of the response. This certainly applies to the intestinal immune system where both the types of antigens present in the lumen and the GALT/MALT display singular attributes resulting in responses entirely different from those that would occur at the systemic level even in response to the same antigen. Because the achievement of a controlled immune response in the gut is largely dependent on the induction of immune tolerance, a comprehensive review of all elements and phenomena that contribute to adaptive immunity in the human intestine is not warranted in view of the goals of this chapter. Instead, we will outline selected features of humoral and cell-mediated immunity that may help in restraining mucosal immune reactivity, reserving a more detailed discussion for the mechanisms of immune unresponsiveness (tolerance) and their contribution to physiological intestinal inflammation.

Active immunity

Humoral immunity

Antibody production at mucosal surface is dominated by sIgA, secretory IgM playing only a supplementary role. The multiple biological activities of IgA are well known and most of them appear to have evolved in order to provide specialized protection at mucosal surfaces [65]. Secretory IgA is a structurally stable molecule, a quality attributed to the linkage with the secretory component that hides the potential site of proteolytic cleavage. This makes sIgA particularly suited to function in the enzymatically rich intestinal mucosa where it can exert its broad protective activities. Prime among these are the inhibition of bacterial adherence [66], a critical first step in bacterial colonization and eventual invasion, the induction of bacterial agglutination, and the ability to trap bacteria within the mucus layer. Secretory IgA has neutralizing activity for viruses, but also for

some enzymes and toxins of bacterial origin [67]. Due to its ability to agglutinate and entrap in the mucus, sIgA decreases the uptake of antigens generated by prior enteric sensitization and thus limits the subsequent antigenic load stimulating the mucosal lymphoid tissue [68]. Another quality of sIgA, distinct from that of most other immunoglobulins, is that of having a weak or no ability to activate the complement system by either the classical or alternative pathway [69], a clearly advantageous property with anti-inflammatory implications. Finally, sIgA synergizes with some non-immune components of humoral defenses including lactoferrin, peroxidases and lysozyme. Given all the above characteristics it is fair to conclude that sIgA plays a major contributory role to intestinal immune homeostasis and the local state of controlled inflammation.

Cell-mediated immunity

In the human intestine T lymphocytes can be found at inductive sites, such as Peyer's patches and lymphoid follicles, where naive CD45RA+ cells are originally primed by antigens, and at effector sites in the intraepithelial compartment and the lamina propria, where memory CD45RO+ cells reside ready to react upon re-encountering the specific antigen to which they were originally primed. Intraepithelial lymphocytes (IEL) and lamina propria T cells (LPT) are both mature effector T cells, but their phenotype and functional properties are quite distinct.

Intraepithelial lymphocytes

The vast majority of human IEL are CD8+ T cells bearing the T cell receptor (TCR) α/β and are oligoclonal in nature [70]. This oligoclonality is present all along the epithelium lining, maybe reflecting a restricted ability to respond to yet-unidentified antigens present in the gut [71]. This restriction may be useful because it diminishes the frequency of specific immune reactivity and decreases the chance of mounting a response potentially injurious to the surrounding epithelial cells. Some T cells in humans display the γ/δ TCR and they are involved in protective immunity against infectious agents [72]. A small number of IEL also display the γ/δ TCR and it is conceivable that they are also involved in a similar protective activity. The functional capacity of human IEL is still controversial. They exhibit a limited proliferative response to mitogens but they respond vigorously to red blood cells, a reaction that probably mimics activation through the CD2 receptor [73]. Some of the morphological features of IEL, e.g. their resemblance to large granular NK lymphocytes, and their CD8[+] phenotype, have long suggested that IEL may be cytotoxic cells, but some reports deny while others support this contention [74, 75]. Recent evidence shows that IEL have potent chemotactic activity in response to IL-8 and RANTES (regulated on activation, normal T cell expressed and secreted) [76], underlying the ability to be mobilized to sites of inflammation where they could mediate a protective function.

Lamina propria T cells

The lamina propria of the small intestine and colon contains a large and more heterogeneous population of T cells, of which 60–70% are CD4[+] and 20–30% are CD8[+]. Their predominant phenotype is that of helper and cytolytic cells [77], and they are also oligoclonal in nature, probably reflecting the selective antigen pressure of the intestinal milieu [78]. Compared to their peripheral blood counterparts, LPT are in a higher state of activation, as shown by their cell surface markers and gene expression patterns [79, 80]. In addition, they express high levels of Fas antigen and Fas ligand, rendering them more susceptible to Fas-mediated apoptosis than circulating T cells [81, 82] (Fig. 2). This aptness to die could be advantageous in limiting undesirable and potentially damaging immune responses. In fact, an inappropriately low rate of cell death could transform the state of physiological intestinal inflammation into a pathological one, as apparently is the case in IBD [83, 84].

Functionally, LPT proliferate to mitogens, bacterial antigens, and LPS [85], but comparatively less than blood T cells, and display various forms of non-specific cytolytic activities including lectin-, cytokine- and anti-CD3-induced cytotoxicity [86–88], but not spontaneous NK-like activity or mixed lymphocyte reaction-induced lympholysis [86, 89]. LPT produce a broad spectrum of cytokines in response to a variety of stimuli including mitogens, cytokines and receptor stimulation [90]. The types of soluble mediators secreted by LPT include Th0, Th1 and Th2 cytokines [91], suggesting that the state of physiological inflammation is independent on an atypically skewed or well-polarized helper T cell response.

An aspect that deserves special attention is the considerable evidence showing that LPT exhibit a distinct differential reactivity when activated through the CD3 or the CD2 receptor pathways. Compared to peripheral blood T cells, LPT prolif-

erative response and IL-2 receptor expression are reduced following activation of the CD3, but not the CD2 receptor [92, 93]. This may be partially explained by down-regulation of protein kinase C in LPT, perhaps induced by unidentified mucosal factors [94, 95]. On the other hand the CD2 pathway is more efficient than the CD3 pathway in inducing cytokine production by LPT, supporting the conclusion that the association of low proliferative reactivity with high cytokine output is a characteristic feature of human mucosal T cells. This could be construed as reflecting a peculiar state of 'selective unresponsiveness' translating an adaptation of T cells to the immunological conditions of the intestine [96]. This notion is strengthened by the proposed role of CD2 signaling in the induction of T cell anergy, which is one of the mechanisms mediating peripheral T cell tolerance [97, 98].

When all the above information is considered together and analyzed in view of results from non-human systems also showing that mucosal T cells provide strong helper function through release of soluble mediators but fail to proliferate in response to antigen-specific stimulation [99], an overall functional phenotype emerges for human LPT. Such phenotype is consistent with a highly differentiated effector cell population with a relatively restricted capacity to clonally expand but very efficient at producing regulatory and effector cytokines. How these singular characteristics of mucosal T cells relate to the induction or maintenance of a controlled state of intestinal inflammation is not readily apparent. However, highly specialized and very capable effector cells are implicitly quicker and more efficient to enact an immune response with a high degree of specificity and able to exert 'damage control' by limiting a number of undesirable collateral effects.

Immunological tolerance

Active immunity is generally regarded as the principal mechanism the body utilizes to ward off offending agents and ensure an effective protection aimed at preserving health. While this view is correct, an immunogenic response is the exception rather than the rule in the mucosal immune system [100]. Faced with the continuous onslaught of luminal antigens the intestine needs very effective mechanisms to prevent the damaging effects of exceedingly strong immune responses while concurrently fostering protection within the limits of a controlled immune response. Cardinal to these mechanisms is *immuno-*

logical tolerance, defined as a state of unresponsiveness that is specific for a particular antigen and is induced by prior exposure to that antigen. The following paragraphs will provide an overview of the various types of immunological tolerance, how they work, and how their breakdown transforms physiological into pathological intestinal inflammation. It should be noted that, in contrast to the reports mentioned so far, the bulk of knowledge on immunological tolerance is based on animal studies to which we will refer for the sake of understanding and completeness.

Mechanisms of tolerance

Immunological tolerance is a fundamental characteristic of the immune system that allows us to discriminate self from non-self, and thus prevents reactions directed at autoantigens that may result in pathogenic events [101]. Two types of immunological tolerance exist: central or thymic tolerance, and peripheral or post-thymic tolerance. *Central tolerance* is developed during maturation in the thymus, where immature T cells that recognize high-affinity self-antigens are deleted (clonal deletion). Since dietary and microbial antigens are not present during fetal development this form of tolerance is less likely to play a significant role in intestinal immunity. *Peripheral tolerance* is developed against antigens not present in the thymus that are met by mature CD4$^+$ T cells later in life. Four different non-exclusive cellular mechanisms mediate peripheral tolerance: *clonal ignorance, anergy, deletion*, and *active suppression*. In clonal ignorance self-reactive lymphocytes fail to recognize peripheral autoantigens such as those sequestered in the eye, thyroid or central nervous system. There is no evidence that this form of tolerance is acting in the intestine and it will not be further considered here.

Anergy

Anergy occurs when antigen recognition occurs under suboptimal costimulatory conditions [98]. This is the case when CD4$^+$ T cells are presented antigens by APC deficient in costimulatory molecules, mainly B7-1 and B7-2, or when T cells use CTLA-4 (cytotoxic T-lymphocyte-associated antigen, the inhibitory receptor for the B7 molecules) to recognize costimulatory molecules on APC during the process of antigen presentation [102]. Under these conditions T cells become incapable of recognizing antigens even if later presented by competent APC, perhaps due to altered TCR signaling [103].

The nature of the APC (professional APC such as macrophages or dendritic cells vs non-professional APC such as epithelial, endothelial or mesenchymal cells), their state of activation (MHC class II antigen positivity or negativity), and the expression repertoire of costimulatory molecules (mainly B7-1/CD80 and B7-2/CD86) are crucial determinants of whether the overall outcome of the immune response will lean toward responsiveness (active immunity) or unresponsiveness (tolerance) [104] (Fig. 3). In addition to lymphoid cells the intestinal mucosa contains epithelial, endothelial and mesenchymal cells that express low or no levels of costimulatory molecules even when MHC class II antigens are up-regulated during inflammation [105]. This results in a limited capacity to respond to local antigens, which further fosters the development of anergy and contributes to restrain immune reactivity and maintain a controlled state of inflammation.

Deletion

Deletion occurs when T cells are repeatedly stimulated by exposure to the same antigen resulting in activation-induced cell death (apoptosis) [106]. As a consequence of activation T cells express on their surface the Fas (CD95) receptor, a member of the TNF receptor family, and the Fas ligand, a molecule homologous to TNF [107]. The binding of Fas by Fas ligand on the same or adjacent T cells triggers a cascade of signaling events leading to the activation of intracellular cysteine proteases (caspases) that ultimately cause cell death by apoptosis, resulting in the elimination of the mature T cell population repeatedly stimulated by the original antigen. Constant antigen exposure is a typical feature of intestinal immunity and mucosal T cells normally express high levels of both Fas and Fas ligand [81], making clonal deletion of T cells a likely mechanism of immune homeostasis in physiological intestinal inflammation.

Active suppression

Of all the mechanisms participating in peripheral tolerance active suppression is probably the most common and effective. Active suppression is a process in which regulatory CD4$^+$ T cells activated by exposure to a sensitizing antigen release cytokines such as IL-14, IL-10 and TGF-β [108]. This release of cytokines by tolerized T cells blocks the activation and function of other effector T cells and induces an important 'bystander suppression' effect in the local microenvironment, resulting in the inhibition of

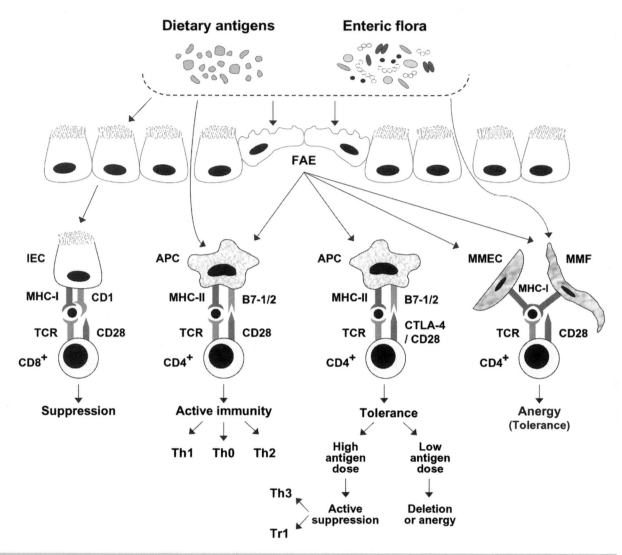

Figure 3. Proposed mechanisms of adaptive immunity involved in the induction and maintenance of physiological inflammation in the normal intestine. Antigens derived from the diet and the commensal enteric flora can access the GALT and MALT through specialized cells forming the follicle-associated epithelium (FAE), intestinal epithelial cells (IEC), or the paracellular route between IEC. Antigens processed by non-professional antigen-presenting IEC bearing major histocompatibility complex (MHC) class I and CD1 molecules will preferentially activate CD8[+] T cells and result in suppression (far left). When antigens are processed by professional antigen-presenting cells (APC) bearing MHC class II antigens and B7-1/2 costimulatory molecules and are presented to CD28[+] CD4[+] T cells this will result in active immunity with a non-polarized (Th0) or polarized (Th1 or Th2) profile depending on the nature of the antigen and the surrounding cytokine milieu (center left). When antigens are processed by professional APC bearing MHC class II antigens but presented through deficient B7-1/2 costimulation or preferentially to CTLA-4[+] CD4[+] T cells this will result in tolerance mediated by active suppression (executed by Th3 or Tr1 cells) or deletion/anergy depending on the dose of the antigen (center right). Antigens processed by non-professional antigen-presenting mucosal microvascular endothelial cells (MMEC) or mucosal myofibroblast (MMF)-bearing major histocompatibility (MHC) class I molecules but no costimulatory molecules will result in the generation of anergic T cells and the induction of tolerance (far right).

immune responses to unrelated, but anatomically co-localized, antigens [109]. Active suppression is probably the most important mechanism of tolerance in the gut, not only because of the high likelihood of local T cells to re-encounter antigens to which they have been previously sensitized, but also because of the abundance of mature effector T cells capable of producing immunosuppressive molecules [110].

Oral tolerance

The tolerance mechanisms discussed so far are based primarily on systemic immune responses to self rather than foreign protein antigens. The nature, dose and way of administration of any foreign protein are key determining factors in deciding whether active immunity or tolerance will ensue. When a foreign protein enters the body via the gastrointestinal tract this usually leads to a marked suppression of systemic humoral and cell-mediated immune responses upon rechallenge by the same protein. This phenomenon is called *oral tolerance*, and is believed to be essential in preventing deleterious immune responses against proteins that need to be absorbed for nutritional purposes, and developing tolerance against the antigens of the normal enteric flora that is indispensable to energy metabolism, nutrient absorption and general health [109, 111, 112]. Various mechanisms mediate oral tolerance but generally, based on experimental animal systems, a high antigen dose induces anergy or deletion [113, 114], whereas a low antigen dose induces active T cell-mediated suppression (Fig. 3). This latter form of regulation is mediated the immunosuppressive cytokines IL-4, IL-10 and TGF-β produced by various types of CD4$^+$ T cells with functional phenotypes of Th2, Th3, Treg (T regulatory cell) or Tr1 (T regulatory cell 1), all of which are involved in systemic or organ-specific autoimmune phenomena [115–117]. There is good evidence that these regulatory T cells exist in the gut of normal humans and animals with experimental intestinal inflammation [118–120], as well as evidence for the anti-inflammatory activity of locally secreted cytokines such as IL-10 and TGF-β [120–122].

Broken tolerance: impact on intestinal immune homeostasis

To be fully protective oral tolerance must be developed for the two main components of the luminal content: food antigens and the endogenous flora. Ingestion of specific proteins and peptides is widely utilized in studies of systemic and organ-specific

immunity and autoimmunity, as well as a form of treatment for autoimmune diseases [123]. Unfortunately, except for classical food allergies, a form of immediate hypersensitivity reaction mediated primarily by mast cells and eosinophils [124], little is known about the role of normal dietary antigen in physiological or pathological intestinal inflammation. In contrast, knowledge on the role of the commensal flora on intestinal immunity and inflammation has greatly expanded in recent years, justifying some discussion on how normal enteric bacteria induce and maintain a controlled state of inflammation in the mucosa, and how loss of tolerance to these bacteria may contribute to chronic intestinal inflammation as observed in IBD.

Gut microbial–immune interactions

The development of a mature intestinal immune system is strictly dependent on the introduction of environmental antigens into the lumen, e.g. food and microorganisms [125]. Immediately after birth the newborn's gastrointestinal tract, previously sterile, is colonized with aerobic and anaerobic bacteria [126]. The ability to induce tolerance requires colonization by Gram-negative bacteria early in life, and germfree conditions or exposure to certain aerobic Gram-positive bacteria may impair development of oral tolerance mechanisms [127]. With advancing age, and feeding of complex diets, the gut acquires a full spectrum of microflora that increases in number and variety from the almost sterile stomach to the luxuriant milieu of the colon, where *Bacteroides*, *Bifidobacteria*, *Peptostreptococcus* and *Eubacterium* spp. predominate. The type of feeding has a significant impact on colonization: for example, distinct from breast-fed infants, *Bacteroides* count increases in formula-fed infants, and anaerobic counts remain high after introduction of solid food [128].

The normal human intestinal biota consists of hundreds of bacterial species that vary considerably from person to person, though the predominant phylogenetic groups do not change [129]. The interdependence of the bacterial and immune systems in the gut is mutual and lifelong, and enteric bacteria exert a wide range of modulatory effects on specific and non-specific immune responses. In animals they range from mitogenic effects on lymphocytes to induction of NK and cytotoxic cell activity, enhanced antibody production, stimulation of macrophage phagocytosis, cytokine production, and induction of oxygen free radicals [128]. In humans the enteric bacteria affect both systemic and mucosal immunity, including modulation of IL-1, IL-2, IL-6, TNF-α, and IFN-γ production, antigen- and mitogen-induced lymphocyte proliferation, and macrophage phagocytic and killing activity [130].

Normal enteric flora and pathological intestinal inflammation

There is compelling evidence for a decisive role of the commensal flora in pathological gut inflammation. Four lines of evidence support this claim. The strongest evidence for a role of the normal enteric flora in IBD comes from experimental models of bowel inflammation in transgenic and gene-deleted rodents [131]. For instance, HLA-B27/human β₂-microglobulin transgenic rats and IL-10-deficient mice fail to develop colitis under germfree conditions, but do so when exposed to normal luminal bacteria, and the load and composition of commensal bacteria influences the degree of inflammation [132–134]. Additional support comes from human studies in which the fecal content has been removed from or put in contact with intestinal mucosa. Crohn's disease patients with fecal stream diversion after ileal resection have no inflammation in the neoterminal ileum, but inflammation quickly reappears after reanastomosis [135]. Furthermore, infusion of intestinal luminal contents into histologically normal excluded ileal loops after ileocolonic resection induces inflammatory changes within a few days [136]. Another example of how luminal content affects the health of the intestinal mucosa derives from ulcerative colitis patients with a reconstructed ileo-anal pouch who develop pouchitis, a recurrent inflammation in the remodeled small bowel loops. This condition is believed to be caused by a bacterial dysbiosis induced by the presence of colonic-type bacteria in the small bowel loops forming the pouch [137]. Finally, antibiotics can be beneficial in the management of IBD and particularly CD [138], and probiotics appear to be a promising new form of treatment for IBD and pouchitis [139, 140].

Loss of tolerance to normal enteric flora in intestinal inflammation

If gut-induced tolerance is crucial to prevent systemic immune responses, the same must be true for local responses, and it seems logical that gut inflammation may result from loss of local tolerance. This concept finds support in a series of human and animal studies. LPMC isolated from the inflamed, but not uninflamed, intestine of adult IBD patients proliferate strongly in response to autologous, but not heterologous, intestinal bacteria [141]. LPMC from control and IBD patients in remission fail to proliferate to autologous bacteria. This suggests that tolerance to commensal flora normally exists in the healthy intestine, and that tolerance is broken during inflammation. Loss of tolerance to commensal flora is also demonstrable in murine hapten-induced colitis, and tolerance can be restored by treatment with IL-10 or neutralization of IL-12 [142]. Gut bacteria-reactive T cells are found in patients with IBD and murine models of IBD [119, 143–145], and the adoptive transfer of bacterial antigen-specific CD4⁺ T cells from diseased into naive animals induces colitis [119, 145]. Taken together, these results indicate that loss of tolerance to autologous enteric flora is instrumental in the pathogenesis of some forms of pathological intestinal inflammation.

Implications of physiological intestinal inflammation for health and disease

Having defined some of the physical and biological control mechanisms responsible for the development and maintenance of a state of controlled inflammation in the intestine, few final considerations are in order to conclude what physiological inflammation really is and what its role might be in health and disease. This may be best done by posing a series of intriguing questions. How much physiological inflammation is enough? Why does the degree of mucosal leukocyte infiltration vary among normal individuals? Why is physiological inflammation symptom-free? Why does a certain degree of mucosal lymphoid cell infiltration represent physiological inflammation in one individual when the same degree may be accompanied by symptoms of pathological inflammation in another? In other words, when does gut inflammation cease to be physiological and become pathological? Clinical experience shows that IBD patients in remission often display significant inflammatory changes at endoscopic or histological examination, and that a routine screening colonoscopy reveals the presence of florid inflammation in an individual totally free of gastrointestinal symptoms. These practical observations indicate that physiological intestinal inflammation cannot be simply equated to a certain number of cells per volume of mucosa just as much as pathological inflammation cannot be defined only by clinical symptoms. Therefore, it is reasonable to assume that, depending on genetic make-up, a healthy subject can have disparate amounts of immunocytes in the gastrointestinal mucosa. This amount is almost certainly modified by the quality of his or her diet, as well as the concentration and type of commensal flora, as shown by differences between individuals living in northern vs tropical areas. While these concepts may be intuitively acceptable, on the other hand they complicate the definition of physiological intestinal inflammation. Since it appears that what is physiological in one person may be pathological in another, perhaps it would be best to assume that what constitutes physiological inflammation in response to normal stimuli is as tailor-made as the response each person puts forward in the face of pathological stimuli.

References

1. Brandtzaeg P, Farstad IN, Haraldsen G. Regional specialization in the mucosal immune system: primed cells do not always home along the same track. Immunol Today 1999; 20: 267–77.
2. Ogra PL, Mestecky J, Lamm ME, Strober W, Bienenstock J, McGhee JR. Mucosal Immunology, 2nd edn. San Diego: Academic Press, 1999.
3. Mayer EA, Raybould H, Koelbel C. Neuropeptides, inflammation and motility. Dig Dis Sci 1988; 33: 71S–7S.
4. Chang S-K, Dohrman AF, Basbaum CB *et al.* Localization of mucin (MUC2 and MUC3) messenger RNA and peptide expression in human normal intestine and colon cancer. Gastroenterology 1994; 107: 28–36.
5. Cone RA. Mucus. In: Ogra PL, Mestecky J, Lamm ME, Strober W, Bienenstock J, McGhee JR, editors. Mucosal Immunity, 2nd edn. San Diego: Academic Press, 1999: 43–64.
6. Kato T, Owen RL. Structure and function of intestinal mucosal epithelium. In: Ogra PL, Mestecky J, Lamm ME, Strober W, Bienenstock J, McGhee JR, editors. Mucosal Immunity, 2nd edn. San Diego: Academic Press, 1999: 115–32.
7. Gebert A, Rothkotter HJ, Pabst R. M cells in Peyer's patches of the intestine. Int Rev Cytol 1996; 167: 91–159.
8. Hecht G. Innate mechanisms of epithelial host defense: spotlight on intestine. Am J Physiol 1999; 277: C351–68.
9. McKay DM, Baird AW. Cytokine regulation of epithelial permeability and ion transport. Gut 1999; 44: 283–9.
10. Jung HC, Eckmann L, Yang S-K, et al. A distinct array of proinflammatory cytokines is expressed in human colon epithelial cells in response to bacterial invasion. J Clin Invest 1995; 95: 55–65.
11. Kagnoff MF, Eckmann L. Epithelial cells as sensors for microbial infection. J Clin Invest 1997; 100: 6–10.
12. Kim JM, Eckmann L, Savidge TC, Lowe DC, Witthoft T, Kagnoff MF. Apoptosis of human intestinal epithelial cells after bacterial invasion. J Clin Invest 1998; 102: 1815–23.
13. Hershberg RM, Mayer LF. Antigen processing and presentation by intestinal epithelial cells – polarity and complexity. Immunol Today 2000; 21: 123–8.
14. Mayer L, Shlien R. Evidence for function of Ia molecules on gut epithelial cells in man. J Exp Med 1987; 166: 1471–83.
15. Madara JL. Maintenance of the macromolecular barrier at cell extrusion sites in intestinal epithelium: physiological rearrangements of tight junctions. J Membr Biol 1990; 116: 177–84.
16. Bjarnason I, MacPherson A, Hollander D. Intestinal permeability: an overview. Gastroenterology 1995; 108: 1566–81.
17. Soderholm JA, Peterson KM, Olaison G et al. Epithelial permeability to proteins in the noninflamed ileum of Crohn's disease? Gastroenterology 1999; 117: 65–72.
18. Butcher EC, Picker LJ. Lymphocyte homing and homeostasis. Science 1996; 272: 60–6.
19. Schieferdecker HL, Ullrich R, Hirseland H, Zeitz M. T cell differentiation antigens on lymphocytes in the human intestinal lamina propria. J Immunol 1992; 149: 2816–22.
20. Springer TA. Traffic signals for lymphocyte recirculation and leukocyte emigration: the multistep paradigm. Cell 1994; 76: 301–14.
21. Akbar AN, Salmon M. Cellular environments and apoptosis: tissue microenvironments control activated T cell death. Immunol Today 1997; 18: 72–6.
22. Frenette PS, Wagner DD. Adhesion molecules – Part I. N Engl J Med 1996; 334: 1526–9.
23. Panes J, Granger DN. Leukocyte–endothelial interactions: molecular mechanisms and implications in gastrointestinal disease. Gastroenterology 1998; 114: 1066–90.
24. Briskin M, Winsor-Hines D, Shyjan A et al. Human mucosal addressin cell adhesion molecule-1 is preferentially expressed in intestinal tract and associated lymphoid tissue. Am J Pathol 1997; 151: 97–110.
25. Salmi M, Jalkanen S. Molecules controlling lymphocyte migration to the gut. Gut 1999; 45: 148–53.
26. Kunkel SL. Through the looking glass: the diverse *in vivo* activities of chemokines. J Clin Invest 1999; 104: 1333–4.
27. Cyster JG. Chemokines and cell migration in secondary lymphoid organs. Science 1999; 286: 2098–102.
28. Luster AD. Chemokines – chemotactic cytokines that mediate inflammation. N Engl J Med 1998; 338: 436–45.
29. Utgaard JO, Jahnsen FL, Bakka A, Brandtzaeg P. Rapid secretion of prestored interleukin 8 from Weibel-Palade bodies of microvascular endothelial cells. J Exp Med 1998; 188: 1751–6.
30. Premack BA, Schall TJ. Chemokine receptors: gateways to inflammation and infection. Nature Med 1996; 2: 1174–8.
31. Ward SG, Bacon K, Westwick J. Chemokines and T-lymphocytes: more than an attraction. Immunity 1998; 9: 1–11.
32. Campbell JJ, Haraldson G, Pan J et al. The chemokine receptor CCR4 in vascular recognition by cutaneous but not intestinal memeory T cells. Nature 1999; 400: 776–80.
33. Mackay CR. Dual personality of memory T cells. Nature 1999; 401: 659–60.
34. Zabel BA, Agace WA, Campbell JJ et al. Human G protein-coupled receptor GPR-9-6/CC chemokine receptor 9 is selectively expressed on intestinal homing T lymphocytes, mucosal lymphocytes, and thymocytes and is required for thymus-expressed chemokine-mediated chemotaxis. J Exp Med 1999; 190: 1241–55.
35. Papadakis KA, Prehn J, Nelson V et al. The role of thymus-expressed chemokine and its receptor CCR9 in the regional specialization of the mucosal immune system. J Immunol 2000; 165: 5069–76.
36. Bonecchi R, Bianchi G, Bordignon PP et al. Differential expression of chemokine receptors and chemotactic responsiveness of type 1 T helper cells (Th1s) and Th2s. J Exp Med 1998; 187: 129–34.
37. Agace WW, Roberts AI, Wu L, Greineder C, Ebert EC, Parker CM. Human intestinal lamina propria and intraepithelial lymphocytes express receptors specific for chemo-

kines induced by inflammation. Eur J Immunol 2000; 30: 819–26.

38. Salmi M, Granfors K, MacDermott RP, Jalkanen S. Aberrant binding of lamina propria lymphocytes to vascular endothelium in inflammatory bowel disease. Gastroenterology 1994; 106: 596–605.

39. MacDermott RP, Sanderson IR, Reinecker H-C. The central role of chemokines (chemotactic cytokines) in the immunopathogenesis of ulcerative colitis and Crohn's disease. Inflamm Bowel Dis 1998; 4: 54–67.

40. Selsted ME, Oullette AJ. Defensins in granules of phagocytic and phagocytic cells. Trends Cell Biol 1995; 5: 114–19.

41. Ouellette AJ. Paneth cells and innate immunity in the crypt microenvironment. Gastroenterology 1997; 113: 1779–84.

42. Lehrer RI, Bevins CL, Ganz T. Defensins and other antimicrobial peptides. In: Ogra PL, Mestecky J, Lamm ME, Strober W, Bienenstock J, McGhee JR, editors. Mucosal Immunity, 2nd edn. San Diego: Academic Press, 1999: 89–99.

43. Yang D, Chertov O, Bykovskaia SN et al. β-Defensins: linking innate and adaptive immunity through dendritic and T cell CCR6. Science 1999; 286: 525–8.

44. Tomita M, Takase M, Bellamy W, Shimamura S. A review: the active peptide of lactoferrin. Acta Paediatr Jpn 1994; 36: 585–91.

45. Fearon DT, Locksley RM. The instructive role of innate immunity in the acquired immune response. Science 1996; 272: 50–3.

46. Medzhitov R, Janeway C. Innate immunity. N Engl J Med 2000; 343: 338–44.

47. Medzhitov R, Janeway CA. Innate immunity: impact on the adaptive immune response. Curr Opin Immunol 1997; 9: 4–9.

48. Rock FL, Hardiman G, Timans JC, Kastelein RA, Bazan JF. A family of human receptors structurally related to *Drosophila* Toll. Proc Natl Acad Sci USA 1998; 95: 588–93.

49. Selby WS, Poulter LW, Hobbs S, Jewell D, Janossy G. Heterogeneity of HLA-DR positive histiocytes of human intestinal lamina propria: a combined histochemical and immunological analysis. J Clin Pathol 1983; 36: 379–84.

50. Allison MC, Cornwall S, Poulter LW, Dhillon AP, Pounder RE. Macrophage heterogeneity in normal colonic mucosa and in inflammatory bowel disease. Gut 1988; 29: 1531–8.

51. Hara J, Ohtani H, Matsumoto T et al. Expression of costimulatory molecules B7-1 anf B7-1 in macrophages and granulomas of Crohn's disease: demonstration of cell-to-cell contact with T lymphocytes. Lab Invest 1997; 77: 175–84.

52. Golder JP, Doe WF. Isolation and preliminary characterization of human intestinal macrophages. Gastroenterology 1983; 84: 795–802.

53. Mahida YR, Wu KC, Jewell DP. Respiratory burst activity of intestinal macrophages in normal and inflammatory bowel disease. Gut 1989; 30: 1362–70.

54. Rugtveit J, Nilsen EM, Bakka A, Carlsen H, Brandtzaeg P, Scott H. Cytokine profiles differ in newly recruited and resident subsets of mucosal macrophages from inflammatory bowel disease. Gastroenterology 1997; 112: 1493–505.

55. Abbas AK, Lichtman AH, Pober JS, editors. Cellular and Molecular Immunology, 4th edn. Philadelphia: W.B. Saunders, 2000.

56. Simmonds NJ, Allen RE, Stevens TRJ et al. Chemiluminescence assay of mucosal reactive oxygen metabolites in inflammatory bowel disease. Gastroenterology 1992; 103: 186–96.

57. Oshitani N, Kitano A, Okabe H, Nakamura S, Matsumoto T, Kobayashi K. Location of superoxide anion generation in human colonic mucosa obtained by biopsy. Gut 1993; 34: 936–8.

58. Buffington GD, Doe WF. Depleted mucosal antioxidant defences in inflammatory bowel disease. Free Radical Biol Med 1995; 19: 911–18.

59. Dijkstra G, Moshage H, VanDulleman HM et al. Expression of nitric oxide synthases and formation of nitrotyrosine and reactive oxygen species in inflammatory bowel disease. J Pathol 1998; 186: 416–21.

60. Singer II, Kawka DW, Scott S et al. Expression of inducible nitric oxide synthase and nitrotyrosine in colonic epithelium in inflammatory bowel disease. Gastroenterology 1996; 111: 871–85.

61. Wallace JL, Miller MJS. Nitric oxide in mucosal defense: a little goes a long way. Gastroenterology 2000; 119: 512–20.

62. Carroll MC. The role of complement and complement receptors in induction and regulation of immunity. Annu Rev Immunol 1998; 16: 545–68.

63. Halstensen TS, Mollnes TE, Brandtzaeg P. Persistent complement activation in submucosal vessels of active inflammatory bowel disease: immunohistochemical evidence. Gastroenterology 1989; 97: 10–19.

64. Ahrenstedt O, Knutson L, Nilsson B, Nilsson-Ekdahl K, Odlind B, Hallgren R. Enhanced local production of complement components in the small intestines of patients with Crohn's disease. N Engl J Med 1990; 322: 1345–9.

65. Russell MW, Kilian M, Lamm ME. Biological activities of IgA. In: Ogra PL, Mestecky J, Lamm ME, Strober W, Bienenstock J, McGhee JR, editors. Mucosal Immunology, 2nd edn. San Diego: Academic Press, 1999.

66. Carbonare SB, Silva MLM, Trabulsi LR, Carneiro-Sampaio MMS. Inhibition of HEp-2 cell invasion by entroinvasive Escherichia coli by human colostrum IgA. Int Arch Allergy Immunol 1995; 198: 113–18.

67. Childers NK, Bruce MG, McGhee JR. Molecular mechanisms of immunoglobulin A defense. Annu Rev Microbiol 1989; 43: 503–36.

68. Walker WA, Isselbacher KJ, Bloch KJ. Intestinal uptake of macromolecules: effect of oral immunization. Science 1972; 177: 608–10.

69. Nikolova EB, Tomana M, Russell MW. All forms of human IgA antibodies bound to antigen interfere with complement (C3) fixation induced by IgG or by antigen alone. Scand J Immunol 1994; 39: 275–80.

70. VanKerckhove C, Russell GJ, Deusch K et al. Oligoclonality of human intestinal intraepithelial T cells. J Exp Med 1992; 175: 57–63.

71. Gross GC, Schwartz VL, Stevens C, Ebert EC, Blumberg RS, Balk SP. Distribution of dominant T cell receptor β chain in human intestinal mucosa. J Exp Med 1994; 180: 1337–44.

72. Ladel CH, Blum C, Dreher A, Reifenberg K, Kaufmann SH. Protective role of γ/δ T cells and α/β T cells in tuberculosis. Eur J Immunol 1995; 25: 2877–81.

73. Ebert EC. Proliferative responses of human intraepithelial lymphocytes to various T cell stimuli. Gastroenterology 1989; 97: 1372–81.

74. Cerf-Bensussan N, Guy-Grand D, Griscelli C. Intraepithelial lymphocytes of human gut: isolation, characterization and study of natural killer activity. Gut 1985; 26: 81–8.

75. Taunk J, Roberts AI, Ebert EC. Spontaneous cytotoxicity of human intrapithelial lymphocytes against epithelial cell tumors. Gastroenterology 1992; 102: 69–75.

76. Ebert EC. Human intestinal intraepithelial lymphocytes have potent chemotactic activity. Gastroenterology 1996; 109: 1154–9.

77. James SP, Fiocchi C, Graeff AS, Strober W. Phenotypic analysis of lamina propria lymphocytes. Predominance of helper-inducer and cytolytic T cell phenotype and deficiency of suppressor-inducer phenotype in Crohn's disease and control patients. Gastroenterology 1986; 91: 1483–9.

78. Saubermann LJ, Probert CSJ, Christ AD *et al.* Evidence of T cell receptor β-chain patterns in inflammatory and noninflammatory bowel disease states. Am J Physiol 1999; 276: G613–21.

79. Pallone F, Fais S, Squarcia O, Biancone L, Pozzilli P, Boirivant M. Activation of peripheral blood and intestinal lamina propria lymphocytes in Crohn's disease. *In vivo* state of activation and *in vitro* response to stimulation as defined by the expression of early activation antigens. Gut 1987; 28: 745–53.

80. Matsuura T, West GA, Youngman KR, Klein JS, Fiocchi C. Immune activation genes in inflammatory bowel disease. Gastroenterology 1993; 104: 448–58.

81. DeMaria R, Boirivant M, Cifone MG *et al.* Functional expression of Fas and Fas ligand on human gut lamina propria T lymphocytes. J Clin Invest 1996; 97: 316–22.

82. Boirivant M, Pica R, DeMaria R, Testi R, Pallone F, Strober W. Stimulated human lamina propria T cells manifest enhanced Fas-mediated apoptosis. J Clin Invest 1996; 98: 2616-22.

83. Ina K, Itoh J, Fukushima K *et al.* Resistance of Crohn's disease T cells to multiple apoptotic stimuli is associated with a Bcl-2/Bax mucosal imbalance. J Immunol 1999; 163: 1081–90.

84. Boirivant M, Marini M, DiFelice G *et al.* Lamina propria T cells in Crohn's disease and other gastrointestinal inflammation show defective CD2 pathway-induced apoptosis. Gastroenterology 1999; 116: 557–65.

85. Fiocchi C, Battisto JR, Farmer RG. Studies on isolated gut mucosal lymphocytes in inflammatory bowel disease. Detection of activated T cells and enhanced proliferation to *Staphylococcus areus* and lipopolysaccharides. Dig Dis Sci 1981; 26: 728–36.

86. MacDermott RP, Franklin GO, Jenkins KM, Kodner IJ, Nash GS, Weinrieb IJ. Human intestinal mononuclear cells. I. Investigation of antibody-dependent, lectin-induced, and spontaneous cell-mediated cytotoxic capabilities as Gastroenterology 1980; 78: 47–56.

87. Fiocchi C, Tubbs RR, Youngman KR. Human intestinal mucosal mononuclear cells exhibit lymphokine-activated killer cell activity. Gastroenterology 1985; 88: 625–37.

88. Shanahan S, Brogan M, Targan S. Human mucosal cytotoxic effector cells. Gastroenterology 1987; 92: 1951–7.

89. MacDermott RP, Bragdon MJ, Jenkins KM, Franklin GO, Shedlofsky S, Kodner IJ. Human intestinal mononuclear cells. II. Demonstration of a naturally occurring subclass of T cells which respond in the allogeneic mixed lymphocyte reaction but do not effect cell-mediated lympholysis. Gastroenterology 1981; 80: 748–57.

90. Fiocchi C. Cytokines. In: Targan SR, Shanahan F, editors. Inflammatory Bowel Disease. From Bench to Bedside. Baltimore: Williams & Wilkins, 1994: 106–22.

91. Fuss IJ, Neurath M, Boirivant M *et al.* Disparate CD4+ lamina propria lymphokine secretion profiles in inflammatory bowel disease. J Immunol 1996; 157: 1261–70.

92. Pirzer UC, Schurmann G, Post S, Betzler M, Meuer SC. Differential responsiveness to CD3-Ti vs CD2-dependent activation of human intestinal lymphocytes. Eur J Immunol 1990; 20: 2339–42.

93. Qiao L, Schurmann G, Betzler M, Meuer SC. Activation and signaling status of human lamina propria T lymphocytes. Gastroenterology 1991; 101: 1529–36.

94. Qiao L, Schurmann G, Betzler M, Meuer SC. Downregulation of protein kinase C activation in human lamina propria T lymphocytes: influence of intestinal mucosa on T cell reactivity. Eur J Immunol 1991; 21: 2385–9.

95. Qiao L, Schurmann G, Autschbach F, Wallich R, Meuer SC. Human intestinal mucosa alters T cell reactivities. Gastroenterology 1993; 105: 814–19.

96. Meuer SC, Autschbach F, Schurmann G, Golling M, Braunstein J, Qiao L. Molecular mechanisms securing 'unresponsiveness' in lamina propria T lymphocytes. NY Acad Sci 1996; 778: 174–84.

97. Bell GM, Imboden JB. CD2 and the regulation of T cell anergy. J Immunol 1995; 154: 2805–6.

98. Quill H. Anergy as a mechanims of peripheral T cell tolerance. J Immunol 1996; 156: 1325–7.

99. Zeitz M, Quinn TC, Graeff AS, James SP. Mucosal T cells provide helper function but do not proliferate when stimulated by specific antigen in lymphogranuloma venereum proctitis in nonhuman primates. Gastroenterology 1988; 94: 353–66.

100. McGhee JR, Lamm ME, Strober W. Mucosal immune responses. In: Ogra PL, Mestecky J, Lamm ME, Strober W, Bienenstock J, McGhee JR, editors. Mucosal Immunity, 2nd edn. San Diego: Academic Press, 1999: 485–506.

101. VanParijs L, Abbas AK. Homeostasis and self-tolerance in the immune system: turning lymphocytes off. Science 1998; 280: 243–8.

102. Bluestone JA. Is CTLA-4 a master switch for peripheral T cell tolerance? J Immunol 1997; 158: 1989–93.

103. Salojin KV, Zhang J, Madrenas J, Delovitch TL. T cell anergy and altered T cell receptor signaling: effects on autoimmune disease. Immunol Today 1998; 19: 468–73.

104. Reiser H, Stadecker MJ. Costimulatory B7 molecules in the pathogenesis of infections and autoimmune diseases. N Engl J Med 1996; 335: 1369–77.

105. Marelli-Berg FM, Lechler RI. Antigen presentation by parenchymal cells: a route to peripheral tolerance? Immunol Rev 1999; 172: 297–314.

106. Kabelitz D, Pohl T, Pechhold K. Activation-induced cell death (apoptosis) of mature peripheral blood T lymphocytes. Immunol Today 1993; 14: 338–9.

107. Lynch DH, Ramsdell F, Alderson MR. Fas and FasL in the homeostatic regulation of immune responses. Immunol Today 1995; 16: 569–74.

108. Shevach EA. Regulatory T cells in autoimmunity. Annu Rev Immunol 2000; 18: 423–49.

109. Strobel S, Mowat AM. Immune responses to dietary antigens: oral tolerance. Immunol Today 1998; 19: 173–81.

110. Podolsky DK, Fiocchi C. Cytokines, chemokines, growth factors, eicosanoids and other bioactive molecules in IBD. In: Kirsner JB, editor. Inflammatory Bowel Disease. Philadelphia: W.B. Saunders, 1999: 191–207.

111. Husby S. Normal immune responses to ingested foods. J Pediatr Gastroenterol Nutr 2000; 30: S13–19.

112. Simecka JW. Mucosal immunity of the gastrointestinal tract and oral tolerance. Adv Drug Deliv Rev 1998; 34: 235–59.

113. Whitaker CC, Gienapp IE, Orosz CG, Bitar D. Oral tolerance in experimental autoimmune encephalomyelitis. III. Evidence for clonal anergy. J Immunol 1991; 147: 2155–63.

114. Chen Y, Inobe J-I, Marks R, Gonnella P, Kuchroo VK, Weiner HL. Peripheral deletion of antigen-reactive T cells in oral tolerance. Science 1995; 376: 177–80.

115. Saoudi A, Seddon B, Heath V, Fowell D, Mason D. The physiological role of regulatory T cells in the prevention of autoimmunity: the function of the thymus in the generation of the regulatory T cell subset. Immunol Rev 1996; 149: 195–216.

116. Chen Y, Kuchroo VK, Inobe J-I, Hafler DA, Weiner HL. Regulatory T cell clones induced by oral tolerance: suppression of autoimmune encephalomyelitis. Science 1994; 265: 1237–40.

117. Groux H, O'Garra A, Bigler M *et al.* A CD4$^+$ T cell subset inhibits antigen-specific T cell responses and prevents colitis. Nature 1997; 389: 737–42.

118. Khoo UY, Proctor IE, Macpherson AJS. CD4$^+$ T cell down-regulation in human intestinal mucosa. Evidence for intestinal tolerance to luminal bacterial antigens. J Immunol 1997; 158: 3626–34.

119. Cong BY, Brandwein SL, McCabe RP *et al.* CD4+ T cells reactive to enteric bacterial antigens in spontaneously colitic C3H/HeJBir mice: increased T helper cell type 1 response and ability to transfer disease. J Exp Med 1998; 187: 855–64.

120. Read S, Malmstrom V, Powrie F. Cytotoxic T lymphocyte-associated antigen 4 plays an essential role in the function of CD25+CD4+ regulatory cells that control intestinal inflammation. J Exp Med 2000; 192: 295–302.

121. Asseman C, Mauze S, Leach MW, Coffman RL, Powrie F. An essential role for interleukin 10 in the function of regulatory T cells that inhibit intestinal inflammation. J Exp Med 1999; 190: 995–1003.

122. Gorelik L, Flavell RA. Abrogation of TGFβ signaling in T cells leads to spontaneous T cell differentiation and autoimmune disease. Immunity 2000; 12: 171–81.

123. Weiner HL. Oral tolerance: immune mechanisms and treatment of autoimmune diseases. Immunol Today 1997; 18: 335–43.

124. Crowe SE. Food allergies. In: Ogra PL, Mestecky J, Lamm ME, Strober W, Bienenstock J, McGhee JR, editors. Mucosal Immunity, 2nd edn. San Diego: Academic Press, 1999: 1129–39.

125. Fiocchi C. The immunological resources of the large bowel. In: Kirsner JB, Shorter RG, editors. Diseases of the Colon, Rectum, and Anal Canal. Baltimore: Williams & Wilkins, 1988: 95–117.

126. Fuller R. A review: Probiotics in man and animals. J Appl Bacteriol 1989; 66: 365–78.

127. Kolb H, Pozzilli P. Cow's milk and type I diabetes: the gut immune system deserves attention. Immunol Today 1999; 20: 108–110.

128. Naidu AS, Bidlack WR, Clemens RA. Probiotic spectra of lactic acid bacteria (LAB). Critical Rev Food Sci Nutr 1999; 38: 13–126.

129. Wilson KH, Ikeda JS, Blitchington RB. Phylogenetic placement of community members in human colonic biota. Clin Infect Dis 1997; 25: S114–16.

130. Famularo G, Moretti S, Marcellini S, DeSimone C. Stimulation of immunity by probiotics. In: Fuller R, editor. Probiotics 2. Applications and Practical Aspects. London: Chapman & Hall, 1997: 133–61.

131. Elson CO, Sartor RB, Tennyson GS, Riddell RH. Experimental models of inflammatory bowel disease. Gastroenterology 1995; 109: 1344–67.

132. Rath HC, Herfarth HH, Ikeda JS *et al.* Normal luminal bacteria, especially *Bacteroides* species, mediate chronic colitis, gastritis, and arthritis in HLA-B27/human β2 microglobulin transgenic rats. J Clin Invest 1996; 98: 945–53.

133. Rath HC, Ikeda JS, Linde H-J, Scholmerich J, Wilson KH, Sartor RB. Varying cecal bacterial loads influences colitis and gastritis in HLA-B27 transgenic rats. Gastroenterology 1999; 116: 310–19.

134. Sellon RK, Tonkonogy S, Schultz M *et al.* Resident enteric bacteria are necessary for development of spontaneous colitis and immune system activation in interleukin-10-deficient mice. Infect Immun 1998; 66: 5224–31.

135. Rutgeerts P, Geboes K, Peeters M *et al.* Effect of faecal stream diversion on recurrence of Crohn's disease in the neoterminal ileum. Lancet 1991; 2: 771–4.

136. D'Haens G, Geboes K, Peeters M, Baert F, Penninckx F, Rutgeerts P. Early lesions caused by infusion of intestinal contents in excluded ileum of Crohn's disease. Gastroenterology 1998; 114: 262–7.

137. Ruseler-van-Embden JGH, Schouten WR, van Lieshout LMC. Pouchitis: result of microbial imbalance? Gut 1994; 35: 658–64.

138. Prantera C, Scribano ML, Berto E, Zannoni F. Antibiotic use in Crohn's disease – why and how? Biodrugs 1997; 8: 293–306.

139. Turunen UM, Farkkila MA, Hakala K *et al.* Long-term treatment of ulcerative colitis with ciprofloxacin: a prospective, double-blind, placebo-controlled study. Gastroenterology 1998; 115: 1072–8.

140. Gionchetti P, Rizzello F, Venturi A *et al.* Oral bacteriotherapy as maintenance treatment in patients with chronic pouchitis: a double-blind, placebo-controlled trial. Gastroenterology 2000; 119: 305–9.

141. Duchmann R, Kaiser I, Hermann E, Mayet W, Ewe K, Meyer zum Buschenfelde KH. Tolerance exists towards resident intestinal flora but it is broken in active inflammatory bowel disease (IBD). Clin Exp Immunol 1995; 102: 448–55.

142. Duchmann R, Schmitt E, Knolle P, Meyer zum Buschenfelde KH, Neurath M. Tolerance towards resident intestinal flora in mice is abrogated in experimental colitis and restored by treatment with interlukin-10 or antibodies to interleukin-12. Eur J Immunol 1996; 26: 934–8.

143. Pirzer U, Schonhaar A, Fleischer B, Hermann E, Meyer zum Buschenfelde KH. Reactivity of infiltrating T lymphocytes with microbial antigens in Crohn's disease. Lancet 1991; 338: 1238–9.

144. Takahashi I, Iijima H, Katashima R, Itakura M, Kiyono H. Clonal expansion of CD4$^+$ T cells in TCR α-chain-deficient mice by gut-derived antigens. J Immunol 1999; 162: 1843–50.

145. Wirtz S, Finotto S, Kanzler S *et al.* Chronic intestinal inflammation in STAT-4 transgenic mice: characterization of disease and adoptive transfer by TNF- plus IFN-γ-producing CD4+ T cells that respond to bacterial antigens. J Immunol 1999; 162: 1884–8.

6 | The lymphocyte–epithelial–bacterial interface

ROBERT HERSHBERG AND RICHARD S. BLUMBERG

Introduction

The immunologic and antigenic challenge faced along the gastrointestinal tract is truly extraordinary. Across a surface area that approximates a tennis court, it is here that we separate the highest concentration of foreign antigen (mostly food and bacteria) from the largest complement of lymphocytes in the body by a single cell layer of polarized epithelium. The gut-associated lymphoid tissue (or GALT) has evolved highly complex mechanisms to permit life in this 'open ecosystem'. Although the dominant 'response' of the GALT to orally administered antigen or non-invasive microbes is that of immunologic tolerance (or oral tolerance), the GALT can also initiate both regional and systemic responses to certain antigens and pathogens. The precise molecular mechanisms by which the mucosal immune system regulates this intricate balance between tolerance and responsiveness remain incompletely understood [1, 2].

While most individuals can maintain 'homeostasis' and health in the face of this extreme immunologic challenge, others cannot. Indeed, the clinical entities collectively known as inflammatory bowel disease, or IBD (i.e. Crohn's disease and ulcerative colitis) are conditions in which inflammation persists at various anatomic sites along the gastrointestinal tract [3]. IBD is the second most common disease of potential autoimmune etiology in the United States – affecting approximately 1 in 2 to 1 in 10 individuals [4]. Although many details regarding the etiology of IBD remain unclear, a central hypothesis has emerged. Specifically, IBD can be said to represent an aberrant immune response to bacteria from the lumen of the intestinal tract in a subset of individuals with a genetic predispostion or propensity to develop chronic, mucosal inflammation.

This is a broad hypothesis that needs to be viewed within the context of the current genetic data describing the marked heterogeneity of human IBD. Still, the microbial focus inherent to the hypothesis highlights a series of important cell types at the mucosal interface (T lymphocytes and antigen-presenting cells including intestinal epithelial cells) and their associated questions. For example, what is the nature of the bacterial species that are responsible? Do the predisposing genes relate to immunologic function within the GALT or to intrinsic properties of the gastrointestinal tract (e.g. intestinal barrier function)? What are the immune effector cells that mediate IBD and how are they modulated by bacteria? In this chapter we address these and other questions and early events relevant to the central hypothesis outlined; in particular, those involving interaction between bacteria and the lymphocytes of the GALT at the epithelial interface.

The microbial ecosystem

We live in a complex microbial environment, with the diversity and number of prokaryotic cells far outnumbering the eukaryotic cells of their hosts. In no instance of human health or disease is this fact more important than in a discussion of immunity at mucosal surfaces and the pathogenesis of IBD. Indeed, we exist in a completely open ecosystem – with the anatomy of the entire gastrointestinal tract from the mouth to the rectum in continuity with the external environment. In this context one might consider the gastrointestinal tract as 'outside-in' – with an extensive microbiota derived from the *outside* world resident *inside* the body, generally with highly beneficial consequences [5].

Studies from both humans and mice have underscored the critical nature of the intestinal microbiota in the establishment and maintenance of IBD. The data from human studies include the potential efficacy of antibiotics in treating patients with IBD [6], the resolution of inflammation distal to fecal diversion [7], and the recent data showing a beneficial effect of 'probiotic' therapy [8]. The mouse data are even more compelling with data from many labora-

Stephan R. Targan, Fergus Shanahan and Loren C. Karp (eds.), Inflammatory Bowel Disease: From Bench to Bedside, 2nd Edition, 121–146.
© 2003 *Kluwer Academic Publishers. Printed in Great Britain*

tories demonstrating a lack of mucosal inflammation in established mouse models of IBD raised in either a 'germfree' (GF) or a clean 'specific pathogen free' (SPF) environment. These data have extended across the spectrum of mouse models described [3], including models dominated by 'Th1' responses (e.g. IL-$10^{-/-}$, IL-$2^{-/-}$, CD45RB^{hi} transfer model, SAMP1/Yit) models dominated by 'Th2' responses (e.g. TCRα$^{-/-}$, WASP$^{-/-}$) and models characterized by intrinsic 'barrier' defects (e.g. mdr1a$^{-/-}$) (reviewed in ref. 9 and Chapter 4). Recent data from a number of laboratories indicate that repopulation of these mice with limited numbers of organisms (e.g. murine *Helicobacter*) in these 'clean' mice can trigger the inflammation previously seen when the mice were housed in conventional ('dirty') colonies [10, 11]. Interestingly, the same bacterial challenge in normal mice has no untoward consequences. Although the molecular details as to how these bacteria induce mucosal inflammation in these genetically susceptible hosts remain to be determined, the mounting evidence favors the 'bacterial hypothesis'. Given the estimates of there being approximately 10^9 organisms per milliliter of fecal material (closely approximating the maximum packing density), it is perhaps surprising that more individuals do not develop chronic mucosal inflammation.

Clearly, the mucosal immune system has evolved to balance the need to respond to pathogens while maintaining active 'tolerance' to commensal bacteria (and food antigens) [2]. Consistent with the data from mice and family studies in humans highlighting the genetic basis of susceptibility to IBD in certain individuals (addressed in more detail in Chapter 3), most individuals exist in a homeostatic balance with the complex microbiota in their intestinal tract [12]. Understanding why and how certain people show a 'dysregulated' (or pathogenic) response to bacteria that are not universally pathogenic remains central to our detailed understanding of IBD pathogenesis. Still, the microbiota itself can be considered a dynamic, living, organism – and is likely to shape the host mucosal immune response and balance [13]. Hence, a more detailed understanding of the bacterial populations of the gastrointestinal tract is likely also to offer important and critical clues to the cause(s) of IBD.

The microbiota of the gastrointestinal tract have been the topic of several recent thorough and insightful reviews from authors with extensive experience in this area [5, 13–16]. In this portion of the current chapter we focus on microbial aspects most relevant to IBD, and not on providing the comprehensive microbiological overview seen in these recent summaries.

General considerations

Although precise estimates are difficult, there appear to be > 350 different species of bacteria present in the colon of the normal human. In actuality the number is likely to be dramatically higher when viewed in the context that conventional culture techniques result in growth of less than 50% of the organisms present [17]. There are clear regional differences in bacterial populations identified along the cephalocaudal axis of the gastrointestinal tract (see below), but the overall representation of bacterial genera is extremely broad. In the colon, where bacterial counts are four to five orders of magnitude higher than proximal to the ileocecal valve, all major groups of bacterial species are present (Table 1). Specifically, one finds a diverse mixture of Gram-positive, Gram-negative, and atypical bacteria (e.g. mycobacteria) that grow under varying conditions (e.g. aerobic, facultatively anaerobic and obligate anaerobic conditions).

Hence, in order to interpret the literature in this complex area, and its potential relationship to IBD, one needs to consider a few important technical considerations. First, what are the conditions used to culture the organisms? For example, culture conditions for aerobes or facultative anaerobes are widely available, while anaerobic culture is still difficult and problematic. Second, what is the nature of the patient sampling? Certainly, the clinical and medication history (e.g. bowel preparation for surgery or endoscopy) will bias the results obtained from microbiological analysis. In addition, there are likely to be marked differences when biopsies and/or surgical specimens are used as a source for culture compared to stool samples. Finally, what is the cost of such detailed analysis? Given the biodiversity present, the answer is likely to be high. This final consideration has limited the detailed analysis of large numbers of individual patients and detailed 'species' analysis. The increasing widespread use of 16S rRNA sequence analysis for microbial detection and analysis [18] is a promising approach now being extended to studies of the gastrointestinal tract [19].

In this context it should not be surprising that there are few data on the 'complete' analysis of the gastrointestinal mucosal microbiota – either in normal individuals or individuals with IBD. The 'best' data set now dates back to the seminal work of

Table 1. Common bacteria in human large intestine

Organism	Description	Range in log scale
Bacterioides	Anaerobic Gram-negative rods, most common species include *B. thetaiotaomicron*, *B. vulgatus*, *B. ovatus* and *B. fragilis*	9–12
Fusobacterium	Anaerobic Gram-negative rods, most common species include *F. mortiferum* and *F. necrophorum*	7–12
Peptostreptococcus	Anaerobic Gram-positive cocci, most common species is *Ps. productus*	5–12
Bifidobacterium	Anaerobic Gram-positive, non-spore-forming rods, most common species include *B. adolescentis*, *B. infantis* and *B. longum*	6–12
Eubacterium	Anaerobic Gram-positive, non-spore-forming rods, most common species include *E. aerofaciens*, *E. lentum* and *E. contortum*	9–12
Lactobacillus	Facultative and obligately anaerobic Gram-positive rods, most common species include *L. acidophilus*, *L. fermentum* and *L. plantarum*	4–12
Clostridium	Anaerobic, spore-forming, Gram-positive rods, most common species include *C. perfringens*, *C. bifermentans* and *C. ramosum*	7–12
Enterococcus	Facultative Gram-positive cocci; *E. faecalis* and *E. faecium* are most common species	5–10
Streptococcus	Facultative Gram-positive cocci; *S. lactis* and *S. intermedius* are most common species	5–9
Staphylococcus	Facultative Gram-positive cocci	3–6
Eschericha coli	Facultative Gram-negative cocci	3–9
Enterobacter	Facultative Gram-negative cocci	3–9
Klebsiella	Facultative Gram-negative cocci	3–9

Reproduced with permission from ref. 14

Gorbach and colleagues [20], i.e. over 20 years. The current consensus will be briefly summarized.

Stomach/small intestine

Previously thought to be 'sterile', the stomach and small intestine harbor considerable microbiologic diversity. The proximal gastrointestinal tract contains abundant flora, derived predominantly from the mouth. These include, but are not limited to, alpha-hemolytic *Streptococcus*, *Staphylococcus epidermidis*, and various yeast species. The hostile acidic environment of the stomach results in a rapid decline of culturable organisms. Still, the obvious presence and functional consequences of *Helicobacter pylori* infection in the stomach and proximal small intestine highlight the importance of bacterially-driven mucosal inflammation even in the proximal gastrointestinal tract [21].

The small intestine is marked by a 'transition' from oral to colonic flora. It is here that one needs to consider ingested food as a microbiological reservoir and source for colonization. For example, dairy products, meats and fruits/vegetables are rich sources of bacteria. The substantial antimicrobial effect of low gastric pH is likely responsible for the fact that bacterial counts are not higher in the proximal gastrointestinal tract. Still, as one moves more distally, one sees increasing concentrations of bacterial counts and increasing numbers of Gram-negative species (e.g. Enterobacteriaceae, *Bacteroides*, Enterococci species) as one approaches the terminal ileum. The total counts in the jejunum are 10^3–10^4 times higher than in the jejunum, and one study has estimated the counts at the terminal ileum approximating those seen in the proximal colon [22].

Table 2. Comparison of human MHC class I, MHC class II, and CD1

	MHC class I	MHC class II	CD1
Structure			
Gene locus	Chromosome 6	Chromosome 6	Chromosome 1
N-glycosylation	Yes	Yes	Yes; No (37 kDa CD1d)
Cytoplasmic tail	Long: 3 exons	Variable lengths: 1 exon	Short: 2 exons with motif for endosomal targeting in CD1b,c,d*
Genomic structure	Exons 2–4 encode the $\alpha 1$, $\alpha 2$, $\alpha 3$ domains	Exons 2–3 encode the $\alpha 1$, $\alpha 2$ (or $\beta 1$, $\beta 2$) domains	Exons 2–4 encode the $\alpha 1$, $\alpha 2$, $\alpha 3$ domains
Homology in $\alpha 1$, $\alpha 2$, $\alpha 3$ domains	–	–	25–30% with $\alpha 2$ domain of MHC class I; 30–35% with $\beta 2$ domain of MHC Class II
Allelic polymorphism in $\alpha 1$–$\alpha 2$ domains	Polymorphic	Polymorphic	Nonpolymorphic
Biosynthesis/assembly			
β_2-microglobulin dependence	Yes	No	Yes (CD1a–c); yes/no (CD1d)
TAP dependence	Yes	No	No
Associated chaperones	Calnexin, calreticulin, tapasin	Invariant chain, HLA-DM	Calnexin (CD1b) prolyl-4-hydroxylase (CD1d)
Function			
Cellular expression	Ubiquitous	B-cells, dendritic cells, Langerhans cells, activated monocytes, IEC	CD1a–c: thymocytes, B cells, Langerhans cells, activated monocytes, IELs (?); CD1d: IEC, hepatocytes, B cells, monocytes, dendritic cells
Peptide presentation	9 amino acids	14–22 amino acids	22 amino acids (murine CD1d)
Lipid presentation	No	No	Lipoglycan: CD1b,c; glycosylceramide and glyco-phosphatidylinositol: CD1d
T cell recognition	CD8$^+$, TCR $\alpha\beta^+$	CD4$^+$, TCR $\alpha\beta^+$	CD8$^-$CD4$^-$TCR $\alpha\beta^+$ (CD1a,b,c,d); CD8$^-$CD4$^-$TCR $\gamma\delta^+$ (CD1c); CD8$^+$ TCR $\alpha\beta^+$ iIELs (CD1a,c,d); CD8$^-$CD4$^+$TCR$\alpha\beta^+$ (CD1d)

*YXXZ → Tyrosine–amino acid–amino acid–hydrophobic amino acid.

is orders of magnitude greater than that of the FAE, and that many bacteria adhere to and invade columnar epithelial cells, it is likely that bacterial entry is not restricted to lymphoid follicles. Indeed, in the colon, 'classical' lymphoid follicles (PP) are absent, although small lymphoid aggregates, presumably with modified FAE, can be seen (see below), yet

bacteria are able to cross the mucosal barrier and trigger IBD.

The barriers to bacterial entry across the intestinal mucosal surface are numerous and varied. From an anatomical standpoint there is an extensive mucinous glycocalyx extending from the apical (i.e. luminal) surface of epithelial cells that can trap bacteria and prevent adherance [42]. In addition, epithelial cells are connected to one another by so-called tight junctions which effectively limit the paracellular transport of macromolecules across the epithelial barrier [43]. Furthermore, various populations of cells along the gastrointestinal tract (e.g. Paneth cells) are capable of secreting small peptides (e.g. defensins) that have potent, local, antimicrobial properties (see below).

How do bacteria breach this formidable barrier and stimulate mucosal inflammation? The answer is complex, but derives in part from the growing realization that alterations in intestinal barrier function are seen in IBD – and that this 'dysregulation' of barrier function may contribute to the establishment of IBD. Indeed, the term 'dysregulation' (and not simply disruption) underscores the fact that the barrier is a dynamic structure that is actively regulated and maintained. Based on seminal studies using polarized monolayers of intestinal epithelial cells *in vitro*, it is clear that various cytokines present in the intestinal mucosa regulate intestinal barrier function. Notably, interferon gamma (IFN-γ), IL-4, and IL-13 all attenuate barrier function [44, 45], while IL-10 appears to 'enhance' the barrier [46]. While the precise mechanisms underlying this regulation are not known, recent data suggest that alterations in the apical actin cytoskeleton might disrupt the structural integrity of the tight junction [47]. As the molecular architecture of the tight junction becomes more clear, establishing the direct link(s) between signaling events resulting from proinflammatory cytokines (for example, IFN-γ) and specific tight junction proteins will be possible. These proteins are likely to include the growing number of MAGUK-like molecules (Z0-1, -2, -3, claudins, occludins) that are concentrated at these junctions [48].

Finally, it is important to consider how alterations in intestinal barrier function (with the untoward effect of increased transit of bacteria into mucosal tissues) may contribute to an underlying genetic predisposition to the development of IBD. As noted, decreased barrier function is a hallmark of established IBD [49]. Interestingly, some investigators have suggested that alterations in barrier function actually precede the appearance of IBD, and are seen to a greater degree in healthy, first-degree relatives of patients with IBD [50]. These human data are supported by mouse data showing alterations in barrier function preceding histological inflammation in the IL-10 knockout mice [51] and the enhanced mucosal inflammation that could be induced in mice deficient

for intestinal trefoil factor, a molecule important in intestinal epithelial repair and restitution [52]. Taken together, the information suggests that subtle alterations in barrier function (e.g. abnormal regulation of tight junctions, impaired epithelial restitution) may contribute to the underlying genetic susceptibility to IBD seen in humans and some experimental animals. One might predict that the function of one of more of the IBD susceptibility genes being mapped by various groups will relate to intestinal barrier maintenance.

Immune cell populations

Phenotype of T cells

Exemplary of the fact that the mucosal surfaces of the intestine must confront a large microbial antigenic burden, it is not surprising that it has been estimated that approximately 10% of the T lymphocytes in the normal host are associated with the GALT. These GALT-associated T cells are organized into three compartments connected by distinctive and highly regulated trafficking pathways. These include Peyer's patches (PP) and related isolated lymphoid follicles that are considered important sites of immune response induction and the loosely affiliated lamina propria and intraepithelial lymphocyte compartments, which are considered effector compartments [53]. Consistent with this, the vast majority of T cells within the PP are naive, thymically derived T cells that are characterized as $CD3^+$ $TCR\alpha\beta^+$ $CD45RA^+$ $\alpha^4\beta_7^{hi}$ L-selectin $(CD62L)^+$ $CD44^{lo}$ $\alpha^E\beta_7^-$ with a CD4:CD8 ratio of 3.5:1. These naive T cells, as well as their naive $(IgM^+ IgD^+)$ B cell counterparts, are directed to the PP via interactions between $\alpha^4\beta_7$ and L-selectin on the T cell and the protein and carbohydrate constituents of Mad-CAM1 on the high endothelial venule (HEV), respectively. In addition, contributions are provided from interactions between LFA1 ($\alpha^L\beta_2$, CD11a/CD18) and either ICAM1 (CD54) or ICAM2 (CD120) on the lymphocyte and HEV, respectively. Consistent with this naivety, most of the T cells possess a diverse array of TCR-$\alpha\beta$ chains [54]. Few TCR-$\gamma\delta^+$ T cells can be observed within the PP, consistent with the notion that they have received their priming earlier in ontogeny within the thymus [55].

At any one time a significant subset of these naive T cells within the PP are likely the recipients of their cognate antigen-derived signal from the luminal milieu as transported to the lymphoreticular structures of the PP by specialized microfold villous (M) cells. This is based upon the fact that the ratio of CD45RA:CD45RO within the organized GALT is 1:1 and the majority of these CD40RO$^+$ (memory) cells are congregated within the M cell pocket immediately adjacent to the lumen in the context of professional APC [56]. The range of luminal antigens, including antigens from commensal bacteria, that are specifically sampled by the M cell and/or breach the M cell barrier through pathologic mechanisms (e.g. pathogenic microbes) thus dictates the generation of antigen-specific B and T cell blasts which emigrate from the PP via efferent lymphatics.

The antigen-specific CD4$^+$ and CD8$^+$ T cell blasts including memory populations, which are largely $\alpha^4\beta_7^{hi}$ L-selectin^{lo} CD45RO$^+$, presumably migrate from the PP and disseminate widely to the loosely affiliated tissues associated with the lamina propria and epithelium. This occurs through interactions between protein components of MadCAM1 on the postcapillary venule (PCV) and $\alpha^4\beta_7$ on the T cell together with interactions between LFA-1 on the T cell and ICAM1/ICAM2 on the PCV. Whereas both CD4$^+$ and CD8$^+$ memory cells and blasts populate the lamina propria, the epithelium is preferentially populated by CD8$^+$ T cells. The basis for this is unclear, but presumably reflects differences in the presumed effector functions of the T cells within the lamina propria and epithelium [57].

Lamina propria lymphocytes (LPL)

LPL represent a tightly regulated effector compartment. The vast majority of these T cells express the memory marker, CD45RO ($>80\%$), with a ratio of CD4:CD8 cells which approximates peripheral blood (2:1) [32, 53]. Based upon TCR repertoire analysis the CD4$^+$ LPL are directed at a broad range of antigens with evidence of a limited number of clonally expanded cell populations [36]. Although the nature of the antigens to which these small numbers of clonal expansions is directed is unknown, it is presumed that they relate to secondary responses to previously remote antigenic encounters. This is consistent with the fact that LPL, which are responsive to remote enteral viral infections and presumably microbial infections, for example, can be identified [58]. The CD8$^+$ LPL, on the other hand, exhibit a significantly greater proportion of clonal expansions as defined by complementarity determining region 3 (CDR3) analyses suggesting, perhaps, either a larger number of secondary exposures for this subset and/or differences in their susceptibility to activation-induced cell death in comparison to the CD4$^+$ T cell subset [36].

The entire LPL compartment, both CD4 and CD8, are highly activated. This activation is manifest by a phenotype which is uniformly L-selectin^{lo} CD44^{hi} CD69$^+$. Yet, at the same time, the activation LPL is restrained since only a limited proportion of these cells express the high-affinity IL-2 receptor α chain, CD25 ($<20–25\%$) [53]. Moreover, LPL exhibit a limited evidence of spontaneous proliferation based upon expression of Ki67, a nuclear marker of proliferation, or uptake of bromodeoxyuridine. Additionally, LPL are hypoproliferative to TCR/CD3 complex-mediated signals *in vitro* [59]. However, at the same time, LPL respond to antigenic signals with significant cytokine production (as measured by IL-2). These characteristics suggest that, under physiologic circumstances, LPL are chronically stimulated by antigens ubiquitously present in the intestinal environment but which elicit predominantly cytokine production and little proliferation. This maintains a tight control on LPL T cell numbers. The cytokines produced are consistent with a predominantly T helper (Th) 2-tone under normal physiologic conditions [60]. In the physiologic context it is likely that the antigens responsible for this unique state of T cell activation are derived from the intestinal microenvironment and, presumably, components of the normal microbiota. Specifically, mice expressing a transgenic T cell receptor specific for ovalbumin in the context of MHC class II I-A^d do not exhibit this activated LPL phenotype when the transgenic animal is back-crossed onto a recombinase activating gene (RAG)-deficient background [61]. In the absence of the RAG gene the expression of non-allelically excluded T cell receptor (TCR)-α chains is prevented. Thus, it can be argued that the LPL are maintained at a certain level of restrained activation by components of the normal microbiota; poised for a pathologic assault.

The loosely affiliated lamina propria also contains varieties of organized structures: lymphocyte filled villi (LFV), isolated lymphoid follicles (ILF) and cryptopatches. LFV are congregations of predominantly CD4$^+$ CD45RO$^+$ T cells with variable numbers of B cells and MHC class II$^+$ dendritic cells with an overlying epithelium similar to FAE [62]. ILF are submucosal lymphoid aggregates that contain a B cell follicle and memory T cells, suggesting a region undergoing a cognate immune response. Finally, cryptopatches, which are present in rodent but not adult human intestinal tissues, consist of lamina propria structures that appear to be the source of extrathymic T cell lymphopoiesis within the intestine. These structures are independent of luminal bacteria (occur in germfree animals) and a thymus (occur in nu/nu mice) but are dependent on IL-7 and consist of a limited number (2000–5000) of c-kit$^+$IL7R$^+$CD44$^+$Thy1$^{+/-}$CD4$^{+/-}$CD25$^{+/-}$α^E-β$_7$Lin$^-$ (lineage markers such as CD3, B220, Mac-1 and Gr-1 associated with T cell, B cell, macrophage and granulocyte development, respectively) cells which give rise to TCR-αβ and TCR-γδ cells [63].

iIEL

Intestinal intraepithelial lymphocytes (iIEL) are predominantly T cells with few, if any, B cells [57]. Although IEL are present in the epithelium during antenatal life as early as 11 weeks of gestation, suggesting an initial antigen-independent origin, their numbers increase rapidly postnatally. This massive increase (more than 10-fold) appears to be driven by the luminal microbiota as it is not evident in germfree mice and rats [64]. Although it is possible that these developmental changes may be due to the induction of phenotypic changes in the epithelium and associated structures, there is some reason to believe that these changes are antigen-driven as the effects of the microbiota on IEL are also reflected in changes in TCR repertoire [65].

Most IEL of mouse and human origin are CD45RO$^+$ (memory) CD8$^+$ T cells which express a limited array of αβ TCR, suggesting restriction to a narrow range of MHC class I-related molecules and their antigenic ligands. Whether these putative antigens are derived from the normal luminal microbiota, and thus reflect important immunoregulatory functions of these cells such as the MHC class I chain-related genes [MICA; 66] or are directed to either non-cognate 'stress signals' on altered intestinal epithelial cells or remote pathogenic exposures remains to be defined. It is likely that all these possibilities are operative, although their relative contributions at any given time are unknown. IEL have been shown to have immunoregulatory functions associated with oral tolerance, to exhibit recognition of non-classical MHC-like molecules (see below) and to exhibit antigen-specific, MHC recognition of remote viral antigens, for example [57].

Like LPL, IEL are in a unique state of activation. They are almost uniformly CD69$^+$, CD44^{hi} and L-sel^{lo} consistent with previous exposure to an activation signal delivered presumably through the TCR [53]. Given that this phenotype is evident in the 'physiologically' inflamed intestine, it seems plausible to suggest that these antigenic signals are derived from the luminal microbiota. Whether the oligoclonality normally associated with human and rodent IEL is related to these same antigenic signals is unknown [67–69].

In addition to these activation markers, IEL also express a unique constellation of homing markers consistent with their mucosal localization within the epithelium (α^{E}β$_7$$^+$, CCR9$^+$) and natural killer markers [70–72]. The latter are quite interesting as this group of molecules (killer inhibitory and activatory receptors) affect the regulation and activation state of cells. This suggests one possible mechanism by which IEL may be tightly controlled despite a constant exposure to their cognate, perhaps luminal bacterial, antigens as reflected by their anatomic location and activation state. Control of IEL and likely LPL is also likely mediated by a large array of soluble mediators including TGF-β and unknown factors many of which are derived from the IEC itself [73]. Whether these factors are directly regulated by the luminal microbiota is unknown.

Regulation of lymphocyte populations by luminal microbiota

Given the apparent central role of the normal luminal microbiota in regulating the development of IBD, and that colonization of the mammalian intestine occurs prior to the onset of disease in genetically susceptible animals (rodent and human), it is important to consider how the phenotype and function of mucosal lymphocyte populations are regulated by such factors. There are two potential roles of the luminal microbiota: promoting the development of the normal GALT and maintenance of the state of physiologic inflammation. Given that both of these are likely operative in the normal mammalian host, it is possible that, in the genetically susceptible host, abnormalities of one and/or the other process may be existent. It is therefore important to consider the supportive evidence for these processes in the normal host and what is known in the genetically susceptible host.

Most of the work in this area has been performed with respect to the development and responses of B lymphocytes [74]. Germfree rodents exhibit functional hypotrophy of the cells and tissues associated with the GALT. The PP are small, poorly developed structures that primarily contain B cells which exhibit diminished responses to B cell mitogens and antigens. Most of the B cells which are present have a naive (IgM$^+$IgD$^+$) phenotype with few or no IgG$^+$ or IgA$^+$ cells, indicating that these cells have switched their immunoglobulin locus under stimulation of cognate antigen. Consistent with this, IgA$^+$ antibody secreting plasma cells are markedly diminished in the spleen and lamina propria. In comparison, rodents raised in conventional conditions exhibit PP with secondary lymphoid follicles with reactive germinal centers as would be observed in an antigen-activated peripheral lymph node, high levels of switched B cells (IgG$^+$ and IgA$^+$) in the PP and significant number of IgA-secreting plasma cells in the spleen and lamina propria. Interestingly, when adult rodents which had previously been raised under germfree conditions are later colonized with non-pathogenic microorganisms, their immune responses are often augmented [75]. This suggests that, if mucosal priming does not occur either at the correct time of life or with the appropriate microbial antigen, hyperresponsiveness to the microbial antigen may ensue; a phenomenon of obvious relevance to IBD.

It is also important to recognize that not all organisms have the ability to drive the development and activation state of the GALT. Some organisms which are components of the normal microbiota elicit no detectable immune response as assessed by the presence of IgA antibodies. Such organisms are considered part of the authochthonous microbiota which have presumably coevolved with the host to such a degree that they are truly tolerated non-pathogens. Other organisms, on the other hand, which are also components of the normal microbiota, elicit a non-pathogenic secretory IgA immune response. This immune response is, however, self-limited in that secondary exposures with the same microorganism are muted. At the same time the immunizing microorganism can be found intraluminally coated with IgA. Thus the normal microbiota of the mammalian intestine stimulates a state of tolerance that is manifest by the production of specific secretory IgA antibodies that likely prevents the further uptake of the relevant microbe.

Similar regulation of the development and activation of the cellular immune system has also been elucidated [74]. As noted above, the numbers of TCR-$\alpha\beta^+$ IEL, but not TCR-$\gamma\delta^+$ IEL, increase dramatically with bacterial colonization [64]. Moreover,

the spontaneous cytotoxic activity of these IEL, a characteristic feature of these cells, is also markedly up-regulated. Thus, the cytotoxicity of IEL obtained from conventionally reared animals is markedly elevated over those observed with animals reared under germfree conditions. Not only the CD8$^+$ compartment, but also the CD4$^+$ compartment, is affected. CD4$^+$ T cells from germfree animals exhibit a diminution in the autologous mixed lymphocyte reaction. Consistent with these functional observations, most PP T cells in germfree animals are naive (CD45RB^{hi}), similar to the levels observed in a sterile peripheral lymph node. Upon colonization, increased levels of activated or memory (CD45RB^{lo}) cells are observed. Given that all of these characteristics are observed in healthy animals, it can only be assumed that the normal microbiota establishes a unique state of inflammation which is associated with the health of the host. Moreover, this healthy state not only affects the physiology of the intestine but extends to the whole host [76].

The intestinal epithelial cell as an antigen-presenting cell

The gastrointestinal tract represents a unique immunologic compartment which subserves an important role in host defense against a wide variety of microorganisms and the regulation of responses to foreign antigen [2, 32]. The management of antigen responsiveness is accomplished through complex pathways of antigen uptake and processing by antigen-presenting cells (APC) and their subsequent presentation to T lymphocytes. In the intestine, APC include not only cells of the monocyte–macrophage lineage and B cells, but also potentially non-conventional APC such as the IEC [77]. The gastrointestinal tract epithelial cells may have a unique role in immunoregulation, since luminal events are likely important in normal gut homeostasis and may be prerequisite for the initiation and/or perpetuation of inflammation as occurs in IBD. The IEC are the first host cells to come in contact with dietary and microbial antigens and are therefore in a unique position to function as an early host-signaling system to the immune cells located adjacent to and in the underlying intestinal mucosa. Therefore, antigen-presenting molecules that are expressed on the IEC cell surface may function in the regulation of gut immune responses by presenting specific antigen-containing ligands to T cells which function in the direct activation and/or down-regulation of local T lymphocytes. In the former case this activation may be associated with engagement of regulatory T cells which mediate down-regulatory signals. These MHC-restricted signals which are delivered to local T cells by IEC are geared toward the self-perpetuation of the intestinal barrier, the removal of altered epithelial cells injured by stress (including hypoxia), infection and/or neoplasia and the tight regulation of responses to antigen at the mucosal surfaces [77]. As such the IEC and local gut T cells within the epithelium and lamina propria utilize the fine specificity provided by MHC-related molecules on intestinal epithelia and the T cell receptor (TCR) and costimulatory molecules on T cells to regulate barrier function, antigen absorption and processing, immunosurveillance and local immunoregulation.

Antigen presentation

It is now well established that there are two major pathways of antigen presentation: the MHC class I pathway and the MHC class II pathway (reviewed in ref. 33). T cells recognize processed nominal antigens, usually peptides, derived from proteolytic degradation of a larger polypeptide chain. These processed peptides are recognized in the context of an MHC class I or II molecule on the cell surface of an APC (summarized in Table 2). MHC class I consists of a 43–45 kDa glycosylated heavy chain non-covalently associated with β_2-microglobulin which presents a nonapeptide, acquired from the transporter associated with antigen presentation (TAP), to CD8$^+$ T cells. MHC class II consists of a 32–34 kDa $\alpha\beta$ heterodimer that presents much longer peptides (14–22 amino acids) to CD4$^+$ T cells. Since MHC class I generally presents an array of peptides derived from the degradation of intracellular proteins and MHC class II from extracellular proteins, these antigen-presenting pathways have likely evolved to a large extent for the protection of the host from unforeseen intracellular and extracellular deleterious events, respectively.

As described above, T lymphocytes are abundant in the gastrointestinal tract and are implicated in a wide variety of 'physiological' immune responses (both oral tolerance and responses to invasive pathogens) and 'pathophysiological' responses (for example, the induction/maintenance of chronic inflammation, or IBD). T cells are stimulated by foreign protein antigens via specific molecules on their surface (the so-called T cell receptor, or TCR) which recognize processed nominal fragments of the antigen. These fragments are 'presented' to the T cell by molecules of the MHC complex which are expressed on the surface of so-called antigen-presenting cells, or APC. These APC also express additional surface molecules (e.g. co-stimulatory molecules such as CD80 and/or CD86) that are required for maximal stimulation of T cells via counter-receptor expressed on the surface of the T cell other than the specific TCR. The majority of APC are bone marrow-derived cells (e.g. dendritic cells, or DC) with specialized mechanisms for regulated and efficient antigen uptake, processing and presentation. In addition, within specific anatomical contexts, other 'non-professional' APC exist. These are cells which express MHC antigens and have a limited, but significant, capacity to process and present antigen to T cells.

One such 'non-professional' APC relevant to the gastrointestinal tract is the polarized epithelial cell which separates the extremely high concentration of foreign antigen from the underlying lymphoid tissue. Consistent with a potential role in antigen presentation, these IEC are in intimate contact with the various T cell populations previously described. Specifically, IEC have extensive contact along their lateral and basal surface with IEL, and contact underlying LPL via basolateral projections through the semiporous basement membrane.

As outlined, considerable reactivity against bacterial antigens exists within the T cell compartments of the GALT. The mechanisms underlying the processing of intact bacteria and/or bacterial fragments and the generation of specific bacteria-derived T cell epitopes remain poorly defined, however. The GALT and regional nodes (e.g. mesenteric lymph nodes) are replete with potential APC, including apparently distinct populations of DC, which may be involved in processing of bacterial antigens [78]. In addition, the anatomic considerations noted above, and the fact that IEC of the colon are exposed to the highest concentration (by several orders of magnitude) of luminal bacteria and bacterial antigens of any cell in the gastrointestinal tract highlight the possibility that these cells may participate in the processing and/or presentation of bacterial (or other) antigens to T cells in the GALT. In this section we review some of the recent data consistent with this supposition, focusing on several of the unique features of IEC antigen processing and presentation that distinguish these cells from other more conventional APC.

Antigen presentation by IEC

General features of IEC as antigen-presenting cells

In order for IEC to act as APC, they must be able to internalize and process antigen. The apical mucous layer and glycocalyx in the intestine can restrict the size of particles capable of being internalized by IEC favoring antigen uptake by the modified 'dome' epithelium (M cells) which overlie Peyer's patches [79]. The highly specialized M cells facilitate transport of macromolecules without significant 'cellular processing' to the underlying lymphoid tissue which contains several different types of professional APC including dendritic cells and B cells [80]. However, the surface area of the villous epithelium is extraordinary (the surface area of the human small intestine being approximately equal to that of a tennis court) and IEC have a well-documented role in nutrient and solute uptake. IEC are exposed to a wide variety of antigens of diverse sizes and varying biochemical properties, including some antigens such as gliadin with known pathologic significance. In addition, a wide variety of organisms of various sizes (e.g. rotavirus, *Salmonella*, and spp.) can enter IEC from their luminal (i.e. apical) surface. Collectively, these observations highlight a physiologic role for the IEC in the uptake and processing of luminal antigens and pathogens.

Several unique characteristics related to antigen uptake by the epithelium are worthy of note. First, IEC express a variety of molecules on their apical surface that might serve as 'antigen receptors' (e.g. FcRn [81, 82], DEC-205 [83], ganglioside M1 (GM1), which may enhance antigen processing by directing internalization via receptor-mediated (instead of fluid-phase) endocytosis. The polarized expression of these molecules on IEC is likely to dramatically modulate processing of antigens by enhancing antigen uptake and/or 'targeting' antigens to certain intracellular compartments. In addition, the rate and efficiency of antigen uptake and endocytic processing by IEC can be modulated by a variety of inflammatory mediators, such as interferon (IFN)-γ.

Interaction of IEC with CD4+ T cells — MHC class II processing by IEC

CD4+ T cell responses are critical for both the establishment of oral tolerance [84–86] and in several experimental models of IBD [87]. Two distinct populations of CD4+ T cells are present within the intestinal mucosa and in intimate contact with IEC.

A limited, but significant, number of IEL express CD4 (most notably in the colon [88, 89]) and approximately two-thirds of LPL express CD4 [53]. Because the expression of MHC class II antigens is required on an APC in order to stimulate CD4+ T cells, it is noteworthy that MHC class II expression has been observed on IEC from human, mouse and rat with elevated levels consistently seen in the context of mucosal inflammation [90–92]. Indeed, using a variety of *in-vitro* models, several groups have demonstrated the capacity of IEC to process and present antigen via HLA class II [91, 93].

There are marked regional differences in the composition (and presumably the function) of the GALT along the cephalo-caudal axis of the gastrointestinal tract. Given the limitation of the *in-vitro* models it is difficult to address potential distinctions in MHC class II processing between IEC of the small and large intestine. In fact, little information is available regarding specific regional differences (both crypt to villous, and small intestine to colon) in the co-expression of MHC class II antigens and other molecules (for example, invariant chain and HLA-DM) essential for efficient class II processing in conventional APC (reviewed in ref. 94), which are typically induced along with MHC class II at the transcriptional level following activation of the APC with IFN-γ [95]. Data from IEC cell lines transfected with HLA-DR alone or with Ii and HLA-DM are consistent with the observations that the generation of specific class II peptide epitopes shows a variable dependence on the expression of Ii and HLA-DM in IEC – with some epitopes processed via other class II pathways [96, 97]. Several groups have described one such 'alternative' class II processing pathway that uses MHC class II molecules recycled from the cell surface, which presumably bind peptide antigens in an early endosomal compartment [98, 99]. These alternative pathways may be particularly relevant to MHC class II processing by IEC, especially when MHC class II expression may be limited (i.e. in the absence of inflammation) and the antigen may be denatured or fragmented following luminal 'pre-processing'.

Influence of IEC polarity on antigen presentation by IEC class II molecules

IEC are highly polarized cells, with distinct apical and basolateral domains with very different physicochemical properties. The highly polarized morphology of IEC highlights several important distinctions in class II processing between IEC and other more conventional APC. First, the expression of HLA class II antigens *in vivo* and in cell culture models of polarized IEC is mostly restricted to the basolateral membrane (where the cell contacts both iIEL and LPL) [96, 100, 101]. Hence, antigen presentation occurs in a highly polarized manner. In addition, *in vitro* data suggest that the polarized surface from which antigen is internalized dramatically affects the functional outcome with regard to the generation of T cell epitopes [96]. This notion is consistent with the biochemical differences observed between endocytosis from the apical and basolateral surface of polarized epithelial cells [102, 103].

Consequences of MHC class II expression and processing by IEC

There is limited experimental data regarding the *in vivo* function of MHC class II on IEC. MHC class II-restricted antigen presentation can be identified in uninflamed small intestinal [104] and colonic epithelium [105], and is increased in colonic epithelium in the setting of inflammation as observed in IL-2-deficient animals [105]. It is thus not unreasonable to suggest that, under pathological circumstances, when the balance shifts toward uncontrolled inflammation such as in IBD (for reasons that remain obscure), the IEC functions as an important accessory APC, stimulating mucosal CD4+ T cell responses. Within the setting of the inflamed mucosa the unique features of polarized MHC class II processing may come into play. In particular, the processing of luminal antigens (such as bacterial or food antigens) normally exposed only to the apical surface might have especially untoward effects when these antigens gain access to the basolateral surface of IEC via 'leaky' tight junctions [106]. Conceivably, 'pathogenic epitopes' within an antigen (that normally elicits no significant response or a tolerogenic response when processed apically) may be unmasked via internalization and trafficking from the basolateral surface and presented to underlying CD4+ T cells. Whether IEC can stimulate 'naive' CD4+ T cells or CD28-dependent T cells in the intestinal mucosa (if either of these populations exist in this anatomical location) remains a matter for speculation.

CD4+ T cells have been widely implicated in the development of IBD [87]. Hence the possibility exists that the processing of intact bacteria and/or bacterial fragments by HLA class II positive professional (dendritic cells, macrophages) and non-professional (intestinal epithelial cells) APCs results in the presentation of specific bacterial T cell epitopes to pathogenic CD4+ T cells. This hypothesis, which does not preclude the potential role of bacteria or bacteria-derived products such as LPS in modulating mucosal immune responses, is an attractive explanation for the dependence of mucosal inflammation on a subset of bacteria present in the lumen of the gastrointestinal tract. Data supporting this hypothesis exist in mice and humans. It has recently become appreciated that IBD-like pathology can be initiated by CD4+ T cells with a Th1 cytokine profile which are restricted to MHC class II and specific for peptide antigens associated with the normal luminal microbiota [107]. In a corollary manner, CD4+ regulatory T cells with a cytokine profile consistent with T regulatory 1 cells (IL-10) can be similarly identified and established which can antagonize these effector Th1 cells in adoptive transfer models [108]. Although their site of origin is unclear, based upon studies of oral tolerance induction and work in the TCR-α-deficient animal model of colitis, it can be suggested that these agonist and antagonist cell populations originate within the inductive sites of the distal small intestine (appendix, Peyer's patches) and carry out their effector functions at the epithelial barrier of the colon after subsequent reactivation by either homologous or heterologous microbial antigen at this location [2, 38]. Whether the subsequent encounters are through interaction with the IEC or professional APC subjacent to the epithelium remains unclear. Nonetheless, these studies suggest that MHC class II antigen presentation pathways in the context of the immunologic milieu associated with the inductive sites of the GALT lead to the generation of agonist and antagonist (regulatory) T cell populations. Furthermore, it can be hypothesized that, under normal circumstances, these regulatory populations prevail over the agonist cells leading to homeostasis. In IBD, however, this tolerance to the antigens of the normal microbiota is not established [12].

Interaction of IEC with CD8+ cells

In the earliest studies assessing the capacity of IEC to act as non-professional APC, the T cells activated were predominantly CD8+, which functionally suppressed immune responses in an antigennon-specific fashion [109]. Consistent with the somewhat unusual features of these CD8+ T cells stimulated by IEC (i.e. the lack of cytotoxicity and the ability of these cells to suppress a mixed lymphocyte reaction), recent data have emerged revealing atypical characteristics of

MHC class I function in IEC. For example, although IEC lines have been shown to be good targets for class I-restricted virus-specific cytotoxic T lymphocytes (CTL) and appear to express a normal proteasome repertoire, they fail to prime an antiviral CTL response (K. Becker and L. Mayer, unpublished). These data suggest that MHC class I-mediated processing may be somehow 'altered' in IEC compared to professional APC like dendritic cells, or imply that the lack of conventional costimulation may preclude priming of a naive CD8$^+$ T cell responses [110].

Several lines of evidence point to novel interactions between CD8$^+$ T cells and IEC. One stems from the early observation that antibodies specific for HLA class I did not inhibit the IEC-induced proliferation of CD8$^+$ T cells *in vitro* [109]. One intriguing hypothesis proposes that 'non-classical' or class Ib molecules function in antigen presentation by IEC to CD8$^+$ T cells in the intestinal mucosa. This hypothesis is supported by data demonstrating the expression of these molecules by IEC in mice and humans, often in a pattern highly restricted to the intestinal epithelium [111, 112] (reviewed in ref. 113). In humans, the list includes CD1d [114], MICA and MICB [115], HLA-E [116], and HFE (which is involved in iron metabolism) all of which are expressed by IEC [117].

CD1D, a novel ligand on IEC

CD1 family of proteins

Recent studies have revealed that, in addition to MHC class I and class II, the host also utilizes a third pathway of antigen presentation which is represented by the CD1 gene family. This pathway (or pathways) functions in specific tasks of immunologic recognition distinct from MHC class I and II, yet which draws structural and functional features of both. First identified on cortical thymocytes, the CD1 gene family encodes a group of proteins which are structurally most similar to MHC class I proteins but have several features in common with MHC class II [34]. This suggests that CD1 emerged from an ancient ancestor that diverged into MHC class I, MHC class II, and CD1 (Table 2). The human CD1 locus on chromosome 1 contains five genes, CD1A–E [by convention, CD1 genes are in capital letters (A–E) and CD1 proteins in lower-case letters (a–e)]. The human CD1 gene family falls into two groups based upon sequence homology: CD1A–C (group 1) and

CD1D (group 2). A gene product for CD1E has not been defined. CD1a–c subserves a specific role in presenting lipoglycan antigens from mycobacteria (and bacteria) to discrete subsets of CD8$^+$ and double-negative (CD4$^-$CD8$^-$) T cells [118, 119]. These T cells utilize a wide variety of conventional αβ TCR. CD1a–c are expressed by the majority of immature, double-positive (CD4$^+$CD8$^+$) thymocytes and professional APC such as B cells, dendritic cells and activated monocytes. Rodents do not express group 1 CD1 proteins and appear to have deleted these genes [34].

CD1d and natural killer T cells

CD1d is expressed by the majority of thymocytes and at low levels by resting B cells and monocytes [34, 120–122]. In addition, we have also found that CD1d is expressed by a variety of epithelial cell types including IEC and hepatocytes [120, 121]. CD1d functions in the presentation of lipids. These include glycosylphosphatidyl inositol, which has been eluted from murine CD1d in transfectants [123], and α-galactosylceramide (α-GalCer), which has been extracted from marine sponges [124]. CD1d has also been shown to present hydrophobic peptides [125]. These observations are consistent with the hydrophobic nature of the CD1d groove [126]. Recognition of CD1d appears to be primarily accomplished by a discrete subset of T cells, which share similarities with natural killer (NK) cells [127]. These NK-T cells, which are also commonly called natural T cells, were initially described in mouse systems [128]. Mice express the human homologue of CD1d but not CD1a–c [129, 130]. These murine CD1d-restricted T cells are characterized by their expression of the NK1.1 marker (NKR-P1C or CD161), a C-type lectin, and an invariant TCRα-chain (Vα14-Jα281), which preferentially pairs with Vβ8.2, 7 or 2 in hierarchal order [127, 131, 132]. These cells are also either CD4$^+$CD8$^-$ or double-negative since the forced expression of CD8 in mouse results in the deletion of invariant NK-T cells [133].

NK-T cells represent a major fraction of mature thymocytes, liver-associated T cells and up to 5% of splenic cells [134]. In addition, they have been identified in the epithelium amongst IEL [135] and among LPL at low levels (R.S.B., personal observation). Although their function is not entirely clear, they have been recognized to be the major source of IL-4 and IFN-γ *in vivo* in response to anti-CD3 stimulation, suggesting an important immunoregulatory role during early phases of an immune response [136]. CD1d-deficient mice lack NK-T cells and the early cytokine response associated with anti-CD3 activation, but maintain their ability to mount most T helper (Th2)-type responses [137–139]. Murine NK-T cells are also involved in IL-12-mediated pathways as they express IL-12 receptors and, when stimulated by IL-12, exhibit significant cytolytic activity and regulation of IFN-γ responses; responses which are lacking in CD1d-deficient mice [140, 141]. These observations with murine NK-T cells suggest that they play an important role in immunoregulation of type 1 and type 2 cytokine responses through their ability to generate high levels of cytokines and immunosurveillance through high cytolytic activity.

Similar populations of NK-T cells are also expressed in humans. Analogous to mice, these human NK-T cells express an invariant TCR composed of Vα24-JαQ which preferentially pairs with Vβ11, the human homologue of mouse Vβ8 [142, 143]. Most human NK-T cells are double-negative while a minority express CD4 [144]. They uniformly express NKR-P1A (CD161), the only human homologue of mouse NK1.1, which may provide crucial costimulatory signals [145]. NK-T cells also express two other C-type lectins, CD94 (the ligand for HLA-E) and CD69, but lack expression of most other NK markers including CD16, CD56, CD57 or killer inhibitory receptors [142]. Similar to the mouse NK-T cells, human NK-T cells function as potent cytolytic effectors and secrete cytokines with a Th0 phenotype in response to CD1d-transfected APC [142, 145]. These functional activities are significantly enhanced by the lipid antigen, α-GalCer isolated from marine sponge [146–148].

Although much is known about the cellular immunology of CD1a–d, little is known about the role of CD1d in human diseases. The information to date points toward a crucial role of CD1d in *immunoregulation* to microbial antigens given the vigorous cytokine production of CD1d-responsive, NK-T cells and observations that NK-T cells are significantly diminished in diabetes mellitus [149], systemic lupus erythematosus [150] and systemic sclerosis [151] and *immunosurveillance* to microbial antigens functions given the potent anti-tumor responses of NK-T cells in mouse models [152].

The CD1d pathway is particularly relevant to IBD pathogenesis given its biologic relevance to the central hypothesis raised above. CD1d is expressed by IEC [153, 154] and professional APC [122], and on

IEC is able to present model glycolipid antigens to NK-T cells [155]. This presentation is polarized in that it is most efficient basally relative to apically, suggesting a role for CD1d in presenting glycolipid antigens from luminal microbial antigens to subepithelial CD1d-restricted T cells such as the NK-T cells [155]. Indeed, activation of NK-T cells in a CD1d-restricted manner leads to the amelioration of colitis in the dextran sodium sulfate colitis model [156] and promotion of Th2-mediated colitis [W. Strober and R. Blumberg, unpublished observation] suggesting complex interactions of NK-T cells in mucosal tissues relative to IBD induction.

Mechanisms of innate immunity throughout the intestinal mucosa

The intestinal lumen, particularly that of the colon, contains a large variety of bacteria and bacterially derived products [157, 158]. As a consequence a number of 'broadly specific' defense mechanisms have evolved to guard against the risk of attack from invasive microorganisms. These factors are important because they can be mobilized rapidly in comparison to the time taken for mobilization of the adaptive responses described in the sections above. These mechanisms can be classified as intrinsic or extrinsic in nature. Intrinsic mechanisms of immunity are derived from the physical presence of an epithelial barrier and are dependent upon the unique structural properties exhibited by the IEC. Extrinsic defenses are defined as those processes which act outside of the monolayer to resist microbial interaction with the mucosa. In addition to these two mechanisms, cells constituting the epithelial monolayer have developed an ability to interact with immune cell populations of the underlying intestinal mucosa, thereby alerting the immune system to the presence of luminal pathogens. These three levels of innate immunity are described below.

Intrinsic barriers

The formation of a selectively permeable epithelial barrier is essential in preventing the uncontrolled passage of pathogenic antigens from the external environment to the internal tissue. Establishment of the epithelial monolayer by contributing IEC is dependent upon a considerably high degree of intracellular and intercellular organization [159]. Besides allowing the formation of tight intercellular junctions, IEC exhibit a number of structural and functional features that help physically restrict the passage of potentially harmful microorganisms into the underlying mucosa. Interaction of macromolecules with the apical surface of IEC is reduced by the presence of large heavily glycosylated proteins, or mucins, anchored to the epithelial plasma membrane [160]. In addition, the organization of the apical membrane into microvilli is thought to minimize the contact area available to luminal macromolecular antigens [161]. Cell trafficking processes within the IEC may also reduce the amount of intact microbial antigen crossing the monolayer. The contents of epithelial cell endocytic vesicles are, for example, primarily directed to proteolytic lysosomal compartments. Thus, internalization of many microorganisms is liable to lead to their degradation.

Extrinsic barriers

Mucus

The surface of the intestinal epithelium is lined with a layer of mucus produced as a result of mucin secretion by goblet cells [162, 163]. Mucins, a group of glycoproteins of which the mucus lining is composed, protect the epithelium in several ways. By creating a hydrated viscous layer they act as a physical barrier, separating IEC from the turbulent luminal environment of the intestinal tract [164, 165]. In addition, the carbohydrate moieties present in mucins display the ability to adhere to the surfaces of many microoganisms, preventing microbial association with the monolayer [166–168]. With time, mucus is propelled down the intestinal tract thereby facilitating the removal of bound microbial components away from the epithelia. The mucus lining is therefore considered to contribute to innate immune responses within the intestine. In support of this role it has been observed that mucus secretion is induced in the presence of agents potentially harmful to the epithelium including noxious chemical and bacterial toxins [169–171]. Such a response may act to counter the presence of these agents by reducing their capacity to interact with the monolayer.

Defensins

A second extrinsic mechanism of mucosal defense occurs by the secretion of agents that directly exhibit microbicidal or antiviral activities. Investigations performed on sections of the mouse epithelium have revealed the presence of mRNA encoding cyptdins or α-defensins, molecules sharing a conserved cysteine-rich motif with the family of antimicrobial peptides known as defensins [172]. Expression of cryptdin mRNA was confined to Paneth cells, located within intestinal crypts. Further studies revealed the presence of two peptides in these cells, termed cryptdin 1 and cryptdin 2 [173]. Both these peptides display a high degree of sequence homology to the defensins secreted by polymorphonuclear leukocytes and exhibit potent microbicidal activity on a variety of bacteria including strains of *Escherichia coli*, *Salmonella typhimurium* and *Listeria monocytogenes*. The potential importance of cryptdins in conferring resistance to bacterial infection is highlighted by the observation that, while avirulent strains of *S. typhimurium* are susceptible to the antimicrobial properties of cryptdins, the growth of pathogenic *S. typhimurium* is not affected by these peptides [173]. Although unclear, it remains possible that the loss of cryptdin sensitivity in the pathogenic strain contributes to its enhanced virulence.

Intestinal epithelial cells also express defensins. Recent studies have revealed that human IEC express two functionally related peptides termed β-defensin 1 and β-defensin 2 (hBD1 and hBD2 respectively) [174]. hBD1 was shown to be constitutively expressed while hBD2 was induced following stimulation with the cytokine IL-1. Like the α-defensins, both hBD1 and hBD2 exhibit antimicrobial activity against a range of bacteria including *E. coli* and strains of *Salmonella* spp. and *Pseudomonas* spp.

Lysozyme and lactoferrin

Lysozyme and lactoferrin represent two proteins which, like defensins, are thought to contribute to the innate defense of mucosal surfaces [175]. Both lysozyme and lactoferrin are found in exocrine secretions and can be detected within the lumen of the human gastrointestinal tract. Lactoferrin (Lf), a molecule that is thought to facilitate iron transport across the epithelium of suckling infants, is cleaved by gastric pepsin to form a peptide exhibiting potent antimicrobial properties [176]. *In vitro*, Lf inhibits replication of a number of viruses including cytomegalovirus (CMV), herpes simplex virus (HSV) and members of the rotavirus family [177, 178]. Lf interacts with both the lipoglycan-coated cell wall of Gram-positive bacteria and the outer membrane of Gram-negative bacteria, processes that are thought to mediate its bactericidal function. In addition, Lf inhibits the adhesion of enterotoxigenic *E. coli* to human epithelial cells, thereby preventing its colonization of the surface monolayer [179]. Lactoferrin is also capable of inhibiting fungal growth, and has been shown to be cytotoxic to several protozoan parasites such as trophozoites of *Giardia lamblia* and *Toxoplasma gondii* [180, 181].

Human lysozyme consists of a single polypeptide chain of 129 amino acids, which is crosslinked by four stabilizing disulfide interactions. The polypeptide is a constituent of both saliva and pancreatic juice. Luminal concentrations within the intestinal tract range from 43 to 106 micrograms per milliliter [175]. Lysozyme exerts its microbicidal activity at a number of levels. These include the hydrolysis of bacterial cell wall peptidoglycans, the activation of bacterial autolysins, the induction of bacterial cell aggregation and the abrogation of bacterial adhesion to host epithelial cells. However, while lysozyme may possess multiple enzymatic activities, it is thought that its cationic properties are primarily responsible for its ability to interact strongly with bacterial membranes and may contribute to the disruption of membrane processes [182]. In many cases lysozyme alone does not alter bacterial viability but does render the bacteria more susceptible to lysis by other environmental factors. In this regard a combination of lysozyme with lactoferrin is microbicidal for *Streptococcus mutans* while lysozyme alone has no visible effect on the growth of this bacterial strain [183]. Similarly, lysozyme synergizes with peroxides in preventing glucose uptake by *S. mutans* [175]. *In vivo* therefore, lysozyme is likely to function in association with additional antimicrobial agents.

Other microbicidal factors, which function as innate mechanisms of defense at mucosal surface, include peroxidases and components of the complement pathway. Studies using the human epithelial cell line Caco-2 have demonstrated that these cells express and secrete complement components including C3, C4 and factor B [184]. Peroxidases, secreted from exocrine glands onto mucosal surfaces, catalyze the peroxidation of halides such as chloride, bromide and thiocyanide into oxidative products, which exhibit potent antimicrobial activity.

Epithelial cell–immune cell cross-talk

The exposed location of the epithelia implies that IEC are likely to play an important role in alerting components of the mucosal immune system to the presence of foreign antigen. Intestinal epithelial cells coexist with immune cell populations present along the epithelium itself and those localized to the lamina propria. iIEL reside at the basolateral surface of the epithelium. Immune cell populations within the lamina propria include lymphocytes, macrophages, granulocytes and mast cells. Within this environment IEC have developed an ability to communicate with regional immune cell populations in a manner proposed to directly influence their growth, migration and state of responsiveness to antigenic stimuli. Some of the methods by which IEC affect the mucosal immune system are categorized and discussed below.

Chemokines

Under conditions that promote infection or insult to the epithelial monolayer, an influx of immune and inflammatory cells into the mucosa is observed as these cells are recruited to the site of injury. This recruitment can occur within hours of infection and is mediated, partly, by a group of chemotactic cytokines known as chemokines [185, 186]. Several studies have revealed the ability for IEC to express and secrete chemokines including IL-8, ENA 78, gro-α, MIP-1α, and MCP-1 [187]. Infection of the epithelial cell lines T84, HT29 and Caco-2 with *Salmonella dublin*, *Yersinia enterocolitica* or *Shigella dysentariae*, for example, selectively induces expression of IL-8 and MCP-1 [188–191]. Following cellular invasion by *S. typhimurium*, IL-8 is secreted from the basolateral surface establishing a chemical gradient and facilitating the migration of neutrophils into the paracellular spaces of the monolayer [189]. IL-8 expression is also induced in gastric epithelial cells in response to *Helicobacter pylori* infection [192, 193]. Taken together, these data demonstrate the ability of IEC to actively participate in recruiting immune cells, to sites of infection, through the release of chemotactic factors upon exposure to luminal pathogens.

Cytokines

Cytokines are a group of factors that exert profound influence on the functional state of immune cell populations through inducing an altered pattern of gene expression upon binding to specific cellular receptors [194]. Intestinal epithelial cells are capable of expressing a number of cytokines, thereby possessing the ability to affect local immune responses. The cell lines T84 and Caco-2 constitutively express mRNA for the proinflammatory cytokines, IL-1α, IL-1β, IL-8, IL-15 and TNF-α [187, 191, 195, 196]. These cells also express TGF-β, a cytokine thought to play a role both in promoting IEC growth and in regulating IEC barrier function and responses of IEL to antigenic stimuli [197–199]. IL-6, a cytokine thought to be important in generating IgA-secreting plasma cells, has been shown to be expressed in freshly isolated human IEC, and can be induced in a variety of epithelial cell lines by cholera toxin secreted from *Vibrio cholerae* [2]. IL-6 release by IEC may therefore contribute to the production of secretory IgA.

IL-10 represents another cytokine expressed by IEC [46]. Like IL-6 it is thought to promote IgA secretion by B cells [201]. In addition to this, IL-10 acts as a suppressor of Th1 responses through inhibiting macrophage function and cytokine secretion from Th1 cells [202]. Recently, studies have shown that IL-10 secretion from T84 cells can protect the epithelial monolayer from IFN-γ-induced permeabilization [46, 203, 204]. Its ability both to suppress Th1 responses and to maintain epithelial barrier function implicates IL-10 as a regulator of intestinal inflammation. The production of IL-10 from IEC may therefore act to protect the barrier against injury resulting from an influx of inflammatory effector cells.

A number of additional factors secreted from IEC are thought to be important in influencing the growth and development of surrounding iIEL. Mice lacking the functional gene encoding IL-7 exhibit reduced levels of $\gamma\delta^+$ T cells in the epithelia, while IL-7 receptor knockout mice do not possess any intestinal $\gamma\delta^+$ T cells [205, 206]. IL-7 has also been shown to play a role in activating T cell cytolytic function against various intracellular parasites including HIV [207, 208]. Such findings, together with the observation that freshly isolated IEC produce IL-7 [209], suggest that epithelial-derived IL-7 may contribute to maintaining iIEL growth and responsiveness to foreign antigens. In addition to IL-7, two other molecules secreted from epithelial cells are important in influencing iIEL activity. Stem cell factor, or SCF, is required for sustaining levels of $\gamma\delta^+$ T cells in the intestine [210]. Furthermore, *in vitro* studies suggest that SCF can protect IEC from bacterial infection [211]. Murine epithelial cells have also been shown to express thyroid-stimulating hormone (TSH) [212]. Secreted following the action of thyrotropin-releasing hormone on its receptor, TSH is critical in maintaining normal levels of $CD8\alpha\beta^+$ T cells within IEL populations [212, 213].

Intestinal epithelial cells are also able to synthesize a variety of prostanoids. Rabbit colonic IEC consti-

tutively express prostaglandin E2 (PGE_2), 6-keto-prostaglandin F1α (6-keto $PDF_{1\alpha}$), prostaglandin D2 (PGD_2) and prostaglandin F2α ($PGF_{2\alpha}$) [214]. PGE_2 has been shown to reduce IL-3 secretion from lamina propria mononuclear cells, inhibit the effects of local T cells on the epithelial barrier and reduce IL-2 secretion by activated T cell lines [214, 215]. Based on such data it seems likely that the release of PGE_2 from IEC functions to regulate leukocyte responses within the intestinal mucosa.

Cytokine receptors

Besides exhibiting an ability to influence mucosal immune responses, IEC are also able to alter their own phenotype in response to cytokines released from local immune cell populations. Freshly isolated human IEC, as well as a number of IEC lines, express mRNA for the common gamma chain and specific alpha chains of the receptors for IL-2, IL-4, IL-7, IL-9, and IL-15 [196, 197, 216]. Northern blot analysis has further revealed the presence of the IL-2 receptor β chain while studies of rat IEC demonstrate the expression of the IL-1 receptor (IL-1R), a molecule homologous to the human type I IL-1R [216, 217]. Through the expression of cytokine receptors the epithelium is sensitive to immunologic changes within its environment and can subsequently respond in a way that either facilitates or regulates those responses. In the presence of IL-4, IFN-γ or TNF-α, for example, IEC respond by enhancing levels of the polymeric immunoglobulin receptor, thus facilitating the release of secretory IgA [218–220]. IFN-γ also induces the expression of MHC class II molecules and the epithelial cell adhesion molecule, ICAM1 [221–224]. IFN-γ is capable of stimulating cell surface expression of the co-stimulatory factor CD86 while IL-6 and IL-1 trigger the release of complement components C3, C4 and factor B from IEC [184, 225, 226]. Receptiveness of the epithelium to the local cytokine environment, therefore, allows the mucosal immune system to enhance both the epithelial cells' innate capacity for defense and their ability to interact with and influence local immune cell populations.

Toll-like receptors

The mucosal immune system represents a dominant interface between the two main arms of the immune system – so-called 'innate' and 'adaptive' immunity. We have outlined the various cellular components of the adaptive immune system, in particular, the diverse T cell populations with somatically rear-

Table 3. Mechanisms of bacteria-driven IBD

Pathogenic category	Functional category	Organism, molecule or cellular subset	Mechanism of action
Microbial virulence factors	IEC adherence	ETEC EPEC *Yersinia enterocolitica*	Specific colonization factors Attachment and effacement via Bfp pili Intimin binds to $\alpha 4\beta 1$ integrin
	IEC invasion	*Shigella* spp. *Salmonella* spp.	Type III secretion system Type III secretion system
	Cytotoxins	*Clostridium difficile* EHEC	*C. difficile* toxins A and B *Shiga*-like toxins
Luminal dysbiosis	Abnormal metabolism	*Eubacteria* spp.	Hydrogen-sulfide inhibition of SCFA utilization
Pattern recognition molecules of innate immune system	Microbial poly-saccharide recognition	C-reactive protein Serum amyloid protein Mannose binding protein	Activates complement and phagocytosis Facilitates phagocytosis Binds C19 receptor and promotes phagocytosis
	Microbial glyco-lipid recognition	DEC-205 Lipipolysaccharide binding protein Soluble CD14 and CD14 Surfactant protein A	Cell surface protein that targets MHC class II pathway Inactivates LPS Binds and regulates proinflammatory response to LPS Binds and aggregates lipids
Adaptive (specific immune responses	Cellular	$CD4^+$ T cell	Recognition of bacterial peptide antigens on APC in context of MHC class II leading to excess proinflammmatory (TNF-α, IFN-γ) relative to anti-inflammatory (TGF-β) cytokines
	Humoral	B cell	Production of autoantibodies that cross-react with microbial antigens (e.g. ANCA cross-reactivity with I2 sequence of *Pseudomonas* spp.

Adapted from refs 15, 27, 30. ETEC, enterotoxygenic *E. coli*; EHEC, enterohemorrhagic *E. coli*; EPEC, enteropathogenic *E. coli*; ANCA, anti-neutrophil cytoplasmic antibody.

ranged T cell receptors that recognize specific processed protein fragments displayed by histocompatibility molecules on the surface of APC. While it is likely that 'specific' T cell (and B cell) responses to bacteria and other luminal microorganisms will be increasingly implicated in the pathogenesis of IBD, a growing body of literature suggests that 'innate' responses to the mucosal microbiota are likely to have a dramatic influence on the immunological tone at mucosal surfaces.

As detailed, the mucosal microbiota is extremely diverse, with most major classes of bacteria, yeast and, often, helminthes represented. In this complex microbiological ecosystem the challenge of the innate system is daunting. It has become increasingly clear that, in order for the innate immune system to be able to recognize and respond to such a large number of diverse microbial stimuli, it has evolved an intricate system of 'pattern recognition' [30]. Specifically, this involves the ability to respond to structural motifs shared by diverse groups of organisms (e.g. lipid A from Gram-negative bacteria, peptidoglycans from Gram-positive bacteria (Table 3).

Recent data on the Toll-like receptors (TLR) in humans and mice have provided keen insight regarding the mechanisms by which this diverse pattern recognition occurs [227, 228]. The term Toll-like derives from structural homology to the gene product of the Toll locus in the fruitfly *Drosophila melanogaster* [229]. Mutations in Toll, and genes relevant to the signaling events downstream from this surface receptor (with homology to the receptor for IL-1), result in marked defects in innate immunity (particularly to yeast and Gram-positive bacteria). Homologues to *Drosophila* Toll have been found in mice and humans, with a growing family of proteins with homology to Toll, currently with 10 distinct members comprising the list of TLR. Interestingly, the different TLR appear to have distinct ligand specificity – in the cases so far determined, representing structural disparate 'bioactive' components of microorganisms. This rapidly changing area of scientific inquiry has been the topic of several recent insightful reviews [230, 231].

One particular example of TLR biology illustrates both the importance of these molecules in innate immunity and the potential relevance to inflammatory responses of the gastrointestinal tract. First, in an elegant series of genetic studies in mouse strains hyporesponsive to bacterial LPS (e.g. C3H/HeJ), mutations were identified in a conserved region of TLR4 [232]. Subsequent studies from a number of laboratories have demonstrated that (in concert with LPS binding protein, LBP and surface or soluble CD14) TLR4 is the 'dominant' surface molecule that confers a signal by LPS [233]. Recent data are emerging to indicate that TLR2 may be involved in signaling by LPS of certain bacteria, for example, *Porphomonas gingivalis*. The pattern of expression of TLR4 is variable, and includes macrophages and dendritic cells. Interestingly, functional TLR4 has also been shown to be expressed on non-hematopoietic cells, including IEC [234]. Recently it has been demonstrated that TLR4 is selectively upregulated on IEC from patients with IBD. Based on these studies one might predict an 'exaggerated' response to LPS (a potent immunomodulatory molecule driving 'proinflammatory' responses) in IBD. Additionally, these studies highlight TLR4 as a potential target for antagonism therapeutically in IBD. The complexity is likely to increase further as one considers the role of other bacterially derived immunomodulators (e.g. CpG islands in bacterial DNA that signal via TLR9 [235]) and potential interactions between the TLR within the anatomically varied sites along the gastrointestinal tract. This is likely to be an extremely important area with considerable therapeutic relevance in the coming years.

References

1. McGhee JR, Lamm ME, Strober W. Mucosal immune responses: an overview. In: Ogra RL, Mestecky J, Lamm ME, Strober W, Bienenstock J, McGhee JR, eds. Mucosal Immunology, 2nd edn. San Diego: Academic Press, 1999: 485–506.
2. Strobel S, Mowat AM. Immune responses to dietary antigens: oral tolerance. Immunol Today 1998; 19: 173–81.
3. Blumberg RS, Saubermann LJ, Strober W. Animal models of mucosal inflammation and their relation to human inflammatory bowel disease. Curr Opin Gastroenterol 1999; 11: 648–56.
4. Strober W, Blumberg RS. Inflammatory bowel diseases. J Am Med Assoc 2001; 285: 643–7.
5. Drasar BS, Barrow PA. Intestinal microbiology. In: Aspects of microbiology 10 [monograph]. Am Soc Microbiol. Berkshire, UK, 1985.
6. Sutherland L, Singleton J, Sessions J *et al.* Double blind, placebo-controlled trial of metronidazole in Crohn's disease. Gut 1991; 32: 1071.
7. Rutgeerts P, Geboes K, Peeters M *et al.* Effect of faecal stream diversion on recurrence of Crohn's disease in the neoterminal ileum. Lancet 1991; 338: 771.
8. Shanahan F. Probiotics and inflammatory bowel disease: is there a scientific rationale? Inflam Bowel Dis 20; 6: 107–15.
9. Sartor RB. Enteric microflora in IBD: pathogens or commensals? Inflam Bowel Dis 1997; 3: 230.
10. Fox J. Enterohepatic helicobacters: natural and experimental models. Ital J Gastroenterol Hepatol 1998; 30: S264–9.
11. Dielman LA, Arends A, Tonkonogy SL *et al. Helicobacter hepaticus* does not induce or potentiate colitis in interleukin-10-deficient mice. Infect Immun 20; 68: 5107–13.
12. Duchman R, Kaiser I, Hermann E, Mayet W, Ewe K, Meyer zum Buschenfelde K-H. Tolerance exists towards resident intestinal flora but is broken in active inflammatory bowel disease (IBD). Clin Exp Immunol 1995; 102: 448–55.
13. Savage DC. Mucosal microbiota. In: Ogra RL, Mestecky J, Lamm ME, Strober W, Bienenstock J, McGhee JR, eds. Mucosal Immunology, 2nd edn. San Diego: Academic Press, 1999: 19–30.
14. Onderdonk AB. Intestinal microflora and inflammatory bowel disease. In: Kirsner, J and Shorter RG, eds. Inflammatory Bowel Disease, 5th edn. Baltimore: Williams & Wilkins, 2000: 144–52.
15. Sartor RB. Microbial factors in the pathogenesis of Crohn's Disease, ulcerative colitis, and experimental intestinal inflammation. In: Kirsner, J and Shorter RG, eds. Inflammatory Bowel Disease, 5th edn. Baltimore: Williams & Wilkins, 2000: 153–78.
16. Theron J, Cloete TE. Molecular techniques for determining microbial diversity and community structure in natural environments. Crit Rev Microbiol 20; 26: 37–57.
17. Schmidt TM, Relman DA. Phylogenetic identification of uncultured pathogens using ribosomal RNA sequences. Methods Enzymol 1994; 235: 205–22.
18. Kolbert CP, Persing DH. Ribosomal DNA sequencing as a tool for identification of bacterial pathogens. Curr Opin Microbiol 1999; 2: 299–305.
19. Tannock GW. Analysis of the intestinal microflora: a renaissance. Antonie Van Leeuwenhoek 1999; 76: 265–78.

20. Gorbach SL, Plaut AG, Nahas L *et al*. Studies of intestinal microflora. II. Microorganisms of the small intestine and theirrelations to oral and fecal flora. Gastroenterology 1967; 73: 856.

21. Warren JR, Marshall BJ. Unidentified curved bacilli on gastric epithelium in active gastritis. Lancet. 1983; 1: 1273–5.

22. Drasar BS, Shiner M, McLeod GM. Studies on the intestinal flora. I. The bacterial flora of the gastrointestinal tract in healthy and achlorhydric persons. Gastroenterology 1969; 56: 71–9.

23. Banerjee S, LaMont JT. Treatment of gastrointestinal infections. Gastroenterology 20; 118: 548–67.

24. Onderdonk AB, Hermos JA, Bartlett JG. The role of the intestinal microflora in experimental colitis. Am J Clin Nutr 1977; 30: 1819.

25. Van de Merwe JP, Schroder AM, Wesninck F *et al*. The obligate anaerobic faecal flora of patients with Crohn's disease and their first-degree relatives. Scand J Gastroenterol 1988; 23: 1125.

26. Burke DA, Axon ATR. Adhesive *Escherichia coli* in inflammatory bowel disease and infective diarrhea. Br Med J 1988; 297: 102.

27. Lee C, Mekalanos J. Bacterial interactions with intestinal epithelial cells. In: Ogra RL, Mestecky J, Lamm ME, Strober W, Bienenstock J, McGhee JR, eds. Mucosal Immunology, 2nd edn. San Diego: Academic Press, 1999: 657–69.

28. Roediger WEW, Duncanb A, Kapaniris OK *et al*. Reducing sulfur compounds of the colon impair colonocyte nutrition: implications for ulcerative colitis. Gastroenterology 1993; 104: 803.

29. Breuer RI, Soergel KH, Lashner B *et al*. Short chain fatty acid rectal irrigation for left-sided ulcerative colitis: a randomized, placebo controlled trial. Gut 1997; 40: 485.

30. Fearon DT, Locksley RM. The instructive role of innate immunity in the acquired immune response. Science. 1996; 272: 50–4.

31. Sartor RB, Rath HC, Sellon RK. Microbial factors in chronic intestinal inflammation. Curr Opin Gastroenterol 1996; 12: 327.

32. Abreu-Martin MT, Targan SR. Regulation of immune responses of the intestinal mucosa. Crit Rev Immunol 1996; 16: 277–309.

33. Germain R. MHC-dependent antigen processing and peptide presentation: providing ligands for T lymphocyte activation. Cell. 1994; 76: 287–99.

34. Blumberg R, Gerdes D, Chott A, Porcelli S, Balk S. Structure and function of the CD1 family of MHC-like cell surface proteins. Immunol Rev. 1995; 147: 5–29.

35. Fiocchi C. Inflammatory bowel disease: etiology and pathogenesis. Gastroenterology 1998; 115: 182–205.

36. Chott A, Gross GG, Probert C, Schwartz VL, Blumberg RS, Balk SP. Analysis of T cell antigen receptor expression by intestinal mucosa lymphocytes demonstrates a common junctional motif among CD8$^+$ T cells in ulcerative colitis. J Immunol 1996a; 156: 3024–35.

37. Probert CS, Chott A, Turner JR, Bodinaku K, Elson CO, Balk SP, Blumberg RS. Persistent clonal expansions of peripheral blood CD4$^+$ lymphocytes in chronic inflammatory bowel disease. J Immunol 1996b; 157: 3182–91.

38. Mizoguchi A, Mizoguchi E, Saubermann SJ, Higaki K, Blumberg RS, Bhan AK. Limited CD4$^+$ T cell diversity associated with colitis in T cell receptor α mutant mice requires a T helper 2 environment. Gastroenterology 20; 119: 983–95.

39. Cohavy O, Harth G, Horwitz M *et al*. Identification of a novel mycobacterial histone H1 homologue (HupB) as an antigenic target of pANCA monoclonal antibody and serum

immunoglobulin A from patients with Crohn's disease. Infect Immun 1999; 67: 7510–17.

40. Kraehenbuhl JP, Neutra MR. Epithelial M cells: differentiation and function. Annu Rev Cell Dev Biol 20; 16: 301–32.

41. Davis IC, Owen RL. The immunopathology of M cells. Springer Sem Immunopathol 1997; 18: 421–48.

42. Cone RA. Mucus. In: Ogra RL, Mestecky J, Lamm ME, Strober W, Bienenstock J, McGhee JR, eds. Mucosal Immunology, 2nd edn. San Diego: Academic Press, 1999: 43–64.

43. Mitic LL, Van Itallie CM, Anderson JM. Molecular physiology and pathophysiology of tight junctions I. Tight junction structure and function: lessons from mutant animals and proteins. Am J Physiol Gastrointest Liver Physiol 120; 279: G250–4.

44. Colgan SP, Parkos CA, Matthews JB *et al*. Interferon-γ induces a cell surface phenotype switch on T84 intestinal epithelial cells. Am J Physiol 1994; 267: C402–10.

45. Zund G, Madara JL, Dzus AL, Awtrey CS, Colgan SP. Interleukin-4 and interleukin-13 differentially regulate epithelial chloride secretion. J Biol Chem 1996; 271: 7460–4.

46. Colgan SP, Hershberg RM, Furuta GT, Blumberg RS. Ligation of epithelial CD1d by antibody crosslinking induces bioactive IL-10; critical role of the cytoplasmic tail in autocrine signaling. Proc Natl Acad Sci USA 1999; 96: 13938–43.

47. Liu Y, Nusrat A, Schnell FJ *et al*. Human junction adhesion molecule regulates tight junction resealing in epithelia. J Cell Sci 20; 113: 2363–74.

48. Kinugasa T, Sakaguchi T, Gu X, Reinecker HC. Claudins regulate the intestinal barrier in responseto immune mediators. Gastroenterology 20; 118: 1001–11.

49. Miki K, Moore DJ, Butler RN, Southcott E, Couper RTG, Davidson GP. The sugar permeability test reflects disease activity in children and adolescents with inflammatory bowel disease. J Pediatr 1998; 133: 750–4.

50. Munkholm P, Langholz E, Hollander D *et al*. Intestinal permeability in patients with Crohn's disease and ulcerative colitis and their first degree relatives. Gut 1994; 35: 68–72.

51. Madsen KL, Malfair D, Gray D, Doyle JS, Jewell LD, Fedorak RN. Interleukin-10 gene-deficient mice develop a primary intestinal permeability defect in response to enteric microflora. Inflam Bowel Dis 1999; 5: 262-70.

52. Mashimo H, Wu DC, Podolsky DK, Fishman MC. Impaired defense of intestinal mucosa in mice lacking intestinal trefoil factor. Science 1996; 274: 262–5.

53. Brandtzaeg P, Farstad IN, Helgeland L. Phenotypes of T cells in the gut. Chem Immunol. 1998; 71: 1–26.

54. Dogan A, Dunn-Walters DK, MacDonald TT. Demonstration of local clonality of mucosal T cells in human colon using DNA obtained by microdissection of immunohistochemically stained tissue sections. Eur J Immunol 1996; 26: 1240-5.

55. Itohara S, Farr AG, Lafaille JJ *et al*. Homing of γδ thymocyte subset with homogeneous T-cell receptors to mucosal epithelia. Nature 1990; 343: 754–7.

56. Farstad IN, Norstein J, Brandtzeg P. Phenotypes of B and T cells in human intestinal and mesenteric lymph. Gastroenterology 1997; 112: 163–73.

57. Lefrancois L, Fuller B, Huleatt JW, Olson S, Puddington L. On the front lines: intraepithelial lymphocytes as primary effectors of intestinal immunity. Springer Sem Immunopathol. 1997; 18: 463–76.

58. Molberg O, Nilsen EM, Sollid LM *et al*. CD4$^+$ T cells with specific reactivity against astrovirus isolated from normal human small intestine. Gastroenterology 1998; 114: 115–22.

59. James SP, Graeff AS, Zeitz M. Predominance of helper–inducer T cells in mesenteric lymph nodes and intestinal

lamina propria of normal nonhuman primates. Cell Immunol 1987; 107: 372–83.

60. Brandtzaeg P, Haraldsen G, Rugtveit J. Immunopathology of human inflammatory bowel disease. Springer Sem Immunopathol. 1997; 18: 555–89.

61. Hurst SD, Sitterding SM, Ji S, Barrett TA. Functional differentiation of T cells in the intestine of T cell receptor transgenic mice. Proc Natl Acad Sci USA 1997; 94: 3920–5.

62. Moghaddami M, Cummins A, Mayrhofer G. Lymphocyte-filled villi: comparison with other lymphoid aggregations in the mucosa of the human small intestine. Gastroenterology 1998; 115: 1558.

63. Suzuki K, Oida T, Hamada H *et al.* Gut cryptopatches: direct evidence of extrathymic anatomical sites for intestinal T lymphopoiesis. Immunity 20; 13: 691–702.

64. Umesaki Y, Setoyama H, Matsumoto S, Okada Y. Expansion of $\alpha\beta$ T-cell receptor-bearing intestinal intraepithelial lymphocytes after microbial colonization in germfree mice and its independence from thymus. Immunology 1993; 79: 32–7.

65. Helgeland L, Vaage JT, Rolstad B, Midtvedt T, Brandtzaeg P. Microbial colonization influences composition and T-cell receptor Vβ repertoire of intraepithelial lymphocytes in rat intestine. Immunology 1996; 89: 494–501.

66. Bahram S, Bresnahan M, Geraghty DE, Spies T. A second lineage of mammalian major histocompatibility complex class I genes. Proc Natl Acad Sci USA 1994; 91: 6259–63.

67. Balk S, Ebert E, Blumenthal R *et al.* Oligoclonal expansion and CD1 recognition by human intestinal intraepithelial lymphocytes. Science 1991; 253: 1411–15.

68. Blumberg RS, Yockey CE, Gross GG, Ebert EC, Balk SP. Human intestinal intraepithelial lymphocytes are derived from a limited number of T cell clones that utilize multiple Vβ T cell receptor genes. J Immunol. 1993; 150: 5144–53.

69. Gross GG, Schwartz VL, Stevens C, Ebert EC, Blumberg RS, Balk SP. Distribution of dominant T cell receptor β chains in human intestinal mucosa. J Exp Med. 1994; 180: 1337–44.

70. Cepek KL, Parker CM, Madara JL, Brenner MB. Integrin $\alpha^E\beta_7$ mediates adhesion of T lymphocytes to epithelial cells. J Immunol 1993; 150: 3459–70.

71. Papadakis KA, Prehn J, Nelson V *et al.* The role of thymus-expressed chemokine and its receptor CCR9 on lymphocytes in the regional specialization of the mucosal immune system. J Immunol 20; 165: 5069–76.

72. Jabri B, de Serre NP, Cellier C *et al.* Selective expansion of intraepithelial lymphocytes expressing the HLA-E-specific natural killer receptor CD94 in celiac disease. Gastroenterology 20; 118: 867–79.

73. Christ AD, Colgan SP, Balk SP, Blumberg RS. Human intestinal epithelial cell lines produce factor(s) that inhibit CD3-mediated T-lymphocyte proliferation. Immunol Lett 1997; 58: 159–65.

74. Cebra JJ, Jiang H-Q, Sterzl J, Tlaskalova-Hogenova H. The role of mucosal microbiota in the development and maintenance of the mucosal immune system. In: Ogra RL, Mestecky J, Lamm ME, Strober W, Bienenstock J, McGhee JR, eds. Mucosal Immunology, 2nd edn. San Diego: Academic Press, 1999: 267–80.

75. Berg RD, Savage DC . Immune responses of specific pathogen-free and gnotobiotic mice to antigens of indigenous and nonindigenous microorganisms. Infect Immun 1975; 11: 320–9.

76. Nieuwenhuis ESS, Visser MR, Kavelaars A *et al.* Oral antibiotics as a novel therapy forarthritis; evidence of a beneficial effect of intestinal *Escherichia coli*. Arthritis Rheum 20; 43: 2583–9.

77. Christ AD, Blumberg RS. The intestinal epithelial cell: immunological aspects. Springer Sem Immunopathol. 1997; 18: 449–62.

78. Kelsall BL, Strober W. Dendritic cells of the gastrointestinal tract. Springer Sem Immunopathol. 1997; 18: 409–20.

79. Frey A, Giannasca KT, Weltzin R *et al.* Role of the glycocalyx in regulating access of microparticles to apical plasma membranes of intestinal epithelial cells: implications for microbial attachment and oral vaccine targeting. J Exp Med 1996; 184,1045-59.

80. Neutra MR. Current concepts in mucosal immunity. V. Role of M cells in transepithelial transport of antigens and pathogens to the mucosal immune system. Am J Physiol 1998; 274, G785–91.

81. Dickinson BL, Badizadegan K, Wu Z *et al.* Bidirectional FcRn-dependent IgG transport in a polarized human intestinal epithelial cell line. J Clin Invest 1999; 104: 903-11.

82. Zhu X, Meng G, Dickinson BL *et al.* MHC class I-related neonatal Fc receptor for IgG is functionally expressed in monocytes, macrophages and dendritic cells. J Immunol 2001; 166: 3266–76.

83. Witmer-Pack MD *et al.* Tissue distribution of the DEC-205 protein that is detected by the monoclonal antibody NLDC-145. II. Expression *in situ* in lymphoid and nonlymphoid tissues. Cell Immunol 1995; 163: 157–62.

84. Barone KS, Jain SL, Michael JG *et al.* Effect of *in vivo* depletion of CD4$^+$ and CD8$^+$ cells on the induction and maintenance of oral tolerance. Cell Immunol . 1995; 163: 19–29.

85. Chen Y, Inobe J, Weiner HL. Induction of oral tolerance to myelin basic protein in CD8-depleted mice: both CD4$^+$ and CD8$^+$ cells mediate active suppression. J Immunol 1995; 155: 910–16.

86. Garside P, Steel M, Liew FY, Mowat AM. CD4$^+$ but not CD8$^+$ T cells are required for the induction of oral tolerance. Int Immunol 1995; 7: 501–4.

87. Powrie F. T cells in inflammatory bowel disease: protective and pathogenic roles. Immunity 1995; 3: 171–4.

88. Beagley KW, Fujihashi K, Lagoo AS *et al.* Differences in intraepithelial lymphocyte T cell subsets isolated from murine small versus large intestine. J Immunol 1995; 154: 5611–19.

89. Camerini V, Panwala C, Kronenberg M. Regional specialization of the mucosal immune system. J Immunol 1993; 151: 1765–76.

90. Bland PW, Whiting CV. Induction of MHC class II gene products in rat intestinal epithelium during graft-versus-host disease and effects on the immune function of the epithelium. Immunology 1992; 75: 366–71.

91. Kaiserlian D, Vidal K, Revillard JP. Murine enterocytes can present soluble antigen to specific class II-restricted CD4$^+$ T cells. Eur J Immunol. 1989; 19: 1513–16.

92. Mayer L, Eisenhardt D, Salomon P *et al.* Expression of class II molecules on intestinal epithelial cells in humans. Differences between normal and inflammatory bowel disease. Gastroenterology 1991; 1: 3–12.

93. Hershberg RM, Framson PE, Cho DH *et al.* Intestinal epithelial cells utilize two distinct pathways for HLA class II antigen processing. J Clin Invest. 1997; 1: 204–15.

94. Wolf PR, Ploegh HL. How MHC class II molecules acquire peptide cargo: biosynthesis and trafficking through the endocytic pathway. Annu Rev Cell Dev Biol 1995; 11: 267–306.

95. Chang C-H, Flavell RA. Class II transactivator regulates the expression of multiple genes involved in antigen presentation. J Exp Med 1995; 181: 765–7.

96. Hershberg RM, Cho DH, Youakim A *et al.* Highly polarized HLA class II antigen processing and presentation by human intestinal epithelial cells. J Clin Invest 1998; 102: 792–803.

97. Katz JF, Stebbins C, Appella E, Sant AJ. Invariant chain and DM edit self-peptide presentation by major histocompatibility complex (MHC) class II molecules. J. Exp. Med. 1996; 184: 1747–53.

98. Pinet V, Vergelli M, Martin R *et al*. Antigen presentation mediated by recycling of surface HLA-DR molecules. Nature 1995; 375: 603–6.

99. Zhong G, Romagnoli P, Germain RN. Related leucine-based cytoplasmic targeting signals in invariant chain and major histocompatibility complex class II molecules control endocytic presentation of distinct determinants in a single protein. J Exp Med 1997; 185: 429–38.

100. Hirata I, Austin LL, Blackwell WH *et al*. Immunoelectron microscopic localization of HLA-DR antigen in control small intestine and colon and in inflammatory bowel disease. Dig Dis Sci 1986; 31: 1317–30.

101. Mayrhofer G, Spargo LD. Distribution of class II major histocompatibility antigens in enterocytes of the rat jejunum and their association with organelles of the endocytic pathway. Immunology 1990; 70: 11–19.

102. Gottlieb TA, Ivanov IE, Adesnik M, Sabatini DD. Actin microfilaments play a critical role in endocytosis at the apical but not the basolateral surface of polarized epithelial cells. J Cell Biol 1993; 120: 695–710.

103. Jackman MR, Shurety W, Ellis JA, Luzio JP. Inhibition of apical but not basolateral endocytosis of ricin and folate in Caco-2 cells by cytochalasin D. J Cell Sci 1994; 107: 2547–56.

104. Brandeis JM, Sayegh, Gallon L, Blumberg RS, Carpenter CB. Rat intestinal epithelial cells present major histocompatibility complex allopeptides to primed T cells. Gastroenterology 1994; 107: 1537–42.

105. Telega GW, Baumgart DC, Carding SR. Uptake and presentation of antigen to T cells by primary colonic epithelial cells in normal and diseased states. Gastroenterology 20; 119: 1548–59.

106. Madara J L, Stafford J. Interferon-gamma directly affects barrier function of cultured intestinal epithelial monolayers. J Clin Invest 1989; 83: 724–7.

107. Cong J, Brandwein SL, McCabe RP *et al*. CD4$^+$ T cells reactive to enteric bacterial antigens in spontaneous colitis C3H/HeJBir mice: increased T helper cell type 1 response and ability to transfer disease. J Exp Med 1998; 187: 855–64.

108. Groux H, O'Garra A, Bigler M *et al*. A CD4$^+$ T-cell subset inhibits antigen-specific T-cell responses and prevents colitis. Nature 1997; 389: 737–42.

109. Mayer L, Shlien R. Evidence for function of Ia molecules on gut epithelial cells in man. J. Exp. Med. 1987; 166: 1471–83.

110. Hershberg R, Blumberg RS. What's so (co)stimulating about the intestinal epithelium? Gastroenterology. 1999; 117: 726–36.

111. Bleicher PA, Balk SP, Hagen SJ *et al*. Expression of murine CD1 on gastrointestinal epithelium. Science 1990; 250: 679–82.

112. Hershberg R, Eghtesady P, Sydora B *et al*. Expression of the thymus leukemia antigen in mouse intestinal epithelium. Proc Natl Acad Sci USA 1990; 87: 9727–31.

113. Blumberg RS. Current concepts in mucosal immunity. II. One size fits all: nonclassical MHC molecules fulfill multiple roles in epithelial cell function. Am J Physiol 1998; 274: G227–31.

114. Balk SP, Burke S, Polischuk JE *et al*. Beta 2-microglobulin-independent MHC class Ib molecule expressed by human intestinal epithelium. Science 1994; 265: 259–62.

115. Groh V, Bahram S, Bauer S *et al*. Cell stress-regulated human major histocompatibility complex class I gene expressed in gastrointestinal epithelium. Proc Natl Acad Sci USA 1996; 93: 12445–50.

116. Braud VM, Allan DS, McMichael AJ. Functions of non-classical MHC and non-MHC-encoded class I molecules. Curr Opin Immunol 1999; 11: 100–8.

117. Parkkila S, Waheed A, Britton RS *et al*. Immunohistochemistry of HLA-H, the protein defective in patients with hereditary hemochromatosis, reveals unique pattern of expression in gastrointestinal tract. Proc Natl Acad Sci USA 1997; 94: 2534–9.

118. Beckman E, Porcelli S, Morita C, Behar S, Furlong S, Brenner M. Recognition of a lipid antigen by CD1-restricted αβ$^+$ T cells. Nature 1994; 372: 691–4.

119. Sieling PA, Chatterjee D, Porcelli SA *et al*. CD1-restricted T cell recognition of microbial ligoplycan antigens. Science 1995; 269: 227–30.

120. Blumberg R, Terhorst C, Bleicher P *et al*. Expression of a nonpolymorphic MHC class I-like molecule, CD1d by human intestinal epithelial cells. J Immunol 1991; 147: 2518–24.

121. Canchis P, Bhan A, Landau S, Yang L, Balk S, Blumberg R. Tissue distribution of the non-polymorphic major histocompatibility complex class I-like molecule, CD1d. Immunology 1993; 80: 561–5.

122. Exley M, Garcia J, Wilson SB *et al*. Developmental and activation regulated expression of CD1d in human lymphoid and myeloid lineages. Immunology 20; 1: 37–47.

123. Joyce S, Woods AS, Yewdell JW *et al*. Natural ligand of mouse CD1d1: cellular glycosylphosphatidylinositol. Science 1998; 279: 1541–4.

124. Kawano T, Cui J, Koezuka Y *et al*. CD1d-restricted and TCR-mediated activation of Vα14 NKT cells by glycosylceramides. Science 1997; 278: 1626–9.

125. Castano A, Tangri S, Miller S *et al*. Peptide binding and presentation by mouse CD1. Science 1995; 269: 223–6.

126. Zeng A-H, Castano AR, Segelke BW, Stura EA, Peterson PA, Wilson IA. Crystal structure of mouse CD1: an MHC-like fold with a large hydrophobic binding groove. Science 1997; 277: 339–45.

127. Bendelac A, Lantz O, Quimby M, Yewdell J, Bennink J, Brutkiewicz R. CD1d recognition by mouse NK1$^+$ lymphocytes. Science. 1995; 268: 863–5.

128. Bendelac A, Rivera MN, Park S-H, Roark JH. Mouse CD1-specific NK1 T cells: development, specificity, and function. Annu Rev Immunol 1997; 15: 535–62.

129. Balk S, Bleicher P, Terhorst C. Isolation and expression of cDNA encoding the murine homologues of CD1. J Immunol. 1991; 146: 768–74.

130. Calabi R, Bradbury A. A review. The CD1 system. Tissue Antigens. 1991; 37: 1–9.

131. MacDonald HR. NK1.1$^+$ T cell receptor-α/β$^+$ cells: new clues to their origin, specificity, and function. J Exp Med 1995; 182: ; 633–8.

132. Chen H, Paul WE. Cultured NK1.1$^+$CD4$^+$ T cells produce large amounts of IL-4 and IFN-γ upon activation by anti-CD3 or CD1. J Immunol 1997; 159: 2240–9.

133. Lantz O, Bendelac A. An invariant T cell receptor α chain is used by a unique subset of MHC class I-specific CD4$^+$ and CD4$^-$CD8$^-$ T cells in mice and humans. J Exp Med 1994; 180: 1097–106.

134. Toyabe S, Seki S, Liai T *et al*. Requirement of IL-4 and liver NK1$^+$ T cells for concanavalin A-induced hepatic injury in mice. J Immunol 1997; 159: 1537–42.

135. Matsuda JL, Naidenko OV, Gapin L *et al*. Tracking the response of natural killer T cells to a glycolipid antigen using CD1d tetramers. J Exp Med 2000; 192: 741–54.

136. Yoshimoto T, Bendelac A, Watson C, Hu-Li J, Paul WE. Role of NK1.1$^+$ T cells in a T$_H$2 response and in immunoglobulin E production. Science 1995; 270: 1845–7.

137. Smiley ST, Kaplan MH, Grusby MJ. Immunoglobulin E production in the absence of interleukin-4-secreting CD1d-dependent cells. Science 1997; 275: 977–9.

138. Mendiratta SK, Martin WD, Hong S, Boesteanu A, Joyce S, Van Kaer L. CD1d1 mutant mice are deficient in natural T cells that promptly produce IL-4. Immunity 1997; 6: 469–77.

139. Chen YH, Chiu MM, Mandel M, Wang CR. Impaired NK-T cells development and early IL-4 production in CD1-deficient mice. Immunity 1997; 459–67.

140. Kawamura T, Takeda K, Mendiratta SK et al. Cutting edge: critical role of NK1⁺ T cells in IL-12-induced immune responses *in vivo*. J Immunol 1998; 160: 16.

141. Seki S, Hashimoto W, Ogasawara K et al. Antimetastatic effect of NK1 T cells on experimental haematogenous tumour metastases in the liver and lungs of mice. Immunology 1997; 92: 561.

142. Exley M, Garcia J, Balk SP, Porcelli S. Requirements for CD1d recognition by human invariant Vα24⁺ CD4⁻CD8⁻ T cells. J Exp Med 1997; 186: 1.

143. Prussin C, Foster B. TCR Vα24 and Vβ11 coexpression defines a human NK1 T cell analog containing a unique Th0 subpopulation. J Immunol 1997; 159: 5862–70.

144. Porcelli S, Gerdes D, Fertig A, Balk SP. Human T cells expressing an invariant Vα24-JαQ TCRα are CD4⁻ and heterogeneous with respect to TCRβ expression. Human Immunol 1996; 48: 63.

145. Exley M, Porcelli S, Furman M, Garcia J, Balk S. CD161 (NKR-P1A) costimulation of CD1d-dependent activation of human T cells expressing invariant Vα24JαQ T cell receptor α chains. J Exp Med 1998; 188: 867.

146. Brossay L, Chioda M, Burdin N et al. CD1d-mediated recognition of an α-galactosylceramide by natural killer T cells is highly conserved through mammalian evolution. J Exp Med 1998; 188: 1521–8.

147. Nieda M, Nicol A, Koezuka Y et al. Activation of human VαNKT cells by α-glycosylceramide in a CD1d-restricted and Vα24 TCR-mediated manner. Human Immunol 1999; 60: 10–19.

148. Spada FM, Koezuka Y, Porcelli SA. CD1d-restricted recognition of synthetic glycolipid antigens by human natural killer T cells. J Exp Med 1998; 188: 1529–34.

149. Wilson SB, Kent SC, Patton KT et al. Extreme Th1 bias of invariant Vα2JαQ T cells in type 1 diabetes. Nature 1998; 391: 177.

150. Mieza MA, Itoh T, Cui JQ et al. Selective reduction of Vα14⁺ NK T cells associated with disease development in aujtoimmune-prone mice. J Immunol 1996; 156: 4035.

151. Sumida T, Sakamoto A, Murata H et al. Selective reduction of T cells bearing invariant Vα24JαQ antigen receptor in patients with systemic sclerosis. J Exp Med 1995: 182: 1163.

152. Cui J, Shin T, Kawano T et al. Requirement for Vα14 NKT cells in IL-12-mediated rejection of tumors. Science 1997; 278: 1623–9.

153. Somnay-Wadgaonkar K, Nusrat A, Kim HS et al. Immuno-localization of CD1d in human intestinal epithelial cells and identification of a β2-microglobulin associated form. Int Immunol 1999; 383–92.

154. Blumberg RS, Terhorst C, Bleicher P et al. Expression of human CD1d on gastrointestinal epithelium. J Immunol 1991; 147: 2518–24.

155. van de Wal Y, Pitman RS, Hershberg RM et al. Human and mouse intestinal epithelial cells (IEC) present glycolipid antigens to natural killer (NK)-T cells in a CD1d-restricted manner. Gastroenterology 2001 (in press).

156. Saubermann LJ, Beck P, de Jong YP et al. Natural killer-T cells activated by α-galactosylceramide in the presence of CD1d provide protection against colitis in mice. Gastroenterology 20; 119: 119–28.

157. Bleday R, Braidt J, Ruoff K, Shellito PC, Ackroyd FW. Quantitative cultures of the mucosal-associated bacteria in the mechanically prepared colon and rectum. Dis Colon Rectum 1993; 36: 844–9.

158. Roediger WE. Anaerobic bacteria, the colon and colitis. Aust NZ J Surg 1980; 50: 73–5.

159. Madara JL. Epithelia: biologic principles of organization. In: Yamada T, ed. Textbook of Gastroenterology. Philadelphia: Lippincott, 1995: 141.

160. Perez-Vilar J, Hill RL. The structure and assembly of secreted mucins. J Biol Chem 1999; 274: 31751–4.

161. Sanderson IR, Walker A. Mucosal barrier: an overview. In: Ogra RL, Mestecky J, Lamm ME, Strober W, Bienenstock J, McGhee JR, eds. Mucosal Immunology, 2nd edn. San Diego: Academic Press, 1999: 5.

162. Jabbal I, Kells DI, Forstner G, Forstner J. Human intestinal goblet cell mucin. Can J Biochem 1976; 54: 707–16.

163. Gum JR Jr. Mucin genes and the proteins they encode: structure, diversity, and regulation. Am J Respir Cell Mol Biol 1992; 7: 557–64.

164. Loomes KM, Senior HE, West PM, Roberton AM. Functional protective role for mucin glycosylated repetitive domains. Eur J Biochem 1999; 266: 105–11.

165. Kindon H, Pothoulakis C, Thim L, Lynch-Devaney K, Podolsky DK. Trefoil peptide protection of intestinal epithelial barrier function: cooperative interaction with mucin glycoprotein. Gastroenterology 1995; 109: 516–23.

166. Lindahl M, Carlstedt I. Binding of pig small intestinal mucin glycopeptides to fimbriated enterotoxigenic *Escherichia coli*. Symp Soc Exp Biol 1989; 43: 423–8.

167. Piotrowski J, Slomiany A, Murty VL, Fekete Z, Slomiany BL. Inhibition of *Helicobacter pylori* colonization by sulfated gastric mucin. Biochem Int 1991; 24: 749–56.

168. Smith C J, Kaper JB, Mack DR. Intestinal mucin inhibits adhesion of human enteropathogenic *Escherichia coli* to HEp-2 cells. J Pediatr Gastroenterol Nutr 1995; 21: 269–76.

169. Epple HJ, Kreusel KM, Hanski C, Schulzke JD, Riecken EO, Fromm M. Differential stimulation of intestinal mucin secretion by cholera toxin and carbachol. Pflugers Arch 1997; 433: 638–47.

170. Choi J, Klinkspoor JH, Yoshida T, Lee SP. Lipopolysaccharide from *Escherichia coli* stimulates mucin secretion by cultured dog gallbladder epithelial cells. Hepatology 1999; 29: 1352–7.

171. McCool DJ, Marcon MA, Forstner JF, Forstner GG. The T84 human colonic adenocarcinoma cell line produces mucin in culture and releases it in response to various secretagogues. Biochem J 1990; 267: 491–500.

172. Ouellette, AJ, Greco RM, James M, Frederick D, Naftilan J, Fallon JT. Developmental regulation of cryptdin, a corticostatin/defensin precursor mRNA in mouse small intestinal crypt epithelium. J Cell Biol 1989; 108: 1687–95.

173. Eisenhauer PB, Harwig SS, Lehrer RI. Cryptdins: antimicrobial defensins of the murine small intestine. Infect Immun 1992; 60: 3556–65.

174. O'Neil DA, Porter EM, Elewaut D et al. Expression and regulation of the human beta-defensins hBD-1 and hBD-2 in intestinal epithelium. J Immunol 1999; 163: 6718–24.

175. Pruitt KM, Rahemtulla B, Rahemtula F, Russel MW. Innate humoral factors. In: Ogra RL, Mestecky J, Lamm ME, Strober W, Bienenstock J, McGhee JR, eds. Mucosal Immunology, 2nd edn. San Diego: Academic Press, 1999: 65.

176. Bellamy W, Takase M, Wakabayashi H, Kawase K, Tomita M. Antibacterial spectrum of lactoferricin B, a potent bactericidal peptide derived from the N-terminal region of bovine lactoferrin. J Appl Bacteriol 1992; 73: 472–9.

177. Harmsen MC, Swart PJ, de Bethune MP et al. Antiviral effects of plasma and milk proteins: lactoferrin shows potent

activity against both human immunodeficiency virus and human cytomegalovirus replication *in vitro*. J Infect Dis 1995; 172: 380–8.

178. Fujihara T, Hayashi K. Lactoferrin inhibits herpes simplex virus type-1 (HSV-1) infection to mouse cornea. Arch Virol 1995; 140: 1469–72.

179. Kawasaki Y, Tazume S, Shimizu K *et al*. Inhibitory effects of bovine lactoferrin on the adherence of enterotoxigenic *Escherichia coli* to host cells (In process citation). Biosci Biotechnol Biochem 2000; 64: 348–54.

180. Turchany JM, Aley SB, Gillin FD. Giardicidal activity of lactoferrin and N-terminal peptides. Infect Immun 1995; 63: 4550–2.

181. Tanaka T, Omata Y, Saito A, Shimazaki K, Igarashi I, Suzuki N. Growth inhibitory effects of bovine lactoferrin to *Toxoplasma gondii* parasites in murine somatic cells. J Vet Med Sci 1996; 58: 61–5.

182. Wang YB, Germaine GR. Effect of lysozyme on glucose fermentation, cytoplasmic pH, and intracellular potassium concentrations in *Streptococcus mutans* 10449. Infect Immun 1991; 59: 638–44.

183. Soukka T, Lumikari M, Tenovuo J. Combined inhibitory effect of lactoferrin and lactoperoxidase system on the viability of *Streptococcus mutans*, serotype c. Scand J Dent Res 1991; 99: 390–6.

184. Andoh A, Fujiyama Y, Bamba T, Hosoda S. Differential cytokine regulation of complement C3, C4, and factor B synthesis in human intestinal epithelial cell line, Caco-2. J Immunol 1993; 151: 4239–47.

185. MacDermott RP, Sanderson IR, Reinecker HC. The central role of chemokines (chemotactic cytokines) in the immunopathogenesis of ulcerative colitis and Crohn's disease. Inflam Bowel Dis 1998; 4: 54–67.

186. MacDermott RP. Chemokines in the inflammatory bowel diseases. J Clin Immunol 1999; 19: 266–72.

187. Eckmann L, Jung HC, Schurer-Maly C, Panja A, Morzycka-Wroblewska E, Kagnoff MF. Differential cytokine expression by human intestinal epithelial cell lines: regulated expression of interleukin 8. Gastroenterology 1993; 105: 1689–97.

188. Eckmann L, Kagnoff MF, Fierer J. Epithelial cells secrete the chemokine interleukin-8 in response to bacterial entry. Infect Immun 1993; 61: 4569–74.

189. McCormick BA, Hofman PM, Kim J, Carnes DK, Miller SI, Madara JL. Surface attachment of *Salmonella typhimurium* to intestinal epithelia imprints the subepithelial matrix with gradients chemotactic for neutrophils. J Cell Biol 1995; 131: 1599–608.

190. Schulte R, Autenrieth IB. *Yersinia enterocolitica*-induced interleukin-8 secretion by human intestinal epithelial cells depends on cell differentiation. Infect Immun 1998; 66: 1216–24.

191. Jung HC, Eckmann L, Yang SK *et al*. A distinct array of proinflammatory cytokines is expressed in human colon epithelial cells in response to bacterial invasion. J Clin Invest 1995; 95: 55–65.

192. Crowe SE, Alvarez L, Dytoc M *et al*. Expression of interleukin 8 and CD54 by human gastric epithelium after *Helicobacter pylori* infection *in vitro*. Gastroenterology 1995; 108: 65–74.

193. Jung HC, Kim JM, Song IS, Kim CY. *Helicobacter pylori* induces an array of pro-inflammatory cytokines in human gastric epithelial cells: quantification of mRNA for interleukin-8, -1 alpha/beta, granulocyte-macrophage colony-stimulating factor, monocyte chemoattractant protein-1 and tumour necrosis factor-alpha. J Gastroenterol Hepatol 1997; 12: 473–80.

194. Husband AJ, Beagley KW, McGhee JR. Mucosal Cytokines. In: Ogra RL, Mestecky J, Lamm ME, Strober W,

Bienenstock J, McGhee JR, eds. Mucosal Immunology, 2nd edn. San Diego: Academic Press, 1999: 541.

195. Schuerer-Maly CC, Eckmann L, Kagnoff MF, Falco MT, Maly FE. Colonic epithelial cell lines as a source of interleukin-8: stimulation by inflammatory cytokines and bacterial lipopolysaccharide. Immunology 1994; 81: 85–91.

196. Reinecker HC, MacDermott RP, Mirau S, Dignass A, Podolsky DK. Intestinal epithelial cells both express and respond to interleukin 15. Gastroenterology 1996; 111: 1706–13.

197. Ciacci C, Mahida YR, Dignass A, Koizumi M, Podolsky DK. Functional interleukin-2 receptors on intestinal epithelial cells. J Clin Invest 1993; 92: 527–32.

198. Ciacci C, Lind SE, Podolsky DK. Transforming growth factor beta regulation of migration in wounded rat intestinal epithelial monolayers. Gastroenterology 1993; 105: 93–101.

199. Kim PH, Kagnoff MF. Transforming growth factor beta 1 increases IgA isotype switching at the clonal level. J Immunol 1990; 145: 3773–8.

200. Bromander AK, Kjerrulf M, Holmgren J, Lycke N. Cholera toxin enhances alloantigen presentation by cultured intestinal epithelial cells. Scand J Immunol 1993; 37: 452–8.

201. Goodrich ME, McGee DW. Effect of intestinal epithelial cell cytokines on mucosal B-cell IgA secretion: enhancing effect of epithelial-derived IL-6 but not TGF-β pm IgA⁺ B cells. Immunol Lett 1999; 67: 11–14.

202. Defrance T, Vanbervliet B, Briere F, Durand I, Rousset F, Banchereau J. Interleukin 10 and transforming growth factor beta cooperate to induce anti-CD40-activated naive human B cells to secrete immunoglobulin A. J Exp Med 1992; 175: 671–82.

203. Moore KW, O'Garra A, de Waal Malefyt R, Vieira P, Mosmann TR. Interleukin-10. Annu Rev Immunol 1993; 11: 165–90.

204. Madsen KL, Lewis SA, Tavernini MM, Hibbard J, Fedorak RN. Interleukin 10 prevents cytokine-induced disruption of T84 monolayer barrier integrity and limits chloride secretion. Gastroenterology 1997; 113: 151–9.

205. Fujihashi K, McGhee JR, Yamamoto M, Peschon JJ, Kiyono H. An interleukin-7 internet for intestinal intraepithelial T cell development: knockout of ligand or receptor reveal differences in the immunodeficient state. Eur J Immunol 1997; 27: 2133–8.

206. He YW, Malek TR. Interleukin-7 receptor alpha is essential for the development of gamma delta + T cells, but not natural killer cells. J Exp Med 1996; 184: 289–93.

207. Maki K, Sunaga S, Komagata Y *et al*. Interleukin 7 receptor-deficient mice lack gammadelta T cells. Proc Natl Acad Sci USA 1996; 93: 7172–7.

208. Carini C, Essex M. Interleukin 2-independent interleukin 7 activity enhances cytotoxic immune response of HIV-1-infected individuals. AIDS Res Hum Retroviruses 1994; 10: 121–30.

209. Kasper LH, Matsuura T, Khan IA. IL-7 stimulates protective immunity in mice against the intracellular pathogen, *Toxoplasma gondii*. J Immunol 1995; 155: 4798–804.

210. Watanabe M, Ueno Y, Yajima T *et al*. Interleukin 7 is produced by human intestinal epithelial cells and regulates the proliferation of intestinal mucosal lymphocytes. J Clin Invest 1995; 95: 2945–53.

211. Puddington L, Olson S, Lefrancois L. Interactions between stem cell factor and c-Kit are required for intestinal immune system homeostasis. Immunity 1994; 1: 733–9.

212. Klimpe, GR, Langley KE, Wypych J, Abrams JS, Chopra AK, Niesel DW. A role for stem cell factor (SCF): c-kit interaction(s) in the intestinal tract response to *Salmonella typhimurium* infection. J Exp Med 1996; 184: 271–6.

213. Wang J, Whetsell M, Klein JR. Local hormone networks and intestinal T cell homeostasis. Science 1997; 275: 1937–9.

214. Hata Y, Ota S, Nagata T, Uehara Y, Terano A, Sugimoto T. Primary colonic epithelial cell culture of the rabbit producing prostaglandins. Prostaglandins 1993; 45: 129–41.

215. Barrera S, Lai J, Fiocchi C, Roche JK. Regulation by prostaglandin E2 of interleukin release by T lymphocytes in mucosa. J Cell Physiol 1996; 166: 130–7.

216. Reinecker HC, Podolsky DK. Human intestinal epithelial cells express functional cytokine receptors sharing the common gamma c chain of the interleukin 2 receptor. Proc Natl Acad Sci USA 1995; 92: 8353–7.

217. Sutherland DB, Varilek GW, Neil GA. Identification and characterization of the rat intestinal epithelial cell (IEC-18) interleukin-1 receptor. Am J Physiol 1994; 266: C1198–203.

218. McGee DW, Vitkus SJ, Lee P. The effect of cytokine stimulation on IL-1 receptor mRNA expression by intestinal epithelial cells. Cell Immunol 1996; 168: 276–80.

219. Sollid LM, Kvale D, Brandtzaeg P, Markussen G, Thorsby E. Interferon-gamma enhances expression of secretory component, the epithelial receptor for polymeric immunoglobulins. J Immunol 1987; 138: 4303–6.

220. Kvale D, Lovhaug D, Sollid LM, Brandtzaeg P. Tumor necrosis factor-alpha up-regulates expression of secretory component, the epithelial receptor for polymeric Ig. J Immunol 1998; 140: 3086–9.

221. Phillips JO, Everson MP, Moldoveanu Z, Lue C, Mestecky J. Synergistic effect of IL-4 and IFN-gamma on the expression of polymeric Ig receptor (secretory component) and IgA binding by human epithelial cells. J Immunol 1990; 145: 1740–4.

222. Cerf-Bensussan N, Quaroni A, Kurnick JT, Bhan AK. Intraepithelial lymphocytes modulate Ia expression by intestinal epithelial cells. J Immunol 1984; 132: 2244–52.

223. Hoang P, Crotty B, Dalton HR, Jewell DP. Epithelial cells bearing class II molecules stimulate allogeneic human colonic intraepithelial lymphocytes. Gut 1992; 33: 1089–93.

224. Lowes JR, Radwan P, Priddle JD, Jewell DP. Characterisation and quantification of mucosal cytokine that induces epithelial histocompatibility locus antigen-DR expression in inflammatory bowel disease. Gut 1993; 33: 315–9.

225. Kvale D, Krajci P, Brandtzaeg P. Expression and regulation of adhesion molecules ICAM-1 (CD54) and LFA-3 (CD58) in human intestinal epithelial cell lines. Scand J Immunol 1992; 35: 669–76.

226. Ye G, Barrera C, Fan X, Gourley WK, Crowe SE, Ernst PB, Reyes VE. Expression of B7-1 and B7-2 costimulatory molecules by human gastric epithelial cells: potential role in CD4$^+$ T cell activation during Helicobacter pylori infection. J Clin Invest 1997; 99: 1628–36.

227. Medzhitov R, Janeway C Jr. The toll receptor family and microbial recognition. Trends Microbiol 20; 8: 452–6.

228. Medzhitov R, Janeway C Jr. Innate immunity. N Engl J Med 20; 343: 338–44.

229. Aderem A, Ulevitch RJ. Toll-like receptors in the induction of the innate immune response. Nature 20; 406: 782–7.

230. Anderson KV. Toll signaling pathways in the innate immune response. Curr Opin Immunol 20; 12: 13–19.

231. Poltorak A, He X, Smirnova I et al. Defective LPS signaling in C3H/HeJ and C57BL/10ScCr mice; mutations in Tlr4 gene. Science 1998; 282: 2085–8.

232. Cario E, Rosenberg IM, Brandwein SL, Beck PL, Reinecker HC, Podolsky DK. Lipopolysaccharide activates distinct signaling pathways in intestinal epithelial cell lines expressing Toll-like receptors. J Immunol 20; 164: 966–72.

233. Beutler B. Tlr4: central component of the sole mammalian LPS sensor. Curr Opin Immunol 20; 12: 20–6.

234. Cario E, Podolsky DK. Differential alteration in intestinal epithelial cell expression of toll-like receptor 3 (TLR3) and TLR4 in inflammatory bowel disease. Infect Immun 20; 68: 7010–17.

235. Hemmi H, Takeuchi O, Kawai T et al. A Toll-like receptor recognizes bacterial DNA. Nature 20; 408: 740–5.

7 | The mucosal inflammatory response. Cytokines and chemokines

FABIO COMINELLI, KRISTEN O. ARSENEAU AND THERESA T. PIZARRO

Introduction

Cytokines and chemokines play an important role in inflammatory bowel disease (IBD) pathogenesis, as demonstrated by the efficacy of cytokine-targeted immunomodulatory therapy in treating IBD. The precise etiology of IBD is unknown, but disease pathogenesis clearly involves genetic, immunologic, and environmental factors. The current hypothesis for IBD etiology suggests that the disease is initiated and perpetuated by a dysregulated immune response to an unknown environmental antigen in a genetically susceptible host. A working hypothesis for the pathogenesis of Crohn's disease, the most debilitating form of IBD, is depicted in Fig. 1.

In order to maintain gut homeostasis, the normal mucosal immune system must maintain a delicate balance between a network of proinflammatory and/or inductive cytokines and anti-inflammatory and/or regulatory cytokines. During bacterial invasion the proinflammatory and inductive type I T-helper cell (Th1)-polarizing cytokines exert pleiotropic effects upon release from antigen-presenting cells (macrophages, dendritic cells, etc.) in the intestinal mucosa. Proinflammatory cytokines (i.e. interleukin [IL]-1, IL-6, and tumor necrosis factor [TNF]) activate immune cells in the lamina propria and stimulate intestinal epithelial cells (IEC) and macrophages to produce chemokines which, when secreted, establish a chemotactic gradient across the intestinal mucosa, promoting leukocyte recruitment and extravasation across the intestinal endothelium. Meanwhile, Th1-polarizing cytokines (i.e. IL-12, IL-18, TNF) released from antigen-presenting cells (primarily macrophages) induce activation of naive intraepithelial and lamina propria T lymphocytes and Th1 differentiation. These activated Th1 cells release Th1 cytokines (i.e. IL-2, interferon gamma [IFN-γ], and lymphotoxin [LT]), which further perpetuate inflammatory and delayed hypersensitivity immune responses in the gut.

In the normal gut mucosa this proinflammatory/inductive immune response is kept in balance by a network of anti-inflammatory and regulatory cytokines. Regulatory cytokines (i.e. IL-10, IL-4, IL-5, IL-13, and transforming growth factor beta [TGF-β]) are derived from many cellular sources within the intestine, including macrophages as well as type II T-helper (Th2) cells and type I T regulatory (Tr1) cells. Along with anti-inflammatory cytokines (i.e. IL-1 receptor antagonist [IL-1ra] and IL-11) derived primarily from IEC and macrophages, these Th2 cytokines serve to counterbalance the proinflammatory effects of Th1-mediated immune responses.

For unknown reasons, patients with IBD cannot maintain normal gut homeostasis. An understanding of the cytokine network and its role in promoting IBD pathogenesis is a crucial step toward finding a cure for this devastating disease. This chapter provides an overview of the cytokines and chemokines that have been implicated in IBD, with specific focus on what is known about each cytokine in relation to IBD pathogenesis and treatment.

Proinflammatory/inductive cytokines

The first broad class of cytokines includes proinflammatory/inductive cytokines. For organizational purposes we have divided this class into Th1-polarizing cytokines, Th1-derived cytokines, and other proinflammatory/inductive cytokines. These cytokines are innately involved in initiating and promoting inflammatory immune responses within the intestinal mucosa after antigen presentation. Over-production of these cytokines leads to a Th1-type inflammatory response characteristic of human Crohn's disease (CD).

Stephan R. Targan, Fergus Shanahan and Loren C. Karp (eds.), *Inflammatory Bowel Disease: From Bench to Bedside, 2nd Edition*, 147–176.
© 2003 *Kluwer Academic Publishers. Printed in Great Britain*

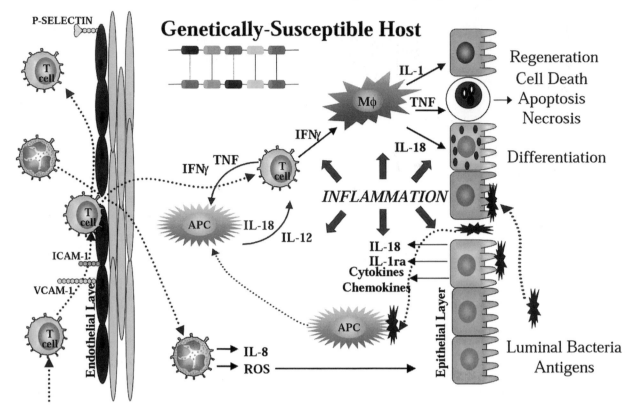

Figure 1. Working hypothesis for the pathogenesis of CD. The disease is initiated and perpetuated by a dysregulated immune response to unknown antigens in a genetically susceptible host. CD4$^+$ T cells and Th1 polarizing cytokines, such as TNF, IL-12, and IL-18, may play an important role in this process. Leukocyte adhesion and trafficking is mediated by specific adhesion molecules, including ICAM1 and VCAM1, which are expressed on endothelial cells and chemotactic chemokines such as IL-8. In this context, intestinal epithelial cells may play a key role in regulating pro- and anti-inflammatory events characteristics of Crohn's disease.

Th1-polarizing cytokines

Th1-polarizing cytokines are a group of inductive proinflammatory cytokines that mediate Th1 CD4$^+$ T cell differentiation. These cytokines are primarily derived from stimulated antigen-presenting cells, and include TNF, IL-12 and IL-18 (Fig. 2).

TNF

TNF classically refers to two closely related cytokines, i.e. TNF-α and TNF-β, which have the ability to bind to the same receptors and trigger a variety of biological effects in human disease. Since the designation of TNF-β has been formally changed to LTβ, it is now widely accepted that TNF-α is simply referred to as TNF. TNF exerts its effects by binding to two distinct receptors, TNFRI and TNFRII, which are expressed on a variety of cell types [1]. Many biological properties of TNF in the intestine are relevant to mucosal inflammation; these include

eliciting chemokine secretion from IEC, disrupting the epithelial barrier and initiating apoptosis of villous epithelial cells [2–4]. In addition, TNF is capable of inducing cytokine and chemokine expression, as well as adhesion molecule production, in endothelial cells [5, 6].

Several studies in animal models of intestinal inflammation have supported the concept that TNF may play a central role in mucosal immune responses. In fact, in animal models of colitis, blockade of TNF significantly ameliorates disease severity [7]. In addition, the severity of colitis is considerably attenuated when colitis is induced in mice that are deficient in TNF. The most compelling evidence that TNF may directly initiate gut mucosal inflammation, in particular a Crohn's-like ileitis, comes from studies in mice carrying a deletion of AU-rich elements (ARE) in the 3'-untranslated region of the TNF gene [8]. Mice carrying this mutation in either a heterozygous or homozygous state are normal at

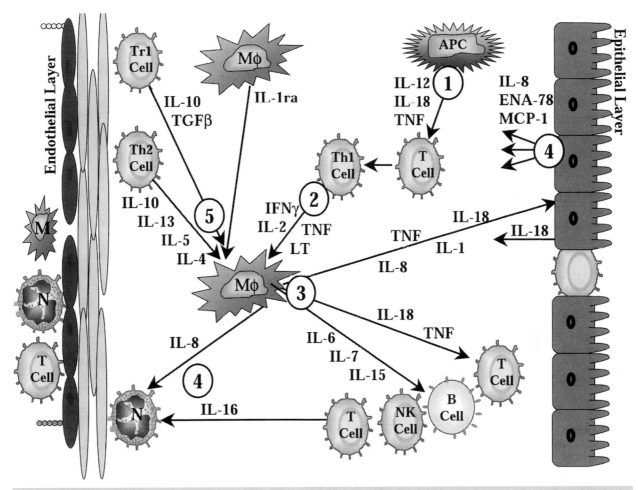

Figure 2. Role of cytokines in the pathogenesis of IBD. Schematic representation of the different groups of cytokines involved in the pathogenesis of intestinal inflammation characteristic of IBD: (1) Th-1 polarizing, (2) Th-1 derived, (3) proinflammatory, (4) chemokines, (5) Th-2 derived/anti-inflammatory cytokines.

birth but soon develop two organ-specific pathologies, namely arthritis and a Crohn's-like enteritis. Another feature of these mice is that high levels of circulating TNF are present and the mice eventually succumb with a multi-organ failure syndrome. Interestingly, the main abnormality of TNF regulation in these mutant mice relates to the increased stability of TNF mRNA which consequently results in an increased production of TNF protein. In a series of elegant studies, Kontoyiannis *et al.* demonstrated that Crohn's-like ileitis is dependent on T cells and requires the presence of TNFRI and II (Fig. 3). In recent studies the same group has demonstrated that overexpression of TNF in macrophages is sufficient to cause the Crohn's-like phenotype, and that IL-12 appears to mediate the effects of TNF in this model [9]. These findings are further supported by work done by Corazza *et al.* in which this group demonstrated that TNF produced by resident non-T cells, but not by transferred T cells, was sufficient to cause colitis in the CD45Rb[hi] transfer model of colitis.

In a recently described mouse model of Crohn's-like disease (i.e. the SAMP1/Yit model), TNF also appears to mediate the spontaneous ileitis characteristic of these mice [10]. In fact, administration of monoclonal antibodies against TNF to SCID mice adoptively transferred with CD4[+] T cells from SAMP1/Yit mice markedly diminished disease severity in recipient animals. The SAMP1/Yit model is of particular interest due to the spontaneous nature of the intestinal lesions in these mice, as well as the close resemblance to the human disease. As such, this model offers great promise to understand the precise

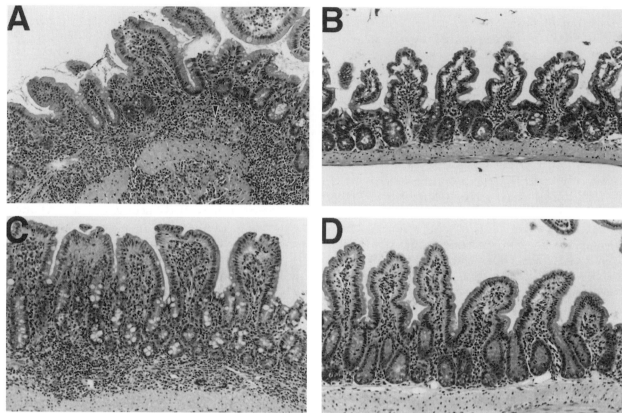

Figure 3. Role of TNF receptors and lymphocytes in the pathogenesis of ileitis in TNF$^{\Delta ARE}$ mice. **A**: TNF$^{\Delta ARE/+}$ heterozygote at 16 weeks. There is typical villous blunting with marked acute and chronic inflammatory cells infiltrating transmurally. An ill-defined non-caseating granuloma is present in the submucosa (arrowhead). **B**: TNF$^{\Delta ARE/\Delta ARE}$/TNFRI$^{-/-}$ double homozygote at 12 weeks. There is normal intestinal appearance with preserved villi, minimal chronic inflammation confined to the mucosa, and an unremarkable muscularis. **C**: TNF$^{\Delta ARE/+}$/TNFRII$^{-/-}$ at 16 weeks. There is modest villous blunting with mild chronic inflammation and few neutrophils in the lamina propria without transmural inflammation. **D**: TNF$^{\Delta ARE/+}$/RAG1$^{-/-}$ at 12 weeks. There is mild patchy villous blunting and widening with a modest, almost normal chronic inflammatory infiltrate in the lamina propria only. There is no acute inflammation (H&E staining; original magnification × 150).

mechanism by which anti-TNF treatment amelio-rates disease severity in patients with CD.

Studies performed in patients with either CD or ulcerative colitis (UC) aimed at measuring TNF in the circulation and/or gut lesions have generated controversial initial results. Although some studies have shown increased TNF mRNA or protein levels in tissue specimens, isolated mucosal cells, stool, and the systemic circulation of patients with IBD, others have not [11–14]. However, the demonstration that approximately two-thirds of patients with CD treated with a single infusion of a chimeric mono-clonal antibody to TNF (infliximab) experience a dramatic improvement in disease activity unques-tionably proves the central role of TNF in CD. Another monoclonal antibody to TNF, CDP571, has been tested in patients with CD with encouraging

results [15]. Since this compound is a humanized antibody consisting of the complementary-determin-ing regions of a mouse anti-human TNF antibody fused to human IGg4, it is likely that less adverse reactions will be observed with infusion [16]. Another potential biological therapy for patients with IBD is etanercept (Enbrel), which is a chimeric TNF inhibitory molecule consisting of the extra-cellular domain of the p75 TNFR spliced to an Ig heavy-chain molecule [16, 17]. Although this compound is approved for the treatment of rheuma-toid arthritis, a preliminary study showed no effect in patients with CD using doses recommended for the treatment of rheumatoid arthritis [18]. It is interest-ing that etanercept, unique from other anti-TNF therapies such as infliximab and CDP571, neutra-lizes LTα in addition to TNF, thus preventing the activation of both TNF receptors. The precise reasons for these differences in efficacy are unknown at the present time. Several other TNF inhibitors have been tested in patients with IBD. In recent pilot trials thalidomide, a synthetic inhibitor of TNF, showed promising results for the treatment of mild to moderate CD [19, 20]. Unfortunately, the well-known side-effects of thalidomide represent a serious limitation to the widespread use of this drug in IBD.

The role of TNF in UC has been less clear, with an initial multi-center trial showing disappointing results [21]. However, a recent study from Chey *et al.* has shown a dramatic improvement in 14–16 patients with severe UC (Chey W, personal communication). A double-blind placebo-controlled multi-center trial in patients with moderate to severe UC is under way at the present time.

Altogether, these studies demonstrate the central role of TNF in the pathogenesis of CD. The ability to generate safe, orally active compounds with TNF-inhibitory activity will represent a major advance in the treatment of IBD and will allow better therapeutic options for the disease.

IL-12

IL-12 is a macrophage-derived heterodimeric cytokine that plays a critical role in T cell differentiation. During chronic intestinal inflammation, IL-12 is a potent inducer of Th1 polarization and has the ability to elicit secretion of Th1 cytokines, particularly IFN-γ. IL-12 exerts these effects through a high-affinity receptor complex composed of two subunits, designated $\beta1$ and $\beta2$. The $\beta2$ subunit is more tightly regulated than $\beta1$ and may serve as a regulatory mechanism for IL-12 signaling [22]. IL-12 is primarily secreted by antigen-presenting cells in response to stimulation by bacterial antigens, and induces the production of Th1 cytokines, such as IFN-γ and TNF, and initiates NK and T cell cytolytic activity [23, 24]. IL-12 production is modulated by interactions between the surface marker CD40 located on stimulated antigen-presenting cells and the CD40 ligand expressed on CD4$^+$ T cells [25–27]. Because of the primary role IL-12 plays in inducing Th1 polarization characteristic of CD, IL-12 is considered a primary target for therapy in CD patients.

Animal models of colitis have helped to elucidate the critical role of IL-12 in promoting Th1-mediated intestinal inflammation. In two chemically induced models of colitis, administration of recombinant (r)IL-12 leads to severe exacerbation of disease [25,

28]. This effect is further aggravated in mice co-administered both rIL-12 and rIL-18, which synergistically leads to lethal toxicity and elevated IFN-γ serum levels [29]. Likewise, administration of anti-IL-12 antibodies to mice with hapten-induced colitis leads to marked improvement in the clinical and histopathological features of disease, complete normalization of IFN-γ levels, as well as induction of Fas-mediated apoptosis of Th1 T cells in the lamina propria and spleen [30, 31]. A similar effect is seen in both IL-10-deficient and TGϵ26 transgenic mice administered anti-IL-12 antibodies [32, 33]. In IL-10-deficient mice, IL-12 neutralization ameliorates colitis in adult mice and completely prevents colitis in young mice. The effect seen in adult mice appears to be specific for IL-12 blockade and is not seen with treatment of antibodies targeting IFN-γ. In contrast, IL-12 neutralization does not appear to possess beneficial effects in colitic models dominated by Th2 immune responses. For example, administration of anti-IL-12 antibodies in oxazolone-induced colitis, a model of Th2-mediated disease that resembles UC, does not appear to be efficacious for disease progression, and may in fact exacerbate disease [34].

Animal models of colitis have also revealed a reciprocal relationship between IL-12 and TGF-β. In the hapten-induced model of colitis, mice rectally administered 2,4,6-trinitrobenzene sulfonic acid (TNBS) develop a Th1-dominated distal colitis. However, if hapten colonic proteins are fed prior to the induction of colitis, these mice appear to develop oral tolerance to the disease. This tolerance is associated with elevated levels of TGF-β and Th2 cytokines, and decreased levels of the Th1 cytokines, IL-12 and IFN-γ. If treated with antibodies targeting TGF-β or rIL-12 during oral tolerance, these mice remain susceptible to colitis [35]. Further evidence for this reciprocal relationship has been reported in studies using intranasal administration of a novel pCMV vector encoding TGF-β_1, which has also been shown to prevent TNBS-induced colitis by down-regulating IL-12, IL-12Rβ_2, and IFN-γ production, while up-regulating TGF-β and IL-10 [36].

The expression of IL-12 in IBD has been recently investigated by Monteleone *et al.*, who reported increased expression of IL-12 in lamina propria mononuclear cells (LPMC) isolated from patients with IBD. In this study IL-12 expression was associated with CD, but not UC or healthy individuals [37]. In addition, the same group has demonstrated that certain chemokines, as well as IFN-γ and prostaglandin E2, can also modulate IL-12 production by activated LPMC [38, 39].

Taken together, these findings indicate that IL-12 may play a critical role in Th1-mediated intestinal inflammation and may have strong therapeutic potential for the treatment of CD. However, the results obtained in chemically induced or immunodeficient mice need to be confirmed in more relevant mouse models of IBD, and ultimately in patients with CD. The results of a multi-center, double blind placebo-controlled clinical trial using monoclonal antibodies against IL-12 that is currently under way will shed light on the efficacy of IL-12 neutralization in treating patients with CD.

IL-18

IL-18 was initially characterized as a novel IFN-γ stimulating factor in mice infected with *Propionibacterium acnes* and subsequently challenged with a sublethal dose of lipopolysaccharide (LPS); as such this factor was originally coined IFN-γ-inducing factor or IGIF [40]. Using degenerate oligonucleotides derived from amino acid sequences of IGIF purified from liver homogenates, the murine form of IGIF was subsequently cloned [41]. The resulting recombinant protein was shown to induce IFN-γ in the presence of a mitogen or IL-2 and these effects were shown to be independent of IL-12 [42]. Cloning of human IGIF followed and the previously reported effects of the naturally occurring molecule were confirmed using recombinant human IGIF [43]. Since the IGIF amino acid sequence showed similarity to human IL-1 (19% positional identity with hIL-1β and 12% with hIL-1α), it was suggested that the name 'IGIF' be changed to IL-1γ [44]. However, since there was no evidence that IGIF binds to the IL-1 receptor type I (IL-1RI) [45], the signaling receptor for IL-1, the name IL-18 was finally chosen [43]. Other similarities exist between IL-18 and IL-1β. Like the precursor form of IL-1β (proIL-1β), the precursor form of IL-18 (proIL-18) does not contain a signal peptide required for the cellular secretion of mature bioactive protein [44]. In addition, similar to the conversion of proIL-1β to mature IL-1β, the IL-1β-converting enzyme (ICE or caspase-1) cleaves the 23 kDa pro form of IL-18, thus generating the mature and bioactive 18.3 kDa IL-18 protein [46]. Finally, IL-18 has been shown to bind to the IL-1R-related protein (IL-1Rrp), a member of the IL-1 receptor family and an essential component of IL-1 and IL-18 signaling [47]. Altogether, these results suggest that IL-18 may be considered a related member of the IL-1 family, including IL-1α, IL-1β and the IL-1 receptor antagonist [48].

In addition to its ability to act as a co-stimulant for IFN-γ production, IL-18 possesses several other biological activities that underscore the potential for IL-18 to be a key proinflammatory cytokine [48]. In fact, IL-18 can induce TNF, IL-1β and both C-C and C-X-C chemokines in peripheral blood mononuclear cells (PBMC) [49]. IL-18 has also been reported to induce Fas ligand as well as nuclear translocation of NF-κB in activated T cells [50, 51]. IL-18 is produced primarily by macrophages, but also other cell types including keratinocytes and other epithelial-like cells [52–54].

Following the cloning of both the murine and human forms of IL-18 and their biological characterization [41, 42], it has been suggested that IL-18 may play a primary role in Th1-mediated immune responses [53, 55]. To support this concept, IL-18 has recently been observed to possess proinflammatory properties, exemplified by its ability to directly stimulate TNF gene expression and synthesis from CD3$^+$/CD4$^+$ and NK cells, which subsequently results in production of IL-1β and IL-8 from the CD14$^+$ population of PBMC [49]. Taken together, these results support the concept that IL-18 is a pleiotropic cytokine, which may play a primary role in Th1-mediated inflammatory disorders, including CD.

Pizarro *et al.* were the first to report that IL-18 is up-regulated in CD patients compared to UC and control patients, and that IL-18 is primarily produced by three main cellular sources within the gut mucosa, i.e. intestinal epithelial cells (IEC), tissue macrophages (histiocytes), and dendritic cells [52]. In this study more abundant IL-18 mRNA transcripts were found in IEC compared to LPMC regardless of the patient source. However, increased IL-18 steady-state mRNA levels were observed in both IEC and LPMC obtained from CD compared to UC and control patients. Immunolocalization studies uncovered one interesting finding. In CD patients, although there is an overall increase in gut IL-18 expression as disease severity increases, there is a dramatic shift in the cellular source of IL-18, from the epithelium to LPMC, with IEC being the prevalent producer of IL-18 in non-involved areas, and macrophages and dendritic cells in more severely involved lesions [52]. These results were supported by Monteleone *et al.*, who also confirmed that IL-18 produced in CD tissues was functionally active. In this study IL-18, as well as IFN-γ, production was decreased in LPMC derived from CD patients following treatment with an anti-sense oligonucleotide specific for IL-18 [56]. Furthermore, Kanai *et al.* showed that LPMC possess IL-18 receptors, and in CD this cell population expresses increased IL-2 receptor and proliferates more potently in response to IL-18 than those isolated from normal non-inflamed control patients [57]. These effects can be potentiated with the addition of IL-12 to CD LPMC; however, proliferation of LPMC isolated from both UC and control patients also increased upon stimulation with IL-18 plus IL-12. Similarly, BALB/c mice given IL-18 and IL-12 resulted in more prominent intestinal mucosal inflammation when these Th1-polarizing cytokines were administered together than alone [58].

Taken together, these data indicate that IL-18 may play a pivotal role in the pathogenesis of CD. IL-18 is not only produced by antigen-presenting cells (i.e. tissue histiocytes and dendritic cells) and IEC to mount a Th1-polarized immune response in synergy with, and independently of, IL-12 through IFN-γ production (Th1 inductive phase), but it also stimulates TNF gene expression and secretion from activated T cells (effector phase) [49]. In addition, IL-18 is capable of stimulating IL-1β as well as IL-8 from activated macrophages, thus affecting the final common pathway of CD immunopathogenesis [49]. Therefore, it is conceivable that IL-18 may, in fact, fulfill the specific requirements to be considered a primary initiating cytokine in Th1-mediated diseases, such as CD. Recent animal studies using monoclonal antibody neutralization against IL-18 in organ-specific autoimmune diseases have supported this concept [48]. Clinical trials using monoclonal antibodies against IL-18 or other IL-18 antagonists are anticipated in the near future for the treatment of Th1-mediated immune disorders, including CD.

Th1-derived cytokines

Th1 cytokines, including IL-2, IFN-γ, and lymphotoxin (LT) are derived from Th1 CD4+ T cells and promote chronic inflammation associated with a variety of disease states, including human CD (Fig. 2).

IL-2

IL-2 is a prototypic Th1 cytokine primarily involved in lymphocyte proliferation and differentiation. In intraepithelial lymphocytes (IEL), IL-2 is produced predominantly by cells expressing the αβ+ T cell receptor (TCRαβ+ IEL), while IL-2 receptors are localized on the surface membranes of TCRγδ+ IEL. IL-2 carefully regulates TCRγδ+ IEL by promoting activation and differentiation, and by also inducing apoptosis after re-stimulation through the TCR [59–61]. In contrast, IL-2 has a protective effect against apoptosis of unstimulated lamina propria lymphocytes (LPL) [62]. IL-2 signaling requires formation of IL-2 receptor (IL-2R) heterodimers composed of a β-chain and a common γ-chain. In IEC, IL-2 signaling leads to enhanced epithelial cell restitution *in vitro*, suggesting that IL-2 may be involved in maintaining epithelial barrier function [63–65].

A useful tool for understanding the functional role of IL-2 in IBD pathogenesis has been the creation of IL-2-deficient mice. These mice develop colitis that is mediated by cytotoxic CD4+ TCRαβ+ T cells, which accumulate in the colon prior to the onset of macroscopic inflammation [66, 67]. The mechanism for this accumulation may involve α4β7 integrins [68]. IL-2-deficient mice also exhibit enhanced expression of the proinflammatory cytokines IL-1, IL-6, and TNF, inducible nitric oxide synthase, the transcription factor NF-κB, and IL-12-driven IFN-γ production [69–72]. In addition, colonic epithelial cells from IL-2-deficient mice express increased levels of IL-15, TGF-β, and the surface marker CD14 [73]. It has also been reported that IL-2-deficient mice develop a chronic Th1-mediated colitis when reared in conventional conditions. A similar colitis develops in specific pathogen-free conditions when mice are immunized with 2,4,6-trinitrophenol-conjugated keyhole limpet hemocyanin (TNP-KLH). Interestingly, in germfree conditions only a mild focal colitis with delayed onset is seen, despite the fact that the mice retain their extraintestinal pathologies, including anemia and extraintestinal lymphoid hyperplasia. Thus, this model system clearly associates environmental antigens with chronic intestinal inflammation, but not with other pathological conditions that develop in IL-2-deficient mice [74–77].

In humans, IL-2 production is increased in the intestines of patients with CD, but not in UC. Mucosal biopsies from patients with CD contain elevated levels of IL-2 in areas of active inflammation. However, no increase is seen in areas of either active or inactive UC. In fact, concentrations in UC have been reported as inversely correlated with the degree of inflammation [78–81]. Patterns of IL-2 production in isolated LPMC are less clear, with some studies reporting an increase in IL-2 levels among CD patients and others a reduction [82–84]. Several drugs used to treat IBD appear to alter IL-2 production in the gut. Variations in IL-2 and soluble IL-2R plasma levels, as well as the percentage of IL-2-secreting cells, have been reported in CD patients following treatment with cyclosporine and corticosteroids [85, 86]. Reductions in IL-2 production have also been observed in UC and CD patients treated with sulfasalazine, as well as in PBMC isolated from healthy volunteers after treatment with transdermal nicotine, a possible new therapeutic approach for UC [87, 88]. Finally, more recent preliminary studies have shown possible therapeutic potential for an IL-2IgG2b fusion protein, which is capable of decreasing wasting and histopathological signs of colitis in TNBS-treated mice [89].

IFN-γ

IFN-γ is a Th1 cytokine and is secreted in response to various stimuli, including IL-12. It exerts its inductive effects on a variety of cell types, including IEC, monocytes, endothelial cells, and lymphocytes. IFN-γ induces changes in epithelial permeability in a dose- and time-dependent fashion, possibly through disruption of tight junctions, and promotes polarized polymorphonuclear cell transmigration through the epithelial barrier [90–92]. IFN-γ is also capable of mediating chemokine expression by IEC and monocytes *in vitro* [93, 94]. In IEL populations TCRαβ$^+$ IEL subsets appear to be more efficient producers of IFN-γ than TCRγδ$^+$ IEL [95]. Like IL-12, IFN-γ appears to share a reciprocal relationship with the regulatory cytokine TGF-β [96]. However, more information is warranted to understand whether the role of IFN-γ in this reciprocal relationship is direct or indirect.

The relative correlation between IFN-γ and IL-4 levels has been used extensively to characterize animal models of intestinal inflammation as being mediated by either Th1 or Th2 immune responses. For example, in several Th1-mediated models, mucosal levels of IFN-γ, but not IL-4, are elevated; these include IL-10, Gα$_{i2}$, and IL-2-deficient mice, CD4$^+$ and CD8$^+$ TCRαβ$^+$ T cells from TGε26 transgenic mice, and SCID mice with intestinal tissue grafts from immunocompetent mice [97–101]. Recently, a spontaneous mouse model of ileitis (i.e, the SAMP1/Yit model) has been characterized as being mediated by Th1 immune responses with high levels of IFN-γ production but no increased IL-4 production from mesenteric lymph node cells [10]. Conversely, Th2-mediated models of intestinal

inflammation display elevated mucosal levels of IL-4, including TCR-deficient mice and the oxazolone model of colitis [34, 102, 103]. Other chemically induced models of colitis are less straightforward. Chronic dextran sodium sulfate (DSS)-induced colitis exhibits both a Th1 and Th2 profile as evidenced by focal increases in both IFN-γ and IL-4 levels in areas of active inflammation [104]. Similarly, activated CD4$^+$ T cells from TNBS-treated mice produce 20–50-fold increases in IFN-γ secretion, suggesting a Th1 phenotype. These mice, however, also have elevated IL-4 and IL-5 levels, and blockade of IL-4 has a greater effect on ameliorating disease than blockade of IFN-γ, suggesting that TNBS colitis may be dominated by Th2 responses [30, 105]. Nonetheless, the relationship between IFN-γ and IL-4 has been a useful marker of inflammatory phenotype in many animal models of IBD.

Animal models have also provided several lines of evidence associating IFN-γ with chronic intestinal inflammation. SCID mice reconstituted with activated CD4$^+$ T cells from IFN-γ-deficient mice develop a less severe colitis than SCID mice reconstituted with cells from wild-type mice. In addition, SCID/IFN-γ-deficient mice have a 2–3-fold increase in the number of IL-4-producing cells, suggesting that the absence of IFN-γ leads to an elevated Th2 response and thus a milder form of colitis [106]. In the CD45Rb^{hi} T cell transfer model, adoptive transfer of pathogenic T cells into SCID mice induces colitis. Neutralization of IFN-γ results in improved colitis. The same result is seen in chronic, but not acute, DSS-induced colitis [28, 107, 108]. The IL-10-deficient model of colitis is also dependent, in part, on IFN-γ production. IFN-γ is essential for the onset of colitis in recombinant activating gene-2 (RAG2)-deficient mice (which lack both B and T cells) reconstituted with CD4$^+$ T cells from IL-10-deficient mice [109]. Blockade of IFN-γ in IL-10-deficient mice completely ameliorates disease in young mice, but cannot reverse established disease in adult mice. Blockade of IL-12, a potent inducer of IFN-γ, is able to reduce colitis in adult mice and simultaneously reduce the number of IFN-γ-producing cells in the colon and mesenteric lymph nodes [32]. In contrast, IFN-γ does not appear to be necessary for the development of colitis in TCR-deficient mice [103].

With the exception of one study, IFN-γ concentrations in humans are consistently elevated in the intestinal mucosa of CD, but not UC, patients [78, 80, 81, 110, 111]. The same results are consistently observed for IFN-γ secretion from intestinal LPL isolated from CD and UC patients [82, 112, 113]. However, studies evaluating cytokine production from early (acute) and late (chronic) CD lesions reveal that early lesions are, in fact, associated with a Th2 response, and exhibit increased IL-4 and decreased IFN-γ production, while late CD lesions display the characteristic Th1 immune response. Therefore, in humans, different cytokine profiles may be associated with acute versus chronic phases of disease [114].

IFN-γ is currently not a strong candidate as a target for immunomodulatory therapy. Although IFN-γ-deficient mice do display abnormalities in their immune system, they do not develop colitis resembling IBD. However, to date, monoclonal antibodies against IFN-γ have not been tested in patients with either CD or UC.

Lymphotoxin

Lymphotoxin is a Th1 cytokine and member of the TNF family that is primarily involved in the early development of lymphoid tissue. It exists as both as a membrane-bound heterotrimer composed of α and β subunits (LTαβ), and as a soluble homotrimer consisting of the α subunit (LTα3) (previously known as TNF-β). LTαβ is expressed on the surface of activated CD4$^+$ T cells, particularly Th1 cells; exposure to IL-4 or a Th2 environment leads to loss of LTαβ surface expression, as well as down-regulation of soluble LTα3 and TNF [115]. Soluble LTα3 has the ability to bind to both the p55 and p75 TNF receptors, while surface LTαβ binds to a LTβ receptor. LTα may exert its effects on lymphoid organ development through the p55 TNF receptor, which is known to mediate TNF-induced Peyer's patch organogenesis [116].

Animal models deficient in either LTα or β have provided useful information in understanding the role of this molecule in the intestinal immune system. LTα-deficient mice display splenic disorganization and non-segregating T/B cell zones. These mice lack Peyer's patches, peripheral lymph nodes, B cell follicles, germinal centers, and follicular dendritic networks. LTβ-deficient mice possess a similar phenotype, but retain some ability to develop limited germinal centers and follicular dendritic networks, and have some segregation of T/B cell zones [117, 118]. Studies in both LTα transgenic and LTα-deficient mice have revealed that LTα3 promotes Th1 immune responses, in part, by up-regulating chemokine expression by endothelial cells, as well as peripheral node addressin and mucosal addressin

adhesion molecule-1 (MAdCAM-1) [119, 120]. Finally, LTβ receptor-deficient mice display distinct abnormalities when compared with both LTα LTβ-deficient mice. These studies suggest that LTβR may transduce signals from other members of the TNF family in addition to membrane-bound LTαβ [121].

Given the success of therapeutics targeting TNF, its plausible that LT would be a strong candidate for immunomodulatory therapy in IBD. Evidence for this therapeutic potential can be seen in the CD45Rb^{hi}/SCID adoptive transfer as well as the TGε26 transgenic mouse models of colitis. In both of these models, fusion proteins, which bind to the LTβR and inhibit LTαβ signaling, are able to improve clinical features of disease [122]. These findings suggest that LT may play an important role in IBD pathogenesis, similar to its close relative TNF. However, as mentioned earlier (see TNF), blockade of LTα together with TNF by etanercept does not appear to have beneficial effects in a recently reported pilot study [18].

Other proinflammatory/inductive cytokines

This subgroup of proinflammatory/inductive cytokines includes IL-1, IL-6, IL-7 and IL-15. These cytokines have been implicated in mediating the non-specific inflammatory phase of chronic intestinal inflammation and are produced primarily by macrophages, and in some cases other cell types (Fig. 2).

IL-1

IL-1 is a pleiotropic proinflammatory cytokine produced in two forms, IL-1α and IL-1β, which have the ability to bind to the same cell surface receptor and possess identical biological activities [123]. In contrast to IL-1α, which remains largely intracellular or is expressed on cell surface membranes, the IL-1β precursor molecule is cleaved intracellularly by the IL-1β-converting enzyme to its mature form and is subsequently secreted. Two IL-1 receptors exist, IL-1 receptor type I and type II (IL-1RI and IL-1RII, respectively). The IL-1RI is present on IEC, hepatocytes, fibroblasts, endothelial cells, T lymphocytes and keratinocytes, whereas the IL-1RII is found primarily on B lymphocytes, neutrophils and monocytes [123]. Several of the biological properties of IL-1, which is produced by many cell types, including activated monocytes, macrophages, fibroblasts, smooth muscle cells, and endothelial cells, are relevant to IBD [124]. Within the inflamed intestinal mucosa of IBD patients, IL-1 expression is markedly increased primarily in LPMC [125]. Other cell types, however, including intestinal smooth muscle cells and fibroblasts, may also contribute to IL-1 production in IBD [126]. Locally, IL-1 induces the production of a variety of proinflammatory and immunoregulatory cytokines as well as arachidonic acid metabolites by lamina propria immune and mesenchymal cells, thereby amplifying gut inflammatory responses. IL-1 has also been shown to increase expression of adhesion molecules on endothelial and immune cells, up-regulate IL-2 receptors on T lymphocytes, stimulate proliferation of intestinal fibroblasts and smooth muscle cells, and enhance collagen synthesis by fibroblasts [127]. Thus, IL-1 appears to play a central role during gut inflammatory responses characteristic of IBD by recruiting inflammatory cells to the site of injury and by activating not only immune cells, but also mesenchymal and epithelial cells.

A primary role of IL-1 has been proposed in the pathogenesis of intestinal inflammation and is demonstrated by three studies. Specifically, IL-1 regulates the production of PGE_2, 6-keto-PGI_2, and TXB_2 in the normal and inflamed rabbit colon [128]. In addition, IL-1 gene expression and synthesis occurs early in the course of immune complex-induced colitis and precedes the appearance of colonic PGE_2 and LTB_4; moreover, tissue levels of IL-1 correlate with the degree of tissue inflammation and necrosis [129]. Finally, specific blockade of IL-1 by recombinant IL-1ra dose-dependently suppresses the inflammatory response and the production of PGE_2 and LTB_2 associated with experimental rabbit colitis [130]. The latter results have been confirmed in other animal models of intestinal inflammation and injury, suggesting that IL-1 may, in fact, play a role of paramount importance in gut inflammation [131–133]. Additional evidence that IL-1 may be an important inflammatory mediator in patients with IBD is also provided by the fact that compounds that are routinely used in the treatment of symptoms, such as sulfasalazine, corticosteroids and other immunosuppressive drugs, may exert some of their effects through the inhibition of IL-1 synthesis and/or activity [134, 135].

The expression of IL-1 in patients with IBD has been extensively investigated in different cell types. Early studies have focused on determining whether PBMC isolated from active UC and CD patients produced more IL-1 than PBMC isolated from control patients. Satsangi *et al.* originally demonstrated that cultured PBMC, isolated from patients with CD, produced increased amounts of bioactive IL-1 when compared to PBMC isolated from controls [136]. These results have subsequently been confirmed using specific immunoassays in patients with active IBD [123, 137, 138]. Since PBMC may not truly represent the LPMC population found in the inflamed tissues of IBD patients, interest has focused more recently on measuring levels of IL-1 in freshly isolated LPMC from these patients. Elevated IL-1 levels in these cells have been reported in patients with IBD compared to controls [139]. Interestingly, freshly isolated IEC do not express IL-1 mRNA transcripts or protein, supporting the hypothesis that production of IL-1 is localized to LPMC [125].

These studies, taken together, have generated great enthusiasm for IL-1 as a key pathogenic cytokine in IBD. Despite this potential for IL-1 as a candidate for therapeutic targeting, no control studies in patients with either UC or CD have been performed using monoclonal antibodies against IL-1 or other specific IL-1 inhibitors.

IL-6

IL-6, in addition to IL-1 and TNF, is part of a group of prototypic macrophage-derived proinflammatory cytokines secreted into the intestinal mucosa in response to antigen stimulation or induction by Th1 cytokines. IL-6 has several functions, including regulation of apoptosis, activation of mesenchymal cells, and possibly wound healing after intestinal anastamosis [126, 140, 141]. IL-6 may also play a critical role in B cell terminal differentiation, proliferation, and immunoglobulin secretion, although conflicting reports using IL-6-deficient mice have made this finding somewhat controversial [142–145]. IL-6 has the ability to bind to both membrane-bound IL-6 receptors (IL-6R) as well as soluble IL-6 receptors (sIL-6R). In fact, IL-6 can interact with cells not expressing IL-6R by a process known as trans-signaling in which IL-6 forms a complex with sIL-6R, which can then transduce signal to target cells [146]. In addition to macrophages, IEC also have the ability to secrete IL-6, and IL-6R have been detected on both the apical and basal surfaces of IEC in culture [147, 148]. A variety of molecules are capable of inducing or potentiating IL-6 production from IEC, including other proinflammatory and regulatory cytokines (i.e. IL-1, IFN-γ and TGF-β), heat-shock proteins, endotoxins, and prostaglandins (PGE_2) [149–152].

IL-6 expression and secretion in patients with IBD has been well studied. Within the intestinal mucosa, IL-6 has been detected in both T and B lymphocytes, macrophages, and IEC [153–155]. IL-6 can be detected in normal mucosa, with elevated levels in areas of active inflammation; this increase appears to correlate with the degree of inflammation [156–159]. It is less clear whether serum levels, which are also elevated in IBD patients, correlate with disease activity. Serum concentrations of IL-6 have been reported to be higher in patients with CD compared to UC, but patients with UC have higher levels than healthy individuals [160, 161]. Soluble IL-6R levels are also elevated in patients with active IBD compared to inactive IBD, other types of intestinal inflammation or healthy individuals [162].

The IL-6 system has been evaluated for therapeutic potential in several animal models of colitis. Like in humans, IL-6 levels are elevated in the inflamed colons of IL-10-deficient mice and after acetic acid-induced tissue injury [163, 164]. Furthermore, Yamamoto *et al.* have shown that blockade of IL-6R ameliorates disease in the CD45Rb^{hi}/SCID adoptive transfer model of colitis, as evidenced by normal growth, decreased T cell expansion, and a down-regulation of adhesion molecules and proinflammatory cytokines [165]. This result has been confirmed in several models of Th1-mediated colitis. The mechanism of action may involve induction of lamina propria T cell apoptosis. Similar results are seen after neutralization of sIL-6R, which results in improved colitis and an increase in lamina propria T cell apoptosis, suggesting that sIL-6R may prevent T cell apoptosis. As further support for this mechanism, Atreya *et al.* showed that mucosal T cells isolated from patients with CD show evidence of trans-signaling through the IL-6/sIL-6R complex, and blockade of trans-signaling induces T cell apoptosis [166]. Therefore, increased mucosal levels of IL-6 and sIL-6R have the potential to inhibit apoptosis of pathogenic T cells, which have been associated with the development and perpetuation of IBD. This possibility needs further investigation, but could lead to new therapeutic approaches.

IL-7

IL-7, an important mediator of B and T cell growth and differentiation, is produced by a variety of cell types, including bone marrow stromal cells, B cells, monocytes, macrophages, dendritic cells, keratino-

cytes, and IEC. IL-7 shares many functions with IL-2 and has the ability to stimulate proliferation of IEL and LPL through an IL-2-dependent CD3 pathway. In addition, IL-7, along with IL-2 and IL-15, plays an essential role in IEL development, which is dependent on signaling through the IL-2R common γ chain [61, 167]. Likewise, IL-7 and IL-2 exhibit a reciprocal relationship in promoting IEL growth and differentiation. IL-7 derived from neighboring TCRαβ$^+$ T cells and IEC has the ability to induce expression of IL-2R on the surface of TCRγδ$^+$ T cells. Conversely, IL-2 has been shown to increase expression of the IL-7 receptor (IL-7R) [59, 168]. Lastly, IEC express both the IL-7R and IL-2R common γ chain *in vivo*, both of which are required for IL-7 signaling [64].

IL-7 preferentially targets development of TCRγδ$^+$ T cell subsets. For example, although IL-7 and IL-7R-deficient mice both have reduced numbers of B cells and retarded growth of TCRαβ$^+$ T cells, they have few or no TCRγδ+ T cells [169–171]. Moreover, IL-7 administration to IL-7-deficient mice results in restoration of TCRγδ$^+$ T cell populations, as well as the formation of Peyer's patches and crypt abscesses [172]. These findings suggest that the IL-7/IL-7R system is essential for TCRγδ$^+$ T cell growth and development.

Evidence also supports a role for IL-7 in mediating colitis. Mice-deficient in both T and B cells develop colitis when exposed to certain bacterial flora. However, when these mice are crossed with IL-7-deficient mice and colonized with the same flora, they do not develop colitis. This model demonstrates that IL-7 can modulate the onset of colitis, independent of B and T cells [173]. In a second model, mice that are genetically manipulated to overexpress IL-7 develop acute and chronic colitis similar to that observed in human UC. The resulting disease appears to be primarily mediated by a dysregulated colonic epithelium, driven by elevated levels of IL-7 [174]. Therefore, IL-7 appears to play a role in intestinal inflammation, but it remains unclear whether or not this role is specific to IBD pathogenesis.

IL-15

IL-15 is derived from mainly non-lymphoid cells and, like IL-7, shares many similarities to IL-2. IL-15, however, is produced by intestinal macrophages and other cell types in response to antigen and plays an important role in growth and differentiation of immune cells within the intestinal mucosa, including T and B lymphocytes, NK cells, macrophages and monocytes. In IEC, IL-15 activates the signal transducer and activator of transcription-3 (STAT-3) pathway and induces proliferation; it can also alter epithelial permeability and down-regulate chemokine production [175–177]. In contrast, IL-15 has the ability to stimulate chemokine production from monocytes [178]. In LPL, IL-15 potentiates IL-12-induced secretion of IFN-γ [179]. IL-15 exerts most of these effects by binding to a heterotrimeric complex composed of the IL-2R β chain, the IL-2R common γ chain, and the IL-15 receptor α chain (IL-15Rα) [180].

IL-15 is an important mediator of IEL proliferation and survival. Like IL-7, IL-15 appears to preferentially target $TCR\gamma\delta^+$ IEL over $TCR\alpha\beta^+$ cells. $TCR\gamma\delta^+$ IEL constitutively express IL-15 and exhibit a greater proliferative response to IL-15 than $TCR\alpha\beta^+$ IEL [181]. Moreover, like IL-2, IL-15 induces re-stimulation of $CD8^+$ $TCR\gamma\delta^+$ IEL. However, upon re-stimulation, these two cytokines differentially regulate cell survival. IL-15 promotes survival after re-stimulation by protecting against apoptosis of this IEL population, as well as in other TCR-specific intraepithelial $CD8^+$ T cell subsets, while IL-2 induces programmed cell death in these populations [60, 182]. Furthermore, IL-15-deficient mice display a marked reduction of $CD8^+$ T cells, as well as certain IEL subsets. Incidentally, these mice also lack NK cells, suggesting that IL-15 may also be involved in expansion and survival of NK cells [183]. Therefore, IL-15 appears to be capable of maintaining a unique reserve of IEL.

Few studies have investigated the role of IL-15 in IBD pathogenesis. Elevated levels of IL-15 have been detected in the intestinal mucosa of patients with IBD, and LPMC isolated from IBD patients appear to be hyper-responsive to IL-15, inducing T cell activation, proliferation, and proinflammatory cytokine production [184, 185]. Further studies are needed to identify whether IL-15 is involved in promoting IBD.

Anti-inflammatory/regulatory cytokines

A second class of cytokines are known as anti-inflammatory/regulatory cytokines, so named for their role in mediating inflammatory responses and restoring gut homeostasis (Fig. 2).

Th2 regulatory cytokines

Th2 cytokines are a subset of immune mediators derived from Th2 $CD4^+$ T cells; these include IL-10, IL-4, IL-5 and IL-13. Th2 immune responses are associated with allergic reactions and atopic disorders, as well as intestinal nematode infections. Although it is well accepted that human IBD is associated with a dysregulated Th1/Th2 immune response, it is currently unclear, in humans, whether up- or down-regulation of Th2 responses plays a critical role in CD or UC, respectively. However, as will be described below, it is clear that Th2 cytokines, IL-10 in particular, may play a central role in IBD pathogenesis (Fig. 2).

IL-10

IL-10 is a potent anti-inflammatory Th2 cytokine that has the ability to suppress production of proinflammatory cytokines secreted from macrophages, dendritic cells, T cells, and NK cells within the inflamed intestinal mucosa [186]. This inhibitory effect is potentiated by synergism with IL-4 and IL-13 in monocytes and epithelial cells [187, 188]. IL-10 also acts to counterbalance many of the proinflammatory functions of Th1-polarizing cytokines and suppresses proinflammatory cytokine and chemokine production by intestinal macrophages [189]. IL-10 regulates human intestinal T cells by blocking proliferation and activation of $CD8^+$ T cells and inhibiting production of Th1-polarizing cytokines (i.e. IL-2, IFN-γ, and TNF), while concurrently enhancing IL-2-induced cytotoxicity, thereby maintaining a basal level of host defense [190].

IL-10 also appears to promote differentiation of a unique subset of immunoregulatory T cells, deemed Tr1-type T cells. Tr1 T lymphocytes display reduced proliferative capabilities and secrete large amounts of IL-10, along with low levels of IL-2 and IL-4 [191]. These cells can prevent colitis in the $CD45Rb^{hi}$/SCID adoptive transfer model of colitis. Similar efficacy is observed with administration of recombinant IL-10 (rIL-10) [191, 192]. In wild-type animals, co-transfer of $CD45Rb^{lo}$ T cells can prevent the pathogenic effects of $CD45Rb^{hi}$ T cells [108]. These protective effects, however, are not observed with transfer of $CD45Rb^{lo}$ T cells from IL-10-deficient mice are transferred into recipient mice [193]. In addition, $CD45Rb^{lo}$ T cells from IL-4-deficient mice are also able to prevent colitis in recipient mice [194]. All of these functions suggest that IL-10 plays an important role in maintaining gut homeostasis.

Studies in IL-10-deficient mice clearly support this concept. These mice spontaneously develop colitis similar to human IBD when raised under conventional conditions [195]. Colitis first develops in the cecum, ascending, and transverse colon around 3 weeks of age. The inflammation spreads through the entire colon and parts of the ileum as the mice age. A majority of IL-10-deficient mice develop colorectal adenocarcinomas by 60 weeks of age.

The development of colitis in IL-10-deficient mice appears to be dependent on a combination of genetics, immunoregulatory, and environmental factors. The genetic background of IL-10-deficient mice can influence the severity of resulting intestinal lesions. The intestinal inflammatory infiltrate in these mice is characterized by increased numbers of macrophages, B cells, plasma cells, and $CD4^+$ $TCR\alpha\beta^+$ T cells, in addition to a dysregulated Th1 cytokine profile [196]. IL-1, IL-6, TNF, IFN-γ, LTβ, and TGF-β mRNA levels are 10–35-fold higher in the intestinal mucosa of IL-10-deficient mice compared to wild-type controls; adhesion molecules intracellular adhesion molecule-1 (ICAM-1), vascular cell adhesion molecule-1 (VCAM-1), and MAdCAM-1 mRNA and protein levels are also elevated 5–23-fold [164]. Furthermore, as noted above, treatment with anti-IL-12 antibodies completely abolishes colitis in young IL-10-deficient mice, and significantly improves disease in adult mice, suggesting that the inflammation in these mice is indeed Th1-mediated. Antibodies against IFN-γ can prevent colitis in young mice but, unlike anti-IL-12 antibodies, do not appear to be efficacious in treating established disease in adult mice [32, 196]. The development of colitis in IL-10-deficient mice is also believed to be mediated by pathogenic T cell subsets. IEL and LPL from IL-10-deficient mice are capable of inducing colitis upon transfer to RAG2 knockout mice. The disease severity of the resulting colitis is dependent on the number of cells that are transferred [197]. Moreover, these cells are predominantly $CD4^+$ $TCR\alpha\beta^+$ $CD44^+$ $CD45Rb^{lo}$ T cells, implicating a subset of activated memory cells.

The normal enteric bacterial flora is also an important factor that influences the development of colitis in IL-10-deficient mice. IL-10-deficient mice raised under germfree conditions do not develop colitis. However, colitis does result when these mice are populated with specific bacterial strains found in the normal intestinal flora, indicating that the resident bacterial flora is necessary for the induction of colitis [198]. Moreover, the appearance and number of mucosal adherent colonic bacteria is altered in IL-10-deficient mice prior to the onset of colitis, and antibiotic therapy is able to attenuate intestinal inflammation [199]. These invasive bacteria may gain access to the intestinal mucosa through increased intestinal permeability, which can be detected in IL-10-deficient mice by 2 weeks of age [200]. Although it still remains unclear which strains harbor pathogenic potential, studies have implicated novel *Helicobacter* species as well as *Bacteroides vulgatus* [198, 201, 202]. Conversely, some enteric bacteria may protect against colitis, including *Lactobacillus* species. IL-10-deficient neonates have reduced levels of colonic *Lactobacillus* species and elevated levels of mucosal adherent and translocated bacteria. When levels are normalized through rectal delivery of bacteria under specific-pathogen free conditions, colitis is prevented [203]. Taken together, these observations support the role of the bacterial flora in initiating colitis in IL-10-deficient mice.

In humans, IL-10 is constitutively produced within the intestinal mucosa. Elevated levels of IL-10 mRNA and protein are seen in areas of active inflammation in the intestinal mucosa of IBD patients compared to non-inflamed areas as well as mucosa from healthy patients [78, 81, 111]. IL-10 mRNA and protein concentrations in IEC are similar among CD, UC, and healthy mucosa; however, IBD samples have an increased number of IL-10-producing mononuclear cells (mainly macrophages) in the submucosa of inflamed tissue [204]. IL-10 production in the lamina propria of samples from patients with active IBD is relatively low compared to that seen in the submucosa, suggesting that IBD patients may not be deficient in IL-10, but rather may have differential local IL-10 distribution within the mucosa. Since IL-10 appears to be an important mediator involved in IBD pathogenesis, studies have begun to focus on its therapeutic potential in humans.

Human recombinant (hr) IL-10 has been tested in clinical trials as a new therapy for patients with CD. Animal studies have demonstrated that a high dose of rIL-10 can ameliorate macroscopic formalin-induced colitis in rabbits and DSS-induced colitis in mice [205, 206]. Preliminary clinical trials in humans have shown hrIL-10 to be safe and potentially efficacious. Daily subcutaneous hrIL-10 injections can induce remission in up to 50% of steroid refractory CD patients after 3 weeks of treatment, compared to 23% of patients receiving placebo [207]. However, larger clinical trials to directly evaluate the efficacy of subcutaneous IL-10 administration in patients with CD have shown a marginal beneficial effect [208, 209]. The lack of efficacy of IL-10 has also been demonstrated in a subsequent large, double blind, placebo-controlled study yet to be published [210].

IL-4

IL-4 is a CD4$^+$ T cell-derived Th2-polarizing cytokine that exhibits many regulatory functions within the intestinal mucosa. It elicits these effects primarily through activation of STAT-6 and STAT-1, and works synergistically with both IL-10 and IL-13 [211]. IL-4 and IL-13 mediate *in vitro* production of chemokines (i.e. IL-8, RANTES, and MCP-1) by IEC lines, and inhibit inducible nitric oxide synthase expression in inflamed areas of the intestinal mucosa in response to elevated levels of proinflammatory cytokines [188, 212–215]. Both IL-4 and IL-13 are capable of synergizing with IL-10 to block the release of lysosomal enzymes from PBMC and LPMC, thereby inhibiting mucosal cytotoxic activity [216]. These three cytokines also work together to inhibit release of proinflammatory cytokines from intestinal monocytes [187, 217]. However, monocytes isolated from IBD patients appear to be less responsive to IL-13 inhibition than monocytes derived from patients without IBD [216, 217]. IL-4 and IL-13 also appear to play a role in mediating intestinal epithelial barrier function [218]. In mast cells, IL-4 works synergistically with stem cell factor to enhance histamine, leukotriene C4, as well as IL-5 secretion.[219]

As discussed above (see IFN-γ), IL-4 levels have been used extensively in conjunction with IFN-γ levels to characterize animal models of intestinal inflammation as either mediated by Th1 or Th2 immune responses. Animal models have also been useful in evaluating the therapeutic potential of IL-4. Two injections of retrovirally encoded IL-4 cause an overexpression of IL-4 in TNBS-treated rats and significantly attenuate tissue damage, as well as circulating and local levels of IFN-γ, inducible calcium-independent nitric oxide synthase gene expression, nitric oxide synthesis, and myeloperoxidase activity in the distal colon [220].

In humans, different IL-4 secretion patterns are associated with UC and CD. Overall, isolated LPMC from intestinal biopsies of patients with IBD produce reduced levels of IL-4 mRNA and protein compared to normal LPMC [82, 221, 222]. Likewise, reduced numbers of IL-4-secreting cells are found in diverted versus non-diverted areas of intestine from IBD

patients who have undergone surgery [223]. In addition, peripheral monocytes and intestinal macrophages from IBD patients appear to be less responsive to the inhibitory effects of IL-4 [224]. These differences, however, are seen when IL-4 levels are analyzed separately in patients with CD and UC. In UC, IL-4 levels in the intestinal mucosa are similar to those found in normal mucosa; in intestinal biopsies from patients with CD, IL-4 levels are low to undetectable [112, 225]. These effects, however, may be dependent on early versus late phases of disease. In fact, increased levels of IL-4 can be detected in early CD lesions along with decreased levels of IFN-γ, while chronic lesions display a Th1 cytokine profile, suggesting that Th2 responses are associated with acute inflammation in CD, whereas Th1 responses are more predominant in chronic inflammation [114].

IL-5 and IL-13

Comparatively less is known regarding the role of the Th2 cytokines, IL-5 and IL-13, in IBD. IL-4 and IL-13 share many similarities in structure and function [226]. Genes encoding both cytokines are located in close proximity to each other on chromosome 5 and contain identical major transcriptional regulatory elements. They also share certain receptors and receptor subchains, as well as exhibiting similar signal transduction pathways. As a result of these similarities, IL-4 and IL-13 appear to have overlapping functions and work in synergy as described above (see IL-4).

IL-5 has mainly been implicated in chronic parasitic and allergic diseases. However, increased levels of IL-5 have been detected in colonic patch T cells in hapten-induced colitis [105]. Elevated IL-5 production is also seen in stimulated T cells isolated from intestinal lesion in mice with oxazolone-induced colitis [34]. Finally, purified lamina propria CD4$^+$ T cells from the inflamed intestinal mucosa of patients with UC produce increased concentrations of IL-5 after stimulation when compared to normal controls [82]. The possible role of IL-5 and IL-13 pharmacological modulation in the treatment with IBD has not yet been explored and may be a potential target for the treatment of this disease.

Other anti-inflammatory cytokines

IL-1ra

Several inhibitory activities of IL-1 have been described for many years and have been identified to originate from a variety of sources, such as urine and serum from febrile patients, as well as supernatants from a variety of cell types [227]. The IL-1 inhibitor isolated from human urine was partially purified as a 23 kDa protein and the mechanism of its action was shown to be at the level of blocking the binding of IL-1 to T cells and fibroblasts, with a subsequent reduction in biological responses to IL-1 [227, 228]. In 1990 the cDNA for an IL-1 inhibitor produced by human PBMC and a human monocytic cell line was cloned and expressed, and termed the IL-1 receptor antagonist (IL-1ra) [229, 230]. These functional inhibitors are components of a homeostatic mechanism that has the ability to regulate IL-1 activity physiologically, thereby controlling inflammation. Since IBD is characterized by an inflammatory response that is not appropriately down-regulated, an imbalance between the production of IL-1 and its natural antagonist, IL-1ra, has been proposed as an important mechanism in perpetuating immune responses in IBD. Casini-Raggi et al. initially investigated the balance of IL-1 and IL-1ra in freshly isolated intestinal mucosal cells from patients with UC, CD, and surgical controls [231]. IL-1 levels were markedly increased in freshly isolated mucosal cells from CD and UC patients compared to controls. In contrast, IL-1ra levels were slightly elevated in CD, and significantly increased in UC, compared to controls. The ratio of IL-1ra to IL-1, however, was significantly decreased in intestinal mucosal cells from IBD patients compared to controls. These data suggest that an insufficient amount of intestinal IL-1ra may be produced during inflammation in IBD patients. The specificity of these findings for IBD was investigated comparing the IL-1/IL-1ra ratio in intestinal mucosal biopsies obtained from IBD patients with the ratio in biopsies obtained from patients with self-limited acute colitis (inflammatory controls). The results of these studies showed that an imbalance of IL-1ra to IL-1 is present in inflamed tissues from IBD patients, whereas inflammatory controls have an intestinal IL-1 to IL-1ra ratio comparable with that present in intestinal tissues from normal surgical controls [231]. These data are in agreement with results from studies performed by other groups showing decreased intestinal IL-1ra mRNA transcripts or protein levels in IBD patients

compared to inflammatory controls [232, 233]. The discovery of IL-1ra genetic polymorphisms and the association of allele 2 of the IL-1ra gene with the incidence of UC have suggested the interesting hypothesis that IL-1ra production may be genetically regulated [234]. Thus, a deficit of IL-1ra mucosal production may exist in patients carrying a specific IL-1ra polymorphism. Tountas et al. have recently demonstrated the association between allele 2 and UC in Hispanic and Jewish populations from the Los Angeles area, and that individuals carrying allele 2 have the ability to produce decreased amounts of IL-1ra protein from stimulated PBMC obtained from these individuals [235]. However, this association has not been detected in Caucasian northern European patients, although trends toward an association have been observed [236, 237]. In a recent study, Carter et al. reassessed the presence of a significant association in a large independent set of well-characterized Caucasian patients and performed a meta-analysis of reported patients series. Using this methodology the association between IL-1ra allele 2 and UC was confirmed and shown to be weak, conferring only a small risk in this patient population [238].

Taken together, these findings strongly support the hypothesis that the imbalance of IL-1ra to IL-1 may be important in the pathophysiology of IBD. Therefore, providing exogenous IL-1ra or increasing the synthesis of endogenous IL-1ra has been proposed as a potential treatment for patients with IBD. Unfortunately, no reliable clinical trials have been performed using administration of recombinant of IL-1ra to patients with either CD or UC. Therefore, the precise pathogenic role of either IL-1 or IL-1ra in IBD remains poorly understood.

IL-11

IL-11 is a stromal cell-derived growth factor with many functions, both extra-intestinally and within the gut. IL-11 is a hematopoietic agent that can stimulate peripheral platelet counts, and is approved as a treatment for chemotherapy-induced thrombocytopenia. IL-11 is also involved in the induction of acute phase reactants from the liver, and appears to have a trophic effect for the damaged intestinal epithelium [239]. IL-11 plays an important role in gut tissue repair, especially with regard to small intestinal villi. It appears to regulate normal growth control and proliferation of intestinal epithelial crypt cells, as well as partial suppression of apoptosis and extension of villous length [240]. These effects promote epithelial restitution in irradiated mice treated with rhIL-11, and may be mediated by TGF-β via the transcription factor activating protein-1 [241, 242]. IL-11 also exhibits anti-inflammatory properties by blocking production of IL-1, IL-6, IL-12, TNF, and nitric oxide by macrophages through inhibition of NF-κB, as well as by down-regulating Th1 cytokine production by CD4⁺ T cells, while inducing Th2 cytokine production [243, 244].

Notably, these anti-inflammatory properties of rhIL-11 also induce improvement of macroscopic and microscopic intestinal tissue damage in several animal models of IBD, including the acetic acid model of acute colitis, the TNBS model of colitis, and HLAB27 rats [245–247]. The same effect is seen in rats that have undergone massive intestinal resections. These animals have increased intestinal absorption and mucosal mass after treatment with rhIL-11, indicating that rhIL-11 may be a potential therapy for patients with short-bowel syndrome [248–250]. Taken together, IL-11 appears to have strong therapeutic potential for human IBD. Clinical trials are currently under way to investigate the safety and efficacy of subcutaneous rhIL-11 injections in patients with CD. In initial human trials, short-term treatment with rhIL-11 was well tolerated and efficacious, with 42% of CD patients experiencing a clinical response after five weekly injections of rhIL-11, compared to 7% of patients treated with placebo [251].

TGF-β

TGF-β is a pleiotropic growth factor with immunoregulatory properties important to intestinal inflammation. TGF-β enhances epithelial restitution in IEC lines, and inhibits growth and proliferation in both IEC lines and primary cultures by down-regulating cellular division [252–255]. TGF-β has also been shown to enhance IL-1 and TNF-induced IL-6 secretion from IEC *in vitro*, and is able to maintain colonic epithelial barrier function in the presence of T cell-derived cytokines that promote intestinal permeability (IFN-γ, IL-4, and IL-10) [256, 257]. Certain strains of bacteria that are part of the normal intestinal flora stimulate TGF-β-induced collagen deposition, possibly supporting a role for TGF-β in the formation of intestinal strictures [258]. TGF-β may also be involved in regulating IgA production since TGF-β-deficient mice lack IgA-committed B cells in the intestine [259].

In the intestine, TGF-β is derived primarily from regulatory T cells and IEC. Animal models have localized TGF-β to the surface epithelium of the murine small intestine, with expression predominantly in the villous tips, but not in the crypts [260]. Unstimulated human intestinal endothelial cells also express TGF-β in culture [6]. In addition, TGF-β receptors have been detected on the apical and basal colonic crypt surfaces [256]. The kinetics of TGF-β production appear to be different in the IEC versus lamina propria T cells. TGF-β mRNA is constitutively expressed by colonic and small intestinal epithelium of IL-2-deficient mice, and increased concentrations can be detected in areas of active inflammation. Unlike in lamina propria T cells, elevated levels of TGF-β in the epithelium can be detected before the development of clinical symptoms, suggesting that TGF-β may indeed play a role in the early phases of disease pathogenesis [73].

As discussed earlier, TGF-β may share a reciprocal relationship with IL-12 and IFN-γ (see sections on IL-12 and IFN-γ) [96]. Lamina propria T lymphocytes from TNP-KLH-immunized IL-2-deficient mice do not produce TGF-β during early stages of colitis, compared to an 8-fold increase in TGF-β protein production in wild-type mice. Induction of TGF-β in these mice inhibits IFN-γ production by lamina propria T cell and the development of colitis. Likewise, blocking TGF-β with neutralizing antibodies restores IFN-γ production and the resulting colitis, supporting a reciprocal relationship between these two cytokines [74].

Studies involving TGF-β have complicated the accepted Th1/Th2 paradigm in animal models of intestinal inflammation. As seen with IL-10-deficient mice, antibodies targeting TGF-β can reverse the protective effects of CD45Rb^lo T cells in the CD45Rb^hi/SCID adoptive transfer model of colitis, suggesting that both IL-10 and TGF-β are essential in the regulation of pathogenic T cells [193, 194]. Since this effect is independent of IL-4, these results suggest a more complicated relationship than the proposed Th1/Th2 paradigm, perhaps involving Tr1 T cell subsets. TGF-β has also shown therapeutic potential in other animal models of colitis. In gene therapy studies 50% of rats administered TNBS and injected with an expression vector encoding the TGF-β gene developed minimal or no ulceration compared to controls, 83% of which had scores indicating maximal tissue damage [261]. As mentioned earlier, oral feeding of haptenized colonic proteins can suppress sensitivity to TNBS. This effect is associated with a marked increase in TGF-β production, and is abolished upon treatment with neutralizing antibodies against TGF-β [35]. Therefore, TGF-β is an important regulator of immune responses in animal models of colitis.

TGF-β has been directly implicated in human IBD. In the inflamed mucosa of IBD patients, increased levels of TGF-β and increased numbers of TGF-β-producing T cells, neutrophils, monocytes, and macrophages can be found in close proximity to luminal surfaces in the lamina propria, but expression is unchanged in the epithelium [262, 263]. IBD patients also have abnormal expression patterns of TGF-β receptors type I and II. Receptors are found on IEC and on fibroblasts during early stages of fibrosis [264]. Increases in both TGF-β type I and II receptors can be seen in surgically resected intestinal specimens from CD patients, as well as striking increases in TGF-β; both TGF-β and its signaling receptor appear to be co-expressed in the intestinal mucosa of patients with CD [265]. In contrast, mucosal samples from patients with UC have lower levels of TGF-β compared to normal mucosa, possibly reflecting differential mechanisms of disease pathogenesis for CD versus UC [266].

Chemokines

Chemokines are chemotactic cytokines that play an important role in mucosal inflammation. These low molecular weight proteins consist of two subfamilies primarily based on their structure. The CXC chemokines, or α subfamily, have a single amino acid located between the first two of four cysteine residues; this amino acid is absent in the CC chemokines, or β subfamily. Chemokines, along with their abundant receptors, are expressed by a variety of cells types, including epithelial cells, macrophages, T and B lymphocytes, endothelial cells, and neutrophils. Many of their effects are overlapping. In fact, one chemokine receptor can bind up to eight chemokines, while a single chemokine can bind up to four receptors. Chemokines have a variety of functions in the mucosal immune system. They activate immune cells and induce enzyme production and granule exocytosis. They also act as chemoattractants for infiltrating granulocytes, monocytes, and lymphocytes. Chemokines regulate leukocyte cell trafficking to the gut, adherence to the endothelial lining of blood vessels, and migration into the intestinal mucosa. They are secreted upon stimulation into the lamina propria and mucosa where they establish a chemotactic gradient, which attracts infiltrating leukocytes to sites of inflammation. This process normally leads to enhanced leukocyte extravasation and an increase in the number of infiltrating immune cells into the gut mucosa; however, similar to cytokine production during disease pathogenesis, dysregulated chemokine production may result in acute and chronic inflammation as well as tissue damage. Therefore, dysregulation of chemokines may play an important role in the pathogenesis of IBD (Fig. 2).

CXC chemokines (α subfamily)

IL-8

IL-8, the prototypic CXC chemokine, is a potent neutrophil chemoattractant and activator of polymorphonuclear cells. *In vitro*, IL-8 is secreted in a polarized fashion from the apical surface of IEC lines in response to stimulation by bacteria and their products, as well as TNF, and IL-1β [267–269]. *In vivo* studies have demonstrated that IL-8 is expressed primarily by macrophages, epithelial cells, and neutrophils in areas of active inflammation within the intestinal mucosa of IBD patients [270]. IL-8 mRNA is consistently detected in macrophages and neutrophils in the inflamed lamina propria [271–273]. Transcripts have also been detected in IEC located at the base of intestinal ulcers, in crypt abscesses, and along the border of fistulas and mucosal surfaces [270]. A differential distribution of IL-8 mRNA within the intestinal mucosa of patients with UC and CD reflects characteristic histological differences between these two diseases. In UC, IL-8 mRNA is diffusely distributed throughout the entire affected mucosa, while IL-8 mRNA transcripts have a more focal distribution in inflamed tissue from CD patients [270].

Levels of IL-8 mRNA and protein concentrations are increased in inflamed tissue from IBD patients. Significantly high levels of mRNA are found in involved areas of both CD and UC intestinal mucosa compared to uninvolved areas [274]. Increased IL-8 protein concentrations are found in homogenates of colonic biopsies from patients with active CD and UC, but not in samples from inactive CD and UC, tissue from other inflammatory intestinal diseases, or normal mucosa. This increase correlates extremely well with the macroscopic grade of inflammation, the number of invading neutrophils in the mucosa, as well as tissue levels of TNF and IL-1β, all of which are associated with IL-8 activity [275].

Furthermore, the number of IL-8-producing cells in the colonic and small intestinal mucosa of patients with IBD also correlates well with the histological grade of disease severity [270]. Colorectal perfusates from patients with active ulcerative proctosigmoiditis also contain enhanced concentrations of IL-8, which correlate well with several measures of inflammation [276]. These data strongly support an association between enhanced IL-8 production and disease pathogenesis in IBD.

Although IL-8 is implicated in both UC and CD, the evidence suggests a somewhat stronger association with UC pathogenesis. It has been reported that enhanced production of IL-8 in the inflamed mucosa of patients with IBD is significantly greater in patients with UC compared to CD [277–279]. Similarly, organ cultures of mucosal biopsies from IBD patients secrete higher levels of IL-8 compared to normal biopsies, but the effect is more pronounced in patients with UC [280]. In this system, increased IL-8 secretion results in enhanced chemotactic activity and an increase in neutrophil binding capacity, both of which are inhibited by pretreatment with anti-IL-8 antibodies, thereby confirming the functional role of IL-8 [280]. Taken together, these findings suggest that IL-8 may be a non-specific mediator of inflammation with a distinct role in IBD, particularly in UC.

ENA-78

Epithelial cell-derived neutrophil-activating peptide-78 (ENA-78) is also a potent neutrophil chemoattractant and immune cell activator that shares 22% sequence homology with IL-8. Like IL-8, ENA-78 is a CXC chemokine produced by IEC lines and monocytes in response to stimulations with bacteria, bacterial products (such as LPS), IL-1β and TNF [94, 281–284]. ENA-78 and IL-8 secretion by human monocytes is drastically reduced by IFNα and IFN-γ, both of which can also inhibit the function of ENA-78 and IL-8 in neutrophil activation, suggesting that IFNα and IFN-γ may regulate neutrophil chemotaxis [94].

Although these two chemokines share many common properties, differences in their kinetic profiles suggest they are differentially regulated. After stimulation with IL-1β and TNF, IEC lines produce IL-8 as early as 4 h before ENA-78, with peak levels observed by 12 h before maximal levels of ENA-78 [284]. Similar results are seen in freshly isolated colonic epithelial cells from patients with CD and UC, with rapid and transient bursts of IL-8 secretion, but delayed and steady production of ENA-78

[4]. A similar pattern is seen in monocytes following LPS stimulation, wherein ENA-78 displays a biphasic kinetics profile after stimulation with IL-1β and TNF, with an initial peak between 8 and 12 h post-stimulation and a second peak between 20 and 28 h [283]. This biphasic pattern may suggest differential regulation in acute and chronic inflammation. Of note, ENA-78 expression in monocytes or epithelial cells does not begin until after IL-8 expression has ceased, further supporting differential regulation for these two neutrophil chemoattractants. Also, ENA-78 and IL-8 bind to chemokine receptors with different affinities. Both efficiently bind to CXCR2 but, unlike IL-8, higher concentrations of ENA-78 are needed for binding to CXCR1 [285]. Thus, receptor binding affinities may represent another layer of differential regulation.

ENA-78 production is enhanced in IBD. ENA-78 mRNA levels are 24-fold higher in tissues from UC compared to normal mucosa, and protein levels are 4-fold higher [284]. Immunoreactivity is primarily associated with the crypt epithelium. Similar levels of ENA-78 mRNA are expressed by IEC from patients with either CD and UC, and over 90% of epithelial cells from IBD patients stain positive for ENA-78 protein [286]. Little or no ENA-78 mRNA is detected in normal mucosa, and protein is produced by less than 30% of IEC from patients not afflicted with IBD [284, 286].

Other CXC chemokines

Although IL-8 and ENA-78 are the primary CXC chemokines that have been implicated in IBD pathogenesis, other CXC chemokines have also been associated with IBD. Interferon-inducible protein 10 (IP-10) is a potent chemoattractant for NK cells *in vitro*, and mediates NK cell cytolytic responses by inducing degranulation [287]. Unlike other CXC chemokines, IP-10 can bind to receptors that are highly expressed on IL-2-activated T lymphocytes, but is incapable of inducing transendothelial migration among T cell subsets [288–290]. In addition, IP-10 is markedly expressed in normal intestinal mucosa, and the number of IP-10-expressing cells in colonic biopsies from patients with UC is significantly elevated compared to normal tissue [291].

Fractalkine is a CX3C chemokine that also acts as an adhesion molecule on the surface of activated endothelial cells. Fractalkine induces adhesion between circulating monocytes and the intestinal endothelium through interactions with integrins and their ligands [291, 292]. IEC and endothelial cells have been shown to produce fractalkine in the normal mucosa, with fractalkine protein levels up-regulated in inflamed areas of mucosa obtained from patients with active CD [293]. However, more recent studies have suggested the possibility that fractalkine is specifically expressed by IEC [294]. Subpopulations of IEL express CX3CR1, a receptor for fractalkine, and migrate in response to a fractalkine chemotactic gradient following activation with IL-2, suggesting that fractalkine may also function as a lymphocyte chemoattractant [293].

Overall, the role of CXC chemokines in the pathogenesis of IBD and the potential role of their pharmacological modulation remains to be tested in patients with both CD and UC.

CC chemokines (β subfamily)

MCP-1

Monocyte chemoattractant peptide (MCP)-1 is a CC chemokine and an important inducer of monocyte chemotaxis and transendothelial migration. Similar to other chemokines, MCP-1 elicits migration by establishing a chemotactic gradient across the vascular endothelium, which is inhibited by neutralizing antibodies against MCP-1, as well as by disruption of the chemotactic gradient [295]. In addition to inducing monocytes chemotaxis, MCP-1 is also capable of promoting transmigration of specific T cell subsets, including TCRαβ$^+$ and γδ$^+$ T lymphocytes [290]. Other CC chemokines, such as RANTES, IL-16, and MIP-1α, are also capable of inducing chemotaxis of these T cell populations; however, the CXC chemokines IL-8 and IP-10 are not. More recently, MCP-1 has been implicated as a mediator of Th2 polarization. MCP-1-deficient mice are incapable of mounting Th2 responses [296]. These mice produce low levels of IL-4, IL-5 and IL-10 in their lymph nodes, but have normal levels of IFN-γ and IL-12. MCP-1-deficient mice also have normal trafficking of naïve T cells, suggesting that defective polarization is a direct effect of MCP-1, rather than due to abnormal cell migration. MCP-1-deficient mice lack the ability to recruit monocytes [297]. Therefore, MCP-1 functions both as a monocyte chemoattractant in response to cytokine stimulation and as a mediator of T cell polarization.

MCP-1 gene expression and protein production are mediated by cytokines. IEC lines do not constitutively secrete MCP-1, which is released in response to stimulation with IL-1β or TNF [93]. IFN-γ and IL-4 potentiate IL-1β-induced MCP-1 mRNA expression and protein production by IEC lines, but with different kinetics [298]. IL-15 down-regulates production of MCP-1 in both IEC lines and freshly isolated human colonic epithelial cells; this effect is inhibited almost entirely by antibodies against specific IL-2 receptors, which also bind IL-15 [177]. In monocytes, IL-15 stimulation results in monocyte chemotaxis, which is blocked by neutralizing antibodies against MCP-1 [178]. MCP-1 secretion can be detected in culture after IL-15 stimulation, and secretion is enhanced by co-stimulation with IFN-γ and IL-15. Unlike in epithelial cells, this effect is inhibited by IL-4. Cytokines can also regulate expression of chemokine receptors on cell surfaces. The MCP-1 receptor, CCR2, is expressed on the cell surface of monocyte cell lines, and its expression is down-regulated by incubation with either TNF or IL-1β [299]. Since these two proinflammatory cytokines also stimulate MCP-1 expression and secretion from epithelial cells, chemokine receptors may function as an additional level of chemokine regulation for maintaining tissue homeostasis.

Increased levels of MCP-1 have been associated with IBD. In the normal intestinal mucosa, MCP-1 mRNA is present in surface epithelial cells. However, in IBD, many cell types have MCP-1 immunoreactivity, including spindle cells, mononuclear cells, and endothelial cells. In addition, MCP-1 mRNA levels are elevated in IBD mucosa compared to normal tissue [300]. The number of MCP-1-expressing cells is also increased in the intestinal endothelium and lamina propria of tissues from IBD patients, but not in the intestinal epithelium [291, 300]. Moreover, isolated IEC from IBD patients are capable of inducing monocyte chemotaxis, which is inhibited by anti-MCP-1 antibodies. Facilitating its role as a potent mediator of chemotaxis, MCP-1 is produced by several cell types that surround the intestinal vasculature in IBD patients, including newly recruited infiltrating macrophages, medial smooth muscle cells, intraluminal cells, as well as endothelial cells [301, 302]. Based on these studies it is evident that MCP-1 represents a logical target for anti-inflammatory therapy and immunomodulation in patients with IBD.

IL-16

IL-16 is a 56-kDa C-C chemokine originally identified as lymphocyte chemoattractant factor. The protein consists of four non-covalently linked monomers, which are initially synthesized as inactive precursor proteins (pro-IL-16) and cleaved by caspase-3 to form mature, biologically active IL-16 monomers [303–305]. IL-16 is primarily produced by $CD8^+$ T lymphocytes, as well as eosinophils, mast cells, and pulmonary epithelial cells [306–308]. With regard to function, IL-16 is a unique proinflammatory chemoattractant that appears to play an important role in T cell recruitment, growth, and proliferation. It binds to CD4 and subsequently induces migration in $CD4^+$ immune cells, including T cells, macrophages, and eosinophils [309–311]. In addition to its chemoattrant properties, IL-16 can also induce expression of IL-2 receptors and MHC class II molecules in target cells, thereby promoting T cell growth and proliferation [310, 312].

IL-16 has recently been associated with intestinal inflammation in patients with CD. In a recent study by Keates *et al.*, colonic IL-16 protein levels were found to be significantly increased in patients with CD, but not in UC [313]. Furthermore, the study demonstrated that monoclonal antibody blockade of IL-16 in mice attenuates hapten-induced colitis, resulting in decreased levels of mucosal ulceration, weight loss, and myeloperoxidase activity, as well as reduced mucosal levels of IL-1β and TNF. A second recent study has reported elevated levels of IL-16 in the colonic mucosa of IBD patients (CD and UC) compared to normal controls, but suggests that increased IL-16 production may be limited to areas of active inflammation in patients with UC [314].

Other CC chemokines

There is some evidence that other CC chemokines may have a role in IBD pathogenesis. These CC chemokines induce monocyte, lymphocyte, NK cell, and possibly dendritic cell migration, and include RANTES (regulated on activation, normal T cell expressed and secreted), MCP-2, MCP-3, macrophage inflammatory protein (MIP)-1α, and MIP-1β [287, 289, 290, 315–317]. Elevated levels of RANTES expression are seen in IEL and in the subepithelial lamina propria of intestinal mucosal samples obtained from IBD patients compared to normal controls [301]. Freshly isolated IEC from patients with UC and CD also secrete RANTES, MIP-1α, and MIP-1β [4]. Finally, colonic biopsies from IBD patients contain an increased number of cells that express MCP-3 compared to normal tissues. Taken together, these findings suggest a possible role for CC

chemokines in acute as well as chronic inflammation associated with IBD.

New interleukins: 'cytokines 2002'

To date there are currently 23 interleukins officially reported and classified. This section will describe the initial characterization of IL-20, IL-21, IL-22, and IL-23, all of which have been recently discovered.

IL-20

IL-20 was identified as a novel IL-10 homologue using a structural, profile-based algorithm [318]. Overexpression of IL-20 in transgenic mice caused neonatal lethality with skin abnormalities including aberrant epidermal differentiation. As such, a role for IL-20 in epidermal function and psoriasis has been proposed. Because of the important role of other cytokines produced by keratinocytes, such as IL-1, IL-1ra and IL-18, the role of IL-20 in intestinal inflammation and IBD warrants further investigation.

IL-21

IL-21 was originally described as IL-10-related T cell-derived inducible factor (IL-TIF). This is a new cytokine originally identified in mice as a gene induced by IL-9 in both T cells and mast cells [319]. The human homologue of IL-21 was recently cloned and functionally characterized as a hepatocyte-stimulating factor [320]. IL-21 shares the same receptor with IL-10 and is capable of inducing the production of acute-phase reactants both *in vitro* and *in vivo*. In addition, IL-21 expression was found to be rapidly increased after LPS injection. The proinflammatory actions of this novel cytokine suggest that IL-21 may have a potential role in the pathogenesis of intestinal inflammation.

IL-22

IL-22 was recently discovered as a novel human cytokine produced by activated T cells and distantly related to IL-10 [321]. It signals through a specific receptor that is a member of the interferon receptor-related proteins CRF2-4 without binding to the IL-10 receptor. In contrast to IL-10, IL-22 does not suppress the production of proinflammatory cytokines by monocytes or interfere with IL-10 function of monocytes. The precise biological function of IL-22 is poorly understood and its role in diseases, including IBD, remains to be determined.

IL-23

IL-23 was discovered as a novel p19 protein that, when combined with the p40 subunit of IL-12, forms a new biologically active composite cytokine [322]. Activated dendritic T cells secrete detectable levels of this complex. IL-23 has been shown to share several biological activities with IL-12 including the ability to stimulate IFN-γ production and proliferation of PHA blast T cells, as well as CD45RO (memory) T cells. A unique activity of IL-23, distinct from IL-12, is the induction of a potent proliferation of mouse memory (CD4$^+$ CD45Rb^{lo}) T cells. Because of the very important role of IL-12 in Th1 polarization and possibly CD, IL-23 expression has been recently investigated in the intestinal mucosa of patients with CD and was shown to be specifically elevated compared to patients with UC and normal controls (unpublished results).

The rapid progress in the field of cytokine gene discovery will generate new information on a variety of cytokines, whose biological function needs to be carefully investigated both using *in-vitro* and *in-vivo* models, and ultimately in patients with IBD. We anticipate that a variety of novel therapeutic cytokine targets will be developed in order to continue to improve the therapeutic modalities and quality of life in patients affected by IBD. Therefore, the scientific approach of taking information at the bench to the patient's bedside remains the most important approach for the treatment of chronic inflammatory diseases, including CD and UC.

References

1. Bazzoni F, Beutler B. The tumor necrosis factor ligand and receptor families. N Engl J Med 1996; 334: 1717–25.
2. Guy-Grand D, DiSanto JP, Hencholz P, Malassis-Seris M, Vassali P. Small bowel enteropathy: role of intraepithelial lymphocytes and of cytokines (IL-12, IFN-y, TNF) in the induction of epithelial cell death and renewal. Eur J Immunol 1998; 28: 730–44.
3. Abreu-Martin MT, Vidrich A, Lynch DH, Targan SR. Divergent induction of apoptosis and IL-8 secretion in HT-29 cells in response to TNF-α and ligation of Fas antigen. J Immunol 1995; 155: 4147–54.
4. Yang SK, Eckmann L, Panja A, Kagnoff MF. Differential and regulated expression of C-X-C, C-C, and C-chemokines by human colon epithelial cells. Gastroenterology 1997; 113: 1214–23.
5. Feldmann M, Elliott MJ, Woody JN, Maini RN. Anti-tumor necrosis factor-α therapy of rheumatoid arthritis. Adv Immunol 1997; 61: 283–350.
6. Nilsen EM, Johansen FE, Jahnsen FL *et al.* Cytokine profiles of cultured microvascular endothelial cells from the human intestine. Gut 1998; 42: 635–42.
7. Neurath MF, Fuss I, Pasparakis M *et al.* Predominant pathogenic role of tumor necrosis factor in experimental colitis in mice. Eur J Immunol 1997; 27: 1743–50.
8. Kontoyiannis D, Pasparakis M, Pizarro TT, Cominelli F, Kollias G. Impaired on/off regulation of TNF biosynthesis in mice lacking TNF AU-rich elements: implications for joint and gut-associated immunopathologies. Immunity 1999; 10: 387–98.
9. Cominelli F, Kontoyiannis D, Pasparaki M, Pizarro TT, Nast CC, Kollias GA. Contribution of TNF receptor (TNFR) types and T lymphocyte populations to the pathogenesis of experimental Crohn's disease (CD) in TNF deltaARE mutant mice. Gastroenterology 1999; 116: G3005.
10. Kosiewicz MM, Nast CC, Krishnan A *et al.* Th1-type responses mediate spontaneous ileitis in a novel murine model of Crohn's disease. J Clin Invest 2001; 107: 695–702.
11. Braegger CP, Nicholls S, Murch SH, Stephens S, MacDonald TT. Tumour necrosis factor alpha in stool as a marker of intestinal inflammation. Lancet 1992; 339: 89–91.
12. Nicholls S, Stephens S, Braegger CP, Walker-Smith JA, MacDonald TT. Cytokines in stools of children with inflammatory bowel disease or infective diarrhoea. J Clin Pathol 1993; 46: 757–60.
13. Saiki T, Mitsuyama K, Toyonaga A, Ishida H, Tanikawa K. Detection of pro- and anti-inflammatory cytokines in stools of patients with inflammatory bowel disease. Scand J Gastroenterol 1998; 33: 616–22.
14. Dionne S, Hiscott J, D'Agata I, Duhaime A, Seidman EG. Quantitative PCR analysis of TNF-alpha and IL-1 beta mRNA levels in pediatric IBD mucosal biopsies. Dig Dis Sci 1997; 42: 1557–66.
15. Sandborn WJ, Feagan BG, Hanauer SB *et al.* An engineered human antibody to TNF (CDP571) for active Crohn's disease: a randomized double-blind placebo-controlled trial. Gastroenterology 2001; 120: 1330-8.
16. Sandborn WJ, Hanauer SB. Antitumor necrosis factor therapy for inflammatory bowel disease: a review of agents, pharmacology, clinical results, and safety. Inflamm Bowel Dis 1999; 5: 119–33.
17. Kam LY, Targan SR. Cytokine-based therapies in inflammatory bowel disease. Curr Opin Gastroenterol 1999; 15: 302-7.
18. Sandborn WJ, Hanauer SB, Katz S *et al.* A randomized double-blind, placebo-controlled trial of subcutaneous etanercept (p75 soluble tumor necrosis factor: FC fusion protein) in the treatment of moderate to severe Crohn's disease. Gastroenterology 2001; 120: A20.
19. Ehrenpreis ED, Kane SVl, Cohen LB, Hanauer SB. Thalidomide therapy for patients with refractory Crohn's disease: an open-label trial. Gastroenterology 1999; 117: 1271-7.
20. Vasiliauskas EA, Kam LY, Abreu-Martin MT *et al.* An open-label pilot study of low-dose thalidomide in chronically active, steroid-dependent Crohn's disease. Gastroenterology 1999; 117: 1278–87.
21. Sands BE, Podolsky DK, Tremaine WJ *et al.* Chimeric monoclonal anti-tumor necrosis factor antibody (cA2) in the treatment of severe, steroid refractory ulcerative colitis. Gastroenterology 1996; 110: A1008.
22. Gately MK, Renzetti LM, Magram J *et al.* The interleukin-12/interleukin-12-receptor system: role in normal and pathologic immune responses. Annu Rev Immunol 1998; 16: 495–521.
23. Hessle C, Hanson LA, Wold AE. Lactobacilli from human gastrointestinal mucosa are strong stimulators of IL-12 production. Clin Exp Immunol 1999; 116: 276–82.
24. Monteleone G, MacDonald TT, Wathen NC, Pallone F, Pender SL. Enhancing lamina propria Th1 cell responses

with interleukin 12 produces severe tissue injury. Gastroenterology 1999; 117: 1069–77.

25. Stuber E, Strober W, Neurath M. Blocking the CD40L–CD40 interaction *in vivo* specifically prevents the priming of T helper 1 cells through the inhibition of interleukin 12 secretion. J Exp Med 1996; 183: 693–8.

26. Cong Y, Weaver CT, Lazenby A, Elson CO. Colitis induced by enteric bacterial antigen-specific CD4$^+$ T cells requires CD40–CD40 ligand interactions for a sustained increase in mucosal IL-12. J Immunol 2000; 165: 2173–82.

27. Liu Z, Colpaert S, D'Haens GR *et al.* Hyperexpression of CD40 ligand (CD154) in inflammatory bowel disease and its contribution to pathogenic cytokine production. J Immunol 1999; 163: 4049–57.

28. Hans W, Scholmerich J, Gross V, Falk W. Interleukin-12 induced interferon-gamma increases inflammation in acute dextran sulfate sodium induced colitis in mice. Eur Cytokine Netw. 2000; 11: 67–74.

29. Nakamura S, Otani T, Ijiri Y, Motoda R, Kurimoto M, Orita K. IFN-gamma-dependent and -independent mechanisms in adverse effects caused by concomitant administration of IL-18 and IL-12. J Immunol 2000; 164: 3330–6.

30. Neurath MF, Fuss I, Kelsall BL, Stuber E, Strober W. Antibodies to interleukin 12 abrogate established experimental colitis in mice. J Exp Med 1995; 182: 1281–90.

31. Fuss IJ, Marth T, Neurath MF, Pearlstein GR, Jain A, Strober W. Anti-interleukin 12 treatment regulates apoptosis of Th1 T cells in experimental colitis in mice. Gastroenterology 1999; 117: 1078–88.

32. Davidson NJ, Hudak SA, Lesley RE, Menon S, Leach MW, Rennick DM. IL-12, but not IFN-gamma, plays a major role in sustaining the chronic phase of colitis in IL-10-deficient mice. J Immunol 1998; 161: 3143–9.

33. Simpson SJ, Shah S, Comiskey M *et al.* T cell-mediated pathology in two models of experimental colitis depends predominantly on the interleukin 12/Signal transducer and activator of transcription (Stat)-4 pathway, but is not conditional on interferon gamma expression by T cells. J Exp Med 1998; 187: 1225–34.

34. Boirivant M, Fuss IJ, Chu A, Strober W. Oxazolone colitis: a murine model of T helper cell type 2 colitis treatable with antibodies to interleukin 4. J Exp Med 1998; 188: 1929–39.

35. Neurath MF, Fuss I, Kelsall BL, Presky DH, Waegell W, Strober W. Experimental granulomatous colitis in mice is abrogated by induction of TGF-beta-mediated oral tolerance. J Exp Med 1996; 183: 2605–16.

36. Kitani A, Fuss IJ, Nakamura K, Schwartz OM, Usui T, Strober W. Treatment of experimental (trinitrobenzene sulfonic acid) colitis by intranasal administration of transforming growth factor (TGF)-beta1 plasmid. TGF-beta1-mediated suppression of T helper cell type 1 response occurs by interleukin (IL)-10 induction and IL-12 receptor beta2 chain downregulation. J Exp Med 2000; 192: 41–52.

37. Monteleone G, Biancone L, Marasco R *et al.* Interleukin 12 is expressed and actively released by Crohn's disease intestinal lamina propria mononuclear cells. Gastroenterology 1997; 112: 1169–78.

38. Braun MC, Lahey E, Kelsall BL. Selective suppression of IL-12 production by chemoattractants. J Immunol 2000; 164: 3009–17.

39. Monteleone G, Parrello T, Monteleone I, Tammaro S, Luzza F, Pallone F. Interferon-gamma (IFN-gamma) and prostaglandin E2 (PGE2) regulate differently IL-12 production in human intestinal lamina propria mononuclear cells (LPMC). Clin Exp Immunol 1999; 117: 469–75.

40. Okamura H, Nagata K, Komatsu T *et al.* A novel costimulatory factor for gamma interferon induction found in the livers of mice causes endotoxic shock. Infect Immun 1995; 63: 3966–72.

41. Okamura H, Tsutsi H, Komatsu T *et al.* Cloning of a new cytokine that induces IFN-gamma production by T cells. Nature 1995; 378: 88–91.

42. Kohno K, Kataoka J, Ohtsuki T *et al.* IFN-gamma-inducing factor (IGIF) is a costimulatory factor on the activation of Th1 but not Th2 cells and exerts its effect independently of IL-12. J Immunol 1997; 158: 1541–50.

43. Ushio S, Namba M, Okura T *et al.* Cloning of the cDNA for human IFN-gamma-inducing factor, expression in *Escherichia coli*, and studies on the biologic activities of the protein. J Immunol 1996; 156: 4274–9.

44. Bazan JF, Timans JC, Kastelein RA. A newly defined interleukin-1?. Nature 1996; 379: 591.

45. Udagawa N, Horwood NJ, Elliott J *et al.* Interleukin-18 (interferon-gamma-inducing factor) is produced by osteoblasts and acts via granulocyte/macrophage colony-stimulating factor and not via interferon-gamma to inhibit osteoclast formation. J Exp Med 1997; 185: 1005–12.

46. Gu Y, Kuida K, Tsutsui H *et al.* Activation of interferon-gamma inducing factor mediated by interleukin-1beta converting enzyme. Science 1997; 275: 206-9.

47. Torigoe K, Ushio S, Okura T *et al.* Purification and characterization of the human interleukin-18 receptor. J Biol Chem 1997; 272: 25737–42.

48. Dinarello CA, Novick D, Puren AJ *et al.* Overview of interleukin-18: more than an interferon-gamma inducing factor. J Leuk Biol 1998; 63: 658–64.

49. Puren AJ, Fantuzzi G, Gu Y, Su MS, Dinarello CA. Interleukin-18 (IFNgamma-inducing factor) induces IL-8 and IL-1beta via TNFalpha production from non-CD14$^+$ human blood mononuclear cells. J Clin Invest 1998; 101: 711–21.

50. Matsumoto S, Tsuji-Takayama K, Aizawa Y *et al.* Interleukin-18 activates NF-kappaB in murine T helper type 1 cells. Biochem Biophys Res Commun 1997; 234: 454–7.

51. Dao T, Ohashi K, Kayano T, Kurimoto M, Okamura H. Interferon-gamma-inducing factor, a novel cytokine, enhances Fas ligand-mediated cytotoxicity of murine T helper 1 cells. Cell Immunol 1996; 173: 230–5.

52. Pizarro TT, Michie MH, Bentz M *et al.* IL-18, a novel immunoregulatory cytokine, is up-regulated in Crohn's disease: expression and localization in intestinal mucosal cells. J Immunol 1999; 162: 6829–35.

53. Matsui K, Yoshimoto T, Tsutsui H *et al. Propionibacterium acnes* treatment diminishes CD4$^+$ NK1.1+ T cells but induces type I T cells in the liver by induction of IL-12 and IL-18 production from Kupffer cells. J Immunol 1997; 159: 97–106.

54. Stoll S, Muller G, Kurimoto M *et al.* Production of IL-18 (IFN-gamma-inducing factor) messenger RNA and functional protein by murine keratinocytes. J Immunol 1997; 159: 298–302.

55. Micallef MJ, Ohtsuki T, Kohno K *et al.* Interferon-gamma-inducing factor enhances T helper 1 cytokine production by stimulated human T cells: synergism with interleukin-12 for interferon-gamma production. Eur J Immunol 1996; 26: 1647–51.

56. Monteleone G, Trapasso F, Parrello T *et al.* Bioactive IL-18 expression is up-regulated in Crohn's disease. J Immunol 1999; 163: 143–7.

57. Kanai T, Watanabe M, Okazawa A, Sato T, Hibi T. Interleukin-18 and Crohn's disease. Digestion 2001; 63(Suppl. 1): 37–42.

58. Chikano S, Sawada K, Shimoyama T *et al.* IL-18 and IL-12 induce intestinal inflammation and fatty liver in mice in an IFN-gamma dependent manner. Gut. 2000; 47: 779–86.

59. Fujihashi K, Kawabata S, Hiroi T *et al.* Interleukin 2 (IL-2) and interleukin 7 (IL-7) reciprocally induce IL-7 and IL-2 receptors on gamma delta T-cell receptor-positive intrae-

pithelial lymphocytes. Proc Natl Acad Sci USA 1996; 93: 3613–18.

60. Chu CL, Chen SS, Wu TS, Kuo SC, Liao NS. Differential effects of IL-2 and IL-15 on the death and survival of activated TCR gamma delta+ intestinal intraepithelial lymphocytes. J Immunol 1999; 162: 1896–903.

61. Porter BO, Malek TR. IL-2Rbeta/IL-7Ralpha doubly deficient mice recapitulate the thymic and intraepithelial lymphocyte (IEL) developmental defects of gammac–/– mice: roles for both IL-2 and IL-15 in CD8alphaalpha IEL development. J Immunol 1999; 163: 5906–12.

62. Boirivant M, Pica R, DeMaria R, Testi R, Pallone F, Strober W. Stimulated human lamina propria T cells manifest enhanced Fas-mediated apoptosis. J Clin Invest 1996; 98: 2616–22.

63. Ciacci C, Mahida YR, Dignass A, Koizumi M, Podolsky DK. Functional interleukin-2 receptors on intestinal epithelial cells. J Clin Invest 1993; 92: 527–32.

64. Reinecker HC, Podolsky DK. Human intestinal epithelial cells express functional cytokine receptors sharing the common gamma c chain of the interleukin 2 receptor. Proc Natl Acad Sci USA 1995; 92: 8353–7.

65. Dignass AU, Podolsky DK. Interleukin 2 modulates intestinal epithelial cell function *in vitro*. Exp Cell Res 1996; 225: 422–9.

66. Simpson SJ, Mizoguchi E, Allen D, Bhan AK, Terhorst C. Evidence that CD4+, but not CD8+ T cells are responsible for murine interleukin-2-deficient colitis. Eur J Immunol 1995; 25: 2618–25.

67. Ma A, Datta M, Margosian E, Chen J, Horak I. T cells, but not B cells, are required for bowel inflammation in interleukin 2-deficient mice. J Exp Med 1995; 182: 1567–72.

68. Ludviksson BR, Strober W, Nishikomori R, Hasan SK, Ehrhardt RO. Administration of mAb against alpha E beta 7 prevents and ameliorates immunization-induced colitis in IL-2-/– mice. J Immunol 1999; 162: 4975–82.

69. Ehrhardt RO, Ludviksson BR, Gray B, Neurath M, Strober W. Induction and prevention of colonic inflammation in IL-2-deficient mice. J Immunol 1997; 158: 566–73.

70. Autenrieth IB, Bucheler N, Bohn E, Heinze G, Horak I. Cytokine mRNA expression in intestinal tissue of interleukin-2 deficient mice with bowel inflammation. Gut 1997; 41: 793–800.

71. Yang F, de Villiers WJ, Lee EY, McClain CJ, Varilek GW. Increased nuclear factor-kappaB activation in colitis of interleukin-2-deficient mice. J Lab Clin Med 1999; 134: 378–85.

72. Harren M, Schonfelder G, Paul M et al. High expression of inducible nitric oxide synthase correlates with intestinal inflammation of interleukin-2-deficient mice. Ann NY Acad Sci 1998; 859: 210–15.

73. Meijssen MA, Brandwein SL, Reinecker HC, Bhan AK, Podolsky DK. Alteration of gene expression by intestinal epithelial cells precedes colitis in interleukin-2-deficient mice. Am J Physiol 1998; 274: G472–9.

74. Ludviksson BR, Ehrhardt RO, Strober W. TGF-beta production regulates the development of the 2,4,6-trinitrophenol-conjugated keyhole limpet hemocyanin-induced colonic inflammation in IL-2-deficient mice. J Immunol 1997; 159: 3622–8.

75. Ludviksson BR, Gray B, Strober W, Ehrhardt RO. Dysregulated intrathymic development in the IL-2-deficient mouse leads to colitis-inducing thymocytes. J Immunol 1997; 158: 104–11.

76. Schultz M, Tonkonogy SL, Sellon RK et al. IL-2-deficient mice raised under germfree conditions develop delayed mild focal intestinal inflammation. Am J Physiol 1999; 276: G1461–72.

77. Contractor NV, Bassiri H, Reya T et al. Lymphoid hyperplasia, autoimmunity, and compromised intestinal intraepithelial lymphocyte development in colitis-free gnotobiotic IL-2-deficient mice. J Immunol 1998; 160: 385–94.

78. Murata Y, Ishiguro Y, Itoh J, Munakata A, Yoshida Y. The role of proinflammatory and immunoregulatory cytokines in the pathogenesis of ulcerative colitis. J Gastroenterol 1995; 30(Suppl. 8): 56–60.

79. Mullin GE, Lazenby AJ, Harris ML, Bayless TM, James SP. Increased interleukin-2 messenger RNA in the intestinal mucosal lesions of Crohn's disease but not ulcerative colitis. Gastroenterology 1992; 102: 1620–7.

80. Breese E, Braegger CP, Corrigan CJ, Walker-Smith JA, MacDonald TT. Interleukin-2- and interferon-gamma-secreting T cells in normal and diseased human intestinal mucosa. Immunology 1993; 78: 127–31.

81. Niessner M, Volk BA. Altered Th1/Th2 cytokine profiles in the intestinal mucosa of patients with inflammatory bowel disease as assessed by quantitative reversed transcribed polymerase chain reaction (RT-PCR). Clin Exp Immunol 1995; 101: 428–35.

82. Fuss IJ, Neurath M, Boirivant M et al. Disparate CD4+ lamina propria (LP) lymphokine secretion profiles in inflammatory bowel disease. Crohn's disease LP cells manifest increased secretion of IFN-gamma, whereas ulcerative colitis LP cells manifest increased secretion of IL-5. J Immunol 1996; 157: 1261–70.

83. Gurbindo C, Sabbah S, Menezes J, Justinich C, Marchand R, Seidman EG. Interleukin-2 production in pediatric inflammatory bowel disease: evidence for dissimilar mononuclear cell function in Crohn's disease and ulcerative colitis. J Pediatr Gastroenterol Nutr 1993; 17: 247–54.

84. Shinoda M, Haruta J, Tanimoto M et al. Lamina propria mononuclear cells express and respond to interleukin-2 differently in Crohn's disease and ulcerative colitis. Intern Med 1996; 35: 679–85.

85. Brynskov J, Tvede N. Plasma interleukin-2 and a soluble/shed interleukin-2 receptor in serum of patients with Crohn's disease. Effect of cyclosporin. Gut 1990; 31: 795–9.

86. Breese EJ, Michie CA, Nicholls SW et al. The effect of treatment on lymphokine-secreting cells in the intestinal mucosa of children with Crohn's disease. Aliment Pharmacol Ther 1995; 9: 547–52.

87. van Dijk AP, Meijssen MA, Brouwer AJ et al. Transdermal nicotine inhibits interleukin 2 synthesis by mononuclear cells derived from healthy volunteers. Eur J Clin Invest 1998; 28: 664–71.

88. Elsasser-Beile U, von Kleist S, Gerlach S, Gallati H, Monting JS. Cytokine production in whole blood cell cultures of patients with Crohn's disease and ulcerative colitis. J Clin Lab Anal 1994; 8: 447–51.

89. Stallmach A, Wittig B, Giese T et al. Protection of trinitrobenzene sulfonic acid-induced colitis by an interleukin 2-IgG2b fusion protein in mice. Gastroenterology 1999; 117: 866–76.

90. Adams RB, Planchon SM, Roche JK. IFN-gamma modulation of epithelial barrier function. Time course, reversibility, and site of cytokine binding. J Immunol 1993; 150: 2356–63.

91. Youakim A, Ahdieh M. Interferon-gamma decreases barrier function in T84 cells by reducing ZO-1 levels and disrupting apical actin. Am J Physiol 1999; 276: G1279–88.

92. Colgan SP, Parkos CA, Delp C, Arnaout MA, Madara JL. Neutrophil migration across cultured intestinal epithelial monolayers is modulated by epithelial exposure to IFN-gamma in a highly polarized fashion. J Cell Biol 1993; 120: 785–98.

93. Warhurst AC, Hopkins SJ, Warhurst G. Interferon gamma induces differential upregulation of alpha and beta chemo-

kine secretion in colonic epithelial cell lines. Gut 1998; 42: 208–13.

94. Schnyder-Candrian S, Strieter RM, Kunkel SL, Walz A. Interferon-alpha and interferon-gamma down-regulate the production of interleukin-8 and ENA-78 in human monocytes. J Leuk Biol 1995; 57: 929–35.

95. Kohyama M, Hachimura S, Nanno M, Ishikawa H, Kaminogawa S. Analysis of cytokine producing activity of intestinal intraepithelial T cells from TCR beta-chain and delta-chain mutant mice. Microbiol Immunol 1997; 41: 353–9.

96. Strober W, Kelsall B, Fuss I et al. Reciprocal IFN-gamma and TGF-beta responses regulate the occurrence of mucosal inflammation. Immunol Today 1997; 18: 61–4.

97. Bregenholt S, Claesson MH. Increased intracellular Th1 cytokines in scid mice with inflammatory bowel disease. Eur J Immunol 1998; 28: 379–89.

98. Hornquist CE, Lu X, Rogers-Fani PM et al. G(alpha)i2-deficient mice with colitis exhibit a local increase in memory CD4+ T cells and proinflammatory Th1-type cytokines. J Immunol 1997; 158: 1068–77.

99. McDonald SA, Palmen MJ, Van Rees EP, MacDonald TT. Characterization of the mucosal cell-mediated immune response in IL-2 knockout mice before and after the onset of colitis. Immunology 1997; 91: 73–80.

100. Simpson SJ, Hollander GA, Mizoguchi E et al. Expression of pro-inflammatory cytokines by TCR alpha beta+ and TCR gamma delta+ T cells in an experimental model of colitis. Eur J Immunol 1997; 27: 17–25.

101. Rennick DM, Fort MM, Davidson NJ. Studies with IL-10-/- mice: an overview. J Leuk Biol 1997; 61: 389–96.

102. Iijima H, Takahashi I, Kishi D et al. Alteration of interleukin 4 production results in the inhibition of T helper type 2 cell-dominated inflammatory bowel disease in T cell receptor alpha chain-deficient mice. J Exp Med 1999; 190: 607–15.

103. Mizoguchi A, Mizoguchi E, Bhan AK. The critical role of interleukin 4 but not interferon gamma in the pathogenesis of colitis in T-cell receptor alpha mutant mice. Gastroenterology 1999; 116: 320–6.

104. Dieleman LA, Palmen MJ, Akol H et al. Chronic experimental colitis induced by dextran sulphate sodium (DSS) is characterized by Th1 and Th2 cytokines. Clin Exp Immunol 1998; 114: 385–91.

105. Dohi T, Fujihashi K, Rennert PD, Iwatani K, Kiyono H, McGhee JR. Hapten-induced colitis is associated with colonic patch hypertrophy and T helper cell 2-type responses. J Exp Med 1999; 189: 1169–80.

106. Bregenholt S, Brimnes J, Nissen MH, Claesson MH. In vitro activated CD4+ T cells from interferon-gamma (IFN-gamma)-deficient mice induce intestinal inflammation in immunodeficient hosts. Clin Exp Immunol 1999; 118: 228–34.

107. Obermeier F, Kojouharoff G, Hans W, Scholmerich J, Gross V, Falk W. Interferon-gamma (IFN-gamma)- and tumour necrosis factor (TNF)-induced nitric oxide as toxic effector molecule in chronic dextran sulphate sodium (DSS)-induced colitis in mice. Clin Exp Immunol 1999; 116: 238–45.

108. Powrie F, Leach MW, Mauze S, Menon S, Caddle LB, Coffman RL. Inhibition of Th1 responses prevents inflammatory bowel disease in scid mice reconstituted with CD45RBhi CD4+ T cells. Immunity 1994; 1: 553–62.

109. Fort MM, Leach MW, Rennick DM. A role for NK cells as regulators of CD4+ T cells in a transfer model of colitis. J Immunol 1998; 161: 3256–61.

110. Noguchi M, Hiwatashi N, Liu Z, Toyota T. Enhanced interferon-gamma production and B7-2 expression in isolated intestinal mononuclear cells from patients with Crohn's disease. J Gastroenterol 1995; 30(Suppl. 8): 52–5.

111. Akagi S, Hiyama E, Imamura Y, Takesue Y, Matsuura Y, Yokoyama T. Interleukin-10 expression in intestine of Crohn disease. Int J Mol Med 2000; 5: 389–95.

112. Parronchi P, Romagnani P, Annunziato F et al. Type 1 T-helper cell predominance and interleukin-12 expression in the gut of patients with Crohn's disease. Am J Pathol 1997; 150: 823–32.

113. Fais S, Capobianchi MR, Silvestri M, Mercuri F, Pallone F, Dianzani F. Interferon expression in Crohn's disease patients: increased interferon-gamma and -alpha mRNA in the intestinal lamina propria mononuclear cells. J Interferon Res 1994; 14: 235–8.

114. Desreumaux P, Brandt E, Gambiez L et al. Distinct cytokine patterns in early and chronic ileal lesions of Crohn's disease. Gastroenterology 1997; 113: 118–26.

115. Gramaglia I, Mauri DN, Miner KT, Ware CF, Croft M. Lymphotoxin alphabeta is expressed on recently activated naive and Th1-like CD4 cells but is down-regulated by IL-4 during Th2 differentiation. J Immunol 1999; 162: 1333–8.

116. Neumann B, Luz A, Pfeffer K, Holzmann B. Defective Peyer's patch organogenesis in mice lacking the 55-kD receptor for tumor necrosis factor. J Exp Med 1996; 184: 259–64.

117. Alexopoulou L, Pasparakis M, Kollias G. Complementation of lymphotoxin alpha knockout mice with tumor necrosis factor-expressing transgenes rectifies defective splenic structure and function. J Exp Med 1998; 188: 745–54.

118. Koni PA, Sacca R, Lawton P, Browning JL, Ruddle NH, Flavell RA. Distinct roles in lymphoid organogenesis for lymphotoxins alpha and beta revealed in lymphotoxin beta-deficient mice. Immunity 1997; 6: 491–500.

119. Cuff CA, Sacca R, Ruddle NH. Differential induction of adhesion molecule and chemokine expression by LTalpha3 and LTalphabeta in inflammation elucidates potential mechanisms of mesenteric and peripheral lymph node development. J Immunol 1999; 162: 5965–72.

120. Cuff CA, Schwartz J, Bergman CM, Russell KS, Bender JR, Ruddle NH. Lymphotoxin alpha3 induces chemokines and adhesion molecules: insight into the role of LT alpha in inflammation and lymphoid organ development. J Immunol 1998; 161: 6853–60.

121. Futterer A, Mink K, Luz A, Kosco-Vilbois MH, Pfeffer K. The lymphotoxin beta receptor controls organogenesis and affinity maturation in peripheral lymphoid tissues. Immunity 1998; 9: 59–70.

122. Mackay F, Browning JL, Lawton P et al. Both the lymphotoxin and tumor necrosis factor pathways are involved in experimental murine models of colitis. Gastroenterology 1998; 115: 1464–75.

123. Dinarello CA, Thompson RC. Blocking IL-1: interleukin 1 receptor antagonist in vivo and in vitro. Immunol Today 1991; 12: 404–10.

124. Dinarello CA. Interleukin-1 and interleukin-1 antagonism. Blood 1991; 77: 1627–52.

125. Youngman KR, Simon PL, West GA et al. Localization of intestinal interleukin 1 activity and protein and gene expression to lamina propria cells. Gastroenterology 1993; 104: 749–58.

126. Strong SA, Pizarro TT, Klein JS, Cominelli F, Fiocchi C. Proinflammatory cytokines differentially modulate their own expression in human intestinal mucosal mesenchymal cells. Gastroenterology 1998; 114: 1244–56.

127. Dinarello CA, Wolff SM. The role of interleukin-1 in disease. N Engl J Med 1993; 328: 106–113.

128. Cominelli F, Nast CC, Dinarello CA, Gentilini P, Zipser RD. Regulation of eicosanoid production by interleukin-1 in normal rabbit colon. Gastroenterology 1989; 97: 1400–5.

129. Cominelli F, Nast CC, Clark BD et al. Interleukin 1 (IL-1) gene expression, synthesis, and effect of specific IL-1 recep-

tor blockade in rabbit immune complex colitis. J Clin Invest 1990; 86: 972–80.

130. Cominelli F, Nast CC, Duchini A, Lee M. Recombinant interleukin-1 receptor antagonist blocks the proinflammatory activity of endogenous interleukin-1 in rabbit immune colitis. Gastroenterology 1992; 103: 65–71.

131. McCall RD, Haskill S, Zimmermann EM, Lund PK, Thompson RC, Sartor RB. Tissue interleukin 1 and interleukin-1 receptor antagonist expression in enterocolitis in resistant and susceptible rats. Gastroenterology 1994; 106: 960–72.

132. Thomas TK, Will PC, Srivastava A *et al.* Evaluation of an interleukin-1 receptor antagonist in the rat acetic acid-induced colitis model. Agents Actions 1991; 34: 187–90.

133. Jacobson K, McHugh K, Collins SM. The mechanism of altered neural function in a rat model of acute colitis. Gastroenterology 1997; 112: 156–62.

134. Ligumsky M, Simon PL, Karmeli F, Rachmilewitz D. Role of interleukin 1 in inflammatory bowel disease – enhanced production with active disease. Gut 1990; 31: 686–9.

135. Kern JA, Lamb RJ, Reed JC, Daniele RP, Nowell PC. Dexamethasone inhibition of interleukin 1 beta production by human monocytes. Posttranscriptional mechanisms. J Clin Invest 1988; 81: 237–44.

136. Satsangi J, Wolstencroft RA, Cason J, Ainley CC, Dumonde DC, Thompson RP. Interleukin 1 in Crohn's disease. Clin ExpImmunol 1987; 67: 594–605.

137. Nakamura M, Saito H, Kasanuki J, Tamura Y, Yoshida S. Cytokine production in patients with inflammatory bowel disease. Gut 1992; 33: 933–7.

138. Mazlam MZ, Hodgson HJ. Interrelations between interleukin-6, interleukin-1 beta, plasma C-reactive protein values, and *in vitro* C-reactive protein generation in patients with inflammatory bowel disease. Gut 1994; 35: 77–83.

139. Mahida YR, Wu K, Jewell DP. Enhanced production of interleukin 1-beta by mononuclear cells isolated from mucosa with active ulcerative colitis of Crohn's disease. Gut 1989; 30: 835–8.

140. Ishimura K, Tsubouchi T, Okano K, Maeba T, Maeta H. Wound healing of intestinal anastomosis after digestive surgery under septic conditions: participation of local interleukin-6 expression. World J Surg 1998; 22: 1069–75; discussion 1076.

141. Swank GM, Lu Q, Xu DZ, Michalsky M, Deitch EA. Effect of acute-phase and heat-shock stress on apoptosis in intestinal epithelial cells (Caco-2). Crit Care Med 1998; 26: 1213–17.

142. Bromander AK, Ekman L, Kopf M, Nedrud JG, Lycke NY. IL-6-deficient mice exhibit normal mucosal IgA responses to local immunizations and Helicobacter felis infection. J Immunol 1996; 156: 4290–7.

143. Ramsay AJ, Husband AJ, Ramshaw IA *et al.* The role of interleukin-6 in mucosal IgA antibody responses *in vivo*. Science 1994; 264: 561–3.

144. Bao S, Beagley KW, Allanson M, Husband AJ. Exogenous IL-6 promotes enhanced intestinal antibody responses *in vivo*. Immunol Cell Biol 1998; 76: 560–2.

145. Bao S, Husband AJ, Beagley KW. B1 B cell numbers and antibodies against phosphorylcholine and LPS are increased in IL-6 gene knockout mice. Cell Immunol 1999; 198: 139–42.

146. Ward LD, Hammacher A, Howlett GJ *et al.* Influence of interleukin-6 (IL-6) dimerization on formation of the high affinity hexameric IL-6.receptor complex. J Biol Chem 1996; 271: 20138–44.

147. Panja A, Goldberg S, Eckmann L, Krishen P, Mayer L. The regulation and functional consequence of proinflammatory cytokine binding on human intestinal epithelial cells. J Immunol 1998; 161: 3675–84.

148. Molmenti EP, Ziambaras T, Perlmutter DH. Evidence for an acute phase response in human intestinal epithelial cells. J Biol Chem 1993; 268: 14116–24.

149. McGee DW, Beagley KW, Aicher WK, McGhee JR. Transforming growth factor-beta enhances interleukin-6 secretion by intestinal epithelial cells. Immunology 1992; 77: 7–12.

150. McGee DW, Beagley KW, Aicher WK, McGhee JR. Transforming growth factor-beta and IL-1 beta act in synergy to enhance IL-6 secretion by the intestinal epithelial cell line, IEC-6. J Immunol 1993; 151: 970–8.

151. Parikh AA, Moon MR, Kane CD, Salzman AL, Fischer JE, Hasselgren PO. Interleukin-6 production in human intestinal epithelial cells increases in association with the heat shock response. J Surg Res 1998; 77: 40–4.

152. Parikh AA, Salzman AL, Fischer JE, Szabo C, Hasselgren PO. Interleukin-1 beta and interferon-gamma regulate interleukin-6 production in cultured human intestinal epithelial cells. Shock 1997; 8: 249–55.

153. Jones SC, Trejdosiewicz LK, Banks RE *et al.* Expression of interleukin-6 by intestinal enterocytes. J Clin Pathol 1993; 46: 1097–100.

154. Kusugami K, Fukatsu A, Tanimoto M *et al.* Elevation of interleukin-6 in inflammatory bowel disease is macrophage- and epithelial cell-dependent. Digestive Dis Sci 1995; 40: 949–59.

155. Stevens C, Walz G, Singaram C *et al.* Tumor necrosis factor-alpha, interleukin-1 beta, and interleukin-6 expression in inflammatory bowel disease. Dig Dis Sci 1992; 37: 818–26.

156. Reinecker HC, Steffen M, Witthoeft T *et al.* Enhanced secretion of tumour necrosis factor-alpha, IL-6, and IL-1 beta by isolated lamina propria mononuclear cells from patients with ulcerative colitis and Crohn's disease. Clin Exp Immunol 1993; 94: 174–81.

157. Daig R, Rogler G, Aschenbrenner E *et al.* Human intestinal epithelial cells secrete interleukin-1 receptor antagonist and interleukin-8 but not interleukin-1 or interleukin-6. Gut 2000; 46: 350–8.

158. Grottrup-Wolfers E, Moeller J, Karbach U, Muller-Lissner S, Endres S. Elevated cell-associated levels of interleukin 1beta and interleukin 6 in inflamed mucosa of inflammatory bowel disease. Eur J Clin Invest 1996; 26: 115–22.

159. Reimund JM, Wittersheim C, Dumont S *et al.* Increased production of tumour necrosis factor-alpha interleukin-1 beta, and interleukin-6 by morphologically normal intestinal biopsies from patients with Crohn's disease. Gut 1996; 39: 684–9.

160. Hyams JS, Fitzgerald JE, Treem WR, Wyzga N, Kreutzer DL. Relationship of functional and antigenic interleukin 6 to disease activity in inflammatory bowel disease. Gastroenterology 1993; 104: 1285–92.

161. Gross V, Andus T, Caesar I, Roth M, Scholmerich J. Evidence for continuous stimulation of interleukin-6 production in Crohn's disease. Gastroenterology 1992; 102: 514–9.

162. Mitsuyama K, Toyonaga A, Sasaki E *et al.* Soluble interleukin-6 receptors in inflammatory bowel disease: relation to circulating interleukin-6. Gut 1995; 36: 45–9.

163. Dieleman LA, Elson CO, Tennyson GS, Beagley KW. Kinetics of cytokine expression during healing of acute colitis in mice. Am J Physiol 1996; 271: G130–6.

164. Kawachi S, Jennings S, Panes J *et al.* Cytokine and endothelial cell adhesion molecule expression in interleukin-10-deficient mice. Am J Physiol Gastrointest Liver Physiol 2000; 278: G734–43.

165. Yamamoto M, Yoshizaki K, Kishimoto T, Ito H. IL-6 is required for the development of Th1 cell-mediated murine colitis. J Immunol 2000; 164: 4878–82.

166. Atreya R, Mudter J, Finotto S *et al.* Blockade of interleukin 6 trans signaling suppresses T-cell resistance against apop-

and epithelial effects of interleukin-11. Leukemia 1999; 13: 1307–15.

240. Leng SX, Elias JA. Interleukin-11. Int J Biochem Cell Biol 1997; 29: 1059–62.

241. Orazi A, Du X, Yang Z, Kashai M, Williams DA. Interleukin-11 prevents apoptosis and accelerates recovery of small intestinal mucosa in mice treated with combined chemotherapy and radiation. Lab Invest 1996; 75: 33–42.

242. Tang W, Yang L, Yang YC, Leng SX, Elias JA. Transforming growth factor-beta stimulates interleukin-11 transcription via complex activating protein-1-dependent pathways. J Biol Chem 1998; 273: 5506–13.

243. Hill GR, Cooke KR, Teshima T *et al.* Interleukin-11 promotes T cell polarization and prevents acute graft-versus-host disease after allogeneic bone marrow transplantation. J Clin Invest 1998; 102: 115–23.

244. Trepicchio WL, Wang L, Bozza M, Dorner AJ. IL-11 regulates macrophage effector function through the inhibition of nuclear factor-kappaB. J Immunol 1997; 159: 5661–70.

245. Qiu BS, Pfeiffer CJ, Keith JC, Jr. Protection by recombinant human interleukin-11 against experimental TNB-induced colitis in rats. Dig Dis Sci 1996; 41: 1625–30.

246. Peterson RL, Wang L, Albert L, Keith JC, Jr., Dorner AJ. Molecular effects of recombinant human interleukin-11 in the HLA-B27 rat model of inflammatory bowel disease. Lab Invest 1998; 78: 1503–12.

247. Keith JC, Jr, Albert L, Sonis ST, Pfeiffer CJ, Schaub RG. IL-11, a pleiotropic cytokine: exciting new effects of IL-11 on gastrointestinal mucosal biology. Stem Cells 1994; 12(Suppl. 1): 79–89; discussion 89–90.

248. Alavi K, Prasad R, Lundgren K, Schwartz MZ. Interleukin-11 enhances small intestine absorptive function and mucosal mass after intestinal adaptation. J Pediatr Surg 2000; 35: 371–4.

249. Fiore NF, Ledniczky G, Liu Q *et al.* Comparison of interleukin-11 and epidermal growth factor on residual small intestine after massive small bowel resection. J Pediatr Surg 1998; 33: 24–9.

250. Liu Q, Du XX, Schindel DT *et al.* Trophic effects of interleukin-11 in rats with experimental short bowel syndrome. J Pediatr Surg 1996; 31: 1047–50; discussion 1050–1.

251. Sands BE, Bank S, Sninsky CA *et al.* Preliminary evaluation of safety and activity of recombinant human interleukin 11 in patients with active Crohn's disease. Gastroenterology 1999; 117: 58–64.

252. Migdalska A, Molineux G, Demuynck H, Evans GS, Ruscetti F, Dexter TM. Growth inhibitory effects of transforming growth factor-beta 1 *in vivo.* Growth Factors 1991; 4: 239–45.

253. Dignass AU, Podolsky DK. Cytokine modulation of intestinal epithelial cell restitution: central role of transforming growth factor beta. Gastroenterology 1993; 105: 1323–32.

254. Booth C, Evans GS, Potten CS. Growth factor regulation of proliferation in primary cultures of small intestinal epithelium. In Vitro Cell Dev Biol Anim 1995; 31: 234–43.

255. Ebert EC. Inhibitory effects of transforming growth factor-beta (TGF-beta) on certain functions of intraepithelial lymphocytes. Clin Exp Immunol 1999; 115: 415–20.

256. Planchon S, Fiocchi C, Takafuji V, Roche JK. Transforming growth factor-beta1 preserves epithelial barrier function: identification of receptors, biochemical intermediates, and cytokine antagonists. J Cell Physiol 1999; 181: 55–66.

257. McGee DW, Bamberg T, Vitkus SJ, McGhee JR. A synergistic relationship between TNF-αlpha, IL-1 beta, and TGF-beta 1 on IL-6 secretion by the IEC-6 intestinal epithelial cell line. Immunology 1995; 86: 6–11.

258. Mourelle M, Salas A, Guarner F, Crespo E, Garcia-Lafuente A, Malagelada JR. Stimulation of transforming growth factor beta1 by enteric bacteria in the pathogenesis of rat intestinal fibrosis. Gastroenterology 1998; 114: 519–26.

259. van Ginkel FW, Wahl SM, Kearney JF *et al.* Partial IgA-deficiency with increased Th2-type cytokines in TGF-beta 1 knockout mice. J Immunol 1999; 163: 1951–7.

260. Barnard JA, Warwick GJ, Gold LI. Localization of transforming growth factor beta isoforms in the normal murine small intestine and colon. Gastroenterology 1993; 105: 67–73.

261. Giladi E, Raz E, Karmeli F, Okon E, Rachmilewitz D. Transforming growth factor-beta gene therapy ameliorates experimental colitis in rats. Eur J Gastroenterol Hepatol 1995; 7: 341–7.

262. Babyatsky MW, Rossiter G, Podolsky DK. Expression of transforming growth factors alpha and beta in colonic mucosa in inflammatory bowel disease. Gastroenterology 1996; 110: 975–84.

263. Xian CJ, Xu X, Mardell CE *et al.* Site-specific changes in transforming growth factor-alpha and -beta1 expression in colonic mucosa of adolescents with inflammatory bowel disease. Scand J Gastroenterol 1999; 34: 591–600.

264. Ohtani H, Kagaya H, Nagura H. Immunohistochemical localization of transforming growth factor-beta receptors I and II in inflammatory bowel disease. J Gastroenterol 1995; 30(Suppl. 8): 76–7.

265. Friess H, di Mola FF, Egger B *et al.* Transforming growth factor-beta controls pathogenesis of Crohn disease. Langenbecks Arch Chir Suppl Kongressbd 1998; 115: 994–7.

266. Chowdhury A, Fukuda R, Fukumoto S. Growth factor mRNA expression in normal colorectal mucosa and in uninvolved mucosa from ulcerative colitis patients. J Gastroenterol 1996; 31: 353–60.

267. Eckmann L, Kagnoff MF, Fierer J. Epithelial cells secrete the chemokine interleukin-8 in response to bacterial entry. Infect Immun 1993; 61: 4569–74.

268. Schuerer-Maly CC, Eckmann L, Kagnoff MF, Falco MT, Maly FE. Colonic epithelial cell lines as a source of interleukin-8: stimulation by inflammatory cytokines and bacterial lipopolysaccharide. Immunology 1994; 81: 85–91.

269. McCormick BA, Colgan SP, Delp-Archer C, Miller SI, Madara JL. *Salmonella typhimurium* attachment to human intestinal epithelial monolayers: transcellular signalling to subepithelial neutrophils. J Cell Biology 1993; 123: 895–907.

270. Mazzuchelli L, Hauser C, Zgraggen K *et al.* Expression of interleukin-8 gene in inflammatory bowel disease is related to the histological grade of active inflammation. Am J Pathol 1994; 144: 997–1007.

271. Daig R, Andus T, Aschenbrenner E, Falk W, Scholmerich J, Gross V. Increased interleukin 8 expression in the colon mucosa of patients with inflammatory bowel disease. Gut 1996; 38: 216–22.

272. Grimm MC, Elsbury SK, Pavli P, Doe WF. Interleukin 8: cells of origin in inflammatory bowel disease. Gut 1996; 38: 90–8.

273. Arai F, Takahashi T, Furukawa K, Matsushima K, Asakura H. Mucosal expression of interleukin-6 and interleukin-8 messenger RNA in ulcerative colitis and in Crohn's disease. Dig Dis Sci 1998; 43: 2071–9.

274. Izutani R, Ohyanagi H, MacDermott RP. Quantitative PCR for detection of femtogram quantities of interleukin-8 mRNA expression. Microbiol Immunol 1994; 38: 233–7.

275. Mitsuyama K, Toyonaga A, Sasaki E *et al.* IL-8 as an important chemoattractant for neutrophils in ulcerative colitis and Crohn's disease. Clin Exp Immunol 1994; 96: 432–6.

276. Raab Y, Gerdin B, Ahlstedt S, Hallgren R. Neutrophil mucosal involvement is accompanied by enhanced local

production of interleukin-8 in ulcerative colitis. Gut 1993; 34: 1203–6.

277. Mahida YR, Ceska M, Effenberger F, Kurlak L, Lindley I, Hawkey CJ. Enhanced synthesis of neutrophil-activating peptide-1/interleukin-8 in active ulcerative colitis. Clin Sci 1992; 82: 273–5.

278. Izzo RS, Witkon K, Chen AI, Hadjiyane C, Weinstein MI, Pellecchia C. Interleukin-8 and neutrophil markers in colonic mucosa from patients with ulcerative colitis. Am J Gastroenterol 1992; 87: 1447–52.

279. Izzo RS, Witkon K, Chen AI, Hadjiyane C, Weinstein MI, Pellecchia C. Neutrophil-activating peptide (interleukin-8) in colonic mucosa from patients with Crohn's disease. Scand J Gastroenterology 1993; 28: 296–300.

280. Ina K, Kusugami K, Yamaguchi T et al. Mucosal interleukin-8 is involved in neutrophil migration and binding to extracellular matrix in inflammatory bowel disease. Am J Gastroenterol 1997; 92: 1342–6.

281. Chang MS, McNinch J, Basu R, Simonet S. Cloning and characterization of the human neutrophil-activating peptide (ENA-78) gene. J Biol Chem 1994; 269: 25277–82.

282. Walz A, Burgener R, Car B, Baggiolini M, Kunkel SL, Strieter RM. Structure and neutrophil-activating properties of a novel inflammatory peptide (ENA-78) with homology to interleukin 8. J Exp Med 1991; 174: 1355–62.

283. Schnyder-Candrian S, Walz A. Neutrophil-activating protein ENA-78 and IL-8 exhibit different patterns of expression in lipopolysaccharide- and cytokine-stimulated human monocytes. J Immunol 1997; 158: 3888–94.

284. Keates S, Keates AC, Mizoguchi E, Bhan A, Kelly CP. Enterocytes are the primary source of the chemokine ENA-78 in normal colon and ulcerative colitis. Am J Physiol 1997; 273: G75–82.

285. Wuyts A, Proost P, Lenaerts JP, Ben-Baruch A, Van Damme J, Wang JM. Differential usage of the CXC chemokine receptors 1 and 2 by interleukin-8, granulocyte chemotactic protein-2 and epithelial-cell-derived neutrophil attractant-78. Eur J Biochem 1998; 255: 67–73.

286. Z'Graggen K, Walz A, Mazzucchelli L, Strieter RM, Mueller C. The C-X-C chemokine ENA-78 is preferentially expressed in intestinal epithelium in inflammatory bowel disease. Gastroenterology 1997; 113: 808–16.

287. Taub DD, Sayers TJ, Carter CR, Ortaldo JR. Alpha and beta chemokines induce NK cell migration and enhance NK-mediated cytolysis. J Immunol 1995; 155: 3877–88.

288. Loetscher M, Gerber B, Loetscher P et al. Chemokine receptor specific for IP10 and mig: structure, function, and expression in activated T-lymphocytes. J Exp Med 1996; 184: 963–9.

289. Roth SJ, Carr MW, Springer TA. C-C chemokines, but not the C-X-C chemokines interleukin-8 and interferon-gamma inducible protein-10, stimulate transendothelial chemotaxis of T lymphocytes. Eur J Immunol 1995; 25: 3482–8.

290. Roth SJ, Diacovo TG, Brenner MB et al. Transendothelial chemotaxis of human alpha/beta and gamma/delta T lymphocytes to chemokines. European J Immunol 1998; 28: 104–13.

291. Uguccioni M, Gionchetti P, Robbiani DF et al. Increased expression of IP-10, IL-8, MCP-1, and MCP-3 in ulcerative colitis. Am J Pathol 1999; 155: 331–6.

292. Chapman GA, Moores KE, Gohil J et al. The role of fractalkine in the recruitment of monocytes to the endothelium. Eur J Pharmacol. 2000; 392: 189–95.

293. Muehlhoefer A, Saubermann LJ, Gu X et al. Fractalkine is an epithelial and endothelial cell-derived chemoattractant for intraepithelial lymphocytes in the small intestinal mucosa. J Immunol 2000; 164: 3368–76.

294. Lucas AD, Chadwick N, Warren BF et al. The transmembrane form of the CX3CL1 chemokine fractalkine is expressed predominantly by epithelial cells in vivo. Am J Pathol 2001; 158: 855–66.

295. Randolph GJ, Furie MB. A soluble gradient of endogenous monocyte chemoattractant protein-1 promotes the transendothelial migration of monocytes in vitro. J Immunol 1995; 155: 3610–18.

296. Gu L, Tseng S, Horner RM, Tam C, Loda M, Rollins BJ. Control of TH2 polarization by the chemokine monocyte chemoattractant protein-1. Nature 2000; 404: 407–11.

297. Lu B, Rutledge BJ, Gu L et al. Abnormalities in monocyte recruitment and cytokine expression in monocyte chemoattractant protein 1-deficient mice. J Exp Med 1998; 187: 601–8.

298. Winsor GL, Waterhouse CC, MacLellan RL, Stadnyk AW. Interleukin-4 and IFN-gamma differentially stimulate macrophage chemoattractant protein-1 (MCP-1) and eotaxin production by intestinal epithelial cells. J Interferon Cytokine Res 2000; 20: 299–308.

299. Tangirala RK, Murao K, Quehenberger O. Regulation of expression of the human monocyte chemotactic protein-1 receptor (hCCR2) by cytokines. J Biol Chem 1997; 272: 8050–6.

300. Reinecker HC, Loh EY, Ringler DJ, Mehta A, Rombeau JL, MacDermott RP. Monocyte-chemoattractant protein 1 gene expression in intestinal epithelial cells and inflammatory bowel disease mucosa. Gastroenterology 1995; 108: 40–50.

301. Mazzucchelli L, Hauser C, Zgraggen K et al. Differential in situ expression of the genes encoding the chemokines MCP-1 and RANTES in human inflammatory bowel disease. J Pathol 1996; 178: 201–6.

302. Grimm MC, Elsbury SK, Pavli P, Doe WF. Enhanced expression and production of monocyte chemoattractant protein-1 in inflammatory bowel disease mucosa. J Leuk Biol 1996; 59: 804–12.

303. Keane J, Nicoll J, Kim S et al. Conservation of structure and function between human and murine IL-16. J Immunol 1998; 160: 5945–54.

304. Baier M, Bannert N, Werner A, Lang K, Kurth R. Molecular cloning, sequence, expression, and processing of the interleukin 16 precursor. Proc Natl Acad Sci USA 1997; 94: 5273–7.

305. Zhang Y, Center DM, Wu DM et al. Processing and activation of pro-interleukin-16 by caspase-3. J Biol Chem 1998; 273: 1144–9.

306. Bellini A, Yoshimura H, Vittori E, Marini M, Mattoli S. Bronchial epithelial cells of patients with asthma release chemoattractant factors for T lymphocytes. J Allergy Clin Immunol 1993; 92: 412–24.

307. Laberge S, Cruikshank WW, Kornfeld H, Center DM. Histamine-induced secretion of lymphocyte chemoattractant factor from CD8+ T cells is independent of transcription and translation. Evidence for constitutive protein synthesis and storage. J Immunol 1995; 155: 2902–10.

308. Lim KG, Wan HC, Bozza PT et al. Human eosinophils elaborate the lymphocyte chemoattractants. IL-16 (lymphocyte chemoattractant factor) and RANTES. J Immunol 1996; 156: 2566–70.

309. Cruikshank WW, Center DM, Nisar N et al. Molecular and functional analysis of a lymphocyte chemoattractant factor: association of biologic function with CD4 expression. Proc Natl Acad Sci USA 1994; 91: 5109–13.

310. Cruikshank WW, Berman JS, Theodore AC, Bernardo J, Center DM. Lymphokine activation of T4+ T lymphocytes and monocytes. J Immunol 1987; 138: 3817–23.

311. Rand TH, Cruikshank WW, Center DM, Weller PF. CD4-mediated stimulation of human eosinophils: lymphocyte chemoattractant factor and other CD4-binding ligands elicit eosinophil migration. J Exp Med 1991; 173: 1521–8.

312. Cruikshank WW, Greenstein JL, Theodore AC, Center DM. Lymphocyte chemoattractant factor induces CD4-dependent intracytoplasmic signaling in lymphocytes. J Immunol 1991; 146: 2928–34.

313. Keates AC, Castagliuolo I, Cruickshank WW *et al*. Interleukin 16 is up-regulated in Crohn's disease and participates in TNBS colitis in mice. Gastroenterology 2000; 119: 972–82.

314. Seegert D, Rosenstiel P, Pfahler H, Pfefferkorn P, Nikolaus S, Schreiber S. Increased expression of IL-16 in inflammatory bowel disease. Gut 2001; 48: 326–32.

315. Uguccioni M, D'Apuzzo M, Loetscher M, Dewald B, Baggiolini M. Actions of the chemotactic cytokines MCP-1, MCP-2, MCP-3, RANTES, MIP-1 alpha and MIP-1 beta on human monocytes. Eur J Immunol 1995; 25: 64–8.

316. Taub DD, Proost P, Murphy WJ *et al*. Monocyte chemotactic protein-1 (MCP-1), -2, and -3 are chemotactic for human T lymphocytes. J Clin Invest 1995; 95: 1370–6.

317. Xu LL, Warren MK, Rose WL, Gong W, Wang JM. Human recombinant monocyte chemotactic protein and other C-C chemokines bind and induce directional migration of dendritic cells *in vitro*. J Leuk Biol 1996; 60: 365–71.

318. Blumberg H, Conklin D, Xu WF *et al*. Interleukin 20: discovery, receptor identification, and role in epidermal function. Cell 2001; 104: 9–19.

319. Dumoutier L, Louahed J, Renauld JC. Cloning and characterization of IL-10-related T cell-derived inducible factor (IL-TIF), a novel cytokine structurally related to IL-10 and inducible by IL-9. J Immunol 2000; 164: 1814–9.

320. Dumoutier L, Van Roost E, Colau D, Renauld JC. Human interleukin-10-related T cell-derived inducible factor: molecular cloning and functional characterization as an hepatocyte-stimulating factor. Proc Nat Acad Sci USA 2000; 97: 10144–9.

321. Xie MH, Aggarwal S, Ho WH *et al*. Interleukin (IL)-22, a novel human cytokine that signals through the interferon receptor-related proteins CRF2-4 and IL-22R. J Biol Chem 2000; 275: 31335–9.

322. Oppmann B, Lesley R, Blom B *et al*. Novel p19 protein engages IL-12p40 to form a cytokine, IL-23, with biological activities similar as well as distinct from IL-12. Immunity 2000; 13: 715–25.

8 Role of the microcirculation in chronic gut inflammation

Matthew B. Grisham, F. Stephen Laroux and D. Neil Granger

Introduction

Active episodes of inflammatory bowel disease (IBD; Crohn's disease (CD), ulcerative colitis (UC)) are characterized by rectal bleeding, severe diarrhea, exudation, fever, abdominal pain, and weight loss. Histopathological inspection of tissue obtained from the involved segment of the small and/or large bowel reveals vasodilation, venocongestion, edema, infiltration of large numbers of inflammatory cells and erosions and ulcerations [1]. Although the pathogenetic mechanisms responsible for the microvascular dysfunction, mucosal inflammation and injury are not entirely clear at the present time, there is an accumulating body of experimental and clinical data to suggest that IBD may result from the dysregulated immune response to components of the normal gut flora [1–5]. It has been proposed that the inability to regulate the normally protective cell-mediated immune response results in activation of the $CD4^+$ T cells with subsequent release of interleukin-2 (IL-2), interferon-γ (IFN-γ) and tumor necrosis factor-α (TNF-α) [6]. These Th1-type cytokines in turn activate tissue macrophages to release a variety of proinflammatory mediators including TNF-α, IL-1β, IL-12, platelet-activating factor (PAF), leukotriene B4 (LTB4), reactive oxygen species (ROS), nitric oxide (NO) and prostaglandins [6–8]. Some of these inflammatory mediators (e.g. histamine, bradykinin, nitric oxide, prostaglandins) will increase blood flow (hyperemia), thereby producing erythema. Another consequence of enhanced arteriolar blood flow is an increased hydrostatic pressure in the downstream capillaries resulting in fluid movement across intestinal capillaries and interstitial edema. Certain proinflammatory cytokines (TNF, IFN-γ, IL-12) released by activated mast cells, macrophages and lymphocytes activate venular endothelial cells and increase expression of endothelial cell adhesion molecules that mediate leukocyte–endothelial cell adhesion and eventual emigration (tissue infiltration) of leukocytes. Leukocyte emigration is often associated with vascular protein leak (extravasation) and the accumulation of albumin and other plasma proteins in the gut interstitium. The resultant increase in interstitial oncotic pressure further promotes fluid filtration across capillaries and accelerates the development of interstitial edema. Taken together, these pathophysiological considerations suggest that the intestinal microcirculation contributes, in a large part, to much of the pathophysiology of chronic gut inflammation (Fig. 1).

This chapter reviews the current state of knowledge regarding the mechanisms that regulate the three structurally and functionally important elements of the microcirculation, i.e. the arterioles, capillaries and venules. This discussion will focus on the potential role of the microvasculature in inflammatory bowel disease.

Anatomical and functional organization of the gut microcirculation

The microcirculation consists of arterioles, capillaries, and venules, which form a branching, tapered network of approximately circular tubes (Fig. 1). The fundamental inter-organ variations in microvascular anatomy relate primarily to branching patterns, vessel densities, and the fine structure of capillaries. Each small artery can give rise to several (one to four) arterioles as its diameter decreases toward the tissue core (or periphery). Arterioles are usually less than 500 μm in diameter, with an external muscular coat that consists of two to four circumferentially arranged smooth muscle cells. As arteriolar diameter decreases, so does the number of smooth muscle

Stephan R. Targan, Fergus Shanahan and Loren C. Karp (eds.), Inflammatory Bowel Disease: From Bench to Bedside, 2nd Edition, 177–196.

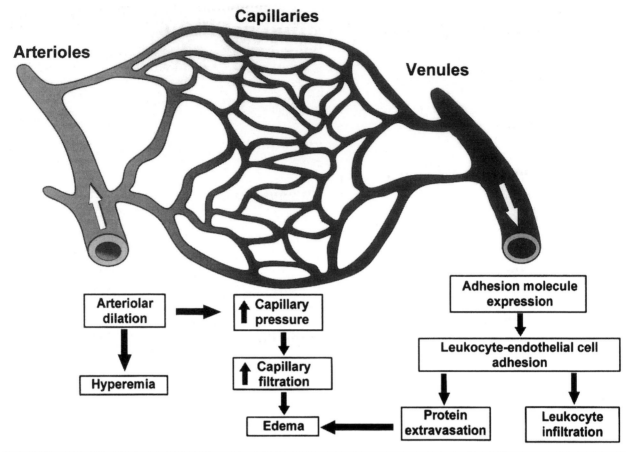

Figure 1. All segments of the microcirculation contribute to the pathophysiology of chronic gut inflammation. A variety of inflammatory mediators (e.g. histamine, bradykinin, nitric oxide, prostaglandins) produced by the affected tissue relax the vascular smooth muscle surrounding arterioles. The consequent dilation of arterioles leads to an increased blood flow (hyperemia) thereby producing erythema. Another consequence of arteriolar dilation is an increased hydrostatic pressure in the downstream capillaries. The increased capillary hydrostatic pressure alters the balance of forces that govern fluid movement across intestinal capillaries to favor net fluid filtration. The increased capillary filtration rate contributes to the interstitial edema associated with gut inflammation. Proinflammatory cytokines (TNF, IFN-γ, IL-12) released by activated mast cells, macrophages and lymphocytes, activate venular endothelial cells and increase expression of endothelial cell adhesion molecules that mediate leukocyte–endothelial cell adhesion and eventual emigration (tissue infiltration) of leukocytes. Leukocyte emigration is often associated with vascular protein leak (extravasation). Consequently, inflammation generally results in a diminished endothelial barrier function in venules that promotes the accumulation of albumin and other plasma proteins in the interstitium. The resultant increase in interstitial oncotic pressure further promotes fluid filtration across capillaries and accelerates the development of interstitial edema.

layers. The terminal (precapillary) arterioles have an internal diameter of 15–20 μm and are surrounded by only one layer of smooth muscle cells. Arterioles, like their parent vessels (large and small arteries), have an inner lining of endothelial cells, and the periphery of the vessel may be invested by fibroblasts as well as a network of non-myelinated nerves. Arterioles can undergo active changes in diameter, about 2–3-fold in the smallest vessels and 20–40% in the larger arterioles, depending on the initial state of vascular tone.

The majority of capillaries are derived from terminal arterioles with capillaries consisting of a tube of 4–10 μm in internal diameter and lined by a single layer of endothelial cells and a thin basement membrane. The ultrastructure and endothelial thickness of capillaries varies considerably between and within different organs [9, 10]. Based on the fine structure of their endothelium, capillaries are generally divided into the following categories: (a) fenestrated, (b) continuous, and (c) discontinuous. In many tissues, including the gut, only a fraction (e.g. 20–30%) of the capillaries are open to perfusion

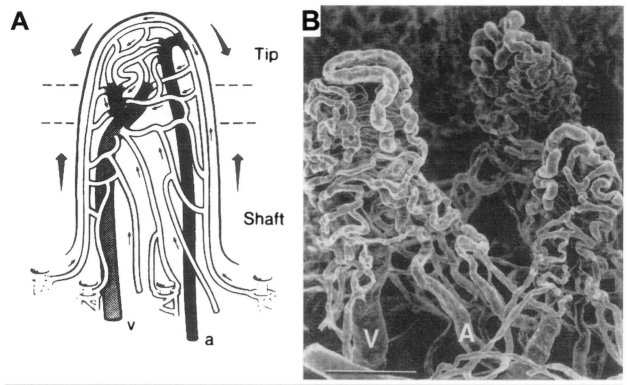

Figure 2. Microcirculatory pattern of the small intestinal mucosa. **A**: Fountain-like pattern of blood flow to the villus *a* represents arteriole and *v* represents venule. **B**: Cast of the microvasculature of the small intestinal villus. The pattern of arterioles (A) and venules (V) conforms to the shape of the villus. This capillary plexus immediately underlies the base of the epithelium (reproduced from ref. 14, with permission).

under resting conditions [11]. The ability of tissues to recruit additional perfused capillaries during periods of stress (e.g. hypoxia) has been attributed to the existence of precapillary sphincters, which may represent one or two layers of smooth muscle that surround the entrance of a capillary. The capillary network, with its large surface area and an endothelial barrier that is highly permeable to lipid-soluble and small water-soluble molecules, appears well suited for the exchange of gases, nutrients, and water between the blood stream and tissues.

Capillaries drain into larger vessels that are also devoid of a smooth muscle cells. These postcapillary venules represent the segment of the microvasculature that is most reactive to inflammation and contain intercellular endothelial junctions that can open to allow plasma proteins and circulating leukocytes to escape from the blood [12]. Smooth muscle appears on the media of larger venules (muscular venules) that drain the postcapillary venules [10]. The organization of the venular network is similar to that of the arterioles except that venules are two to

three times wider and are somewhat more numerous than the arterioles. Furthermore, smooth muscle is more abundant on arterioles than on muscular venules. The passive, distensible nature of the post-capillary and muscular venules accounts for the ability of these microvessels to store and mobilize significant quantities of blood in certain organs, particularly tissues perfused by the splanchnic circulation.

Examples of the interorgan variation in the micro-vascular anatomy can be seen in the small and large intestine (Figs. 2 and 3). For example, the arteriolar supply from the submucosal arterial plexus passes directly to the villus tip of the small intestine where this vessel then branches at the tip of the villus into a fountain-like formation of capillaries (Fig. 2) [13, 14]. This dense plexus of subepithelial capillaries is drained by a single venule. The capillaries of the colonic mucosa, on the other hand, are arrayed in a honeycomb-like plexus or ring pattern in which each ring of capillaries surrounds the openings to the colonic crypts (Fig. 3) [13, 14].

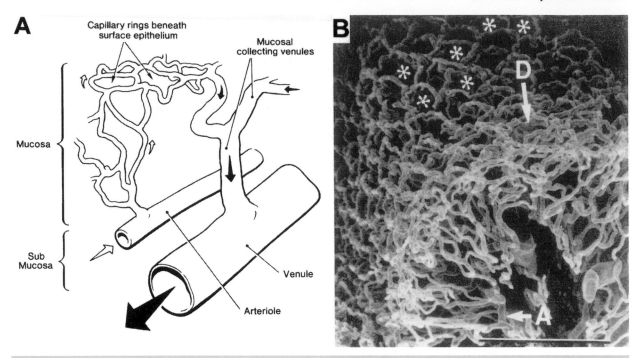

Figure 3. Microcirculatory pattern of the colonic mucosa. **A**: Capillaries nearest the mucosa are arranged in a honeycomb-like plexus of interconnecting rings in which each ring of capillaries surrounds the openings of the colonic crypts. **B**: Cast of the colonic capillary plexus illustrating the interacting rings of capillaries surrounding each colonic gland (*) (reproduced from ref. 14, with permission). Also evident is an arteriole (A) as well as the site where the mucosal drainage begins (D).

Endothelial cells and smooth muscle cells represent the major functional elements of the blood vessel wall that allow arterioles, capillaries and venules to carry out their functions. While the two cell types are clearly capable of functioning independently, there are processes that enable one cell type to influence the other. The phenomenon of endothelium-dependent vasodilation (discussed below) perhaps best exemplifies how endothelial cells can exert control over the tone of adjacent vascular smooth muscle cells through the production and liberation of vasoactive substances. There are, however, other cells that are either in contact with or adjacent to the blood vessel wall that can exert an influence on the activity of endothelial cells and/or vascular smooth muscle (VSM). Pericytes and mast cells are examples of such auxiliary cells that can exert a profound influence on the function of arterioles, capillaries and/or venules.

Pericytes are amoeba-shaped, actin-containing cells that are associated abluminally with capillaries and postcapillary venules [15]. These cells extend long, slender processes that are embedded within the basement membrane to directly contact the underlying endothelium. The density of pericytes in a vascular bed varies among tissues and between different-sized vessels. Pericytes are more numerous and have more extensive processes (more contact with endothelium) on venous capillaries and post-capillary venules. Studies on individually cultured and co-cultured (with endothelial cells) pericytes reveal an ability of these cells to contract and to produce substances that modulate the development and function of endothelial cells (and vice versa). Accordingly, pericytes have been invoked in the regulation of capillary blood flow, capillary growth, and vascular permeability, as well as precursors to VSM [15].

Mast cells are also found closely apposed to the microvasculature, particularly the postcapillary venules. These cells are exquisitely sensitive to activation by a variety of stimuli, including neuropeptides (e.g. substance P), ROS, lipid mediators (PAF, LTB4), and bacterial peptides. Upon activation, mast cells release a number of substances that can influence the function of endothelial cells and vascular smooth muscle in all segments of the microvasculature. Mast cell-derived modulators of microvascular function include histamine, adenosine, nitric oxide, cytokines (e.g. TNF, IL-1), proteases (e.g. cathepsin G), and oxidants [10, 11].

There is also evidence that propagation of electrical impulses along the endothelial cell monolayer, as well as between endothelial cells and VSM, may contribute to the coordination of microvessel responses to physiological stimuli [16]. Vasoactive agents applied directly onto capillaries have been shown to elicit dilation of upstream arterioles via a process that appears to involve electrical communication between the endothelial cells of capillaries and arterioles. Similar evidence has been presented to support the possibility of upstream propagation of an endothelial response from venules to capillaries. Measurements of intracellular potentials in endothelial cells and VSM of arterioles suggest that these cells also function as an electrical syncytium. Gap junctional tracers appear to move bidirectionally between adjacent smooth muscle or adjacent endothelial cells, as well as between endothelial cells and VSM, but not in the reverse direction. These observations indicate that the anatomical configuration of gap junctions in microvessels allows for ready communication of electrical and perhaps chemical signals among the different control elements of the microcirculation, i.e. arterioles, capillaries and venules.

Arterioles

Contribution of different-sized vessels to total vascular resistance

The profile of pressures within different segments of the microcirculation provides valuable insight into the distribution of resistances within a vascular bed, as well as the impact of a change in the caliber of specific vessels on total vascular resistance. In most tissues studied to date, it appears that vascular resistance primarily lies in arterioles with diameters less than 200 μm. Approximately 30% of basal vascular resistance in a regional circulation can be attributed to 150–250 μm diameter arterioles, with an additional 40% of the total resistance to flow generated by arterioles of smaller caliber (<150 μm) [16, 17]. Capillaries and veins account for only 25% of the total resistance. These observations support the view that a major portion of the resistance in most vascular beds is controlled by the arterioles. This characteristic imparts a dominant role for the smallest arterioles in the regulation of blood flow

under resting conditions. However, this role can be shifted toward larger arterioles as well large conducting arteries under conditions of intense vasodilation and in inflammatory diseases [16, 17]. There is also mounting evidence that the various factors that act to regulate blood flow in tissues exert their actions at discrete sites along the arterial tree. This site-specificity of microvessels' responsiveness to physiological stimuli suggests that regulatory mechanisms are not uniform throughout the vascular tree [10, 18].

Factors governing the tone of resistance microvessels

Role of endothelial cells

The resting tone of arterioles appears to result from a complex interaction of metabolic, myogenic, neurohumoral and physical (e.g. stretch or shear) signals received by the blood vessel wall. Until recently the responses of arterioles to physiological stimuli were believed to be initiated almost exclusively by signals sensed by VSM cells. There is now clear evidence that endothelial cells play an important role in maintaining vascular tone by releasing substances that modulate the delicate balance between vasodilation and vasoconstriction. An appreciation for the contribution of endothelial cells to vascular tone comes from studies demonstrating that acetylcholine dilates arterial smooth muscle only if the endothelium is intact and viable [19]. Indeed, the loss of endothelial cell integrity can result in the transformation of potent dilators (e.g. acetylcholine, substance P) to vasoconstrictors. This mechanism may also account for the asymmetrical responses of human arteries to acetylcholine; it is a dilator when applied intraluminally but a constrictor when applied abluminally.

Further investigations of the phenomenon of endothelium-dependent vasodilation have implicated a short-lived (biological half-life = 30 s) substance that resembles nitrosovasodilators in that it activates VSM cell-soluble guanylate cyclase, producing a rise in cGMP [20, 21]. Furthermore, this substance, termed endothelial-derived relaxing factor (EDRF) is inactivated by superoxide anions and protected by superoxide dismutase (SOD). Nitric oxide (NO), a potent VSM relaxant that is produced in endothelial cells through the oxidation of L-arginine by the enzyme NO synthase, is now generally recognized to be EDRF. A role for NO in modulating arteriolar tone is supported by studies employing L-arginine analogs that inhibit NO synthase as well as L-arginine supplementation to enhance NO production. For example, the NO synthase inhibitor N^G-nitro-L-arginine methyl ester (L-NAME) has been shown to constrict microvessels and to inhibit the vasodilation normally elicited by inflammation [16].

Endothelial cells produce a variety of substances, in addition to nitric oxide, that can contribute to basal vascular tone [20, 21]. Prostacyclin (PGI_2) and adenosine are both potent VSM relaxants that are produced by endothelial cells. However, endothelial cells are equally capable of producing vasoconstrictor agents, the most powerful of which is endothelin (ET). The endothelin family of vasoactive peptides (ET-1, ET-2, ET-3) can interact with receptors found on VSM (ET_A) or endothelial cells (ET_B), with the former receptors accounting for ET-induced constriction of arterioles. Angiotensin-converting enzyme (ACE) is produced by, and expressed on the luminal surface of, endothelial cells, thereby allowing these cells to make a local contribution to the powerful renin–angiotensin system. Other vasoconstrictor agents generated by endothelial cells include thromboxane A_2 and superoxide. Indeed, it has been suggested that under normal conditions a balance exists between the production of PGI_2 and TxA_2, and between NO and superoxide, which allows for the maintenance of normal arteriolar tone. Conditions that upset this balance between endothelial cell-derived vasodilators and vasoconstrictors can result in profound alterations in tissue perfusion [19].

Metabolic control

It is widely held that factors (metabolites and tissue pO_2) that are linked to oxidative metabolism may represent the most important mechanism for blood flow regulation in metabolically active tissues [22]. When metabolic activity increases, tissue pO_2 falls and metabolites accumulate in the tissue. Arterioles dilate in response to either a reduction in tissue pO_2 or upon exposure to metabolites such as adenosine. Hence, it has been proposed that the changes in tissue milieu that are associated with an increased oxygen consumption result in vasodilation and a consequent increase in blood flow, which serves to deliver more oxygen to the tissue [22].

Myogenic control

Arteriolar smooth muscle intrinsically responds to stretch by contracting and it relaxes when smooth muscle tension is reduced [22]. An extension of this phenomenon is the myogenic mechanism which enables arterioles to contract when transmural pressure is increased and relax when transmural pressure falls. This mechanism invokes a role for arteriolar wall tension, rather than blood flow, as the controlled variable in the vasculature. According to the Laplace relationship ($T = P \times r$), when intravascular pressure (P) is doubled, arteriolar radius (r) must decrease to half its initial value in order to restore tension (T) to its original value. By its nature the myogenic mechanism tends to maintain a constant intravascular pressure at the microvascular level. Myogenic responses have been demonstrated in arterioles of the intestine, heart, kidney coronary, renal, intestinal and other vascular beds.

Flow-dependent dilation

Increases in blood flow through various vascular beds is accompanied by dilation of small arteries and arterioles [18]. This response is endothelium-dependent and may be explained by the action of shear stress on endothelial cells. Increased shear stress has been shown to elicit a calcium-dependent activation of endothelial cell NO synthase and to activate phospholipase A_2. These changes likely result in an increased endothelial production of NO and PGI_2, and consequently lead to relaxation of the underlying VSM cells. A role for NO in flow-dependent dilation of isolated coronary arterioles is supported by the observation that NO synthase inhibitors abolish the response.

Spatial heterogeneity of vasoregulatory mechanisms

The technique of intravital microscopy has enabled investigators to assess the importance of each of the aforementioned regulatory mechanisms in arterial microvessels of varying sizes. These studies have revealed that different segments of the arterial tree can respond in profoundly different ways to various physiological and pharmacological stimuli. The observed patterns of vascular responsiveness indicate the following: (1) while small arteries (>200 μm diameter) do not respond to a myogenic stimulus, arterioles (<200 μm diameter) respond with powerful contractions; (2) flow-induced (endothelium-dependent) dilation is observed throughout most of the arterial tree with large arterioles exhibiting the most intense response to flow changes; (3) the responsiveness to metabolic factors increases as arterial diameter decreases, such that metabolic control is a dominant influence on the tone of terminal arterioles; and (4) there is considerable redundancy of blood flow control mechanisms within those segments of the arterial tree (arterioles) that normally contribute most to total vascular resistance. These patterns of vascular responsiveness suggest that the potent vasodilatory stimuli that accumulate in inflamed tissue would result in compensatory changes in the caliber of arterial vessels, a likely consequence of which is a blunted hyperemic response.

Arteriolar alterations associated with IBD

The vascular changes associated with IBD are often remarkable, but vary considerably and appear to be related to the severity of the inflammation. In active UC, for example, the submucosal arteries display a tortuous course and dilation and congestion of the mucosal and submucosal microvessels is often striking. Studies employing microangiography, vascular casts, and mesenteric angiography have demonstrated widened arteries and a rapid venous return, suggesting that an increase in colonic blood flow occurs with active UC [23–29]. Another frequent vascular abnormality is vasodilation of the lymph node vasculature, including vessels of the nodal medulla, paracortex, cortex and perinodal connective tissue [30].

In CD, the morphologial alterations are less uniform than those described for UC and the vascular changes show considerable variation from one patient to another. For example, angiographic examination of the small bowel in CD indicates that the degree of dilation and engorgement of ileal and colonic microvessels may be as conspicuous as in active UC, although a reduced vascularity is also commonly reported [23–25, 27, 31, 32]. In addition, in areas with mild alteration (deep lymphocytic infiltration but not ulcerative lesions of fissures), there is a distinct focal hypervascularity in the submucosa evidenced by numerous dilated arterial vessels which have a straight 'broom-like' course. The functional significance of these morphological alterations is largely unknown, although the results have been interpreted as suggesting an increase in blood flow to the inflamed tissue. Bacaneer provided the first quantitative evidence that flow was dramatically altered in different stages of UC [33]. Hulten and co-workers confirmed and extended these observations by employing an isotope washout technique to estimate regional intestinal blood flow and its intramural distribution in patients with UC and CD [26]. Their results indicate that, in patients with IBD, blood flow in affected regions may increase 2–6-fold. In addition, determination of the intramural distribution of blood flow indicated that this increase is confined largely to the mucosa–submucosal layer. Based on these observations, Hulten and associates estimated that blood flow in the inflamed colon corresponds to 25–30% of the resting cardiac output and suggested that these high flows may represent an important factor contributing to the physical deterioration often observed in these patients.

In contrast to the results obtained in active and exudative stages of UC and CD, colonic blood flow decreases below normal in the late fibrosing stage [26]. A similar pattern is observed for the ileum in patients with CD affecting this segment of the bowel. These findings correlate well with the observed reduction in vascularity in this stage of disease progression. Hulten and co-workers also correlated their blood-flow measurements with the degree of vascular dilation and engorgement and found agreement between the alterations of blood flow and vascular morphology [26]. In addition to these changes, a characteristic distension or clubbing of the villi occurs and, in a later phase, epithelial denudation and destruction of the villi. Although the mechanisms underlying these alterations in colonic blood flow are unknown, sustained overproduction of NO and/or arachidonic acid metabolites may be important.

Interstitial edema–arterioles

Interstitial edema and mucosal exudation are cardinal histopathological signs of inflammatory bowel disease [34]. All three segments of the intestinal microvasculature, i.e. arterioles, capillaries and venules, contribute to the interstitial edema associated with IBD. The arteriolar dilation that accounts for the intense hyperemia during inflammation may represent a major pathway for enhanced filtration of fluid across the walls of downstream capillaries [35, 36]. This arteriole dilation-dependent enhancement of capillary fluid filtration results from an increased capillary hydrostatic pressure. Capillary pressure (P_c) rises when arterioles dilate because a larger fraction of the prevailing arterial pressure is transmitted to the downstream capillaries. An elevated P_c alters the balance of hydrostatic and oncotic forces that govern fluid movement across capillaries. If the increment in P_c is of sufficient magnitude, the rate of fluid filtration is accelerated to an extent that produces interstitial edema, i.e. the rate of fluid entry into the mucosal or submucosal interstitium exceeds the capacity of lymphatics to drain the interstitial compartment. That capillary filtration is elevated in the intestinal vasculature during IBD is supported by reports describing increased intestinal lymph flow [37]. While the magnitude of the increase in P_c during IBD has not been determined experimentally, published reports of blood flow changes in human subjects provide some insights into this potential P_c elevation during the inflammatory response [26].

Angiographic studies in patients with UC or CD demonstrate widened splanchnic arteries [38]. However, estimates of colonic blood flow (using an isotope washout technique) in patients with inflammatory bowel disorders indicate a 2–6-fold increase in colon blood flow that is largely confined to the mucosa–submucosa layers [37]. As mentioned previously, Hulten and associates [26] have estimated that the inflamed colon, in the early 'exudative' stage, may be supplied by approximately 1500 ml/min of blood, corresponding to 25–30% of the resting cardiac output. Assuming that the decrease in colonic vascular resistance occurs predominantly at the arteriolar level, it can be estimated that microvascular pressure may rise by 10–40 mmHg. An increase in capillary pressure of this magnitude should profoundly increase the rate of capillary fluid filtration and promote a massive accumulation of interstitial fluid. Similarly, the fluid filtration that results from such a large increase in P_c should lead to disruption of the mucosal barrier and exudation of interstitial fluid into the lumen [39].

Capillaries

Role of capillaries as exchange vessels

There are several anatomical and physiological properties of a typical capillary bed that enable this segment of the microcirculation to serve as the major site of exchange of gases (O_2, CO_2), nutrients (glucose) and water between blood and parenchymal cells [10]. The numbers of capillaries, capillary luminal volume (internal diameter), as well as the dimensions and frequency of pores that pierce capillary endothelium, determine the effective surface area available for exchange across capillaries. The low red blood cell velocity and low intravascular pressure in capillaries also serve to optimize the rates of O_2

transport and fluid filtration, respectively. The capacity for pore-bound diffusion of small water-soluble nutrients (e.g. glucose) across capillaries varies according to ultrastructural classification of capillaries, with the smaller pores of continuous-type capillaries allowing lower exchange rates than capillaries of the fenestrated and discontinuous type. Nonetheless, under physiological conditions the capacity for transcapillary nutrient diffusion is several times the rate of delivery of these nutrients to the tissue by blood flow. There is a substantial organ-to-organ variability in capillary exchange parameters that reflects the specific functional and metabolic demands placed on the microvasculature by different tissues. For example, pulmonary microcirculation, with its unique role as a gas exchange membrane, has a capillary surface area that is nearly 30 times larger than the small intestine, which in turn has twice the capillary surface area of skeletal muscle (Table 1).

Table 1. Regional differences in capillary density (cm^2/g)

Organ	Capillary density (cm^2/g)
Lung	3000
Heart	500
Brain	240
Small intestine	125
Skeletal muscle	70

Modulation of functional and anatomical capillary density

Most vascular beds, including the intestine, have only a small fraction (e.g. 20–30%) of the total capillary population open for blood perfusion. Physiological stresses such as an increased metabolic demand and/or reduced blood flow in these tissues are generally associated with the recruitment of additional perfused capillaries. Consequently, the classic concept has been that alterations in functional capillary density allow for local modulation of O_2 exchange area and capillary-to-cell diffusion distances [22]. The structural element that governs the patency of exchange vessels (so-called 'precapillary sphincters') has not been clearly defined in many vascular beds. This has led to the proposal that terminal arterioles (10–15 μm diameter) regulate functional capillary density because these microvessels exhibit vasomotion (entrained fluctuations in microvessel diameter and flow) and account for only a fraction of total microvascular resistance [22]. Alternatively, local alterations in capillary lumen diameter mediated by contractile elements in or around capillaries could provide extremely fine spatial control of the number of perfused capillaries. Pericytes may represent the contractile element that mediates subtle narrowing of the capillary lumen that is sufficient to hinder the passage of red blood cells [15]. Although the structural equivalent of the 'precapillary sphincter' remains undefined, it is clear that this element exerts its influence on capillary patency by responding to sudden changes in the tissue environment (e.g. decreased oxygen tension) that necessitate an appropriate change in perfused capillary surface area.

Capillary proliferation represents another mechanism whereby tissues can compensate for chronic alterations in oxygen delivery and/or metabolic demand, and to restore organ function after injury [40]. The endothelium that lines normal capillaries is an extremely stable population of cells with very low mitotic activity; only 0.01% of endothelial cells in the body are dividing at any given time [41]. Hence, capillary growth and proliferation is rarely observed in normal adult tissues except during wound healing and cyclical events in the female reproductive cycle (ovulation, menstruation) [41]. In the presence of appropriate stimuli the process of angiogenesis (development of new blood vessels from an existing vascular network) can be initiated. Endothelial cells exposed to such stimuli first release proteases that degrade the underlying basement membrane and surrounding structural elements. The cells then migrate toward the angiogenic (chemotactic) stimulus within the extravascular space, with a concomitant proliferation of the endothelial cells lining the vessel wall to replace the previously migrated cells. The migrating and proliferating endothelial cells form cord-like structures in target tissues that later canalize to form functional vessels, that are further stabilized by surrounding pericytes. The initiation of angiogenesis is often associated with an increased capillary permeability that serves to enrich the adjacent interstitial compartment with plasma components [42].

A variety of physiological factors have been implicated in the modulation of angiogenesis (Table 2) [41, 42]. These factors have been shown to exert an influence on the angiogenic process through actions on the migration and/or proliferation of endothelial cells and/or smooth muscle cells. VEGF, one of the best-studied angiogenic factors, is produced by nor-

mal as well as many tumor cells, and can be found at elevated levels in the serum and urine of cancer patients. This angiogenic peptide increases capillary permeability and stimulates both the migration and proliferation of capillary endothelium *in vivo*. Transgenic animals with a null mutation for the VEGF gene exhibit embryonic lethality, characterized by absent or delayed endothelial cell differentiation and impaired angiogenesis. *In vitro*, VEGF is a potent and selective mitogen for endothelial cells, and this effect appears to be mediated by nitric oxide since NO synthase inhibitors block VEGF-induced endothelial cell proliferation.

Less is known about endogenous inhibitors of angiogenesis (Table 2). Thrombospondin, which is secreted by normal cells, is believed to contribute to capillary quiescence observed in healthy tissue. There is also a growing body of evidence that implicates proteolytic fragments of the extracellular matrix as inhibitors of angiogenesis. These factors may play an important role in the resolution of transitory angiogenic responses, such as wound healing.

Table 2. Modulators of capillary proliferation

Inducers	Inhibitors
Basic fibroblast growth factor (bFGF)	Thrombospondin
Vascular endothelial growth factor (VEGF)	Angiostatin*
Platelet-derived growth factor (PDGF)	Proteolytic fragments of laminin, fibronectin and collagen
Transforming growth factor-β (TGF-β)	Interleukin-12

*circulating proteolytic fragment of plasminogen

Pathological alterations in functional capillary density

Alterations in perfused capillary density have been implicated in the adaptive responses of tissues to prolonged hypoxia (e.g. exercise) and as a critical step in the pathogenesis of certain disease states (diabetes mellitus, cancer). Such alterations in capillary perfusion can result from intravascular events that lead to the acute obstruction of microvessels or from long-term changes in total capillary density that reflect either the dissolution or proliferation of capillaries. Acute capillary obstruction may result from the lodging of activated, less deformable leukocytes, endothelial cell swelling or both. Hemorrhagic shock and ischemia are conditions that exemplify the potential complications that can arise from acute capillary obstruction that results from microthrombi (aggregates of leukocytes and platelets with fibrin) that lodge within the capillary lumen, thereby preventing the flow of blood through these vessels [43]. It remains unclear whether the intense activation of leukocytes that occurs as these cells transit through inflamed tissue alters cell deformability sufficiently to cause significant capillary obstruction.

Capillary proliferation provides a mechanism for tissues to compensate for an inadequate delivery of oxygen that is associated with chronic hypoxia, ischemia and/or an increased metabolic demand. Capillary growth has been demonstrated in heart, brain and skeletal muscle during exposure to high-altitude hypoxia, and in the heart and skeletal muscles during some types of exercise [40]. The mechanisms involved in these conditions of enhanced capillary proliferation remain poorly defined, but it seems likely that the hypoxic stimulus and/or chronically elevated blood flow (via flow-dependent production of nitric oxide) contributes to the angiogenic response.

The adaptive responses to a reduced capillary density in injured tissue appear rather slow and inefficient. Dramatic increases in the expression of VEGF and its receptors on endothelial cells have been noted in experimental models of tissue injury as well as in serum and mucosa of patients with IBD [44]. Similarly, it has been shown that the concentration of basic fibroblast growth factor (bFGF) in the lumen of patients with UC is nearly 10 times higher than in control subjects [45]. There are also reports that implicate bFGF release as an important mediator of the angiogenesis and wound healing seen in pediatric CD [46]. Since exogenously administered bFGF, as well as other angiogenic factors (PDGF (platelet-derived growth factor) and VEGF,) have been shown to increase capillary density and induce vessel regrowth in different animal models of tissue injury [42], the concept 'therapeutic angiogenesis' has been proposed whereby growth factor production in damaged tissues is stimulated using drugs or gene therapy [42]. However, it remains unclear whether vascular proliferation is a rate-limiting determinant of the mucosal repair process that occurs during the healing phases of IBD.

Venules

Postcapillary venules and small venules have long been appreciated for their contribution to the capacitance function of the cardiovascular system [10].

These distensible microvessels serve as the major storage site for blood in many tissues, particularly in splanchnic organs. To certain physiological stimuli the venules respond with intense constriction, which expels the stored blood into the central circulation. This mechanism accounts in part for the ability of sympathetic activation to maintain adequate levels of cardiac output during periods of exercise or following hemorrhage.

The application of intravital videomicroscopic techniques to the field of microvascular research has led to the recognition that venules represent the major site of transvascular protein exchange (vascular permeability to plasma proteins) and leukocyte trafficking (leukocyte–endothelial cell adhesion) [9]. The localization of these inflammatory functions in venules is believed to reflect the unique characteristics of endothelial cells in this segment of the microcirculation [47]. Consequently, the literature is replete with reports that describe the responses of cultured venous endothelial cells (usually derived from human umbilical vein) to various inflammatory stimuli. These *in-vitro* studies, coupled to data derived from experiments utilizing intravital microscopy, have improved our understanding of the potential contribution of venules to the pathogenesis of certain inflammatory diseases.

Leukocyte–endothelial cell adhesion

Circulating leukocytes are recruited to sites of inflammation and tissue injury by a highly coordinated process that occurs primarily in postcapillary venules. As leukocytes exit capillaries, hemodynamic forces give rise to an outward radial movement of leukocytes toward the venular endothelium. This margination process is generally attributed to red blood cells (which normally pile up behind the larger leukocyte in capillaries) that overtake the leukocyte and tend to push it toward the venular wall. The initial adhesive interaction between the leukocyte and venular endothelium is rolling. This low-affinity (weak) interaction is subsequently strengthened such that the leukocytes attach to endothelium and remain stationary. The leukocytes are then able to migrate into the interstitium through spaces between adjacent endothelial cells. These interactions are regulated by sequential activation of different families of adhesion molecules expressed on the surface of neutrophils and endothelial cells [48] (Fig. 4).

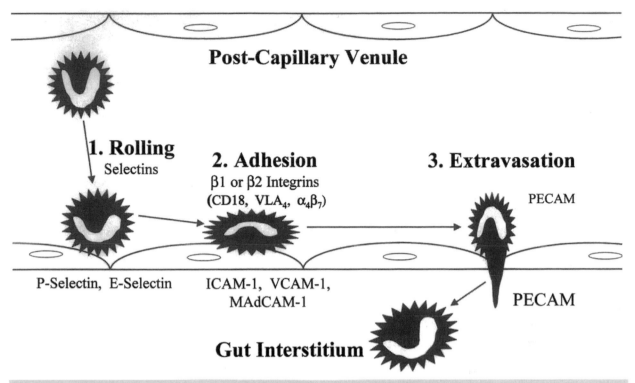

Figure 4. Leukocyte–endothelial cell interactions in the postcapillary venule. Infiltration of leukocytes into the intestinal interstitium requires the coordinated interaction of different adhesion molecules on the leukocyte and microvascular endothelial cell.

Table 3 summarizes some of the adhesion molecules expressed on the surface of endothelial cells and their respective counter-receptors on circulating leukocytes. Lectin-like adhesion glycoproteins called the selectins mediate leukocyte rolling. Both P- and E-selectin expression are increased on endothelial cells when the appropriate stimuli are present in inflamed tissue. P-selectin, which is stored in endothelial cells as a preformed pool, can be rapidly mobilized to the cell surface by stimuli such as histamine, hydrogen peroxide and leukotrienes. A slower, more prolonged (transcription-dependent) expression of P-selectin can also be demonstrated (peaking at 4 h) after cytokine or endotoxin stimulation. E-selectin, which does not exist in a preformed pool, is entirely under transcriptional regulation and requires about 3 h to reach peak expression on intestinal endothelial cells. Endothelial cell adhesion molecules that mediate firm adhesion of leukocytes include intercellular adhesion molecule-1 (ICAM1), vascular cell adhesion molecule-1 (VCAM1) and mucosal cell addressin adhesion molecule-1 (MAd-CAM1). All three of these glycoproteins are constitutively expressed on venular endothelial cells, but

Table 3. Endothelial cell adhesion molecules: ligands and functions

Adhesion molecule	Leukocyte receptors	Adhesion response
P-selectin	L-selectin PSGL-1	Rolling
E-selectin	L-selectin	Rolling
ICAM1	CD11/CD18	Adherence, emigration
VCAM1	VLA_4	Adherence, emigration
MAdCAM1	$\alpha_4\beta_7$	Adherence, emigration
PECAM	PECAM	Emigration

PSGL = P-selectin glycoprotein ligand; VLA_4= very late antigen-4.

the density of expression can be profoundly increased following challenge with cytokines or bacterial endotoxin. The expression of P-selectin, E-selectin, ICAM1, VCAM1 and MAdCAM1 on vascular endothelial cells is temporally coordinated to ensure that the processes of leukocyte rolling and firm adhesion/emigration can occur for several hours after the initiation of an inflammatory response. The importance of these endothelial cell adhesion molecules and their counter-receptors on leukocytes in different animal models of inflammation has been demonstrated using either adhesion molecule-specific blocking monoclonal antibodies (mAbs) or mice that are genetically deficient in one or more adhesion molecules [48].

There are several other factors that influence leukocyte–endothelial cell adhesion in postcapillary venules. Nitric oxide, adenosine and prostacyclin produced by endothelial cells tend to prevent adhesion, while the oxygen radicals (superoxide, hydrogen peroxide) generated by activated leukocytes and endothelial cells promote leukocyte adhesion [48]. These agents appear to exert their actions by interfering either with the production of inflammatory mediators (e.g. platelet-activating factor) that induce leukocyte adhesion or with the induction of adhesion molecule expression on endothelial cells and/or leukocytes. Auxiliary cells, such mast cells (histamine), macrophages (cytokines) and platelets (leukotrienes), also produce substances that can promote leukocyte–endothelial cell adhesion [11]. Agents that promote the accumulation of endogenous anti-adhesion molecules (e.g. nitric oxide), as well as agents that either neutralize adhesion glycoproteins (mAbs) or prevent the accumulation of proinflammatory factors (e.g. cytokines) provide therapeutic avenues for inhibition of leukocyte recruitment in postcapillary venules.

The physical forces generated by the movement (flow) of blood in the microcirculation also play an important role in the modulation of leukocyte–endothelial cell adhesion [48]. The prevailing shear rate exerted on the walls of postcapillary venules determines the level of leukocyte rolling and firm adherence, and it dictates the contact area between leukocytes and the endothelial cell surface. Even in the absence of an inflammatory stimulus, graded reductions in venular shear rate for brief periods (<2 min) elicit progressive recruitment of both rolling and firmly adherent leukocytes. Similarly, it has been noted that the number of adherent leukocytes recruited into venules by an inflammatory stimulus is inversely proportional to the wall shear rate, suggesting that it is easier for leukocytes to create strong adhesive bonds with endothelial cells at low shear rates and that high shear rates may prevent the creation of such bonds. While the higher wall shear rates experienced by endothelial cells in arterioles (compared to venules) have been invoked to explain the rarity of leukocyte adhesion in arterioles, recent evidence suggests that the leukocyte's preference for venular endothelium reflects the higher density of adhesion molecules expressed by these cells [47].

Vascular permeability to plasma proteins

Vascular endothelial cells normally serve as a barrier that minimizes the movement of fluid and proteins from blood to interstitium. When this barrier function is lost, either as a consequence of endothelial cell damage or contraction of adjacent endothelial cells, plasma proteins gain greater access to the interstitial compartment, which results in an elevated oncotic pressure and excess fluid accumulation, i.e. interstitial edema. While capillaries are the major source of fluid that is filtered into the interstitial spaces, postcapillary venules represent the major site of vascular protein leakage (extravasation) [12]. The role of venules in protein extravasation is particularly evident in inflamed tissue because the accumulated inflammatory mediators and immune cells can act on venules to diminish endothelial barrier function [12].

There are several characteristics of postcapillary venules that allow this segment of the microvasculature to regulate vascular permeability to plasma proteins. Ultrastructural analyses of the pathways for transvascular exchange have revealed that both the size and frequency of interendothelial junctions and endothelial fenestrae are higher in postcapillary venules than in either arterioles or capillaries [9]. These pathways are normally large enough to allow for a low basal level of plasma protein leakage that is driven by both diffusive and convective (coupled to fluid filtration) mechanisms. Venular endothelium also appears to possess a higher density of cell surface receptors for inflammatory mediators than their counterparts in arterioles and capillaries [12]. Engagement of certain inflammatory mediators (e.g. histamine, platelet-activating factor) with their receptors on venular endothelial cells elicit cell contraction, which results in a widening of the junctions (gaps) between adjacent endothelial cells and a consequent increase in protein extravasation. Furthermore, since postcapillary venules are the preferred site for leukocyte trafficking (due to the high density of leukocyte adhesion receptors), these endothelial cells are more frequently exposed to neutrophil products (proteases, oxidants), which can diminish barrier function, than are their counterparts in arterioles and capillaries. The process of leukocyte emigration also appears to render venular endothelial cells more vulnerable to barrier dysfunction. In some models of inflammation a strong positive correlation has been shown between venular albumin leakage and the rate of transendothelial migration of leukocytes [48].

Interstitial edema – venules

Another mechanism that could explain the interstitial edema that is associated with IBD is an increased vascular permeability. This response of the vasculature to inflammation is generally localized in the postcapillary venules, which is the normal site of plasma protein extravasation in most vascular beds. An increased vascular permeability can result from the contraction of cytoskeletal elements of venular endothelial cells which creates larger channels (pores) for protein extravasation [39]. Alternatively, endothelial cell damage and detachment to the underlying basement membrane can yield a similar reduction in endothelial barrier function. It is likely, however, that the endothelial cell contraction, mediated by the variety of inflammatory mediators that are detected in diseased tissue, is responsible for the increased vascular permeability of IBD. Histamine, serotonin, bradykinin, substance P, cytokines, and other biogenic amines that are released in the inflamed bowel can elicit endothelial cell contraction and an increased permeability [1]. The mucosal ulceration accompanying IBD allows bacterial toxins to gain access to the interstitial space, where the toxins can elicit the release of cytokines and other mediators from macrophages, and subsequently increase vascular permeability. A role for bacterial endotoxins in producing an increased vascular permeability in inflammatory bowel disease is supported by reports that approximately 50% of patients with these diseases have elevated titers of antibody to antigens derived from *Escherichia coli* or other bacteria [1, 49]. Since leukocyte infiltration is another histopathological feature of IBD, these cells may also contribute to the increased vascular permeability. There is evidence that the adhesion and emigration of leukocytes in inflamed postcapillary venules can result in an increased plasma protein extravasation

at the sites of leukocyte transendothelial migration [39]. Whether this relationship between vascular permeability and leukocyte trafficking represents physical disruption of endothelial junctions by the transmigrating leukocytes or results from the release of reactive oxygen metabolites and/or proteases from the activated adherent leukocytes, remains unclear [39].

While the magnitude and underlying mechanisms of the increased intestinal vascular permeability in IBD are poorly defined, the impact and consequences of such a leakage of plasma proteins from venules can be predicted from existing principles of capillary fluid exchange [35]. When plasma proteins accumulate in the mucosal interstitium there is a resultant increase in interstitial oncotic pressure (πt), which alters the balance of forces governing capillary fluid exchange to favor enhanced filtration. Another consequence of the diminished endothelial barrier function in inflamed venules is a greater capacity of these vessels to transport water for a given intravascular pressure. Hence, the combined effects of increased vascular pressures, resulting from arteriolar dilation, and an increased hydraulic conductance, which reflects the endothelial barrier dysfunction, likely lead to a profound enhancement of vascular fluid filtration in the inflamed bowel.

The amount of fluid that accumulates in the intestinal interstitium is determined by the balance between the rates of capillary fluid filtration and lymph flow. In CD, dilated lymphatic vessels are frequently present, and it has generally been considered that lymphatic obstruction plays a prominent part in the submucosal edema observed in the inflamed bowel [50, 51]. The results of a morphological study suggest that structural changes in the walls of lymphatic capillaries may result in a decreased permeability of these vessels that diminishes the drainage of fluid and protein from the interstitium [50]. The changes described include a lack of open intercellular junctions seen in normal lymphatics, development of a more extensive basement membrane, and accumulation of protein-rich fluid at the abluminal surface of the lymphatic capillaries. A causal role for lymphatic obstruction in the pathogenesis of IBD has been proposed based on the observation that chronic lymphatic obstruction (either surgically or with sclerosing agents) results in intestinal inflammation (including the infiltration of lymphocytes and monocytes), interstitial edema and hyperemia [50]. These changes were most marked in animals with no demonstrable reorganization of the lymphatic system (due to lymphaneogenesis) and bear some resemblance to the vascular and tissue responses seen in CD.

Endothelial cell adhesion molecule expression and leukocyte infiltration in IBD

It is well appreciated that Th1- or macrophage-derived cytokines such as IL-1β, TNF-α, lympho-toxin-α, or IL-12 promote leukocyte adhesion and extravasation *in vitro* and *in vivo* [52]. The mechanisms by which this diverse group of proinflammatory agents promote leukocyte recruitment *in vivo* are not entirely clear; however, recent data suggest that cytokine-receptor interaction transcriptionally activates the expression of certain ECAMs via NF-κB.

L-selectin of leukocytes and the P- and E-selectins of endothelial cells have been implicated as the major ECAM involved in rolling of leukocytes along the endothelium [48, 53–55]. L-selectin is constitutively expressed on quiescent PMN and lymphocytes, whereas P- and E-selectins appear only on the surface of cytokine-activated endothelium. E-selectin mobilization to the surface of the endothelial cell is stimulated by certain Th1 and/or macrophage-derived cytokines (e.g. IFN-γ, lymphotoxin, TNF-α) and maximum surface levels are achieved several hours after activation with a return to basal levels within 12–24 h. Koizumi *et al.* [56] and Nakamura *et al.* [57] have demonstrated that E-selectin is significantly upregulated on the surface of endothelial cells in mucosa obtained from patients with active but not quiescent ulcerative or Crohn's colitis. We have recently shown that colonic E-selectin expression is significantly enhanced with the onset of chronic colitis in SCID mice which have been reconstituted with CD45RB^{hi} T cells or in colons of IL-10-deficient (IL-10$^{-/-}$) mice with colitis [58–61]. One study demonstrates that two different antibodies to E-selectin did not attenuate the spontaneous colitis that develops in cottontop tamarins, suggesting that E-selectin-dependent leukocyte adhesion may not represent an important interaction to sustain the inflammatory response in this model of colitis [62]. The authors suggested that if E-selectin is not necessary to promote leukocyte migration into the colonic mucosa, then other pathways for leukocyte adhesion must exist in the inflamed colon. P-selectin, on the other hand, is rapidly mobilized to the endothelial cell surface, reaching peak levels within 10–30 min. The expression of P-selectin is very

transient, decreasing to negligible levels within minutes due to internalization of the selectin via endocytosis. Interestingly, some stimuli (e.g. reactive oxygen species, bacterial products species) can activate endothelial cells in such a manner that P-selectin expression is prolonged for several hours [63]. Nakamura *et al.* [57] and Schurmann *et al.* [64] have shown that P-selectin is up-regulated in venules of mucosa obtained from patients with active IBD. The ligands for the selectins have not been firmly established, but are thought to be Sialyl–Lewis × and other fucosylated carbohydrates [53]. A direct interaction between the selectins is also possible, i.e. PMN or lymphocyte L-selectin may interact with the P- or E-selectin on the endothelium. L-selectin has been shown to be important for PMN or lympho-cyte–endothelial rolling [65].

It is believed that the rolling of leukocytes along the venular endothelium keeps these cells in close apposition to the endothelium, thereby facilitating their activation by inflammatory mediators generated by the endothelium or interstitial cells (e.g. lymphocytes, macrophages, mast cells). For example, activated PMN (or monocytes), and to a lesser extent lymphocytes, adhere to venular endothelium (despite the shear stress of flowing blood) by virtue of the strong adhesive interactions between β₂ integrins (CD11/CD18) on these leukocytes and ICAM1 on endothelial cells.

Upon activation, PMN and lymphocytes shed their L-selectin and up-regulate and/or activate their integrins [48, 54]. The β₂ integrins on PMN are heterodimers consisting of a common subunit (CD18) non-covalently linked to one of three immunologically distinct subunits designated CD11a, CD11b and CD11c. CD11a/CD18 is basally expressed on the surface of PMN and lymphocytes and interacts with ICAM1 and ICAM2 on endothelial cells to promote adhesive interactions [66, 67]. Although it has been generally assumed that CD11/CD18-dependent adhesion is essential for mediating much of the tissue injury and dysfunction during acute flares of colitis, a recent report by D'Agata *et al.* [68] suggests that this concept may need to be reexamined. They report a case of CD11/CD18 deficiency characterized by a chronic ileocolitis in which bone marrow transplantation completely resolved the intestinal inflammation, suggesting that marrow-derived leukocyte dysfunction may contribute to disease. These data are similar to those recently reported demonstrating that four of five CD patients given allogenic marrow transplantation remained disease-free for several years post-transplantation [69].

ICAM1 and ICAM2 are endothelial cell adhesion molecules which are members of the immuno-globulin supergene family [65, 67, 70, 71]. ICAM1 is basally expressed on endothelial cells and its expression is increased in response to activation of endothelial cells with certain Th1- or macrophage-derived cytokines. ICAM2 is a truncated form of ICAM1and is also basally expressed on endothelial cells, but its level of expression is higher (10-fold) than that of ICAM1 [71]. In contrast to ICAM1, ICAM2 expression is not increased on cytokine-activated endothelial cells. Several different reports have demonstrated enhanced staining for ICAM1 on mucosal mononuclear or endothelial cells in biopsies obtained from patients with active UC and CD [57, 72, 73]. We have shown that colonic ICAM1 but not ICAM2 expression is significantly enhanced in colitic SCID mice reconstituted with CD45RB^{hi} T cells or in colons from IL-10$^{-/-}$ mice with active enterocolitis [58–61]. A recent series of experimental and clinical studies have demonstrated that infusion of an antisense oligonucleotide, directed against ICAM1 message, produces clinical improvement in a mouse model of colitis and in steroid-resistant CD patients, respectively [74, 75]. These data raise the exciting possibility that ICAM1 may represent a new therapeutic target for the treatment of IBD.

PMN–endothelial cell interactions predominate in acute flares of IBD, whereas lymphocyte, monocyte and, in some cases, eosinophil interactions with the microvascular endothelium are more prevalent during the chronic stages of gut inflammation. The mononuclear leukocytes possess a β_1 integrin called very-late activation antigen-4 (VLA-4; $\alpha_4\beta_1$) which binds to the inducible VCAM1and MAdCAM1 expressed on the surface of cytokine-activated endothelial cells. Recent studies from our laboratory demonstrate a significant enhancement in colonic VCAM1 expression with the onset of chronic colitis in the SCID/CD45RB^{hi} or IL-10$^{-/-}$ models of chronic colitis [58–60]. A great deal of interest has been generated regarding the possibility that VCAM1 may be important in promoting chronic gut inflammation however, several different laboratories have failed to consistently demonstrate enhanced expression of VCAM1 in biopsies obtained from patients with active colitis [56, 57, 72]. These observations are somewhat surprising in view of two recent reports demonstrating that primary cultures of microvascular endothelial cells

isolated from human intestine and colon respond to different proinflammatory cytokines with enhanced surface expression of VCAM1 [76, 77]. The reasons for these differences between experimental and human IBD are not known but may represent the inherent variability known to be associated with immunohistochemistry compared to the objective, more qualitative method to quantify ECAM expression *in vivo* [58–61, 78]. Alternatively, the quality of the antibodies used for the immunolocalization studies may also represent an important determinant for accurate determination of VCAM1.

Lymphocytes possess an additional ligand/counter-receptor pair which is important in cell–cell adhesion, signaling, trafficking and regulation of the immune responses in mucosal tissues, especially in the gastrointestinal tract [79, 80]. MAdCAM1 is a member of the Ig supergene family that is expressed on gastrointestinal mucosal endothelial cells and high endothelial cells in lymph nodes and Peyer's patches, and is involved in the selective homing of lymphocytes to mucosal tissue [79, 80]. Surface expression of MAdCAM1 is induced by certain Th1- or macrophage-derived cytokines and bacterial products and may last for several days [81]. Its lymphocyte-associated counter-receptor, $\alpha_4\beta_7$, is found primarily on a subpopulation of memory lymphocytes involved in mucosal immunity. Briskin *et al.* [82] recently reported that MAdCAM1 surface expression on venular endothelial cells in the lamina propria of the gut is enhanced in foci of inflammation in biopsies obtained from patients with active UC or CD. We have demonstrated that colonic and cecal but not ileal MAdCAM1 expression increases dramatically (11-fold) with the onset of colitis in the SCID/CD45RB^{hi} and IL-10$^{-/-}$ models of colitis [58, 60, 78, 81]. Three recent studies using small molecular weight antagonists or immunoneutralizing monoclonal antibodies to either $\alpha_4\beta_7$ or MAdCAM1 demonstrate that the $\alpha_4\beta_7$/MAdCAM1 interaction plays an important role in the pathophysiology in three different models of colitis [83–85]. Future studies may reveal that MAdCAM1 represents a potentially important therapeutic target for the treatment of IBD.

Once leukocytes adhere to the endothelium they send pseudopodia between endothelial cells, and migrate into the interstitium. Based on studies using blocking antibodies, PMN transmigration across endothelial cell monolayers appears to require CD18–ICAM1 interactions as well as platelet–endothelial cell adhesion molecule-1 (PECAM1)

[86]. PECAM1 is preferentially distributed between endothelial cells (intercellular junctions) and the transmigration process appears to involve homotypic adhesive interactions between PECAM1 on PMN and endothelial cells. A report by Shuermann *et al.* demonstrated a significant increase in PECAM expression on venules in mucosa obtained from patients with active UC [87]. Future work may elucidate the precise adhesive interactions involved in the transendothelial migration of PMN. Taken together, these studies suggest that the colonic and/or intestinal microvasculature regulates chronic gut inflammation by virtue of its ability to modulate the infiltration of different populations of leukocytes into the interstitium.

Extravasated PMN as well as other phagocytic leukocytes, migrate through the interstitium in response to certain chemotactic stimuli including bacterial products and proinflammatory mediators released by the inflamed and/or injured tissue, as well as by bacterial products that have made their way into the tissue from the lumen. It is probably this directed migration through the interstitium that ultimately allows the PMN to emigrate out of the tissue and into the crypt lumen to form crypt abscesses. Relatively little information is available regarding the movement of PMN through the interstitium. The interstitial matrix is composed primarily of a fibrous network of collagen, elastin and glycosaminoglycans. Depending upon the degree of hydration this matrix has been estimated to contain pores with dimensions of 250–10 Å. These estimates would suggest that PMN, even with their ability to readily deform and elongate, would enervate significant resistance to movement through the interstitial matrix. Bienvenu *et al.* [88] have shown, using intravitalmicroscopic examination of the rat mesentery, that exposure of the mesentery to the chemotactic bacterial peptide N-formyl-methionyl-leucyl-phenylalanine (FMLP), leukotriene B$_4$ (LTB$_4$), or platelet-activating factor (PAF) enhanced rates of neutrophil interstitial migration from a mean value of 3.0 μm/min in the unstimulated state to rates of 6–8 μm/min. The mechanisms by which PMN negotiate their way through this interstitial meshwork remain to be defined.

The formation of crypt abscesses represents the terminal step in PMN migration out of the circulation. In order for PMN to be present within the lumen of the crypts these inflammatory cells must not only have had to extravasate from the circulation and move through the interstitial matrix, but they must have also have had to interact with the basement membrane and basolateral surface of the crypt epithelium and emigrated out of the gut and into the lumen. The driving force for this directed migration out of the tissue into the lumen is provided by the bacterial gradient present in the distal bowel. Transendothelial as well as transepithelial migration of PMN and other leukocytes may account for some of the fluid accumulation (edema) and enhanced mucosal (i.e. epithelial) permeability observed in patients with active IBD.

Interstitial phagocytic leukocytes will interact with a variety of proinflammatory agents such as TNF-α, IL-1-β, LTB$_4$, PAF, immune complexes, complement components, or bacterial products (e.g. FMLP, lipopolysaccharide) to activate the membrane-associated NADPH oxidase located on the surface of these leukocytes [89]. Activation of this multicomponent, flavoprotein results in the production and release of large amounts of reactive oxygen metabolites including superoxide (O$_2^-$) and hydrogen peroxide (H$_2$O$_2$) as well the myeloperoxidase (MPO)-derived oxidants hypochlorous acid (HOCl) and N-chloramines (Fig. 5). Reactive oxidants may also be generated at sites of inflammation by the interaction between phagocyte-generated O$_2^-$ and the free radical nitric oxide (NO) to produce peroxynitrite (ONNO$^-$) and peroxynitrous acid (ONOOH) [90]:

$$O_2^- + NO \rightarrow ONOO^- + H^+ \rightarrow ONOOH$$

Several recent studies have demonstrated that active episodes of colonic inflammation in humans or animal models of IBD are associated with enhanced NO production [91]. In fact, NO or NO-derived metabolites may play an important role in mediating some of the pathophysiology associated with some but not all models of experimental IBD [89, 91].

Many of these reactive oxygen and nitrogen species are capable of damaging surrounding tissue directly due to their potent oxidizing activity. However, most tissue and extracellular fluids contain ample amounts of antioxidants such as ascorbate, α-tocopherol, reduced glutathione and protein-associated thiols that would effectively limit bystander tissue injury during a normal inflammatory response. However, these protective agents may be consumed during times of sustained inflammation, thereby allowing reactive oxygen and nitrogen species to damage the epithelium and mucosal interstitium either directly or by altering the finely tuned

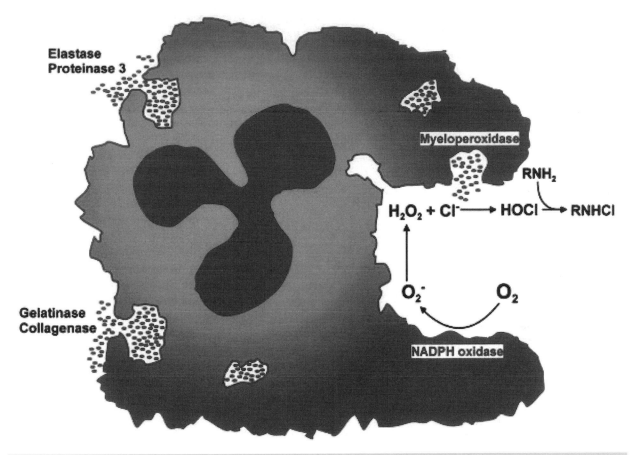

Figure 5. Oxidative metabolism of activated granulocytes (PMNs, monocytes). Activation of membrane-associated NADPH oxidase and secretion of myeloperoxidase results in the production of large amounts of superoxide (O_2^-), hydrogen peroxide (H_2O_2), hypochlorous acid (HOCl) and N-chloramines (RNHCl). In addition, acitvated PMN secrete a variety of proteinases.

proteinase/antiproteinase balance that normally exists within the intestinal interstitium. For example, HOCl (and possibly other lipophilic RNHCl and reactive nitrogen intermediates) inactivates proteinase inhibitors such as α_1-proteinase inhibitor and α_2-macroglobulin present in the extracellular fluid (plasma, lymph) thus allowing for uncontrolled proteolysis by elastase, collagenase, and/or gelatinase [92]. In addition, *in-vitro* studies suggest that the extracellular MPO system (HOCl) activates the latent collagenase and gelatinase secreted by neutrophils [92]. Taken together, these data suggest that oxidative inactivation of important proteinase inhibitors coupled to the oxidant-mediated activation of latent proteases creates an environment favorable for elastase, collagenase and gelatinase-mediated degradation of the mucosal interstitial matrix and epithelial cells.

In addition to these injurious effects of reactive oxygen and nitrogen metabolites, it is important to note that non-toxic concentrations of these oxidants have been shown to promote intestinal chloride secretion, enhance mucosal permeability and alter smooth muscle contractility [89]. Furthermore, sublethal doses of certain reactive oxygen and nitrogen species promote mutagenesis using a variety of different cell systems [89, 90]. It is not difficult to understand how the uncontrolled infiltration and activation of phagocytic leukocytes may contribute to diarrhea, mucosal ulcerations, motility disturbances and colorectal malignancies associated with IBD.

Acknowledgements

Some of this work was supported by grants from the NIH (DK47663 and DK43785), the Crohn's and Colitis Foundation of America, and the Arthritis Center of Excellence of LSU Health Sciences Center.

Reference

1. Kirsner JB. Inflammatory Bowel Disease, 5th edn. Philadelphia: Saunders, 2000.
2. Fiocchi C. Inflammatory bowel disease: etiology and pathogenesis. Gastroenterology 1998; 115: 182–2.
3. Elson CO, Cong Y, Brandwein S *et al.* Experimental models to study molecular mechanisms underlying intestinal inflammation. Ann NY Acad Sci 1998; 859: 85–95.
4. Strober W, Fuss IJ, Ehrhardt RO, Neurath M, Boirivant M, Ludviksson BR. Mucosal immunoregulation and inflammatory bowel disease: new insights from murine models of inflammation. Scand J Immunol 1998; 48: 453–8.
5. Elson CO, Sartor RB, Tennyson GS, Riddell RH. Experimental models of inflammatory bowel disease. Gastroenterology 1995; 109: 1344–67.
6. Powrie F, Leach MW, Mauze S, Menon S, Caddle LB, Coffman RL. Inhibition of Th1 responses prevents inflammatory bowel disease in scid mice reconstituted with CD45RBhi CD4$^+$ T cells. Immunity 1994; 1: 553–62.
7. Powrie F, Mauze S, Coffman RL. CD4+ T cells in the regulation of inflammatory responses in the intestine. Res Immunol 1997; 148: 576–81.
8. Powrie F, Correa-Oliveira R, Mauze S, Coffman RL. Regulatory interactions between CD45RBhigh and CD45RBlow CD4+ T cells are important for the balance between protective and pathogenic cell-mediated immunity. J Exp Med 1994; 179: 589–600.
9. Palade GE, Simionescu M, Simionescu N. Structural aspects of the permeability of the microvascular endothelium. Acta Physiol Scand 1979; 463(Suppl.): 11–32.
10. Granger DN. Physiology and pathophysiology of the microcirculation. Dialogues Cardiovasc Med 1998; 3: 123–40.
11. Kubes P, Granger DN. Leukocyte–endothelial cell interactions evoked by mast cells. Cardiovasc Res 1996; 32: 699–708.
12. Arfors KE, Rutili G, Svensjo E. Microvascular transport of macromolecules in normal and inflammatory conditions. Acta Physiol Scand 1979; 463(Suppl.): 93–103.
13. Kessel RG, Kardon RH. Tissues and Organs: A Text-Atlas of Scanning Electron Microscopy. San Francisco: W.H. Freeman, 1979.
14. Gannon, B.J., Perry, M.A. Histoanatomy and ultrastructure of vasculature of alimentary tract. In: Schultz SG, Rauner BB, Wood JD, eds. American Physiological Society – The Gastrointestinal System. Section 6. Bethesda, MD: American Physiological Society, 1989: 1301–34.
15. Hirschi KK, D'Amore PA. Pericytes in the microvasculature. Cardiovasc Res 1996; 32: 687–98.
16. Chilian WM. Coronary microcirculation in health and disease. Summary of an NHLBI workshop. Circulation 1997; 95: 522–8.
17. Laughlin MH. Endothelium-mediated control of coronary vascular tone after chronic exercise training. Med Sci Sports Exerc 1995; 27: 1135–44.
18. Jones CJ, Kuo L, Davis MJ, Chilian WM. Regulation of coronary blood flow: coordination of heterogeneous control mechanisms in vascular microdomains. Cardiovasc Res 1995; 29: 585–96.
19. Davies MG, Hagen PO. The vascular endothelium. A new horizon. Ann Surg 1993; 218: 593–609.
20. Sellke FW, Boyle EM, Jr, Verrier ED. Endothelial cell injury in cardiovascular surgery: the pathophysiology of vasomotor dysfunction. Ann Thorac Surg 1996; 62: 1222–8.
21. Drexler H. Endothelial dysfunction: clinical implications. Prog Cardiovasc Dis 1997; 39: 287–324.
22. Granger HJ, Shepherd AP, Jr. Intrinsic microvascular control of tissue oxygen delivery. Microvasc Res 1973; 5: 49–72.
23. Allen AC. A unified concept of the vascular pathogenesis of enterocolitis of varied etiology. A pathophysiologic analysis. Am J Gastroenterol 1971; 55: 347–78.
24. Brahme F, Lindstrom C. A comparative radiographic and pathological study of intestinal vaso-architecture in Crohn's disease and in ulcerative colitis. Gut 1970; 11: 928–40.
25. Erikson U, Fagerberg S, Krause U, Olding L. Angiographic studies in Crohn's disease and ulcerative colitis. Am J Roentgenol Radium Ther Nucl Med 1970; 110: 385–92.
26. Hulten L, Lindhagen J, Lundgren O, Fasth S, Ahren C. Regional intestinal blood flow in ulcerative colitis and Crohn's disease. Gastroenterology 1977; 72: 388–96.
27. Johansson H, Krause U, Olding L. Microangiographic studies in Crohn's disease and ulcerative colitis. Acta Chir Scand 1972; 138: 409–14.
28. Tsuchiya M, Miura S, Asakura H *et al.* Angiographic evaluation of vascular changes in ulcerative colitis. Angiology 1980; 31: 147–53.
29. Bolondi L, Gaiani S, Brignola C *et al.* Changes in splanchnic hemodynamics in inflammatory bowel disease. Noninvasive assessment by Doppler ultrasound flowmetry. Scand J Gastroenterol 1992; 27: 501–7.
30. Lott MF, Davies JD. Lymph node hypervascularity: haemangiomatoid lesions and pan-nodal vasodilatation. J Pathol 1983; 140: 209–19.
31. Knutson H, Lunderquist A, Lunderquist A. Vascular changes in Crohn's disease. Am J Roentgenol Radium Ther Nucl Med 1968; 103: 380–5.
32. Lunderquist A, Knutsson H. Angiography in Crohn's disease of the small bowel and colon. Am J Roentgenol Radium Ther Nucl Med 1967; 101: 338–44.
33. Bacaner MB. Quantitative measurement of regional colon blood flow in the normal and pathological human bowel. Gastroenterology 1966; 51: 764–77.
34. Kirsner JB. Inflammatory bowel disease. Considerations of etiology and pathogenesis. Am J Gastroenterol 1978; 69: 253–71.
35. Granger DN, Barrowman JA. Microcirculation of the alimentary tract. I. Physiology of transcapillary fluid and solute exchange. Gastroenterology 1983; 84: 846–68.
36. Granger DN, Barrowman JA. Microcirculation of the alimentary tract. II. Pathophysiology of edema. Gastroenterology 1983; 84: 1035–49.
37. Nicoll PA, Taylor AE. Lymph formation and flow. Annu Rev Physiol 1977; 39: 73–95.
38. Boijsen E, Hartel M. [Contrast flow rates in the superior mesenteric arterial territory]. Fortschr Geb Rontgenstr Nuklearmed 1973; 118: 491–8.
39. Johnson LR. Physiology of the Gastrointestinal Tract, 3rd edn. New York: Raven Press, 1994.
40. Hudlicka O, Brown M, Egginton S. Angiogenesis in skeletal and cardiac muscle. Physiol Rev 1992; 72: 369–417.
41. Hanahan D, Folkman J. Patterns and emerging mechanisms of the angiogenic switch during tumorigenesis. Cell 1996; 86: 353–64.
42. Waltenberger J. Modulation of growth factor action: implications for the treatment of cardiovascular diseases. Circulation 1997; 96: 4083–94.

43. Granger DN, Korthuis RJ. Physiologic mechanisms of postischemic tissue injury. Annu Rev Physiol 1995; 57: 311–32.

44. Griga T, Voigt E, Gretzer B, Brasch F, May B. Increased production of vascular endothelial growth factor by intestinal mucosa of patients with inflammatory bowel disease. Hepatogastroenterology 1999; 46: 920–3.

45. Thorn M, Raab Y, Larsson A, Gerdin B, Hallgren R. Intestinal mucosal secretion of basic fibroblast growth factor in patients with ulcerative colitis. Scand J Gastroenterol 2000; 35: 408–12.

46. Bousvaros A, Zurakowski D, Fishman SJ et al. Serum basic fibroblast growth factor in pediatric Crohn's disease. Implications for wound healing. Dig Dis Sci 1997; 42: 378–86.

47. Iigo Y, Suematsu M, Higashida T et al. Constitutive expression of ICAM-1 in rat microvascular systems analyzed by laser confocal microscopy. Am J Physiol 1997; 273: H138–47.

48. Granger DN, Kubes P. The microcirculation and inflammation: modulation of leukocyte endothelial cell adhesion. J Leuk Biol 1994; 55: 662–75.

49. Kirsner JB. Inflammatory bowel disease. Part I: Nature and pathogenesis. Dis Mon 1991; 37: 6–666.

50. Kalima TV. The structure and function of intestinal lymphatics and the influence of impaired lymph flow on the ileum of rats. Scand J Gastroenterol 1971; 10(Suppl.): 1–87.

51. Del Gaudio A, Bragaglia RB, Boschi L, Del Gaudio GA, Accorsi D. A new approach in the management of Crohn's disease: observations in 20 consecutive cases. Hepatogastroenterology 1997; 44: 1095–103.

52. Winn R, Vedder N, Ramamoorthy C, Sharar S, Harlan J. Endothelial and leukocyte adhesion molecules in inflammation and disease. Blood Coagul Fibrinolysis 1998; 9(Suppl. 2): S17–23.

53. Granger DN. Cell adhesion and migration. II. Leukocyte–endothelial cell adhesion in the digestive system. Am J Physiol 1997; 273: G982–6.

54. Panes J, Granger DN. Leukocyte–endothelial cell interactions: molecular mechanisms and implications in gastrointestinal disease. Gastroenterology 1998; 114: 1066–90.

55. Kishimoto TK, Rothlein R. Integrins, ICAMs, and selectins: role and regulation of adhesion molecules in neutrophil recruitment to inflammatory sites. Adv Pharmacol 1994; 25: 117–69.

56. Koizumi M, King N, Lobb R, Benjamin C, Podolsky DK. Expression of vascular adhesion molecules in inflammatory bowel disease. Gastroenterology 1992; 103: 840–7.

57. Nakamura S, Ohtani H, Watanabe Y et al. In situ expression of the cell adhesion molecules in inflammatory bowel disease. Evidence of immunologic activation of vascular endothelial cells. Lab Invest 1993; 69: 77–85.

58. Kawachi S, Jennings S, Panes J et al. Cytokine and endothelial cell adhesion molecule expression in interleukin-10-deficient mice. Am J Physiol Gastrointest Liver Physiol 2000; 278: G734–43.

59. Morise Z, Eppihimer M, Granger DN, Anderson DC, Grisham MB. Effects of lipopolysaccharide on endothelial cell adhesion molecule expression in interleukin-10 deficient mice. Inflammation 1999; 23: 99–110.

60. Kawachi S, Morise Z, Conner E et al. E-Selectin expression in a murine model of chronic colitis. Biochem Biophys Res Commun 2000; 268: 547–52.

61. Kawachi S, Morise Z, Jennings SR et al. Cytokine and adhesion molecule expression in SCID mice reconstituted with CD4+ T cells. Inflam Bowel Dis 2000; 6: 171–80.

62. Podolsky DK, Lobb R, King N et al. Attenuation of colitis in the cotton-top tamarin by anti-alpha 4 integrin monoclonal antibody. J Clin Invest 1993; 92: 372–80.

63. Eppihimer MJ, Wolitzky B, Anderson DC, Labow MA, Granger DN. Heterogeneity of expression. Circ Res 1996; 79: 560–69.

64. Schurmann GM, Bishop AE, Facer P et al. Increased expression of cell adhesion molecule P-selectin in active inflammatory bowel disease. Gut 1995; 36: 411–18.

65. Springer TA. Traffic signals on endothelium for lymphocyte recirculation and leukocyte emigration. Annu Rev Physiol 1995; 57: 827–72.

66. Smith CW, Marlin SD, Rothlein R, Toman C, Anderson DC. Cooperative interactions of LFA-1 and Mac-1 with intercellular adhesion molecule-1 in facilitating adherence and transendothelial migration of human neutrophils in vitro. J Clin Invest 1989; 83: 2008–17.

67. Carlos TM, Harlan JM. Membrane proteins involved in phagocyte adherence to endothelium. Immunol Rev 1990; 114: 5–28.

68. D'Agata ID, Paradis K, Chad Z, Bonny Y, Seidman E. Leucocyte adhesion deficiency presenting as a chronic ileocolitis. Gut 1996; 39: 605–8.

69. Lopez-Cubero SO, Sullivan KM, McDonald GB. Course of Crohn's disease after allogeneic marrow transplantation. Gastroenterology 1998; 114: 433–40.

70. Diamond MS, Staunton DE, Marlin SD, Springer TA. Binding of the integrin Mac-1 (CD11b/CD18) to the third immunoglobulin-like domain of ICAM-1 (CD54) and its regulation by glycosylation. Cell 1991; 65: 961–71.

71. Staunton DE, Dustin ML, Springer TA. Functional cloning of ICAM-2, a cell adhesion ligand for LFA-1 homologous to ICAM-1. Nature 1989; 339: 61–4.

72. Jones SC, Banks RE, Haidar A et al. Adhesion molecules in inflammatory bowel disease. Gut 1995; 36: 724–30.

73. Oshitani N, Campbell A, Bloom S, Kitano A, Kobayashi K, Jewell DP. Adhesion molecule expression on vascular endothelium and nitroblue tetrazolium reducing activity in human colonic mucosa. Scand J Gastroenterol 1995; 30: 915–20.

74. Bennett CF, Kornbrust D, Henry S et al. An ICAM-1 antisense oligonucleotide prevents and reverses dextran sulfate sodium-induced colitis in mice. J Pharmacol Exp Ther 1997; 280: 988–1000.

75. Yacyshyn BR, Bowen-Yacyshyn MB, Jewell L et al. A placebo-controlled trial of ICAM-1 antisense oligonucleotide in the treatment of Crohn's disease. Gastroenterology 1998; 114: 1133–42.

76. Binion DG, West GA, Ina K, Ziats NP, Emancipator SN, Fiocchi C. Enhanced leukocyte binding by intestinal microvascular endothelial cells in inflammatory bowel disease. Gastroenterology 1997; 112: 1895–907.

77. Haraldsen G, Kvale D, Lien B, Farstad IN, Brandtzaeg P. Cytokine-regulated expression of E-selectin, intercellular adhesion molecule-1 (ICAM-1), and vascular cell adhesion molecule-1 (VCAM-1) in human microvascular endothelial cells. J Immunol 1996; 156: 2558–65.

78. Kawachi S, Cockrell A, Laroux FS et al. Role of inducible nitric oxide synthase in the regulation of VCAM-1 expression in gut inflammation. Am J Physiol 1999; 277: G572-6.

79. Butcher EC, Picker LJ. Lymphocyte homing and homeostasis. Science 1996; 272: 60–6.

80. Butcher EC, Williams M, Youngman K, Rott L, Briskin M. Lymphocyte trafficking and regional immunity. Adv Immunol 1999; 72: 209–53.

81. Connor EM, Eppihimer MJ, Morise Z, Granger DN, Grisham MB. Expression of mucosal addressin cell adhesion molecule-1 (MAdCAM-1) in acute and chronic inflammation. J Leuk Biol 1999; 65: 349–55.

82. Briskin M, Winsor-Hines D, Shyjan A et al. Human mucosal addressin cell adhesion molecule-1 is preferentially ex-

pressed in intestinal tract and associated lymphoid tissue. Am J Pathol 1997; 151: 97–110.

83. Picarella D, Hurlbut P, Rottman J, Shi X, Butcher E, Ringler DJ. Monoclonal antibodies specific for beta 7 integrin and mucosal addressin cell adhesion molecule-1 (MAdCAM-1) reduce inflammation in the colon of scid mice reconstituted with CD45RBhigh CD4+ T cells. J Immunol 1997; 158: 2099–106.

84. Viney JL, Jones S, Chiu HH *et al.* Mucosal addressin cell adhesion molecule-1: a structural and functional analysis demarcates the integrin binding motif. J Immunol 1996; 157: 2488–97.

85. Hesterberg PE, Winsor-Hines D, Briskin MJ *et al.* Rapid resolution of chronic colitis in the cotton-top tamarin with an antibody to a gut-homing integrin alpha 4 beta 7. Gastroenterology 1996; 111: 1373-80.

86. Muller WA, Weigl SA, Deng X, Phillips DM. PECAM-1 is required for transendothelial migration of leukocytes. J Exp Med 1993; 178: 449–60.

87. Schuermann GM, Aber-Bishop AE, Facer P *et al.* Altered expression of cell adhesion molecules in uninvolved gut in inflammatory bowel disease. Clin Exp Immunol 1993; 94: 341–7.

88. Bienvenu K, Harris N, Granger DN. Modulation of leukocyte migration in mesenteric interstitium. Am J Physiol 1994; 267: H1573–7.

89. Grisham MB. Oxidants and free radicals in inflammatory bowel disease. Lancet 1994; 344: 859–61.

90. Beckman JS, Koppenol WH. Nitric oxide, superoxide, and peroxynitrite: the good, the bad, and ugly. Am J Physiol 1996; 271: C1424–37.

91. Grisham MB, Jourd'Heuil D, Wink DA. Nitric oxide. I. Physiological chemistry of nitric oxide and its metabolites: implications in inflammation. Am J Physiol 1999; 276: G315–21.

92. Weiss SJ. Tissue destruction by neutrophils. N Engl J Med 1989; 320: 365–76.

9 | Remission, relapse, intestinal healing and repair

MICHAEL N. GÖKE AND DANIEL K. PODOLSKY

Introduction

Preservation of structural and functional integrity of the intestinal mucosa depends on its ability to defend itself from noxious luminal agents and to effect repair when injury occurred. Coordinated healing of mucosal injury in the intestine is determined by depth of injury and dynamic balance between ongoing destructive and reparative mechanisms. Repair after intestinal injury usually involves a cascade of events: up-regulation of the immune system, leukocyte accumulation and activation, stimulation of cell migration, proliferation, and differentiation. Angiogenesis and extracellular matrix formation also contribute to mucosal tissue remodeling.

Re-establishing epithelial surface continuity is the first requirement of mucosal wound healing. This is initially accomplished by rapid migration of intestinal epithelial cells from the wound margin, a process termed restitution. Restitution prevents deeper mucosal damage and effects closure of shallow defects of the mucosal epithelium within minutes to hours, a much shorter time frame than that required for cell proliferation [1–3]. Cell migration depends on coordinated extension of lamellopodia and filopodia, formation and breaking of focal contacts at the leading edge of the cell as well as cytoskeletal-mediated retraction at the trailing edge [4, 5]. Following restitution, cell proliferation accomplishes replacement of lost epithelial cell populations.

While resealing surface epithelial continuity is a first priority, injury associated with inflammatory bowel diseases and other intestinal disorders is typically accompanied by deeper damage. The processes which reconstitute normal intestinal architecture in the context of transmural inflammatory injury remain incompletely understood. However, the heterogeneous populations of connective tissue fibroblasts, myofibroblasts and smooth muscle cells, as well as other cell types present in the intestine, also make substantial contributions to mucosal wound healing. Of note, eventual down-regulation of the inflammatory responses associated with mucosal injury is necessary to prevent pathological fibrosis which may lead to the clinical manifestations of intestinal stenosis or stricture formation.

Recent research has improved understanding of the factors regulating mucosal wound healing in the intestine. This progress has been made possible largely by use of *in-vitro* cell culture models as well as chemically and genetically induced animal models. This chapter summarizes recent advances in understanding of the regulation of mucosal repair processes as well as intrinsic protective key mechanisms essential for maintaining mucosal surface integrity and normal mucosal function in the intestine.

Factors regulating mucosal repair and protecting from injury in the intestine

Over the past several years it has become clear that the factors which play a critical role in epithelial healing after injury are essentially the same as those protecting the intestinal mucosa from damage. In a simplified view these regulatory factors can be classified as non-peptidyl factors, classic cytokines and peptide growth factors, members of the trefoil peptide family as well as extracellular matrix and integrin molecules.

Non-peptidyl factors

While the importance of polyamines for cell growth has been well recognized, these molecules are also critical for migration of intestinal epithelial cells since α-difluoromethyl-ornithine, a compound which inhibits ornithine decarboxylase, a rate-limiting enzyme in polyamine synthesis, results in depletion of polyamines, disruption of actin filaments and

Stephan R. Targan, Fergus Shanahan and Loren C. Karp (eds.), Inflammatory Bowel Disease: From Bench to Bedside, 2nd Edition, 197–209.

decreased restitution *in vitro* [6]. It has recently been shown that the polyamine putrescine is not itself essential for intestinal epithelial migration and growth, but is effective after conversion into spermidine and/or spermine [7]. Prostaglandins and short-chain fatty acids have also been shown to promote intestinal epithelial restitution [3, 8–11]. Furthermore, the products of cyclooxygenase (COX)-2 appear to be important for intestinal epithelial restitution since a selective COX-2 inhibitor significantly delayed growth factor-mediated restitution *in vitro* [12]. Moreover, COX-1 and COX-2 appear to be important for protection of the intestinal mucosa since COX-1- and COX-2-deficient mice were more susceptible to dextran sodium sulfate-induced colonic epithelial injury than wild-type mice [13]. Intestinal restitution is a pH-dependent process which appears to be optimal in a slightly alkaline milieu [6]. Rho subfamily GTPase proteins appear to play a key role in cytoskeletal reorganization processes important for epithelial cell migration during the restitution phase after injury in the intestinal mucosa [14].

Peptide growth factors and cytokines

Transforming growth factor (TGF)-α and TGF-β are both expressed in intestinal epithelial cells and differentially regulate intestinal epithelial cell growth [15–18]. TGF-α promotes and TGF-β$_1$ strongly inhibits proliferation of intestinal epithelial cells. In addition, epidermal growth factor (EGF), insulin-like growth factor (IGF)-I and -II, hepatocyte growth factor (HGF) and members of the fibroblast growth factor (FGF) family, including acidic and basic FGF as well as keratinocyte growth factor (KGF), increase intestinal epithelial cell proliferation *in vitro* and *in vivo* [19–29]. Recent reports indicate that another factor, glucagon-like peptide-2 (GLP-2) secreted by intestinal epithelia, may also regulate intestinal epithelial cell growth since it has been shown to enhance proliferation and inhibit apoptosis of intestinal epithelial cells [30, 31]. GLP-2 plasma levels have been found elevated in patients with either active Crohn's disease (CD) or ulcerative colitis (UC) [32]. In a murine indomethacin-induced enteritis model, GLP-2 significantly improved survival. GLP-2-treated mice exhibited reduced histological evidence of disease activity, fewer intestinal ulcerations, enhanced epithelial proliferation, reduced apoptosis in the crypts, and decreased myeloperoxidase activity in the small bowel [33].

Interestingly, GLP-2 also significantly reduced cytokine induction and bacteremia [33].

In contrast to predominant autocrine modulation of intestinal epithelial cell function by TGF-α and TGF-β, subepithelial myofibroblast-derived HGF may effect paracrine stimulation of intestinal epithelial cell proliferation through binding to and phosphorylation of its cognate receptor c-Met [34]. Fibroblast-derived IGF-II has also been shown to stimulate intestinal epithelial cell growth in a paracrine fashion [35].

In a mouse intestinal epithelial cell line the proinflammatory cytokine tumor necrosis factor (TNF)-α has been found to enhance proliferation at physiological concentrations and inhibit proliferation at pathological concentrations. Intestinal epithelial mitogenesis appears to be differentially regulated by the two TNF-α receptors, with the TNF-α R1 (55-kDa) receptor inhibiting proliferation and the TNF-α R2 (75-kDa) receptor stimulating proliferation [36].

An *in-vitro* assay using wounded confluent monolayers of non-transformed rat small intestinal epithelial crypt cells (IEC-6) has been a useful tool to study intestinal epithelial restitution [37]. Using the IEC-6 restitution model TGF-β$_1$ was found to enhance intestinal epithelial cell migration [37]. Addition of neutralizing anti-TGF-β antibodies to wounded monolayers suppressed the baseline migration rate, suggesting that TGF-β may indeed be an important intrinsic factor promoting intestinal epithelial restitution.

Still, other growth factors and cytokines present in the mucosa or deeper layers of the intestinal wall also modulate epithelial cell migration. TGF-α, EGF, interleukin (IL)-1β, and interferon (IFN)-γ significantly enhanced epithelial restitution [38] and increased production of bioactive TGF-β$_1$ peptide in wounded IEC-6 monolayers. In contrast, IL-6, TNF-α, platelet-derived growth factor, and the endotoxin lipopolysaccharide (LPS) did not significantly affect intestinal epithelial cell migration [38]. The observation that the stimulatory effects of TGF-α, EGF, IL-1β and IFN-γ on intestinal epithelial restitution were abrogated in the presence of neutralizing anti-TGF-β$_1$ antibodies suggests that these effects are mediated through a TGF-β$_1$-dependent pathway by increasing cellular production and secretion of bioactive TGF-β$_1$. The importance of TGF-β$_1$ was supported by the finding that TGF-β$_1$ also enhanced intestinal epithelial barrier function in a T-84 cell model as reflected by increased transepithelial electrical resistance and diminished macromolecule permeability [39]. Similarly, basic FGF, KGF and HGF all stimulated intestinal epithelial cell migration [23, 26], an effect which was independent of cell proliferation.

Increased expression of TGF-α has been found in a rat TNBS colitis model [40] and up-regulation of TGF-α binding sites has been observed in an experimental rabbit immune complex–formalin colitis model [41]. Enhanced TGF-α expression has been found in the colonic mucosa of patients with inactive UC compared to active UC, CD, or normal controls [42]. The importance of TGF-α for healing and/or protection of mucosal healing in the intestine is underscored by the observation that mice lacking TGF-α were more susceptible to dextran sodium sulphate (DSS)-induced colitis compared to wild-type mice and that intraperitoneal administration of TGF-α reduced the severity of mucosal injury in TGF-α-deficient mice [43]. Conversely, mice over-expressing TGF-α showed a reduced susceptibility to DSS-induced colitis [44]. TGF-α likely also plays a role in promoting proliferation of colonic malignant epithelial cells [45–48].

Expression of EGF in the intestine distal from the duodenum has been reported but this finding has been inconsistent. EGF has been found in goblet-like cells surrounding areas of ulceration and inflammation in the small and large bowel, while other studies did not confirm these observations [15, 40, 49, 50]. EGF is a potent mitogen; when administered orally it reduces the intestinal atrophy associated with parenteral nutrition [51, 52] and ameliorates methotrexate-induced intestinal damage [53]. The role of EGF in IBD is controversial. Intraperitoneal and subcutaneously administered EGF, but not intracolonically given EGF, has been observed to reduce the severity of TNBS-induced colitis [54, 55]. Intestinal EGF-receptor expression has also been found to be increased in TNBS colitis. The observation that only small amounts of EGF mRNA and no EGF protein are present in TNBS colitis in contrast to strong up-regulation of TGF-α mRNA and protein content [40] supports the concept that TGF-α but not EGF is the most important 'physiological' ligand for EGF-receptor in this animal model of colitis. In human IBD, EGF expression does not appear to be dramatically induced [49]. In contrast to TGF-α and EGF, the roles of EGF family members including amphiregulin, cripto, heparin-binding EGF (HB-EGF), betacellulin, and heregulin in IBD are not fully understood.

TGF-β expression is increased in patients with both UC and CD with active disease [42]. It has been been shown that increased TGF-β_1 expression precedes colitis in IL-2-deficient mice [56]. In addition to its effects on cell migration, proliferation, differentiation and extracellular matrix production, TGF-β has chemotactic proinflammatory effects. Most notably, TGF-β exerts potent immunoregulatory effects. Targeted disruption of the TGF-β_1 gene in mice results in multifocal inflammatory disease and early death [57]. Animal studies suggest a role of TGF-β in IBD. In mice with Th1 T cell-mediated colitis induced by the haptenizing reagent 2,4,6-trinitrobenzene sulfonic acid (TNBS), TGF-β-producing cells inhibit the inflammatory response and anti-TGF-β antibodies aggravate the disease [58]. Recent studies demonstrated that intestinal epithelial cell expression of TGF-β dominant negative receptor II results in decreased wound healing *in vitro* and increased susceptibility to colonic injury *in vivo* [59]. As in other organ systems TGF-β appears to be involved in the pathogenesis of intestinal fibrosis and muscle hypertrophy found in IBD [60–62]. The role of other members of the TGF-β superfamiliy in mucosal inflammation, repair, and protection in the intestine is largely unknown.

KGF (also termed FGF-7) is the most abundant member of the large FGF family in the gastrointestinal tract. KGF expression is substantially increased in mesenchymal cells in the inflamed intestine of patients with either CD or UC [63, 64]. In another study, KGF mRNA expression was observed to be greater in UC than in CD because of increased production by mucosal myofibroblasts [65]. In addition to mesenchymal cells of the intestinal mucosa, intraepithelial lymphocytes (IEL) can express KGF [66] although the amounts found in IEL in inflamed IBD tissue appear to be low [67]. In a rat TNBS colitis model, intraperitoneal administration of KGF after but not before induction of colitis significantly ameliorated tissue damage [68]. Recently, it has been reported that oral administration of KGF resulted in a significant reduction of mucosal injury in DSS-induced colitis in mice [69]. Intraperitoneal and subcutaneous KGF-2 (syn. FGF-10) reduced mortality and weight loss and improved histology and stool scores [70]. The expression and functional role of other members of the FGF family in IBD is still not characterized [29].

Increased IGF-I expression has been found in several animal colitis and injury models and administration of IGF-I reduced the severity of colitis [29,

71–73]. In pediatric CD patients, reduced IGF-I serum concentrations have been found in active disease, while serum levels increased with corticosteroid treatment [74]. Besides its wound healing promoting effects, IGF-I increases type I collagen synthesis in rat intestinal smooth muscle cells [75]. Interestingly, IGF-I was detected in intestinal lavage fluid in a high percentage of CD patients with strictures, while IGF-I was found in only a few patients without strictures [76]. In addition to IGF-I, fibroblast-derived IGF-II may also play a role in IBD. However, its role still remains to be defined.

Although it appears plausible that HGF also plays a role in protection and repair of the intestinal epithelium, its role in IBD is largely unknown. Few data are available concerning expression of HGF and its receptor, c-met, in IBD [49, 77]. Increased blood levels of HGF have been detected in mice after acetic acid-induced colitis and in active UC [78, 79].

Recent studies have yielded some insights into the intracellular signaling pathways controlling growth factor-mediated epithelial wound healing in the intestine. Mitogen-activated protein (MAP) kinase pathways have been recognized as a major signaling system by which cells transduce extracellular signals. Several distinct MAP kinase cascades have been identified [80–87]. Among the extracellular signal-regulated Erk-, c-Jun- and p38-kinase pathways, Erk-1 and Erk-2 are known to be activated by growth factors, including TGF-α, EGF, TGF-β, FGF and HGF. Erk-1/-2 kinases are activated by MAP kinase kinase 1 (MEK-1) through Ras or Raf dependent mechanisms [80, 81, 87]. Subsequently, Erk-1 and Erk-2 phosphorylate various downstream substrates including ternary complex factor-1/Elk, fos, and early growth response-1 (Egr-1) nuclear phosphoprotein resulting in activation of transcription factors that control cellular growth, differentiation, transformation and development. Since several growth factors promoting epithelial wound repair, including TGF-α, EGF, HGF and TGF-β, activate both Erk-1 and Erk-2 MAP kinases, repair mechanisms after intestinal epithelial wounding may be mediated by activation of MAP kinase signal transduction pathways. In the IEC-6 *in-vitro* wound assay a rapid increase of Erk-1 and Erk-2 tyrosine phosphorylation as well as kinase activity was observed after wounding [88]. Erk-1 and Erk-2 kinase activation was mediated by a paracrine mechanism in part by TGF-α. Wounding of immortalized mouse intestinal epithelial cells results in a rapid increase in tyrosine phosphorylation of the EGF-receptor

(EGF-R), the receptor for EGF and TGF-α [89]. Increased phosphorylation of phospholipase C-γ_1 appears to be essential for EGF-EGF-R-mediated signaling after injury [89]. Increased EGF-R phosphorylation and Erk-1/Erk-2 activity have also been observed in the mucosa during gastric ulcer healing in rats *in vivo* [90]. In addition to TGF-α mediated Erk-1/-2 activation in association with increased proliferation of intestinal epithelial cells after wounding, MAP kinase activation may be involved in mediating the effects of other protective peptide growth factors including HGF. HGF ('scatter factor') binds to its receptor c-Met, resulting in activation of Erk-1 and Erk-2 MAP kinases in HT-29 model colon epithelial cells [91] and HGF-induced scattering of HT29 cells was blocked by a MEK-1 inhibitor. The importance of Erk-1/-2 MAP kinases in epithelial wound healing in the intestine is consistent with increased Erk-1/-2 activation and enhanced fos and early growth response-1 (Egr-1) nuclear phosphoprotein mRNA expression in wounded IEC-6 cells [92]. Addition of the MAP kinase inhibitor PD98959 inhibited Erk activity in a dose-dependent manner and substantially blocked restitution. Restitution was also inhibited after transfection of IEC-6 cells with a dominant negative Egr-1 construct [92]. Collectively, these data indicate that MAP kinase activation and the resulting downstream events are pivotal for cell migration in the restitution phase after intestinal epithelial injury *in vitro* in addition to their effects on proliferation. Full elucidation of the intracellular signaling and transcriptional events downstream of Erk MAP kinases after mucosal injury in the intestine is still needed. Better understanding of these processes may provide the basis for pharmacological modulation of intestinal epithelial restitution and proliferation in intestinal diseases characterized by epithelial defects.

In addition to Erk-1/Erk-2 activation, disruption of intestinal epithelial cell monolayers also activates c-Jun-N-terminal protein kinase-1 (JNK-1) and p38 MAP kinases [88, 93]. The role of these signaling events in intestinal epithelial wound healing remains to be clarified.

Trefoil peptides

Trefoil peptides encompass a family of several proteins composed of the intestinal trefoil factor (ITF) and the gastric peptides SP (previously termed spasmolytic polypeptide) and pS2 [94], also designated TFF-3, -2, and -1, respectively. These small [7–12 kDa] proteins are abundantly expressed by specialized mucus-producing cells throughout the gastrointestinal tract in a regional selective manner. They are secreted onto the gastrointestinal mucosal surface. pS2 expression is found in mucin-secreting cells of the proximal stomach, and human SP is expressed in the distal stomach and biliary tree. ITF is secreted by goblet cells of the small and large intestine. Trefoil peptides share a distinctive motif of six cysteine residues, designated trefoil domain, which leads to formation of three intrachain loops through disulfide bonding. Trefoil peptides are resistant to both acidic and enzymatic degradation.

In-vitro and *in-vivo* studies have demonstrated that trefoil peptides play an essential role in repair after gastrointestinal mucosal injury. Addition of trefoil proteins to wounded monolayers of intestinal epithelial cells increases restitution *in vitro* [95]. In contrast to cytokine-mediated stimulation of intestinal epithelial cell restitution, trefoil peptide stimulation of intestinal epithelial restitution was not associated with significant changes in production of bioactive TGF-β_1 and was not affected by neutralizing anti-TGF-β antibodies. These observations indicate that trefoil factors found at the apical surface of the gastrointestinal epithelium exert their effects through a pathway distinct from that used by growth factors and cytokines which may act at the basolateral cell surface of the epithelial monolayer. The essential role of trefoil peptides in repair of gastrointestinal mucosal injury is underscored by the absence of colonic epithelial restitution in mice made ITF deficient by targeted gene deletion [96] despite the presence of all other peptides which enhance restitution *in vitro*.

The mechanisms through which trefoil peptides promote intestinal epithelial restitution is incompletely understood. ITF stimulates rapid tyrosine phosphorylation of beta-catenin, reduces membranous E-cadherin expression and effects perturbation of intercellular adhesion in HT29 cells [97] which may facilitate cell motility by dissociating cells from attachment to adjacent cells. The inference that E-cadherin modulates repair functions in the intestinal epithelium is supported by observations made in mice expressing increased E-cadherin in the intestinal epithelium under the control of a fatty-acid binding protein gene promoter [98]. In these mice, epithelial cell proliferation was suppressed and apoptosis increased in the crypt and cell movement up the villus was slowed. Although anchored epithelial cells are generally protected from apoptosis by maintenance of cell–matrix and cell–cell interactions [99, 100], epithelial detachment normally results in apoptosis (anoikis). Since epithelial restitution after injury involves detachment of cells from cell–substratum and cell–cell contacts, mechanisms preventing programmed cell death must exist *in vivo*. It is of interest that recent studies demonstrated that either endogenous or exogenous ITF can prevent p53-dependent and p53-independent apoptosis in transformed and non-transformed intestinal epithelial cell lines [101]. This effect was abrogated by wortmannin and tyrphostin A25, indicating the potential involvement of phosphatidylinositol-3-kinase and EGF-R activation.

Several *in-vitro* and *in-vivo* studies have shown that mammalian trefoil peptides not only promote restitution but can also protect the gastrointestinal epithelium from a variety of noxious agents, including bacterial toxins, chemicals and drugs [102–105]. In studies with T-84 colon epithelial cells which form tight polarized monolayers, addition of trefoil factors alone resulted in as much as 50% attenuation of damage to monolayer integrity from various forms of injury [102]. Up to 95% protection was achieved when trefoil peptides were added together with mucin glycoproteins.

Trefoil peptides also exert substantial mucosal protective effects *in vivo*. Oral recombinant human SP and ITF markedly protected against both ethanol- and indomethacin-induced gastric injury in rats [103]. The functional importance of ITF is underscored by the effects of ITF observed in animal colitis models. In ITF null mice, topical administration of recombinant ITF diminished the extent of acetic acid-induced colitis and improved healing [96]. Recent observations indicate that exogenous ITF decreases chemotherapy- and radiotherapy-induced intestinal mucositis in ITF-null mice [104]. Furthermore, overexpression of another trefoil factor (pS2) in mice resulted in decreased susceptibility to NSAID-induced mucosal damage [105].

In the gastrointestinal tract, production of trefoil peptides is markedly enhanced in close proximity to sites of ulceration, irrespective of the nature of the underlying injury. Increased trefoil peptide expression has been observed in animal models of colitis as well as in the mucosa of patients with IBD adjacent to sites of ulceration. Enhanced trefoil peptide expression has been observed during initial periods of mucosal healing and in association with, or prior to, EGF or TGF-α [106–108]. Up-regulation of trefoil peptides at sites of ulceration is not confined to the specific trefoil peptide normally present in that region of the gastrointestinal tract but all three may be induced [109]. In gastric epithelial cell lines, trefoil peptides were capable of auto- and cross-induction. Trefoil-mediated transcriptional cross-regulation requires activation of the Ras/MEK/MAP kinase signal transduction pathway and EGF receptor activation. The latter is reflected by tyrosine phosphorylation of EGF-receptor after trefoil peptide stimulation [109]. Since EGF receptor expression is itself strongly induced after mucosal damage, the trefoil/EGF receptor relationship may play a key role in generating and maintaining mucosal repair.

Neuropeptides including somatostatin and vasoactive intestinal polypeptide, as well as the synthetic acetylcholine homolog, carbachol, stimulate ITF mRNA expression [110], while cytokines, arachidonic acid metabolites, and growth factors with the exception of keratinocyte growth factor have generally not been found to regulate ITF production by the HT-29 colon cancer epithelial cell line. This suggests that enteric neurons may contribute to mucosal wound healing by release of neuropeptides which increase trefoil peptide synthesis and secretion.

The presence of trefoil peptides in goblet cells and surface gel of the gastrointestinal tract [94, 111, 112] and the observation that characteristic trefoil peptide domains are integral parts of frog integumentary mucins [113, 114] led to speculation that trefoil peptides may link mucins and modulate production, stability or function of mucus. This concept is supported by the finding of increased viscosity of mucin preparations in the presence of SP and ITF [94] and absent gastric antral mucus in pS2 null mice [115]. Furthermore, studies using intestinal epithelial model cell lines demonstrated that the protective as well as the restitution-promoting effects of SP and ITF are enhanced by the concurrent presence of mucin glycoproteins [95, 102]. Use of the yeast two-hybrid system in order to identify trefoil peptide-interacting proteins by screening stomach and duodenum expression cDNA libraries has recently demonstrated that pS2 interacts with cysteine-rich domains of mucins MUC2 and MUC5AC providing confirmation of the concept of an interaction between trefoil factors and mucin glycoproteins [116].

In addition to functions on gastrointestinal epithelia, a recent report described SP and ITF expression in rat lymphoid tissues [117]. In rat spleen, increased trefoil peptide expression was found after stimulation with LPS. Furthermore, SP and ITF both stimulated migration of monocytes [117]. These data indicate that trefoil peptides may also be involved in the immunological response following tissue injury. Intrarectal application of SP not only accelerated healing but also reduced local inflammation in a rat model of colitis induced by intracolonic administration of dinitrobenzene sulphonic acid [118]. A still-unresolved question is whether trefoil peptides modulate growth of gastrointestinal epithelia and whether they play a role in the development and progression of colon cancer [95, 96, 115, 119–122].

Extracellular matrix (ECM) molecules

It is known that epithelial cell adhesion, proliferation, morphogenesis, and differentiation of intestinal epithelial cells are modulated by ECM [123–129]. Basement membranes are composed predominantly of laminin, type IV collagen, nidogen/entactin, and heparan sulfate proteoglycans [130]. In addition, fibronectin has been found in the basement membrane of the intestine. Small amounts of fibronectin have been detected in adult intestinal basement membranes underlying villi [131, 132], while abundant expression has been found in crypt basement membranes [132]. Although intestinal fibroblasts are presumed to be the principal source of the basement membrane in the intestine, intestinal epithelial cells have also been shown to contribute to basement membrane synthesis. Non-transformed rat intestinal crypt epithelial cells express fibronectin, laminin β_1 and laminin γ_1 transcripts and proteins as well as low levels of collagen IV (α_1/α_2), but not laminin α_1 [133]. Epithelial–mesenchymal interactions are thought to be important in formation of a complete basement membrane in the intestine [134–136].

Basement membrane turnover studies suggest that intestinal epithelial cells migrate over the basement membrane and that synchronous migration of epithelium, basement membrane, and mesenchyme as a unit from crypt to villus tip does not occur [137]. RGD peptides which specifically compete with the major cell attachment site on fibronectin strongly inhibit restitution of wounded IEC-6 monolayers [133], consistent with effects of fibronectin on other epithelial cell populations [138, 139]. Among ECM components, collagens type I, and especially types III and IV, also appear to stimulate intestinal epithelial restitution [133, 140, 141]. In contrast, neutralizing anti-laminin antisera had no significant effect on restitution [133]. Collectively, these observations support the concept that fibronectin and collagens type I, III and IV but not laminin promote intestinal epithelial cell restitution.

In the context of the apparent importance of the ECM for intestinal epithelial restitution, it is noteworthy that TGF-β_1 stimulates ECM expression by intestinal epithelial cells as well as mesenchymal cells [133]. Thus TGF-β may mediate its restitution-enhancing effects, at least in part, through enhanced expression of fibronectin and collagen type IV, and perhaps other ECM components in intestinal epithelial cells. Although heterotrimeric laminin ($\alpha_1/\beta_1/\gamma_1$) does not appear to play a significant role in restitution, it may contribute to other processes involved in tissue repair, e.g. differentiation and organization of intestinal epithelial cells as reported in model small intestinal and colonic epithelial cell lines (IEC-6, Caco-2) and fetal intestinal epithelial cells in vitro [123–125, 129]. The functional effects of other intestinal basement membrane components (e.g. entactin/nidogen and heparan sulfate) in intestinal epithelial homeostasis needs to be defined by future studies. The proteoglycan perlecan is a potent inducer of high-affinity basic FGF binding to its receptor to promote its bioactivities [142–145] and collagens in the liver ECM bind HGF [146], suggesting that ECM molecules may exert an even broader range of functional effects in mucosal (patho)physiology.

ECM is degraded by a family of Zn^{2+}-dependent matrix metalloproteinases (MMP) proteolytic enzymes which are inhibited by tissue inhibitors of metalloproteinases (TIMP) [147]. Expression of MMP-1, -2, -3, -9, -10, -12, and -13 as well as TIMP-1 and TIMP-3 is increased in involved intestinal mucosa of patients with UC and CD [147–150]. It is of interest that a recent report indicates that orally given marimastat, a broad-spectrum matrix metalloproteinase inhibitor, significantly reduced tissue injury and inflammation in the rat TNBS colitis model [151].

Regulation of mucosal repair by subepithelial cell populations and development of fibrosis

Lamina propria cell populations are present in close proximity to the epithelium [152, 153]. Despite increasing knowledge concerning the effects of regulatory factors, there is currently still limited information available on regulation of epithelial wound healing by subepithelial cell populations in the intestinal wall. In addition to the 'indirect' effects of subepithelial cell populations on surface repair mediated by production of soluble factors and ECM molecules, these cells may also have direct involvement through numerous discrete, uniformly distributed pores of 0.2–3.3 μm in the intestinal basement membrane of the small and large intestine [154]. In vitro studies have demonstrated that various lamina propria cells can migrate through pores and tunnels of the intestinal basement membrane [154–156].

Intestinal myofibroblasts encompass a family of heterogeneous cells which serve as integral components of a complex network of immune and non-immune cells in the intestinal mucosa. For many years intestinal fibroblasts have been viewed as purely structural elements of the intestinal mucosa responsible for production and deposition of ECM molecules. However, recent data indicate a substantially broader spectrum of mesenchymal cell function [34, 157, 158]. In addition to bidirectional effects on other subepithelial cells of the intestinal wall, they modulate epithelial repair. These cells may promote intestinal epithelial restitution by release of several peptide growth factors including HGF and IGF-II as described, and both by TGF-β and FGF. All of these growth factors except TGF-β enhance proliferation of intestinal epithelial cells.

While ECM contributes to re-establishing surface epithelial continuity and reconstruction of normal mucosal architecture after transmural intestinal injury, excessive ECM production may result in pathological fibrosis and scarring. Reports have demonstrated increased collagen content and relative amounts of type III and V collagens in intestinal strictures of patients with CD [159]. These changes were associated with typical thickening of the bowel wall and increased proliferation of smooth muscle cells. Increased collagen type III synthesis has been documented in fibroblasts isolated from strictures of patients with CD [160]. Increased collagen production has also been observed in intestinal smooth muscle cells of IBD patients [161]. Human intestinal mucosal mesenchymal cells (muscularis mucosae cells and fibroblasts) proliferate in response to proinflammatory cytokines IL-1β, IL-6, and TNF-α [162, 163]. Moreover, stimulation of intestinal mucosal mesenchymal cells with proinflammatory cytokines resulted in increased mRNA encoding their proinflammatory gene products [162]. Therefore, intestinal mucosal mesenchymal cell populations may not only facilitate mucosal healing and intestinal tissue remodeling by release of growth factors and ECM production, they may also amplify intestinal inflammation by increased expression of proinflammatory cytokines and increased proliferation which may eventually result in excessive fibrosis and scarring. Increased IGF-I and TGF-β expression in IBD mucosa may further stimulate myofibroblast and smooth muscle cell proliferation and production of ECM, most notably collagens. Recent observations suggest that intestinal subepithelial myofibroblasts in different regions of the intestine exhibit distinct phenotypes. For example, myofibroblasts isolated from the distal ileum and colon differ in their relative

expression of HGF and TGF-β [164]. While TGF-β is the predominant product of myofibroblasts from the distal ileum, HGF was the predominant factor expressed by colonic myofibroblasts. Parallel differences in the ability of myofibroblasts to support epithelial cell growth were observed. Myofibroblasts expressing more HGF were more effective in promoting epithelial growth, while those myofibroblasts expressing more TGF-β did not support epithelial cell growth. However, the latter myofibroblasts may stimulate cellular extracellular matrix (ECM) production more effectively.

Summary and perspectives

Wound healing after intestinal injury is regulated by a variety of factors, including non-peptidyl factors, cytokines and growth factors, members of the recently identified trefoil peptide family, and extracellular matrix molecules. It is likely that MMP and TIMP also contribute to mucosal protection and modulate tissue repair in IBD. Furthermore, other molecules may be pivotal for regulation of mucosal

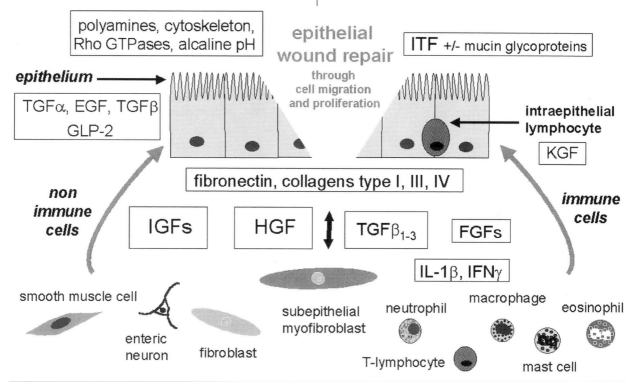

Figure 1. Healing of the intestinal epithelium is regulated by cytokines, growth factors and trefoil peptides as well as ECM molecules and non-peptidyl factors. While intestinal myofibroblasts appear to be important for epithelial repair, the roles of many other subepithelial populations still need to be defined.

wound healing in the intestine, e.g. activin A, another member of the TGF-β superfamily [165], connective tissue growth factor [166] and growth hormone [167] as well as molecules regulating the cytoskeleton including the focal adhesion-associated molecule PTEN [168] may modulate mucosal wound repair. Reduced mucosal wound healing in the intestine of telomerase-deficient mice suggests that cell aging and telomerase may have an impact on these processes [169]. A complete understanding of transcription factors which orchestrate proinflammatory or immunoregulatory cytokine responses in IBD mucosa is also essential. In addition to the identification and characterization of new factors regulating mucosal homeostasis and wound repair in the intestine, future efforts may delineate contributions of intraepithelial lymphocytes [170] and subepithelial cell populations [171] on mucosal integrity and repair, including lamina propria lymphocytes, mononuclear cells, mast cells, eosinophils and enteric neurons (see Fig. 1). While inflammation may be a response of the intestine to initiate mucosal healing after injury, eventual down-regulation of the inflammatory process is necessary in order to prevent development of pathological fibrosis. Better understanding of these processes, i.e. the responsible cell types and key regulatory molecules as well as the timing for these on/off processes, should allow modulation to assure reconstitution of normal physiological structure, and with that an opportunity to remove continued stimulation of inflammatory injury by the complex milieu of luminal agents.

References

1. Silen W. Gastric mucosal defense and repair. In: Johnson LR, ed. Physiology of the Gastrointestinal Tract, 2nd edn. New York: Raven Press, 1987: 1055–69.
2. Göke M, Podolsky DK. Regulation of the mucosal epithelial barrier. Baillière's Clin Gastroenterol 1996; 10: 393–405.
3. Wilson AJ, Gibson PR. Epithelial migration in the colon: filling in the gaps. Clin Sci 1997; 93: 97–108.
4. Gumbiner BM. Cell adhesion: the molecular basis of tissue architecture and morphogenesis. Cell 1996; 84: 345–57.
5. Mitchison TJ, Cramer LP. Actin-based cell motility and cell locomotion. Cell 1996; 84: 371–9.
6. McCormack SA, Viar MJ, Johnson LR. Migration of IEC-6 cells: a model for mucosal healing. Am J Physiol 1992; 263: G426–35.
7. Yuan Q, Viar MJ, Ray RM, Johnson LR. Putrescine does not support the migration and growth of IEC-6 cells. Am J Physiol 2000; 278: G49–56.
8. Zushi S, Shinomura Y, Kiyohara T et al. Role of prostaglandins in intestinal epithelial restitution stimulated by growth factors. Am J Physiol 1996; 270: G757–62.
9. Blikslager AT, Roberts MC, Rhoads JM, Argenzio RA. Prostaglandins I2 and E2 have a synergistic role in rescuing epithelial barrier function in porcine ileum. J Clin Invest 1997; 100: 1928–33.
10. Wilson AJ, Gibson PR. Short-chain fatty acids promote the migration of colonic epithelial cells *in vitro*. Gastroenterology 1997; 113: 487–96.
11. Ruthig DJ, Meckling-Gill KA. Both (n-3) and (n-6) fatty acids stimulate wound healing in the rat intestinal epithelial cell line, IEC-6. J Nutr 1999; 129: 1791–8.
12. Horie-Sakata K, Shimada T, Hiraishi H, Terano A. Role of cyclooxygenase 2 in hepatocyte growth factor-mediated gastric epithelial restitution. J Clin Gastroenterol 1998; 27(Suppl. 1): S40–6.
13. Morteau O, Morham SG, Sellon R et al. Impaired mucosal defense to acute colonic injury in mice lacking cyclooxygenase-1 or cyclooxygenase-2. J Clin Invest 2000; 105: 469–78.
14. Santos MF, McCormack SA, Guo Z et al. Rho proteins play a critical role in cell migration during the early phase of mucosal restitution. J Clin Invest 1997; 100: 216–25.
15. Koyama S, Podolsky DK. Differential expression of transforming growth factors α and β in rat intestinal epithelial cells. J Clin Invest 1989; 83: 1768–73.
16. Kurokawa M, Lynch K, Podolsky DK. Effects of growth factors on an intestinal epithelial cell line: transforming growth factor β inhibits proliferation and stimulates differentiation. Biochem Biophys Res Commun 1987; 42: 775–82.
17. Podolsky DK, Babyatsky MW. Growth and development of the gastrointestinal tract. In: Yamada T, ed. Textbook of Gastroenterology, 2nd edn. Philadelphia: JB Lippincott,1995: 546–77.
18. Suemori S, Ciacci C, Podolsky DK. Regulation of transforming growth factor expression in rat intestinal epithelial cell lines. J Clin Invest 1991; 87: 2216–221.
19. Ohneda K, Ulshen MH, Fuller CR, D'Ercole AJ, Lund PK. Enhanced growth of small bowel in transgenic mice expressing human insulin-like growth factor I. Gastroenterology 1997; 112: 444–54.
20. Guo YS, Narayan S, Yallampalli C, Singh P. Characterization of insulin-like growth factor I receptors in human colon cancer. Gastroenterology 1992; 102: 1101–8.
21. Park JHY, McCusker RH, Vanderhoof JA, Mohammadpour H, Harty RF, MacDonald RG. Secretion of insulin-like growth factor II (IGF-II) and IGF-binding protein-2 by intestinal epithelial (IEC-6) cells: implications for autocrine growth regulation. Endocrinology 1992; 131: 1359–68.
22. Steeb CB, Trahair JF, Read LC. Administration of insulin-like growth factor-I (IGF-I) peptides for three days stimulates proliferation of the small intestinal epithelium in rats. Gut 1995; 37: 630–8.
23. Dignass AU, Lynch-Devaney K, Podolsky DK. Hepatocyte growth factor/scatter factor modulates intestinal epithelial proliferation and migration. Biochem Biophys Res Commun 1994; 202: 701–9.
24. Fukamachi H, Ichinose M, Tsukada S et al. Hepatocyte growth factor region specifically stimulates gastrointestinal epithelial growth in primary culture. Biochem Biophys Res Commun 1994; 205: 1445–51.
25. Göke M, Kanai M, Podolsky DK. Intestinal fibroblasts regulate intestinal epithelial cell proliferation via hepatocyte growth factor. Am J Physiol 1998; 274: G809–18.
26. Dignass AU, Tsunekawa S, Podolsky DK. Fibroblast growth factors modulate intestinal epithelial cell growth and migration. Gastroenterology 1994; 106: 1254–62.
27. Housley RM, Morris CF, Boyle W et al. Keratinocyte growth factor induces proliferation of hepatocytes and epithelial cells throughout the rat gastrointestinal tract. J Clin Invest 1994; 94: 1764–77.
28. Potten CS, Owen G, Hewitt D et al. Stimulation and inhibition of proliferation in the small intestinal crypts of

the mouse after *in-vivo* administration of growth factors. Gut 1995; 36: 864–73.

29. Beck PL, Podolsky DK. Growth factors in inflammatory bowel disease. Inflam Bowel Dis 1999; 5: 44–60.

30. Tsai CH, Hill M, Asa SL, Brubaker PL, Drucker DJ. Intestinal growth-promoting properties of glucagon-like peptide-2 in mice. Am J Physiol 1997; 273: E77–84.

31. Brubaker PL, Izzo A, Hill M, Drucker DJ. Intestinal function in mice with small bowel growth induced by glucagon-like peptide-2. Am J Physiol 1997; 272: G559–63.

32. Xiao Q, Boushey RP, Cino M, Drucker DJ, Brubaker PL. Circulating levels of glucagon-like peptide-2 in human subjects with inflammatory bowel disease. Am J Physiol Regul Integr Comp Physiol 2000; 278: R1057–63.

33. Boushey RP, Yusta B, Drucker DJ. Glucagon-like peptide 2 decreases mortality and reduces the severity of indomethacin-induced murine enteritis. Am J Physiol 1999; 277: E937–47.

34. Göke M, Kanai M, Podolsky DK. Intestinal fibroblasts regulate intestinal epithelial cell proliferation via hepatocyte growth factor. Am J Physiol 1998; 274: G809–18.

35. Simmons JG, Pucilowska JB, Lund PK. Autocrine and paracrine actions of intestinal fibroblast-derived insulin-like growth factors. Am J Physiol 1999; 276: G817–27.

36. Kaiser GC, Polk DB. Tumor necrosis factor alpha regulates proliferation in a mouse intestinal cell line. Gastroenterology 1997; 112: 1231–40.

37. Ciacci C, Lind SE, Podolsky DK. Transforming growth factor β regulation of migration in wounded rat intestinal epithelial monolayers. Gastroenterology 1993; 105: 93–101.

38. Dignass AU, Podolsky DK. Cytokine modulation of intestinal epithelial cell restitution: central role of transforming growth factor β. Gastroenterology 1993; 105: 1323–32.

39. Planchon SM, Martins CAP, Guerrant RL, Roche JK. Regulation of intestinal epithelial barrier function by TGF-β_1. J Immunol 1994; 153: 5730–9.

40. Hoffmann P, Zeeh JM, Lakshmanan J et al. Increased expression of transforming growth factor alpha precursors in acute experimental colitis in rats. Gut 1997; 41: 195–202.

41. Sottili M, Sternini C, Reinshagen M et al. Up-regulation of transforming growth factor alpha binding sites in experimental rabbit colitis. Gastroenterology 1995; 109: 24–31.

42. Babyatsky MW, Rossiter G, Podolsky DK. Expression of transforming growth factors alpha and beta in colonic mucosa in inflammatory bowel disease. Gastroenterology 1996; 110: 975–84.

43. Egger B, Procaccino F, Lakshmanan J et al. Mice lacking transforming growth factor alpha have an increased susceptibility to dextran sulfate-induced colitis. Gastroenterology 1997; 113: 825–32.

44. Egger B, Carey HV, Procaccino F et al. Reduced susceptibility of mice overexpressing transforming growth factor alpha to dextran sodium sulphate induced colitis. Gut 1998; 43: 64–70.

45. Filipe MI, Osborn M, Linehan J, Sanidas E, Brito MJ, Jankowski J. Expression of transforming growth factor alpha, epidermal growth factor receptor and epidermal growth factor in precursor lesions to gastric carcinoma. Br J Cancer 1995; 71: 30–6.

46. Sharp R, Babyatsky MW, Takagi H et al. Transforming growth factor alpha disrupts the normal program of cellular differentiation in the gastric mucosa of transgenic mice. Development 1995; 121: 149–61.

47. Messa C, Russo F, Caruso MG, DiLeo A. EGF, TGF-αlpha, and EGF-R in human colorectal adenocarcinoma. Acta Oncol 1998; 37: 285–9.

48. Barnard JA, Beauchamp RD, Russell WE, Dubois RN, Coffey RJ. Epidermal growth factor-related peptides and their relevance to gastrointestinal pathophysiology. Gastroenterology 1995; 108: 564–80.

49. Chowdhury A, Fukuda R, Fukumoto S. Growth factor mRNA expression in normal colorectal mucosa and in uninvolved mucosa from ulcerative colitis patients. J Gastroenterol 1996; 31: 353–60.

50. Wright NA, Pike CM, Elia G. Induction of a novel epidermal growth factor-secreting cell lineage by mucosal ulceration in human gastrointestinal stem cells. Nature 1990; 343: 82–5.

51. Bragg LE, Hollingsed TC, Thompson JS. Urogastrone reduces gut atrophy during parenteral alimentation. J Parenter Enteral Nutr 1990; 14: 283–6.

52. Ardawi MS. Effects of epidermal growth factor and glutamine-supplemented parenteral nutrition on the small bowel of septic rats. Clin Sci 1992; 82: 573–80.

53. Petschow BW, Carter DL, Hutton GD. Influence of orally administered epidermal growth factor on normal and damaged intestinal mucosa in rats. J Pediatr Gastroenterol Nutr 1993; 17: 49–58.

54. Procaccino F, Reinshagen M, Hoffmann P et al. Protective effect of epidermal growth factor in an experimental model of colitis in rats. Gastroenterology 1994; 107: 12–17.

55. Luck MS, Bass P. Effect of epidermal growth factor on experimental colitis in the rat. J Pharmacol Exp Ther 1993; 264: 984–90.

56. Meijssen MA, Brandwein SL, Reinecker HC, Bhan AK, Podolsky DK Alteration of gene expression by intestinal epithelial cells precedes colitis in interleukin-2-deficient mice. Am J Physiol 1998; 274: G472–9.

57. Shull MM, Ormsby I, Kier AB et al. Targeted disruption of the mouse transforming growth factor-beta 1 gene results in multifocal inflammatory disease. Nature 1992; 359: 693–9.

58. Neurath MF, Fuss I, Kelsall BL, Presky DH, Waegell W, Strober W. Experimental granulomatous colitis in mice is abrogated by induction of TGF-βeta-mediated oral tolerance. J Exp Med 1996; 183: 2605–16.

59. Beck PL, Xavier RJ, Rosenberg I, Podolsky DK. Intestinal epithelial cell expression of TGF-β dominant negative receptor II (DNRII) results in decreased wound healing *in vitro* and increased susceptibility to colonic injury *in vivo*. Gastroenterology 2000; 118: A4843.

60. Ohtani H, Kagaya H, Nagura H. Immunohistochemical localization of transforming growth factor-beta. J Gastroenterol Suppl 1995; 30: 76–7.

61. Graham MF, Bryson GR, Diegelmann RF. Transforming growth factor β_1 selectively augments collagen synthesis by human intestinal smooth muscle cells. Gastroenterology 1990; 99: 447–53.

62. Mourelle M, Salas A, Guarner F, Crespo E, Garcia-Lafuente A, Malagelada JR. Stimulation of transforming growth factor-beta-1 by enteric bacteria in the pathogenesis of rat intestinal fibrosis. Gastroenterology 1998; 114: 519–26.

63. Finch PW, Pricolo V, Wu A, Finkelstein SD. Increased expression of keratinocyte growth factor messenger RNA associated with inflammatory bowel disease. Gastroenterology 1996; 110: 441–51.

64. Brauchle M, Madlener M, Wagner AD et al. Keratinocyte growth factor is highly overexpressed in inflammatory bowel disease. Am J Pathol 1996; 149: 521–9.

65. Bajaj-Elliott M, Breese E, Poulsom R, Fairclough PD, MacDonald TT. Keratinocyte growth factor in inflammatory bowel disease. Increased mRNA transcripts in ulcerative colitis compared with CD in biopsies and isolated mucosal myofibroblasts. Am J Pathol 1997; 151: 1469–76.

66. Boismenu R, Havran WL. Modulation of epithelial cell growth by intraepithelial gamma delta T cells. Science 1994; 266: 1253–5.

67. Finch PW, Cheng AL. Analysis of the cellular basis of keratinocyte growth factor overexpression in inflammatory bowel disease. Gut 1999: 45: 848–55.

68. Zeeh JM, Procaccino F, Hoffmann P *et al*. Keratinocyte growth factor ameliorates mucosal injury in an experimental model of colitis in rats. Gastroenterology 1996; 110: 1077–83.

69. Egger B, Procaccino F, Sarosi I, Tolmos J, Buchler MW, Eysselein VE. Keratinocyte growth factor ameliorates dextran sodium sulfate colitis in mice. Dig Dis Sci 1999; 44: 836–44.

70. Miceli R, Hubert M, Santiago G *et al*. Efficacy of keratinocyte growth factor-2 in dextran sulfate sodium-induced murine colitis. J Pharmacol Exp Ther 1999; 290: 464–71.

71. Zimmermann EM, Sartor RB, McCall RD, Pardo M, Bender D, Lund PK. Insulinlike growth factor I and interleukin 1 beta messenger RNA in a rat model of granulomatous enterocolitis and hepatitis. Gastroenterology 1993; 105: 399–409.

72. Zeeh JM, Hoffmann P, Sottili M, Eysselein VE, McRoberts JA. Up-regulation of insulinlike growth factor I binding sites in experimental colitis in rats. Gastroenterology 1995; 108: 644–52.

73. Howarth GS, Xian CJ, Read LC. Insulin-like growth factor-I partially attenuates colonic damage in rats with experimental colitis induced by oral dextran sulphate soium. Scand J Gastroenterol 1998; 33: 180–90.

74. Thomas AG, Holly JM, Taylor F, Miller V. Insulin like growth factor-I, insulin like growth factor binding protein-1, and insulin in childhood Crohn's disease. Gut 1993; 34: 944–7.

75. Zimmermann EM, Li L, Hou YT, Cannon M, Christman GM, Bitar KN. IGF-I induces collagen and IGFBP-5 mRNA in rat intestinal smooth muscle. Am J Physiol 1997; 273: G875–82.

76. Gosh S, Humphreys K, Papachrysostomou M, Ferguson A. Detection of insulin-like growth factor-I and transforming growth factor-beta in whole gut lavage fluid: a novel method of studying intestinal fibrosis. Eur J Gastroenterol Hepatol 1997; 9: 505–8.

77. Alexander RJ, Panja A, Kaplan-Liss E, Mayer L, Raicht RF. Expression of growth factor receptor-encoded mRNA by colonic epithelial cells is altered in inflammatory bowel disease. Dig Dis Sci 1995; 40: 485–94.

78. Matsumo M, Shiota G, Umeki K, Kawasaki H, Kojo H, Miura K. Induction of plasma hepatocyte growth factor in acute colitis of mice. Inflam Res 1997; 46: 166–7.

79. Matsumo M, Shiota G, Umeki K, Kawasaki H, Kojo H, Miura K. Clinical evaluation of hepatocyte growth factor in patients with gastrointestinal and pancreatic diseases with special reference to inflammatory bowel disease. Res Commun Mol Pathol Pharmacol 1997; 97: 25–37.

80. Boulton TG, Nye SH, Robins DJ *et al*. ERKs: a family of protein–serine/threonine kinases that are activated and tyrosine phosphorylated in response to insulin and NGF. Cell 1991; 65: 663–75.

81. Bogoyevitch MA, Ketterman AJ, Sugden PH. Cellular stresses differentially activate c-Jun N-terminal protein kinases and extracellular signal-regulated protein kinases in cultured ventricular myocytes. J Biol Chem 1995; 270: 29710–17.

82. Sanchez I, Hughes RT, Mayer BJ *et al*. Role of SAPK/ERK kinase-1 in the stress-activated pathway regulating transcription factor c-Jun. Nature 1994; 72: 794–8.

83. Derijard B, Hibi M, Wu IH *et al*. JNK1. A protein kinase stimulated by UV light and Ha-Ras that binds and phosphorylates the c-Jun activation domain. Cell 1994; 76: 1025–37.

84. Kyriakis JM, Banerjee P, Nikolakaki E *et al*. The stress-activated protein kinase subfamily of c-Jun kinases. Nature 1994; 369: 156–60.

85. Rouse J, Cohen P, Trigon S *et al*. A novel kinase cascade triggered by stress and heat shock that stimulates MAPKAP kinase-2 and phosphorylation of the small heat shock proteins. Cell 1994; 78: 1027–37.

86. Han J, Lee JD, Bibbs L, Ulevitch RJ. A MAP kinase targeted by endotoxin and hyperosmolarity in mammalian cells. Science 1994; 265: 808–11.

87. Robinson MJ, Cobb MH. Mitogen-activated protein kinase pathways. Curr Opin Cell Biol 1997; 9: 180–6.

88. Göke M, Kanai M, Lynch-Devaney K, Podolsky DK. Rapid mitogen-activated protein kinase activation by transforming growth factor alpha in wounded rat intestinal epithelial cells. Gastroenterology 1998; 114: 697–705.

89. Polk DB. Epidermal growth factor receptor-stimulated intestinal epithelial cell migration requires phospholipase C activity. Gastroenterology 1998; 114: 493–502.

90. Pai R, Ohta M, Itani RM, Safreh IJ, Tarnawski AS. Induction of mitogen-activated protein kinase signal transduction pathway during gastric ulcer healing in rats. Gastroenterology 1998; 114: 706–13.

91. Sebolt-Leopold JS, Dudley DT, Herrera R *et al*. Blockade of the MAP kinase pathway suppresses growth of colon tumors *in vivo*. Nat Med 1999; 5: 810–16.

92. Dieckgraefe BK, Weems DM. Epithelial injury induces Egr-1 and Fos expression by a pathway involving protein kinase C and ERK. Am J Physiol 1999; 276: G322–30.

93. Dieckgraefe BK, Weems DM, Santoro SA, Alpers DH. ERK and p38 MAP kinase pathways are mediators of intestinal epithelial wound-induced signal transduction. Biochem Biophys Res Commun 1997; 233: 389–94.

94. Sands BE, Podolsky DK. The trefoil peptide family. Annu Rev Physiol 1996; 58: 253–73.

95. Dignass A, Lynch-Devaney K, Kindon H, Thim L, Podolsky DK. Trefoil peptides promote epithelial migration through a transforming growth factor b-independent pathway. J Clin Invest 1994; 94: 376–83.

96. Mashimo H, Wu DC, Podolsky DK, Fishman MC. Impaired defence of intestinal mucosa in mice lacking intestinal trefoil factor. Science 1996; 274: 262–5.

97. Liu D, el-Hariry I, Karayiannakis AJ *et al*. Phosphorylation of beta-catenin and epidermal growth factor receptor by intestinal trefoil factor. Lab Invest 1997; 77: 557–63.

98. Hermiston ML, Wong MH, Gordon JI. Forced expression of E-cadherin in the mouse intestinal epithelium slows cell migration and provides evidence for nonautonomous regulation of cell fate in a self-renewing system. Genes Dev 1996; 10: 985–96

99. Frisch SM, Francis H. Disruption of epithelial cel-matrix interactions induces apoptosis. J Cell Biol 1994; 124: 619–26.

100. Hague A, Hicks DJ, Bracey TS, Paraskeva C. Cell–cell contact and specific cytokines inhibit apoptosis of colonic epithelial cells: growth factors protect against c-myc-independent apoptosis. Br J Cancer 1997; 75: 960–8.

101. Taupin DR, Kinoshita K, Podolsky DK. Intestinal trefoil factor confers colonic epithelial resistance to apoptosis. Proc Natl Acad Sci USA 2000; 97: 799–804.

102. Kindon H, Pothoulakis C, Thim L, Lynch-Devaney K, Podolsky DK. Trefoil peptide protection of intestinal epithelial barrier function: cooperative interaction with mucin glycoprotein. Gastroenterology 1995; 109: 516–23.

103. Babyatsky MW, deBeaumont M, Thim L, Podolsky DK. Oral trefoil peptides protect against ethanol- and indomethacin-induced gastric injury in rats. Gastroenterology 1996; 110: 489–97.

104. Beck PL, Podolsky DK. Intestinal trefoil factor reduces the severity of chemotherapy- and radiotherapy-induced intestinal mucositis. Gastroenterology 1999; 116: A486.

105. Playford RJ, Marchbank T, Goodlad RA *et al.* Transgenic mice that overexpress the human trefoil peptide pS2 have an increased resistance to intestinal damage. Proc Natl Acad Sci USA 1996; 93: 2137–42.

106. Wright NA, Poulsom R, Stamp GW *et al.* Epidermal growth factor (EGF/URO) induces expression of regulatory peptides in damaged human gastrointestinal tissues. J Pathol 1990; 162: 279–84

107. Wright NA, Poulsom R, Stamp G *et al.* Trefoil peptide gene expression in gastrointestinal epithelial cells in inflammatory bowel disease. Gastroenterology 1993; 104: 12–20.

108. Itoh H, Tomita M, Uchino H *et al.* cDNA cloning of rat pS2 peptide and expression in acetic acid-induced colitis. Biochem J 1996; 318: 939–44.

109. Taupin DR, Wu DC, Jeon WK, Devaney K, Wang TC, Podolsky DK. The trefoil gene family are co-ordinately expressed immediate-early genes: EGF receptor- and MAP kinase-dependent interregulation. J Clin Invest 1999; 103: R31–8.

110. Ogata H, Podolsky DK. Trefoil peptide expression and secretion is regulated by neuropeptides and acetylcholine. Am J Physiol 1997; 273: G348–54.

111. Podolsky DK, Lynch-Devaney K, Stow JL *et al.* Identification of human intestinal trefoil factor. Goblet-cell specific expression of a peptide targeted for apical secretion. J Biol Chem 1993; 268: 6694–702.

112. Newton JL, Allen A, Westley BR, May FE. The human trefoil peptide, TFF1, is present in different molecular forms that are intimately associated with mucus in normal stomach. Gut 2000; 46: 312–20

113. Hoffmann W. A new repetitive protein from *Xenopus laevis* skin highly homologous to pancreatic spasmolytic polypeptide. J Biol Chem 1988; 263: 7686–90.

114. Hauser F, Hoffmann W. P-domains as shuffled cysteine-rich modules in in integumentary mucin C.1 (FIM-C.1) from *Xenopus laevis*. J Biol Chem 1992; 267: 24620–4.

115. Lefebvre O, Chenard MP, Masson R *et al.* Gastric mucosa abnormalities in mice lacking the pS2 trefoil protein. Science 1996; 274: 259–62.

116. Tomasetto C, Masson R, Linares JL *et al.* pS2/TFF1 interacts directly with the VWFC cysteine-rich domains of mucins. Gastroenterology 2000; 118: 70–80.

117. Cook GA, Familari M, Thim L, Giraud AS. The trefoil peptides TFF2 and TFF3 are expressed in rat lymphoid tissues and participate in the immune response. FEBS Lett 1999; 456: 155–9.

118. Tran CP, Cook GA, Yeomans ND, Thim L, Giraud AS. Trefoil peptide TFF2 (spasmolytic polypeptide) potently accelerates healing and reduces inflammation in a rat model of colitis. Gut 1999; 44: 636–42.

119. Hoosein NM, Thim L, Jørgensen KH, Brattain MG. Growth stimulatory effect of pancreatic spasmolytic polypeptide on cultured colon and breast tumor cells. FEBS Lett 1989; 247: 303–6.

120. Thim L. A new family of growth factor-like peptides: 'trefoil' disulphide loop structures as a common feature in breast cancer associated peptide (pS2), pancreatic spasmolytic polypeptide (PSP), and frog skin peptides (spasmolysins). FEBS Lett 1989; 250: 85–90.

121. Kato K, Chen MC, Nguyen M, Lehmann FS, Podolsky DK, Soll AH. Effects of growth factors and trefoil peptides on migration and replication in primary oxyntic cultures. Am J Physiol 1999; 276: G1105–16.

122. Uchino H, Kataoka H, Itoh H, Hamasuna R, Koono M. Overexpression of intestinal trefoil factor in human colon carcinoma cells reduces cellular growth *in vitro* and *in vivo*. Gastroenterology 2000; 118: 60–9.

123. Carroll KM, Wong TT, Drabik DL, Chang EB. Differentiation of rat small intestinal epithelial cells by extracellular matrix. Am J Physiol 1988; 254: G355–60.

124. Hahn U, Stallmach A, Hahn EG, Riecken EO. Basement membrane components are potent promoters of rat intestinal epithelial cell differentiation *in vitro*. Gastroenterology 1990; 98: 322–35.

125. Olson AD, Pysher T, Bienkowski RS. Organization of intestinal epithelial cells into multicellular structures requires laminin and functional actin microfilaments. Exp Cell Res 1991; 192: 543–9.

126. Simo P, Simon-Assmann P, Arnold C, Kedinger M. Mesenchyme-mediated effect of dexamethasone on laminin in cocultures of embryonic gut epithelial cells and mesenchyme-derived cells. J Cell Sci 1992; 101: 161–71.

127. Moore R, Madara JL, MacLeod RJ. Enterocytes adhere preferentially to collagen IV in a differentially regulated divalent cation-dependent manner. Am J Physiol 1994; 266: G1099–107.

128. Turowski GA, Rashid Z, Hong F, Madri JA, Basson MD. Glutamine modulates phenotype and stimulates proliferation in human colon cancer cell lines. Cancer Res 1994; 54: 5974–80.

129. Vachon PH, Beaulieu JF. Extracellular heterotrimeric laminin promotes differentiation in human enterocytes. Am J Physiol 1995; 268: G857–67.

130. Timpl R, Dziadek M. Structure, development, and molecular pathology of basement membranes. Int Rev Exp Pathol 1986; 29: 1–112.

131. Laurie GW, Leblond CP, Martin GR. Localization of type IV collagen, laminin, heparan sulfate proteoglycan, and fibronectin to the basal lamina of basement membranes. J Cell Biol 1982; 95: 340–4.

132. Quaroni A, Isselbacher KJ, Ruoshlahti E. Fibronectin synthesis by epithelial crypt cells of rat small intestine. Proc Natl Acad Sci USA 1978; 75: 5548–52.

133. Göke M, Zuk A, Podolsky DK. Regulation and function of extracellular matrix in intestinal epithelial restitution *in vitro*. Am J Physiol 1996; 271: G729–40.

134. Hahn U, Schuppan D, Hahn EG, Merker HJ, Riecken EO. Intestinal cells produce basement membrane proteins *in vitro*. Gut 1987; 28: S143–51.

135. Simo P, Bouziges F, Lissitzky JC, Sorokin L, Kedinger M, Simon-Assmann P. Dual and asynchronous deposition of laminin chains at the epithelial–mesenchymal interface in the gut. Gastroenterology 1992; 102: 1835–45.

136. Weiser MM, Sykes DE, Killen PD. Rat intestinal basement membrane synthesis. Epithelial versus non epithelial contributions. Lab Invest. 1990;62:325–30.

137. Trier JS, Allan CH, Abrahamson DR, Hagen SJ. Epithelial basement membrane of mouse jejunum. Evidence for laminin turnover along the entire crypt–villus axis. J Clin Invest 1990; 86: 87–95.

138. O'Keefe EJ, Payne RE, Russell N, Woodley DT. Spreading and enhanced motility of human keratinocytes on fibronectin. J Invest Dermatol 1985; 85: 125–30.

139. Sarret Y, Stamm C, Jullien D, Schmitt D. Keratinocyte migration is partially supported by the cell-binding domain of fibronectin and is RGDS-dependent. J Invest Dermatol 1992; 99: 656–9.

140. Basson MD, Modlin IM, Flynn SD, Jena BP, Madri JA. Independent modulation of enterocyte migration and proliferation by growth factors, matrix proteins, and pharmacologic agents in an *in vitro* model of mucosal healing. Surgery 1992; 112: 299–307.

141. Moore R, Madri J, Carlson S, Madara JL. Collagens facilitate epithelial migration in restitution of native Guinea

pig intestinal epithelium. Gastroenterology 1992; 102: 119–30.

142. Burgess WH, Maciag T. The heparin-binding (fibroblast) growth factor family of proteins. Annu Rev Biochem 1989; 58: 575–606.

143. Ruoslahti E, Yamaguchi Y. Proteoglycans as modulators of growth factor activities. Cell 1991; 64: 867–9.

144. Yayon A, Klagsbrun M, Esko JD, Leder P, Ornitz DM. Cell surface, heparin-like molecules are required for binding of basic fibroblast growth factor to its high affinity receptor. Cell 1991; 64: 841–8.

145. Aviezer D, Hecht D, Safran M, Eisinger M, David G, Yayon A. Perlecan, basal lamina proteoglycan, promotes basic fibroblast growth factor-receptor binding, mitogenesis, and angiogenesis. Cell 1994; 79: 1005–13.

146. Schuppan D, Schmid M, Somasundaram R *et al.* Collagens in the liver extracellular matrix bind hepatocyte growth factor. Gastroenterology 1998; 114: 139–52.

147. MacDonald TT, Pender SL. Proteolytic enzymes in inflammatory bowel disease. Inflam Bowel Dis 1998; 4: 157–64.

148. Vaalamo M, Karjalainen-Lindsberg ML, Puolakkainen P, Kere J, Saarialho-Kere U. Distinct expression profiles of stromelysin-2 (MMP-10), collagenase-3 (MMP-13), macrophage metalloelastase (MMP-12), and tissue inhibitor of metalloproteinases-3 (TIMP-3) in intestinal ulcerations. Am J Pathol 1998; 152: 1005–14.

149. Baugh MD, Perry MJ, Hollander AP *et al.* Matrix metalloproteinase levels are elevated in inflammatory bowel disease. Gastroenterology 1999; 117: 814–22.

150. Louis E, Ribbens C, Godon A *et al.* Increased production of matrix metalloproteinase-3 and tissue inhibitor of metalloproteinase-1 by inflamed mucosa in inflammatory bowel disease. Clin Exp Immunol 2000; 120: 241–6.

151. Sykes AP, Bhogal R, Brampton C *et al.* The effect of an inhibitor of matrix metalloproteinases on colonic inflammation in a trinitrobenzenesulphonic acid rat model of inflammatory bowel disease. Aliment Pharmacol Ther 1999; 13: 1535–1542.

152. Deane HW. Some electron microscopic observations on the lamina propria of the gut, with some comments on the close association of macrophages, plasma cells and eosinophils. Anat Rec 1964; 149: 453–73.

153. Donellan WL. The structure of the colonic mucosa. The epithelium and subepithelial reticulo-histiocytic complex. Gastroenterology 1965; 49: 496–514.

154. Mahida YR, Galvin AM, Gray T et al. Migration of human intestinal lamina propria lymphocytes, macrophages and eosinophils following the loss of surface epithelial cells. Clin Exp Immunol 1997; 109: 377–86.

155. McAlindon ME, Gray T, Galvin A, Sewell HF, Podolsky DK, Mahida YR. Differential lamina propria cell migration via basement membrane pores of inflammatory bowel disease mucosa. Gastroenterology 1998; 115: 841–8.

156. Mahida YR, Beltinger J, Makh S *et al.* Adult human colonic subepithelial myofibroblasts express extracellular matrix proteins and cyclooxygenase-1 and -2. Am J Physiol 1997; 273: G1341–8.

157. Powell DW, Mifflin RC, Valentich JD, Crowe SE, Saada JI, West AB. Myofibroblasts. I. Paracrine cells important in health and disease. Am J Physiol 1999; 277: C1–9.

158. Powell DW, Mifflin RC, Valentich JD, Crowe SE, Saada JI, West AB. Myofibroblasts. II. Intestinal subepithelial myofibroblasts. Am J Physiol 1999; 277: C183–201.

159. Graham MF, Diegelmann RF, Elson CO *et al.* Collagen content and types in the intestinal strictures of Crohn's disease. Gastroenterology 1988; 94: 257–65.

160. Stallmach A, Schuppan D, Matthes H, Riecken EO. Increased collagen type III synthesis in fibroblasts isolated from strictures of patients with Crohn's disease. Gastroenterology 1992; 102: 1920–9.

161. Graham MF, Drucker DEM, Diegelmann RF, Elson CO. Collagen synthesis by human intestinal smooth muscle cells in culture. Gastroenterology 1987; 92: 400–5.

162. Strong SA, Pizarro TT, Klein JS, Cominelli F, Fiocchi C. Proinflammatory cytokines differentially modulate their own expression in human intestinal mucosal mesenchymal cells. Gastroenterology 1998; 114: 1244–56.

163. Jobson TM, Billington CK, Hall IP. Regulation of proliferation of human colonic subepithelial myofibroblasts by mediators important in intestinal inflammation. J Clin Invest 1998; 101: 2650–7.

164. Plateroti M, Rubin DC, Duluc I *et al.* Subepithelial fibroblast cell lines from different levels of gut axis display regional characteristics. Am J Physiol 1998; 274: G945–54.

165. Munz B, Smola H, Engelhardt F *et al.* Overexpression of activin A in the skin of transgenic mice reveals new activities of activin in epidermal morphogenesis, dermal fibrosis and wound repair. EMBO J 1999; 18: 5205–15.

166. Dammeier J, Brauchle M, Falk W, Grotendorst GR, Werner S. Connective tissue growth factor: a novel regulator of mucosal repair and fibrosis in inflammatory bowel disease? Int J Biochem Cell Biol 1998; 30: 909–22.

167. Slonim AE, Bulone L, Damore MB, Goldberg T, Wingertzahn MA, McKinley MJ. A preliminary study of growth hormone therapy for Crohn's disease. N Engl J Med 2000; 342: 1633–7.

168. Ali IU, Schriml LM, Dean M. Mutational spectra of PTEN/MMAC1 gene: a tumor suppressor with lipid phosphatase activity. J Natl Cancer Inst 1999; 91: 1922–32.

169. Rudolph KL, Chang S, Lee HW *et al.* Longevity, stress response, and cancer in aging telomerase-deficient mice. Cell 1999; 96: 701–12.

170. Kagnoff MF. Current concepts in mucosal immunity. III. Ontogeny and function of γ/δ T cell in the intestine. Am J Physiol 1998; 274: G455–8.

171. Fiocchi C. Inflammatory bowel disease: etiology and pathogenesis. Gastroenterology 1998; 115: 182–205.

10 | Antibodies in the exploration of inflammatory bowel disease pathogenesis and disease stratification

JONATHAN BRAUN, OFFER COHAVY AND MARK EGGENA

Introduction

Normal mucosal homeostasis is the interdependent relationship of epithelium, luminal microorganisms, and the regional immune system (Fig. 1). This tripartite relationship has particularly evolved during the eutherian period, due to the emergence of a dynamic, antigen-specific immune system [1, 2]. The mammalian immune system has an exceptional capacity for specific antigen recognition and immunologic memory to microibal antigens, and for powerful amplification of effector mechanisms against such antigenic targets [3, 4]. These properties obviously require special adaptation to preserve the mucosal–microbial interrelationship essential for normal intestinal function. It is widely understood that inflammatory bowel disease (IBD) involves a chronic disturbance in this homeostasis.

In recent years there has been a particular effort to understand this homeostatic disturbance in the context of immunologic activation and tissue damage. In particular, this effort has been informed by the emerging understanding of *Helicobacter pylori* pathogenesis in peptic ulcer disease. From this precedent we have learned that the manifestation of clinical disease reflects the interplay of commensal bacterial and host traits, which together affect levels of colonization, and the nature and intensity of inflammation and tissue damage [5, 6]. Our review focuses on the insights provided by IBD-associated antibodies on disease pathogenesis and clinical stratification. We will first consider the nature of immunologic quiescence in the mucosa. We will then assess the concepts and experimental issues regarding disease-related antibodies and their antigenic targets. This will be followed by an analysis of the

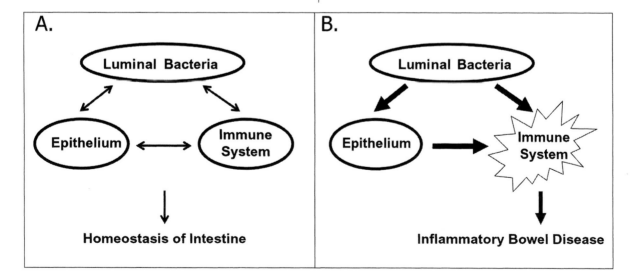

Figure 1. Immune activation as a phenotype of disturbed mucosal homeostasis in IBD.

Stephan R. Targan, Fergus Shanahan and Loren C. Karp (eds.), Inflammatory Bowel Disease: From Bench to Bedside, 2nd Edition, 211–222.

microbial antigens and autoantigens identified by IBD-related antibodies. Finally, we will discuss how these antibodies and antigens are being applied to issues of disease diagnosis, clinical stratification, and strategies for treatment.

The quiescence of the mucosal immune system to local microbial antigens and autoantigens

The immune system is classically understood to launch strong responses upon encounter with micro-organisms. It is likely that such proinflammatory responses reflect programming of nascent lympho-cyte and antigen-presenting populations by micro-bial products [3]. The mechanism of this program-ming is multifaceted, but clearly includes elements of the innate immunity [4, 7–9]. In contrast, immune responses to microbial products by gastrointestinal lymphocytes are remarkably curtailed. For example, in the human it is difficult to detect native or induced T cell or antibody responses to abundant commensal bacteria, either in the mucosal or peripheral sites [10–14]. Moreover, such studies indicate that this immunologic quiescence may be relatively restricted to autologous bacterial strains, since experimental challenge with heterologous (but not autologous) strains is relatively immunogenic. These findings suggest a state of immune tolerance to antigens encountered in the gastrointestinal environment, including those expressed by commensal bacteria. Indeed, the apparent tolerogenic consequence of gastrointestinal antigen exposure has been inten-sively studied from the standpoint of therapeutic applications of oral tolerance [15].

The mechanism of immunologic quiescence in the mucosa is a fascinating and still unresolved issue (see Chapter 5). Conceptually, this quiescence probably reflects the coordinated contribution of each of the three mucosal elements. For example, certain chemokines and the Gαi2-linked signaling cascade suppress IL-12 expression by macrophages and dendritic cells, hence polarizing immune responses away from TH1 differentiation [16–19]. Among these, MCP-1 and MIP-1α are constitutively produced by colonic epithelial cells [20], and may thereby contribute to the blunted TH1 mucosal phenotype. Within the lymphoid compartment itself, subsets of dendritic cells and intraepithelial lympho-cytes are likely to play a role, through their multi-faceted regulation of αβ T cell function, and production of growth factors preserving epithelial integrity [21–23].

Bacterial traits also contribute to this quiescent environment, presumably reflecting the coevolution of intestinal colonists with immunologic discretion. Thus *Bacteroides* and *Bifidobacter* species, while the numerically most abundant genera of intestinal (colonic) colonists, are subject to minimal or modest T cell and antibody activity in healthy individuals. Such responses are typically genus- rather than species-specific, further indicating the absence of specific immune activity elicited by these intestinal colonists [24–27]. Secretory IgA activity can be substantial to some abundant colonic species, and this appears in part to reflect a primitive innate immune recognition [28, 29].

Stable colonization indicates that commensal bacteria are well adapted to such recognition, and emerging evidence indicates that this adaptation includes active bacterial regulation of the innate bacterial recognition process [30–34]. These observa-

Table 1. Autoantigens in IBD

Antigen	Disease	References
pANCA	UC, CD subset	75, 83, 161–163
Tropomyosin	UC	164–168
Anti-endothelial IgG	UC, CD subset	169–171
50 kDa myeloid-specific nuclear protein	UC, hepatobiliary disease	172
Neutrophil granule proteins (cathepsin G, lactoferrin, BPI, catalase, alpha-enolase)	Various	173–178
HMG-1 and HMG-2	UC	179, 180
Histone H1	Various	181–183
24,28 kDa protein	UC subset	184, 185
Hsp60	CD	186, 187
Pancreatic acinar cell antigen	CD subset	188, 189

tions focus on three important issues for further investigation: (a) bacterial products involved in host recognition; (b) intrinsic bacterial resistance mechanisms to recognition-induced host effector processes; (c) extrinsic bacterial traits which modify specific and innate immune recognition in the intestine. Resolution of these issues is central to important new anti-inflammatory therapeutic strategies, notably probiotics [35].

Tolerance to autoantigens is a parallel immunologic issue to such antibacterial quiescence. A variety of processes contribute to self-tolerance, including central and peripheral clonal deletion, blunted activity of stimulatory receptor pathways, and deviation of effector function [36–38]. These processes relate to IBD pathogenesis in two general ways. First, mechanisms of these tolerance processes should encompass the mechanisms of immune quiescence to commensal bacteria. Indeed, there is substantial evidence that peripheral tolerance in many cases arises through activation and differentiation of autoreactive lymphocytes in the mucosal environment [39–41]. Second, the recurrent observation of autoimmunity to mucosal antigens in IBD suggests a direct contribution of such activity to intestinal damage.

Disordered mucosal immunity in IBD-susceptibility, stimuli, and marker antibodies

At the tissue level the hallmark of ulcerative colitis (UC) and Crohn's disease (CD) is aberrant immune activity, and the mucosal damage caused by the resultant inflammatory processes (Fig. 2). Accordingly, the core issues in IBD pathogenesis are the identity of the stimuli driving the disordered immune function, and the host traits promoting aberrant responses to these stimuli. Genetic approaches have identified a series of loci and candidate genes modifying host susceptibility [42–50]. While the identity of the relevant genes at these loci is unknown, it is likely that some will function directly or indirectly to modify the recognition or effector processes induced by the immunologic stimuli. CD4+ T cell activity (and its disease-specific effector heterogeneity) is presently accepted as the focal point of the immunopathogenic process in IBD, initiating and organizing the effector processes leading to mucosal damage [51–55]. However, T cells pose a formidable chal-

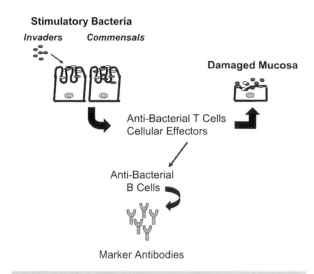

Figure 2. Relationship between stimulatory bacteria, tissue-destructive effector mechanisms, and marker antibody production in IBD.

lenge in the identification of their cognate antigenic stimuli. Identification approaches generally require cell-based assays, with the attendant complexities of clonal heterogeneity and assay insensitivity with mixed populations. Some innovations have been developed, using TCR polymorphism analysis and expression cloning technologies [56–59]. However, these have not yet reached the robustness required for evaluation of undefined antigenic systems.

Fortunately, immune responses typically include recruitment of antigen-specific B lymphocytes (Fig. 2). Such recruitment is a consequence of membrane immunoglobulin expression by the B cell, and the highly efficient antigen uptake and presentation mediated by this receptor in antigen-specific B cells [60, 60–65]. As a result, antibodies specific for the major antigenic stimuli of an immune response are commonly produced, even when the humoral response is not central to the immune effector mechanism (e.g. responses predominating with TH1- or CTL-dependent processes). Such antibodies are initially recognized as disease-associated 'marker' antibodies, often detected adventitiously with crossreactive laboratory antigens. However, antibodies are superb analytic reagents, providing a powerful tool for identification of disease-related tissue antigen. The precedent of diabetes mellitus is a striking case where the isolation and use of disease-specific marker antibodies propelled the characterization of antigenic stimuli central to this complex immunologic disease [66, 67].

Technologically, there are several issues to consider in isolating disease-related marker antibodies. First, the antibody composition of patient sera is complex, and the relevant marker antibodies typically must be isolated to reduce background seroreactivity and increase titer to analytically useful levels. This is most commonly achieved by affinity purification of antigen-specific antibodies from individuals with high-titer antibody levels. The conventional approach is hampered by limited antibody yield (particularly with low-titer antibodies), and reproducibility with different donors due to heterogeneity in fine antigen specificity.

Alternatively, monoclonal antibodies can be produced, using hybridoma or phage-display technology [68–73]. Such reagents are analytically superior because of renewability and consistency. Use of these clonal approaches requires efficient localization and isolation of marker antibody-producing cells. These requirements are significant challenges for hybridoma preparation, and are compounded by the need for cells which are biologically suitable as fusion partners. The powerful cloning and selection features of phage-display technology overcome some of these difficulties. However, phage-display methods can suffer from unfavorable reassortment of heavy and light chain genes, and donor and avidity skewing of fine specificity in the course of clonal selection.

In the following sections we will review the use of such isolated marker antibodies to identify and characterize their cognate autoantigens and microbial antigens. Together, these molecules and cell types comprise the set of candidate immunologic stimuli predominant in IBD-associated immunity. Several criteria have been used to assess the significance of these antigens in disease pathogenesis: specificity and sensitivity of expression in IBD; expression in relevant tissue sites; and targeting by regulatory and effector T cells. While these criteria can associate the antigens with IBD, they leave open the critical issue of causation. This issue is addressed by demonstration of these criteria in animal disease models, and direct studies in which immune responses induced by these antigens might elicit disease. At this writing, no antigens have reached this level of experimental validation. We will denote those antigens which fulfill multiple criteria of disease association, and thus can be considered high-priority candidates for an immunologic role in disease.

Autoantigens

pANCA

Perhaps the most widely studied marker antibody in IBD is pANCA – antibodies to a perinuclear neutrophil antigen [74–76]. These antibodies are distinguished from other cANCA and pANCA by sensitivity of their antigen to DNAse I treatment, and localization to the inner nuclear membrane leaflet [77, 78]. Reliable detection of this UC-associated pANCA depends on proper fixation procedures, IgG isotype specificity, and DNAse I sensitivity. Using these criteria, 60–70% of UC patients are antibody-positive. Antibody levels are relatively stable over time regardless of disease activity, and uncommonly occur in patients with other gastrointestinal diseases. This indicates that they do not represent non-specific markers of general colonic inflammation. In fact, pANCA expression is elevated in unaffected family members, concordant in monozygotic twins, and associated with a distinct MHC II haplotype [79–83]. These observations indicate that pANCA expression is a phenotype associated with immunogenetic susceptibility for UC.

The close association of pANCA expression with disease susceptibility is emphasized by their occurrence in the $TCR\alpha^{-/-}$ and C3H/HeJBir colitis-prone mouse strains [84, 85]. It is also notable that pANCA antibodies are characteristic of patients with primary sclerosing cholangitis, in which UC is highly concordant [77, 86, 87]. About 20–25% of CD patients also express pANCA, and analyses of these individuals reveal a CD subset with distinctive genetics and UC-like clinical features [83, 88–93]. The use of pANCA for disease stratification is addressed in the final section.

pANCA-related autoantigens

The search for the pANCA antigen(s) has been a challenging one. The first candidates were granule proteins of the neutrophil, particularly cathepsin G and lactoferrin [88, 89, 94, 95]. Some reports have also described other granule proteins, including bactericidal/permeability-increasing protein (BPI), catalase, and alpha-enolase [96, 97]. Disease association studies of these antigens using ELISA and Western analysis indicate a distinct pattern compared with pANCA, notably their discordance with pANCA levels, correlation with disease activity, relatively high occurrence in CD compared to UC, and association with other rheumatologic diseases. Biochemically, these antigens also would not appear to fulfill the subcellular localization criterion of the pANCA antigen [78]. However, it is notable that antibody levels to granule proteins appear to identify patient subsets with distinct clinical courses, and may thus be a phenotype of the corresponding immunologic traits underlying these clinical manifestations.

A recent study employed high-titer pANCA sera to isolate a myeloid-specific 50 kDa nuclear envelope protein [98]. Western analysis of a large patient serum panel discriminated most patients with UC, primary sclerosing cholangitis, and autoimmune hepatitis. It will be important for this intriguing report to be validated for disease specificity in other laboratories, and further defined biochemically and in colitis model systems.

Nuclear high-mobility group proteins (HMG-1 and 2) [99, 100] and members of the histone H1 family [81, 101, 102] are a second category of pANCA antigen candidates. These structurally related nuclear proteins associate with distinct chromatin domains that are localized to the nuclear envelope region, explaining their pANCA staining pattern, and fulfilling this pANCA antigen criterion [103–105]. A core epitope (PKKAK) was identified using a UC-related anti-histone H1 monoclonal (phage-display) antibody [102]. Structurally, this epitope is present in both families of nuclear proteins, and is distinct from the C-terminal histone H1 epitopes predominating in anti-H1 antibodies associated with SLE, HIV, and rheumatoid arthritis [106–108]. Anti-H1 and anti-HMG antibodies are each expressed in 15–25% of pANCA$^+$ ulcerative patients, suggesting that these two specificities could account for as much as half of the pANCA antibody response. However, these antibodies do not correlate well with pANCA levels or UC specificity, indicating that they are probably distinct from the predominant UC–pANCA seroreactivity. It is interesting to note that antibodies to HMG-1 and -2 are highly correlated with autoimmune hepatitis, and an epitopically distinct pANCA typical of this disease [77, 109].

A 24,28 kDa antigen has been identified with the 5-3 pANCA human monoclonal antibody [110], and found to be expressed in mast cells (including those of mucosal origin), certain ganglionic cells, and pancreatic islets [111, 112]. Seroreactivity to these antigens was observed by Western analysis in UC patients, but this evaluation was limited by the lack of biochemically isolated and defined antigen for comprehensive studies. This protein(s) does not appear to represent the predominant pANCA antigen, since it is localized intracellularly as a cytoplasmic granule.

Other autoantigens

Antiepithelial antibodies have been a recurrent focus of investigation in IBD [113]. In recent years tropomyosin has received substantial support as a candidate epithelial antigen [114–118]. Antibodies to this antigen are expressed in the majority of UC patients, and are uncommon in control gastrointestinal disease patients. A tropomyosin epitope, HIAE-DADRK, provided excellent discrimination for this disease-related antibody activity, and such antibodies mediated antibody-dependent cytotoxicity in a tissue culture cell line [114, 118]. Antitropomyosin antibodies have also been identified in TCRα$^{-/-}$ and Gαi2$^{-/-}$ colitis-prone mice, and in the latter case precede clinical disease [52, 117, 119]. Using a representative monoclonal antibody, a crossreactive epitope of the appropriate molecular weight (40 kDa) was detected in epithelial cells of tissues involved with extracolonic manifestations of UC (skin, biliary). These observations are striking, and the role of this autoantigenic target in UC pathogenesis clearly deserves broader investigation.

Antibodies to heat-shock proteins, notably hsp60, are elevated in certain CD patients [120]. In the mouse a clonal hsp60-specific CD8 T cell line induced colitis when transferred to recipient mice. The disease process was TNF-α-dependent, and inflamed mucosa showed increased hsp60 expression. These findings are provocative, due to the following implications: hsp60 may be a colitis autoantigen, an amplification loop may occur for pathogenesis through inflammation-mediated antigen up-regulation; and CD8 T cells may function in regulatory or effector roles for chronic colitis [121].

An anti-acinar cytoplasmic granule pancreatic autoantibody has been reported by Seibold and colleagues in about 25% of CD patients [122, 123]. While no biochemical definition of this antigen has been reported, it is apparently distinguished from the 24,28 kDa antigen by pancreatic cell type and IBD subtype (CD versus UC). Antiendothelial antibodies have been reported in about 75% of UC patients and 25% of CD patients [124–126]. Antibody levels were correlated with disease activity, although the antibodies themselves did not appear to be cytotoxic.

While the antigen remains undefined, the appropriate microanatomic localization and strong disease association recommend them for further study.

Microbial antigens

For more than 15 years investigators have observed elevated IgG seroreactivity in CD patients to a variety of bacterial taxa [10, 127–130]. This is also an immunologic feature of at least one IBD animal model C3H/HeJBir [24]. In that model the antibody response cecal bacteria is accompanied by corresponding antibacterial CD4$^+$ T cell activity, and such T cell lines can transfer colitis [131]. It is interesting to note that absorption experiments revealed cross-reactivity between antibacterial IgG and pANCA activity [85].

Several interpretations have been suggested to explain the diversity of antibacterial recognition in CD. First, formation of such antibodies might be a secondary consequence of disease-related epithelial permeability and excessive luminal bacterial exposure [132, 133]. As will be illustrated in the following examples, detailed analysis of antibody levels and familial patterns does not support this model of antibody formation. Second, bacteria-dependent inflammation may be elicited in IBD by innate immunity to conserved bacterial products such as LPS and cell wall peptidoglycans [134]. However, this mechanism is not a sufficient factor, since mono-association studies with bacteria expressing proinflammatory molecules have in almost all cases been unsuccessful. A provisional conclusion is that the pertinent colitigenic traits of luminal bacteria, whether targeting antigenic or innate effector processes, are expressed in only a subset of bacterial species. A plausible goal of the marker antibody studies is to identify candidate bacteria to be evaluated for these traits.

ASCA

Antibodies to the cell wall mannan polysaccharide of *Saccharomyces cerevisiae* (ASCA) are detectable in about 60% of patients with CD and may fluctuate with disease activity [83, 135–140]. ASCA is highly specific for CD, with minimal seroreactivity of patients with UC, other colitides, or non-gastrointestinal diseases. To our knowledge ASCA levels have not been evaluated in IBD animal models. The origin of the antigenic stimulus for this ASCA response is uncertain, since the core epitope of this response is recurrent among taxa of plants and bacteria [141]. Thus, while ASCA levels are consistent with a CD-related bacterial cell wall-specific response, it is conceivable that dietary antigens may also play a stimulatory role [142, 143].

A substantial fraction of CD patients are seronegative despite similar clinical activity. This observation suggests that mucosal disruption and antigenic overexposure is not in itself a predominant factor. Concordance and intraclass correlation of ASCA levels in affected and unaffected first-degree relatives indicate that seronegative and seropositive phenotypes are distinct familial and perhaps genetic traits [144, 145]. The use of ASCA for disease stratification and preclinical risk assessment is discussed in the final section.

Mycobacterium

Antibodies to mycobacterial antigens are selectively associated with CD [11, 146, 147]. Recombinant proteins (p35 and p36) have been characterized from *M. paratuberculosis*, which in a tandem IgG immunoassay showed high specificity and sensitivity to CD ($\sim 75\%$ and $\sim 90\%$) compared to normals and UC patients [148–150]. This species specificity has been independently confirmed using a conventional absorption strategy [147]. IgA ELISA seroreactivity was also observed with a conserved mycobacterial

Table 2. Microbial and environmental antigens in IBD

Microorganism	Antigen	Disease	References
Undefined	ASCA	CD	190–194
M. paratuberculosis	p35, p36, HupB	CD	195–200
B. caccae, B. thetaiotaomicron	OmpW, SusC (?)	CD	201, 202
E. coli	OmpC	CD, UC subset	201
P. fluorescens	I2	CD	203
	Dietary	CD	204–207

protein, HupB [151]. It is interesting to add that the latter antigen was initially identified by its antigenic crossreactivity with a pANCA histone H1-related epitope.

These observations comprise one line of evidence implicating mycobacteria, particularly *M. paratuberculosis*, in CD pathogenesis. This hypothesis stems from the role of this organism as an etiologic agent in Johne's disease, a granulomatous colitis of cattle [152]. To this point, studies with species-specific PCR are inconsistent in localizing mycobacterial sequences to CD lesions; mycobacterial antibiotic therapy also has not yet demonstrated efficacy (reviewed in reference 153). Several mycobacterial antigens appear useful for CD serodiagnosis, but further lines of experimentation are required to resolve or refine the pathogenesis hypothesis.

OmpC and OmpW

Using a monoclonal pANCA antibody, libraries of colonic bacteria were generated and screened for crossreactive antigens by immunoblot analysis [154]. Three major bacterial species were identified: *Escherichia coli*, *Bacteroides caccae*, and *B. thetaiotaomicron*. The *E. coli* protein was cloned and confirmed by recombinant expression and genetic analysis as the outer membrane porin OmpC. IgG ELISA demonstrated elevated IgG anti-OmpC in high-titered pANCA UC patients, and IgA anti-OmpC in approximately half of CD patients. Similarly, a newly described outer membrane protein, OmpW, was identified as the antigen for *B. caccae*, and IgA anti-OmpW was elevated in the same subset of CD patients [155]. Based on size and close sequence homology, the antigen in *B. thetaiotaomicron* is expected to be SusC. These findings identify a set of antigenically related bacterial outer membrane proteins as immunologic targets in CD, and reveal a structural relationship between them. Notably, these proteins are homologous to RagA of *Porphyromonas gingivalis*, and hence reveal their structural relationship to a bacterial virulence factor in periodontal disease.

Pseudomonas I2

Representational difference analysis was used to isolate microbial DNA segments specific for CD lesional mucosa versus adjacent uninvolved mucosa [156]. This search resulted in the isolation of I2, a tetR bacterial transcription factor family member, derived from *Pseudomonas fluorescens* (Wei *et al.*, in preparation). In the large intestine, quantitative PCR established that the I2 sequence was present in ~50% of CD lesions (compared to 5–10% of histologically uninvolved CD mucosa, or other inflammatory controls). In the small intestine, I2 was detectable in the ileum of both patients and healthy controls, indicating commensal colonization of this compartment. Serum IgA anti-I2 ELISA with recombinant I2 detected ~60% of CD patients, and ~5% of non-CD controls. In the mouse the I2 sequence is also localized at sites homologous to the human (distal small intestine). Immunologically, I2 is the target of a strong proliferative and IL-10 cytokine response mediated by murine CD4$^+$ splenic T cells. Several lines of evidence indicate that this response to I2 is a T cell superantigen [157]. In contrast, the T cell response to I2 in colitis-prone mouse strains predominated with IFN-γ production. The microanatomic localization of I2 and its unique immunostimulatory activity reflect traits of *P. fluorescens* which may be pertinent to proinflammatory activity in susceptible hosts.

Diagnosis and disease stratification

The strong association of the pANCA and ASCA expression with UC and CD, respectively, has prompted efforts to use these marker antibodies to define more biologically homogeneous patient subsets for IBD diagnosis, prognosis, and treatment planning. With regard to diagnosis, combined testing for these two analytes increases sensitivity for overall IBD serodiagnosis, due to the occurrence of an ASCA$^-$/pANCA$^+$ CD subset, and the greater lability of ASCA but not pANCA levels to disease activity [83, 90, 91]. High pANCA levels predict a more aggressive disease phenotype, including elevated disease activity and pouchitis [88, 93, 158–160]. Conversely, pANCA$^+$ CD patients are distinguished by later onset and more UC-like features, including resistance to anti-TNF-α therapy. This distinctive biology is correlated with differential allelism at the MHC locus, indicating that pANCA expression is an intermediate marker for the genetics of disease susceptibility. In CD, high ASCA levels are independently associated with aggressive disease (early onset, perforation, and fibrostenosing disease [91], although this was not observed in the pediatric population [90].

As noted previously, seronegative and seropositive ASCA phenotypes are each distinct familial traits in CD, and are observed in clinical unaffected family members [144, 145]. Similarly, pANCA-positive and negative family phenotypes define UC and CD subsets [79, 80, 83, 91]. This presumably reflects biologically important differences in host genetics, bacterial exposure, or both. Accordingly, ASCA and pANCA are promising immunologic parameters to identify family members at risk for disease for early, preventative intervention. No prospective studies have yet addressed whether any of the known ser-omarkers is indeed a preclinical disease susceptibility marker. However, this issue is an important opportunity to develop, in view of the clinical progress on early intervention in immunologic diseases such as diabetes mellitis [67].

As elaborated in this chapter, distinctive genetics and microbiology are likely to underlie the expression of the emerging panel of antigen-defined, disease-related autoantibodies and microbial antibodies. Moreover, levels of these antibodies are generally independent of ASCA and pANCA, indicating that they may complement these established disease markers in patient stratification.

In the near term, realization of these opportunities will most critically require further validation of disease-related antigens and organisms, using animal model systems. Moreover, mechanistic characterization of their action should permit the design of novel therapies at an antigen-specific or microbial level. At the clinical level systematic studies will be required to identify new combinations of marker antibodies, in concert with emerging genetic markers which most effectively discriminate patient subpopulations. This homogenization of patient subsets will be useful for empirically refining diagnosis and treatment planning. In addition, homogeneous subsets should permit more powerful analysis of genetic traits and biologic processes responsible for disease pathogenesis, and ultimately the incorporation of sophisticated therapeutic and preventative interventions.

Acknowledgements

This work was supported by NIH DK46763, the UCLA Clinical and Fundamental Immunology Training Grant (AI 07126-23), the Crohn's and Colitis Foundation, UCLA CURE, and the Jonsson Comprehensive Cancer Center.

References

1. Zinkernagel RM, Bachmann MF, Kundig TM, Oehen S, Pirchet H, Hengartner H. On immunological memory. Annu Rev Immunol 1996; 14: 333–67.
2. Litman GW, Anderson MK, Rast JP. Evolution of antigen binding receptors. Annu Rev Immunol 1999; 17: 109–47.
3. Matzinger P. Tolerance, danger, and the extended family. Annu Rev Immunol 1994; 12: 991–1045.
4. Hoffmann JA, Kafatos FC, Janeway CA, Ezekowitz RAB. Phylogenetic perspectives in innate immunity. Science 1999; 284: 1313–18.
5. Blanchard TG, Czinn SJ, Nedrud JG. Host response and vaccine development to *Helicobacter pylori* infection. Curr Top Microbiol Immunol 1999; 241: 181–213.
6. Covacci A, Telford JL, Del Giudice G, Parsonnet J, Rappuoli R. *Helicobacter pylori* virulence and genetic geography. Science 1999; 284: 1328–33.
7. Yuk MH, Harvill ET, Cotter PA, Miller JF. Modulation of host immune responses, induction of apoptosis and inhibition of NF-kappaB activation by the *Bordetella* type III secretion system. Mol Microbiol 2000; 35: 991–1004.
8. Sousa CR, Hieny S, Scharton-Kersten T *et al. In vivo* microbial stimulation induces rapid CD40 ligand-independent production of interleukin 12 by dendritic cells and their redistribution to T cell areas [See comments]. J Exp Med 1997; 186: 1819–29.
9. Fearon DT, Locksley RM. Elements of immunity: the instructive role of innate immunity in the acquired immune response. Science 1996; 272: 50–4.
10. Blaser MJ, Miller RA, Lacher J, Singleton JW. Patients with active Crohn's disease have elevated serum antibodies to antigens of seven enteric bacterial pathogens. Gastroenterology 1984; 87: 888–94.
11. Wayne LG, Hollander D, Anderson B, Sramek HA, Vadheim CM, Rotter JI. Immunoglobulin A (IgA) and IgG serum antibodies to mycobacterial antigens in Crohn's disease patients and their relatives. J Clin Microbiol 1992; 30: 2013–18.
12. Khoo UY, Proctor IE, Macpherson AJ. CD4+ T cell down-regulation in human intestinal mucosa: evidence for intestinal tolerance to luminal bacterial antigens. J Immunol 1997; 158: 3626–34.
13. Duchmann R, May E, Heike M, Knolle P, Neurath M, Meyer zum Buschenfelde KH. T cell specificity and cross reactivity towards enterobacteria, *Bacteroides*, *Bifidobacterium*, and antigens from resident intestinal flora in humans. Gut 1999; 44: 812–18.
14. Duchmann R, Neurath MF, Meyer zum Buschenfelde KH. Responses to self and non-self intestinal microflora in health and inflammatory bowel disease. Res Immunol 1997; 148): 589–94.
15. Weiner HL, Friedman A, Miller A, Khoury SJ, Al-Sabbagh A, Santos L *et al.* Oral tolerance: immunologic mechanisms and treatment of animal and human organ-specific autoimmune diseases by oral administration of autoantigens. Annu Rev Immunol 1994; 12: 809–37.
16. Braun MC, Lahey E, Kelsall BL. Selective suppression of IL-12 production by chemoattractants. J Immunol 2000; 164: 3009–17.
17. Gu L, Tseng S, Horner RM, Tam C, Loda M, Rollins BJ. Control of TH2 polarization by the chemokine monocyte chemoattractant protein-1. Nature 2000; 404: 407–11.
18. Lu B, Rutledge BJ, Gu L, Fiorillo J, Lukacs NW, Kunkel SL *et al.* Abnormalities in monocyte recruitment and cytokine expression in monocyte chemoattractant protein 1-deficient mice. J Exp Med 1998; 187: 601–8.
19. He J, Gurunathan S, Iwasaki A, Ash-Shaheed B, Kelsall BL. Primary role for Gi protein signaling in the regulation of

interleukin 12 production and the induction of T helper cell type 1 responses. J Exp Med 2000; 191: 1605–10.

20. Uguccioni M, Gionchetti P, Robbiani DF *et al.* Increased expression of IP-10, IL-8, MCP-1, and MCP-3 in ulcerative colitis. Am J Pathol 1999; 155: 331–6.

21. Viney JL, Mowat AM, O'Malley JM, Williamson E, Fanger NA. Expanding dendritic cells *in vivo* enhances the induction of oral tolerance. J Immunol 1998; 160: 5815–25.

22. Banchereau J, Briere F, Caux C, Davoust J, Lebecque S, Liu YJ *et al.* Immunobiology of dendritic cells. Annu Rev Immunol 2000; 18: 767–811.

23. Hayday AC. [gamma][delta] cells: a right time and a right place for a conserved third way of protection. Annu Rev Immunol 2000; 18: 975–1026.

24. Brandwein SL, McCabe RP, Cong Y *et al.* Spontaneously colitic C3H/HeJBir mice demonstrate selective antibody reactivity to antigens of the enteric bacterial flora. J Immunol 1997; 159: 44–52.

25. Rath HC, Herfarth HH, Ikeda JS *et al.* Normal luminal bacteria, especially *Bacteroides* species, mediate chronic colitis, gastritis, and arthritis in HLA-B27/human beta2 microglobulin transgenic rats. J Clin Invest 1996; 98: 945–53.

26. Kimura K, McCartney AL, McConnell MA, Tannock GW. Analysis of fecal populations of bifidobacteria and lactobacilli and investigation of the immunological responses of their human hosts to the predominant strains. Appl Environ Microbiol 1997; 63: 3394–8.

27. Duchmann R, Kaiser I, Hermann E, Mayet W, Ewe K, Meyer zum Buschenfelde KH. Tolerance exists towards resident intestinal flora but is broken in active inflammatory bowel disease (IBD). Clin Exp Immunol 1995; 102: 448–55.

28. Klaasen HL, Van der Heijden PJ, Stok W *et al.* Apathogenic, intestinal, segmented, filamentous bacteria stimulate the mucosal immune system of mice. Infect Immun 1993; 61: 303–6.

29. Macpherson AJ, Gatto D, Sainsbury E, Harriman GR, Hengartner H, Zinkernagel RM. A primitive T cell-independent mechanism of intestinal mucosal IgA responses to commensal bacteria. Science 2000; 288: 2222–6.

30. Gewirtz AT, McCormick B, Neish AS *et al.* Pathogen-induced chemokine secretion from model intestinal epithelium is inhibited by lipoxin A4 analogs. J Clin Invest 1998; 101: 1860–9.

31. Gao Y, Lecker S, Post MJ *et al.* Inhibition of ubiquitin-proteasome pathway-mediated I kappa B alpha degradation by a naturally occurring antibacterial peptide. J Clin Invest 2000; 106: 439–48.

32. Maksymowych WP, Ikawa T, Yamaguchi A *et al.* Invasion by *Salmonella typhimurium* induces increased expression of the LMP, MECL, and PA28 proteasome genes and changes in the peptide repertoire of HLA-B27. Infect Immun 1998; 66: 4624–32.

33. VanCott JL, Chatfield SN, Roberts M *et al.* Regulation of host immune responses by modification of *Salmonella* virulence genes. Nature Med 1998; 4: 1247–52.

34. Neish AS, Gewirtz AT, Zeng H *et al.* Prokaryotic regulation of epithelial responses by inhibition of IkappaB-alpha ubiquitination [See comments]. Science 2000; 289: 1560–3.

35. Dunne C, Murphy L, Flynn S *et al.* Probiotics: from myth to reality. Demonstration of functionality in animal models of disease and in human clinical trials. Antonie Van Leeuwenhoek 1999; 76: 279–92.

36. Shevach EM. Regulatory T Cells in autoimmmunity. Annu Rev Immunol 2000; 18: 423–49.

37. Healy JI, Goodnow CC. Positive versus negative signaling by lymphocyte antigen receptors. Annu Rev Immunol 1998; 16: 645–70.

38. Cobbold S, Waldmann H. Infectious tolerance. Curr Opin Immunol 1998; 10: 518–24.

39. Gutgemann I, Fahrer AM, Altman JD, Davis MM, Chien YH. Induction of rapid T cell activation and tolerance by systemic presentation of an orally administered antigen. Immunity 1998; 8: 667–73.

40. Mowat AM, Viney JL. The anatomical basis of intestinal immunity. Immunol Rev 1997; 156: 145–66.

41. Naftzger C, Takechi Y, Kohda H, Hara I, Vijayasaradhi S, Houghton AN. Immune response to a differentiation antigen induced by altered antigen: a study of tumor rejection and autoimmunity. Proc Natl Acad Sci USA 1996; 93: 14809–14.

42. Hugot J-P, Laurent-Puig P, Gower-Rousseau C *et al.* Mapping of a susceptibility locus for Crohn's disease on chromosome 16. Nature 1996; 379: 821–3.

43. Ohmen JD, Yang H-Y, Yamamoto KK *et al.* Susceptibility locus for inflammatory bowel disease on chromosome 16 has a role in Crohn's disease, but not in ulcerative colitis. Hum Mol Genet 1996; 5: 1679–83.

44. Satsangi J, Parkes M, Jewell DP, Bell JI. Genetics of inflammatory bowel disease. Clin Sci 1998; 94: 473–8.

45. Cavanaugh JA, Callen DF, Wilson SR *et al.* Analysis of Australian Crohn's disease pedigrees refines the localization for susceptibility to inflammatory bowel disease on chromosome 16. Ann Hum Genet 1998; 62: 291–8.

46. Hampe J, Lynch NJ, Daniels S *et al.* Fine mapping of the chromosome 3p susceptibility locus in inflammatory bowel disease. Gut 2001; 48: 191–7.

47. Annese V, Latiano A, Bovio P *et al.* Genetic analysis in Italian families with inflammatory bowel disease supports linkage to the IBD1 locus – a GISC study. Eur J Hum Genet 1999; 7: 567–73.

48. Duerr RH, Barmada MM, Zhang L, Pfutzer R, Weeks DE. High-density genome scan in Crohn disease shows confirmed linkage to chromosome 14q11-12. Am J Hum Genet 2000; 66: 1857–62.

49. Lesage S, Zouali H, Colombel JF *et al.* Genetic analyses of chromosome 12 loci in Crohn's disease. Gut 2000; 47: 787–91.

50. Stokkers PC, Huibregtse K, Jr, Leegwater AC, Reitsma PH, Tytgat GN, van Deventer SJ. Analysis of a positional candidate gene for inflammatory bowel disease: NRAMP2. Inflam Bowel Dis 2000; 6: 92–8.

51. Dohi T, Fujihashi K, Kiyono H, Elson CO, McGhee JR. Mice deficient in Th1- and Th2-type cytokines develop distinct forms of hapten-induced colitis. Gastroenterology 2000; 119: 724–33.

52. Bhan AK, Mizoguchi E, Smith RN, Mizoguchi A. Colitis in transgenic and knockout animals as models of human inflammatory bowel disease. Immunol Rev 1999; 169: 195–207.

53. De Winter H, Cheroutre H, Kronenberg M. Mucosal immunity and inflammation. II. The yin and yang of T cells in intestinal inflammation: pathogenic and protective roles in a mouse colitis model. Am J Physiol 1999; 276: G1317-21.

54. MacDonald TT. Effector and regulatory lymphoid cells and cytokines in mucosal sites. Curr Top Microbiol Immunol 1999; 236: 113–35.

55. Sartor RB. Pathogenesis and immune mechanisms of chronic inflammatory bowel diseases. Am J Gastroenterol 1997; 92: 5S–11S.

56. Mizoguchi A, Mizoguchi E, Saubermann LJ, Higaki K, Blumberg RS, Bhan AK. Limited CD4 T-cell diversity associated with colitis in T-cell receptor alpha mutant mice requires a T helper 2 environment. Gastroenterology 2000; 119: 983–95.

57. Rees W, Bender J, Teague TK *et al.* An inverse relationship between T cell receptor affinity and antigen dose during CD4+ T cell responses *in vivo* and *in vitro*. Proc Natl Acad Sci USA 2000; 96: 9781–6.

58. Saubermann LJ, Probert CS, Christ AD *et al.* Evidence of T cell receptor beta-chain patterns in inflammatory and non-inflammatory bowel disease states. Am J Physiol 1999; 276: G613–21.

59. Sanderson S, Campbell DJ, Shastri N. Identification of a CD4+ T cell-stimulating antigen of pathogenic bacteria by expression cloning. J Exp Med 1995; 182: 1751–7.

60. Casten LA, Pierce SK. Receptor-mediated B cell antigen processing. Increased antigenicity of a globular protein covalently coupled to antibodies specific for B cell surface structures. J Immunol 1988; 140: 404–10.

61. Bottomly K, Janeway CA Jr. Antigen presentation by B cells. Nature 1989; 337: 24.

62. Liu KJ, Parikh VS, Tucker PW, Kim BS. Role of the B cell antigen receptor in antigen processing and presentation: involvement of the transmembrane region in intracellular trafficking of receptor/ligand complexes. J Immunol 1993; 151: 6143–54.

63. Schultze JL, Gribben JG, Nadler LM. Tumor-specific adoptive T-cell therapy for CD40+ B-cell malignancies. Curr Opin Oncol 1998; 10: 542–7.

64. Tony H-P, Phillips N, Parker D. Role of membrane immunoglobulin (Ig) crosslinking in membrane Ig-mediated, major histocompatibility-restricted T cell-B cell cooperation. J Exp Med 1985; 162: 1695–708.

65. Lanzavecchia A. Receptor-mediated antigen uptake and its effect on antigen presentation to class-II-restricted T lymphocytes. Annu Rev Immunol 1990; 8: 773–94.

66. Korganow AS, Ji H, Mangialaio S *et al.* From systemic T cell self-reactivity to organ-specific autoimmune disease via immunoglobulins. Immunity 1999; 10: 451–61.

67. Abiru N, Eisenbarth GS. Multiple genes/multiple autoantigens role in type 1 diabetes. Clin Rev Allergy Immunol 2000; 18: 27–40.

68. Burton DR. A vaccine for HIV type 1: the antibody perspective. Proc Natl Acad Sci USA 1997; 94: 10018–23.

69. Winter G, Griffiths AD, Hawkins RE, Hoogenboom HR. Making antibodies by phage display technology. Annu Rev Immunol 1994; 12: 433–55.

70. De Wildt RMT, Steenbakkers PG, Pennings AHM, Van den Hoogen FHJ, Van Venrooij WJ, Hoet RMA. A new method for the analysis and production of monoclonal antibody fragments originating from single human B cells. J Immunol Meth 1997; 207: 61–7.

71. Siegel DL, Chang TY, Russell SL, Bunya VY. Isolation of cell surface-specific human monoclonal antibodies using phage display and magnetically-activated cell sorting: applications in immunohematology. J Immunol Meth 1997; 206: 73–85.

72. Jespers LS, Roberts A, Mahler SM, Winter G, Hoogenboom HR. Guiding the selection of human antibodies from phage display repertoires to a single epitope of an antigen. Biotechnology 1994; 12: 899–903.

73. Vaughn TJ, Williams AJ, Pritchard K *et al.* Human antibodies with sub-nanomolar affinities isolated from a large non-immunized phage display library. Nature Biotechnol 1996; 14: 309–14.

74. Saxon A, Shanahan F, Landers C, Ganz T, Targan SR. A distinct subset of antineutrophil cytoplasmic antibodies is associated with inflammatory bowel disease. J Allergy Clin Immunol 1990; 86: 202–10.

75. Rump JA, Scholmerich J, Gross V *et al.* A new type of perinuclear anti-neutrophil cytoplasmic antibody (p-ANCA) in active ulcerative colitis but not in Crohn's disease. Immunobiology 1990; 181: 406–13.

76. Duerr RH, Targan SR, Landers CJ, Sutherland LR, Shanahan F. Anti-neutrophil cytoplasmic antibodies in ulcerative colitis. Comparison with other colitides/diarrheal illnesses. Gastroenterology 1991; 100: 1590–6.

77. Vidrich A, Lee J, James E, Cobb L, Targan SR. Segregation of pANCA antigenic recognition by DNase treatment of neutrophils: ulcerative colitis, type 1 autoimmune hepatitis, and primary sclerosing cholangitis. J Clin Immunol 1995; 15: 293–9.

78. Billing P, Tahir S, Calfin B *et al.* Nuclear localization of the antigen detected by ulcerative colitis-associated perinuclear antineutrophil cytoplasmic antibodies. Am J Pathol 1995; 147: 979–87.

79. Shanahan F, Duerr RH, Rotter JI *et al.* Neutrophil autoantibodies in ulcerative colitis: familial aggregation and genetic heterogeneity. Gastroenterology 1992; 103: 456–61.

80. Yang H-Y, Rotter JI, Toyoda H *et al.* Ulcerative colitis: a genetically heterogeneous disorder defined by genetic (HLA class II) and subclinical (antineutrophil cytoplasmic antibodies) markers. J Clin Invest 1993; 92: 1080–4.

81. Folwaczny C, Noehl N, Endres SP, Heldwein W, Loeschke K, Fricke H. Antinuclear autoantibodies in patients with inflammatory bowel disease – high prevalence in first-degree relatives. Dig Dis Sci 1997; 42: 1593–7.

82. Yang P, Jarnerot G, Danielsson D, Tysk C, Lindberg E. P-ANCA in monozygotic twins with inflammatory bowel disease. Gut 1995; 36: 887–90.

83. Quinton JF, Sendid B, Reumaux D *et al.* Anti-*Saccharomyces cerevisiae* mannan antibodies combined with antineutrophil cytoplasmic autoantibodies in inflammatory bowel disease: prevalence and diagnostic role. Gut 1998; 42: 788–91.

84. Mizoguchi E, Mizoguchi A, Chiba C, Niles JL, Bhan AK. Antineutrophil cytoplasmic antibodies in T-cell receptor alpha-deficient mice with chronic colitis. Gastroenterology 1997; 113: 1828–35.

85. Seibold F, Brandwein S, Simpson S, Terhorst C, Elson CO. pANCA represents a cross-reactivity to enteric bacterial antigens. J Clin Immunol 1998; 18: 153–60.

86. Seibold F, Slametschka D, Gregor M, Weber P. Neutrophil autoantibodies: a genetic marker in primary sclerosing cholangitis and ulcerative colitis. Gastroenterology 1994; 107: 532–6.

87. Gahl WA, Brantly M, Kaiser-Kupfer MI *et al.* Genetic defects and clinical characteristics of patients with a form of oculocutaneous albinism (Hermansky–Pudlak syndrome). N Engl J Med 1998; 338: 1258–64.

88. Vecchi M, Bianchi MB, Sinico RA *et al.* Antibodies to neutrophil cytoplasm in Italian patients with ulcerative colitis: sensitivity, specificity and recognition of putative antigens. Digestion 1994; 5: 34–9.

89. Mulder AH, Broekroelofs J, Horst G, Limburg PC, Nelis GF, Kallenberg CG. Anti-neutrophil cytoplasmic antibodies (ANCA) in inflammatory bowel disease: characterization and clinical correlates. Clin Exp Immunol 1994; 95: 490–7.

90. Ruemmele FM, Targan SR, Levy G, Dubinsky M, Braun J, Seidman EG. Diagnostic accuracy of serological assays in pediatric inflammatory bowel disease. Gastroenterology 1998; 115: 822–9.

91. Vasiliauskas EA, Kam LY, Karp LC, Gaiennie J, Yang H, Targan SR. Marker antibody expression stratifies Crohn's disease into immunologically homogeneous subgroups with distinct clinical characteristics. Gut 2000; 47: 487–96.

92. Sandborn WJ, Landers CJ, Tremaine WJ, Targan SR. Association of antineutrophil cytoplasmic antibodies with resistance to treatment of left-sided ulcerative colitis: results of a pilot study. Mayo Clin Proc 1996; 71: 431–6.

93. Vasiliauskas EA, Plevy SE, Landers CJ *et al.* Perinuclear antineutrophil cytoplasmic antibodies in patients with Crohn's disease define a clinical subgroup. Gastroenterology 1996; 110: 1810–19.

94. Sobajima J, Ozaki S, Okazaki T *et al.* Anti-neutrophil cytoplasmic antibodies (ANCA) in ulcerative colitis: anti-cathepsin G and a novel antibody correlate with refractory type. Clin Exp Immunol 1996; 105: 120–5.

95. Sugi K, Saitoh O, Matsuse R *et al.* Antineutrophil cytoplasmic antibodies in Japanese patients with inflammatory bowel disease: prevalence and recognition of putative antigens. Am J Gastroenterol 1999; 94: 1304–12.

96. Roozendaal C, Zhao MH, Horst G, Lockwood CM, Kleibeuker JH, Limburg PC *et al.* Catalase and alpha-enolase: two novel granulocyte autoantigens in inflammatory bowel disease (IBD). Clin Exp Immunol 1998; 112: 10–16.

97. Walmsley RS, Zhao MH, Hamilton MI *et al.* Antineutrophil cytoplasm autoantibodies against bactericidal/permeability-increasing protein in inflammatory bowel disease. Gut 1997; 40: 105–9.

98. Terjung B, Spengler U, Sauerbruch T, Worman HJ. 'Atypical p-ANCA' in IBD and hepatobiliary disorders react with a 50-kilodalton nuclear envelope protein of neutrophils and myeloid cell lines. Gastroenterology 2000; 119: 310–22.

99. Sobajima J, Ozaki S, Osakada F, Uesugi H, Shirakawa H, Yoshida M *et al.* Novel autoantigens of perinuclear anti-neutrophil cytoplasmic antibodies (p-ANCA) in ulcerative colitis: non-histone chromosomal proteins, HMG1 and HMG2. Clin Exp Immunol 1997; 107: 135–40.

100. Sobajima J, Ozaki S, Uesugi H *et al.* Prevalence and characterization of perinuclear anti-neutrophil cytoplasmic antibodies (P-ANCA) directed against HMG1 and HMG2 in ulcerative colitis (UC). Clin Exp Immunol 1998; 111: 402–7.

101. Reumaux D, Meziere C, Colombel J-F, Duthilleul P, Muller S. Distinct production of autoantibodies to nuclear components in ulcerative colitis and in Crohn's disease. Clin Immunol Immunopathol 1995; 77: 349–57.

102. Eggena M, Cohavy O, Parseghian M *et al.* Identification of histone H1 as a cognate antigen of the ulcerative colitis-associated marker antibody pANCA. J Autoimmun 2000; 14: 83–97.

103. Giese K, Cox J, Grosschedl R. The HMG domain of lymphoid enhancer factor 1 bends DNA and facilitates assembly of functional nucleoprotein structures. Cell 1992; 69: 185–95.

104. Yoshida M, Shimura K. Unwinding of DNA by nonhistone chromosomal protein HMG (1+2) from pig thymus as determined with endonuclease. J Biochem 1984; 95: 117–24.

105. Parseghian M, Harris DA, Rishwain DR, Hamkalo BA. Characterization of a set of antibodies specific for three human histone H1 subtypes. Chromosoma 1994; 103: 198–208.

106. Muller S, Richalet P, Laurent-Crawford A *et al.* Autoantibodies typical of non-organ-specific autoimmune diseases in HIV-seropositive patients. AIDS 1992; 6: 933–42.

107. Morino N, Sakurai H, Yamada A, Yazaki Y, Minota S. Rabbit anti-chromatin antibodies recognize similar epitopes on a histone H1 molecule as lupus autoantibodies. Clin Immunol Immunopathol 1995; 77: 52–8.

108. Stemmer C, Briand J-P, Muller S. Mapping of linear epitopes of human histone H1 recognized by rabbit anti-H1/H5 antisera and antibodies from autoimmune patients. Mol Immunol 1994; 31: 1037–46.

109. Sobajima J, Ozaki S, Uesugi H *et al.* High mobility group (HMG) non-histone chromosomal proteins HMG1 and HMG2 are significant target antigens of perinuclear anti-neutrophil cytoplasmic antibodies in autoimmune hepatitis [See comments]. Gut 1999; 44: 867–73.

110. Eggena M, Targan SR, Iwanczyk L, Vidrich A, Gordon LK, Braun J. Phage display cloning and characterization of an immunogenetic marker (perinuclear anti-neutrophil cytoplasmic antibody) in ulcerative colitis. J Immunol 1996; 156: 4005–11.

111. Gordon LK, Eggena M, Targan SR, Braun J. Definition of ocular antigens in ciliary body and retinal ganglion cells by the marker antibody pANCA. Invest Ophthalmol Vis Sci 1999; 40: 1250–5.

112. Gordon LK, Eggena M, Targan SR, Braun J. Mast cell and neuroendocrine cytoplasmic autoantigen(s) detected by monoclonal pANCA antibodies. Clin Immunol 2000; 94: 42–50.

113. Fiocchi C, Roche JK, Michener WM. High prevalence of antibodies to intestinal epithelial antigens in patients with inflammatory bowel disease and their relatives. Ann Intern Med 1989; 110: 786–94.

114. Halstensen TS, Das KM, Brandtzaeg P. Epithelial deposits of immunoglobulin G1 and activated complement co-localize with the M(r) 40 kD putative autoantigen in ulcerative colitis. Gut 1993; 34: 650–7.

115. Das KM, Vecchi M, Sakamaki S. A shared and unique epitope(s) on human colon, skin, and biliary epithelium detected by a monoclonal antibody. Gastroenterology 1990; 98: 464–9.

116. Geng X, Biancone L, Dai HH *et al.* Tropomyosin isoforms in intestinal mucosa: production of autoantibodies to tropomyosin isoforms in ulcerative colitis. Gastroenterology 1998; 114: 912–22.

117. Ohman L, Franzen L, Rudolph U, Harriman GR, Hultgren HE. Immune activation in the intestinal mucosa before the onset of colitis in Galphai2-deficient mice. Scand J Immunol 2000; 52: 80–90.

118. Sakamaki S, Takayanagi N, Yoshizaki N *et al.* Autoantibodies against the specific epitope of human tropomyosin(s) detected by a peptide based enzyme immunoassay in sera of patients with ulcerative colitis show antibody dependent cell mediated cytotoxicity against HLA-DPw9 transfected L cells. Gut 2000; 47: 236–41.

119. Mizoguchi A, Mizoguchi E, Smith RN, Preffer FI, Bhan AK. Suppressive role of B cells in chronic colitis of T cell receptor alpha mutant mice. J Exp Med 1997; 186: 1749–56.

120. Stevens TR, Winrow VR, Blake DR, Rampton DS. Circulating antibodies to heat-shock protein 60 in Crohn's disease and ulcerative colitis. Clin Exp Immunol 1992; 90: 271–4.

121. Steinhoff U, Brinkmann V, Klemm U *et al.* Autoimmune intestinal pathology induced by hsp60-specific CD8 T cells. Immunity 1999; 11: 349–358.

122. Seibold F, Mork HJ, Tanza S *et al.* Pancreatic autoantibodies in Crohn's disease: a family study. Gut 1997; 40: 481–4.

123. Seibold F, Weber P, Henss H, Widmann KH. Antibodies to a trypsin sensitive pancreatic antigen in chronic inflammatory bowel disease. Specific markers for a subgroup of patients with Crohn's disease. Gut 1991; 32: 1192–7.

124. Stevens TR, Harley SL, Groom JS *et al.* Anti-endothelial cell antibodies in inflammatory bowel disease. Dig Dis Sci 1993; 38: 426–32.

125. Romas E, Paspaliaris B, d'Apice AJ, Elliott PR. Autoantibodies to neutrophil cytoplasmic (ANCA) and endothelial cells. Austr NZ J Med 1992; 22: 652–9.

126. Aldebert D, Masy E, Reumaux D, Lion G, Colombel J-F, Duthilleul P. Immunoglobulin G subclass distribution of anti-endothelial cell antibodies (AECA) in patients with ulcerative colitis and Crohn's disease. Dig Dis Sci 1997; 42: 2350–5.

127. Auer IO, Roder A, Wensinck F, van de Merwe JP, Schmidt H. Selected bacterial antibodies in Crohn's disease and ulcerative colitis. Scand J Gastroenterol 1983; 18: 217–23.

128. O'Mahony S, Anderson N, Nuki G, Ferguson A. Systemic and mucosal antibodies to *Klebsiella* in patients with ankylosing spondylitis and Crohn's disease. Ann Rheum Dis 1992; 51: 1296–300.

129. Liu Y, Van Kruiningen HJ, West AB, Cartun RW, Cortot A, Colombel J-F. Immunocytochemical evidence of *Listeria*, *Escherichia coli*, and *Streptococcus* antigens in Crohn's disease. Gastroenterology 1995; 108: 1396–404.

130. Walmsley RS, Anthony A, Sim R, Pounder RE, Wakefield AJ. Absence of *Escherichia coli*, *Listeria monocytogenes*, and *Klebsiella pneumoniae* antigens within inflammatory bowel disease tissues. J Clin Pathol 1998; 51: 657–61.

131. Cong Y, Brandwein SL, McCabe RP et al. CD4+ T cells reactive to enteric bacterial antigens in spontaneously colitic C3H/HeJBir mice: increased T helper cell type 1 response and ability to transfer disease. J Exp Med 1998; 187: 855–64.

132. Peeters M, Geypens B, Claus D et al. Clustering of increased small intestinal permeability in families with Crohn's disease. Gastroenterology 1997; 113: 802–7.

133. Hollander D, Vadheim CM, Brettholz E, Petersen GM, Delahunty T, Rotter JI. Increased intestinal permeability in Crohn's patients and their relatives: an etiologic factor? Ann Intern Med 1986; 105: 883–5.

134. Sartor RB. The influence of normal microbial flora on the development of chronic mucosal inflammation. Res Immunol 1997; 148: 567–76.

135. Main J, McKenzie H, Yeaman GR, Kerr MA, Robson DPCR, Parratt D. Antibody to *Saccharomyces cerevisiae* (bakers' yeast) in Crohn's disease. Br Med J 1988; 297: 1105–6.

136. McKenzie H, Main J, Pennington CR, Parratt D. Antibody to selected strains of *Saccharomyces cerevisiae* (baker's and brewer's yeast) and *Candida albicans* in Crohn's disease. Gut 1990; 31: 536–8.

137. Barnes RMR, Allan S, Taylor-Robinson CH, Finn R, Johnson PM. Serum antibodies reactive with *Saccharomyces cerevisiae* in inflammatory bowel disease: is IgA antibody a marker for Crohn's disease. Int Arch Allergy Appl Immunol 1990; 92: 9–15.

138. Giaffer MH, Clark A, Holdsworth CD. Antibodies to *Saccharomyces cerevisiae* in patients with Crohn's disease and their possible pathogenic importance. Gut 1992; 33: 1071–5.

139. Lindberg E, Magnusson KE, Tysk C, Jarnerot G. Antibody (IgG, IgA, and IgM) to baker's yeast (*Saccharomyces cerevisiae*), yeast mannan, gliadin, ovalbumin, and betalactoglobulin in monozygotic twins with inflammatory bowel disease. Gut 1992; 33: 909–13.

140. Colombel J-F, Sendid B, Jacquinor PM, Cortot A, Camus D, Poulain D. Evidence for a specific antibody response to *Saccharomyces cerevisiae* oligomannosidic epitopes in Crohn's disease. Gastroenterology 1994; 108: 800A.

141. Sendid B, Colombel JF, Jacquinot PM et al. Specific antibody response to oligomannosidic epitopes in Crohn's disease. Clin Diag Lab Immunol 1996; 3: 219–26.

142. Davidson IW, Lloyd RS, Whorewell PJ, Wright R. Antibodies to maize in patients with Crohn's disease, ulcerative colitis, and coeliac disease. Clin Exp Immunol 1979; 35: 147–8.

143. Sonnenberg A. Occupational distribution of inflammatory bowel disease among German employees. Gut 1990; 31: 1037–40.

144. Sendid B, Quinton JF, Charrier G et al. Anti-*Saccharomyces cerevisiae* mannan antibodies in familial Crohn's disease. Am J Gastroenterol 1998; 93: 1306–10.

145. Sutton C, Yang H-Y, Rotter JI, Targan SR, Braun J. Familial expression of anti-*Saccharomyces cerevisiae* mannan antibodies (ASCA) in affected and unaffected relatives of Crohn's disease patients. Gut 2000; 46: 58–63.

146. Elsaghier A, Prantera C, Moreno C, Ivanyi J. Antibodies to *Mycobacterium paratuberculosis*-specific protein antigens in Crohn's disease. Clin Exp Immunol 1992; 90: 503–8.

147. Suenaga K, Yokoyama Y, Nishimori I et al. Serum antibodies to *Mycobacterium paratuberculosis* in patients with Crohn's disease. Dig Dis Sci 1999; 44: 1202–7.

148. Vannuffel P, Dieterich C, Naerhuyzen B et al. Occurrence, in Crohn's disease, of antibodies directed against a species-specific recombinant polypeptide of *Mycobacterium paratuberculosis*. Clin Diag Lab Immunol 1994; 1: 241–3.

149. El-Zaatari FA, Naser SA, Engstrand L, Hachem CY, Graham DY. Identification and characterization of *Mycobacterium paratuberculosis* recombinant proteins expressed in *E. coli*. Curr Microbiol 1994; 29: 177–84.

150. Naser SA, Hulten K, Shafran I, Graham DY, El Zaatari FA. Specific seroreactivity of Crohn's disease patients against p35 and p36 antigens of *M. avium* subsp. *paratuberculosis*. Vet Microbiol 2000; 77: 497–504.

151. Cohavy O, Harth G, Horwitz MA et al. Identification of a novel mycobacterial histone H1 homologue (HupB) as an antigenic target of pANCA monoclonal antibody and serum IgA from patients with Crohn's disease. Infect Immun 1999; 67: 6510–17.

152. Cocito C, Gilot P, Coene M, De Kesel M, Poupart P, Vannuffel P. Paratuberculosis. Clin Microbiol Rev 1994; 7: 328–45.

153. Van Kruiningen HJ. Lack of support for a common etiology in Johne's disease of animals and Crohn's disease in humans. Inflam Bowel Dis 1999; 5: 183–91.

154. Cohavy O, Bruckner D, Eggena ME, Targan SR, Gordon LK, Braun J. Colonic bacteria express an ulcerative colitis pANCA-related protein epitope. Infect Immun 2000; 68: 1542–8.

155. Wei B, Dalwadi H, Gordon LK et al. Molecular cloning of a *Bacteroides caccae* TonB-linked outer membrane protein associated with inflammatory bowel disease. Infect Immun 2001 (In press).

156. Sutton CL, Kim J, Yamane A et al. Identification of a novel bacterial sequence associated with Crohn's disease. Gastroenterology 2000; 119: 23–8.

157. Dalwadi H, Kronenberg M, Sutton CL, Braun J. The Crohn's disease-associated bacterial protein, I2, is a novel enteric T cell superantigen. Immunity 2001 (submitted).

158. Lombardi G, Annese V, Piepoli A et al. Antineutrophil cytoplasmic antibodies in inflammatory bowel disease: clinical role and review of the literature. Dis Colon Rectum 2000; 43: 999–1007.

159. Fleshner PR, Vasiliauskas EA, Kam LY, Abreu-Martin MT, Targan SR. High level perinuclear antineutrophil cytoplasmic antibody (pANCA) in ulcerative colitis patients before colectomy predicts the development of chronic pouchitis after ileal pouch anal anastomosis. Gastroenterology 1999; 116: A716.

160. Vecchi M, Bianchi MB, Calabresi C, Meucci G, Tatarella M, de Franchis R. Long–term observation of the perinuclear anti-neutrophil cytoplasmic antibody status in ulcerative colitis patients. Scand J Gastroenterol 1998; 33: 170–3.

11 | Pathophysiology of inflammatory bowel disease: the effect of inflammation on intestinal function

STEPHEN M. COLLINS AND KENNETH CROITORU

Introduction

Many symptoms of inflammatory bowel disease (IBD) arise as a result of alterations in gut physiology. For example diarrhea reflects changes in epithelial transport as well as changes in gastrointestinal motility. These changes may reflect the actions of inflammatory mediators on target cells that include the epithelial cell, smooth muscle cell and nerves. The changes may also arise as a result of phenotypic shifts in these cells induced by inflammation or immune activation; such shifts enable these cell types to produce mediators that, in an autocrine or paracrine fashion, alter the physiological role of the cell; an example is the production of cytokines by smooth muscle or epithelial cells.

Gut physiology is highly integrated and is controlled via a hierarchy of mechanisms that include local factors involving cell-to-cell contact, the paracrine secretion of humoral substances such as prostaglandins and regulatory peptides, the endocrine secretion of peptide hormones such as cholecystokinin (CCK) or 5-hydroxytryptamine (5-HT), or through neural networks. The latter may be intrinsic to the gut or may involve extrinsic nerves including those of the autonomic or central nervous systems.

Finally, gut physiology may be perturbed indirectly through inflammation-induced structural changes in the gut. Examples of this include the effects of bacterial overgrowth resulting from strictures or fistulas or the effects of obstructing strictures on the physiology of cells in the prestenotic regions of the gut.

It follows, therefore, that inflammation, albeit restricted to one region of the gut, may produce widespread perturbations of gut function by altering a variety of cell types, in non-inflamed regions as well as inflamed regions of the gut, through the involvement of endocrine or neural networks.

The effect of inflammation on epithelial cells

Clinical observations

The intestinal epithelium is responsible for the absorption of nutrients and the regulation of water and ion transport. Changes in these functions contribute to the diarrhea associated with IBD. The net accumulation of fluid into the intestinal lumen leads to increased stool number and volume. Inflammation and ulceration of the epithelium leads to loss of the digestive enzymes required for the breakdown and absorption of protein and fat, and loss of the large surface area required for nutrient absorption. The clinical result is diarrhea, weight loss, malnutrition and changes in fluid and electrolyte homeostasis. The inflammatory destruction of the mucosa is also associated with blood and protein losses manifest by iron deficiency anemia, and in severe cases, hypoalbuminemia. In addition, disruption of the integrity of the intestinal epithelial layer, an important barrier to macromolecules, allows for stimulation of the local immune system by luminal antigens [1, 2]. The issue of whether all intestinal permeability changes are acquired or inherited remains controversial [3].

Chronic mucosal inflammation has a significant influence on the physiological function of the intestinal epithelium. In addition, the intestinal epithelial cell is actively involved in regulating and influencing the inflammatory process and the mucosal immune function of the intestine. In addition, there is new appreciation of the direct effect of the non-pathogenic gut flora on epithelial cell function. These findings are supported by the clinical observation that broad-spectrum antibiotics may have therapeutic value in specific clinical situations in IBD patients [4]. The advances made in our understanding of the mechanisms underlying these observed changes in

Stephan R. Targan, Fergus Shanahan and Loren C. Karp (eds.), *Inflammatory Bowel Disease: From Bench to Bedside, 2nd Edition*, 223–234.

epithelial cell function in IBD are critical to our management of the disease.

Insights into underlying mechanisms from animal studies

Epithelial cell growth, differentiation and apoptosis

Epithelial cell (EC) proliferation, differentiation and death are significantly altered during inflammation. In the small bowel of rodents and humans parasite-induced inflammation can lead to villous atrophy and crypt hyperplasia. The loss of the large mucosal surface area provided by the intestinal villi leads to loss of normal absorptive capacities [5]. Similar changes can be initiated by immune activation with food antigen in patients with celiac disease [5]. The immune activation leads to release of mediators and cytokines that participate in the initiation of mucosal damage [6]. Direct T cell activation *in vivo* in mice leads to loss of normal epithelial structure with loss of villi and crypt epithelial cells due to apoptosis [7]. T cell activation in human fetal intestinal explants also caused loss of villi and increased proliferation of crypt cells [8]. Although cytokines such as tumor necrosis factor α (TNF-α) can directly cause these changes *in vivo* [9], T cell-mediated damage involves the interplay of Perforin and Fas/FasL, with TNF-α playing a non-essential role (Croitoru, unpublished observation). Other factors influencing epithelial cell turnover include cytokines such as transforming growth factor β (TGF-β) and interferon gamma (IFN-γ) and growth factors such as growth hormone, glucagon-like peptides and trefoil factor peptides [10–14]. It is evident that these molecules influence the normal growth and development of intestinal epithelial cells in addition to participating in the immune-mediated damage of the mucosa.

Permeability changes

An important function of the epithelial layer in the intestine is that of a barrier to macromolecules. Inflammation alters the barrier function of the intestine, as can be measured by change in permeability or leakiness of the mucosal epithelium to radiolabeled macromolecules of varying sizes [15, 16]. The mechanisms underlying this loss of barrier function have been examined in a number of animal models of inflammation as well as in humans. Antigenic challenge of sensitized rats, with increases in mucosal mast cell numbers, leads to a localized anaphylactic reaction associated with an increase in epithelial permeability [17–19]. Mediators released from mucosal mast cells, which include histamine, serotonin, proteases and various cytokines, contribute to these changes in epithelial barrier function [20]. The molecular elements that result in altered permeability include IFN-γ and TNF-α. These cytokines synergistically alter the integrity of epithelial tight junctions through mechanisms that remain to be identified [21, 22]. *In-vitro* studies have shown that incubation of an epithelial cell line monolayer, T84, with neutrophils leads to permeability changes of the monolayer correlated with neutrophil transmigration [23]. These studies identify cellular and molecular mechanisms by which immune cells alter intestinal epithelial barrier function.

Fluid and ion transport

Epithelial cell chloride secretion is reflected by measured changes in the short-circuit current generated across intestinal mucosa mounted in an Ussing chamber [24]. Ion transport measured in this way reflects the ability of intestinal epithelial cells to regulate fluid and electrolyte absorption and secretion. Rodents undergoing inflammatory events such as infection with parasites such as *Nippostrongylus brasiliensis* and *Trichinella spiralis*, as well as food antigen-induced hypersensitivities (e.g. egg albumin and cow's milk protein) have altered chloride secretion [25]. *In-vitro* studies extend our understanding of how inflammatory cells and cytokines can alter epithelial cell ion transport [7, 25–28]. Studies in human tissue confirm many of these findings e.g. TNF-α induces chloride secretion [15]. Specific changes that occur in patients with IBD are now being defined [25, 29, 15].

Epithelial cells and cytokines

As described, a number of cytokines such as TNF-α and IFN-γ can alter chloride secretion in the intestine [28, 30–32]. Thus immune cells such as lymphocytes and mast cells, rich in cytokines, influence epithelial cell function [33]. Intraepithelial lymphocytes, which lie between epithelial cells, also produce cytokines including IL-2, -3, -5, -6, TGF-β and IFN-γ that may influence chloride secretion [34]. These observations highlight the importance of lymphocyte-derived cytokines and lymphocyte–epithelial cell interactions in altering the intestinal epithelial function.

Epithelial cell as a participant in the immune response

The discussion above illustrates how the inflammatory and immune response can alter intestinal epithelial cell function, contributing to the pathophysiology of the clinical syndrome of IBD. At the same time it has become clear that the intestinal epithelial cell can contribute to the local immune and inflammatory response in the intestine.

Antigen presentation

Intestinal epithelial cells express the MHC class II molecule in both rodents and humans [35, 36]. This cell surface molecule is associated with the ability of cells such as macrophages, B cells and dendritic cells to present antigen to T cells. *In-vitro* evidence suggests that intestinal epithelial cells can also serve in antigen presentation [37, 38]. MHC class II expression on intestinal epithelial cells is stimulated by IFN-γ [39]. Intestinal epithelial cells preferentially stimulate CD8 T cells, i.e. the suppressor/cytotoxic T cell subset. In this way one can speculate that epithelial cells help down-regulate the mucosal immune response [40]. Epithelial cell interaction with CD8 T cells leads to CD8-associated p56lck activation [41] and the CD8 binding ligand is a 180 kDa glycoprotein that has homology with carcinoembryonic antigen [42]. In patients with IBD the type of MHC class II molecules expressed is altered [43] as is the antigen-presenting ability of epithelial cells. IBD derived epithelial cells preferentially stimulate CD4 helper T cells, which might contribute to the inflammatory response [44]. Other accessory molecules identified on colonic epithelial cells may contribute to this stimulation of CD4 T cell proliferation [45]. Therefore, in IBD the epithelial cell contributes to the initiation and possibly the perpetuation of the local inflammation.

Interaction between epithelial cells and lymphocytes

Mucosal mast cells have a unique mediator content and function differently than connective tissue mast cells [46]. Mucosal tissue also attracts unique subsets of T cells such as the γ/δ T cell receptor bearing intraepithelial lymphocytes (IEL) [47, 48]. In addition, mucosal B cells also include unusal populations that preferentially produce and secrete IgA selectively recognizing gut flora-related antigen [49]. These unusual phenotypes are a result of local influences in which cytokines and growth factors favor the development of immune effector cells especially adapted to the mucosa. For example, epithelial cells express cell surface markers that allow for specific interactions with local lymphocytes. In addition to MHC class II molecules, these include CD1 [38, 50] accessory molecules such as CD86 [45] and adhesion molecules such as ICAM1 [51]. In addition, the IEL adhesion molecule ligand CD105 serves to maintain epithelial integrity [52, 53].

In addition to the ability of epithelial cells to influence local lymphocyte traffic and function, epithelial cells also influence local T cell differentiation. The gut mucosal immune system has long been considered a primary lymphoid organ, primarily for B cell development [54]. It is also evident that interactions between epithelial cells and lymphocytes derived from Peyer's patches induce the differentiation of epithelial cells into M cells [55]. This is in keeping with the notion that the intestine is an important site for T cell development [56–58]. Evidence has shown that intestinal T cell subsets can develop extrathymically [48, 58] and that *in-vitro* epithleial cell lines can influence bone marrow-derived T cell differentiation [59]. The presence of intestinal T cells with similar phenotypic characteristics in humans suggest the possible existence of a similar thymus-independent lineage [60]. The significance of an intestinal-derived T cell lineage is that the intestinal environment would control the development of the T cell repertoire. Changes in this environment might then alter T cell repertoires with potential increases in autoreactivity.

Cytokine production

Epithelial cells produce and secrete a myriad of cytokines, which could influence the local immune response. Cytokine production by epithelial cells of the thymus, lung, nasal passageways and kidney suggests a functional potential of epithelial cells in general. Some of these cytokines are produced in response to inflammation or normal bacterial products and others reflect constitutive abilities. The list of cytokines produced by gastrointestinal epithelial cells include IL-1α, ILβ, TNF-α [61, 62], granulocyte–macrophage colony-stimulating factor (GM-CSF), G-CSF and IL-6 [63], IL-8 [64, 65]. The ability of epithelial cells to produce IL-8 has been of particular interest because of the role IL-8 plays as a chemotactic factor for neutrophils. It is probable that this cytokine is involved in the pathogenesis of crypt abscess as well as lamina propria inflammation. Other cytokines shown to be produced by epithelial cells include IL-7, an important regulator of mucosal lymphocytes [66]. Loss of IL-7 function in mice leads to the development of colitis [67]. Clearly epithelial cells have a significant potential to influence the local inflammatory and immune response.

Immunoglobulin receptors

Secretory component (SC) is an epithelial cell receptor for IgA and IgM and functions in the directional transport of polymeric Ig from lamina propria to the intestinal lumenal side of epithelial cells. SC is up-regulated by IFN-γ [68] and TNF-α [69]. Presumably, the increased SC expression would allow for increased transport of protective IgA into the intestinal lumen in response to inflammation [70]. More recent work has shown that other Ig receptors on epithelial cells can serve as an antigen-specific receptor and lead to selective and specific recognition and uptake of luminal proteins [20].

Epithelial–bacterial interactions

Invasive bacteria induce the expression of ICAM1 on epithelial cells leading to an increase in neutrophil adhesion [71]. In addition, bacterial infection leads to an increase in the expression of a host of epithelial-derived cytokines [72]. Bacterial pathogens such as *Helicobacter pylori* induce epithelial cell production of cytokines such as IL-8 [64, 73]. The induction of cytokine production by epithelial cells is in part a result of direct bacterial adhesion and in part due to soluble bacterial factors such as bacterial chemotactic peptide N-formyl-methionine-leucine-phenylalanine (FMLP). Receptors for FMLP have been identified in the subepithelial layer of the gastrointestinal mucosa [74]. Recent studies have shown that pathogens such as *H. pylori* and *E. coli* strains can inject bacterial proteins via type IV secretory mechanisms in host epithelial cells [75]. The injected protein, in the case of *H. pylori* cagA, undergoes tyrosine phosphorylation within the host cells allowing for changes in host cell intracellular signaling [75].

Human and animal studies suggest that non-pathogenic gut bacteria are involved in the pathogenesis of IBD [76, 77]. Intestinal epithelial cell responses to luminal bacterial flora may contribute to inflammation through the release of proinflammatory cytokines [78, 79]. Epithelial cells constitutively express Toll-like receptors (TLR), which are key regulators of innate immune response to bacteria. Changes in the profile of these receptors in patients with IBD may explain differences in responses to normal gut flora in patients with IBD [80]. More recently, mutations in a non-TLR receptor for LPS induced NF-κB activation has been identified as the

IBD1 locus gene in Crohn's patients with a strong familial history [81, 82]. Whether changes in this gene alter the innate immune response of epithelial cells to normal gut flora remains to be defined. Other epithelial-derived mechanisms involved in the innate response to gut flora include defensins, a series of antibacterial peptides produced by Paneth cells and other epithelial cells [83–85]. Future studies are required to define the role of these peptides in the pathogenesis of IBD.

Clinical implications of altered epithelial function in IBD.

The mechanisms by which cells of the immune system and the intestinal epithelial cell interact have given us new avenues to explore in our attempt to understand the pathophysiology of IBD, as well as in our attempt to design new forms of treatment. The challenge is to define which alterations in cytokines are important for the development of IBD (reviewed in ref. 86). Such studies will allow for the development of new therapeutic strategies. The potential for treatment of IBD patients with biological reagents such as infliximab (anti-TNF-α) has already stimulated rapid development in this area. For example, recent work on the epithelial derived cytokine, IL-18 in Crohn's disease (CD) [87–90] has led to the development of neutralizing antibodies for clinical studies [91].

The effect of inflammation on the sensory-motor apparatus of the gut
Clinical observations

It has long been recognized that motility is altered in IBD. Initial reports were restricted to studies on patients with active colitis and showed a generalized decrease in contractile activity [92]. However, the pharmacologic sensitivity of the colon to opiates was exaggerated and the authors believed this was associated with the development of toxic megacolon [93]. However, the normal physiologic response to a meal is suppressed in patients with active colitis [94, 95]. Under normal conditions contractions in the proximal colon are largely segmental and serve to retard transit, allowing time for water absorption and solidification of the stool. In ulcerative colitis (UC) these contractions are reduced and there is an increase in propagated contractile activity [96, 97] resulting in increased colonic transit, particularly in the distal colon. There is also a reduction in anal sphincter function in the presence of active colitis, and this may contribute to episodes of fecal incontinence seen in some patients [96]. Changes in contractility are not restricted to the colon in UC. Changes have also been observed in the small intestine [98] and in the gallbladder of patients after colectomy, a finding which may result [99] in increased gallstone formation in these patients [100]. In severe colitis a loss of motor activity, which is likely mediated by increased nitric oxide generation, results in toxic megacolon and may lead to multiple organ failure [101, 102].

Motility changes in ulcerative colitis

Studies on tissue from patients with UC provide some insight into mechanisms underlying the reduction in motility in patients with active disease. *In vitro* there is evidence of impaired contractility of smooth muscle from UC patients [103]. Immunohistochemical studies have identified a dominance on inhibitory nerves, including nerves containing vasoactive intestinal peptide (VIP) and a reduction in excitatory transmitters including substance P [104]. This is corroborated by functional studies on muscle strips from patients with colitis; there is a large neural inhibitory component compared to responses from non-inflamed tissues and these responses could be blocked through inhibition of nitric oxide synthase (NOS), implicating nitric oxide as the mediator [105]. Similarly, the responses to the excitatory neurotransmitters such as substance P were reduced by 17–33% in muscle from patients with UC compared to controls [106]. There is an increase in iNOS in the nerves of the myenteric plexus as well as in smooth muscle cells in the colon in UC [107], and these are the likely sources of NO. Prostanoids and leukotrienes may also contribute to altered motility in IBD as inducible cyclo-oxygenase (COX-2) has been identified in colonic nerves and muscle cells of patients with active colitis [99]. The cell types involved in the altered motor pattern include smooth muscle and enteric and autonomic nerves in the gut wall and interstitial cells of Cajal [108].

Motility changes in Crohn's disease

Because of limited access, studies on small intestinal motility are few, but there is evidence of altered interdigestive motility in the small intestine in CD in almost 80% of patients studied [109]. This may result in changes in oro-cecal transit that could lead to bacterial overgrowth [110] or to altered drug delivery in these patients [111]. A reduction in gastric emptying has been identified in patients with non-obstructive CD using radioscintigraphy [112] but not using real-time ultrasonography [113]. Gallbladder emptying is decreased in patients with CD but, unlike UC, it is not related to colectomy [114].

The effect of inflammation on smooth muscle contraction

In-vitro studies have shown an increase in the contractile response of intestinal muscle to agonists such as acetylcholine and histamine in CD [115]. In UC there is a decrease in muscle contractility due in part to altered neural input to the gut from both enteric and autonomic nerves [116, 117].

Mechanisms underlying inflammation-induced altered muscle contraction have been reviewed [118]. From work performed largely in models of acute inflammation, in many cases based on nematode infection or hapten-induced colitis, the following concepts have emerged. Changes in muscle contractility occur with superficial inflammation and without overt infiltration of the neuromuscular layers. [119]. Changes in muscle function occur at non-inflamed sites distant from the site of inflammation [120]; this is important considering the extensive motility changes that have been identified in IBD described above. Changes may persist after resolution of the inflammation [121]. Numerous cell types and their products have been shown to influence muscle contractility and these include polymorph leukocytes [122], mast cells [123] and T lymphocytes [124]. Th1 and Th2 cytokines appear to have opposing effects on smooth muscle contractility [125], but this concept needs to be examined in models of Th1- and Th2-mediated inflammation. Certainly, in Th2-driven inflammation associated with nematode infection, there is hypercontractility of muscle similar to that seen on exposure to IL-4 or IL-13 and is dependent on signal transducer and activator of transcription factor 6 (STAT-6) which is necessary for the effect of many Th2 cytokines [126].

More recent work has examined the impact of chronic inflammation on muscle contractility and has shown changes in ileal muscle evident after 12 weeks of inflammation induced by *Schistosoma mansoni* in mice [127] and time-dependent changes have also been shown in a rat model of colitis [128]. Others have examined the effects of repeated episodes of acute inflammation and have shown that the impact of an acute inflammatory response occurring in a naive intestine differs from that occurring in a previously inflamed intestine [129, 130]. These findings are important in our understanding of motility changes seen in chronic relapsing IBD in humans and merit further investigation.

Several mechanisms contribute to altered muscle contractility. While some changes are receptor-mediated, post-receptor mechanisms are likely to be more important given the broad range of agonists involved. Thus, described changes in the sodium–potassium ATPase [131] and in contractile proteins [132] are the probable basis for hypercontractility, whereas changes in ion channels may contribute to hypocontractility of muscle [133].

The effect of inflammation on efferent nerves

The enteric nervous system plays a crucial role in regulating and coordinating gut physiology. Inflammation-induced changes in enteric nerves are likely to have a widespread effect on gut function, and this is evident from studies in animal models. The human literature contains numerous reports of changes in the structure, appearance or neurotransmitter content of the gut in IBD but the data are often conflicting (for a comprehensive review the reader is directed to ref. 134). These discrepancies may be attributed to two factors. The first is the wide difference in techniques used to identify and quantitate nerves in inflamed tissue, and the second is the fact that the involvement of nerves by the inflammatory process is patchy and depends on the severity and probably the nature of the inflammatory infiltrate [104, 135–137]. Studies in animal models provide clear demonstrations that various cell types in the inflammatory response confer different changes in neuromuscular function [138, 139]. It is therefore difficult to generalize about the profile of neurotransmitter changes in IBD. There appears to be an increase in inhibitory nerves in UC, resulting in the observed decrease in motor activity. While reports on the role of vasoactive intestinal peptide (VIP) are conflicting, there appears to be some agreement that nitric oxide is an important mediator of this increased inhibition [105]. With respect to excitatory neurotransmitters there appears to be agreement on a reduction in cholinergic innervation,

in agreement with animal models, but changes in other transmitters such as substance P (SP) are unclear. There are conflicting reports of decreases [104] or increases [140] in SP, as well as of increased SP binding sites in IBD [141].

Neurally-mediated alterations in gut physiology in IBD may also be due to remodeling rather than injury to nerves. There is growing appreciation of the plasticity of the nervous system and the ability of inflammatory or immune mediators to modulate this [142]. Work in animal models suggests that this occurs during intestinal inflammation [143] and there are a number of observations that provide functional correlation of this plasticity, an example of which is provided in the spot-inflammatory remodeling of the enteric nervous system following experimental colitis in the rat [129].

It is important to recognize that there is bidirectional communication between the nervous and immune systems, and while it is clearly established that nerves are altered by inflammatory processes, it is also now evident that nerves may influence the inflammatory response. While a full covering of this is beyond the scope of this chapter, the reader should be aware of data from animal models that provide clear demonstrations of the role of several components of the nervous system to modulate intestinal inflammation, in either a deleterious or protective manner. For example, sensory neural circuits are protective, as reflected by the deleterious effect of ablation of primary afferent nerves using capsaicin [144, 145]. In contrast, sympathetic nerves appear to be proinflammatory, as reflected by the amelioration of inflammation following chemical sympathectomy [145]. The latter observation may explain the reported benefit of clonidine in colitis [146]. The apparent benefit of local anesthetics in colitis [147] is not, however, explained on the basis of animal studies showing a protective role of sensory nerves [57, 148].

The modulatory effect of nerves is not restricted to the enteric and autonomic systems. There is evidence that the central nervous system also influences intestinal inflammation in the context of stress. It is generally acknowledged that stress plays a role in relapses of IBD [149, 150] and recent work in animal models shows that stress may enhance inflammatory responses [151] or reactivate inflammation in mice which had recovered from previous colitis [152]. A discussion of underlying mechanisms is beyond the scope of this review but the reader is referred to a recent review of the subject [153].

The effect of inflammation on enteroglia

There is increasing acknowledgement of the role of glial cells in mediating neural changes in inflammatory processes in the gut. This was prompted by the report of Geboes *et al.* showing MHC II expression by glial cells in the enteric nervous system in IBD, suggesting immune-mediated injury [154]. Studies using isolated enteroglia demonstrate their ability to respond to, as well as produce, cytokines [155, 156]. This cell type is therefore strategically important in mediating neuroimmune interactions in the inflamed gut.

The effect of inflammation on sensory nerves in IBD

Although abdominal pain is common in IBD patients in the absence of obstructing lesions, underlying mechanisms are unclear. While inflammation is a generally accepted mechanism for the induction of hyperalgesia in a variety of diseases, and is readily demonstrable in animal model systems, the literature with respect to IBD is conflicting. The inability of patients with active colitis to tolerate balloon distension of the rectum is a long-standing observation [157] and has been interpreted to represent visceral hyperalgesia. However, more recent work from one group using graded distension protocols has identified increased thresholds for pain perception in both the intact colon and in patients with ileo-anal pouches [158–160]. In addition IBD patients exhibit a greater tolerance of somatic pain [161] and do not have features of chronic widespread pain [162]. The basis for this apparent discrepancy between demonstrations of visceral hyperalgesia and increased visceral pain thresholds is not immediately clear, but may reflect differences in experimental protocol as well as the fact that hyperalgesia was demonstrated in patients with active disease, whereas more recent studies have focused on patients with less active chronic disease. The authors have interpreted the increased pain threshold on the basis of increased descending spinal inhibitory pathways [160]. It is also entirely possible that certain types of inflammation may reduce pain sensitivity [163], via the production of endorphins at the site of injury [164, 165].

The effect of inflammation on the autonomic and central nervous systems

The autonomic nervous system modulates all aspects of gut physiology and available evidence indicates that this regulation is altered in IBD. First, there are morphological data demonstrating changes in sympathetic and parasympathetic nerves in IBD (for review see ref. 134). Second, functional studies have shown that in CD there is sympathetic dysfunction whereas in UC there is evidence of vagal dysfunction and consequent sympathetic dominance [166, 167]. Preliminary work suggests that sympathetic dominance in UC is more prominent in patients with limited distal disease [168]. It is possible that the apparent benefit of nicotine in UC is due to balancing of autonomic input to the inflamed colon in the face of sympathetic dominance, as data from experimental models suggest that sympathetic nerves play a proinflammatory role [145].

With respect to the central nervous system, there is a report of small structural defects in the white matter in some patients with IBD [169]. The nature and significance of this finding, however, remain unclear.

The effect of inflammation on interstitial cells of Cajal

It is apparent that the interstitial cell of Cajal (ICC) plays an important role in the control of gastrointestinal motility; these cells serve as pacemaker cells [170]. The absence of these cells results in a major disruption of motility in animals [171, 172] and in humans [173]. In animal models of intestinal inflammation there is evidence of structural damage and functional impairment of these cells [174]. Recent observations have shown that there is structural damage to the ICC in the colon of patients with UC, and this almost certainly contributes to altered colonic motility seen in these patients [175]. Because of their strategic role in the control of motility these cells would be ideal targets for therapy aimed at directly correcting motility patterns in IBD.

The effect of inflammation on enteroendocrine cells (EEC)

Local and systemically produced hormones constitute another mechanism by which gut physiology is regulated. Important among these hormones is serotonin, the highest concentration of which is found in the gut, and in the colon in particular. One report in patients with UC suggests a significant decrease in the enterochromaffin cells in the colonic mucosa [86]. There is a single report of an increase in enterochromaffin cells in an animal model of colitis [87]. Recent reports of 'ischemic' colitis occurring in patients receiving serotonin antagonists for the treatment of irritable bowel syndrome raise the possibility of a linkage between serotonin and gut defense. Thus, studies on EEC cells and serotonin metabolism in IBD warrant further study.

References

1. Olaison G, Sjödahl R, Tagesson C. Abnormal intestinal permeability in Crohn's disease. A possible pathogenic factor. Scand J Gastroenterol 1990; 25: 321–8.
2. Sartor RB. Postoperative recurrence of Crohn's disease: the enemy is within the fecal stream. Gastroenterology 1998; 114: 398–400.
3. Meddings J. Barrier dysfunction and Crohn's disease. Ann NY Acad Sci 2000; 915: 333–8.
4. Colombel JF, Cortot A, Van Kruiningen HJ. Antibiotics in Crohn's disease. Gut 2001; 48: 647.
5. Perdue MH, McKay DM. Integrative immunophysiology in the intestinal mucosa. Am J Physiol 1994; 267: G151–6.
6. Mowat AMcI, Sprent J. Induction of intestinal graft-versus-host reactions across mutant major histocompatibility complex antigens by T lymphocyte subsets in mice. Transplantation 1989; 47: 857–63.
7. Radojevic NR, McKay DM, Merger M, Vallance B, Collins SM, Croitoru K. Characterization of enteric functional changes evoked by *in vivo* anti-CD3 T cell activation. Am J Physiol Regul Integr Compar Physiol 1999; 45: R715–23.
8. Evans CM, Phillips AD, Walker-Smith JA, MacDonald TT. Activation of lamina propria T cells induces crypt epithelial proliferation and goblet cell depletion in cultured human fetal colon. Gut 1992; 33: 230–5.
9. Garside P, Mowat AM. Natural killer cells and tumour necrosis factor-a-mediated enteropathy in mice. Immunology 1993; 78:335–7.
10. Kurokowa M, Lynch K, Podolsky DK. Effects of growth factors on an intestinal epithelial cell line: transforming growth factor beta inhibits proliferation and stimulates differentiation. Biochem Biophys Res Commun 1987; 142: 775–82.
11. Deem RL, Shanahan F, Targan SR. Triggered human mucosal T cells release tumour necrosis factor-alpha and interferon-gamma which kill human colonic epithelial cells. Clin Exper Immunol 1991; 83: 79–84.
12. Williams KL, Fuller CR, Dieleman LA et al. Enhanced survival and mucosal repair after dextran sodium sulfate-induced colitis in transgenic mice that over-express growth hormone. Gastroenterology 2001; 120: 925–37.
13. Tsai CH, Hill M, Asa SL, Brubaker PL, Drucker DJ. Intestinal growth-promoting properties of glucagon-like peptide-2 in mice. Am J Physiol Endocrinol Metab 1997; 273: E77–84.
14. Tomita K, Taupin DR, Itoh H, Podolsky DK. Distinct pathways of cell migration and antiapoptotic response to epithelial injury: structure-function analysis of human intestinal trefoil factor. Mol Cell Biol 2000; 20: 4680–90.
15. Schmitz H, Barmeyer C, Gitter AH et al. Epithelial barrier and transport function of the colon in ulcerative colitis. Ann NY Acad Sci 2000; 915: 312–26.
16. Schmitz H, Barmeyer C, Fromm M et al. Altered tight junction structure contributes to the impaired epithelial barrier function in ulcerative colitis. Gastroenterology 1999; 116: 301–9.
17. D'Inca R, Ernst P, Hunt RH, Perdue MH. Role of T lymphocytes in intestinal mucosal injury. Inflammatory changes in athymic nude rats. Dig Dis Sci 1992; 37: 33–9.
18. Turner MW, Boulton P, Shields JG et al. Intestinal hypersensitivity reactions in the rat. I. Uptake of intact protein, permeability to sugars and their correlation with mucosal mast-cell activation. Immunology 1988; 63: 119–24.
19. Ramage JK, Hunt RH, Perdue MH. Changes in intestinal permeability and epithelial differentiation during inflammation in the rat. Gut 1988; 29: 57–61.
20. Yu LC, Perdue MH. Immunologically mediated transport of ions and macromolecules. Ann NY Acad Sci 2000; 915: 247–59.
21. Madara JL, Stafford J. Interferon-gamma directly affects barrier function of cultured intestinal epithelial monolayers. J Clin Invest 1989; 83: 724–7.
22. Fish SM, Proujansky R, Reenstra WW. Synergistic effects of interferon gamma and tumour necrosis factor alpha on T84 cell function. Gut 1999; 45: 191–8.
23. Madara JL. Review article: Pathobiology of neutrophil interactions with intestinal epithelia. Aliment Pharmacol Ther 1997; 11(Suppl. 3): 57–62.
24. Turnberg LA, Fordtran JS, Carter NW, Rector FC. Mechanism of bicarbonate absorption and its relation to sodium absorption in the human jejunum. J Clin Invest 1970; 49: 548–58.
25. Crowe SE, Perdue MH. Gastrointestinal food hypersensitivity: basic mechanisms of pathophysiology. Gastroenterology 1992; 103:075–95.
26. Shaw SK, Hermanowski-Vosatka A, Shibahara T et al. Migration of intestinal intraepithelial lymphocytes into a polarized epithelial monolayer. Am J Physiol Gastrointest Liver Physiol 1998; 275: G584–91.
27. McKay DM, Croitoru K, Perdue MH. T cell–monocyte interactions regulate epithelial physiology in a co-culture model of inflammation. Am J Physiol 1996; 270: C418–28.
28. Zund G, Madara JL, Dzus AL, Awtrey CS, Colgan SP. Interleukin-4 and interleukin-13 differentially regulate epithelial chloride secretion. J Biol Chem 1996; 271: 7460–4.
29. Soderholm JD, Peterson KH, Olaison G et al. Epithelial permeability to proteins in the non-inflamed ileum of Crohn's disease? Gastroenterology 1999; 117: 65–72.
30. Holmgren J, Fryklund J, Larsson H. Gamma-interferon-mediated down-regulation of electrolyte secretion by intestinal epithelial cells: a local immune mechanism? Scand J Immunology 1989; 30: 499–503.
31. Oprins JC, Meijer HP, Groot JA. Tumor necrosis factor-alpha potentiates ion secretion induced by muscarinic receptor activation in the human intestinal epithelial cell line HT29cl.19A. Ann NY Acad Sci 2000; 915: 102–6.
32. Chang EB, Musch MW, Mayer L. Interleukins 1 and 3 stimulate anion secretion in chicken intestine. Gastroenterology 1990; 98: 1518–24.
33. Gordon JR, Galli SJ. Release of both preformed and newly synthesised tumour necrosis factor a (TNF-α)/cachectin by mouse mast cells stimulated via the FceRO/ A mechanism for the sustained action of mast cell-derived TNF-α during IgE-dependent biological responses. J Exp Med 1991; 174: 103–7.
34. Mowat AM. Human intraepithelial lymphocytes. Springer Semin Immunopathol 1990; 12: 165–90.

35. Mayer L, Eisenhardt D, Salomon P, Bauer W, Plous R, Piccinini L. Expression of class II molecules on intestinal epithelial cells in humans. Differences between normal and inflammatory bowel disease. Gastroenterology 1991; 100: 3–12.

36. Bland PW. MHC class II expression by the gut epithelium. Immunol Today 1988; 9: 174–8.

37. Kaiserlian D, Vidal K, Revillard J-P. Murine enterocytes can present soluble antigen to specific class II-restricted CD4$^+$ T cells. Eur J Immunol 1989; 19: 1513–6.

38. Blumberg RS. Current concepts in mucosal immunity. II. One size fits all: nonclassical MHC molecules fulfill multiple roles in epithelial cell function. Am J Physiol Gastrointest Liver Physiol 1998; 274: G227–31.

39. Cerf-Bensussan N, Quaroni A, Kurnick JT, Bhan A. K. Intraepithelial lymphocytes modulate Ia expression by intestinal epithelial cells. J Immunol 1984; 132: 224-5.

40. Mayer L, Shlien R. Evidence for function of Ia molecules on gut epithelial cells in man. J Exp Med 1987; 166: 1471–83.

41. Li Y, Yio XY, Mayer, L. Human intestinal epithelial cell-induced CD8+ T cell activation is mediated through CD8 and the activation of CD8- associated p56^{lck}. J Exp Med 1995; 182: 1079–88.

42. Yio XY, Mayer L. Characterization of a 180-kDa intestinal epithelial cell membrane glycoprotein, gp180 – a candidate molecule mediating T cell epithelial cell interactions. J Biol Chem 1997; 272: 12786–92.

43. Salomon P, Pizzimenti A, Panja A, Reisman A, Mayer L. The expression and regulation of class II antigens in normal and inflammatory bowel disease peripheral blood monocytes and intestinal epithelium. Autoimmunity 1991; 9: 141–9.

44. Mayer L, Eisenhardt D. Lack of induction of suppressor T cells by intestinal epithelial cells from patients with inflammatory bowel disease. J Clin Invest 1990; 86: 1255–60.

45. Nakazawa A, Watanabe M, Kanai T et al. Functional expression of co-stimulatory molecule CD86 on epithelial cells in the inflamed colonic mucosa. Gastroenterology 1999; 117: 536–45.

46. Befus AD, Goodacre R, Dyck N, Bienenstock J. Mast cell heterogeneity in man. 1. Histological studies of the intestine. Int Arch Allergy Appl Immunol 1985; 76: 232–6.

47. Goodman T, Lefrancois L. Expression of the gamma-delta T-cell receptor on intestinal CD8+ intraepithelial lymphocytes. Nature 1988; 333: 855–8.

48. Croitoru K, Ernst PB. Leukocytes in the intestinal epithelium: An unusual immunological compartment revisited. Reg Immunol 1992; 4: 63–9.

49. Macpherson AJ, Gatto D, Sainsbury E, Harriman GR, Hengartner H, Zinkernagel RM. A primitive T cell-independent mechanism of intestinal mucosal IgA responses to commensal bacteria. Science 2000; 288: 2222–6.

50. Colgan SP, Morales VM, Madara JL, Polischuk JE, Balk SP, Blumberg RS. IFN-gamma modulates CD1d surface expression on intestinal epithelia. Am J Physiol Cell Physiol 1996; 271: C276–83.

51. Kaiserlian D, Rigal D, Abello J, Revillard JP. Expression, function and regulation of the intercellular adhesion molecule-1 (ICAM-1) on human intestinal epithelial cell lines. Eur J Immunol 1991; 21: 2415–21.

52. Cepek KL, Shaw SK, Parker CM et al. Adhesion between epithelial cells and T lymphocytes mediated by E-cadherin and the aEb7 integrin. Nature 1994; 372: 190–3.

53. Dogan A, Wang ZD, Spencer J. E-cadherin expression in intestinal epithelium. J Clin Pathol 1995; 48: 143–6.

54. Perey DYE, Bienenstock J. Effects of bursectomy and thymectomy on ontogeny of fowl IgA, IgG and IgM. J Immunol 1973; 111: 633–7.

55. Kernéis S, Bogdanova A, Kraehenbuhl JP, Pringault E. Conversion by Peyer's patch lymphocytes of human enterocytes into M cells that transport bacteria. Science 1997; 277: 949–52.

56. Poussier P, Julius M. Intestinal intraepithelial lymphocytes: the plot thickens. J Exp Med 1994; 180: 1185–9.

57. Lefrancois L. Extrathymic differentiation of intraepithelial lymphocytes: generation of a separate and unequal T-cell repertoire? Immunol Today 12:36-38, 1991.

58. Poussier, P. and Julius, M. Thymus independent T cell development and selection in the intestinal epithelium. Annu Rev Immunol 1994; 12: 521–53.

59. Maric D, Kaiserlian D, Croitoru K. Intestinal epithelial cell line induction of T cell differentiation from bone marrow precursors. Cell Immunol 1996; 172: 172–9.

60. Lundqvist C, Baranov V, Hammarström S, Athlin L, Hammarström ML. Intra-epithelial lymphocytes. Evidence for regional specialization and extrathymic T cell maturation in the human gut epithelium. Int Immunol 1995; 7: 1473–87.

61. Stashenko P, Jandinski JJ, Fujiyoshi P, Rynar J, Socransky SS. Tissue levels of bone resorptive cytokines in periodontal disease. J Periodontol 1991; 62: 504–9.

62. Spriggs, D. R, Imamura, K, Rodriguez, C et al. Tumor necrosis factor expression in human epithelial tumor cell lines. J Clin Invest 1988; 81: 455–60.

63. Ohtoshi T, Vancheri C, Cox G et al. Monocyte–macrophage differentiation induced by human upper airway epithelial cells. Am J Respir Cell Mol Biol 1991; 4: 255–63.

64. Crowe SE, Alvarez L, Dytoc M et al. Expression of interleukin 8 and CD54 by human gastric epithelium after *Helicobacter pylori* infection *in vitro*. Gastroenterology 1995; 108: 65–74.

65. Standiford TJ, Kunkel SL, Basha MA et al. Interleukin-8 gene expression by a pulmonary epithelial cell line. A model for cytokine networks in the lung. J Clin Invest 1990; 86: 1945–53.

66. Watanabe M, Ueno Y, Yajima T et al. Interleukin 7 is produced by human intestinal epithelial cells and regulates the proliferation of intestinal mucosal lymphocytes. J Clin Invest 1995; 95: 2945–53.

67. Watanabe M, Ueno Y, Yajima T et al. Interleukin 7 transgenic mice develop chronic colitis with decreased interleukin 7 protein accumulation in the colonic mucosa. J Exp Med 1998; 187: 389–402.

68. Sollid LM, Kvale D, Brandtzaeg P, Markussen G, Thorsby E. Interferon-gamma enhances expression of secretory component, the epithelial receptor for polymeric immunoglobulins. J Immunol 1987; 138: 4303–6.

69. Kvale D, Lovhaug D, Sollid LM, Brandtzaeg P. Tumour necrosis factor-alpha up-regulates expression of secretory component, the epithelial receptor for polymeric Ig. J Immunol 1988; 140: 3086–9.

70. Kaetzel CS, Robinson JK, Lamm ME. Epithelial transcytosis of monomeric IgA and IgG cross-linked through antigen to polymeric IgA: a role for monomeric antibodies in the mucosal immune system. J Immunol 1994; 152: 72–6.

71. Huang GTJ, Eckmann L, Savidge TC, Kagnoff MF. Infection of human intestinal epithelial cells with invasive bacteria upregulates apical intercellular adhesion molecule-1 (ICAM-1) expression and neutrophil adhesion. J Clin Invest 1996; 98: 572–83.

72. Jung HC, Eckmann L, Yang S-K et al. A distinct array of proinflammatory cytokines is expressed in human colon epithelial cells in response to bacterial invasion. J Clin Invest 1995; 95: 55–65.

73. Aihara M, Tsuchimoto D, Takizawa H et al. Mechanisms involved in Helicobacter pylori-induced interleukin- 8 pro-

151. Gue M, Bonbonne C, Fioramonti J *et al*. Stress-induced enhancement of colitis in rats: CRF and arginine vasopressin are not involved. Am J Physiol 1997; 272: G84–91.

152. Qiu B, Vallance B, Blennerhassett P, Collins SM. The role of CD4+ve lymphocytes in the susceptibility of the mice to stress-induced relapse of colitis. Nature Med 1999; 5, 1178–82.

153. Collins SM. Stress and the gastrointestinal tract. IV. Modulation of intestinal inflammation by stress: basic mechanisms and clinical relevance. Am J Physiol Gastrointest Liver Physiol 2001; 280: G315–8.

154. Geboes K, Rutgeerts P, Ectors N *et al*. Major histocompatibility class II expression on the small intestinal nervous system in Crohn's disease. Gastroenterology 1992; 103: 439–47.

155. Ruhl A, Franzke S, Collins SM, Stremmel W. Interleukin-6 expression and regulation in rat enteric glial cells. Am J Physiol Gastrointest Liver Physiol 2001; 280: G1163–71.

156. Ruhl A, Franzke S, Stremmel W. IL-1beta and IL-10 have dual effects on enteric glial cell proliferation. Neurogastroenterol Motil 2001; 13: 89–94.

157. Farthing MJG, Lennard-Jones JE. Sensitivity of the rectum to distension and the anorectal distension reflex in ulcerative colitis. Gut 1978; 19: 64–9.

158. Chang L, Munakata J, Mayer EA *et al*. Perceptual responses in patients with inflammatory and functional bowel disease. Gut 2000; 47: 497–505.

159. Bernstein CN, Rollandelli R, Niazi N *et al*. Characterization of afferent mechanisms in ileoanal pouches. Am J Gastroenterol 1997; 92: 103–8.

160. Bernstein CN, Niazi N, Robert M *et al*. Rectal afferent function in patients with inflammatory and functional intestinal disorders. Pain 1996; 66: 151–61.

161. Cook IJ, van Eeden A, Collins SM. Patients with irritable bowel syndrome have greater pain tolerance than normal subjects. Gastroenterology 1987; 93: 727–33.

162. Palm O, Moum B, Jahnsen J, Gran JT. Fibromyalgia and chronic widespread pain in patients with inflammatory bowel disease: a cross sectional population survey. J Rheumatol 2001; 28: 590–4.

163. Porreca F, Lai J, Malan TP, Jr. Can inflammation relieve pain? Nat Med 1998; 4: 1359–60.

164. Mousa SA, Zhang Q, Sitte N, Ji R, Stein C. beta-Endorphin-containing memory-cells and mu-opioid receptors undergo transport to peripheral inflamed tissue. J Neuroimmunol 2001; 115: 71–8.

165. Sharp B, Yaksh T. Pain killers of the immune system. Nat Med 1997; 3: 831–2.

166. Lindgren S, Stewenius J, Sjolund K, Lilja B, Sundkvist G. Autonomic vagal nerve dysfunction in patients with ulcerative colitis. Scand J Gastroenterol 1993; 28: 638–42.

167. Lindgren S, Lilja B, Rosen I, Sundkvist G. Disturbed autonomic nerve function in patients with Crohn's disease. Scand J Gastroenterol 1991; 26: 361–6.

168. Ganguli SC, Kamath MV, Mohammed M *et al*. Patients with inflammatory bowel disease demonstrate distinct abnormalities of autonomic function. Can J Gastroenterol 2001; 15(Suppl. A): 15A.

169. Geissler A, Andus T, Roth M *et al*. Focal white-matter lesions in brain of patients with inflammatory bowel disease. Lancet 1995; 345: 897–8.

170. Thomsen L, Robinson TR, Lee JC *et al*. Interstitial cells of Cajal generate arrhythmia pacemaker current. Nature Med 1998; 4: 1–4.

171. Malysz J, Thuneberg L, Mikkelsen HB, Huizinga JD. Action potential generation in the small intestine of W mutant mice that lack interstitial cells of Cajal. Am J Physiol 1996; 271: G387–99.

172. Sato D, Lai ZF, Tokutomi N *et al*. Impairment of Kit-dependent development of interstitial cells alters contractile responses of murine intestinal tract. Am J Physiol 1996; 271: G762–71.

173. Isozaki K, Hirota S, Miyagawa J, Taniguchi M, Shinomura Y, Matsuzawa Y. Deficiency of c-kit+ cells in patients with a myopathic form of chronic idiopathic intestinal pseudo-obstruction. Am J Gastroenterol 1997; 92: 332–4.

174. Der T, Bercik P, Donnelly G *et al*. Interstitial cells of Cajal and inflammation-induced motor dysfunction in the mouse small intestine. Gastroenterology 2000; 119: 1590–9.

175. Rumessen JJ. Ultrastructure of interstitial cells of Cajal at the colonic submuscular border in patients with ulcerative colitis. Gastroenterology 1996; 111: 1447–55.

12 | Systemic consequences of intestinal inflammation

KONSTANTINOS A. PAPADAKIS AND MARIA T. ABREU

Introduction

A large number of changes, distant from the intestinal mucosa and involving many organ systems, may accompany the inflammatory process in ulcerative colitis (UC) or Crohn's disease (CD). The systemic response to inflammation includes changes in the concentration of many plasma proteins, known as the acute-phase proteins, and several neuro-endocrine, metabolic, and hematopoietic alterations collectively termed the acute-phase response [1]. The acute-phase response occurs in many clinical situations characterized by tissue injury, such as trauma, ischemia, burns, infections, malignancy, and autoimmune diseases. At the molecular level these symptoms correlate with changes in the levels of proinflammatory cytokines such as tumor necrosis factor (TNF), interleukin (IL)-1, and IL-6, although other cytokines and chemokines also mediate the acute phase response. Many constitutional symptoms such as anorexia, malaise, fatigue, fever, myalgias, arthralgias, night sweats, weight loss and cachexia are directly or indirectly attributed to the effects of these proinflammatory cytokines.

During inflammation the inflammatory cytokines TNF, IL-1 and IL-6 are secreted in that order [2, 3]. Although many cytokine effects are predominantly paracrine and autocrine, they do mediate systemic effects [4]. For example, central infusion of TNF led to predominant anorexia whereas peripheral production of TNF produced predominant metabolic losses of protein [5, 6].

TNF is a 17 kDa protein that is produced by cells of hematopoietic lineage in response to several stimuli such as bacterial pathogens and lipopolysaccharide. It is first produced as a maebrane-bound protein of 26 kDa, which is cleaved to the mature form by the TNF-α converting enzyme. It has several biological effects depending on the amount and the rapidity with which it is produced in response to a specific stimulus. High levels of TNF that are produced acutely lead to shock and tissue injury, vascular leakage syndrome, acute respiratory distress syndrome (ARDS), gastrointestinal necrosis, acute tubular necrosis, adrenal hemorrhage, disseminated intravascular coagulation, and fever. Chronic low-dose exposure to TNF leads to weight loss, anorexia, protein catabolism, lipid depletion, hepatosplenomegaly, insulin resistance, acute-phase protein release, and endothelial activation [6–8].

IL-1 is a family of three proteins, IL-1α, IL-1β, and the IL-1 receptor antagonist (IL-1ra); the latter acts as inhibitor of IL-1 signaling [9, 10]. IL-1α and IL-1β are synthesized as precursors and are cleaved to the mature forms by the action of interleukin-1β-converting enzyme (ICE) (caspase-1). IL-1 function as a lymphocyte-activating factor by enhancing the production of IL-2, and IL-2 receptors by T lymphocytes. It synergizes with various colony-stimulating factors to stimulate early bone marrow hematopoietic progenitor cell proliferation. IL-1 and TNF share numerous biologic activities and frequently act in synergism. IL-1 stimulates the catabolism of muscle, and in joints stimulates synovial cell proliferation, cartilage and bone resorption, and collagen deposition. The effects of IL-1 on muscles and joints contribute to the myalgias and arthralgias associated with illness. Many of the proinflammatory activities of IL-1 relate to the generation of small mediator molecules, frequently in synergy with TNF, such as platelet-activating factor and leukotrienes, prostanoids, nitric oxide, and chemokines. IL-1 has several proinflammatory activities, such as induction of fever, slow-wave sleep, anorexia, and neuropeptide release. Hypotension, myocardial suppression, septic shock, and death can all be physiologic responses to overwhelming expression of IL-1 and other proinflammatory cytokines [11]. Humans injected with IL-1 experience fever, headache, myalgias, and arthralgias, each of which is reduced by the coadministration of COX inhibitors [12].

IL-6 is a 26-kDa protein produced by a wide variety of cells. IL-6 is one of the principal mediators

Stephan R. Targan, Fergus Shanahan and Loren C. Karp (eds.), Inflammatory Bowel Disease: From Bench to Bedside, 2nd Edition, 235–250.
© 2003 *Kluwer Academic Publishers. Printed in Great Britain*

of the clinical manifestations of tissue injury, including fever, cachexia, leukocytosis, thrombocytosis, increased plasma levels of acute-phase proteins, and decreased plasma levels of albumin. It is a pleiotropic cytokine with both proinflammatory and anti-inflammatory properties. IL-6 also stimulates plasmacytosis and hypergammaglobulinemia and activates the hypothalamic–pituitary–adrenal axis [2]. In addition to differentiating B cells, IL-6 stimulates proliferation of thymic and peripheral T cells. Along with IL-1, IL-6 induces T cell differentiation to cytolytic T cells and activates natural killer cells. These observations emphasize the importance of IL-6 in both innate and adaptive immunity. In addition to its immunologic/inflammatory role, IL-6 may play an important role in bone metabolism, spermatogenesis, epidermal proliferation, megakaryocytopoiesis, and neural cell differentiation and proliferation. The age-associated rise in IL-6 has been linked to lymphoproliferative disorders, multiple myeloma, osteoporosis, and Alzheimer's disease [13]. Recently IL-6/IL-6 receptor (IL-6R) signaling has been shown to be crucial in liver regeneration following hepatectomy [14, 15]. The IL-6 family of cytokines, apart from IL-6 itself, comprises IL-11, ciliary neurotrophic factor, cardiotropin, oncostatin M, leukemia inhibitory factor, and neurotrophin 1/B cell stimulating factor 3, which all share the common signal transducer gp130 as part of their receptors [15].

Elevated mucosal and serum levels of several proinflammatory cytokines have been observed in patients with CD and UC, including IL-1 and TNF. IL-6 serum levels have been reported to be elevated in active CD but not in UC, whereas elevated circulating levels of IL-6R have been detected in active stages of both diseases [16]. Increased serum levels of IL-8 have also been reported in active UC but not in CD [17]. Approximately 90% of patients with CD have a triad of features that are persistent and progressive, namely diarrhea, abdominal pain, and *weight loss* [18]. As many as 40% of patients with UC may experience noticeable weight loss [19]. *Cachexia*, the loss of body mass that occurs in severe chronic inflammatory disease, results from decreases in skeletal muscle, fat tissue, and bone mass [20]. Cytokines such as IL-1, IL-6, TNF, and interferon gamma (IFN-γ) contribute to these processes [21]. Investigators have found a link between inflammatory cytokines and muscle damage. TNF-α and IFN-γ are both activators of nuclear factor kappa B (NF-κB) in muscle. Activation of NF-κB results in the

decreased expression of MyoD, a transcription factor that is essential for repair of damaged skeletal muscle. Thus, the net effect of TNF-α and IFN-γ is defective muscle repair which may explain the cachexia that develops in patients with cancer and other high TNF-α states. Although cachexia is characterized by hypermetabolism, defined as an elevation in resting energy expenditure, in CD patients without malabsorption, short-term weight change is more closely related to decreased caloric intake rather than to increased resting energy expenditure. Although 'sitophobia' – in anticipation of abdominal pain – may contribute to weight loss, it usually relates to the severity of anorexia. *Anorexia* is one of the most common symptoms associated with acute illness, results from proinflammatory cytokine activity and has both central and peripheral elements [4]. Several cytokines affect food intake directly or indirectly with effects on other mediators such as corticotrophin-releasing hormone, serotonin, cholecystokinin, neuropeptide Y, insulin or leptin. A number of hypothalamic nuclei involved in eating behavior contain binding sites for cytokines [22]. In animals endotoxin increases the plasma levels of leptin and white fat leptin mRNA suggesting that leptin may be a mediator of anorexia in inflammatory states [4, 23]. Several alterations in gastrointestinal function that indirectly affect nutritional status have been ascribed to proinflammatory cytokines, including altered gastric emptying, decreases in intestinal blood flow, changes in small bowel motility and cellular proliferation, and altered ion fluxes [4].

A significant percentage of patients with active CD and UC have *fever*, usually low-grade [19, 24]. Several cytokines, including IL-1α, IL-1β, TNF, lymphotoxin α (LT-α), IFN-α and IL-6, are intrinsically pyrogenic in that they produce a rapid-onset fever by acting directly on the hypothalamus without the requirement for the formation of another cytokine. Several other cytokines that use the gp130 signal transducer as part of their receptor, as mentioned earlier, may also contribute to the febrile response [25]. Pyrogenic cytokines released during the inflammatory response interact with a rich vascular network close to the cluster of neurons in the preoptic/anterior hypothalamus. These sites, called the circumventricular organs or organum vasculosum laminae terminalis (OVLT), possess little if any blood–brain barrier. It is likely that endothelial cells lining the OVLT either offer no resistance to the movement of pyrogenic cytokines into the brain or release arachidonic acid metabolites which then may diffuse into the preoptic/anterior hypothalamic region to induce fever. Alternatively, prostaglandin E2 (PGE_2) and other prostaglandins may be produced by the endothelial cells which, in turn, induce a neurotransmitter-like substance, such as cAMP, that acts to raise the set-point [25].

Acute phase proteins

An acute-phase protein has been defined as one whose plasma concentration increases (positive acute-phase proteins, such as C-reactive protein (CRP) and serum amino acids (SAA) or decreases (negative acute-phase proteins, such as albumin) by at least 25 % during inflammation. The changes in the concentration of acute-phase proteins are due largely to changes in their production by hepatocytes [20]. Inflammatory cytokines, which operate both as a cascade and as a network in stimulating the production of acute-phase proteins, include IL-6, IL-1β, TNF, IFN-γ, TGF-β, and IL-8 [20] (Table 1). IL-6 is a major hepatocyte stimulator and produces a variety of acute-phase proteins in the liver of experimental animals and in cultured human hepatocytes, SAA and CRP being most induced [26]. Glucocorticoids act synergistically with IL-6 in stimulating the production of acute-phase proteins. Synthesis of acute-phase proteins in IL-6 knockout mice is greatly impaired in response to non-specific irritants, such as turpentine, but is normal when bacterial lipopolysaccharide is the inflammatory stimulus [27]. Inactivation of gp130 in adult mice decreases the ability of these mice to synthesize acute-phase response proteins similarly to the IL-6 knockout mice [28]. The acute-phase proteins include several components of the complement system, which are involved in the accumulation of phagocytes at an inflammatory site and the killing of microbial pathogens. CRP binds various pathogens and materials from damaged cells, promotes opsonization of these materials, and activates the complement system. Recently it has been shown that CRP enhanced opsonization and phagocytosis of apoptotic cells by macrophages associated with the expression of the anti-inflammatory cytokine TGF-β. These observations demonstrate that CRP and the classical complement components act in concert to promote non-inflammatory clearance of apoptotic cells [29]. In this context, production of acute-phase proteins by proinflammatory cytokines can be viewed as a protective host defense mechanism that limits tissue injury [2]. How-

ever, acute-phase protein production is not uniformly beneficial. For example, secondary amyloidosis has long been recognized as a deleterious consequence of elevated SAA concentrations in some patients with chronic inflammatory conditions, including IBD [30]. Several acute-phase proteins have been measured in IBD, including CRP, oromucoid ($α_1$-acid glycoprotein), serum and fecal $α_1$-antitrypsin, $β_2$-microglobulin, phospholipase A2, as well as the erythrocyte sedimentation rate (ESR), and have been shown to correlate with disease activity [16].

The systemic effects of several proinflammatory cytokines have been substantiated by inhibiting their action in several human diseases. For example, Castleman's disease, an atypical lymphoproliferative disorder, is characterized by dysregulated overproduction of IL-6. Patients with this disease frequently have systemic manifestations such as fever, anemia, leukocytosis, thrombocytosis, hypergammaglobulinemia, hypoalbuminemia, and an increase in acute-phase proteins. Administration of a humanized anti-IL-6R antibody in patients with Castleman's disease led to immediate disappearance of fever and fatigue and gradual improvement of anemia, as well as serum levels of CRP, fibrinogen, and albumin, thus confirming the role of IL-6 in the systemic manifestations of the disease. Similarly patients with lymphoma who experience fever, weight loss, and night sweats (B symptoms) exhibit significantly higher levels of serum IL-6 levels compared to patients without B symptoms [31]. Anti-TNF treatment in CD and rheumatoid arthritis has been associated with a decrease in the levels of CRP and IL-6 respectively.

Table 1. Relationship of cytokines to systemic manifestations

Inflammatory mediator	Systemic manifestations
TNF	Fever, cachexia, anorexia, protein catabolism, insulin resistance, activation of HPA axis
IL-1	Fever, myalgias, arthralgias, bone resorption, anorexia, induction of acute-phase proteins, activation of HPA axis
IL-6	Fever, fatigue, leukocytosis, thrombocytosis, induction of acute-phase proteins, activation of HPA axis

HPA = hypothalamic–pituitary–adrenal axis

Hematologic consequences of intestinal inflammation

Anemia

Anemia in patients with inflammatory bowel disease (IBD) is multifactorial and can contribute to the fatigue and poor quality of life experienced in this patient group [32, 33] (Table 2). Between one-third and one-half of patients with IBD are anemic [34–36] and the anemia may occasionally predate the development of gastrointestinal symptoms, especially in children [37–39]. Studies performed in CD patients with anemia reveal that correction of the underlying anemia improves quality-of-life scores, especially the feeling of well-being, mood, physical ability, and ability to perform social activities, supporting the idea that anemia is an important cause of constitutional symptoms [33]. This section will focus on the effect of chronic intestinal inflammation on red blood cell homeostasis and treatment of the common causes of anemia.

Intestinal ulceration, whether related to UC or CD is associated with increased intestinal blood loss, both microscopic and macroscopic, and iron deficiency anemia [35]. Iron-deficiency anemia can be assessed by measuring iron and total iron binding capacity (TIBC) levels which should reflect low iron saturation, $<15\%$. Ferritin levels may be falsely elevated because of inflammation but low levels (<5 µg/L) are indicative of iron deficiency [40]. Poor iron absorption in the proximal gastrointestinal tract can contribute to the anemia of patients with CD and rapid intestinal transit in both CD and UC can impair oral iron replacement therapy. Because oral iron supplementation is often poorly tolerated and poorly absorbed, patients may require administration of parenteral iron. In an open-label study performed in patients with UC and anemia, defined as hemoglobin <10.5 g/dl, investigators administered iron saccharate over an 8-week period [41]. Mean hemoglobin increased by 3.6 g/dl. Only four patients out of 22 did not respond to intravenous iron. This latter group was given erythropoietin and achieved a mean hemoglobin increase of 3.3 g/dl. Similar results have been observed in patients with CD. Specifically, patients with CD and anemia who fail oral iron replacement, or are intolerant of oral iron, who are then given intravenous iron have a 75% response rate with mean hemoglobin increases of 3.3 g/dl [33]. Intravenous iron is associated with a low ($<1\%$) but significant risk of anaphylactoid reaction which manifests during the first few minutes of an infusion and resembles a type I (IgE-mediated) allergic reaction [42, 43]. More commonly up to 30% of patients given iron dextran develop arthralgias and fever within 24–48 h of initiation of intravenous iron therapy.

Ileal disease and resections in patients with CD result in impaired vitamin B_{12} absorption leading to a megaloblastic anemia. Indeed, up to three-fifths of patients with ileal CD who have never had an intestinal resection have evidence of vitamin B_{12} deficiency and megaloblastosis [44, 45]. As little as 30 cm of terminal ileum resected can lead to vitamin B_{12} malabsorption, but in general greater than 60 cm of terminal ileum must be resected for vitamin B_{12} malabsorption [46, 47]. These patients require monthly injections of vitamin B_{12} (cyanocobalamin) (1000 µg) or weekly nasal delivery of topical B_{12} once stores have been replenished [48]. Rarely, patients with CD and short bowel who are dependent on total parenteral nutrition (TPN) may develop anemia and pancytopenia as a result of copper deficiency [49].

The anemia experienced by patients with IBD is generally mixed and may have features of anemia of chronic disease. Anemia of chronic disease can be attributed to the increased production of the cytokines that contribute to the underlying IBD including TNF-α, IL–1, and the interferons [50, 51]. These cytokines have the effect of shortening red cell survival, blunting the erythropoietin response to anemia, impairing erythroid colony formation in response to erythropoietin, and abnormal mobilization of reticuloendothelial iron stores. Not surprisingly, the degree of anemia in patients with IBD correlates with underlying disease activity as well as systemic levels of IL-1β [52]. In addition to iron-deficiency anemia from increased blood loss, patients with IBD have inappropriately low levels of erythropoietin for their degree of anemia and therefore cannot utilize iron appropriately [50, 52]. Erythropoietin is a renally produced hormone that regulates red blood cell mass by preventing apoptosis of erythroid precursors [53]. The reason for low erythropoietin levels in patients with IBD may be elevated systemic inflammatory cytokines, especially TNF-α, IL-1, IL-6 and the interferons which have been shown to decrease mRNA expression of erythropoietin [54–56]. In addition to causing lower than expected levels of erythropoietin, systemic inflammation leads to relative hyporesponsiveness to erythropoietin [57, 58]. A study performed in UC and CD patients failing oral iron therapy has shown that supplemental erythropoietin (150 U per kilogram of body weight twice per week) in combination with oral iron replacement (100 mg/day) resulted in an average hemoglobin increase of 1.7 g/dl over a 12-week period whereas the placebo-controlled, iron-only group experienced a decline in hemoglobin levels (–0.9 g/dl) [52]. Another study performed in patients with CD and anemia has shown that intravenous iron alone, or in combination with erythropoietin, is effective at increasing hemoglobin levels [33]. Patients receiving erythropoietin had greater increases in hemoglobin levels than the placebo group (4.9 g/dl compared with 3.3 g/dl). Importantly, patients whose anemia responded to therapy had an improved quality of life, suggesting that anemia does contribute to the constitutional symptoms experienced by these patients. Thus in patients with IBD and anemia who have not responded to oral iron replacement, iron levels should be evaluated. Erythropoietin is not effective in patients whose iron stores are not replete, and is the most common cause of erythropoietin resistance [59]. If iron stores are normal, patients should be treated empirically with weekly erythropoietin. A response to oral iron with or without supplemental erythropoietin is generally obtained within 8 weeks of therapy. If iron stores are reduced, intravenous iron can be used alone or in combination with erythropoietin to achieve a clinical effect.

In addition to these physiologic causes of anemia, the treatment of IBD may also result in anemia. Antimetabolites such as azathioprine (AZA) and 6-mercaptopurine (6-MP) are purine antagonists and are thought to exert their beneficial effects by interfering with DNA synthesis. As a result, these drugs can cause a megaloblastic anemia that is generally dose-related [60]. Both can cause dose-dependent bone marrow suppression by inhibiting DNA and RNA synthesis. Thiopurine methyltransferase (TPMT) converts 6-MP to 6-methylmercaptopurine. TPMT is inherited in an autosomal co-dominant fashion such that patients who are heterozygous (14% of Caucasians) or homozygous (1% of Caucasians) for a mutant TPMT gene have diminished or absent ability to metabolize azathioprine or 6-mercaptopurine and are therefore at increased risk for developing hematologic toxicity [61–63]. In addition to an inherited inability to metabolize 6-MP/AZA, certain mesalamine-containing compounds have been described to inhibit the TPMT enzyme, leading to bone marrow suppression [64–66]. For this reason, patients who are initiating 6-MP/AZA

therapy, or who are on a stable dose but have a recent addition of a 5-ASA product, should be followed for the development of hematologic toxicity.

Sulfa and methotrexate (MTX) both interfere with folate metabolism which is required for nucleotide synthesis. Folate supplementation is required in patients taking either sulfasalazine or MTX. MTX acts by inhibiting dihydrofolate reductase. 5-Formal tetrahydrofolate (calcium leucovorin, citrovorum factor or folinic acid) administered 24 h after the administration of MTX can rescue normal cells from the effects of MTX by providing a reduced form of folic acid to the cells. Folate deficiency has been detected in patients receiving sulfasalazine for IBD and may be due to impaired absorption of folate [67]. Red cell folate levels correlate inversely with the dose of sulfasalazine [68]. Patients who are slow acetylators are also at increased risk for sulfasalazine-induced anemia [69]. In addition to the antimetabolite effect of drugs for IBD, mesalamine and sulfasalazine have been associated with rare cases of aplastic anemia, thrombocytopenia or neutropenia [70–73].

Perhaps the least common reason for anemia in a patient with IBD is hemolytic anemia [74–76]. Hemolytic anemia develops in an animal model of UC in which animals are genetically unable to produce IL-2 (IL-2 $^{-/-}$). Whereas the colitis in these animals is mediated by T cells, B cells are required for the anemia [77]. Although there are many case reports in the literature of UC associated with hemolytic anemia, it is not clear that this complication is more common in patients with IBD than in the general population [74, 78]. In the largest series of patients reported from the Mount Sinai School of Medicine only eight patients out of 1150 hospitalized patients with UC (0.7%) were identified with autoimmune hemolytic anemia [74]. The highest incidence of hemolytic anemia was found in a prospective study performed in 302 Greek patients with UC in which 1.7% developed autoimmune hemolytic anemia [79]. Some studies have found a correlation of the hemolysis with disease activity [79] but others have not [74]. The reasons for hemolytic anemia include idiopathic immune-mediated destruction or drugs, especially sulfasalazine [80–82]. Mononuclear cells extracted from the colon of a patient with severe hemolytic anemia and UC, but not peripheral blood cells, were able to transfer IgG with anti-red cell activity, suggesting that in certain cases the colon is the source of hemolysis-inducing antibodies [83]. Characteristics of hemolysis including high lactate dehydrogenase (LDH) and low haptoglobin levels should prompt a Coombs's test for the presence of anti-red blood cell (RBC) antibodies. The hemolysis generally responds to steroids but may require colectomy or splenectomy in patients who fail medical therapy [74, 79, 84].

Hemolytic anemia secondary to sulfasalazine can occur as a result of immune-mediated hemolysis associated with Coombs' positivity, or may be due to glucose-6-phosphate dehydrogenase deficiency [80, 81, 85]. Patients who develop Coombs' positive hemolytic anemia secondary to sulfasalazine may have been taking sulfasalazine for several years prior to the development of this type of anemia [80]. In addition to Coombs testing, agglutination studies may be done wherein sulfasalazine can be added to the patient's serum in the presence of normal erythrocytes and may demonstrate abnormal agglutination.

Disorders of coagulation

An estimated one in 1000 people in the general population experience a thrombotic episode [86] compared with approximately 1–7% of patients with IBD [87–91]; thus hypercoagulability is an important systemic consequence of IBD (Fig. 1). In addition to deep venous thromboses or life-threatening pulmonary emboli, other manifestations of hyper-coagulability in patients with IBD include cerebral venous thromboses [92–98], portal vein thromboses [99, 100], hepatic vein thromboses (Budd–Chiari) [101–104] and arterial thromboses [105]. The reasons for hypercoagulability include inherited disorders of coagulation and acquired disorders of coagulation often due to inflammation-associated changes in hemostatic factors. Most thrombotic events are coincident with flares of IBD [87, 89]. In a study of 52 patients with IBD who experienced thrombo-embolic events, 45% of patients with UC and 89% of patients with CD had active disease at the time of the event [90].

Table 2. Evaluation of anemia in patients with inflammatory bowel disease

Cause of anemia	Characteristics of anemia	Disease prevalence	Diagnostic tests	Treatment
Increased intestinal blood loss	Iron deficiency/ microcytic	Ulcerative colitis > Crohn's disease	Serum Fe, TIBC ratio <15%; ferritin <5 µg/L (may be confounded by acute inflammation)	Oral iron replacement (ferrous sulfate 300 mg t.i.d.); if no response within 4 weeks, parenteral iron replacement*
Diminished iron absorption	Iron deficiency/ microcytic	Crohn's disease > ulcerative colitis	Serum Fe, TIBC ratio <15%	Parenteral iron replacement*
Drug-induced	Ineffective erythropoeisis/ megaloblastic	Both	Normal iron stores, B_{12} and folate; drug withdrawal or dose adjustment improves anemia within 4 weeks	Reduce dose of anti-metabolite; supplement with folate (sulfasalazine or MTX); leucovorin (MTX)
Anemia of chronic disease	Normocytic or microcytic if mixed	Crohn's disease > ulcerative colitis	Serum Fe, TIBC ratio >15% (serum erythropoietin levels are not useful)	Supplement with recombinant erythropoietin (150 U/kg t.i.w. subq for up to 12 weeks or 10 000 U subq q week)
Vitamin B_{12} deficiency	Megaloblastic	Crohn's disease (ileal disease or ileal resection)	Vitamin B_{12} levels	Monthly IM B12 injections 1000 µg dose
Anti-RBC antibodies	Hemolytic anemia	Ulcerative colitis > Crohn's disease	Coombs test positive	Corticosteroids, usually self-limited

*Parenteral iron dextran replacement is based on the following formula: $0.0476 \times$ (normal hemoglobin − observed hemoglobin in g/dl) ($\pm$) 1 ml/5 kg body weight (up to maximum of 14 ml) which accounts for storage iron = total dosage of iron-dextran in ml.

Active IBD is associated with changes in hemostatic factors which may lead to hypercoagulability. Increases in coagulation factors are known risk factors for the development of thromboembolic disease [106]. The most common hemostatic abnormality identified in patients with IBD is thrombocytosis, which correlates with underlying bowel disease activity [107] (Table 3). In a study of 92 thromboembolic events occurring in 7199 (1.3%) patients with IBD, 60% of patients had thrombocytosis and 73% had elevated ESR values, suggesting active IBD [89]. Patients with IBD have increased levels of thrombin generation (prothrombin fragment 1 + 2 and thrombin–antithrombin III complex) compared with control populations, and these levels correlate with disease activity [107–110]. Fibrinogen, factor V and factor VIII are also commonly elevated in patients with IBD whereas the anticoagulant factors antithrombin III, and proteins S and C, are decreased, which may contribute to the propensity for thrombosis [89, 107, 110–119]. Other platelet-related abnormalities identified in patients with IBD are increased spontaneous and induced platelet aggregation which correlated with a history of thromboembolism in seven of eight patients [107, 120]. Surgical resections in patients with CD result in significant decreases in platelet counts, fibrinogen levels and spontaneous platelet aggregation supporting the concept that the underlying bowel disease contributes to the hypercoagulable state [121]. Increased platelet mass in IBD is due to systemic increases in thrombopoietin and IL-6 [122]. Specifically, patients with active IBD have significantly increased levels of thrombopoietin compared with patients in remission and this increase in thrombopoietin is associated with increased platelet counts. Increased megakaryocyte maturation occurs in response to endogenous production of IL-11 and increases with IL-11 therapy for IBD [123]. Acute inflammation can also result in increased hepatic production of fibrinogen and increased platelet aggregation, which is another risk factor in thrombosis. A study of thrombotic risk factors in IBD found that patients with IBD had increased plasma factor VII coagulant activity (a marker of thrombin generation), lipoprotein (a) and fibrinogen concentrations compared with a normal population [124].

With respect to acquired disorders of coagulation, anticardiolipin antibodies or the lupus anticoagulant are associated with an increased risk of thromboembolic events, and have been found with increased frequency in patients with IBD [107, 118, 125].

Studies examining the prevalence of anticardiolipin antibodies in patients with IBD found that both CD and UC patients had increased antibody titers compared to a control group, but the presence of anticardiolipin antibodies was not associated with a higher risk of thromboembolic events in these patients [87, 126]. Others, however, have described the presence of a lupus anticoagulant in the setting of severe thrombotic events such as dural sinus thrombosis or hepatic vein thrombosis in patients with IBD [94, 104, 127]. Based on these studies, a screen for a lupus anticoagulant should be part of the evaluation of a patient with IBD and a recognized thrombotic event, but has little predictive value in a patient without demonstrated hypercoagulability.

Patients with hypercoagulability and IBD may have inherited disorders of coagulation. In combination with inflammation-associated changes in hemostasis these inherited disorders may become manifest [128]. Activated protein C resistance from a mutation in the prothrombin gene (factor V Leiden) is the most common inherited disorder leading to thrombosis, and accounts for 30–40% of episodes of idiopathic venous thrombosis [128–130]. Other inherited causes of hypercoagulability include hyperhomocysteinemia and mutations in the prothrombin gene [131]. Since the description of the relatively common factor V Leiden mutation as an inherited cause of thrombophilia, several groups have investigated the frequency of this mutation in IBD patients with and without a history of thromboembolism. A study evaluating the prevalence of factor V Leiden, methylene tetrahydrofolate reductase (resulting in hyperhomocysteinemia) and prothrombin gene mutations in IBD patients without thrombosis compared with an age-matched control group found no increase in these inherited disorders [132]. Several studies examining the prevalence of activated protein C resistance or factor V Leiden mutations in adults or children with IBD and without a history of thrombosis have not found an increased prevalence of these mutations compared with healthy controls [119, 133, 134]. A large Greek series identified factor V Leiden mutations in 8.3% of IBD patients, which was not significantly different when compared with a healthy control group with a 4.9% mutation rate [111]. Two studies found a slightly increased allelic frequency of factor V Leiden mutations in UC [135] or CD patients [136], but the sample sizes were limited. Although the prevalence of factor V Leiden mutations or resistance to activated protein C does not appear to be increased in an unselected population of IBD patients, the frequency of this mutation is increased in those IBD patients with a history of thromboembolic events. An Austrian study evaluated the presence of resistance to activated protein C in patients with IBD compared with healthy controls. In IBD patients without a history of thromboembolism, the frequency of activated protein C resistance was similar to that of healthy controls (7% versus 5.9%) [137]. By contrast, 31.3% of IBD patients with a history of thromboembolism had activated protein C resistance, suggesting that patients with thromboembolism and IBD are just as likely to have activated protein C resistance as patients with thromboembolism in the general population [129]. Similar results were observed in an American study that found four of 11 IBD patients (36%) with thrombosis and two of 51 IBD controls (4%) were heterozygotes for the factor V Leiden mutation [138]. In a group of 20 patients with IBD complicated by thrombosis, a screen for the most common inherited and acquired disorders of coagulation including protein S, protein C levels, and antithrombin III levels, antiphospholipid antibodies, and activated protein C resistance were negative, with only one patient found to be heterozygous for factor V Leiden mutation [90]. In patients with IBD there is an increased prevalence of hyperhomocysteinemia, a risk factor for thrombophilia, which can be corrected by the administration of folate, cobalamin and pyridoxine [139]. Recent data also suggest that patients with IBD have increased prevalence of the C677T variant of the methylenetetrahydrofolate reductase gene (17% versus 7.3% in healthy controls) which is associated with thromboembolic disease [140]. In a retrospective study of 231 patients with IBD, hyperhomocysteinemia was more prevalent in patients than in healthy controls, but was not higher in IBD patients with a history of thromboembolic disease [141]. These studies suggest that the majority of patients with thromboembolic events and IBD have the same risk as the rest of the population for inherited disorders of coagulation, but the majority will have no identifiable risk factor except active inflammation. Although the risk of inherited disorders predisposing to thrombophilia is not increased in IBD patients, there is an epidemiologic study suggesting that hemophilia and Von Willebrand's disease are under-represented in the IBD population [142]. As the molecular mechanisms regulating disorders of coagulation are elucidated, additional patients with IBD and hypercoagulability will be recognized to have an inherited disorder of coagulation.

Management of thromboses in patients with IBD requires a multi-faceted approach (see Fig. 1). Even in patients with active IBD, a search for an underlying disorder of coagulation is required. If active IBD is the only identifiable risk factor for the thrombosis, and it is a single thrombotic event, short-term anticoagulation combined with treatment of the underlying IBD is appropriate [143]. Heparin therapy can generally be given safely, and has a small therapeutic benefit in patients with UC [144]. Thrombolytic therapy may be given cautiously in IBD patients with extensive thromboses or if the condition is life-threatening [145, 146]. In patients with recurrent thrombotic episodes or life-threatening thromboses, long-term anticoagulation is required. This may be difficult in the setting of active IBD because of associated intestinal bleeding.

In addition to hypercoagulability due to inherited genetic mutations in coagulation factors or inflammation, there are multiple case reports of disseminated intravascular coagulation in patients with UC generally associated with a flare of the UC [148–150]. Thrombocytopenia may also complicate IBD, and may be immune-mediated [151, 152] or associated with drug-induced bone marrow suppression as described above. Cases of sulfasalazine-induced and mesalamine-induced immune-mediated thrombocytopenia have been reported [153].

Leukocytosis

As with inflammation of any type, leukocytosis is often present in patients with IBD [122]. Elevated leukocyte counts prior to surgical resection for CD are associated with an increased risk of recurrence [154]. White blood cell counts above 18 000 or the presence of an elevated band count, should prompt an investigation for a septic process. Neutrophil and monocyte maturation and release from the bone marrow is regulated by granulocyte colony-stimulating factor (GCSF) and monocyte colony-stimulating factor (MCSF), respectively. These factors are derived from bone marrow stromal cells and monocytes which are activated by IL-1, TNF-α and LPS to release these trophic factors. In addition, GM-CSF is derived from activated T lymphocytes and IL-1/TNF-α-activated stromal cells and monocytes. In patients with active IBD, leukocytosis correlates with serum concentrations of IL-6 and thrombocytosis [122]. The presence of leukocytosis in patients with active IBD is thus related to increased circulating levels of proinflammatory cytokines or a septic

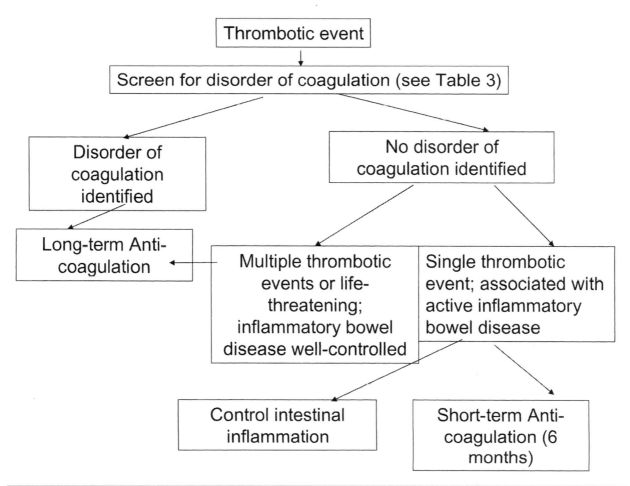

Figure 1. Evaluation of the IBD patient with a thrombotic event.

Table 3. Causes of hypercoagulability in patients with inflammatory bowel disease [128, 147]

Inherited causes of hypercoagulability	Acquired causes of hypercoagulability
Activated protein C resistance (Arg 506 changed to Gln in factor V) (factor V Leiden mutation)	Thrombocytosis (active inflammation)
Prothrombin G20210A polymorphism (results in increased levels of prothrombin)	Increased platelet aggregation
Methylene tetrahydrofolate reductase mutations (hyperhomocysteinemia)	Elevated factor VIII plasma levels
Deficiency or mutations in protein C	Elevated fibrinogen levels
Deficiency or mutations in protein S	Anticardiolipin antibodies
Antithrombin III deficiency	Deficiency in protein S Secondary hyperhomocysteinemia (due to folate, pyridoxine or cobalamin deficiency)

complication such as a microperforation, frank perforation or abscess. Corticosteroids also lead to leukocytosis secondary to down-regulation of intercellular adhesion molecule expression and granulocyte demargination.

Hematologic malignancies

In spite of multiple case reports of leukemias or lymphomas associated with IBD, it remains controversial whether patients with IBD are at increased risk for the development of hematologic malignancies either as a result of chronic inflammatory disease or its treatment [155–157]. Other chronic inflammatory disorders such as rheumatoid arthritis do pose an increased risk of hematologic malignancies [158]. Based on several case series and population-based studies, it seems that patients with CD are at a slightly increased risk for the development of non-Hodgkin's lymphomas than the average population search. A recent study based on Olmstead County, Minnesota, records found a standardized incidence ratio of lymphomas of 2.4 (95% confidence intervals 0.1–13) in patients with CD and no cases of lymphomas occurred in patients with UC [155]. Only three patients out of 61 who developed lymphomas were receiving purine analogs. Few patients with IBD in this study were on immunomodulator therapy thus this may represent the true incidence of lymphomas in IBD patients in the absence of immunosuppressive therapy. There was no increased risk of leukemia in these patients. In another large series of IBD patients, five lymphomas occurred among 1156 patients (0.43%) with UC and four lymphomas among 1480 patients (0.27%) with CD and the risk of lymphomas correlated with disease duration in patients with CD [159]. A recent population-based study performed in Florence, Italy, reported a ninefold increased incidence of Hodgkin's lymphoma in patients with UC compared with the general population [160]. The same study found a reduced risk (standardized incidence ratio 0.6) of respiratory tract cancers in patients with UC and increased risk in patients with CD. Severity of the IBD has not been established as an independent risk factor in the development of lymphomas.

Immunosuppressive therapy has been implicated as a risk factor in the development of hematologic malignancies, but a causal role of immunosuppressive therapy in the development of lymphomas associated with IBD has not been established [161, 162]. To date there have been three published cases of brain lymphomas (one each from three large series) in patients with IBD on long-term AZP or 6-MP in a total of 1701 patients [156, 161, 163]. Although the overall risk of brain lymphomas is low in patients with IBD treated with purine antimetabolites, immunosuppression is clearly a risk factor for this otherwise rare malignancy [164]. In a series of 550 patients with IBD on long-term 6-MP therapy, two patients developed non-Hodgkin's lymphoma, one leukemia and one brain lymphoma [161]. The overall rate of these malignancies was not higher than in the general population. Two other large series of 755 and 396 patients found no excess in the risk of any hematologic malignancies in IBD patients treated with AZP or 6-MP [156, 163]. A decision analysis comparing the efficacy of AZP at maintaining remission in IBD compared with the risk of non-Hodgkin's lymphoma found that AZP was favorable and resulted in improved quality of life [165]. In spite of the encouraging data in patients with IBD, children treated with 6-MP for acute lymphoblastic leukemia have an increased risk of secondary myelodysplasia or acute myeloid leukemia (5/493), and this risk is associated with low TPMT enzymatic activity and high erythrocyte 6-thioguanine nucleotides [166]. 6-MP and AZP have also been associated with rare cases of acute myeloid leukemia in patients with autoimmune diseases including IBD treated for prolonged periods of time [167, 168]. In all the cases a prolonged pancytopenic phase preceded the onset of the leukemia suggesting an antecedent myelodysplastic phase.

Immunocompromised hosts, especially patients who have undergone solid organ transplantation, are at significantly increased risk for the development of B cell lymphomas related to Epstein–Barr virus (EBV) infection [169, 170]. The risk in patients post-transplantation is thought to be high because of the use of multiple immunosuppressive drugs, as well as the long-term nature of the immunosuppression. In a series of four patients with gastrointestinal Hodgkin's lymphoma and IBD, all four lymphomas were found to be EBV-mediated with only two patients on immunomodulator therapy [171]. An additional case of an EBV-driven lymphoproliferative disorder in a CD patient on long-term AZP regressed after discontinuation of the AZP [172, 173]. Finally, one B cell lymphoma and one Hodgkin's lymphoma have been reported in patients with CD after receiving infliximab anti-TNF-α therapy [174]. These lymphomas occurred 3 weeks and 10 months after receiving infliximab. It is too soon to determine the relationship of anti-TNF-α strategies to the development of hematologic malignancies.

Amyloidosis in patients with IBD

An uncommon but morbid systemic consequence of IBD is the development of amyloidosis [30, 175–177]. Amyloidosis is a group of diseases characterized by the extracellular deposition of pathologic insoluble fibrillar proteins in organs and tissues [178, 179]. There are three principal forms of amyloidosis. Systemic AL amyloidosis is associated with blood cell dyscrasias and monoclonal gammopathies. There are multiple familial forms of amyloidosis or type ATTR amyloidosis. As with other chronic inflammatory states such as rheumatoid arthritis, IBD may rarely result in secondary systemic amyloidosis type AA [180, 181]. In general, rheumatologic diseases are more commonly associated with amyloidosis than IBD, and CD is more often complicated by amyloidosis than UC [175, 178, 179, 182]. In a large series of IBD followed at the Mount Sinai Hospital, amyloidosis occurred in 15 of 1709 patients with CD (0.9%) and one of 1341 patients with UC (0.07%) [30]. Amyloidosis was more often associated with CD of the colon than with pure small bowel disease.

The diagnosis of amyloidosis is made by appropriate pathology demonstrating Congo red-positive amyloid deposits on fat-pad biopsy, rectal biopsy or renal biopsy [178, 179]. Scintigraphy has recently been developed as a non-invasive and quantitative alternative to histology. A radioactive tracer ^{123}I-serum amyloid P component is injected and specifically targets amyloid deposits *in vivo*. The technique has almost 100% sensitivity for systemic AA amyloidosis. In four patients with CD and amyloidosis, ^{123}I-serum amyloid P nuclear medicine scanning demonstrated the increased amyloid content and correlated with disease improvement following renal transplantation [180].

In patients with CD and AA amyloidosis, proteinuria is the most common presentation [30, 175, 177, 179, 180, 183]. The overall 5-year mortality for AA amyloidosis is 50% [178, 179]. In one series, one of four patients died prior to renal transplantation demonstrating the high morbidity and mortality from this complication [180]. Nephropathy is the most common lethal manifestation of IBD-associated amyloidosis. Nephrotic syndrome was responsible for 10 deaths out of 25 patients with IBD-associated amyloidosis in a large series [30].

Therapy for type AA amyloidosis is directed at limiting the acute-phase response generating the amyloid protein [178, 179]. Unfortunately, this type of amyloidosis is generally advanced by the time of diagnosis with extensive amyloid deposits and renal failure [175]. Only limited case report information is available on the management of IBD complicated by amyloidosis. Several cases of UC complicated by AA amyloidosis have been effectively treated with colchicine, which led to reduction in proteinuria [182, 184–187]. AZP and colchicine combination therapy has also been effective in improving amyloidosis-induced renal failure and controlling CD in one patient [188]. An elemental diet has been reported as effective in preventing ongoing renal damage in a CD patient with amyloidosis [189]. Regression of amyloid has also been reported in patients with CD after bowel resection or after treatment with dimethylsulfoxide (DMSO) [190, 191]. Based on the limited data, periodic tests of renal function are warranted in patients with IBD to assess nephrotoxicity from medications, as well as the rare occurrence of amyloidosis.

References

1. Chrousos GP. The hypothalamic–pituitary–adrenal axis and immune-mediated inflammation. N Engl J Med 1995; 332: 1351–62.
2. Papanicolaou DA, Wilder RL, Manolagas SC, Chrousos GP. The pathophysiologic roles of interleukin-6 in human disease. Ann Intern Med 1998; 128: 127–37.
3. van Deventer SJ, Buller HR, ten Cate JW, Aarden LA, Hack CE, Sturk A. Experimental endotoxemia in humans: analysis of cytokine release and coagulation, fibrinolytic, and complement pathways. Blood 1990; 76: 2520–6.
4. Kotler D. Cachexia. Annals Intern Med 2000; 133: 622–34.
5. Tracey KJ, Morgello S, Koplin B *et al.* Metabolic effects of cachectin/tumor necrosis factor are modified by site of production. Cachectin/tumor necrosis factor-secreting tumor in skeletal muscle induces chronic cachexia, while implantation in brain induces predominantly acute anorexia. J Clin Invest 1990; 86: 2014–24.
6. Tracey KJ, Cerami A. Tumor necrosis factor: a pleiotropic cytokine and therapeutic target. Annu Review of Med 1994; 45: 491-503.
7. Papadakis KA, Targan SR. Role of cytokines in the pathogenesis of inflammatory bowel disease. Annu Rev Med 2000; 51: 289–98.
8. Papadakis KA, Targan SR. Tumor necrosis factor: biology and therapeutic inhibitors. Gastroenterology 2000; 119: 1148–57.
9. O'Neill LA, Dinarello CA. The IL-1 receptor/toll-like receptor superfamily: crucial receptors for inflammation and host defense. Immunol Today 2000; 21: 206–9.
10. Howard AD, Kostura MJ, Thornberry N *et al.* IL-1-converting enzyme requires aspartic acid residues for processing of the IL-1 beta precursor at two distinct sites and does not cleave 31-kDa IL-1 alpha. J Immunol 1991; 147: 2964–9.

11. Rosenwasser LJ. Biologic activities of IL-1 and its role in human disease. J Allergy Clin Immunol 1998; 102: 344–50.

12. Dinarello CA. Proinflammatory cytokines. Chest 2000; 118: 503–8.

13. Ershler WB, Keller ET. Age-associated increased interleukin-6 gene expression, late-life diseases, and frailty. Annu Rev Med 2000; 51: 245–70.

14. Cressman DE, Greenbaum LE, DeAngelis RA et al. Liver failure and defective hepatocyte regeneration in interleukin-6-deficient mice. Science 1996; 274: 1379–83.

15. Streetz KL, Luedde T, Manns MP, Trautwein C. Interleukin 6 and liver regeneration. Gut 2000; 47: 309–12.

16. Nielsen OH, Vainer B, Madsen SM, Seidelin JB, Heegaard NH. Established and emerging biological activity markers of inflammatory bowel disease. Am J Gastroenterol 2000; 95: 359–67.

17. Mahida YR, Ceska M, Effenberger F, Kurlak L, Lindley I, Hawkey CJ. Enhanced synthesis of neutrophil-activating peptide-1/interleukin-8 in active ulcerative colitis. Clin Sci 1992; 82: 273-5.

18. Farmer RG, Hawk WA, Turnbull RB Jr. Clininical patterns in Crohn's disease: a statistical study of 615 cases. Gastroenterology 1975; 68: 627–35.

19. Sparberg M, Fennessy J, Kirsner JB. Ulcerative proctitis and mild ulcerative colitis: a study of 220 patients. Medicine 1966; 45: 391–412.

20. Gabay C, Kushner I. Acute-phase proteins and other systemic responses to inflammation [published erratum appears in N Engl J Med 1999; 340: 1376]. N Engl J Med 1999; 340: 448–54.

21. Moldawer LL, Copeland EM IIIrd. Proinflammatory cytokines, nutritional support, and the cachexia syndrome: interactions and therapeutic options. Cancer 1997; 79: 1828–39.

22. Plata-Salaman CR. Food intake suppression by growth factors and platelet peptides by direct action in the central nervous system. Neurosci Lett 1988; 94: 161–6.

23. Sarraf P, Frederich RC, Turner EM et al. Multiple cytokines and acute inflammation raise mouse leptin levels: potential role in inflammatory anorexia. J Exp Med 1997; 185: 171–5.

24. Both H, Torp-Pedersen K, Kreiner S, Hendriksen C, Binder V. Clinical appearance at diagnosis of ulcerative colitis and Crohn's disease in a regional patient group. Scand J Gastroenterol 1983; 18: 987–91.

25. Dinarello CA. Cytokines as endogenous pyrogens. J Infect Dis 1999; 179 (Suppl 2): S294–304.

26. Castell JV, Gomez-Lechon MJ, David M et al. Interleukin-6 is the major regulator of acute phase protein synthesis in adult human hepatocytes. FEBS Lett 1989; 242: 237–9.

27. Fattori E, Cappelletti M, Costa P et al. Defective inflammatory response in interleukin 6-deficient mice. J Exp Med 1994; 180: 1243–50.

28. Betz UAK, Bloch W, van den Broek M et al. Postnatally induced inactivation of gp130 in mice results in neurological, cardiac, hematopoietic, immunological, hepatic, and pulmonary defects. J Exp Med 1998; 188: 1955–65.

29. Gershov D, Kim S, Brot N, Elkon K. C-reactive protein binds to apoptotic cells, protects the cells from assembly of the terminal complement components, and sustains an antiinflammatory innate immune response: implications for systemic autoimmunity. J Exp Med 2000; 192: 1353–64.

30. Greenstein AJ, Sachar DB, Panday AK et al.: Amyloidosis and inflammatory bowel disease. A 50-year experience with 25 patients. Medicine 1992; 71: 261–70.

31. Kurzrock R, Redman J, Cabanillas F, Jones D, Rothberg J, Talpaz M. Serum interleukin 6 levels are elevated in lymphoma patients and correlate with survival in advanced Hodgkin's disease and with B symptoms. Cancer Res 1993; 53: 2118–22.

32. Gasche C. Anemia in IBD: the overlooked villain. Inflammat Bowel Dis 2000; 6: 142–50; discussion 151.

33. Gasche C, Dejaco C, Waldhoer T et al. Intravenous iron and erythropoietin for anemia associated with Crohn disease. A randomized, controlled trial. Ann Intern Med 1997; 126: 782–7.

34. Horina JH, Petritsch W, Schmid CR et al. Treatment of anemia in inflammatory bowel disease with recombinant human erythropoietin: results in three patients. Gastroenterology 1993; 104: 1828–31.

35. Gasche C, Reinisch W, Lochs H et al. Anemia in Crohn's disease. Importance of inadequate erythropoietin production and iron deficiency. Dig Dis Sci 1994; 39: 1930–4.

36. Beeken WL. Remediable defects in Crohn disease: a prospective study of 63 patients. Arch Intern Med 1975; 135: 686–90.

37. Gold Y, Reif S. [Aphthous stomatitis as a first manifestation of Crohn's disease in a 5 year-old boy]. Harefuah 1998; 135: 364–6, 407.

38. Froom P, Benbassat J, Kiwelowicz A, Erel J, Davidson B, Ribak J. Significance of low hematocrit levels in asymptomatic young adults: results of 15 years follow-up. Aviat Space Environ Med 1999; 70: 983–6.

39. Menachem Y, Weizman Z, Locker C, Odes S. Clinical characteristics of Crohn's disease in children and adults. Harefuah 1998; 134: 173–5, 247.

40. Smith AD, Cochran KM. Serum ferritin: it may guide the diagnosis of the anaemic patient. Scot Med J 1997; 42: 182–3.

41. Gasche C, Dejaco C, Reinisch W et al.Sequential treatment of anemia in ulcerative colitis with intravenous iron and erythropoietin. Digestion 1999; 60: 262–7.

42. Macdougall IC. Strategies for iron supplementation: oral versus intravenous. Kidney Int (Suppl.) 1999; 69: S61–6.

43. Hamstra RD, Block MH, Schocket AL. Intravenous iron dextran in clinical medicine. J Am Med Assoc 1980; 243: 1726–31.

44. Dyer N, Dawson A: Malnutrition and malabsorption in Crohn's disease with references to the effect of surgery. Br J Surg 1973; 60: 134–40.

45. Dyer NH, Child JA, Mollin DL, Dawson AM. Anaemia in Crohn's disease. Q J Med 1972; 41: 419–36.

46. Thompson W, Wrathell E. The relation between ileal resection and vitamin B12 absorption. Can J Surg 1977; 20: 461–4.

47. Fone D et al. [^{58}]Co B-12 absorption after gastrectomy, ileal resection and in coeliac disorders. Gut 1961; 2: 218.

48. Lee G. Pernicious anemia and other causes of vitamin B12 (cobalamin) deficiency. In: Lee G (ed.), Wintrobe's Clinical Hematology, 10th edn. Baltimore: Lippincott, Williams & Wilkins, 1999; 956.

49. Spiegel JE, Willenbucher RF. Rapid development of severe copper deficiency in a patient with Crohn's disease receiving parenteral nutrition. J Parent Ent Nutr 1999; 23: 169–72.

50. Means RT Jr. Erythropoietin in the treatment of anemia in chronic infectious, inflammatory, and malignant diseases. Curr Opin Hematol 1995; 2: 210–3.

51. Means RT Jr. Advances in the anemia of chronic disease. Int J Hematol 1999; 70: 7–12.

52. Schreiber S, Howaldt S, Schnoor M et al. Recombinant erythropoietin for the treatment of anemia in inflammatory bowel disease. N Engl J Med 1996; 334: 619–23.

53. Koury M, Bondurant M. The molecular mechanism of erythropoietin action. Eur J Biochem 1992; 210: 649–63.

54. Jelkmann WE, Fandrey J, Frede S, Pagel H: Inhibition of erythropoietin production by cytokines. Implications for the anemia involved in inflammatory states. Ann NY Acad Sci 1994; 718: 300–9; discussion 309–11.

55. Jelkmann W. Proinflammatory cytokines lowering erythropoietin production. J Interferon Cytokine Res 1998; 18: 555–9.
56. Faquin WC, Schneider TJ, Goldberg MA. Effect of inflammatory cytokines on hypoxia-induced erythropoietin production. Blood 1992; 79: 1987–94.
57. Gunnell J, Yeun JY, Depner TA, Kaysen GA. Acute-phase response predicts erythropoietin resistance in hemodialysis and peritoneal dialysis patients. Am J Kidney Dis 1999; 33: 63–72.
58. Nordstrom D, Lindroth Y, Marsal L et al. Availability of iron and degree of inflammation modifies the response to recombinant human erythropoietin when treating anemia of chronic disease in patients with rheumatoid arthritis. Rheumatol Int 1997; 17: 67–73.
59. Tarng DC, Huang TP, Chen TW, Yang WC. Erythropoietin hyporesponsiveness: from iron deficiency to iron overload. Kidney Int (Suppl.) 1999; 69: S107–18.
60. Lennard L, Murphy M, Maddocks J: Severe megaloblastic anaemia associated with abnormal azathioprine metabolism. Br J Clin Pharmacol 1984; 17: 171.
61. Weinshilboum RM, Sladek SL. Mercaptopurine pharmacogenetics: monogenic inheritance of erythrocyte thiopurine methyltransferase activity. Am J Hum Genet 1980; 32: 651–62.
62. Schutz E, Gummert J, Armstrong VW, Mohr FW, Oellerich M. Azathioprine pharmacogenetics: the relationship between 6-thioguanine nucleotides and thiopurine methyltransferase in patients after heart and kidney transplantation. Eur J Clin Chem Clin Biochem 1996; 34: 199–205.
63. Lennard L, Van Loon JA, Lilleyman JS, Weinshilboum RM. Thiopurine pharmacogenetics in leukemia: correlation of erythrocyte thiopurine methyltransferase activity and 6-thioguanine nucleotide concentrations. Clin Pharmacol Ther 1987; 41: 18–25.
64. Lowry PW, Szumlanski CL, Weinshilboum RM, Sandborn WJ. Balsalazide and azathiprine or 6-mercaptopurine: evidence for a potentially serious drug interaction [Letter; comment]. Gastroenterology 1999; 116: 1505–6.
65. Lewis LD, Benin A, Szumlanski CL et al. Olsalazine and 6-mercaptopurine-related bone marrow suppression: a possible drug-drug interaction [Published erratum appears in Clin Pharmacol Ther 2000; 67:431]. Clin Pharmacol Ther 1997; 62: 464–75.
66. Szumlanski CL, Weinshilboum RM. Sulphasalazine inhibition of thiopurine methyltransferase: possible mechanism for interaction with 6-mercaptopurine and azathioprine. Br J Clin Pharmacol 1995; 39: 456–9.
67. Swinson CM, Perry J, Lumb M, Levi AJ. Role of sulphasalazine in the aetiology of folate deficiency in ulcerative colitis. Gut 1981; 22: 456–61.
68. Longstreth G, Green R. Folate status in patients receiving maintenance doses of sulfasalazine. Arch Intern Med 1983; 143: 902.
69. Das KM, Eastwood MA, McManus JP, Sircus W. Adverse reactions during salicylazosulfapyridine therapy and the relation with drug metabolism and acetylator phenotype. N Engl J Med 1973; 289: 491–5.
70. Abboudi ZH, Marsh JC, Smith-Laing G, Gordon-Smith EC. Fatal aplastic anaemia after mesalazine [Letter]. Lancet 1994; 343: 542.
71. Dunn AM, Kerr GD. Pure red cell aplasia associated with sulphasalazine [Letter]. Lancet 1981; 2: 1288.
72. Daneshmend T. Mesalazine-associated thrombocytopenia. Lancet 1991; 337: 1297–8.
73. Wyatt S, Joyner M, Daneshmend T. Filgrastim for mesalazine-associated neutropenia. Lancet 1993; 341: 1476.
74. Gumaste V, Greenstein AJ, Meyers R, Sachar DB. Coombs-positive autoimmune hemolytic anemia in ulcerative colitis. Dig Dis Sci 1989; 34: 1457–61.
75. Bell DW, Urban E, Sears DA, Walder AI, Ostrower VS. Ulcerative colitis complicated by autoimmune hemolytic anemia. S Med J 1981; 74: 359–61.
76. Altman AR, Maltz C, Janowitz HD. Autoimmune hemolytic anemia in ulcerative colitis: report of three cases, review of the literature, and evaluation of modes of therapy. Dig Dis Sci 1979; 24: 282–5.
77. Ma A, Datta M, Margosian E, Chen J, Horak I: T cells, but not B cells, are required for bowel inflammation in interleukin 2-deficient mice. J Exp Med 1995; 182: 1567–72.
78. Ramakrishna R, Manoharan A. Auto-immune haemolytic anaemia in ulcerative colitis. Acta Haematol 1994; 91: 99–102.
79. Giannadaki E, Potamianos S, Roussomoustakaki M, Kyriakou D, Fragkiadakis N, Manousos ON. Autoimmune hemolytic anemia and positive Coombs test associated with ulcerative colitis. Am J Gastroenterol 1997; 92: 1872–4.
80. Teplitsky V, Virag I, Halabe A. Immune complex haemolytic anaemia associated with sulfasalazine. Br Med J 2000; 320: 1113.
81. Mechanick JI. Coombs' positive hemolytic anemia following sulfasalazine therapy in ulcerative colitis: case reports, review, and discussion of pathogenesis. Mount Sinai J Med 1985; 52: 667–70.
82. van Hees PA, van Elferen LW, van Rossum JM, van Tongeren JH. Hemolysis during salicylazosulfapyridine therapy. Am J Gastroenterol 1978; 70: 501–5.
83. Yates P, Macht LM, Williams NA, Elson CJ. Red cell autoantibody production by colonic mononuclear cells from a patient with ulcerative colitis and autoimmune haemolytic anaemia. Br J Haematol 1992; 82: 753–6.
84. Murphy PT, Cunney R, Nolan A, O'Donnell JR. Autoimmune haemolytic anaemia associated with ulcerative colitis. Irish Med J 1996; 89: 172–3.
85. Cohen SM, Rosenthal DS, Karp PJ. Ulcerative colitis and erythrocyte G6PD deficiency. Salicylazosulfapyridine-provoked hemolysis. J Am Med Assoc 1968; 205: 528–30.
86. Dahlback B, Blood coagulation. Lancet 2000; 355: 1627–32.
87. Aichbichler BW, Petritsch W, Reicht GA et al. Anti-cardiolipin antibodies in patients with inflammatory bowel disease. Dig Dis Sci 1999; 44: 852–6.
88. Schapira M, Henrion J, Ravoet C et al. Thromboembolism in inflammatory bowel disease. Acta Gastroenterol Belg 1999; 62: 182–6.
89. Talbot RW, Heppell J, Dozois RR, Beart RW, Jr. Vascular complications of inflammatory bowel disease. Mayo Clin Proc 1986; 61: 140–5.
90. Jackson LM, O'Gorman PJ, O'Connell J, Cronin CC, Cotter KP, Shanahan F. Thrombosis in inflammatory bowel disease: clinical setting, procoagulant profile and factor V Leiden. Q J Med 1997; 90: 183–8.
91. Koenigs KP, McPhedran P, Spiro HM. Thrombosis in inflammatory bowel disease. J Clin Gastroenterol 1987; 9: 627–31.
92. Johns DR. Cerebrovascular complications of inflammatory bowel disease. Am J Gastroenterol 1991; 86: 367–70.
93. Carmona MA, Jaume Anselmi F, Ramirez Rivera J. Cerebral thrombosis and vasculitis: an uncommon complication of ulcerative colitis. Bol Asoc Med Puerto Rico 2000; 92: 9–11.
94. Papi C, Ciaco A, Acierno G et al. Severe ulcerative colitis, dural sinus thrombosis, and the lupus anticoagulant. Am J Gastroenterol 1995; 90: 1514–7.
95. Musio F, Older SA, Jenkins T, Gregorie EM. Case report: cerebral venous thrombosis as a manifestation of acute ulcerative colitis. Am J Med Sci 1993; 305: 28–35.

96. Markowitz RL, Ment LR, Gryboski JD. Cerebral thromboembolic disease in pediatric and adult inflammatory bowel disease: case report and review of the literature. J Pediatr Gastroenterol Nutr 1989; 8: 413–20.

97. Bansal R, Goel A. Ulcerative colitis with sagittal sinus thrombosis with normal coagulation profile. Ind J Gastroenterol 2000; 19: 88–9.

98. Derdeyn CP, Powers WJ. Isolated cortical venous thrombosis and ulcerative colitis. Am J Neuroradiol 1998; 19: 488–90.

99. Crowe A, Taffinder N, Layer GT, Irvine A, Nicholls RJ. Portal vein thrombosis in a complicated case of Crohn's disease. Postgrad Med J 1992; 68: 291–3.

100. Miyazaki Y, Shinomura Y, Kitamura S et al. Portal vein thrombosis associated with active ulcerative colitis: percutaneous transhepatic recanalization. Am J Gastroenterol 1995; 90: 1533–4.

101. Chesner IM, Muller S, Newman J. Ulcerative colitis complicated by Budd-Chiari syndrome. Gut 1986; 27: 1096–100.

102. Maccini DM, Berg JC, Bell GA. Budd–Chiari syndrome and Crohn's disease. An unreported association. Dig Dis Sci 1989; 34: 1933–6.

103. Brinson RR, Curtis WD, Schuman BM, Mills LR. Recovery from hepatic vein thrombosis (Budd–Chiari syndrome) complicating ulcerative colitis. Dig Dis Sci 1988; 33: 1615–20.

104. Praderio L, Dagna L, Longhi P, Rubin G, Sabbadini MG. Budd–Chiari syndrome in a patient with ulcerative colitis: association with anticardiolipin antibodies. J Clin Gastroenterol 2000; 30: 203–4.

105. Halliday CE, Farthing MJ. Arterial thrombosis in Crohn's disease. Med J Austr 1988; 149: 559–60.

106. Kyrle PA, Minar E, Hirschl M et al. High plasma levels of factor VIII and the risk of recurrent venous thromboembolism. N Engl J Med 2000; 343: 457–62.

107. Chiarantini E, Valanzano R, Liotta AA. Hemostatic abnormalities in inflammatory bowel disease. Thromb Res 1996; 82: 137–46.

108. Smith CJ, Haire WD, Kaufman SS, Mack DR. Determination of prothrombin activation fragments in young patients with inflammatory bowel disease. Am J Gastroenterol 1996; 91: 1221–5.

109. Chamouard P, Grunebaum L, Wiesel ML et al. Prothrombin fragment 1 + 2 and thrombin–antithrombin III complex as markers of activation of blood coagulation in inflammatory bowel diseases. Eur J Gastroenterol Hepatol 1995; 7: 1183–8.

110. Souto JC, Martinez E, Roca M et al.Prothrombotic state and signs of endothelial lesion in plasma of patients with inflammatory bowel disease. Dig Dis Sci 1995; 40: 1883–9.

111. Koutroubakis IE, Sfiridaki A, Mouzas IA et al. Resistance to activated protein C and low levels of free protein S in Greek patients with inflammatory bowel disease. Am J Gastroenterol 2000; 95: 190–4.

112. Lee LC, Spittell JA, Jr, Sauer WG, Owen CA, Jr, Thompson JH, Jr. Hypercoagulability associated with chronic ulcerative colitis: changes in blood coagulation factors. Gastroenterology 1968; 54: 76–85.

113. Braverman D, Bogoch A. Arterial thrombosis in ulcerative colitis. Am J Dig Dis 1978; 23: 1148–50.

114. Aadland E, Odegaard OR, Roseth A, Try K. Free protein S deficiency in patients with Crohn's disease. Scand J Gastroenterol 1994; 29: 333–5.

115. Talstad I, Rootwelt K, Gjone E. Thrombocytosis in ulcerative colitis and Crohn's disease. Scand J Gastroenterol 1973; 8: 135–8.

116. Lam A, Borda I, Inwood M, Thomson S. Coagulation studies in ulcerative colitis and Crohn's disease. Gastroenterology 1975; 68: 245–51.

117. Morowitz D, Allen L, Kirsner J. Thrombocytosis in chronic inflammatory bowel disease. Ann Intern Med 1968; 68: 1013–21.

118. Vecchi M, Cattaneo M, de Franchis R, Mannucci PM. Risk of thromboembolic complications in patients with inflammatory bowel disease. Study of hemostasis measurements. Int J Clin Lab Res 1991; 21: 165–70.

119. Heneghan MA, Cleary B, Murray M, O'Gorman TA, McCarthy CF. Activated protein C resistance, thrombophilia, and inflammatory bowel disease. Dig Dis Sci 1998; 43: 1356–61.

120. Webberley MJ, Hart MT, Melikian V. Thromboembolism in inflammatory bowel disease: role of platelets. Gut 1993; 34: 247–51.

121. Chiarantini E, Valanzano R, Liotta AA et al. Persistence of hemostatic alterations in patients affected by Crohn's disease after bowel surgery. Thromb Res 1997; 87: 539–46.

122. Heits F, Stahl M, Ludwig D, Stange EF, Jelkmann W. Elevated serum thrombopoietin and interleukin-6 concentrations in thrombocytosis associated with inflammatory bowel disease. J Interferon Cytokine Res 1999; 19: 757–60.

123. Sands BE, Bank S, Sninsky CA et al. Preliminary evaluation of safety and activity of recombinant human interleukin 11 in patients with active Crohn's disease. Gastroenterology 1999; 117: 58–64.

124. Hudson M, Chitolie A, Hutton RA, Smith MS, Pounder RE, Wakefield AJ. Thrombotic vascular risk factors in inflammatory bowel disease. Gut 1996; 38: 733–7.

125. Chamouard P, Grunebaum L, Wiesel ML et al. Prevalence and significance of anticardiolipin antibodies in Crohn's disease. Dig Dis Sci 1994; 39: 1501–4.

126. Koutroubakis IE, Petinaki E, Anagnostopoulou E et al. Anti-cardiolipin and anti-beta2-glycoprotein I antibodies in patients with inflammatory bowel disease. Dig Dis Sci 1998; 43: 2507–12.

127. Vianna JL, D'Cruz DP, Khamashta MA, Asherson RA, Hughes GR. Anticardiolipin antibodies in a patient with Crohn's disease and thrombosis. Clin Exp Rheumatol 1992; 10: 165–8.

128. Olds RJ, Fitches AC, Geary CP. The multigenic basis for venous thrombosis. Br J Haematol 2000; 109: 508–11.

129. Dahlback B. New molecular insights into the genetics of thrombophilia. Resistance to activated protein C caused by Arg (506) to Gln mutation in Factor V as a pathogenic risk factor for venous thrombosis. Thromb Haemostas 1995; 74: 139–48.

130. Sheppard DR. Activated protein C resistance: the most common risk factor for venous thromboembolism. J Am Board Fam Pract 2000; 13: 111–5.

131. De Stefano V, Martinelli I, Mannucci PM, Paciaroni K, Chiusolo P, Casorelli I, Rossi E, Leone G. The risk of recurrent deep venous thrombosis among heterozygous carriers of both factor V Leiden and the G20210A prothrombin mutation. N Engl J Med 1999; 341: 801–6.

132. Vecchi M, Sacchi E, Saibeni S et al. Inflammatory bowel diseases are not associated with major hereditary conditions predisposing to thrombosis. Dig Dis Sci 2000; 45: 1465–9.

133. Zauber NP, Sabbath-Solitare M, Rajoria G, Mogan G. Factor V Leiden mutation is not increased in patients with inflammatory bowel disease. J Clin Gastroenterol 1998; 27: 215–6.

134. Levine A, Lahav J, Zahavi I, Raz A, Dinari G. Activated protein C resistance in pediatric inflammatory bowel disease. J Pediatr Gastroenterol Nutr 1998; 26: 172–4.

135. Haslam N, Standen GR, Probert CS. An investigation of the association of the factor V Leiden mutation and inflammatory bowel disease. Eur J Gastroenterol Hepatol 1999; 11: 1289–91.

136. Over HH, Ulgen S, Tuglular T *et al.* Thrombophilia and inflammatory bowel disease: does factor V mutation have a role? Eur J Gastroenterol Hepatol 1998; 10: 827–9.

137. Novacek G, Miehsler W, Kapiotis S, Katzenschlager R, Speiser W, Vogelsang H. Thromboembolism and resistance to activated protein C in patients with inflammatory bowel disease. Am J Gastroenterol 1999; 94: 685–90.

138. Liebman HA, Kashani N, Sutherland D, McGehee W, Kam AL. The factor V Leiden mutation increases the risk of venous thrombosis in patients with inflammatory bowel disease. Gastroenterology 1998; 115: 830–4.

139. Cattaneo M, Vecchi M, Zighetti ML, *et al.* High prevalence of hyperchomocysteinemia in patients with inflammatory bowel disease: a pathogenic link with thromboembolic complications? Thromb Haemostas 1998; 80: 542–5.

140. Mahmud N, Molloy A, McPartlin J *et al.* Increased prevalence of methylenetetrahydrofolate reductase C677T variant in patients with inflammatory bowel disease, and its clinical implications. Gut 1999; 45: 389–94.

141. Oldenburg B, Fijnheer R, van der Griend R, vanBerge-Henegouwen GP, Koningsberger JC. Homocysteine in inflammatory bowel disease: a risk factor for thromboembolic complications? Am J Gastroenterol 2000; 95: 2825–30.

142. Thompson N, Wakefield A, Pounder R. Inherited disorders of coagulation appear to protect against inflammatory bowel disease. Gastroenterology 1995; 108: 1011–15.

143. Kearon C, Gent M, Hirsh J *et al.* A comparison of three months of anticoagulation with extended anticoagulation for a first episode of idiopathic venous thromboembolism [published erratum appears in N Engl J Med 1999 22; 341: 298]. N Engl J Med 1999; 340: 901–7.

144. Gaffney PR, Doyle CT, Gaffney A, Hogan J, Hayes DP, Annis P. Paradoxical response to heparin in 10 patients with ulcerative colitis. Am J Gastroenterol 1995; 90: 220–3.

145. Van Woert JH, Thompson RC, Cangemi JR, Metzger PP, Blackshear JL, Fleming CR. Streptokinase therapy for extensive venous thromboses in a patient with severe ulcerative colitis. Mayo Clin Proc 1990; 65: 1144–9.

146. Kermode AG, Ives FJ, Taylor B, Davis SJ, Carroll WM. Progressive dural venous sinus thrombosis treated with local streptokinase infusion [Letter]. J Neurol Neurosurg Psychiatry 1995; 58: 107–8.

147. Nguyen A. Prothrombin G20210A polymorphism and thrombophilia. Mayo Clin Proc 2000; 75: 595–604.

148. Muller S, Chesner IM, Sheridan J, Newman J. Ulcerative colitis complicated by disseminated intravascular coagulation. Postgrad Med J 1987; 63: 689–91.

149. Ryan FP, Timperley WR, Preston FE, Holdsworth CD. Cerebral involvement with disseminated intravascular coagulation in intestinal disease. J Clin Pathol 1977; 30: 551–5.

150. Wong TZ, Welch JP, Holt JB. Intraoperative disseminated intravascular coagulation in a patient with ulcerative colitis. Connect Med 1989; 53: 577–8.

151. Zlatanic J, Korelitz BI, Wisch N *et al.* Inflammatory bowel disease and immune thrombocytopenic purpura: is there a correlation? Am J Gastroenterol 1997; 92: 2285–8.

152. Mones RL. Thrombocytopenia and hypofibrinogenemia in association with inflammatory bowel disease. J Pediatr Gastroenterol Nutr 1983; 2: 175–7.

153. Gremse DA, Bancroft J, Moyer MS. Sulfasalazine hypersensitivity with hepatotoxicity, thrombocytopenia, and erythroid hypoplasia. J Pediatr Gastroenterol Nutr 1989; 9: 261–3.

154. Caprilli R, Corrao G, Taddei G, Tonelli F, Torchio P, Viscido A. Prognostic factors for postoperative recurrence of Crohn's disease. Gruppo Italiano per lo Studio del Colon e del Retto (GISC). Dis Colon Rectum 1996; 39: 335–41.

155. Loftus EV, Jr., Tremaine WJ, Habermann TM, Harmsen WS, Zinsmeister AR, Sandborn WJ. Risk of lymphoma in inflammatory bowel disease. Am J Gastroenterol 2000; 95: 2308–12.

156. Connell WR, Kamm MA, Dickson M, Balkwill AM, Ritchie JK, Lennard-Jones JE. Long-term neoplasia risk after azathioprine treatment in inflammatory bowel disease. Lancet 1994; 343: 1249–52.

157. Caspi O, Polliack A, Klar R, Ben-Yehuda D. The association of inflammatory bowel disease and leukemia – coincidence or not? Leukemia Lymphoma 1995; 17: 255–62.

158. Georgescu L, Quinn GC, Schwartzman S, Paget SA. Lymphoma in patients with rheumatoid arthritis: association with the disease state or methotrexate treatment. Semin Arthritis Rheum 1997; 26: 794–804.

159. Greenstein AJ, Mullin GE, Strauchen JA *et al.* Lymphoma in inflammatory bowel disease. Cancer 1992; 69: 1119–23.

160. Palli D, Trallori G, Bagnoli S *et al.* Hodgkin's disease risk is increased in patients with ulcerative colitis. Gastroenterology 2000; 119: 647–53.

161. Korelitz BI, Mirsky FJ, Fleisher MR, Warman JI, Wisch N, Gleim GW. Malignant neoplasms subsequent to treatment of inflammatory bowel disease with 6-mercaptopurine. Am J Gastroenterol 1999; 94: 3248–53.

162. Present DH, Korelitz BI, Wisch N, Glass JL, Sachar DB, Pasternack BS. Treatment of Crohn's disease with 6-mercaptopurine. A long-term, randomized, double-blind study. N Engl J Med 1980; 302: 981–7.

163. Present DH, Meltzer SJ, Krumholz MP, Wolke A, Korelitz BI. 6-Mercaptopurine in the management of inflammatory bowel disease: short- and long-term toxicity. Ann Intern Med 1989; 111: 641–9.

164. Schabet M. Epidemiology of primary CNS lymphoma. J Neuro-Oncol 1999; 43: 199–201.

165. Lewis JD, Schwartz JS, Lichtenstein GR. Azathioprine for maintenance of remission in Crohn's disease: benefits outweigh the risk of lymphoma. Gastroenterology 2000; 118: 1018–24.

166. Bo J, Schroder H, Kristinsson J *et al.* Possible carcinogenic effect of 6-mercaptopurine on bone marrow stem cells: relation to thiopurine metabolism. Cancer 1999; 86: 1080–6.

167. Kwong YL, Au WY, Liang RH. Acute myeloid leukemia after azathioprine treatment for autoimmune diseases: association with –7/7q. Cancer Genet Cytogenet 1998; 104: 94–7.

168. Heizer WD, Peterson JL. Acute myeloblastic leukemia following prolonged treatment of Crohn's disease with 6-mercaptopurine. Dig Dis Sci 1998; 43: 1791–3.

169. DeMario MD, Liebowitz DN. Lymphomas in the immunocompromised patient. Semin Oncol 1998; 25: 492–502.

170. Nalesnik MA. Clinicopathologic features of posttransplant lymphoproliferative disorders. Ann Transplant 1997; 2: 33–40.

171. Kumar S, Fend F, Quintanilla-Martinez L *et al.* Epstein-Barr virus-positive primary gastrointestinal Hodgkin's disease: association with inflammatory bowel disease and immunosuppression. Am J Surg Pathol 2000; 24: 66–73.

172. Calaminici MR, Sheaff MT, Norton AJ, Feakins RM. Ileocaecal Epstein-Barr virus-positive lymphoproliferative disorder complicating Crohn's disease [Letter]. Histopathology 1999; 35: 388–90.

173. Larvol L, Soule JC, Le Tourneau A. Reversible lymphoma in the setting of azathioprine therapy for Crohn's disease [Letter]. N Engl J Med 1994; 331: 883–4.

174. Bickston SJ, Lichtenstein GR, Arseneau KO, Cohen RB, Cominelli F. The relationship between infliximab treatment and lymphoma in Crohn's disease. Gastroenterology 1999; 117: 1433–7.

175. Pardi DS, Tremaine WJ, Sandborn WJ, McCarthy JT. Renal and urologic complications of inflammatory bowel disease. Am J Gastroenterol 1998; 93: 504–14.

176. Kahn E, Markowitz J, Simpser E, Aiges H, Daum F. Amyloidosis in children with inflammatory bowel disease. J Pediatr Gastroenterol Nutr 1989; 8: 447–53.

177. Lowdell CP, Shousha S, Parkins RA. The incidence of amyloidosis complicating inflammatory bowel disease. A prospective survey of 177 patients. Dis Colon Rectum 1986; 29: 351–4.

178. Falk RH, Comenzo RL, Skinner M. The systemic amyloidoses. N Engl J Med 1997; 337: 898–909.

179. Gillmore JD, Hawkins PN, Pepys MB. Amyloidosis. A review of recent diagnostic and therapeutic developments. Br J Haematol 1997; 99: 245–56.

180. Lovat LB, Madhoo S, Pepys MB, Hawkins PN. Long-term survival in systemic amyloid A amyloidosis complicating Crohn's disease. Gastroenterology 1997; 112: 1362–5.

181. Edwards P, Cooper DA, Turner J, O'Connor TJ, Byrnes DJ. Resolution of amyloidosis (AA type) complicating chronic ulcerative colitis. Gastroenterology 1988; 95: 810–15.

182. Gertz MA, Kyle RA. Secondary systemic amyloidosis: response and survival in 64 patients. Medicine 1991; 70: 246–56.

183. Fausa O, Nygaard K, Elgjo K. Amyloidosis and Crohn's disease. Scand J Gastroenterol 1977; 12: 657–62.

184. Meyers S, Janowitz HD, Gumaste VV *et al.* Colchicine therapy of the renal amyloidosis of ulcerative colitis. Gastroenterology 1988; 94: 1503–7.

185. Menges M, Steffen HM. Secondary amyloidosis in ulcerative colitis – successful treatment with colchicine. Z Gastroenterol 1996; 34: 753–6.

186. Gertz MA, Kyle RA. Amyloidosis: prognosis and treatment. Semin Arthritis Rheum 1994; 24: 124–38.

187. Ravid M, Shapira J, Kedar I, Feigl D. Regression of amyloidosis secondary to granulomatous ileitis following surgical resection and colchicine administration. Acta Hepato-Gastroenterol 1979; 26: 513–5.

188. Larvol L, Cervoni J, Besnier M, Dupouet L, Beaufils H, Clauvel J, Levecq H. Reversible nephrotic syndrome in Crohn's disease complicated with renal amyloidosis. Gastroenterol Clin Biol 1998; 22: 639–41.

189. Horie Y, Chiba M, Miura K *et al.* Crohn's disease associated with renal amyloidosis successfully treated with an elemental diet. J Gastroenterol 1997; 32: 663–7.

190. Mandelstam P, Simmons DE, Mitchell B. Regression of amyloid in Crohn's disease after bowel resection. A 19-year follow-up. J Clin Gastroenterol 1989; 11: 324–6.

191. Iwakiri R, Sakemi T, Fujimoto K. Dimethylsulfoxide for renal dysfunction caused by systemic amyloidosis complicating Crohn's disease [Letter; comment]. Gastroenterology 1999; 117: 1031–2.

Section II

THE BEDSIDE

13 | Understanding symptoms and signs in inflammatory bowel disease

CORNELIUS C. CRONIN AND FERGUS SHANAHAN

Introduction

The natural history of Crohn's disease (CD) and ulcerative colitis (UC) is highly variable, but most typically follows a course of relapses and remissions. Some patients have chronically active disease with no or few apparent remissions. In some, the condition appears to 'burn out', and they enter long term remission. Series from specialized centers may tend to over-estimate clinical severity [1]. Generally, symptoms of UC tend to be uniform; most patients complain of abrupt onset passage of blood, diarrhea and weight loss. Each acute relapse typically has similar clinical features. Because of its greater anatomical distribution potentially involving any part of the gastrointestinal tract, its transmural distribution and its propensity to give raise to complications such as strictures and fistulae, CD shows greater variability between patients in clinical features. Also, as the disease evolves involving different parts of the gastrointestinal tract, the clinical features in any one patient may also change through time.

Symptoms and signs of inflammatory bowel disease (IBD) ultimately depend on the extent, distribution and severity of the gastrointestinal inflammation. Many of the clinical features of CD and UC are related to the anatomical location of disease. Abdominal colic is caused by intestinal strictures and diarrhea by intestinal inflammation. Other features such as anorexia, weight loss and malnutrition, anemia and constitutional features are largely due to the systemic consequences of intestinal inflammation. In recent years, the role of soluble mediators of intestinal inflammation in the pathogenesis of non-intestinal features of IBD has been appreciated. Cytokines are produced by many different tissues in response to immune stimulation and mediate a multiplicity of immunologic and non-immunologic functions [2, 3]. As well as local (auto-crine-paracrine) actions, cytokines have systemic (endocrine) effects, many mediated by the central nervous system [4, 5]. While the short-term, local effects of cytokines may be beneficial to the organism in the acute phase of an immune reaction, prolonged systemic cytokine activity as in IBD is often deleterious (Table 1) [6, 7].

Disease vs illness

There is an imperfect association between disease activity and patient disability. The objective assessment of disease activity often provides a poor guide to the subjective impact of the condition on the

Table 1. Adaptions associated with pro-inflammatory cytokines

Behavioral
  Anorexia
  Fatigue
  Malaise
  Altered sleep pattern
  Altered level of consciousness

Physiologic
  Elevated body temperture
  Increased resting energy expenditure
  Stress hormone response
  Skeletal muscle wasting
  Hepatic acute phase response
  Trace mineral sequestration
  Decreased gastric emptying, intestinal transit time
  Bone marrow suppression
  Diuresis

Nutritional
  Weight loss
  Negative nitrogen balance
  Hypoalbuminemia
  Hyperinsulinemia
  Hypertriglyceridemia
  Hypocholesterolemia

Adapted from ref. 7

Stephan R. Targan, Fergus Shanahan and Loren C. Karp (eds.), Inflammatory Bowel Disease: From Bench to Bedside, 2nd Edition, 253–267.
© 2003 *Kluwer Academic Publishers. Printed in Great Britain*

patient: disease does not equate with illness. The biomedical model – the notion that the disease activity determines the clinical outcome – had long been dominant in western medicine. The biopsychosocial model, as described by Engel [8] and further expanded in relation to chronic gastrointestinal disease by Drossman [9], proposes that illness and disease result from simultaneously interacting systems at the cellular, tissue, organism, interpersonal and environmental levels. This approach integrates biological science with the uniqueness of the individual, to determine the degree to which biological and psychosocial factors interact to explain the disease, illness and outcome. Patients with chronic gastrointestinal conditions may develop a variety of psychosociologic responses such as depression, decreased activities, increased illness behaviour, dependent relationships, and decreased responsibilities. Patients often have difficulties in employment, recreation and marital relations. The problems consequent on constitutional symptoms such as malaise and loss of energy may contribute more to patient disability than gastrointestinal symptoms. Illness, particularly that arising from chronic disease, is therefore best understood in terms of a multifactorial model, integrating biologic, psychologic and sociologic variables. Such a model facilitates and optimizes diagnosis, treatment and ultimately patient care. The aphorism 'treat the patient, not the disease' is particularly relevent in the long-term management of chronic IBD.

The unknown primary cause (or causes) of IBD and multiple secondary variables produce the heterogenous pathological and clinical manifestations of the illness. A representative list of such factors is shown in Table 2. The clinical features of IBD are numerous and varied. No symptom or sign exists in isolation. A single mechanism or etiopathogenesis rarely explains any one symptom or sign; nearly all are multifactorial. This chapter reviews aspects of the mechanisms, etiopathogenesis and clinical features of the major clinical features of IBD: abdominal pain, malnutrition and diarrhea.

Pain

Pain is a subjective experience that cannot be accounted for solely by consideration of disturbances in structure and function. The perception of pain involves interaction between pathophysiologic and psychosocial events. The primary pathophysio-

Table 2. A representative list of variables underlying clinical features in inflammatory bowel disease

Demographic factors: age, gender and age of onset

Distribution, extent and severity of inflammation

Disease 'activity' as evidenced by pain, diarrhea, anorexia etc

Anatomical complications such as abscesses, fistulas and obstruction, either mechanical or inflammatory, perianal disease

Nutritional status and related factors

Extraintestinal manifestations affecting the liver, joints, skin, eye etc

Presence of associated diseases

Iatrogenic factors, medical and surgical

Psychological, family and social factors

logic factor is the nature, intensity and extent of the stimulus that causes pain, but the perception of the painful stimulus is also dependent on the type and number of the receptor involved, on the organisation of the anatomical pathways transmitting the stimuli, and also on the complex role of modifying influences on the transmission, interpretation and reaction to the painful stimuli. Psychosocial factors are of particular importance in chronic conditions such as IBD and include the setting in which the pain occurs, personality factors, and family, ethnic and cultural background. All of these factors by influencing the *stoicism* of the patient affect the reaction to, and description of, pain and discomfort.

The goal of management in patients complaining of pain is to identify and treat the underlying cause. This however is often not possible in patients with chronic IBD. Although a multi-disciplinary approach is necessary to help the patient cope with the physical and psychologic manifestations of chronic pain, the central role in long-term management should be taken by a supportive, caring clinician with an unhurried approach. The propensity to addictive behaviour in IBD patients with chronic pain should not be underestimated.

In IBD, pain may arise from non-obstructed inflamed bowel, from bowel distension due to obstruction or from extension of the inflammatory process beyond the bowel wall, from perforation, fistula, or abscess. Temporal aspects, such as its frequency, tempo of onset, duration and its progress over time, often provide a guide to the pathological process causing the pain. Because of the greater extent of inflammation, its transmural distribution, the tendency for stricture formation and obstruction, and involvement of extraintestinal tissues, abdominal pain is more a feature of CD than UC. However, persistent or severe abdominal pain in patients with UC should alert the clinician to the possibility of the presence of complications such as fulminant colitis.

Intermittent, recurrent or chronic pain is a feature of most patients with CD. As a general rule, the degree of pain runs parallel to disease activity, although there are important exceptions. Pain may result from fibrous strictures in the absence of active inflammation. Frequently, irritable bowel syndrome-like symptoms of bloating, gaseous distension and sensation of incomplete evacuation after defecation are present. CD involving the upper gastrointestinal tract may cause odynophagia from esophageal involvement, or when the antrum and duodenum are involved, peptic ulcer disease-like symptoms. Typically, patients with CD of the iliocecal region have steady, mild-to-moderate discomfort in the right iliac fossa. A mass may be palpable. Peritoneal signs are absent. Often, there is superimposed colicky pain, referred to the umbilicus, due to obstruction, or in the absence of obstruction, from hyperalgesia. With bacterial overgrowth, bacterial metabolism of carbohydrate to hydrogen and carbon dioxide may cause abdominal pain from gaseous distension. When obstruction supervenes from either a stricture or from intra-luminal material impacting on a narrowed segment, the classical symptoms of post-prandial colicky cramps, often severe, with nausea and vomiting are found.

With colonic inflammation in either CD or UC, there may be crampy pain in the iliac fossae. Often, the patient has the sensation that bowel opening might provide relief; a similar sensation may be present with small bowel inflammation but is generally less urgent. Inflammation of the distal colon tends to cause tenesmus and pain in the lower back. Fulminant, diffuse abdominal pain with signs of peritoneal inflammation is suggestive of toxic megacolon. Pain and discomfort from perianal CD is mediated by somatic nerves and is sharply localized. Perianal pain usually implies the presence of sepsis.

The extrinsic innervation of the gastrointestinal tract is through the sympathetic and parasympathetic nerves [10, 11]. Although sensory information is carried by both spinal afferent (sympathetic) and vagal (parasympathetic) fibers, pain is mediated primarily by spinal afferents. Free nerve ending mediate both physiological and nociceptive inputs. In health, afferent activity in the gastrointestinal tract seldom reaches the level of consciousness.

In contrast to skin receptors which are highly specialized and complex structures, visceral receptors do not show any morphologic specialization and consist mainly of relatively simple free nerve endings. The abdominal viscera are relatively insensitive to stimuli, such as cutting, tearing and crushing that when applied to, for example, the skin would evoke severe pain. While stimuli from the skin may give raise to a variety of sensations, the only consciously perceived noxious sensation from the viscera is of pain or discomfort. While a range of appropriate and protective reflexes are available to respond to somatic pain, the repetoire of response to visceral pain is limited and generally ineffectual.

Among the stimuli that may give raise to pain in the abdominal viscera are irritation or ulceration of the mucosa or serosa, gross visceral distension, torsion or traction of the mesentery, and forceful contractions, especially when the lumen is obstructed. Receptors are located within the mucosa, submucosa and walls of hollow organs, on the serosal peritoneum and capsules of the solid organs, and in the mesentery. Free nerve endings respond to both mechanical and chemical stimuli.

The principal mechanical signal to which visceral nocioceptors respond is stretch. Tension receptors are in series with the smooth muscle of hollow organs. Pain results when intestinal smooth muscle undergoes a sufficient change in tension.

Pain receptors may be activated by chemical mediators generated or released during intestinal injury and inflammation, tissue hypoxia or necrosis. Mucosal receptors respond primarily to chemical stimuli. After local tissue injury, the release of inflammatory and chemical mediators such as prostaglandins and bradykinin can directly activate nerve endings, and also trigger the release from afferent nerves and other cells of algesic mediators such as histamine, 5-HT, nerve growth factor (NGF) and prostanoids [12, 13]. This assembly of chemicals sensitizes endings of afferent nerve terminals, resulting in an increased response to painful stimuli, and furthermore to a secondary sensitization of nearby nociceptors, in which neuromediators in the extracellular space, such as substance P, histamine, 5-HT and cytokines play a role. Substance P released from nerve endings in intimate contact with mast cells causes degranulation and further histamine release, in turn amplifying release of substance P and NGF. In chronic inflammation, nerve remodelling occurs, increasing nerve sensitivity and lowering the pain

Table 3. Embryologic origin of intestinal innervation

Intestinal structures	Embryologic origin	Spinal segments	Pain location
Distal esophagus, gastric, proximal duodenum	Foregut	T5-6 to T8-9	Epigastric
Small intestine, cecum, ascending and proximal transverse colon	Midgut	T8-11 to L1	Periumbilical
Distal transverse, descending and rectosigmoid colon	Hindgut	T11 to L1	Suprapubic

Adapted from ref. 10.

threshold. Pain may be mediated in part by smooth muscle contraction induced by these mediators.

Somatic structures are densely innervated, and somatic pain is distinct and precisely localized. In contrast, visceral pain is ill-defined and poorly localized. The greater part of the extensive enteric nervous system is involved in local physiological control of secretion, absorption and motility, and does not have a role in the mediation of pain perception. There is no separate visceral sensory pathway. Furthermore, there is a relative paucity of visceral afferent nerves that project to the central nervous system. Also, splanchnic nerves from a single tissue or organ enter the spinal cord through several levels, further diluting the accuracy of localisation. Most abdominal structures are embryologically midline, and receive bilateral and symmetrical innervation. Visceral pain generally localizes to the midline. Clearly lateralized pain arising from the abdominal viscera is usually from those few structures whose innervation is predominantly one-sided; or from structures with somatic rather than visceral innervation. The parietal peritoneum is innervated by somatic nerves, and when involved in the inflammatory process, pain is more precisely localized. In addition, between individuals, there is considerable variability of innervation, and therefore the same stimulus may be differently localized.

The tendency to perceive visceral abdominal pain at a different location from its origin further impairs accurate localisation of visceral pain. In this phenomenon of referred pain, pain is perceived in the skin dermatomes whose afferent nerve roots enter the same levels of the spinal cord as the involved abdominal structure. There are no separate pathways within the spinal cord for visceral and somatic pain. Because somatic afferents are more numerous, the brain tends to associate activation of the second order neurones with a somatic source, irrespective of its origin.

The embryologic origin of abdominal tissues and organs provides a general guide to the localization of gastrointestinal pain [10] (Table 3). Pain arising from foregut structures is generally perceived in the epigastrium, from midgut structures in the periumbilical region, and from the hindgut, suprapubically.

Malnutrition

Malnutrition is common in patients with IBD (Table 4) [14, 15]. Nutritional deficiencies are related to the extent and the activity of disease. Because of small bowel involvement, malnutrition tends to be more common in patients with CD. Many of the studies assessing malnutrition have been in hospitalized patients or in those attending specialized clinics, which may tend to overstate its frequency and severity. In addition, with improved medical and surgical treatment and with the appropriate emphasis on ensuring adequate nutrition in patients with IBD, the prevalence of serious malnutrition may have declined in recent years. Nonetheless, malnutrition remains a major problem in those with IBD, particularly in pediatric patients, and is a major contributer to poor quality of life, morbidity and mortality.

Malnutrition in patients with IBD is multifactorial (Table 5). Several mechanisms may be involved in any one patient, chief among which however in most patients is curtailment of caloric intake due to any combination of anorexia, nausea, post-prandial abdominal pain and vomiting, and dietary restrictions [16]. The importance of poor caloric intake as a cause of weight loss is best illustrated by the sometimes dramatic effect supplemental enteral feeding has on reduced weight in children with IBD [17–19]. Maldigestion and malabsorption of ingested nutrients is likely to be a factor only in those with extensive and chronically active CD or in those who have had major small bowel excisional surgery.

Table 4. Incidence of malnutrition in patients with Crohn's disease

Feature	Percentage
Weight loss	40–80
Growth failure in children	15–88
Muscle wasting	59
Fat depletion	15–30
Hypoalbuminemia	25–76
Iron deficiency	25–50
B_{12} deficiency	20–37
Folate deficiency	13–37
Hypokalemia	33
Hyponatremia	10
Hypomagnesemia	14–88
Zinc deficiency	40
Fat soluble vitamins:	
D	75
K	30–50
A	21
Clinical osteomalacia	36

Adapted from ref. 15.

Table 5. Causes of malnutrition in patients with Crohn's disease

Inadequate intake	Nausea
	Anorexia
	Fear of pain after food
	Fear of diarrhea after food
	Restrictive diets
Malabsorption	Loss of absorptive mucosa (disease/ surgery)
	Stagnant loops/bacterial overgrowth
	Bile salt deficiency after ileal resection
	Rapid GI transit – mucosal disease/ fistulas
	Lymphangiectasia
Increased requirements/ decreased synthesis	Active inflammation
	Increased cell turnover
	Sepsis
Enteric loss of nutrients	Protein-losing enteropathy
	Interrupted enterohepatic circulation
	Gastrointestinal blood loss
	Electrolyte, mineral loss in diarrhea
Drugs	Sulfasalazine
	Corticosteroids
	Cholestyramine
	Immunosuppressives

Inadequate caloric intake

Postprandial symptoms may occasionally be a disincentive to the maintenance of adequate nutritional intake in patients with IBD, particularly the fear of diarrhea or, in patients with stricturing disease, of colicky abdominal pain. Many of the drugs used in the treatment of IBD may themselves cause nausea or anorexia. The use of any nutritionally restrictive dietary therapy is now outmoded. However, the major cause of poor caloric intake is inflammation-related anorexia and loss of appetite. Weight loss often predates the clinical onset of CD and in children, decreased growth velocity precedes diagnosis [20]. Not infrequently, anorexia and weight loss is the predominant initial feature in IBD. Anorexia, particularly in young patients, may occasionally be wrongly attributed to anorexia nervosa. Rapid weight loss is a feature of intra-abdominal sepsis, which may be occult or, less comonly, of intra-abdominal neoplasia.

Physiology of appetite and hunger

Anorexia is the diminution or absence of hunger and appetite. Hunger and appetite both refer to the desire to eat, but whereas the determinants of hunger are related to physiological mechanisms present at a given time, appetite is in addition influenced by ongoing pathophysiological, psychological and environmental processes. Satiety is the gratification of hunger and appetite.

The drive to eat is basic and essential to survival. Its control is complex, multifactorial and ill-understood. The generally accepted working model proposes that eating is regulated by a central feeding drive that is held in check during feeding by a peripheral satiety system. Various gastrointestinal, endocrine/metabolic and neurological stimuli are perceived by peripheral and central receptors and, centrally integrated, ultimately produce the sensations of hunger and satiety, and determine eating behaviour. The hypothalamus plays a key role in interpreting and integrating these signals [21]. From animal experiments, the lateral nucleus of the hypothalamus has been proposed as a center for hunger, and the ventromedial nucleus a center for satiety. Whether such concepts of anatomical centers are applicable to humans is unclear; appetite regulation may be more appropriately viewed as the hypothalmic integration of neurotransmitter-mediated neuropharmacologic systems with opposing effects on hunger/appetite and on satiety.

Many peptides and neurotransmitters acting centrally and peripherally have been proposed as candidates for control of food intake (Table 6) [22–24]. Dopaminergic tracts appear to be vital in initiating feeding, and norepinephric systems and neuropeptide Y (NPY) and peptide YY also promote feeding. NPY, a 36 amino acid peptide is the most potent orexigenic peptide in the hypothalamus, and appears to be of fundamental importance in the regulation of energy homeostasis [25]. Most anorectic peptides exert their effects through interruption of NPY release or action. Among the satiety factors acting on the hypothalamus, serotonin (5-hydroxytryptamine [5-HT]) plays a central role [26]. Most of the clinically available drugs affecting appetite act on serotonin [27]. Injection of serotonin into specific areas of the hypothalamus inhibits feeding in a variety of species. Plasma free tryptophan is the precursor of serotonin, and tryptophan availability parallels synthesis and release of brain serotonin. Carbohydrate ingestion increases circulating tryptophan, mediated in part by insulin. The consequent increased post-prandial brain serotonin levels is a proposed mechanism by which the macronutrient content of a meal is sensed by the brain, promoting satiety. Other proposed appetite-inhibiting neuropeptides are cholecystokinin, corticotrophin-releasing peptide (CRP), calcitonin gene-related peptide and neurotensin.

Several peripheral factors influence appetite, hunger and satiety [22], including the composition of food and not least taste and smell (palatability). Gastric distension is an obvious and important satiety signal, mediated by neural (vagal) and humoral (bombesin) signals, and explains why bulky meals give rise to greater satiety than meals of refined carbohydrates of equal caloric value. Intestinal cholecystokinin (CCK) by sensing intestinal nutrient concentration and the volume and rate of luminal emptying may be an important peripheral regulator of satiety [24]; CCK causes pyloric contraction with resultant gastric distension and binds to the gastric afferent vagus which ultimately courses to the ventromedial hypothalamus. Peripherally released CCK may also exert a central satiety effect. Meal size is reduced by exogenously administered CCK at physiological concentrations, and is increased by specific CCK antagonists, implying that meal size may be physiologically limited by these factors [28, 29]. Ingestion of food presents a large antigen load to the intestine. The substantial amounts of cytokines that are produced in response may also play a role in the control of feeding.

Although these complex neuroendocrine signals may provide a basis for an understanding of how feeding is initiated and terminated, they do not explain how most individuals maintain a stable body weight over long periods of time. The lipostat model hypthesized that signals proportional to the size of body fat stores become integrated with other regulators of food intake [30]. How the size of body fat stores might influence appetite and hunger has been at least in part recently elucidated. Leptin, the protein product of the obese (*ob*) gene, is secreted into the circulation by adipose cells [31]. A rising circulating leptin (from the Greek *leptos*, meaning thin) concentration with increasing adiposity is proposed to serve as a negative feedback signal to the hypothalamus. Mice with a mutated *ob* gene (*ob/ob* mouse) lack functional leptin and develop extreme

Table 6. Neurotransmitters affecting appetite and satiety

Stimulatory
 Norepinephrine
 GABA
 Neuropeptide Y
 Opiods
 Galanin
 Growth-hormone-releasing factor
 Melanin concentrating hormone
 Orexin a and b
 CART

Inhibitory
 5-HT
 Dopamine
 Histamine
 α-Melanocyte-stimulating hormone
 Glucagon-like peptide 1
 Agouti-related protein
 Neurotensin
 Cholecystokinin
 Bombesin
 Calcitonin-gene related peptide
 Amylin
 Adrenomedullin
 Glucagon
 Oxytocin
 Anorectin
 Thyrotropin-releasing hormone
 Pituitary adenylate-cyclase activating polypeptide
 Acidic fibroblast growth factor
 Interleukin 1
 Leptin

obesity at a young age [32]. In humans, plasma leptin concentrations closely correlate with adipose mass. It is proposed that starvation results in a reduction in fat mass and a fall in circulating leptin, promoting appetite and food seeking behaviour, and conversely increasing obesity increases plasma leptin concentration, which acts as a negative signal on the hypothalamus, decreasing appetite. The action of leptin on appetite is independent of its numerous other actions [33]. Insulin as a regulator of adipose tissue mass has many similarities with leptin, including a concentration proportional to adipose tissue mass and receptors in the same key hypothalmic areas. Both when centrally administered reduce food intake and body weight, without producing symptoms of malaise. The hypothalamic effects of leptin and insulin are mediated by a variety of neuropeptides: those that promote feeding and body energy stores include neuropeptide Y and melanin-concentrating hormone, and those that suppress feeding include corticotrophin-releasing factor, the α-melanocyte-stimulating hormone/melanocortin-4 receptor and the cocaine-amphetamine-regulated transcript [34, 35].

The control of feeding is complex, and has variously been described as multiple overlapping systems, each of which may be employed differently under differing circumstances, or as a cascade with the emphasis on driving feeding modulated by a regulatory feedback signals promoting satiety. There may be separate short-term (5HT) and long-term (leptin) satiety signalling systems [36]. Both modulate the action of NPY, which may function as a common output pathway for the expression of appetite [34].

Anorexia of chronic disease

Anorexia accompanies many forms of chronic disease whether due to infection, inflammation, neoplasia or tissue injury. The presence of continuing anorexia despite weight loss implies a failure of the normal compensatory mechanisms which operate after a period of reduced feeding. Increasingly, the anorexia and weight loss of such conditions are attributed to the actions of increased secretion of proinflammatory cytokines [37].

A variety of cytokines inhibits feeding after central or peripheral administration, but IL-1 and TNF-α have the most profound effects. Administration of TNF and IL-1 induces anorexia and weight loss in experimental animals and in humans [38]. The anor-

ectic effect is specific as it is blocked by receptor antagonists or by specific antibodies, and is independent of other systemic effects of these cytokines. Cytokines appear to act by causing a reduction in the body weight set-point, which is then maintained by reduced feeding.

In chronic disease, cytokines are produced mainly in the periphery. To inhibit feeding, cytokines or signals derived from their peripheral actions must influence central mechanisms affecting appetite [38]. Cytokine-mediated visceral afferent nerve activity contributes but is not essential to their action as their effects are not abolished by experimental nerve section experiments [38]. Cytokines increase cholecystokinin and leptin release and activity [39, 40]. Circulating cytokines may also be taken up by the central nervous system – cytokines increase blood brain barrier permeability [4]. In addition, there may be increased *de novo* brain cytokine synthesis [41]. Cytokines have a direct effect on glucose sensitive neurons in the lateral hypothalamus; IL-1 increases central seratonergic activity and other appetite suppressant transmitters such as CRF, histamine and α-MSH and reduces NPY mRNA levels, all features that promote satiety [42].

Anorexia of IBD

Anorexia is the dominant cause of poor nutritional intake and of malnutrition in IBD. The elucidation of the mechanisms is in the early stages of investigation. Most studies thus far have been in experimental models. Classical early experiments showed that the induction of experimental acute colitis by intrarectal administration of trinitrobenzene sulfonic acid (TNBS) causes a 70–80% reduction in food intake, both solid and liquid, during the first three days, which, as the inflammation recedes, reverses within a week [43]. Water consumption and meal frequency are unchanged, but the amount consumed at each meal is reduced, implying that the reduction in intake depends on satiety signals in the brain, and are not due to a state of general malaise.

It is likely that in experimental colitis that alterations in multiple pathways regulating food intake are altered. Increased IL-1 activity may play a pivotal role. The pattern of anorexia with TNBS colitis is similar to that of long-term IL-1 administration; intestinal IL-1 concentrations peak when anorexia is maximal; and administration of IL-1 receptor antagonists significantly attenuates anorexia and weight loss [44]. Immediately after induction of experimental colitis, reduced food intake is associated with hypothalamic IL-1 receptor activation and increases in prostaglandin synthesis. Serotonin release, a potent inhibitor of feeding, from the hypothalamus is stimulated by IL-1. The peak phase of anorexia induced by TNBS-colitis is associated with increased hypothalmic serotonin release, but again serotonin antagonism has only a partial effect on reversal of anorexia [45], suggesting that other factors are also important.

It has been proposed as a mechanism of anorexia and weight loss in chronic IBD that proinflammatory cytokines cause the release of leptin from adipose tissue, giving inappropriately high plasma concentrations for the percentage fat mass. In both animals and human subjects, a number of cytokines, especially tumor necrosis factor (initially termed cachexin), has been shown to increase leptin concentrations [40]. Animal experiments using a variety of methods to induce intestinal inflammation suggest that cytokine-mediated increased circulating leptin during the initial phase of inflammation contributes to the suppression of feeding, and that subsequently as leptin concentration falls, there is an associated and appropriate increase in feeding [46].

There are numerous differences between spontaneously occurring IBD in humans and experimentally induced intestinal inflammation in rodents, including the extent, severity and chronicity of the induced inflammation. Experimental findings in animal models may have limited relevance to human disease. In human IBD, plasma leptin concentration is similar in both patients with active disease and in remission as in control subjects; increased plasma concentrations of soluble TNF-receptor, a marker of intestinal inflammation, are not correlated with plasma leptin [47, 48]. While not excluding a role for disturbed leptin physiology in the causation of intestinal inflammation-related anorexia [35], such mechanisms do not appear to play a similar role in human as in experimental intestinal inflammation.

The study of anorexia and satiety in chronic disease is in its infancy. The unravelling of the mechanisms of anorexia in human disease holds the promise of attenuation or amelioration of the malnutrition associated with chronic IBD, with all its attendent benefits.

Malabsorption

Malabsorption occurs if mucosal inflammation or resection involves a sufficent length of small bowel,

from the combined effects of lack of sufficient absorptive surface, decreased transit time and diminution of the bile salt pool. Less commonly, other mechanisms may be involved, all a consequence of complications of intestinal inflammation.

Each of the three major nutrients – carbohydrate, protein and fat – may be malabsorbed, but clinical symptoms are primarily due to fat malabsorption. In general, malabsorption of carbohydrate and of protein is uncommon and as a factor in decreased energy availability plays only a secondary role to reduced intake. Jejunal function as measured by d-xylose absorption is preserved in most patients, except in patients with extensive small bowel CD [18]. The prevalence of lactose malabsorption is probably not increased in patients with IBD. Albumin concentration, often used as a marker of protein status, may be further reduced from intestinal protein loss, reduced hepatic albumin synthesis, malabsorption and anorexia.

Fat malabsorption occurs in approximately 30% of patients with CD [15]. The most severe steatorrhea and the greatest malnutrition occurs in those with extensive jejunal disease or resection. Normally, because of its large reserve, up to 50% of the small bowel can be resected without serious impairment of nutrition [49]. In CD, however, much of the bowel may be already diseased so that resection of, or extension of inflammation to, even short lengths may be poorly tolerated. Because the small bowel is shorter in women, they may be more prone to develop such problems. Extensive jejunoileal disease or resection is always associated with malabsorption of fluid, electrolyte, calorie and protein intake, whereas an isolated ileal or jejunal disease resection in isolation may be better tolerated.

Transit time through the small bowel is reduced by disease or resection and may occasionally be further compromised by the presence of fistulae, reducing the time available for nutrient absorption.

Bile acids are absorbed in the ileum. If the length of functioning ileum is so compromised that inadequate amounts are reabsorbed, hepatic synthesis may be unable to compensate for bile salt loss. If the concentration of conjugated bile acids falls below the micellar concentration critical for fat absorption, steatorrhoea supervenes.

Other mechanisms may be involved in malabsorption. Small bowel bacterial overgrowth is a syndrome characterized by nutrient malabsorption associated with excessive numbers of bacteria in the small intestine [50]. Small intestinal peristalsis has the major role in preventing bacterial overgrowth. The most common cause of bacterial overgrowth in IBD is stasis from small intestinal strictures. Seedling of colonic bacteria and colonization of the small intestine is further facilitated by resection of the iliocecal valve, and less commonly, by fistulous tracts between the large and small intestines. Other potential factors that may promote bacterial overgrowth are advanced age, hypochlorhydria from gastric atrophy or from surgical resection, drugs, and relative immunodeficiency from malnutrition or drug therapy. Bacterial deconjugation of bile acids is the primary mechanism of fat malabsorption in bacterial overgrowth. In florid cases, malabsorption of fat soluble vitamins A, D and E may occur. Generally, such patients are protected from the coagulopathy of vitamin K deficiency by bacterial vitamin synthesis. Bacterial overgrowth results in carbohydrate malabsorption from reduction of brush border disacharidases and decreased uptake of monosaccharides. Hypoproteinemia is common, arising from a number of mechanisms: bacteria compete for protein substrates; bacteria may induce mucosal injury; and decreased intestinal enzyme activity. Vitamin B_{12} deficiency is a chacteristic finding in bacterial overgrowth. Also, patients with bacterial overgrowth may curtail their nutrient intake to minimize postprandial symptoms from gaseous distension.

Protein losing enteropathy may contribute to malnutrition in patients with IBD. Enteric loss of plasma proteins is normally of minor importance in the metabolism of body proteins. Once plasma proteins pass from the circulation into the gastrointestinal tract, they are degraded in the same manner as orally ingested protein into their constituent amino acids and absorbed. Three mechanisms underlie increased intestinal nutrient loss in IBD: increased mucosal permeability; mucosal erosions or ulceration; and lymphatic obstruction. When excessive amounts of proteins are lost into the gastrointestinal tract, synthetic capacity may not compensate. A new steady state is achieved, characterized by hypoproteinemia, in which the daily losses are balanced by synthesis. Such protein depletion primarily affects proteins with a low turnover rate, with consequent hypoalbuminemia and decreased levels of immunoglobulins, fibrinogen, caeruloplasmin and transferrin. Except for dependent edema, these subnormal protein concentrations infrequently have clinical consequences. Iron, trace elements and lipids may also be lost. If lymphatic obstruction is the major mechanism in the pathogenesis of protein losing enteropathy, as it may be in CD, lymphocytopenia develops.

Growth retardation

Growth retardation represents a specific form of malnutrition in children and adolescents with IBD, particularly in those with CD. Decreased growth velocity often precedes diagnosis [20]. Growth retardation is the presenting symptom in up to a third of young patients with IBD [51] and many others subsequently develop impaired growth. Studies using a variety of definitions of growth impairment based on height for age percentiles have reported frequencies of impaired growth during childhood and adolescence ranging from 13% to 58% in CD patients and from 3% to 21% for UC [52]. Growth retardation may be associated with permanent stunting; as many as 50% of young adults with childhood onset IBD have height percentiles on or less than the 10th percentile [53]. An attendant problem is delayed menarche and lack of development of secondary sexual characteristics.

The final common pathway for growth is the epiphyseal growth plate of long bones. The increase in length of bone is determined by a complex interplay between chondrocyte proliferation, maturation and hypertrophy and matrix synthesis and degradation. Among the factors that may interfere with the process of growth in youngsters with IBD are malnutrition, inflammation and the effects of treatment, particularly corticosteroids [52, 54].

Growth failure in pediatric IBD is primarily due to inadequate caloric intake: estimates of caloric intake have been repeatedly recorded to be between 50% and 75% of recommendations [17]. Rapid and significant height and weight gain have been shown in these patients when they receive oral or enteral caloric supplementation [17–19]. However, optimal growth is not always attained, suggesting factors other than nutritional deprivation may be involved. Maldigestion and malabsorption play a less significant role except in those who have had extensive small bowel inflammation or resection. Zinc deficiency may be associated with growth retardation and delayed bone age in children [55], and has been proposed as a mediator of growth failure with IBD. Zinc deficiency has been documented in some children with IBD and growth retardation [56, 57], arising from malabsorption or from excessive stool losses. There are however no reports of zinc supplementation reversing growth retardation in children with IBD.

As in the human form, growth retardation is a feature of experimental IBD. However, even when adequate nutritional supplementation is administered, animals with experimental colitis do not achieve optimal growth. It has been estimated that up to 40% of growth retardation in experimental colitis may be attributable to the effects, direct or indirect, of inflammation [58], many mediated by cytokines.

A prerequisite for normal linear growth is a functioning growth hormone/insulin-like growth factor-1 axis. Pituitary growth hormone stimulates production of insulin-like growth factor-1 (IGF-1) from the liver, from which most of the circulating IGF-1 is derived, which in turn acts on the epiphyseal growth plate. Young patients with chronic inflammatory states associated with growth retardation (including IBD) have normal growth hormone secretion but suppressed plasma IGF-1 concentrations [59–61]. In animal models of intestinal inflammation, exogenous administration of IGF-1 significantly attenuates growth retardation [58]. The deleterious effects of proinflammatory cytokines on growth may be mediated through interruption of the growth hormone/IGF-1 axis. Transgenic mice overexpressing either IL-1 or TNF have growth retardation [62–64]. Excessive IL-6 activity either by genetic manipulation or by exogenous administration [62] is associated with normal growth hormone levels and with suppression of IGF-1 concentrations, the same pattern as in pediatric IBD. Administration of TNF and IL-1β inhibits IGF-1 production from rat hepatocytes [65]. Immunoneutralization of IL-6 in animal models of intestinal inflammation increases both IGF-1 concentrations and linear growth [58]. In addition to the indirect endocrine-mediated effects of cytokines on bone growth, cytokines may have direct negative effects on the epiphyseal growth plate [64]. Since nutritional supplementation does not fully reverse growth retardation in children with IBD, it may that the achievement of optimal growth may be obtained only by both adequate nutritional and anti-inflammatory therapy.

Corticosteroids used in supraphysiological dosages retard growth in children with a variety of conditions [66]. The use of high dosage steroid therapy is closely linked to disease and inflammatory activity, and it is difficult to separate the effect of one from the other. Dose, type and timing of glucocorticoid exposure each influence the degree of growth

suppression observed. Pre-pubertal children exposed to glucocorticoids may be particularly susceptible.66 Resumption of growth follows discontinution of steroid therapy. However, chronic use of glucocorticoids has a significant effect on final height attained. The pathogenesis of growth suppression by glucocorticoids is complex and multifactorial, involving several steps in the cascade of events leading to linear growth at the epiphyseal growth plate, including the growth hormone/IGF-1 axis [67, 68]. Precisely which effects are most responsible for growth suppression remains unclear (Table 7).

Table 7. Effects of glucocorticoids on linear growth

On bone
> Interfere with the nitrogen and mineral retention required for the growth process
> Inhibition of chondrocyte mitosis
> Inhibition of collagen synthesis
> Inhibition of osteoclastic activity

On calcium metabolism
> Decrease intestinal calcium absorption
> Increase urinary calcium excretion
> Secondary hyperparathyroidism

On endocrine function
> Antagonism of growth hormone
> Reduces growth hormone receptor expression
> Reduces plasma growth hormone-binding protein
> Suppression of IGF-1 activity
> Suppression of sex steroid secretion

Diarrhea

Normal stool frequency varies from between three times a day to three times a week, with formed consistency and a volume of about 100 ml per day. Patients tend to report any increase in their usual frequency, fluidity or volume as diarrhea. Diarrhea is formally defined as an increase in daily stool weight to above 200 g per day. It is important that when a complaint of diarrhea is made that the patient is questioned and the symptom analysed. Diarrhea must be distinguished from hyperdefecation, from urgency and from fecal incontinence. Alterations from the usual bowel habit that are reported as diarrhea but do not fulfill formal diagnostic criteria are still worthy of evaluation and assessment.

The cardinal symptom of IBD and nearly always present in those with active disease, diarrhea varies from being a nuisance to being life-threatening. Diarrhea is related to the severity and extent of intestinal inflammation, and may be used as a marker of activity.

Ulcerative colitis severe enough to cause diarrhea almost always contains blood. If blood is absent, another diagnosis is likely. Patients with colitis typically complain of frequent, small volume stools. If inflammation is confined to the rectum, fresh blood, or blood on the surface of often otherwise normal appearing stool, or blood stained mucus may be passed. Urgency, tenesmus and a sensation of incomplete evacuation are common, and incontinence may occur. Occasional patients with proctitis may complain of constipation. With more extensive colitis, diarrhea is grossly bloody, with pus and fecal matter, sometimes likened to anchovy sauce. Passing clots is unusual and suggests another diagnosis.

Patterns of diarrhea vary in CD, depending on the anatomical distribution. With colonic or rectal involvement, symptoms are similar to those of UC involving the same areas. In disease confined to the small intestine, stools are larger in volume and are not generally associated with tenesmus and urgency and are free of blood. If steatorrhea is present, stools are typically greasy, pale, malodorous and difficult to flush away.

Fluidity of the intestinal contents is essential for digestion, for diffusion of digested nutrients to the absorptive epithelial surface, and for absorption itself. Being critical for a variety of processes, the amount of water in the intestine is closely regulated. The daily intestinal fluid load approximates to 9000 ml. Oral intake is generally about 2000 ml, with saliva, gastric juice, bile, and pancreatic and intestinal secretion accounting for the remainder (Table 8). Of the 9000 ml that enters the duodenum every day, about 7000 ml is absorbed in the small intestine, with 1500–2000 ml reaching the iliocaecal valve. Most of this volume is then reabsorbed in the colon, with the daily stool containing about 100 ml of water [69] (Table 9). The absorptive capacity of the normal small bowel has not been defined, but presumably is considerably greater than the 7000 ml absorbed on average every day. Under experimental conditions, the normal colon has an absorptive capacity of up to 5000 ml per day, but under real life conditions is probably less.

The intestine has a tremendous capacity for both water secretion and absorption. Diarrhea is ulti-

Table 8. Daily fluid load entering duodenum

Origin	ml/24 h
Oral intake	2000
Saliva	1500
Gastric juice	2500
Bile	500
Pancreatic juice	1500
Intestinal secretion	1000
Total	9000

Table 9. Intestinal water and electrolyte distribution

	Water (ml/24 h)	Na (mmol/24 h)	K (mmol/24 h)	Cl (mmol/24 h)
Entering duodenum	80–10 000	800	100	700
Entering colon	1500	200	10	100
Stool	100	3	8	2

Adapted from ref. 69.

mately an expression of deranged intestinal water regulation and may result from increased secretion or reduced absorption or both, originating in either the small or large intestine or both. If small intestinal function is deranged so that its absorptive capacity is reduced, the volume of fluid presented to the colon may exceed that organ's reabsorptive capacity. If the function of the colon is deranged so that it cannot absorb the normal load of 2000 ml presented to it every day, diarrhea will also result. The intestines also have a great potential for secretion of fluid, and abnormal secretion in either the small or large intestine, by overwhelming absorptive capacity, will also result in diarrhea. More commonly in IBD, both functions of the bowel are impaired, and diarrhea results from a combination of impaired absorption and increased secretion, each defect amplifying the effect of the other.

The intestinal epithelium is composed of a single layer of columnar cells, serving as a barrier, absorbing water, electrolytes, and nutrients and secreting water and electrolytes [70]. By convolutions of folds, villi and microvilli, the small intestine has a surface area of greater than 200 m^2, with a tremendous reserve for both absorption and secretion. Water moves passively to maintain isoosmolarity between lumen and tissue. Electrolytes are actively transported, and their movement plays a pivotal role in water regulation. Absorptive and secretory functions are regulated by both intracellular and intercellular mechanisms by an array of endogenous and exogenous factors. Small intracellular molecules act as second messengers, which by controlling the activity of protein kinases, regulate activity of various transport pathways. Intercellular regulatory mechanisms include hormones from endocrine cells, neurotransmitters from nerve cells and mediators released by immune cells [70].

Table 10. Inflammation and diarrhea in inflammatory bowel disease

Decreased absorption of water and electrolytes:
  Reduced surface area – mucosal injury/resection
  Neural/hormonal inhibition of NaCl absorption
  Rapid intestinal transit – increased motor activity
  Increased osmolar load from nutrient malabsorption

Increased secretion of water and electrolytes:
  Inflammation-derived secretagogues
  Loss of mucosal barrier function
  Denuded mucosa leaking plasma and blood

Table 11. Representative list of intestinal absorptive and secretory stimuli

	Absorptive stimuli	Secretory stimuli
Endogenous	α-Adrenergic agonists Dopamine Enkephalins and other opioids Somatostatin Glucocorticoids Angiotensin Peptide YY Neuropeptide Y Prolactin	Acetylcholine Histamine 5-Hydroxytryptamine Substance P Cholecystokinin Prostaglandins Bradykinin Vasoactive intestinal polypeptide Secretin Adenosine Gastrin Motilin
Exogenous	Nutrients: glucose, amino acids	Bacterial enterotoxins Bile salts

Adapted from ref. 70.

Table 12. Causes and mechanisms of diarrhea in inflammatory bowel disease

Consideration	Mechanism	Treatment
Bacterial overgrowth	Deconjugation	Antibiotics
Bile acid diarrhea	Secretion	Cholestyramine
Bile acid deficiency	Steatorrhea	Low fat diet
Lactase deficiency	Osmotic	Avoid lactose
Short bowel	Malabsorption	Low fat diet
Internal fistula	Bypass	Surgery
Antibiotic related	*C. difficile*	Stop antibiotics

Diarrhea in IBD

The physiology of fluid and electrolyte transport in the healthy individual is complex and the relative importance of the various regulatory processes is unclear. When diarrhea results from intestinal inflammation, complexity is increased by an order of magnitude. Diarrhea may be related to the inflammatory process or to specific complications, usually the consequence of inflammation. Pathogenetic processes vary from patient to patient and several mechanisms may be operative in the individual patient.

Inflammation-related diarrhea

Inflammation in the intestinal tract may give raise to diarrhea by inhibiting absorption and/or increasing secretion (Table 10). Loss of absorptive surface area is the major factor in diarrhea in IBD. Diarrhea results when mucosal injury or resection is such that the absorptive capacity of the intestine is diminished or overwhelmed. A major mechanism is inhibition of electrolyte and water absorption by the products of immune and inflammatory processes, mediated by direct effects on enterocytes and by indirect effects on cellular elements in the lamina propria. Immune and inflammatory mediators initiate a cascade of biochemical events that inhibit absorption of sodium and chloride. Inhibition of absorption may also occur in areas where mucosal integrity and structure appear to be intact. In CD, if there is extensive small bowel involvement, malabsorbed and maldigested nutrients increase the osmolarity of the intestinal fluid, exacerbating diarrhea through an osmotic process. Rapid intestinal transit decreases the time available for absorption to occur.

Increased anion secretion is the other major cause of diarrhea in IBD. An ever increasing list of immune and inflammatory mediators have a role in increasing intestinal secretion [70] (Table 11). These mediators directly affect the epithelium, but also stimulate the enteric nervous system. Diarrhea is exacerbated by exudation of plasma-like fluid and blood from denuded epithelium.

Mechanisms other than inflammation-related

Indirect consequences of inflammation may give rise to diarrhea (Table 12). Conjugated bile acids are required for efficient digestion and absorption of dietary fat. Bile acids are actively reabsorbed in the terminal ileum and the bile acid pool is recirculated six times each day – the enterohepatic circulation. In patients with terminal ileal disease or resection, dihydroxy bile salts are not fully absorbed. If a sufficient concentration reaches the colon, net fluid and electrolyte secretion occurs through multiple mechanisms and watery diarrhea ensues. If there is more extensive terminal ileal inflammation or resection (> 100 cm), bile salt loss may be such that hepatic synthesis cannot compensate; bile salt concentration falls below the level critical for adequate fat absorption and steatorrhea ensues.

Bacterial overgrowth may, as outlined above, contribute to malabsorption and weight loss in CD. Diarrhea results through several mechanisms. Bacterial deconjugation of bile acids and consequent malabsorption of fat is the primary mechanism of diarrhea and steatorrhea. Also, bacterial metabolites may have a toxic effect on the small bowel mucosa, acting as secretagogues. Bacterial overgrowth reduces brush border disaccharidases and the increased delivery of osmotically active carbohydrate fragments to the small intestine further exacerbates diarrhea.

In patients with extensive small bowel resection, diarrhea develops as part of the short bowel syndrome. The major mechanism is loss of absorptive surface leading to malabsorption of water, electrolytes and nutrients. Several other factors may be involved: decreased transit time; an osmotic induced diarrhea due to malabsorption of lactose and other carbohydrates; concomitant bacterial overgrowth; and bile acid induced diarrhea from ileal resection. That the diarrhea persists when fasting implies a secretory component, possibly due to absence of signals from the distal small bowel that inhibit proximal intestinal secretion.

References

1. Munkholm P, Langholz E, Davidsen M, Binder V. Disease activity courses in a regional cohort of Crohn's disease patients. Scand J Gastroenterol 1995; 30: 699–706.
2. Curfs JH, Meis JF, Hoogkamf-Korstanje JA. A primer on cytokines: sources, receptors, effects and inducers. Clin Microbiol Rev 1997; 10: 742–80.
3. Lucey DR, Clerici M, Shearer GM. Type 1 and type 2 cytokine dysregulation in human infectious, neoplastic and inflammatory diseases. Clin Microbiol Rev 1996; 9: 532–62.
4. Rivest S, Lacroix S, Vallieres L, Nadeau S, Zhang J, Laflamme N. How the blood talks to the brain parenchyma and the paraventricular nucleus of the hypothalamus during systemic inflammatory and infectious stimuli. Proc Soc Exp Biol Med 2000; 223: 22–38.

5. Faggioni R, Benigni F, Ghezzi P. Proinflammatory cytokines as pathogenetic mediators in the central nervous system: brain-periphery connections. Neuroimmunomodulation 1995; 2: 2–15.
6. Slifka MK, Whitton JL. Clinical implications of dysregulated cytokine production. J Mol Med 2000; 78: 74–80.
7. Kotler DP. Cachexia. Ann Intern Med 2000; 133: 622–34.
8. Engel GL. The need for a new medical model: a challenge for biomedicine. Science 1977; 196: 129–46.
9. Drossman DA. Psychosocial factors in gastrointestinal disorders. In: Feldman M, Scharschmidt BF, Sleisenger MH, eds. Gastrointestinal and Liver Disease, 6th ed. Philadelphia: W.B. Saunders, 1998: 69–79.
10. Klein KB. Approach to the patient with abdominal pain. In: Yamada T, Alpers DH, Owyang C, Powell DW, Silverstein FE, eds. Textbook of Gastroenterology. Philadelphia: J.B. Lippincott, 1995: 750–71.
11. Cervero F, Laird JM. Visceral pain. Lancet 1999; 353: 2145–8.
12. Bueno L, Fioramonti J, Delvaux M, Frexinos J. Mediators and pharmacology of visceral sensitivity: from basic to clinical implications. Gastroenterology 1997; 112: 1714–43.
13. Bueno L, Fioramonti J, Garcia-Villar R. Pathobiology of visceral pain: molecular mechanisms and therapeutic implications – III visceral afferent pathways: a source of new therapeutic targets for abdominal pain. Am J Physiol Gastrointest Liver Physiol 2000; 278: G670–6.
14. Stokes MA. Crohn's disease and nutrition. Br J Surg 1992; 79: 391–4.
15. O'Keefe SJD, Rosser BG. Nutrition and inflammatory bowel disease. In: Targan SR, Shanahan F, eds. Inflammatory Bowel Disease: From Bench to Bedside. Baltimore: Williams & Wilkins, 1994: 461–77.
16. Rigaud D, Angel LA, Cerf M *et al.* Mechanisms of decreased food intake during weight loss in adult Crohn's disease patients without obvious malabsorption. Am J Clin Nutr 1994; 60: 775–81.
17. Kirschner BS, Klich JR, Kalman SS. Reversal of growth retardation in Crohn's disease with therapy emphasizing oral nutritional restitution. Gastroenterology 1981; 80: 10–15.
18. Kelts DG, Grand RJ, Shen G, Watkins JB, Werlin SL, Boehme C. Nutritional basis of growth failure in children and adolescents with Crohn's disease. Gastroenterology 1979; 76: 720–7.
19. Aiges H, Markowitz J, Rosa J, Daum F. Home nocturnal supplemental nasogastric feedings in growth-retarded adolescents with Crohn's disease. Gastroenterology 1989; 97: 905–10.
20. Kanof ME, Lake AM, Bayless TM. Decreased height velocity in children and adolescents before the diagnosis of Crohn's disease. Gastroenterology 1988; 95: 1523–7.
21. Lawrence CB, Turnbull AV, Rothwell NJ. Hypothalamic control of feeding. Curr Opin Neurobiol 1999; 9: 778–83.
22. Stubbs RJ. Peripheral signals affecting food intake. Nutrition 1999; 15: 614–25.
23. Woods SC, Seeley RJ, Porte D, Schwartz MW. Signals that regulate food intake and energy homeostasis. Science 1998; 280: 1378–83.
24. Bray GA. Afferent signals regulating food intake. Proc Nutr Soc 2000; 59: 373–84.
25. Inui A. Neuropeptide Y: a key molecule in anorexia and cachexia in wasting disorders. Mol Med Today 1999; 5: 79–85.
26. Curzon G. Serotonin and appetite. Ann NY Acad Sci 1990; 600: 521–30.
27. Halford JC, Blundell JE. Pharmacology of appetite suppression. Prog Drug Res 2000; 54: 25–58.
28. Lieverse RJ, Jansen JBMJ, Masclee AAM, Lamers CBHW. Satiety effects of cholecystokinin in humans. Gastroenterology 1994; 106: 1451–4.
29. Ballinger A, McLoughlin L, Medbak S, Clark M. Cholecystokinin is a satiety hormone in humans at physiological post-prandial plasma concentrations. Clin Sci (Colch) 1995; 89: 375–81.
30. Kennedy GC. The role of depot fat in the hypothalamic control of food intake in the rat. Proc R Soc Lond 1953; 140: 578–92.
31. Friedman JM, Halaas JL. Leptin and the regulation of body weight in mammals. Nature 1998; 395: 763–70.
32. Zhang Y, Proenca R, Maffei M, Barone M, Leopold L, Friedman J. Positional cloning of the mouse obese gene and its human homologue. Nature 1994; 372: 425–32.
33. Fruhbeck G, Jebb SA, Prentice AM. Leptin: physiology and pathophysiology. Clin Physiol 1998; 18: 399–419.
34. Inui A. Feeding and body-weight regulation by hypothalamic neuropeptides – mediation of the actions of leptin. Trends Neurosci 1999; 22: 62–7.
35. Ballinger A, Farthing M. Intestinal disease, feeding behaviour and leptin – role of the gut-brain axis. CNS 1999; 2: 12–16.
36. Halford JC, Blundell JE. Separate systems for serotonin and leptin in appetite control. Ann Med 2000; 32: 222–32.
37. Plata-Salaman CR. Cytokine-induced anorexia: behavioral, cellular and molecular mechanisms. Ann NY Acad Sci 1998; 856: 160–70.
38. Langhans W, Hrupka B. Interleukins and tumor necrosis factor as inhibitors of food intake. Neuropeptides 1999; 33: 415–24.
39. Daun JM, McCarthy DO. The role of cholecystokinin in interleukin-1 induced anorexia. Physiol Behav 1993; 54: 237–41.
40. Finck BN, Kelley KW, Dantzer R, Johnson RW. *In vivo* and *in vitro* evidence for the involvement of tumor necrosis factor alpha in the induction of leptin by lipopolysaccharide. Endocrinology 1998; 139: 2278–83.
41. Laye S, Gheusi G, Cremona S *et al.* Endogenous brain IL-1 mediates LPS-induced anorexia and hypothalamic cytokine expression. Am J Physiol 2000; 279: R93–8.
42. Laviano A, Cangiano C, Fava A, Muscaritoli M, Mulieri G, Fanelli FR. Peripherally injected IL-1 induces anorexia and increases brain tryptophan concentrations. Adv Exp Med Biol 1999; 467: 105–8.
43. McHugh KJ, Weingarten HP, Keenan C, Wallace JL, Collins SM. On the suppression of food intake in experimental models of colitis in the rat. Am J Physiol 1993; 264: R871–6.
44. McHugh KJ, Collins SM, Weingarten HP. Central interleukin-1 receptors contribute to suppression of feeding after acute colitis in the rat. Am J Physiol 1994; 266: R1659–63.
45. Ballinger A, El-Haj T, Perrett D *et al.* The role of medial hypothalamic serotonin in the suppression of feeding in a rat model of colitis. Gastroenterology 2000; 118: 544-53.
46. Barbier M, Cherbut C, Aube AC, Blottiere HM, Galmiche JP. Elevated plasma leptin concentrations in early stages of experimental intestinal inflammation in rats. Gut 1998; 43: 783–90.
47. Ballinger A, Kelly P, Hallyburton E, Besser R, Farthing M. Plasma leptin in chronic inflammatory bowel disease and HIV: implications for the pathogenesis of anorexia and weight loss. Clin Sci (Colch) 1998; 94: 479–83.
48. Hoppin AG, Kaplan LM, Zurakowski D, Leichtner A, Bousvaros A. Serum leptin in children and young adults with inflammatory bowel disease. J Pediatr Gastroenterol Nutr 1998; 26: 500–5.
49. Williamson RC. Intestinal adaptation. N Engl J Med 1978; 298: 1393–402.

50. Li E. Bacterial overgrowth. In: Yamada T, Alpers DH, Owyang C, Powell DW, Silverstein FE, eds. Textbook of Gastroenterology. Philadelphia: J.B. Lippincott, 1995: 1673–80.

51. Kanof ME, Lake AM, Bayless TM. Decreased height velocity in children and adolescents before the diagnosis of Crohn's disease. Gastroenterology 1988; 95: 10–15.

52. Markowitz J, Daum F. Growth impairment in pediatric inflammatory bowel disease. Am J Gastroenterol 1994; 89: 319–26.

53. Kirschner BS. Growth and development in chronic inflammatory bowel disease. Acta Pediatr Scand 1990; 366(Suppl): 98–104.

54. Ballinger AB, Camacho-Hubner C, Croft NM. Growth failure and intestinal inflammation. Q J Med 2001; 94: 121–5.

55. Solomans NW, Rosenfield RL, Jacobs RA. Growth retardation and zinc deficiency. Pediatr Res 1976; 10: 923–7.

56. Sturniolo GC, Molokhia MM, Shields R, et al . Zinc absorption in Crohn's disease. Gut 1980; 21: 387-3-1.

57. Nishi Y, Lifshitz F, Bayne MA et al. Zinc status and its relation to growth retardation in children with chronic inflammatory bowel disease. Am J Clin Nutr 1980; 33: 2613–21.

58. Ballinger AB, Azooz O, El-Haj T, Poole S, Farthing MJG. Growth failure occurs through a decrease in insulin-like growth factor 1 which is independent of undernutrition in a rat model of colitis. Gut 2000; 46: 694–700.

59. Beattie RM, Camacho-Hubner C, Wacharasindhu S, Cotterill AM, Walker-Smith JA, Savage MO. Responsiveness of IGF-1 and IGFBP-3 to therapeutic intervention in adolescents with Crohn's disease. Clin Endocrinol 1998; 49: 483–9.

60. Tenore A, Berman WF, Parks IS, Bongiovannie AM. Basal and stimulated GH concentrations in inflammatory bowel disease. J Clin Endocrinol Metab 1977; 44: 622–8.

61. Braegger CP, Torresani T, Murch SH, Savage MO, Walker-Smith JA, MacDonald TT. Urinary growth hormone in growth-impaired children with chronic inflammatory bowel disease. J Pediatr Gastroenterol Nutr 1993; 16: 49–52.

62. De Benedetti F, Alonzi T, Moretta A et al. Interleukin-6 causes growth impairment in transgenic mice through a decrease in insulin-like growth factor-1. J Clin Invest 1997; 99: 643–50.

63. Siagel SA, Sheahy DJ, Nakada MT. The mouse human chimeric monoclonal antibody CA2 neutralizes TNF *in vitro* and protects transgenic mice from cachexia and TNF lethality *in vivo*. Cytokine 1995; 7: 15–25.

64. Enomoto M, Pan HO, Kinoshita A, Yutani Y, Suzuki F, Takigawa M. Effects of tumor necrosis factor alpha on proliferation and expression of differentiated phenotypes in rabbit costal chondrocytes in culture. Calcif Tissue Int 1990; 47: 145–51.

65. Wolf M, Bohm S, Brand M, Kreymann C. Pro-inflammatory cytokines interleukin 1 beta and tumor necrosis factor alpha inhibit growth hormone stimulation of insulin-like growth factor-1 synthesis and growth hormone receptor mRNA levels in cultured rat liver cells. Eur J Endocrinol 1996; 35: 729–37.

66. Allen DB. Growth suppression by glucocorticoid therapy. Endocrinol Metabol Clin N Am 1996; 25: 699–717.

67. Guistina A, Wehrenberg WB. The role of glucocorticoids in the regulation of growth hormone secretion – mechanisms and clinical significance. Trends Endocrinol Metab 1992; 3: 306–11.

68. Untermann TG, Phillips LS. Glucocorticoid effects on somatomedins and somatomedin inhibitors. J Clin Endocrinol Metab 1985; 61: 618–26.

69. Powell DW. Approach to the patient with diarrhea. In: Yamada T, Alpers DH, Owyang C, Powell DW, Silverstein FE, eds. Textbook of Gastroenterology, 2nd edn. Philadelphia: J.B. Lippincott, 1995: 813–63.

70. Kaunitz DK, Barrett KE, McRoberts JA. Electrolyte secretion and absorption: small intestine and colon. In: Yamada T, Alpers DH, Owyang C, Powell DW, Silverstein FE, eds. Textbook of Gastroenterology, 2nd edn. Philadelphia: J.B. Lippincott, 1995: 326–61.

14 | Clinical course and complications of ulcerative colitis and ulcerative proctitis

REMO PANACCIONE AND LLOYD R. SUTHERLAND

Introduction

Ulcerative colitis (UC) is a chronic inflammatory condition of the colon that may affect individuals of any age. It generally begins at the anus and extends a variable length from the rectum in a continuous fashion. Patients usually present with a constellation of symptoms including diarrhea (often bloody) and associated with urgency, lower abdominal cramping, and tenesmus. Extensive involvement of the colon is often accompanied by systemic symptoms of anorexia, fatigue, low grade fever, and weight loss.

Knowledge of the natural history of UC and its associated complications forms the cornerstone upon which clinicians can build techniques for the proper education and clinical management of patients with the disease. Questions of interest to most patients include those pertaining to etiology, prognosis, dietary issues, medical and surgical therapy, cancer risk, and genetics. Fortunately, several studies regarding the clinical course of UC and ulcerative proctitis are available to aid the clinician in answering these questions. This chapter will review and highlight the existing literature in UC which will form a foundation upon which clinicians may answer patient inquiries and base management decisions.

Bias

An important concept to understand before reviewing the relevant literature is the problem of bias (Table 1). Decisions regarding patient care are often based on studies that examine patient groups that may have little relevance to physicians in smaller communities. Bias may exist in several forms; however, for the purposes of this discussion, referral, temporal, therapeutic, technological, and statistical biases will be taken into account and examined. A firm understanding of bias will allow the physician to review the studies and decide which are most relevant to his or her patients.

Referral bias

Although patients may have similar diseases, patient populations may differ greatly depending on their source. Differences in population base may alter the clinical course predicted in these different studies. The physician should be aware of the population that most resembles his or her own patient population. Problems in reviewing the literature concerning outcome have been discussed elsewhere [1]. Most of the available data are derived from two major sources, either referral or population-based, and the degree of bias which influences the generalizability of this information varies depending on the source.

The first source of data (referral) is reported by pioneers in inflammatory bowel disease. These studies often reflect the experience of a small number of individuals working in large inflammatory bowel disease referral centers and include series by Kirsner [2], the Mt. Sinai (NY) group, [3], Truelove [4], Lennard-Jones [5, 6] and others [7–9]. The patient population is often biased toward more difficult cases with unusual or rare presentations and complications. Due to the nature of the patient population these series tend to represent the worst-case scenar-

Table 1. Sources of bias

Referral
Temporal
Therapeutic
Technological
Statistical

Stephan R. Targan, Fergus Shanahan and Loren C. Karp (eds.), Inflammatory Bowel Disease: From Bench to Bedside, 2nd Edition, 269–290.
© 2003 *Kluwer Academic Publishers. Printed in Great Britain*

ios with the worst clinical outcomes. These studies will be referred to as non-population-based or referral studies.

The second source of data is derived from population-based studies. These are studies which include all patients within a geographically defined area [10–17]. The clinical outcomes in these studies are often more favorable for several reasons. These populations are not 'contaminated' by excessive numbers of patients with refractory disease who need to be seen by an expert in the field, or by the cases with the unusual presentations or rare complications that gravitate toward tertiary centers. Secondly, the mix of disease tends to be more uniform with a higher proportion of patients with disease limited to the rectum or rectosigmoid. Lastly, follow-up in population-based studies tends to be more complete because these studies originate in countries where the burden of health-care cost is not the responsibility of the patient, and because patients tend to be less mobile and are available for more complete follow-up.

An example of a population-based study comes from Copenhagen where the vast majority (99%) of patients with UC have been followed at one center since 1962 [16]. This center, the Herlev Hospital, serves approximately 10% of the Danish population and is staffed by a small group of gastroenterologists with a dedicated interest in UC. Patient management is quite similar to what would be considered standard gastroenterological practice. Patients with UC are on 5-ASA agents for maintenance of remission purposes. Disease flares are treated with oral or topical corticosteroids, and surgical management with colectomy is reserved for patients who fail medical management. In their latest report [16] the long-term prognosis of 1161 patients is presented. Of the 1161 patients, 44% had rectal involvement, 18% had pancolitis, and the remaining 36% had disease between these extremes. In approximately 2% the localization of disease extent was incomplete. Follow-up was complete and ranged from 1 to 26 years. Patients were assessed annually and the median duration of follow-up was 12 years. This type of data most likely represents the practice of most gastroenterologists.

An example of the differences in prognosis between referred as compared to community-based patients is illustrated in the report of Truelove and Pena [18]. Their study describes the course and prognosis of patients with Crohn's disease (CD) seen at the Radcliffe Infirmary between 1938 and 1970. Of

the 221 patients, 55 (25%) were already diagnosed with CD prior to assessment at the Radcliffe Infirmary; the remainder were patients who lived in the Oxford area. The cumulative mortality for this group utilizing actuarial methods was 21.4% at 15 years, which is much higher than the age-adjusted expected mortality rate of 8.4%. However, when the data are analyzed separately for referred cases and cases within the health district significant differences in the observed mortality are seen (Fig. 1).

Differences in disease extent and severity between population-based and non-population-based studies are shown in Figs 2 and 3. The referral center at Oxford [4] has a higher proportion of patients with pancolitis (Fig. 2) and severe disease activity compared to the population-based studies (Fig. 3). There-

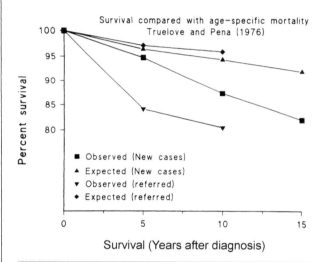

Figure 1. Comparison of life expectancy for patients specifically referred to the Radcliffe Infirmary for treatment of their Crohn's disease compared with those drawn from the local health unit. The life expectancy for the referred patients differs markedly from that of the general population. The difference in mortality for the patients drawn from the local unit compared with the general population is not as marked [18].

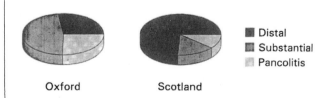

Oxford   Scotland

Figure 2. Comparison of the proportion of patients with pancolitis between a population-based study (Scotland) and a referral-based study (Oxford). The Oxford study contains a greater proportion of patients with extensive disease.

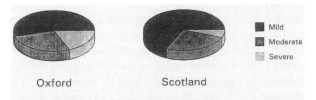

Figure 3. Comparison of the proportion of patients with disease activity characterized as severe in a population-based study (Scotland) and a referral-based study (Oxford). The Oxford study contains a greater proportion of patients characterized as having severe disease.

fore, one can anticipate that outcomes in the Oxford Group would be worse than that of the Scottish group.

Information drawn from non-population-based studies may assist in management decisions for the difficult patient, and better define the range of complications that patients may have. However, information on outcomes is generally more pessimistic and will not aid in counseling individual patients in terms of prognosis.

Temporal bias

Many of the early non-population-based studies which outline the natural course of UC span many decades [3, 4]. During that time advances have occurred in pharmacotherapy, surgical innovation, and postoperative care. If these advances are not taken into account inappropriate conclusions regarding new interventions may be drawn. These early studies are also influenced by referral bias as they originate in centers that are highly specialized and recognized for the excellent care of patients with inflammatory bowel disease.

Therapeutic bias

Therapeutic bias is an important factor to consider when assessing outcomes. Over time there are changes in what is considered to be the standard of care. This standard of care may differ when comparing community-based practices to highly specialized centers. For example, the utility of corticosteroids in the treatment of UC was reported in 1952 [19]. However, corticosteroids did not enter general use until 1958 [4]. This may have arisen due to lack of agreement on patient selection for therapy and controversy regarding dose and duration of therapy. The

same is true regarding sulfasalazine. Although sulfasalazine was available in the United Kingdom as of 1955, a review of the fatalities in the Radcliffe Infirmary study (1953–1962) demonstrates that seven of the 13 were not on any specific therapy at the time of admission [4]. Similarly, although sulfasalazine was shown to be effective for the maintenance of remission in 1965 [20], many of the early long-term prognosis studies included patients who were not on maintenance therapy with a 5-aminosalicylate (5-ASA) agent. The impression that UC is less severe than originally reported may be due to the shift in belief that all patients should be on maintenance therapy [21].

Technological bias

Technological advances have allowed for better characterization of disease severity and extent. Endoscopic evaluation was not available until the late 1960s. Prior to this, extent of disease was based on the findings of rigid sigmoidoscopy combined with a single-contrast enema. Single-contrast studies do not provide the mucosal detail of the air-contrast technique. Disease at presentation and during follow-up may have been underestimated. This is demonstrated in the Ritchie study in which only one of the 269 patients seen between 1969 and 1975 had undergone a full colonoscopic examination [5].

Statistical bias

The technique of life-table analysis, which adjusts for variable lengths of follow-up, has greatly improved our understanding of the natural history of disease. This technique was not used extensively until the 1970s. Data analyzed prior to this in the original natural history studies will therefore contain more limited information.

Presentation of ulcerative colitis and proctititis

Patients with UC present with a variety of symptoms depending on the disease extent and severity. However, it has also been shown that patients may have endoscopic and histological evidence of active disease but be symptom-free. The history and physical examination may assist the physician in differentiating between disease limited to the rectum and more extensive disease. Laboratory evaluation at the time of presentation may be useful in defining severity as well as ruling out other causes of colitis (especially infectious colitis) that may mimic the clinical picture of active UC. Endoscopic evaluation has aided in accurately defining disease extent as well as differentiating between UC and CD in the majority of cases. Despite an increasing effort to educate physicians regarding inflammatory bowel disease the mean and median intervals between onset of symptoms and diagnosis are 1.8 years and 5 months respectively [12].

Presenting symptoms

In the earlier published population-based Copenhagen series of 783 patients 40% had proctitis and 16% had pancolitis, with the remainder having disease extent between these two extremes. In this patient population 75% of the individuals presented with diarrhea and bleeding while 15% had blood-per-rectum alone [22]. The remaining 10% of patients presented with either diarrhea alone or with neither blood nor diarrhea. Fifty-three percent of patients had either abdominal or rectal cramping, 43% described weight loss, and 25% complained of fever. When surveyed, 13% had extracolonic manifestations consisting of joint, eye, or skin manifestations. Joint symptoms were more prevalent in women than men, particularly in those between ages 45 and 59.

Constipation is a well-recognized presentation in those patients with ulcerative proctitis. Of the 100 patients with ulcerative proctitis in the St Mark's series, 30% complained of infrequent stools or passage of hard stools during a flare of their proctitis [6]. The passage of blood alone, or the combination of blood and mucus, was described by the majority of patients (99%). Although systemic complaints are usually associated with more extensive disease, 13% of patients in this series described either fatigue or weight loss.

A few patients with UC may be relatively asymptomatic but have endoscopic evidence of disease. In a study evaluating a screening program for colorectal cancer, six of the 481 patients who tested positive for fecal occult blood had UC at colonoscopy. Four had pancolitis, one had proctosigmoiditis, and the other had proctitis. Two of the patients reported occasional loose stools but otherwise these patients had no intestinal or systemic symptoms [23].

The clinical features at the time of diagnosis may aid in defining patients with so-called acute self-limited colitis and those with true UC. Shumacher and colleagues evaluated 42 patients presenting with acute colitis and followed the patients for at least 5 years [24]. Patients with acute self-limited colitis related to known enteropathogens reported: (1) a shorter duration of symptoms, (2) more bowel motions, and (3) associated fever when compared with those subsequently found to have UC. Patients with UC reported a more insidious onset of symptoms with gradually increasing diarrhea. When symptoms were analyzed using logistic regression analysis this insidious onset of symptoms successfully identified patients with UC. Unfortunately, endoscopic appearance alone could not distinguish between acute self-limited colitis and UC. Histopathological review suggests that basilar plasmacytosis and crypt distortion were found more often in the rectal biopsies of patients with UC. This distinction, based on histopathological features, has been confirmed by others [25].

Physical findings

There have been no studies specifically addressing the physical findings at the time of presentation in patients with UC. The more extensive the disease, and the more severe the symptoms, the more likely the patient will have abnormal findings on physical examination. Patients with ulcerative proctitis often have a completely normal examination except for the digital rectal examination which may reveal bogginess or irregularity of the rectal mucosa or perhaps blood or/and mucus on the examining finger. More extensive and severe disease signs of systemic toxicity may become apparent, including elevated temperature, tachycardia, signs associated with volume depletion, and documented loss of weight. Patients with long-standing symptoms may show signs of malnutrition.

The physical findings associated with the extracolonic manifestations associated with UC are discussed in Chapters 16, 38, 39, and 40. The physical findings of toxic megacolon are discussed later in this chapter.

Laboratory

The laboratory can be used in three distinct areas: first to define disease severity and exclude other diagnoses (infectious colitis, ischemia); second to monitor side-effects of therapeutic agents; and third

Table 2. Truelove and Witts classification of ulcerative colitis

Mild	Moderate	Severe
Less than 5 bowel motions per day	Intermediate between mild and severe	Six or more bowel motions per day
Small amounts of blood in the stool		Large amounts of blood in the stool
No fever		Fever ($> 99.5°$F, $37.5°$C)
No tachycardia		Pulse (> 90 beats/min)
Mild anemia ($> 75\%$, approximately 100 g/L)		Anemia (hemoglobin $> 75\%$)
ESR < 30		ESR > 30

to evaluate new serological markers which may help differentiate between the forms of inflammatory bowel diseases and aid in diagnosis. Laboratory monitoring of therapeutic agents is covered in Chapter 30 and serological markers are discussed in Chapter 20.

At presentation most patients should have a complete blood count, electrolyte profile, blood urea nitrogen, sedimentation rate, and albumin. Stools should be collected for typical pathogens as well as *Clostridium difficile* toxin. Stool studies aid in excluding infectious colitides that may mimic UC. The rest of the blood work serves as a framework to assess the severity of the presentation. Patients with severe or extensive disease may demonstrate anemia, leukocytosis, thrombocytosis, and an elevation of the sedimentation rate. A rise in the blood urea nitrogen and perhaps the creatinine will be present if dehydration exists.

In one study of patients with severe attacks, hypoalbuminemia (< 30 g/L), hypokalemia (< 3.1 mmol/L), and an elevation in the alkaline phosphatase (> 200 units/L) were associated with a poor prognosis [8].

Various laboratory abnormalities may accompany the various extracolonic manifestations and are discussed in Chapters 16, 38, 39, and 40. A complete review of the radiological and pathological features of UC is found in Chapters 19 and 17, respectively.

Assessment of severity

Although there have been numerous disease activity indices to measure disease activity (severity) in CD, this is not the case in UC. There have been two indices developed for clinical trial use but these indices are not informally used [26, 27]. The development of a more precise tool to measure disease severity would greatly improve the ability to compare the various patient populations reported in the literature.

Truelove and Witts developed the first classification of disease activity in 1955 [19] for the trial evaluating the efficacy of corticosteroids in the treatment of UC. The Truelove and Witts classification was developed to describe the severity of presentation for patients with extensive disease. However, it has been used frequently in studies of prognosis to classify severity in patients with variable disease extent including proctitis. The classification scheme proposed by Truelove and Witts characterizes attacks of UC as mild, moderate, or severe, depending on the number of bowel motions per day, presence of blood in the stool, fever, tachycardia, anemia, and the sedimentation rate (Table 2). The classification scheme is easy to use and understand but has never been formally validated. It may lack important variables in defining severity of disease. This is demonstrated in the Oxford series in which several patients classified as having mild or moderate disease at presentation died.

A second scoring system was based on a regression analysis described by the group from Scotland [8]. Different weights are applied to temperature (X_2), number of daily bowel motions (X_4), and sedimentation rate (X_6).

$$Y = 0.84X_2 + 0.12X_4 + 0.35X_6 - 0.59$$

Classification is mild, moderate, or severe according to the value of Y. All patients who died as a result of UC during their first attack were identified as severe by this scoring system according to the authors. However, this tool has not been used extensively outside of Scotland and has also never been validated.

Table 3. Characteristics of population-defined studies that deal with prognosis

Source	No. of patients	Years of entry	Male/female ratio	Rectum/ sigmoid (%)	Intermediate (%)	Pancolitis (%)
Sinclair *et al.* [10]	537	1967–1976	275:262	74	15	11
Hendriksen *et al.* [31]	783	1960–1978	342:441	41	41	16
Brostrom *et al.* [49]	1274	1955–1979	681:593	25	38	37
Stonnington *et al.* [14]	182	1960–1979	75:63	46	18	36
Jones *et al.* [13]	313	1975–1984	160:153	56	25	19
Ekbom *et al.* [15]	2509	1965–1983	1429:1080	42	28	30

Distribution of disease

The distribution of disease at the time of presentation varies widely depending on the study. This is due to the heterogeneity of the populations being studied (i.e. population- or non-population-based). As previously mentioned, the population-based studies give a more accurate reflection of the natural distribution of the disease. The major population-based studies are summarized in Table 3. Despite all these studies being population-based they may not be comparable, for a variety of reasons. The most obvious reason for inability to accurately assess the precise frequencies of disease extent is the lack of uniformity in actually defining the extent of disease. Different investigators have used different definitions to define disease extent. For example, proctitis has been variably defined as affecting 12–14 cm [2], 15 cm [28], or the distal 20 cm [29]. Various studies have found that 14–36.7% of patients have pancolitis, 36–41% have disease extending beyond the rectum, and 44–49% have proctosigmoiditis [30–32]. Moreover, disease extent is most likely underestimated because the extent was determined by a combination of flexible sigmoidoscopy and barium enema instead of complete colonoscopy. In the recent population-based study from southeastern Norway 525 patients were identified as having UC [33]. All patients underwent a colonoscopy at the time of diagnosis. Eighty-four percent had the colon visualized proximal to the splenic flexure and 73% had a complete colonoscopy with visualization to the cecum. Thirty-two percent had proctitis, 33% had left-sided colitis, and 35% had extensive colitis. This is the largest population-based study in which colonoscopy was used to define extent; it therefore should be considered as representing the true distribution of disease at presentation. However, one must also take into account that disease extent has always been defined by the macroscopic changes on endoscopy and alteration of the mucosal pattern on barium enema. The microscopic extent of disease and its influence on disease course, has never been formally studied.

The actual endoscopic margin of disease extent is not always well demarcated. In many instances there may be a gradual transition form abnormal to normal mucosa. In a study by Geboes and Ectors [34], 75% of patients diagnosed as having proctitis or left-sided disease were found to have segmental inflammation extending into the cecum when ileocolonoscopy was performed. This has also been demonstrated by other investigators who have described the 'patchy' nature of untreated UC [35]. The finding of a patch of cecal inflammation adjacent to the appendiceal orifice (cecal patch) in patients with left-sided disease is also well recognized [36]. These patients for all intents and purposes are thought to have UC, but whether there may be a later transition to CD in a few patients is not known.

The number of patients with ulcerative proctitis may be increasing while the number of cases of UC is decreasing or remaining the same. In the Cleveland Clinic series, 124 patients were described as having ulcerative proctitis during the period 1950–1963. However, 32 newly diagnosed cases were described in 1969 alone [28]. This trend was confirmed in the population-based study from Uppsala, Sweden, in which the increase in total cases of UC was found to be due to an increase in the documented cases of ulcerative proctitis [37]. The age-adjusted incidence rate tripled between 1965–1969 and 1975–1978. The exact reason why the incidence of ulcerative proctitis is climbing in these population-based studies is uncertain. One explanation put forward was possibly an increased incidence of sexually transmitted disease. However, in one study the increase in incidence was due to a rise not only in males but also in females.

Diagnostic accuracy

It is reassuring to note that interobserver variability in the assessment of the rectal mucosa is low at the time of endoscopic examination [38]. The accuracy of colonoscopic diagnosis of inflammatory bowel disease is reported to be 80–90% [39, 40]. In the Copenhagen study, of 1161 patients, 36 initially diagnosed as having UC eventually developed definite signs of CD later in the disease course, whereas seven patients initially diagnosed as having CD were later re-classified as having UC [32]. Only 3.7% of patients had a change in their diagnosis. It is uncertain whether this represents inaccuracy in diagnosis or change in disease over time. These findings are consistent with those of Pera and colleagues, in which 357 patients with inflammatory bowel disease were followed prospectively with endoscopic evaluation [41]. The authors found that the diagnosis was correct in 89% of cases, 4% had been misclassified, and 7% were not easily classified as either CD or UC. Difficulties and errors in diagnosis appeared to occur more often when severe inflammation was present.

UC is characteristically a mucosal disease, usually beginning in the rectum and extending proximally in a continuous fashion for a variable length. However, rectal sparing, even in the absence of local enema therapy, is well described [42]. In a series from the Mayo Clinic there appeared to be a higher incidence of rectal sparing in patients with concurrent primary sclerosing cholangitis [43]. Although the mucosa may appear normal, endoscopic biopsies often show histological abnormalities. This is highlighted in a small study in which 12 patients with diarrhea and intermittent blood and mucus per rectum had normal endoscopic appearance in the rectum, but histological examination of rectal biopsies revealed evidence of UC [44].

Prognosis

The prognosis of UC is the single most important issue from a patient perspective. Although many studies have been published which deal with prognosis, there is a lack of uniformity in these studies. Earlier non-population-based studies may be overly pessimistic with respect to prognosis. Once again the best clinically applicable data come from the larger population-based studies. However, even in these studies the clinician must be aware of differences in prognosis based on disease extent, presentation (first attack or relapse), and temporal trends with respect

to therapy. The past four decades have been accompanied by the use of corticosteroids in severe flares, maintenance therapy in the form of aminosalicylates, and more recently increased utilization of immunomodulators. The introduction of corticosteroids has greatly reduced the mortality of severe disease. Most patients will be on maintenance therapy with aminosalicylates. Patient acceptance of surgical therapy has also increased with the introduction of proctocolectomy with ileal pouch–anal anastamosis. Therefore, more recent studies reflect the natural history of what may be deemed as treated UC [45].

Placebo response

Examining the outcomes of patients randomized to the placebo arm of a randomized clinical trial may represent the natural history of patients with untreated UC. However, this concept has recently been challenged with the increasing awareness of the relationship between the neuropsychiatric system and the immune response controlling inflammation.

Ilnyckyj and colleagues recently reviewed in detail the placebo response in patients with active UC [46]. In this study the placebo response in 38 double-blind randomized controlled studies was evaluated. The clinical remission rate in the placebo groups was 9.1% (CI_{95} 6.6–11.6%) and the benefit rate was 26.7% (CI_{95} 24.1–29.2%). This clinical improvement was accompanied by both endoscopic and histological benefits (endoscopic remission 13.5% (CI_{95} 10.0–17.1%), endoscopic improvement 30.3% (CI_{95} 26.6–34.0%), histological remission 8.6% (CI_{95} 5.0–12%), histological improvement 25.2% (CI_{95} 20.8–29.6%)).

Meyers and Janowitz [47] noted similar findings when randomized placebo-controlled trials of maintenance therapy for UC were evaluated. Fifty-one percent (CI_{95} 36–66%) of patients receiving placebo remained in remission when evaluated at 6 months. Patients with less extensive disease and those already in remission for at least 1 year were more likely to remain in remission compared to patients with more extensive disease and those who had recently entered remission.

Prognosis for the first attack

There are a large number of studies that have examined the issue of prognosis in UC following the first attack. These include both population-based and non-population-based studies. Regardless of the source of information, the major determinant of prognosis appears to be extent and severity of disease. The discussion below will include both non-population-based and population-based studies. Non-population-based studies from tertiary centers once again point to a more pessimistic outlook.

Non-population-based studies

There is some consistency in the reports of the early non-population-based studies in that the majority of first attacks were mild and associated with low mortality [4, 8, 10, 48]. Severe disease occurred in 6–25% of patients and affected predominantly patients with pancolitis. These severe cases were associated with a mortality rate of 20–33%.

Edwards and Truelove described the course and prognosis of 624 patients with UC seen in Oxford between 1938 and 1962 [4]. All patients were available for follow-up during the observation period, which ranged from 1 to 24 years. Two hundred and fifty patients were seen during what is described as their first attack. Most of the 250 patients were seen within 6 months of onset of symptoms with only a minority (22%) having had symptoms between 6 and 12 months. The course of these 250 patients is outlined. Using the Truelove and Witts criteria, 54% had mild disease, 27% had moderate disease, and 19% had severe disease. The mortality rate during the first attack was 10%. Mortality was directly related to severity with most deaths occurring in patients with severe disease. Of the 25 reported deaths, 72% of patients were classified as having severe disease, 24% as having moderate disease, and one patient (4%) had mild disease. The mortality rate of those presenting with severe disease was 33%. Overall, mortality declined over the three decades of the study with no deaths occurring in the mild to moderate disease groups after 1952. There was also a trend toward decreased mortality in patients with severe disease, but this did not reach statistical significance.

Prognostic factors for mortality included age at presentation, short duration of symptoms, extent of disease, and severity. Patients over the age of 60 had a mortality rate of 16.3% compared to 8.7% in patients under 60. A small subset of patients who presented with symptoms of less than 1 month and severe disease had a mortality rate of 18.4%. Increased mortality associated with increasing extent of disease. Twenty-five percent of patients with pancolitis died compared to 7% with disease defined as sub-stantial colitis (i.e. left-sided colitis). No deaths were reported in patients with distal disease. Overall, 84% of patients entered clinical remission, 25% died, and two patients underwent colectomy.

Watts and colleagues reported their experience in treating 204 patients for their first attack of UC between 1952 and 1963 [9]. This group was diagnosed early in the course of disease with 90% of patients having had symptoms for 6 months or less. Thirty-six percent of patients were classified as having severe disease according to Truelove and Witts criteria with a mortality rate of 8.2% in this group. The overall mortality rate was 4%. Severe disease, pancolitis, and age over 60 were associated with increased risk of death or surgery. Complete remission was seen in 70% and a clinical improvement seen in an additional 16.2%.

The rate of colectomy in the Leeds series was 11.3%. This is higher than the 0.8% colectomy rate reported in the Oxford series. The reason for this difference is not readily apparent; however, there appeared to be more patients with severe disease in the Leeds series. Alternatively, the threshold for surgical intervention at the time may have been different between the two centers. Overall, death or colectomy was the end-result in 36% of patients with severe disease, 31% of patients over the age of 60, and 37% of patients with pancolitis.

Jalan and colleagues reviewed the prognosis of 184 patients presenting with their first attack of UC at the Western General Hospital in Edinburgh between 1950 and 1967 [8]. Eighteen of the 19 deaths occurred in patients classified as having severe disease. The mortality rate in the group classified as severe was 26.4%. Ten deaths occurred while the patient was under medical supervision and the other nine fatalities followed emergency surgery. Overall, there were significant decreases in mortality rate over time.

Population-based studies

There are only a few population-based studies that deal with prognosis following the first attack of UC [10, 32, 49]. The most detailed of these studies is that of Sinclair and colleagues, who reviewed all 537 patients newly diagnosed with UC in the northeast of Scotland between 1967 and 1976 [10]. Patients' disease severity was mild in 68%, moderate in 26%, and severe in 6% by Truelove and Witts classification. The extent of disease was distal in 74% (rectum and sigmoid), pancolitis in 11%, and substantial involvement in 15% (proximal to sigmoid but not proximal to hepatic flexure). The mortality rate during the initial attack was 3% with 11 of the 17 deaths occurring in patients over the age of 70.

Patient outcome was related to disease extent and severity. In patients with severe disease, 25% died, 31% underwent colectomy, 4% had continuous symptoms, and only 40% entered clinical remission. Outcomes for patients with mild disease were much better: 92% entered clinical remission, 8% had continuous symptoms, and no deaths were reported. In moderate disease 85% entered remission, 8% also had continuous symptoms, and 3% died. Fig. 5 demonstrates the prognosis for patients characterized as having a severe first attack or pancolitis at presentation.

Two additional population-based studies have been published more recently [32, 49]. Moum and colleagues [49] reported the clinical course of 496 newly diagnosed patients with UC in southeastern Norway between 1990 and 1993. The majority of patients (88%) underwent complete colonoscopy and were followed at 1-year intervals (98%) with a mean follow-up of 16.2 months. The overall mortality rate in this population was 2.2% (11/496) but only two deaths were directly attributable to UC. Four percent of patients underwent colectomy. The colectomy rate was higher in patients with extensive colitis compared to patients with disease limited to the left colon or rectum. During the follow-up period 47% of patients remained in clinical remission. In the study from Copenhagen, involving 1161 patients diagnosed between 1962 and 1987, the overall colectomy rate in the year of diagnosis was 9% [32]. The relative risk of death in the year of diagnosis compared to age- and sex-matched population was 2.4.

Prognosis for subsequent attacks

The majority of patients who enter clinical remission will have a recurrence of their disease over time. There is a small subset of patients who have a single episode of colitis and then enter a prolonged remission. It is difficult to tell whether this truly represents a subset of UC patients or simply reflects patients with presumed infectious etiology who were misdiagnosed as having UC.

The most interesting unanswered question is whether the widespread introduction of 5-ASA agents for maintenance of remission purposes will have an impact on long-term prognosis. Intuitively, one would expect that patients on 5-ASA therapy would spend more time in remission and less time in periods of relapse. Similarly one might expect that progression of disease extension would be reduced.

In the Oxford series [4], 64% of patients had a chronic intermittent course and 7% of patients had a chronic continuous course. Eighteen percent of patients had only one attack over the study period. A proportion of these patients probably represented colitis of an infectious etiology. Stonnington and colleagues [14] reported on 182 patients in Olmsted County, Minnesota, followed between 1935 and 1979. They reported that 28% had a transient colitis, 65% had intermittent course, and 5% had a continuous course.

Extension of disease

A major concern of patients, especially those with localized disease, is the risk of disease extension. This is a difficult area to analyze, for a variety of reasons. First, most of the available studies were performed prior to the advent of fibreoptic technology. Initial extent of disease was based on rigid sigmoidoscopy, which may underestimate disease extent. This is well described in the Cleveland Clinic experience with proctosigmoiditis [28]. In this series of 276 patients the upper limit of disease extent could be identified in only 46% of patients (127 of 276 patients). In the remaining 149 patients the examination failed to define disease beyond 15 cm due either to patient discomfort or lack of proper visualization. Second, the importance of microscopic involvement of endoscopically normal mucosa remains unknown. Many physicians do not biopsy normal mucosa, which histologically may be abnormal and therefore may underestimate the initial extent of disease. Third, the extent of disease tends to be underestimated with barium enema. This is demonstrated by the difference in the reported rates of pancolitis in population-based series in which flexible sigmoidoscopy and barium enema were used to define disease extent which range from 11–18% [10, 16] and those in which colonoscopy was utilized in which the rates of pancolitis ranges from 28% to 36% [15, 48, 50, 51]. Fourth, patients may be reassessed only at the time of dramatic change in disease behavior. There are very few studies in which patients undergo procedures to re-evaluate their disease endoscopically and/or radiologically on a regular basis. Finally, various studies, which have reported the proportion of patients with disease extension, did not use actuarial methods, which would deal with the issue of dropouts in analyzing the data.

Table 4. Clinical outcome after the first 10 years of ulcerative colitis and proctitis (%)

Involved area	Surgery at 5 years	Descending colon	Transverse colon	Ascending colon	Mortality
Rectum	2 ± 2%	5 ± 2%	3 ± 2%	0%	0 (0%)
Sigmoid colon	6 ± 3%	18 ± 5%	Not stated	7 ± 3%	1 (2.6%)
Descending to transverse colon	3 ± 3%	–	–	21 ± 8%	0 (0%)
Ascending colon	30 ± 8%	–	–	–	2 (5.4%)

In the Leeds study [9], 50 of the 204 patients seen within the first year of symptom onset had disease limited to the rectum. During a mean follow-up of 3.2 years (range 6 months to 12 years), 18 of these 50 patients (36%) had proximal extension of their disease. Eleven of the 18 had substantial involvement, while seven developed pancolitis. The figure of 36% may be an underestimate, as actuarial methods were not used.

In the largest series, from St. Mark's, 269 patients diagnosed with UC between 1966 and 1975 were reviewed for progression of disease [5]. All patients were initially assessed for disease extent within 6 months of symptom onset. The extent of disease was defined by rigid sigmoidoscopy and the majority of patients also underwent barium enema. Seventy-nine percent of patients had histologically confirmed disease and all but five patients were included in the follow-up. At initial presentation 28% had proctitis, 29% had proctosigmoiditis, 12% had disease extending from the sigmoid colon to the hepatic flexure, and 14% had disease extending proximal to the hepatic flexure. In 17% the exact extent of disease could not be evaluated as the barium enema failed to reveal abnormalities.

The follow-up in this group ranged from 1 to 11 years. Clinical outcome data are shown in Table 4. Of the 76 patients initially diagnosed with proctitis, five were noted to have disease extension (three to the descending colon, two to the hepatic flexure). The cumulative probability after 5 years of extension into the descending colon was 5% and into the transverse colon was 3%. In the 79 patients presenting with proctosigmoiditis progression was noted in 17 (nine to the descending colon, eight to the ascending colon). The cumulative rate of progression at 5 years was 18% to the descending colon and 7% to the right colon. Thirty-three patients had left-sided disease distal to the hepatic flexure with extension occurring in six. The cumulative probability of extension in this group was 21% at 5 years. These data suggest that the cumulative 5-year probability of disease extension is approximately 10% in patients with ulcerative proctitis and 20% in patients with more extensive disease of the left colon.

Farmer reported higher rates of progression in the Cleveland Clinic series [30]. Although this represents data from a tertiary center the data support a high rate of progression. Farmer and colleagues studied the natural history of 1116 patients with UC seen at the Cleveland Clinic between 1960 and 1983. Of these 1116 patients, 46% had proctosigmoiditis, 17% had left-sided colitis (disease distal to the splenic flexure), and 37% had pancolitis. During a mean follow-up of 13 years the disease had progressed in 54% of the patients. In many patients disease progression was evident without a change in symptoms, suggesting that subclinical extension is common. Seventy percent of patients with left-sided colitis and 34% of patients with proctosigmoiditis extended their disease to develop pancolitis. Factors associated with disease extension included severe disease at presentation, disease of the left colon, young age at diagnosis, joint symptoms at diagnosis, and bleeding at the time of diagnosis (most likely related to severity).

Population-based studies also suggest that distal disease may not be as benign as originally thought. In one study 20–30% of patients with initial distal disease came to proctocolectomy over a 20-year follow-up period [12]. Using actuarial techniques, Sinclair and colleagues reported extension of distal disease in 12% of patients at 5 years and 30% of patients at 10 years [10]. The details of exact disease extent are not given. The colectomy rate in the group with distal disease was less than 5% at 10 years of follow-up.

In the largest population-based study to date, using actuarial methods, Langholz and colleagues evaluated progression in 1161 patients in Copenhagen County diagnosed with UC between 1962 and 1987 [32]. Disease extent was evaluated by sigmoidoscopy (rigid or flexible) and barium enema. At the time of initial diagnosis 44% had proctosigmoiditis (mucosal changes on sigmoidoscopy combined with normal-appearing mucosa on barium enema proximal to the rectum), 36% had substantial colitis (which includes both left-sided and extensive colitis; abnormal-appearing mucosa on barium enema proximal to the rectum but not including the cecum), and 18% had pancolitis (signs of colitis throughout the colon including the cecum). In 1.7% of patients the initial disease was not known; therefore these patients were excluded from the analysis. Two hundred (39%) of the patients with proctosigmoiditis had extension of their disease. In 35% the extension was to substantial colitis and in 4% the extension was to pancolitis. The cumulative probability of extension at 10 years in the patients with proctosigmoiditis was 41%. The colectomy rate in these patients was 12%. Interestingly, of the 422 patients with substantial colitis only 9% progressed to pancolitis, while 44% of patients experienced a radiographic regression of their disease. Radiographic regression was also seen in 39% of patients diagnosed initially with pancolitis. This study suggests that inflammation of the colon is a dynamic state and that both progression and regression can be seen.

The previous studies have relied on radiological assessment to define the extent of disease both at diagnosis and in follow-up. In a review of all patients seen in a district health unit in the United Kingdom [13], 48% of patients had more extensive disease at follow-up colonoscopy compared to presentation. Of the patients initially classified as having 'mild disease' (macroscopic changes at sigmoidoscopy but normal-appearing barium enema), 43% undergoing colonoscopy later in their evaluation were found to have colitis extending into the mid-transverse colon. This once again underscores the difficulty of interpreting studies when extent is based on radiological assessment.

Relapse

In educating patients with respect to their disease course it is evident that the disease course will be characterized by periods of remission and relapse.

For most patients the time spent in remission is far greater than the time spent with a relapse or active disease. This is once again illustrated in the population-based study from Copenhagen [32]. Once again older non-population-based studies initially gave a different impression.

DeDombal and colleagues [52] reported that the majority of patients seen in Leeds spent more time in clinical remission than in relapses. Relapses were usually mild by Truelove and Witts criteria. In Leeds the risk of relapse did not alter over time [53], providing little support for the concept that the will disease burn out.

The report from Edwards and Truelove was not as encouraging. In their series of 250 newly referred patients with UC, 80% had a second attack within 1 year of entering remission [54]. Seven percent of patients had continuous disease. The disease activity and extent of disease at presentation did not alter the probability of relapse. However, one must remember that this report predated the widespread introduction of sulfasalazine.

In the Scottish study [10], 28% of patients did not relapse after 5 years of follow-up. The authors speculated that perhaps the high proportion of patients with mild disease localized to the distal colon may have explained this, but there are no other studies to support this. The authors did introduce the concept of the attack and remission year. An attack year was noted if, at any time during the year, the patient had active symptoms suggesting disease activity. A remission year was noted if the patient was free of disease for the entire year. During follow-up 2674 patient-years were accumulated with 68% of these years spent in clinical remission. There were 864 (32%) attack-years of which 84% were characterized by mild disease activity.

The most complete data set relating to the prognosis of subsequent attacks of UC comes from the Copenhagen study by Langholz and colleagues evaluating their 25-year experience in 1161 patients [55]. Patients were treated according to defined protocols using sulfasalazine or 5-ASA for induction or maintenance of remission purposes, corticosteroids for more acute attacks, and proctocolectomy for patients who failed high-dose corticosteroids. Patients had easy access to subspecialty care ensuring rapid and uniform treatment. Among the 1161 patients from Copenhagen who did not require colectomy most patients had subsequent flares. The cumulative probability of a relapsing course was 90% over the 25-year study period. The cumulative probability of a completely relapse free course was 10.6% at 25 years, whereas the probability of a continuous active course was 0.1%. Fig. 4 demonstrates the cumulative probability of a completely relapse-free course, the cumulative probability of a course with continuous activity, and the cumulative probability of an intermittent course. The authors also calculated the probability of remaining in remission by using Markov modeling. Fig. 5 in Chapter 20 shows the probability of remaining in remission from one year to the next. The probability of a patient in clinical remission remaining in remission the following year was 80–90%. The probability was influenced by the previous disease course in that patients with numerous years of remission were more likely to remain in remission. By contrast patients with clinically active disease had a probability of 70% of having a relapse in the subsequent year. The probability of having active disease every year after a relapse decreased over time from 50% at 2 years to 10–15% at 10 years.

Langholz and colleagues also analyzed a subgroup of 600 patients who had been followed for a minimum of 7 years and had not yet died or undergone colectomy. In this group of patients, who were analyzed in the 5-year period 3–7 years after diagnosis, 25% were in continuous remission, 57% had an intermittent course, and 18% had continuous disease activity. During the 5-year period predictors of disease course included initial disease course in the year of diagnosis plus the following 2 years (more disease activity in early disease led to relapse later in the course); the calendar year (patients diagnosed in the 1960s had a more active course than those diagnosed in the 1980s); and the occurrence of systemic symptoms such as fever and weight loss at the time of diagnosis.

Interestingly, in this study the clinical course over the 25-year follow-up was not influenced by anatomic extent of disease at diagnosis (except in patients with more extensive disease who underwent early colectomy), age, sex, presenting symptoms, length of time between onset symptoms and diagnosis, initial treatment, or occurrence of extraintestinal manifestations. Factors which influenced the course of disease were once again the presence of systemic symptoms at diagnosis and development of disease later in the study period. The difference in time of diagnosis suggests that patient outcomes may be improving with advances in medical therapy.

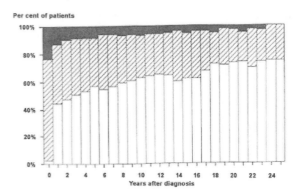

Figure 4. Cumulative probability of remission (□), continuous disease activity (■), and intermittent disease activity (hatched), in all years after diagnosis. Adapted with permission from Ref. 32.

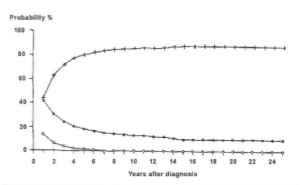

Figure 5. Cumulative probability of having only one disease episode (●), continuous activity (○), or intermittent activity (+) from time of diagnosis. Adapted with permission from Ref. 32.

Risk factors for relapse

A variety of retrospective studies have searched for risk factors that may influence the relapse rate but have been unsuccessful. There are no laboratory markers in UC that consistently warn of the onset of a relapse. Factors that have been put forward as being associated with relapses of UC include viral illnesses [56], seasonality [57–59], and the use of nonsteroidal compounds [60, 61]. Infection with *C. difficile* has also been suggested as possible risk factor [62, 63] but this has not been found consistently [64–66]. Although non-smoking has been associated with an increased risk of developing UC, non-smoking or smoking cessation has never been shown to alter relapse rates.

Surgery

Surgical rates vary from center to center and are influenced by patient preference and individual center bias. Individual centers may have adopted a more aggressive surgical approach to patients and the definition of medical intractability may vary (i.e. the use of cyclosporine in severe UC varies). Surgical outcomes, especially for proctocolectomy with ileal pouch–anal anastamosis, will vary according to the expertise of the surgical center. The decision to proceed to surgery from a patient perspective may relate to impairment of quality of life due to ongoing symptoms, perceived cancer risks, and the efficacy and tolerability of medical therapy. The patient population studied will also influence colectomy rates. Inclusion of a large proportion of patients with distal colitis will obviously lower colectomy rates. Tertiary centers may exhibit higher colectomy rates because of referral bias in which medically refractory cases are referred for either advanced medical management or specifically for surgical intervention.

Surgical colectomy rates are influenced by numerous variables, but the most important factor for subsequent colectomy appears to be the extent and severity of disease at the time of diagnosis. The risk of colectomy is greatest during the first 2 years following diagnosis in both population- and non-population-based studies.

In the non-population-based studies colectomy rates for the first attack of UC range from 0.8% [4] to 11.3% [9]. Subsequent colectomy rates are not available from the early studies because the follow-up period varied and life tables were not generated.

The northeastern Scotland study reported that only 3% of their cohort required colectomy during the first attack [10]. Given the large number of patients with distal colitis this low colectomy rate would be expected. Twenty-nine percent of patients characterized as having severe disease ultimately came to colectomy. The colectomy rate at 10 years for patients initially presenting with extensive disease was approximately 35%.

The factors determining the colectomy rate were studied retrospectively in a population-based cohort of 1586 patients with UC seen in Stockholm between 1955 and 1984 by Leijonmarck and colleagues [12]. During a median observation period of 13 years, 514 patients underwent colectomy. Ten percent had their colectomy during the first year following diagnosis, 4% during the second year, and 1% each during each subsequent year. The 5-year cumulative colectomy rate was 32% (CI_{95} 28–36%) and the 10- and 25-year

cumulative colectomy rates were 42% (CI_{95} 38–46%), and 65% (CI_{95} 58–72%), respectively.

The colectomy rates discussed above are similar to those in the large Danish cohort of 1161 patients which reported a colectomy rate of 9% in the year of diagnosis, 3% per year in the following 4 years and then 1% per year thereafter [32]. The cumulative colectomy rate at 15 years was 30%. The initial extent of disease was associated with higher colectomy rates. Thirty-five percent of patients with extensive colitis underwent colectomy in the first 5 years compared to 19% and 9% with substantial and distal colitis respectively.

The Cleveland Clinic series demonstrates how colectomy rates can be elevated in tertiary referral centers [30]. The colectomy rate in the first 2 years following diagnosis was 38%. Sixty-one percent of those with pancolitis required colectomy. The group with pancolitis included 17% of patients who presented with colonic hemorrhage and 13% with toxic colitis. Primary indications for the entire group were intractability in 40%, fulminant disease in 17%, and colonic dilation in 18%.

The major indications for surgery are complications of UC and medical intractability. An additional consideration for surgery is the risk for colorectal cancer or the finding of dysplasia or malignancy later in the disease course. In a series from St Mark's, 401 patients with pancolitis were entered into a surveillance colonoscopy program over a 22-year period [67]. Thirty-four patients required colectomy for cancer or dysplasia [67].

Overall, population studies confirm the dogma that colectomy rates are the highest in the initial 2 years after diagnosis, and in patients who present with severe or extensive disease. The latter two, as previously outlined, are often related. Later in the course of disease, concerns about the risk of developing cancer or the presence of either dysplasia or cancer are the common indications for surgery.

Additional details regarding surgery in UC pertaining to indications, types of surgery, complications, and patient outcome are discussed in Chapter 31.

Mortality

Mortality as a result of UC has diminished dramatically since the introduction of corticosteroids and the use of maintenance therapy with 5-ASA-containing compounds. In the early report of Edwards and Truelove the excess mortality associated with UC was described as 'formidable' with mortality at 20 years of follow-up at 35% compared to the expected mortality of 5% [4]. This was in the pre-cortico-steroid era and before the introduction of 5-ASA therapy; however, it reminds us that the disease had devastating consequences. Recent data are much more favorable, with the majority of deaths occurring within the first few years following diagnosis. In Stockholm County there appeared to be a trend toward improved survival in patients diagnosed in the period 1970–1985 compared to those diagnosed from 1955–1969 [50]. This trend toward improved mortality was confirmed in the study from Uppsala [68]. Most population-based studies would confirm that overall long-term mortality for patients is minimally different compared with that of the general population.

Ritchie and colleagues [5] did not find any differences between expected and observed mortality during the first 10 years after diagnosis, but their actuarial analysis was confined to the entire patient group; and therefore the impact of disease severity and extent was not examined. It was noted that only three deaths attributable to UC were noted within the first year following diagnosis.

The 10-year survival in northeastern Scotland following diagnosis was 80%, in keeping with that expected in the general population [10]. Differences in mortality were evident only when patients were sub-classified by disease extent or severity. Patients with severe disease at presentation had a mortality of 31% and those with extensive disease had a mortality of 14%, which is above the expected rates (Fig. 5). Most of the excess mortality occurred in the first 4 years following diagnosis, particularly in the first year.

In a detailed Swedish study relative survival was analyzed for 2509 patients diagnosed with UC between 1965 and 1983 [68]. The 10-year survival was 96% of that expected. Patients with ulcerative proctitis, left-sided colitis, and pancolitis had relative survival rates of 98%, 96%, and 93%, respectively. The standardized mortality ratio was increased at 1.4. Inflammatory bowel disease was believed to be responsible for part of this excess mortality. Colorectal cancer was also believed to increase mortality; however, deaths from other cancers were not increased. Interestingly, deaths from obstructive pulmonary diseases were also higher than expected in this cohort. Both the increased mortality from colorectal cancer and from obstructive pulmonary disease was substantiated in the Stockholm study [69].

In the Danish study 149 deaths were observed in the 1161 patients [70]. Twenty-six of the deaths were believed to be attributable to UC or its complications. Once again the mortality was highest in the first year, with the relative risk of death in the first year being 2.4, representing a statistically significant mortality compared with that expected. Overall, the mortality rate attributable to UC was 0.8%. The deaths tended to occur in patients with acute severe colitis. Following the first year there was no statistical difference in mortality between the UC patients and age- and sex-matched controls from the general Danish population.

In the latest data from Olmsted County, Minnesota, Loftus and colleagues did not detect an increase in mortality in their inception cohort of patients followed from 1940 to 1993 [17]. The total observation time was for a total of 4348 person-years with a median duration of follow-up of 14.1 years (range 0.1–51 years). Twenty-year survival was 81% (expected 83%) and 30-year survival was 69% (expected 69%). The normal life expectancy in this population-based trial is consistent with European population-based studies.

Quality of life

UC is a chronic disease, which is highly prevalent, and often affects people at a young age with subsequent impact, not only on physical well-being, but also on emotional and social well-being. Therefore, evaluation of patients with UC should not only include the number of bowel motions or rectal bleeding but should take into the account the impact of the disease on the patients' overall well-being. The concept that inflammatory bowel disease patients required evaluation not only from a physical perspective but also from a psychosocial, cultural, and social perspective, was first introduced by Garret and Drossman [71]. Health related quality of life (HRQOL) represents a patient's perception of his or health status. It differs from other measures of disease activity because it uses the patient's subjective experience of his or her health as the gold standard, and encompasses not only physical symptoms, but also other psychosocial factors.

HRQOL was most likely first measured by Edwards and Truelove in their original work. Using a global assessment (i.e. generic quality-of-life tool) they reported that 69.1% of patients had a normal life and 19.3% of patients led an essentially normal life aside from frequent hospital visits [4]. Michener and colleagues described the quality of life in a group of patients attending the Cleveland Clinic with disease longer than 24 months as good in 10%, fair in 80%, and poor in 10% [72]. These descriptions suggested that UC impacted on HRQOL, but did not identify in which specific areas of daily living were affected.

The impact of UC on a variety of quality-of-life issues including sexual function and impact on employment, have been examined. However, more studies have focused on the influence of procto-colectomy on quality of life.

Drossman and colleagues studied the concerns of patients with inflammatory bowel disease [73]. They found that patients with UC worried most frequently about the impact an ostomy bag would have on their lives. Other concerns (in order of decreasing frequency) were cancer, effects of medication, uncertainty about the course of disease, and the need for surgery. These concerns underscore the importance of patient education regarding the natural history of disease, as most of the concerns did not revolve around UC symptoms.

UC patients were more likely to perceive their health as poor when compared to other patients attending a general gastroenterology clinic [74]. They were also more likely to be concerned with their overall health status. They appeared to be as satisfied with the provision of health care as the general population. However, patients with UC did not rank their health as 'poor' and were not as concerned about their health to the degree of patients with CD administered the same questionnaire. The number of patients who sought the services of an alternative medical practitioner was the same as the general clinic population.

Hjortswang and colleagues [75] studied the HRQOL in 211 Swedish patients using the disease-specific Rating Form of IBD Patient Concerns (RFIPC) [76] and the generic Sickness Impact Profile (SIP). Functional impairment as measured by the SIP was primarily seen in the psychosocial and social domains and to a lesser extent in the physical domains. The most prominent scores in the RFIPC were those related to potential complications similar to those described by Drossman. Patients in relapse had greater concerns, more impairment of functional status, and a reduced subjective sense of well-being than patients in clinical remission.

Several studies have compared HRQOL in patients with inflammatory bowel disease compared to other chronic illnesses. Using the SIP (a generic instrument which measures quality of life), two separate groups have [73, 77] measured HRQOL in referral inflammatory bowel disease centers and ranked them with other chronic diseases. UC patients had poorer HRQOL than patients attending a health maintenance organization [73] but better HRQOL than patients with rheumatoid arthritis [73], multiple sclerosis [77], or amyotrophic lateral sclerosis [73]. The HRQOL was worse in patients with CD compared to those with UC.

Employment prospects of patients with UC have been surveyed in the United Kingdom and Denmark. Wyke and colleagues interviewed a random sample of 75 patients with UC attending the gastroenterology unit in Birmingham, UK, in 1978 [78]. A second questionnaire was mailed in 1985 (response rate 80%). The questionnaire gathered information regarding employment status, type of work, continuity of employment, sick times, and time off work following surgery. Other questions focused on the subjects' attitudes regarding employment options (if they were given a stoma), influence of their illness on promotion, and attitudes of peers and employers regarding their illness. Eighty-six percent of the patients were employed (full-time or part-time), attending school, or characterized themselves as homemakers at the time of the initial survey. Six years later this remained almost unchanged at 83%. The unemployment rate was at 2%, which was lower than the regional unemployment rate of 6%.

Patients appeared to have employment stability. Sixty-seven percent of patients remained with the same employer (57% in the same job capacity, 10% in a different capacity). This may reflect a reluctance either to seek out new employment or lose medical benefits. Half of the patients stated their disease or the need for surgery forced them to change their form of occupation, modify their work hours, ask for lighter work, or seek early retirement. Patients regarded the attitudes of employers to be generally helpful in 80% of cases or neutral in 18%. However, 19% of patients had not informed their employer of their disease or whether or not they had an ileostomy.

In evaluating the Danish UC cohort, 90% of the 1161 patients were fully capable of work with less then 1 month per year of disability [32]. Two percent of patients were partially capable of work with complete disability occurring in only 1.5%. The rest of the cohort was incapacitated for reasons unrelated to their UC. Hospital admissions and physician visits declined annually during follow-up, and after 20 years of disease over 90% of patients had no hospitalizations and not more than two physician visits per year.

Most patients who undergo colectomy for UC have a very good prognosis, and their quality of life is excellent. The two most common operative procedures are proctocolectomy with permanent ileostomy and proctocolectomy with ileal pouch–anal anastamosis (IPAA). Burnham and colleagues surveyed 316 married ileostomists who had undergone ileostomy prior to the age of 45 [79]. Fifteen percent of patients were married after the formation of the ileostomy. Sexual intercourse was reported as being difficult in 10% of patients. However, the stoma appeared to be more bothersome for the patient than for the sexual partner. A small proportion of those with a stoma reported that the ileostomy made them feel less sexually attractive. A minority of patients described their stoma as either 'unpleasant' or 'repulsive'. One third of men with rectal excision reported sexual dysfunction, with men over 45 more likely to suffer dysfunction. Patients were comfortable discussing sexual dysfunction with their physicians; however, most believed that they did not receive helpful advice.

The advent of proctocolectomy with IPAA has increased patient acceptance of proctocolectomy and may also improve quality of life. There are numerous studies that have assessed quality of life issues in patients undergoing proctocolectomy with IPAA. In a small surgical cohort from the Mayo Clinic, 69 of 75 consecutive patients undergoing ileal pouch–anal-anastomosis were assessed 1 and 10 years postoperatively [80]. Eight patients had pouches taken down (11%) and 26% had experienced at least one episode of pouchitis. The median stool frequency remained stable at seven stools per 24-hour period. The Mayo Clinic group also published the results of a large series of 1017 patients undergoing proctocolectomy for either UC or familial polyposis at the Mayo Clinic between 1960 and 1988 [81]. The patients were divided into three groups: those undergoing proctocolectomy with Brooke ileostomy between 1960 and 1980, those undergoing proctocolectomy with continent ileostomy (Kock pouch) in the 1980s, and those undergoing proctocolectomy with IPAA in the 1980s. Patients treated with an IPAA reported less interference with sexual function or sporting activities compared to the other two groups of patients. Performance in general categories including social, recreational, work and family variables, was similar for all groups regardless of the surgical procedure.

McLeod and colleagues studied quality of life of patients with UC preoperatively and 1 year following surgery [82]. The study consisted of two separate groups of patients. The first group of 20 patients was studied prospectively before and after surgery. Disease activity was mild in eight, moderate in seven, and severe in five by physician assessment. Three patients underwent proctocolectomy with Brooke ileostomy, two had a subtotal colectomy followed by rectal excision, one had a continent ileostomy, and 14 had ileal reservoirs (IPAA). There were significant improvements in quality of life postoperatively in all surgical groups as assessed by time trade-off (TTO) and direct questioning of objective techniques which are global quality-of-life tools. A second group of 93 patients was studied retrospectively 1 year after undergoing their surgical procedure. Twenty-eight patients had conventional ileostomies, 28 had continent ileostomies, and 37 had ileal reservoirs. Once again the quality of life was excellent in all patients regardless of surgical procedures using the same quality-of-life techniques.

Most recently Provenzale and colleagues [83] reviewed HRQOL in patients undergoing IPAA at Duke University using the SIP, RFIPC, TTO, and another generic measure, the Short Form 36 (SF-36). HRQOL in patients undergoing IPAA was then compared to previous studies assessing HRQOL in other inflammatory bowel disease patients and the general population. HRQOL in IPAA patients was better than that of inflammatory bowel disease patients in a US national sample when compared by SIP and RFIPC, and similar to that of a normal population when compared by SF-36.

Quality of life is impaired in patients with UC. Many of the patients' worries and concerns surround uncertainty revolving the natural history of their disease. However, quality of life is improved significantly to normal or near-normal levels in those patients undergoing proctocolectomy with Brooke ileostomy or IPAA.

Ulcerative colitis in the elderly

The clinical features in the elderly patient presenting with UC are generally similar to those of patients presenting at a younger age. However, there are certain differences that will be outlined.

In elderly patients with bloody diarrhea the differential diagnosis is broad. It includes infectious colitis, medication-induced colitis (antibiotics, non-steroidal anti-inflammatory agents, chemotherapeutic agents, gold, penicillamine), and Crohn's colitis as in younger patients. However, the entities of ischemic colitis, acute diverticulitis, and radiation proctocolitis are more common in the elderly. Carr and Schofield [84] stressed the importance of careful investigation in patients with left-sided colitis who may in fact have CD, acute diverticulitis, or ischemic colitis rather than UC.

At the time of presentation, patients older than 60 have been shown to have less extensive, predominantly distal, disease. Watts and colleagues [53] found that 42% of older patients presented with proctitis, whereas 12% presented with pancolitis compared to patients younger than 60 where the rates were 33% and 26.5% respectively. This was also demonstrated by Zimmerman and colleagues [85], who noted that older patients had more diarrhea than rectal bleeding, a longer duration of activity following diagnosis, and spent less time in clinical remission. This may have been due in part to a decrease in the response to topical corticosteroids and the subsequent requirement of systemic steroids. However, other studies have shown conflicting data. Gupta and colleagues [86] reported reported that patients over the age of 60 developing UC had a similar spectrum of disease and responded to conventional therapy.

One might expect that the higher frequency of distal disease in elderly patients would translate into less clinical severity. This did not appear to be the case in the population-based northeastern Scotland study, in which Sinclair *et al.* found that 14% of patients presenting after the age of 70 had a severe initial attack, compared to 7% of patients younger than the age of 30, and 3% of patients between the ages of 30 and 69 [10]. This increase in severity resulted in an increased mortality in patients over the age of 70 when compared to the group under the age of 70. Other earlier studies of elderly patients also suggested a more aggressive and ominous course [87–89]. In the Edinburgh study the mortality related to UC in the group of patients over 50 was almost double that of any other age group [89]. However, it has been suggested that referral bias, small numbers, less aggressive medical therapy, and the inclusion of patients with ischemic colitis may have affected these earlier studies.

Not all studies have demonstrated a worse prognosis for elderly patients. More recent studies have suggested that patients older than age 60 respond well to medical management, may have lower rates of relapse than younger patients, and have mortality rates comparable to age-matched controls [90]. Hen-dricksen *et al.* [31] noted only a slight increase in mortality in patients diagnosed over the age of 40 over an 18-year period in the population-based Dutch cohort. The increase in mortality in the older patients was seen within the first 2 years of diagnosis; thereafter, the survival rate was no different than that in younger patients.

Jones and Hoare studied whether UC indeed did behave differently in the elderly [91]. They compared the clinical course of patients diagnosed with UC after the age of 65 with patients diagnosed prior to age 55. Twenty percent of the patients diagnosed were over the age of 65. The proportion of patients admitted to hospital for the first attack was twice that of the younger group (26% vs. 13%, $p < 0.02$). The exact reason for the increase in hospitalization rate could not be determined and physician bias may have played a role. Older patients were more likely to require systemic corticosteroids; however, there was no difference in the requirement for urgent or elective colectomy. The mortality rate in the patients diagnosed after the age of 65 was no different than that of age- and sex-matched controls.

There has been a suggestion that elderly patients are at increased risk of developing toxic dilation of the colon; however, this area has not been well studied and controversy remains. One study reported that 20% of elderly patients developed toxic megacolon [84]; however, this was not detected in two other studies [86, 91].

Complications

UC is associated with various complications that often affect clinical management decisions. The complications of UC can be divided into local or colonic complications and extracolonic complications. The risk of the development of dysplasia and adenocarcinoma are discussed in Chapter 36. Extracolonic complications of UC is discussed in Chapters 38, 39, and 40. The colonic complications of UC, including anorectal lesions, fistulas, toxic dilation, perforation, stricture, and massive hemorrhage are discussed in this section (Table 5).

Anorectal lesions

The presence of anorectal lesions, including hemorrhoids, large perianal skin tags, anal fissures, and perianal abscesses, is much more common in patients with CD than in UC. In extensive perianal involvement a diagnosis of CD should be sought. It is not uncommon for patients with terminal ileal CD to have concurrent isolated proctitis that may be mistaken for ulcerative proctitis. In this situation full radiologic evaluation of the small bowel to rule out CD is recommended. With this in mind, patients with UC may develop perianal lesions, but this is uncommon.

Four percent of patients in the Oxford series [92] gave a history of ischiorectal or perianal abscess. There appeared to be no relationship between the duration of symptoms and the development of an abscess. It is unknown whether any of these patients were later diagnosed as having CD. Twenty percent of patients in the Oxford series had hemorrhoids. Hemorrhoids are best managed conservatively and surgical intervention should be avoided.

Patients with UC may develop fissures in relationship to their disease or possibly as a result of traumatic injury from local therapy. Control of rectal inflammation is essential in aiding in the healing process of these lesions.

Fistulas

The presence of fistula(s) must always bring into mind the diagnosis of CD. Patients diagnosed with UC who develop fistulas during the course of their disease often later have their diagnosis changed to CD after further investigation. These abnormal communications between the gut lumen and the mesentery, another hollow organ, or the skin are rare in UC. Fistula-in-ano was documented in 4% of patients in the Oxford series [92]. Internal fistulas have been rarely documented in UC with the exception of rectovaginal fistulas, which were reported by 3% of women at Oxford [92].

Toxic megacolon

Toxic megacolon refers to the dilation of the colon during the course of severe, usually fulminant extensive involvement or pancolitis. It is a severe complication associated with considerable risk of requiring immediate surgical intervention. The frequency is unknown and differs from series to series. The incidence may be decreasing over time with the improvement of medical therapy. The diagnosis of toxic megacolon is made clinically based on clinical signs of toxic colitis (abdominal distension, peritoneal signs, fever $> 101°F$ ($38°C$), tachycardia

Table 5. Colonic complications of ulcerative colitis

Anorectal lesions
Rectal abscess
Fistula
Toxic megacolon
Perforation
Stricture
Massive hemorrhage

over $120/min$, and leukocytosis over $11 \times 10^9/L$ with radiological or pathological evidence of a dilated colon [93]. The diagnosis is often made on plain radiographs when the colonic diameter exceeds 6 cm with evidence of mucosal or transmural inflammation ('thumb printing') [94].

The frequency of toxic megacolon varies between series. In the Oxford series 10 of 624 patients (1.6%) were described as having acute dilation of the colon [92]. This figure is much lower than that described by Jalan and colleagues, in which study 13% of patients (55 patients) were diagnosed with toxic megacolon between 1950 and 1967 [93]. The development of toxic megacolon in this patient population was associated with a mortality rate of 26%. Approximately 50% of the patients developed their toxic dilation within 3 months of symptom onset. The rest of the patients with toxic megacolon developed the complication as part of a relapse, which varied between 6 months and 10 years from the initial diagnosis.

The vast majority of patients with toxic megacolon will ultimately require surgery. In a review of patients treated medically for toxic megacolon at the Mayo Clinic, 30% had a recurrent episode of toxic megacolon or fulminant colitis. Fifty percent of the patients required proctocolectomy [95].

In an early Mount Sinai Hospital series from New York 61 patients (representing 10% of all UC patients) were admitted for toxic megacolon between 1960 and 1979 [3]. Most of the patients had pancolitis but 10% had disease limited to the left colon (defined as disease distal to the hepatic flexure). Fifty percent of the patients developed toxic megacolon during their first attack of UC. The mortality rate in this group of patients was 16% and was not influenced by: (1) duration of disease, (2) first episode or relapse, or (3) whether the patient underwent medical or surgical management. Mortality was higher in patients over 40 years of age (30% vs. 5%), those undergoing early (less than 5 days) or late (greater than 30 days) surgery (32% vs. 6%). The authors concluded that the difference in the mortality rate and surgical timing was attributed to the presence of perforation in the cases of early surgery and the prolonged severe course in those cases of late surgery. Perforation was associated with the highest mortality with 44% of patients with documented perforation dying. Eleven patients with toxic megacolon improved with medical therapy; however, six of the 11 (55%) eventually required proctocolectomy.

Perforation

Most perforations are associated with the development of toxic megacolon; however, perforation may occur in UC in the absence of toxic dilation. In the Oxford series 3% of patients had a perforation and the majority occurred during the first attack [92]. The most common site for perforation was the sigmoid colon (60%), followed by the descending colon (20%), cecum (10%), and all other sites (10%) [92]. There was no correlation seen between the use of corticosteroids and the frequency of perforations.

In the Mount Sinai series between 1960 and 1979 [3], seven of the 522 patients (1.3%) had a free perforation in the absence of toxic megacolon. Free perforation was associated with a high mortality (57%) in these patients comparable to patients with perforation in the setting of toxic megacolon (44%).

Strictures

Strictures are the most common local complication of UC in most series when pseudopolyposis and hemorrhoids are excluded. The frequency of strictures varies between 6.3% and 11% [92, 96]. For decades it has been thought that these strictures represented fibrous strictures; however, this may not be the case. Goulston and McGovern suggested that the amount of narrowing that is seen is not accounted for pathologically by the degree of fibrosis. They suggest that the narrowing is caused by contraction of the muscularis mucosa rather than irreversible fibrosis [97]. This changes traditional dogma because, based on this theory, a course of medical therapy may be reasonable before proceeding to surgery. However, there is always the concern that strictures in UC may represent an area of dysplasia and/or focus of adenocarcinoma.

Strictures that develop within the first several years following diagnosis presumably have a lower malignant potential than those that develop in patients with long-standing disease. However, neoplasia is always a concern; therefore brushings and biopsies in the area with close surveillance are mandatory if surgery is not performed. However, it has been shown that endoscopic surveillance does not prevent the development of adenocarcinoma [98]. Contrast studies should be performed in conjunction with colonoscopy to define the length of strictures and to exclude any other potential narrowed areas. This is most important in those patients in whom a distal stricture does not allow for complete endoscopic examination of the colon. The authors have a low threshold in recommending surgical intervention among patients with strictures in the setting of UC.

In the Oxford series, 39 of 624 patients (6.3%) developed strictures [92]. Most of these strictures were found distally in the rectum and sigmoid colon. Strictures presented with both constipation, and in many cases diarrhea, giving the impression of active disease. Edwards and Truelove recommended surgery for any stricture in part to ensure its benign nature [92].

Eleven per cent of patients were found to have rectal or colonic strictures in a retrospective review of 465 patients from Leeds [96]. This figure may be high given the usual referral bias. Fifteen percent of patients were documented to have their strictures with their initial attack. The duration of symptoms did not necessarily correlate with the development of a stricture. The strictures were multiple in 25% of cases. Many of the strictures were identified by endoscopic or barium examination, however, a few were only identified intraoperatively. The risk of stricture development was highest in those patients with the most extensive disease.

Massive hemorrhage

Severe gastrointestinal hemorrhage requiring emergency surgical intervention is a rare complication of UC. However, when this rare complication does occur surgery is usually required as endoscopic or radiographic intervention to stop the bleeding is usually unsuccessful.

Robert and colleagues from Mount Sinai Hospital in New York reviewed this topic [99]. The review was drawn from the experience of several large centers with an interest in the medical or surgical management of inflammatory bowel disease. The range of massive hemorrhage was between 0% and 4.5%.

72. Michener WM, Farmer RG, Mortimer EA. Long-term prognosis of ulcerative colitis with onset in childhood or adolescence. J Clin Gastroenterol 1979; 1: 301–5.

73. Drossman DA, Patrick DL, Mitchell CM, Zagami EA, Appelbaum MI. Health-related quality of life in inflammatory bowel disease. Functional status and patient worries and concerns. Dig Dis Sci 1989; 34: 1379–86.

74. Verhoef MJ, Sutherland LR. Outpatient health care utilization of patients with inflammatory bowel disease. Dig Dis Sci 1990; 35: 1276–80.

75. Hjortswang H, Strom M, Almer S. Health-related quality of life in Swedish patients with ulcerative colitis. Am J Gastroenterol 1998; 93: 2203–11.

76. Sullivan M, Ahlmen M, Archenholtz B, Svensson G. Measuring health in rheumatic disorders by means of a Swedish version of the sickness impact profile. Results from a population study. Scand J Rheumatol 1986; 15: 193–200.

77. Farmer RG, Easley KA, Farmer JM. Quality of life assessment by patients with inflammatory bowel disease [See comments]. Cleve Clin J Med 1992; 59: 35–42.

78. Wyke RJ, Edwards FC, Allan RN. Employment problems and prospects for patients with inflammatory bowel disease [Published erratum appears in Gut 1988; 1756]. Gut 1988; 29: 1229–35.

79. Burnham WR, Lennard-Jones JE, Brooke BN. Sexual problems among married ileostomists. Survey conducted by the Ileostomy Association of Great Britain and Ireland. Gut 1977; 18: 673–7.

80. McIntyre PB, Pemberton JH, Wolff BG, Beart RW, Dozois RR. Comparing functional results one year and ten years after ileal pouch–anal anastomosis for chronic ulcerative colitis. Dis Colon Rectum 1994; 37: 303–7.

81. Kohler LW, Pemberton JH, Zinsmeister AR, Kelly KA. Quality of life after proctocolectomy. A comparison of Brooke ileostomy, Kock pouch, and ileal pouch–anal anastomosis [See comments]. Gastroenterology 1991; 101: 679–84.

82. McLeod RS, Churchill DN, Lock AM, Vanderburgh S, Cohen Z. Quality of life of patients with ulcerative colitis preoperatively and postoperatively. Gastroenterology 1991; 101: 1307–13.

83. Provenzale D, Shearin M, Phillips-Bute BG et al. Health-related quality of life after ileoanal pull-through evaluation and assessment of new health status measures. Gastroenterology 1997; 113: 7–14.

84. Carr N, Schofield PF. Inflammatory bowel disease in the older patient. Br J Surg 1982; 69: 223–5.

85. Zimmerman J, Gavish D, Rachmilewitz D. Early and late onset ulcerative colitis: distinct clinical features. J Clin Gastroenterol 1985; 7: 492–8.

86. Gupta S, Saverymuttu SH, Keshavarzian A, Hodgson HJ. Is the pattern of inflammatory bowel disease different in the elderly? Age Ageing 1985; 14: 366–70.

87. Earle E, Rowe RJ. Ulcerative disease of the large intestine in patients more than 50 years old. Dis Colon Rectum 1972; 15: 33–40.

88. Brandt LJ, Boley SJ, Mitsudo S. Clinical characteristics and natural history of colitis in the elderly. Am J Gastroenterol 1982; 77: 382–6.

89. Jalan KN, Prescott RJ, Sircus W et al. An experience of ulcerative colitis. 3. Long term outcome. Gastroenterology 1970; 59: 598–609.

90. Fleischer DE, Grimm IS, Friedman LS. Inflammatory bowel disease in older patients. Med Clin N Am 1994; 78: 1303–19.

91. Jones HW, Hoare AM. Does ulcerative colitis behave differently in the elderly? Age Ageing 1988; 17: 410–4.

92. Edwards F, Truelove SC. The course and prognosis of ulcerative colitis III. Complications. Gut 1964; 5: 1–15.

93. Jalan KN, Sircus W, Card WI et al. An experience of ulcerative colitis. I. Toxic dilation in 55 cases. Gastroenterology 1969; 57: 68–82.

94. Marshak R. Toxic dilatation of the colon in the course of ulcerative colitis. Gastroenterology 1960; 38: 165.

95. Grant CS, Dozois RR. Toxic megacolon: ultimate fate of patients after successful medical management. Am J Surg 1984; 147: 106–10.

96. De Dombal FT, Watts JM, Watkinson G, Goligher JC. Local complications of ulcerative colitis: stricture, pseudopolyposis, and carcinoma of colon and rectum. Br Med J 1966; 5501: 1442–7.

97. Goulston SJ, McGovern VJ. Nature of strictures in chronic ulcerative colitis. Gut 1969; 10: 952.

98. Reiser JR, Waye JD, Janowitz HD, Harpaz N. Adenocarcinoma in strictures of ulcerative colitis without antecedent dysplasia by colonoscopy. Am J Gastroenterol 1994; 89: 119–22.

99. Robert JH, Sachar DB, Aufses AH, Jr., Greenstein AJ. Management of severe hemorrhage in ulcerative colitis. Am J Surg 1990; 159: 550–5.

15 | Clinical features and complications of Crohn's disease

WILLIAM J. TREMAINE

Introduction

The diagnosis of Crohn's disease (CD) is based on an array of clinical findings, as there is no single definitive diagnostic test. The clinical features are many and varied and it is unknown if CD is a single entity or the common presentation of several diseases. Laboratory, radiological and endoscopic studies are helpful, but making the correct diagnosis of CD depends on the skills of a seasoned clinician to assimilate information from the history and physical findings, as well as diagnostic tests. Despite the advances in the development of laboratory studies and imaging, recognition and interpretation of clinical findings is the most important aspect of the management of this disease.

Clinical subtypes

There have been numerous attempts to divide CD into subgroups with common clinical presentations [1–7]. The aim has been to sort out disease characteristics that have more predictable courses than the unpredictable natural history of CD taken as a whole. Genetic associations between the phenotypic subgroups of CD have been noted, although subgroup identification and analysis is still in the state of evolution [8–10]. Current classifications are convenient for description but they are still lacking in prognostic value. Until the etiology of CD is identified, a classification based on genetic findings, the presence or absence of antibodies and clinical phenotype could improve our ability, to target therapy and identify groups at higher risk for complications.

Table 1. Symptoms by anatomic distribution

	Ileocolonic (n = 473) (%)	Ileal (n = 310) (%)	Colonic (n = 320) (%)
Diarrhea	91	89	93
Abdominal pain	66	67	68
Rectal bleeding	19	9	41
Perianal disease (fistula, fissure, abscess)	24	7	27
Weight loss	28	22	38

Adapted from refs 1, 11, and 12.

Anatomical classification

CD has been subcategorized based on the area of anatomic involvement at presentation (Table 1). Farmer *et al.* noted that 41% of patients present with ileocolonic disease, 28.6% present with ileal involvement only, and 27% present with colonic involvement only [1]. The remaining 3.4% of patients presented with perianal disease and all developed more proximal gastrointestinal involvement with CD in follow-up [2]. The relationship between the clinical pattern at presentation and the prognosis for the disease has been sought. In a retrospective study of 615 patients from the Cleveland Clinic, patients with ileocolonic involvement required surgery more commonly than those with small intestinal disease only or colonic or anorectal disease only [1]. Overall, patients with ileocolonic disease had a poorer prognosis then those with other regions of involvement. Although useful for disease description, classifications based only on disease location do not differentiate patients based on disease severity or prognosis. In 1988 a classification based on perforating and non-perforating indications for surgery for CD identified patterns independent of anatomic distribution, with perforating disease following an

Stephan R. Targan, Fergus Shanahan and Loren C. Karp (eds.), *Inflammatory Bowel Disease: From Bench to Bedside, 2nd Edition*, 291–304.
© 2003 *Kluwer Academic Publishers. Printed in Great Britain*

aggressive course and non-perforating disease having a more indolent course [3]. The Rome classification of 1992 combined disease location, behavior (inflammatory, fistulizing, or fibrostenotic disease) and operative history (primary disease or recurrent disease following surgery) to create 756 subgroups so that the practicality was limited [4]. A Vienna classification reduced the variables to 24 subgroups based on age at diagnosis, disease location, and disease behavior. More recently, application of the Vienna classification to a population-based cohort of CD and two aggressive phenotypes, penetrating ileal disease in patients aged less than 40 and penetrating ileal disease in patients greater than 40 years of age, were identified [6]. A retrospective study of 88 patients reported from Philadelphia confirmed that penetrating disease carries a poor prognosis and, in addition, an early postoperative recurrence also does [7].

Serologic classification

Future refinements in the classification of CD will likely include genetic and serologic data. For example, the antineutrophil cytoplasmic antibody is usually positive in patients with CD limited to the colon [8, 9]. The expression of anti-*Saccharomyces cerevisiae* antibody (ASCA) is a marker for familial Crohn's [10]. Higher ASCA levels have been shown to be independently associated with an early age of onset of disease, as well as both fibrostenosing and internal penetrating disease behaviors (Fig. 1) [11].

Disease presentation

It is useful to look at CD from an anatomic distribution, to understand the clinical manifestations, despite the limitations for characterizing disease prognosis (Table 2)

Ileocolonic disease

The most common presentation of CD is involvement of the distal ileum and right colon. Two-thirds of patients have abdominal pain, usually cramping, most prominent in the right lower abdomen [1, 12, 13]. In patients with partial bowel obstruction due to stenosis the pain is usually made worse while eating solids, or within 30–60 min after a meal. About 22% of patients with ileocolonic disease have blood in the bowel movements, usually mixed in with the stool.

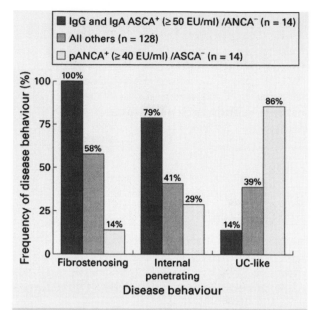

Figure 1. Substratification using selected expression of immune markers. Disease behavior characteristics were examined in more immunologically homogeneous subgroups of patients with Crohn's disease (CD) (those expressing high levels of a single marker antibody) and compared with all other CD study patients. Overall differences in proportions were evaluated using the χ^2 test for trend ($p < 0.001$ for each of the disease behavior characteristics). (From ref. 11, with permission.)

Table 2. Symptomatic Crohn's disease anatomic location

	Adult	Children
Ileocolonic	41–55%	50–60%
Ileal	29–41%	30–35%
Colonic	14–27%	10–15%
Perianal	22–47%	49–50%
Jejunal	4–10%	
Gastroduodenal	5%	30%
Esophageal	Rare	Rare
Oral	Rare	Rare

Adpated from refs. 1 and 42.

About 20% of patients have perianal disease with fistulas. About 12% have clinical features of malnutrition with weight loss and muscle wasting. Extra-intestinal manifestations including pyoderma gangrenosum, colitic arthritis, and spondylitis occur at a lesser frequency than in patients with CD limited to the colon [14]. In a follow-up study from the Cleveland Clinic, 7–13 years after initial observation, 225 of 246 patients (91.5%) with ileocolonic disease had required at least one surgical resection of the distal ileum, the right colon, or both [2]. The most common reasons for surgery, in descending order of frequency, were intestinal obstruction, perianal disease, intestinal perforation with abscess, and toxic megacolon. Long-term survival was similar in patients with ileocolonic disease as compared to those with other presentations, with a 10-year survival of 94% [2].

Ileal disease

Patients with CD limited to the ileum usually have diarrhea, abdominal pain, and weight loss, but have significantly fewer perianal fistulas than patients with colonic or ileocolonic disease and less rectal bleeding than patients with colonic disease [1, 12, 13]. The presentation is variable and onset may be sudden with severe symptoms or insidious with mild symptoms. Diarrhea, the most common symptom, can be intermittent, postprandial, daytime, and mild, resembling irritable bowel syndrome, or it can be severe with frequent nocturnal stools. The abdominal pain is usually localized to the right lower abdominal quadrant and is typically cramping in nature. The pain often occurs during a meal, or within 30 min following a meal, and the pain is worse with a large or high-fiber meal. Weight loss is usually due to a decreased caloric intake, although with extensive disease weight loss may be a combination of diminished intake and malabsorption. Patients may have low-grade fever and may present as a fever of unknown origin (FUO): in a series of 199 consecutive patients who met the classic criteria for FUO, four (2%) had CD [15]. With inflammatory disease there may be a palpable right lower abdominal mass that is firm and mildly tender, and the mass may be of such a size as to cause asymmetry of the lower abdomen, particularly in a thin patient. In women the mass may be palpable on bimanual pelvic examination, extending into the right pelvis. Signs and symptoms of malabsorption can occur with extensive ileal disease, including muscle wasting, edema, vertebral fractures, bruising, and growth impairment in children.

Colonic disease

The most common symptoms of CD isolated to the colon are diarrhea, abdominal pain, and weight loss [1, 12, 13]. Rectal bleeding and perianal disease are

significantly more common than in isolated ileal or ileocolonic disease. The diarrhea may be intermittent and non-bloody. However, there is a subgroup of patients with 'ulcerative colitis-like' CD who have left-sided colonic involvement with rectal bleeding, mucus discharge, fecal urgency, and who respond to treatment with per-rectal therapy with mesalamine or steroids, similar to patients with ulcerative colitis (UC). The serologic profile is the same as in UC, with a positive pANCA antibody and a negative ASCA antibody [8]. In a long-term follow-up study, 24% of 507 patients with colorectal CD subsequently developed small intestinal involvement [16]. Approximately one-half of patients with colonic CD require surgical resection within 10 years of diagnosis and half of those patients ultimately require ileostomy [16].

Perianal disease

Perianal involvement in CD occurs in 22–47% of patients [12, 13, 16, 17], including ulcers, fistulas, abscesses, and strictures. Perianal disease has been classified based on anatomic and pathologic findings and disease severity, initially as the Cardiff Classification, subsequently modified into a simplified clinical classification based on the presence and severity of ulceration, fistula/abscess, and stricture (Table 3) [17]. Involvement is more common with colonic and ileocolonic disease than with small intestinal disease alone. In patients with colonic CD, perianal disease is more common when there is left-sided colonic involvement than when there is only proximal involvement of the colon. In a series from Sweden, 35–45% of patients who had disease involving the left colon had perianal disease compared to 7% of patients who had only proximal disease [16]. Perianal disease may be subclassified as skin lesions, anal canal lesions, and fistulas [18]. Skin lesions include perianal ulceration, abscess, skin tags, and maceration. The skin tags are often edematous and non-tender, and they can cover an ulcer, in which

Table 3. Simplified clinical classification of perianal Crohn's disease

Ulceration	Fistula/abscess	Stricture
Not present	Not present	Not present
Superficial fissure	Low/superficial	Spasm/membranous
Cavitating ulcer	High/complex	Severe fibrotic

case they are known as a sentinel tag. Anal canal disease includes fissures, ulcers, or stenosis. In contrast to anal fissures found in patients who do not have CD, the fissures are usually eccentrically placed laterally, rather than in the midline. The fissures are often non-tender and asymptomatic, and the presence of pain and tenderness may indicate an underlying abscess. There are limited data on the medical therapy of perianal CD. In uncontrolled trials, metronidazole, 6-mercaptopurine, cyclosporine A, and tacrolimus have apparent efficacy. In a controlled trial using 6-mercaptopurine, subgroup analysis showed complete closure of fistulas, including perianal fistulas, in nine of 29 (31%) compared to one of 17 (6%) on placebo [19]. A controlled trial of infliximab given as three intravenous doses over 6 weeks healed cutaneous fistulas, including perianal fistulas, in 55% [20]. The surgical management of perianal disease is usually conservative, to avoid injury to the sphincteric musculature. However, surgical treatment of fissures that have not healed medically may prevent progression to abscess and fistula formation [21]. For more complex disease, seton placement may spare loss of sphincter function [22, 23].

Upper gastrointestinal involvement

CD of the upper gastrointestinal tract is uncommon. The predominant symptom is epigastric, non-radiating pain relieved by acid-blocking therapy, mimicking peptic ulcer disease. Other symptoms include nausea, vomiting, and weight loss [24]. Early satiety, nausea, and vomiting may be due to delayed gastric emptying, even without mechanical obstruction [25].

As in the case of ileal CD, the weight loss is primarily due to decreased caloric intake. Diarrhea is not a prominent symptom and may be due to distal intestinal disease rather than the upper tract involvement. In a recent series from England, 61% of patients required surgery, most for relief of obstruction [26].

The data on prevalence vary widely in series and depend on the criteria for diagnosis. Nugent [43] proposed that one of two criteria must be met to make the diagnosis of upper gastrointestinal tract CD: (1) the presence of non-caseating granulomas in mucosal biopsies, with or without involvement more distally, and without systemic granulomatous disease; or (2) upper gastrointestinal tract disease consistent with CD with documented CD in the ileum, colon, or both ileum and colon. From prevalence

data from a registry of 940 patients with CD at the University Hospital, Leiden, The Netherlands, 72 (8%) of patients had disease in the mouth, esophagus, stomach, duodenum, or jejunum, and all had gastrointestinal symptoms [27]. The age at onset of CD is lower in those with upper gastrointestinal tract involvement than in those patients with only distal intestinal or colonic involvement. [27]. The prevalence is higher in series that include asymptomatic patients and children. For example, in a prospective study of 31 children from France, only 16% had symptoms of upper gastrointestinal involvement, but there were endoscopic abnormalities compatible with CD found at upper gastrointestinal endoscopy in 42% and biopsies revealed granulomas in 39% [28]. Among 32 consecutive children with CD of the distal small intestine or colon, 80% had abnormalities on upper gastrointestinal endoscopy, including 44% with duodenal disease [29]. CD limited to the esophagus, stomach, duodenum, or jejunum without ileocolonic involvement has been reported [30–32].

The prevalence of gastroduodenal granulomas in CD varies in studies from 7% to 83%, with the higher prevalence when serial sections were prepared from multiple biopsies [33]. Although transmural inflammation and epithelioid granulomas are the hallmarks of CD in the lower gastrointestinal tract, an additional characteristic lesion, focally enhanced gastritis, is relatively common in CD of the stomach [34]. The lesion consists of a perifoveolar or periglandular accumulation of $CD68R^+$ histiocytes and $CD3^+$ lymphocytes and, in 80% of cases, granulocytes. In a prospective study of 75 patients with CD the characteristic lesion of focally enhanced gastritis was found in 76% of the *Helicobacter pylori* patients and in only one of 122 (0.8%) of *Helicobacter pylori*-negative controls [34].

The high prevalence of focally enhanced gastritis underscores the systemic nature of CD. Patients with upper gastrointestinal symptoms should be investigated for gastroduodenal involvement. The finding of focally enhanced gastritis could prove useful in confirming the diagnosis of CD in patients with atypical findings in the lower intestinal tract, such as in patients with indeterminate colitis.

Esophageal disease

Esophageal CD is rare and was found in 20 patients (0.2%) of 9900 patients with CD seen at the Mayo Clinic between 1976 and 1998 [35], and in nine of 500 patients in Belgium [36]. CD limited to the esophagus has been described in a few patients [30, 37]. Granulomas were not found in mucosal biopsies from any of the 20 patients in the Mayo series [35] and granulomas were found in five of nine patients in the Belgian series [36]: instead, biopsies usually show non-specific chronic inflammation. Symptoms referable to the esophagus occur in 80–100% of patients [35, 36]. At endoscopy, ulcers are present in 85%, with strictures in 25% [28]. Most patients improve with medical therapy [35, 38], about half respond to acid suppression and corticosteroids, and half required immunosuppressive therapy. In the series of 20 patients from the Mayo Clinic, three patients failed medical therapy including immunosuppression and underwent esophagectomy [35].

Gastric disease

Gastric involvement with CD was found in five (0.5 %) of 940 patients in a series form Leiden, The Netherlands [27]. Abdominal cramping pain is the most common symptom, and less common symptoms are diarrhea, weight loss, and malaise. Nausea and vomiting usually occur as a consequence of gastric outlet obstruction. Endoscopic features include: (1) mucosal nodularity or 'cobblestoned' mucosa; (2) multiple aphthous-like ulcerations and/ or linear ulcerations; (3) thickening of the antral folds; (4) antral narrowing with evidence of hypoperistalsis [39]. Fistulas to the colon [40, 41] and spleen [26] have been reported. Gastric mucosal biopsies in patients with distal CD reveal granulomas in 11% and focal inflammatory infiltrates in the gastric mucosa were present in 23 (63%) of 36 patients [42]. Therapy for inflammatory disease with a combination of an H_2-blocker or proton-pump inhibitor, and an immunosuppressive appear effective, although there are no controlled data. Gastric fistulas usually require partial gastric resection [27, 32, 40].

Duodenal disease

Duodenal CD occurs in 1–7% of cases [39, 43–45]. Usually, the bulb and second portion of the duodenum along with the prepyloric antrum are involved [45]. This is the same distribution of disease seen in *H. pylori* infection, but the prevalence of *H. pylori* infection is no greater than that found in controls with dyspepsia and *H. pylori* does not appear to be the cause of inflammation in these patients [46]. Duodenal disease usually occurs along with ileal or colonic involvement and predominant symptoms are abdominal pain, diarrhea, weight loss, anorexia, and malaise. Early satiety, nausea, and vomiting can occur with or without duodenal obstruction. The endoscopic findings are similar to those seen in CD of the ileum or colon, with aphthous ulcers, linear ulcers, thickened folds, changes, and strictures [47]. The histologic findings may be indistinguishable from peptic ulcer disease [44]. Treatment of duodenal CD has not been tested in prospective trials. It appears that a combination of acid suppression with an H_2-blocker [24] or proton-pump inhibitor [45], along with corticosteroids or an immunosuppressive agent such as 6-mercaptopurine or azathioprine [24, 48], is effective. Up to 40% of patients with gastroduodenal CD require surgery, usually because of obstruction, but is some cases because of bleeding, symptomatic fistulas, or suspicion of malignancy [49]. Gastrojejunal bypass should be performed without vagotomy because of the higher risk of marginal ulcers with vagotomy [24]. Most patients who undergo surgery have good to excellent results, even when reoperation is required [24].

Jejunal disease

Jejunal involvement was found in 4% and 7% of patients in two large clinical series [27, 50]. Disease may involve single or multiple jejunal segments in association with ileal or colonic disease, or as diffuse jejunoileitis. In contrast to ileitis or duodenitis, strictures are more common with jejunal disease at the time of diagnosis [49, 51], with strictures in 69-71% of patients [52–55]. Diffuse jejunoileal involvement was found in 34 (5.7%) of patients with CD from a referral center in Birmingham, UK [55]. Cramping abdominal pain occurred in more than 90%, and the majority had weight loss and diarrhea. Most patients required one or more surgical procedures of relief of obstruction, usually with strictureplasty or limited resection for areas of tight stenosis. Infliximab appears effective in two-thirds of patients [56]. In adults, corticosteroids and immune modulators are the primary medical therapies [57]. The aminosalicylates have not been proven to be of benefit for jejunal or other proximal gastrointestinal involvement with CD. In children, enteral feeding, rather than corticosteroids, is used for diffuse jejunal disease [58].

Oral disease

Oral lesions are found in 4% of patients with CD and in 11% of those with Crohn's colitis [59]. In a series of 75 patients with oral lesions the oral manifestations were the presenting feature in 60%, with lesions found in decreasing order of frequency on the inner lips, gingiva, soft palate, and buccal mucosa [60]. Granulomas are present in about two-thirds of the lesions. Granulomatous oral lesions also occur in the Meldersson–Rosentahl syndrome, but the latter condition also includes a fissured tongue and facial paresis, which do not occur with oral CD [61]. Treatments include corticosteroids by topical, intralesional, or systemic routes, or azathioprine or 6-mercaptopurine, and recent reports show promise using nicotine gum and thalidomide [62].

Extraintestinal manifestations of Crohn's disease

These are reviewed in Chapter 16.

Crohn's disease in older individuals

The onset of CD occurred at age 40 or older in 17% of patients in a population-based study from Olmsted County, Minnesota, with data from 1991 [63]. Patients with onset of disease at age 40 or older ($n = 98$) were compared to younger patients ($n = 347$) in a retrospective study from Leiden University in The Netherlands [27, 61]. The time from onset of symptoms was significantly shorter in the older than in the younger patients (1.8 vs 2.7 years), perhaps because of the greater concern to exclude ischemic colitis, diverticulitis, or malignancy in the elderly [64]. The frequency of diarrhea, rectal bleeding, and weight loss was similar in the two groups, but older individuals have less abdominal pain or cramps [27]. Side-effects of corticosteroids are no more common among patients age 50–65 as compared to those over age 65 years [65]. Mesalamine has the potential to cause interstitial nephritis, and older as well as younger patients should be assessed for renal insufficiency prior to treatment and regularly while on therapy, although the appropriate frequency of monitoring is not well established [66]. Abdominal surgery among older patients has a similar mortality and anastomotic leakage rate, as found in a retrospective study of 33 patients age 55 or older compared to 123 patients younger than age 55 [67]. However, the older patients had significantly more cardiac (18.2% vs 0.8%) and respiratory (18.2% vs 2.4%) complications [67] than younger patients.

Complications

Complications include directs effects of the disease and also side-effects of the medical and surgical treatments.

Strictures

Current classifications of CD include disease behavior, determined by the presence or absence of strictures or fistulas [5]. Strictures were uncommon at presentation in a series of 221 patients from Oxford, UK, with 12 (5%) with intestinal obstruction [68]. In contrast, intestinal obstruction was a presenting feature in 33% of 615 patients at the Cleveland Clinic, and developed in 36% of 592 of the original group of patients followed for a mean of 13 years [2]. Obstruction was more common in patients with ileocolic or isolated small intestinal disease than with isolated colonic disease. The number and length of small intestinal strictures is highly variable. Of 244 patients who underwent exploration for complications of CD, 35 (14%) had short strictures of less than 3 cm up to 10 cm in length, with a mean of two strictures per patient, and as many as eight short strictures in one patient [69]. Twenty-four patients (10%) had resections of longer lengths of bowel, in addition to the strictureplasties [69]. Small intestinal strictures are usually identified by plain abdominal films or by single-contrast, per-oral barium studies. In a patient with obstructive symptoms in whom these studies are unrevealing, small intestinal enteroclysis or transabdominal ultrasonography may be diagnostic [70]. In a prospective trial of 44 patients, both enteroclysis and ultrasound had a diagnostic accuracy for strictures of 80% [71]. Computerize tomography has a sensitivity and specificity of 71% and 98%, respectively, for detecting bowel pathology. In contrast, granulocyte scintigraphy may not identify fibrotic strictures unless there is contiguous active inflammation [72].

Fistulas

In a population-based study from Stockholm County, Sweden, 37% of 507 patients with colonic CD had one or more fistulas [16]. This compares to a frequency of fistulas of 47% in patients with colonic

CD entered into the National Cooperative CD study in the US: the higher frequency in the latter study may reflect a referral bias [12]. Fistulas are most common with ileocolonic disease, occurring in more than one-third of patients [1]. Internal fistulas are usually symptomatic with diarrhea, fever, abdominal pain, and weight loss. In a series of 90 patients with ileosigmoid fistulas, 84 (93%) had specific symptoms [73]. The exception is with a short segment of bypassed bowel, such as from the distal ileum to the proximal colon, bypassing the ileocecal valve, which may be asymptomatic. Internal fistulas are diagnosed preoperatively in 69–77% of patients [6, 74]. In a series of 639 patients from the University of Chicago a fistula was the primary indication for surgery in only 6.3% of patients, and it was one of several indications in the majority [74]. Resection of the fistula and surrounding diseased bowel with primary anastomosis was performed in 73% and the other 27% required a diverting stoma. Postoperative sepsis occurred in 6% [74]. There are limited data on the medical therapy of internal fistulas in CD. Open-label studies of 6-mercaptopurine for CD that included patients with internal fistulas reported closure of the fistula in 39% [75] and improvement in about 65% of patients [76]. In another open-label study, enterovesical fistulas were treated with 6-mercaptopurine with sustained closure in 39% [77]. Methotrexate and cyclosporine have also been reported in open-label studies for treatment of internal fistulas [78, 79]. Management of perianal fistulas has been discussed above.

Abscess

Intra-abdominal and pelvic abscesses occur in 10–30% of patients with CD as a result of localized bowel perforation. Percutaneous drainage under ultrasonographic or computerized tomographic guidance is successful as definitive therapy in some patients and reduces the morbidity of subsequent surgery in others. In one retrospective series of 36 patients with intra-abdominal or pelvic abscesses, percutaneous drainage was attempted in 15 with avoidance of surgery in four patients [80]. Perianal abscesses may be drained by seton or catheter placement [81]. A diverting ileostomy or colostomy is successful in the short-term management of perianal disease, but disease recurrences, including abscess and fistulas, are common with takedown of the temporary stoma [82].

Dysplasia and malignancy

See Chapter 36.

Renal and urologic complications

Renal or urologic complications were identified in 17% of 700 patients with inflammatory bowel disease (IBD), predominantly in those with CD [59]. Kidney stones occurred in 42 of 498 (8.4%) of patients with CD, more commonly with ileocolonic (9%) or isolated ileal disease (8%) than with isolated colonic involvement (3%) [59]. Renal stones are usually found in those with prior intestinal resection, and the more extensive the resection, the higher the risk of stones. Most renal stones are composed of calcium oxalate, and develop as a consequence of bile salt depletion and fat malabsorption, with increased colonic mucosal permeability and increased oxalate absorption, causing enteric hyperoxaluria. The excessive urinary oxalate binds to calcium, forming stones [83]. Uric acid stones are also common in CD as a result of small intestinal and bicarbonate losses due to previous bowel resection or extensively diseased ileum, which results in concentrated urine with a low pH, favoring the precipitation of urate stones [84]. Also, the urinary excretion of citrate, an inhibitor of stone formation, is low in the setting of acidic urine with low urine potassium and magnesium levels [85].

Non-calculous hydronephrosis was demonstrated by intravenous phlebography in 26 of 436 (6%) of patients with ileal involvement, two of 63 (3%) of patients with isolated colonic disease: it usually involves the right ureter due to extrinsic compression by an inflammatory mass, fibrosis, or abscess [59].

Fistulas from the gastrointestinal tract to the urinary system occur in up to 8% of patients with CD. In patients aged less than 40 years, enterovesical fistulas are usually due to CD, but in those of more than 50 years CD accounts for only 1.8%: diverticulitis or cancer is the usual cause in the older group [86].

Glomerulonephritis has been reported in seven patients with CD [87], and this low number may indicate a chance association. Interstitial nephritis has been reported in patients with IBD with and without prior 5-aminosalicylate use and granulomatous interstitial nephritis has been reported in CD [88]. The risk of a reversible rise in serum creatinine levels with mesalamine treatment has been estimated at 1:100, and the risk of clinically significant reduction in renal function was estimated at less than 1:500 [89]. Interstitial nephritis can also be a consequence of chronic hypokalemia due to diarrhea, or to hyperoxaluria [87]. Amyloidosis with renal involvement was present in five of 498 (1%) of patients with CD [59].

Genital involvement with fistulas, abscesses, ulcers, and fibrosis of the genitalia may occur as an extension of perianal disease, and pyoderma gangrenosum, metastatic CD, or Fournier gangrene [87, 90] are other uncommon manifestations

Bone disease

CD carries several risk factors for the development of osteoporosis: cytokine activity, particularly TNF-α, stimulates osteoclast activity, calcium and vitamin D deficiency, corticosteroid use, calcium and vitamin D deficiency, and a low body mass index [91]. Calcium and vitamin D malabsorption plays a minor role, and osteomalacia in uncommon [92]. Osteoporosis also occurs in UC, and corticosteroid use is the most important risk factor in both diseases [93]. However, the prevalence of low bone mineral densities is similar among patients with CD who have never received steroids compared to those who have taken steroids, although patients with severe osteoporosis are more likely to have taken corticosteroids [94]. In IBD, there is a higher prevalence of reduced bone density in the hips (cortical bone) than in the vertebrae (trabecular bone), which is opposite to the pattern found in postmenopausal osteoporosis and following steroid use for other diseases [94]. Cumulative doses of corticosteroids of more than 10 g pose a higher risk than lower cumulative doses [95], the most rapid bone loss occurs in the first 6–12 months of therapy [96]. The diagnosis is usually made using a dual-energy X-ray absorptiometry (DEXA) scan, or with heel ultrasound. The World Health Organization has set the criteria for diagnosis of osteoporosis as a T score of < -2.5 and for osteopenia as a T score of -1.0 to -2.5. Prevention of osteoporosis in CD centers around avoiding or minimizing corticosteroid exposure, assuring adequate calcium and vitamin D intake, and regular physical activity. Estrogen replacement therapy in postmenopausal women and hormone replacement therapy in both women and men with gonadal failure are important measures. Treatment includes the methods used for prevention plus the use of a bisphosphonate [97]. As the oral bisphosphonates are poorly absorbed, patients with extensive resections for CD may require parenteral administration with pamidronate [98]. Calcitonin may also be useful, although there are no studies confirming a reduced fracture risk in steroid-induced osteoporosis [92].

Vascular disease

Thromboembolism developed in 92 (1.3%) of 7199 patients with IBD seen over an 11-year period, including 49 patients with CD. In addition, four patients with CD had temporal arteritis, one had Takayasu's disease, and two had non-specific vasculitis [99]. Patients with vascular disease had a mean age of 46 years, compared to a mean age of 38 years for the entire group [99]. Thromboembolism is more common with active disease, but markers of activation of coagulation are present in both active and quiescent disease [100]. There are several abnormalities in patients with IBD that predispose to thromboembolism. Factor V Leiden mutation is more common in IBD patients: it was present in four of 11 (36%) patients with IBD and a history of thrombosis, including four with CD, as compared to two of 51 (4%) of IBD controls [101]. Factor V Leiden deficiency is the major cause of active protein C resistance (APCR) – the most prevalent cause of inherited thrombophilia with a prevalence of 2–5% in individuals of European descent [101]. Patients with IBD also have an increased prevalence of hyperhomocystinemia, a risk factor for recurrent venous thrombosis [102]. Elevated homocysteine levels may result from low blood levels of folic acid, vitamin B_{12}, or vitamin B_6, which can be corrected with supplementation. The factor V Leiden mutation and hyperhomocystinemia appear to be independent risk factor for thrombosis [103]. Deficiencies of other hemostatic inhibitory proteins, including antithrombin III, protein C, and protein S, do not appear to cause thrombosis in the majority of patients with IBD, although an inherited deficiency of one of these proteins would be an added risk for thrombosis [104].

Pancreatic disease

Pancreatitis may complicate CD by several mechanisms. Medication-induced pancreatitis has been reported as a consequence of the use of mesalamine [105], 6-mercaptopurine [106], azathioprine [107], and metronidazole [108]. There are a few case reports of corticosteroids as a cause of pancreatitis, but the association is unproved. Intravenous fat emulsions given as parenteral nutrition have been associated with pancreatitis [109]. Extensive CD of the duodenum may predispose to pancreatitis, perhaps due to reflux of duodenal contents into the pancreatic duct [110] or due to stenosis of the ampulla of Vater with pancreatic duct obstruction [111]. Primary sclerosing cholangitis is associated with IBD, including CD, and is also associated with chronic pancreatitis [112]. Granulomatous inflammation of the head of the pancreas, duodenum, and stomach has been reported in a 69-year-old woman who presented with cholestasis, presumably due to CD with direct involvement of the pancreas [113]. Hyperamylasemia was found in 11% and hyperlipasemia was found in 7% of 237 patients with IBD: the elevated levels were associated with more extensive and active disease and with primary sclerosing cholangitis [114].

Hepatobiliary disease

See Chapter 38.

Arthropathies and ocular complications

See Chapter 39.

Cutaneous manifestations

See Chapter 40.

Malnutrition

See Chapter 29.

Psychiatric illness

There is controversy in the literature concerning the relationship between psychiatric disease and CD. A number of studies have found no relation between disease activity and psychiatric illness. In a comparison of 50 patients with CD with 50 control subjects with chronic medical illness, there was no evidence of interaction between a psychiatric disorder and CD [115]. However, more patients with CD met the criteria for psychiatric disorder compared with controls [115], and in another study the higher prevalence of psychiatric illness in patients with CD predates the medical illness. In a prospective study of 32 patients with IBD who had at least one relapse during the previous 2 years, there was no evidence

that stressful life events or depressed mood precipitated worsening of disease activity [116]. In a prospective study from Austria of outpatients with IBD, including 72 with CD, disease-related worries and concerns correlated poorly with disease severity or activity [117]. In contrast, some studies have noted a direct relationship between the activity and severity of CD and psychiatric illness. In a study of 162 consecutive outpatients with IBD, including 91 with CD, psychiatric illness was more common with active disease than with disease remission (50% vs 8%); no relationship of psychiatric to physical illness was observed for the patients with UC [118]. In a prospective study of 10 patients with CD there was a direct relation between daily stress and self-rated disease severity [119]. In a survey of 997 members of the Crohn's and Colitis Foundation of America, including 671 people with CD, those with CD had more psychosocial difficulties than patients with UC, related to a greater severity of symptoms [120]. In summary, the current data suggest that psychosocial disorders are not the cause of CD, but an exacerbating factor.

Natural history

The placebo arms of prospective treatment trials for CD provide information regarding the course of the disease. For patients with active disease who are given placebo as single therapy for CD, 25–40% will enter symptomatic remission within 4 months, 20% will remain in remission at 1 year, and 10% will remain in remission after 2 years [121]. For patients in symptomatic remission who enter maintenance studies, regardless of how remission was achieved, 75% will continue in remission at 1 year and 63% will remain in remission at 2 years [121].

The risk of postoperative recurrence can also be assessed from placebo-controlled trials of postoperative maintenance therapy. In a European multicenter trial of 318 patients who underwent resections for CD with primary anastomosis and without placement of a stoma, the symptomatic relapse rate in the placebo group at 18 months was 31% [122]. This compares to a symptomatic relapse rate of 41% (in 131 of 319 patients) in the placebo arms of four studies for the postoperative maintenance of remission from 12 to 36 months noted in a meta-analysis [123]. For Crohn's colitis the risk of small intestinal recurrence is low, at 6–15% with about 15 years follow-up [124, 125]. Segmental resection of the

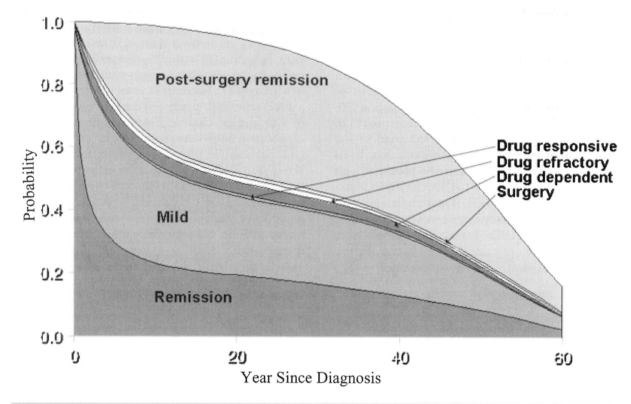

Figure 2. Proportion of Crohn's disease patients in each treatment state by year since diagnosis. (From ref. 128, with permission.)

colon carries a risk of recurrence of 55% with a mean time to recurrence of about 4 years [124].

The rate of endoscopic recurrence of CD is higher than the symptomatic recurrence rate: among 89 patients who underwent distal ileal resection, 70% had lesions in the neoterminal ileum at colonoscopy and only 20% had symptomatic recurrence at 1 year. [126]. A subsequent study showed that endoscopic lesions occur by 3 months after surgery: 22 of 30 (73%) patients had endoscopic lesions just proximal to the ileocolonic anastomosis 3 months post-operatively, and 33% of the patients had recurrent symptoms [127].

Prognosis

The disease course is unpredictable for an individual patient, with periods of active symptoms and period of symptomatic remission of variable length. Estimates of the clinical course have been made based on Markov modeling, using a population-based cohort of 174 patients from Olmsted County,

Minnesota, USA [128]. With a median follow-up of 10 years, 65% of the follow-up time was spent in medical or surgical remission, and the balance of the time spent with medical or surgical treatment (Fig. 2) [128]. For a 30-year-old patient with CD the model predicted 64% of the future life expectancy in remission off medications, with a prediction of 3.2 years (6.9%) of the future life expectancy spent on corticosteroids or immune modulator therapy. The projected future life expectancy based on a mean age at diagnosis of 32.1 years was 42.6 years [128].

Mortality

Several studies have shown a small, but statistically significant, decrease in the survival rate for CD [63]. The relative (actual/expected) survival at 20 years was 92%, 96%, and 94% in the studies from Olmsted County, Minnesota, USA; Uppsala, Sweden; and Stockholm, Sweden, respectively [63, 129, 130]. In contrast, a population-based study from Copenhagen, Denmark, found no difference in survival [131].

In the study from Uppsala [129], IBD was the main reason for the excess mortality, and CD was thought to account for 35% of the mortality in the Olmsted County series [63]. In a population-based study from Italy, the 5-year mortality for UC was lower than expected, and for CD it was higher than expected [132], with the increase in CD due primarily to cancer, including gastric, colonic, respiratory and other solid organ and hematologic malignancies. Sepsis, pulmonary embolism, and hemorrhage were the most common causes of death among operated patients with CD [2].

References

1. Farmer RG, Hawk WA, Turnbull RB. Clinical patterns in Crohn's disease. A statistical study of 615 cases. Gastro enterology 1975; 70: 369–70.
2. Farmer RG, Whelan G, Fazio VW. Long-term follow-up of patients with Crohn's disease: relationships between the clinical pattern and prognosis. Gastroenterology 1985; 88: 1818–25.
3. Greenstein AJ, Lachman P, Sachar DB et al. Perforating and non-perforating indications for repeated operations in Crohn's disease: evidence of two clinical forms. Gut 1988; 29: 588–92.
4. Sachar DB, Andrews HA, Farmer RG et al. Proposed classification of patients subgroups in Crohn's disease. Gastroenterol Intl 1992; 5: 141–54.
5. Gasche C, Scholmerich J, Brynskov J et al. A simple classification of Crohn's disease: report of the working party for the world congresses of gastroenterology, Vienna 1998. Inflam Bowel Dis 2000; 6: 8–15.
6. Panaccione R, Sandborn WJ, Loftus EVL. Phenotype classification of Crohn's disease patients in Olmsted County, Minnesota: application of the Vienna Classification. Gastroenterology 1999; 116: G3515.
7. Lautenbach E, Berlin JA, Lichtenstein GR. Risk factors for early postoperative recurrence of Crohn's disease. Gastroenterology 1998; 115: 259–67.
8. Vasiliauskas EA, Plevy SE, Landers CJ et al. Perinuclear antineutrophil cytoplasmic antibodies in patients with Crohn's disease define a clinical subgroup. Gastroenterology 1996; 110: 1810–19.
9. Satsangi J, Landers CJ, Welsh KI et al. The presence of antineutrophil antibodies reflects clinical and genetic heterogeneity within inflammatory bowel disease. Inflam Bowel Dis 1998; 4: 18–26.
10. Sutton CL, Yang H, Li Z, Rotter JI, Targan SR, Braun J. Familial expression of anti-*Saccharomyces cerevisiae* mannan antibodies in affected and unaffected relatives of patients with Crohn's disease [See comments]. Gut 2000; 46: 58–63.
11. Vasiliauskas EA, Kam LY, Karp LC, Gaiennie J, Yang H, Targan SR. Marker antibody expression stratifies Crohn's disease into immunologically homogeneous subgroups with distinct clinical characteristics. Gut 2000; 47: 487–96.
12. Mekhjian HS, Switz DM, Melnyk CS, Rankin GB, Brooks RK. Clinical features and natural history of Crohn's disease. Gastroenterology 1979; 77: 898–906.
13. Steinhardt HJ, Loeschke K, Kasper H, Holtermuller KH, Schafer H. European cooperative Crohn's disease study (ECCDS): clinical features and natural history. Digestion 1985; 31: 97–108.
14. Rankin GB, Watts D, Melnyk CS et al. National Cooperative Crohn's Disease Study: Extraintestinal manifestations and perianal complications. Gastroenterology 1979; 77: 914–20.
15. Knockaert DC, Vanneste LJ, Vanneste SB et al. Fever of unknown origin in the 1980s: an update of the diagnostic spectrum. Arch Int Med. 1992; 152: 51–5.
16. Lapidus A, Bernell O, Hellers G, Lofberg R. Clinical course of colorectal Crohn's disease: a 35-year follow-up study of 507 patients. Gastroenterology 1998; 114: 1151–60.
17. Hughes LE. Clinical classification of perianal Crohn's disease. Dis Colon Rectum 1992; 35: 928–32.
18. Buchmann P, Keighley MRB, Allan RN, Thompson H, Alexander-Williams J. Natural history of perianal Crohn's disease. Am J Surg 1980; 140: 642–4.
19. Present DH, Korelitz BI, Wisch N, Glass JL, Sachar DB, Pasternack BS. Treatment of Crohn's disease with 6-mercaptopurine. A long-term, randomized, double-blind study. N Engl J Med 1980; 302: 981–7.
20. Present DH, Rutgeerts P, Targan S et al. Infliximab for the treatment of fistulas in patients with Crohn's disease. N Engl J Med 1999; 340: 1398–405.
21. Fleshner PR, Schoetz DJ, Roberts PL, Murray JJ, Coller JA, Veidenheimer MC. Anal fissure in Crohn's disease: a plea for aggressive management. Dis Colon Rectum 1995; 38: 1137–43.
22. Wolff BG. Crohn's disease: the role of surgical treatment. Mayo Clin Proc 1986; 61: 292–5.
23. Faucheron J, Saint-Marc O, Guibert L et al. Long-term seton drainage for high anal fistulas in Crohn's disease: a sphincter saving operation? Dis Colon Rectum 1996; 39: 208–11.
24. Fielding JF, Toye DKM, Beton DC, Cooke WT. Crohn's disease of the stomach and duodenum. Gut 1970; 11: 1001–6.
25. Grill BB, Lange R, Markowitz R, Hillemeier AC, McCallum RW, Gryboski JD. Delayed gastric emptying in children with Crohn's disease. J Clin Gastroenterol 1985; 7: 216–26.
26. Yamamoto T, Allan RN, Keighley MR. An audit of gastroduodenal Crohn's disease: clinicopathologic features and management. Scand J Gastroenterol 1999; 34: 1019–24.
27. Wagtmans AJG, Verspaget HW, Lamers CB, van Hogezand RA. Crohn's disease in the elderly: a comparison with young adults. J Clin Gastroenterol 1998; 27: 129–33.
28. Mashako MN, Cezard JP, Navarro J et al. Crohn's disease lesions in the upper gastrointestinal tract: correlation between clinical, radiological, endoscopic, and histological features in adolescents and children. J Pediatr Gastroenterol Nutr 1989; 8: 442–6.
29. Ruuska T, Vaajalahti P, Arajarvi P, Maki M. Prospective evaluation of upper gastrointestinal mucosal lesions in children with ulcerative colitis and Crohn's disease. J Pediatr Gastroenterol Nutr 1994; 19: 181–6.
30. LiVolsi VA, Jaretzki A. Granulomatous esophagitis: a case of Crohn's disease limited to the esophagus. Gastroenterology 1973; 64: 313–19.
31. Cary ER, Tremaine WJ, Banks PM, Nagorney DM. Isolated Crohn's disease of the stomach. Mayo Clin Proc 1989; 64: 776–9.
32. Ueyama T, Ureshino J, Motooka M, Masuda K. Isolated Crohn's disease of the gastroduodenum: a case report. Rad Med 1993; 11: 167–9.
33. Korelitz BI, Wayne JD, Kreuning J et al. Crohn's disease in endoscopic biopsies of the gastric antrum and duodenum. Am J Gastroenterol 1981; 76: 103–9.

34. Oberhuber G, Puspok A, Oesterreicher C *et al.* Focally enhanced gastritis: a frequent type of gastritis in patients with Crohn's disease. Gastroenterology 1997; 112: 698–706.

35. Decker GA, Loftus EV, Pasha TM, Tremaine WJ, Sandborn WJ. Crohn's disease of the esophagus: clinical features and outcomes. Am J Gastroenterol 1999; 94: 2582.

36. Geboes K, Janssensn J, Rutgeerts P, Vantrappen G. Crohn's disease of the esophagus. J Clin Gastroenterol 1986; 8: 31–7.

37. Madden JL, Raved JM, Haddad JR. Regional esophagitis: a specific entity simulating Crohn's disease. Ann Surg 1969; 170: 351–68.

38. D'Haens G, Rutgeerts P, Geboes K, Vantrappen G. The natural history of esophageal Crohn's disease: three patterns of evolution. Am Soc Gastrointest Endosc 1994; 40: 296–300.

39. Danzi JT, Farger RG, Sullivan BH, Rankin GB. Endoscopic features of gastroduodenal Crohn's disease. Gastroenterology 1976; 70: 9–13.

40. Greenstein AJ, Present DH, Sachar DB *et al.* Gastric fistulas in Crohn's disease. Dis Colon Rectum 1989; 32: 888–92.

41. Jacobson IM, Schapiro RH, Warshaw AL. Gastric and duodenal fistulas in Crohn's disease. Gastroenterology 1985; 89: 1347–52.

42. Meining A, Bayerdorffer E, Bastlein E *et al.* Focal inflammatory infiltrations in gastric biopsy specimens are suggestive of Crohn's disease. Crohn's disease study group, Germany. Scand J Gastroenterol 1997; 32: 813–18.

43. Nugent FW, Roy MA. Duodenal Crohn's disease: an analysis of 89 cases. Am J Gastroenterol 1989; 84: 249–54.

44. Farmer RG, Hawk WA, Turnbull RB. Crohn's disease of the duodenum (transmural duodenitis): clinical manifestations. Report of 11 cases. Am J Dig Dis 1972; 17: 191–8.

45. Fielding JF, Toye DK, Beton DC, Cooke WT. Crohn's disease of the stomach and duodenum. Gut 1970; 11: 1001–6.

46. D'Inca R, Sturniolo G, Cassaro M *et al.* Prevalence of upper gastrointestinal lesions and *Helicobacter pylori* infection in Crohn's disease. Dig Dis Sci 1998; 43: 988–92.

47. Schmitz-Moorman P, Malchow H, Pittner PM. Endoscopic and bioptic study of the upper gastrointestinal tract in Crohn's disease patients. Pathol Res Pract 1985; 179: 377–87.

48. Woolfson K, Greenberg GR. Symptomatic improvement of gastroduodenal Crohn's disease with omeprazole. Can J Gastroenterol 1992; 6: 21–4.

49. Griffiths AM, Alemayehu E, Sherman P. Clinical features of gastroduodenal Crohn's disease in adolescents. J Pediatr Gastroenterol Nutr 1989; 8: 166–71.

50. Goldberg HI, Caruthers SB, Nelson JA. Radiographic findings of the National Cooperative Crohn's Disease Study. Gastroenterology 1979; 77: 925–37.

51. Lamers C. Crohn's disease of the upper gastrointestinal tract. In: Allan, RN, Rhodes JM, Hanauer SB, eds. Inflammatory Bowel Diseases, 3rd edn. New York: Churchill Livingstone, 1997: 583–8.

52. Chrispin AR, Tempany E. Crohn's disease of the jejunum in children. Arch Dis Child 1967; 42: 631–5.

53. Kneppelhout JC, Chandie Shaw P, Pena AS *et al.* Jejuno-ileitis, a subtype of extensive and diffuse Crohn's disease. J Clin Nutr Gastroenterol 1992; 7: 15–21.

54. Zalev AH, Prokipchuk EJ. Crohn's disease of the proximal small intestine: radiologic findings in 55 patients. J Can Assoc Radiol 1992; 43: 170–8.

55. Tan WC, Allan RN. Diffuse jejunoileitis of Crohn's disease. Gut 1993; 34: 1374–8.

56. Ricart E, Panaccione R, Loftus EV, Tremaine WJ, Sandborn WJ. Infliximab for Crohn's disease in clinical practice at the Mayo Clinic: the first 100 patients. Gastroenterology 2000; 118: A2967.

57. Malchow H, Ewe K, Brandes JW *et al.* European Cooperative Crohn's Disease Study (ECCDS): results of drug treatment. Gastroenterology 1984; 86: 249–66.

58. Sanderson IR, Udeen S, Davies PS, Savage MO, Walker-Smith JA. Remission induced by an elemental diet in small bowel Crohn's disease. Arch Dis Child 1987; 62: 123–7.

59. Greenstein AJ, Janowitz HD, Sachar DB. The extraintestinal complications of Crohn's disease and ulcerative colitis: a study of 700 patients. Medicine 1976; 55: 401–12.

60. Plauth M, Jenss H, Meyle J. Oral manifestations of Crohn's disease. An analysis of 79 cases. J Clin Gastroenterol 1991; 13: 29–37.

61. Diamond T, Patterson PG, Emerson TG. Oral Crohn's disease: the distinction from the Melkersson–Rosenthal syndrome. Ulster Med J 1990; 59: 223–4.

62. Tremaine WJ. Treatment of erythema nodosum, aphthous stomatitis, and pyoderma gangrenosum in patients with IBD. Inflam Bowel Dis 1998; 4: 68–9.

63. Loftus EV, Silverstein MD, Sandborn WJ, Tremaine WJ, Harmsen WS, Zinsmeister AR. Crohn's disease in Olmsted County, Minnesota, 1940–1993: incidence, prevalence, and survival. Gastroenterology 1998; 114: 1161–8. Gastroenterology 1999; 116: 1507.

64. Grimm IS, Friedman LS. Inflammatory bowel disease in the elderly. Gastroenterol Clin N Am 1990; 19: 361–89.

65. Akerkar GA, Peppercorn MA. Inflammatory bowel disease in the elderly. Practical treatment guidelines. Drugs Aging 1997; 10: 199–208.

66. Corrigan G, Stevens PE. Review article: Interstitial nephritis associated with the use of mesalazine in inflammatory bowel disease. Aliment Pharmacol Therap 2000; 14: 1–6.

67. Norri B, Solomon MJ, Eyers AA, West RH, Glenn DC, Morgan BP. Abdominal surgery in the older Crohn's population. Austr NZ J Surg 1999; 69: 199–204.

68. Truelove AC, Pena AS. Course and prognosis of Crohn's disease. Gut 1976; 17: 192–201.

69. Spencer MP, Nelson H, Wolff BGF, Dozois RR. Stricturoplasty for obstructive Crohn's disease: the Mayo experience. Mayo Clin Proc 1994; 69: 33–6.

70. Chernish SM, Maglinte DD, O'Connor K. Evaluation of the small intestine by enteroclysis for Crohn's disease. Am J Gastroenterol 1992; 87: 696–701.

71. Kohn A, Cerro P, Milite G, De Angelis E, Prantera C. Prospective evaluation of transabdominal bowel sonography in the diagnosis of intestinal obstruction in Crohn's disease: comparison with plain abdominal film and small bowel enteroclysis. Inflam Bowel Dis 1999; 5: 153–7.

72. Kolkman JJ, Falke TH, Roos JC *et al.* Computed tomography and granulocyte scintigraphy in active inflammatory bowel disease. Comparison with endoscopy and operative findings. Dig Dig Sci 1996; 41: 641–50.

73. Young-Fadok TM, Wolff BG, Meagher A, Benn PL, Dozois RR. Surgical management of ileosigmoid fistulas in Crohn's disease. Dis Colon Rectum 1997; 40: 558–61.

74. Michelassi F, Stella M, Balestracci T, Giuliante F, Marogna P, Block GE. Incidence, diagnosis, and treatment of enteric and colorectal fistuale in patients with Crohn's disease. Ann Surg 1993; 218: 660–6.

75. Korelitz BI, Present DH. Favorable effect of 6-mercaptopurine in fistulas of Crohn's disease. Dig Dis Sci 1985; 30: 58–64.

76. Korelitz BI, O'Brien JJ, Bayless TM, Bayless JA. Use of azathioprine or 6-mercaptopurine in the treatment of Crohn's disease. Gastroenterology 1991; 101: 39–46.

77. Wheeler SC, Marion JF, Present. Medical therapy, not surgery, is the appropriate first line of treatment for Crohn's enterovesical fistula. Gastroenterology 1998; 114: A1113.

78. Mahadevan U, Marion J, Present DH. The place of methotrexate in the treatment of refractory Crohn's disease. Gastroenterology 1997; 112: A1031.

79. Hanauer SB, Smith MD. Rapid closure of Crohn's disease fistula with continuous intravenous cyclosporine. Am J Gastroenterol 1993; 88: 646–9.

80. Jawhari A, Kamm MA, Ong C, Forbes A, Bartram CI, Hawley PR. Intra-abdominal and pelvic abscess in Crohn's disease: results of non-invasive and surgical management. Br J Surg 1998; 85: 367–71.

81. Makowiec F, Jehle EC, Becker HD, Starlinger M. Perianal abscess in Crohn's disease. Dis Colon Rectum 1997; 40: 443–50.

82. Harper PH, Kettlewell MG, Lee EC. The effect of split ileostomy on perianal Crohn's disease. Br J Surg 1982; 69: 608–10.

83. Smith LH. The pathophysiology and medical treatment of urolithiasis. Semin Nephrol 1999; 10: 31–52.

84. Reisner GS, Wilansky DL, Schneiderman C. Uric acid lithiasis in the ileostomy patient. Br J Urol 1973; 45: 340–3.

85. McLeod RS, Churchill DN. Urolithiasis complicating inflammatory bowel disease. J Urol 1992; 148: 974–8.

86. Moisey CU, Williams JL. Vesico-intestinal fistulas. Br J Urol 1972; 44: 662–6.

87. Pardi, DS, Tremaine WJ, Sandborn WJ, McCarthy JT. Renal and urologic complications of inflammatory bowel disease. Am J Gastroenterol 1998; 93: 504–14.

88. Tovbin D, Kachko L, Hilzenrat N. Severe intestinal nephritis in a patient with renal amyloidosis and exacerbation of Crohn's disease. Clin Nephrol 2000; 53: 147–51.

89. Corrigan G, Stevens PE. Review article: Interstitial nephritis associated with the use of mesalazine in inflammatory bowel disease. Aliment Pharmacol Ther 2000; 14: 1–6.

90. Jiang T, Covington JA, Haile CA et al. Fournier gangrene associated with Crohn's disease. Mayo Clin Proc 2000; 75: 647–9.

91. Sliverberg MS, Steinhart AH. Bone density in inflammatory bowel disease. Clin Gastroenterol 2000; 2: 117–24.

92. Adachi JD, Rostom A. Metabolic bone disease in adults with inflammatory bowel disease. Inflam Bowel Dis 1999; 5: 200–11.

93. Bernstein CN, Seeger LL, Sayre JW et al. Decreased bone density in inflammatory bowel disease is related to corticosteroid use and not disease diagnosis. J Bone Miner Res 1995; 10: 250–6.

94. Bjarnason I, Macpherson A, Mackintosh C et al. Reduced bone density in patients with inflammatory bowel disease. Gut 1997; 40: 228–33.

95. Silvennoinen JA, Karttunen TJ, Niemela SE et al. A controlled study of bone mineral density in patients with inflammatory bowel disease. Gut 1995; 37: 71–6.

96. Saito JK, Davis JW, Wasnich RD et al. Users of low dose glucocorticosteroids have increased bone loss rates: a longitudinal study. Calcif Tissue Int 1995; 57: 115–9.

97. Saag KG, Emkey R, Schnitzer TJ et al. Aldendronate for the prevention and treatment of glucocorticoid-induced osteoporosis. N Engl J Med 1998; 339: 292–9.

98. Boutsen Y, Jamart J, Essenlinckx W et al. Primary prevention of glucocorticoid-induced osteoporosis with intermittent intravenous pamidronate: a randomized trial. Calif Tissue Int 1997; 61: 266–71.

99. Talbot RW, Heppell J, Dozois RR, Beart RW. Vascular complications of inflammatory bowel disease. Mayo Clin Proc 1986; 61: 140–5.

100. Hudson M, Hutton RA, Wakefield AJ et al. Evidence for activation of coagulation in Crohn's disease. Blood. Coag Fibrinol 1992; 3: 773–8.

101. Liebman HA, Kashani N, Sutherland D, McGehee W, Kam L. The factor V Leiden mutation increases the risk of venous thrombosis in patients with inflammatory bowel disease. Gastroenterology 1998; 115: 830–4.

102. Cattaneo M, Vecchi M, Zighetti ML et al. High prevalence of hyperchromocysteinemia in patients with inflammatory bowel disease: a pathogenic link with thromboembolic complications? Thromb Haemostas 1998; 80: 542–5.

103. Heijer MD, Koster T, Blom HJ et al. Hyperhomocysteinemia as a risk factor for deep vein thrombosis. N Engl J Med 1996; 334: 759–62.

104. Souto JC, Martinez E, Roca M et al. Prothrombotic state and signs of endothelial lesion in plasma of patients with inflammatory bowel disease. Dig Dis Sci 1995; 40: 1883–9.

105. Radke M, Bartolomaeus G, Muller M, Richter I. Acute pancreatitis in Crohn's disease due to 5-ASA therapy. J Pediatr Gastroenterol Nutr 1993; 16: 337–9.

106. Haber CJ, Meltzer SJ, Present DH, Korelitz BI. Nature and course of pancreatitis caused by 6-mercaptopurine in the treatment of inflammatory bowel disease. Gastroenterology 1986; 91: 982–6.

107. Sturdevant RAL, Singleton JW, Deren JL, Law DH, McCleery JL. Azathioprine-related pancreatitis in patients with Crohn's disease. Gastroenterology 1979; 77: 883–6.

108. Corey WA, Doebbeling BN, DeJong KJ, Britigan BE. Metronidazole-induced acute pancreatitis. Rev Infect Dis 1999; 13: 1213–15.

109. Lashner BA, Kirsner JB, Hanauer SB. Acute pancreatitis associated with high-concentration lipid emulsion during total parenteral nutrition therapy for Crohn's disease. Gastroenterology 1986; 90: 1039–41.

110. Meltzer SJ, Korelitz BI. Pancreatitis and duodenopancreatic reflux in Crohn's disease: case report and review of the literature. J Clin Gastroenterol 1988; 10: 555–8.

111. Newman LH, Wellinger JR, Present DH, Aufses AH. Crohn's disease of the duodenum associated with pancreatitis: a case report and review of the literature. Mt Sinai J Med 1987; 54: 429–32.

112. Borkje B, Betvik K, Odegaard S, Schrumpf E, Larssen TB, Kolmannskog F. Chronic pancreatitis in patients with sclerosing cholangitis and ulcerative colitis. Scand J Gastroenterol 1985; 20: 539–42.

113. Gschwantler M, Kogelbauer G, Klose W, Bibus B, Tscholakoff D, Weiss W. The pancreas as a site of granulomatous inflammation in Crohn's disease. Gastroenterology 1995; 108: 1246–9.

114. Heikius B, Niemela S, Lehtola J, Karttunen TJ. Elevated pancreatic enzymes in inflammatory bowel disease are associated with extensive disease. Am J Gastroenterol 1999; 94: 1062–9.

115. Helzer JE, Chammas S, Norland CC et al. A study of the association between Crohn's disease and psychiatric illness. Gastroenterology 1984; 86: 324–30.

116. North CS, Alpers DH, Helzer JE et al. Do life events or depression exacerbate inflammatory bowel disease? A prospective study. Ann Intern Med 1991; 114: 381–6.

117. Moser G, Tillinger W, Sachs G et al. Disease-related worries and concerns: a study on out-patients with inflammatory bowel disease. Euro J Gastroenterol Hepatol 1995; 7: 853–8.

118. Andrews H, Barczak P, Allan RN. Psychiatric illness in patients with inflammatory bowel disease. Gut 1987; 28: 1600–4.

119. Garrett VD, Brantley PJ, Jones GN et al. The relation between daily stress and Crohn's disease. J Behav Med 1991; 14: 87–96.

120. Drossman DA, Leserman J, Mitchell CM, Li ZM, Zagami EA, Patrick DL. Health status and health care use in persons with inflammatory bowel disease. A national sample. Dig Dis Sci 1991; 36: 1746–55.

121. Meyers S, Janowitz HD. Natural history of Crohn's disease. An analytic review of the placebo lesson. Gastroenterology 1984; 87: 1189–92.
122. Lochs H, Mayer M, Fleig WE. Prophylaxis of postoperative relapse in Crohn's disease with mesalamine: European cooperative Crohn's disease study VI. Gastroenterology 2000; 118: 264–73.
123. Camma C, Giunta M, Rosselli M *et al.* Mesalamine in the maintenance treatment of Crohn's disease: a meta-analysis adjusted for confounding factors. Gastroenterology 1997; 113: 1465–73.
124. Prabhakar LP, Nelson LC, Dozois RR. Avoiding a stoma: role for segmental or abdominal colectomy in Crohn's colitis. Dis Colon Rectum 1997; 40: 71–8.
125. Goligher JC. Surgical treatment of Crohn's disease affecting mainly or entirely the large bowel. World J Surg 1988; 12: 186–90.
126. Rutgeerts P, Geboes K, Vantrappen G, Beyls J, Kerremans R, Hiele M. Predictability of the postoperative course of Crohn's disease. Gastroenterology 1990; 99: 956–63.
127. Olaison G, Smedh K, Sjodahl R. Natural course of Crohn's disease after ileocolonic resection: endoscopically visualized ileal ulcers preceding symptoms. Gut 1992; 33: 331–5.
128. Silverstein MD, Loftus EV, Sandborn WJ *et al.* Clinical course and costs of care for Crohn's disease: Markov model analysis of a population-based cohort. Gastroenterology 1999; 117: 49–57.
129. Ekbom A, Helmick CG, Zack M *et al.* Survival and causes of death in patients with inflammatory bowel disease: a population-based study. Gastroenterology 1992; 103: 954–60.
130. Persson PG, Berness O, Leijonmarck CE *et al.* Survival and cause-specific mortality in inflammatory bowel disease: a population-based cohort study. Gastroenterology 1996; 110: 1339–45.
131. Munkholm P, Langholz E, Davidsen M, Binder V. Disease activity courses in a regional cohort of Crohn's disease patients. Scand J Gastroenterol 1995; 30: 699–706.
132. Cottone M, Maglioco A, Rosselli M *et al.* Mortality in patients with Crohn's disease. Scand J Gastroenterol 1996; 31: 372–5.

16 | Mechanisms of systemic inflammation associated with intestinal injury

R. BALFOUR SARTOR AND STEVEN N. LICHTMAN

Introduction

A characteristic spectrum of systemic inflammation involving the joints, liver, skin, eyes, and hematologic organs is associated with diverse types of intestinal injury (Table 1) [1–12]. Extraintestinal manifestations occur in 20–30% of patients with ulcerative colitis (UC), Crohn's disease (CD), or jejunoileal bypass for obesity but are relatively infrequent or rare in the other listed conditions. Although each of these intestinal disorders has a different pathogenesis, they share common properties of: (1) increased mucosal permeability (UC, CD, and celiac disease); (2) infection (enteric pathogens, Whipple's disease, and diverticulitis); or (3) overgrowth of predominantly anaerobic bacteria (jejunoileal bypass, pouchitis, and bacterial overgrowth associated with gastric or biliary surgery). These insults lead to increased systemic uptake of commensal or pathogenic enteric bacterial products. These clinical associations are supported by experimental observations that jejunal bacterial overgrowth [12, 13], colitis [6, 14], or ileocolitis [15 16] lead to hepatobiliary, joint, and hematologic abnormalities in rodents. Intestinal and systemic inflammation are further linked by finding asymptomatic intestinal inflammation in the majority of patients with primary sclerosing cholangitis (PSC) [17] and spondyloarthropathy [18].

This chapter discusses potential mechanisms and develops a unifying hypothesis explaining the association between intestinal and systemic inflammation. Mechanisms of non-inflammatory and specialized complications of inflammatory bowel diseases (IBD), such as gallstones or renal calculi associated with ileal CD, are discussed in Chapter 15. Clinical and experimental data, which are most extensive for PSC, ankylosing spondylitis, and reactive arthritis, are cited to provide evidence for each potential mechanism.

Clinical clues for pathogenesis of extraintestinal manifestations

Several clinical observations provide important clues to explain the relationship between intestinal and systemic inflammation:

Association with colonic involvement

Extraintestinal manifestations are frequent and approximately equal in UC and CD of the colon but are less commonly associated with isolated ileal disease. In the classic study of Greenstein et al. [4] the incidence of 'colitis-associated' lesions, including joint, skin, eye, and mouth inflammation, was 45% for UC, 55% for granulomatous colitis, 37% for ileocolitis, and 25% for isolated ileitis ($p < 0.001$ vs granulomatous colitis). Liver inflammation, which was considered a non-specific extraintestinal manifestation, occurred in 6% of patients with granulomatous colitis vs 2% of patients with ileitis. In more

Table 1. Association of intestinal and systemic inflammation

	Joint	Hepatobiliary	Skin	Eye	Anemia
Ulcerative colitis	+	+	+	+	+
Crohn's disease	+	+	+	+	+
Celiac disease	+	+	+		
Enteric pathogen*	+		+	+	+
Whipple's disease	+	+	+	+	+
Jejunoileal bypass	+	+	+		+
Pouchitis	+		+		+
Bacterial overgrowth	+		+		+
Diverticulitis	+		+		

*Extraintestinal complications are frequently associated with Yersinia (especially *Y. enterocolitica*), *Shigella*, and *Salmonella* and infrequently with *Campylobacter*, *Clostridium difficile*, *Giardia*, *Ameba*, *Strongyloides*, and *Taenia saginata*.

Stephan R. Targan, Fergus Shanahan and Loren C. Karp (eds.), Inflammatory Bowel Disease: From Bench to Bedside, 2nd Edition, 305–335.
© 2003 *Kluwer Academic Publishers. Printed in Great Britain*

recent studies, PSC complicating CD is confined to patients with extensive colonic involvement [17, 19]. This pattern is also found in peripheral arthritis, which was found in a Korean population to be present in 20% of patients with UC and Crohn's colitis, but in none of the Crohn's patients without colonic involvement [20]. However, fibromyalgia is more common in CD (site of gut inflammation not mentioned) than in UC (49% vs 19%, $p < 0.001$) [21]. Thus most joint, skin, eye, and biliary inflammatory complications are more closely associated with colonic than ileal disease.

Correlation with extent of intestinal inflammation

An increased surface area of inflamed colonic mucosa predisposes to extraintestinal inflammation. The population-based study of Monsen *et al.* [6] described a 21% extraintestinal inflammation rate in non-selected patients with UC. Seventy percent of patients with joint, skin, and eye inflammation had extensive colitis, and only 3% had proctitis. Wright and Watkinson found arthritis in 22.2% of patients with extensive UC (transverse colon or greater extent), in 11.8% with left-sided colitis, but only in 4.7% of isolated proctitis patients [22]. PSC is increased by 11-fold in patients with extensive UC vs those with left-sided disease, whereas only Crohn's patients with pancolitis exhibit PSC [23]. In an Italian population, 68% of UC patients with ankylosing spondylitis had pancolitis [24].

Correlation with disease activity

As outlined in Table 2, systemic manifestations can be categorized based on their response to changes in activity of the underlying bowel disease. In activity-related disorders, activity of extraintestinal inflammation mirrors that of the associated bowel process; onset rarely precedes intestinal symptoms or follows colectomy; and resolves following total proctocolectomy. Activity-unrelated conditions such as PSC and ankylosing spondylitis frequently precede the onset of bowel symptoms, occur after colectomy, and proceed independently of intestinal activity. Pyoderma gangrenosum fits into an intermediate category, as it usually occurs during a flare of IBD but does not universally respond to colectomy. These divergent courses suggest fundamental differences in the pathogenesis of these categories of systemic manifestations.

Table 2. Correlation of activity of systemic and intestinal inflammation

Activity related:	Peripheral arthritis, erythema nodosum, iritis/uveitis, anema
Intermediate:	Pyoderma gangrenosum
Activity unrelated:	Sclerosing cholangitis, ankylosing spondylitis, sacroileitis

Non-random occurrence of systemic manifestations

Certain extraintestinal manifestations, particularly the activity-related conditions (peripheral arthritis, erythema nodosum, and iritis), frequently occur simultaneously in patients with IBD. Monsen *et al.* reported that 39% of patients with activity-related disorders had multiple complications [6]. Seventy percent of patients with iritis had a concurrent condition, most frequently arthritis.

These clinical observations strongly suggest that peripheral arthritis, erythema nodosum, and iritis/uveitis have a common pathogenesis that is dependent on active and extensive colonic inflammation, whereas the mechanisms of ankylosing spondylitis and PSC are distinct from the underlying IBD. Any etiologic theory must account for these associations and explain why only approximately 20–25% of patients with IBD or jejunoileal bypass develop extraintestinal manifestations and why only 1–2% of the general population, but 20% of HLA-B27 patients, develop reactive arthritis following epidemic outbreaks of bacterial enteritis [25].

Mechanisms

Many theories have been advanced to explain the coexistence of injury or infection of the intestine with systemic inflammation. The mechanisms best explaining this association (Table 3) are addressed in the context of current knowledge of IBD pathophysiology. Relevant clinical and experimental evidence supporting each theory is discussed for the major extraintestinal manifestations.

Table 3. Mechanisms of systemic inflammation associated with intestinal injury

Primary or secondary infection
Immunologic
    Autoimmune reaction
    Immune complex deposition
    Systemic distribution of luminal antigens and toxic bacterial
      products
    Systemic distribution of inflammatory mediators and cytokines
      produced by the inflamed intestine
    Local production of cytokines and inflammatory molecules
    Disordered immuoregulation
Genetic
Non-immune injury

Infection with viable commensal or pathogenic organisms

Intestinal and extraintestinal inflammation could be linked by three infectious mechanisms: (1) simultaneous infection of the intestine and systemic organs; (2) translocation of normal microbial flora or pathogens across the more permeable intestinal mucosa; and (3) increased susceptibility of patients with IBD to pathogens with a tropism for systemic organs. Although persistent *Mycobacterium paratuberculosis* or measles infection have been suggested to cause CD [26, 27] these agents have not been associated with systemic complications resembling IBD. Translocation of viable commensal or pathogenic bacteria from the ulcerated distal intestine to the portal vein and the rich presacral lymphatic/venous plexus is a more plausible theory. Enteric bacteria have been cultured from the serosa or mesenteric lymph nodes of 56% of resected CD intestines vs 17% of control intestines [28] and from the portal veins of 27% of patients with UC undergoing colectomy [29]. Although subsequent studies suggest that portal bacteremia occurs substantially less often, portal and lymphatic uptake of viable enteric commensal bacteria are relatively frequent events that expose systemic organs to replicating organisms and their toxic products.

Sclerosing cholangitis

Chronic portal vein bacteremia was studied in calves by continuously infusing *Escherichia coli* into the portal vein for 4–51 days [30]. Although lethal doses of *E. coli* produced periportal inflammation, Kupffer cell hyperplasia, and elevated alkaline phosphatase and transaminase levels, sublethal doses of *E. coli*

caused no hepatobiliary inflammation. Biliary sepsis is relatively frequent with high-grade obstruction, particularly after endoscopic manipulation, but the lack of polymorphonuclear neutrophil leukocyte (PMN) infiltration suggests that chronic bacterial cholangitis is not a prominent feature of early PSC. However, chronic bacterial infection in end-stage PSC was demonstrated by positive bacterial cultures in 58% of cirrhotic livers removed at transplantation [31]. No patients with primary biliary cirrhosis (PBC) had positive cultures. Streptococci were present in 46% of cases and enterococci accounted for 20%. The authors noted an inverse correlation to the interval from last endoscopic retrograde cholangiopancreatography (ERCP). A possible role for streptococci in PSC is supported by the report of three children with PSC responding to oral vancomycin therapy [32]. *Helicobacter pylori* has been found in liver biopsies of 20/24 patients with PSC and PBC vs 1/23 controls [33]. Paradoxically, *H. pylori* is negatively associated with CD [34] and intestinal *Helicobacter* species, such as *H. hepaticus* and *H. bilis* which are implicated in experimental colitis and hepatitis [35], were not found in the liver samples [33]. *H. hepaticus* serum antibodies were not increased in patients with PSC [36].

Likewise, neonatal viral infections and opportunistic infections which produce biliary lesions that resemble PSC in patients with AIDS are not frequently found in IBD patients. Cytomegalovirus and reovirus type III infections cause obliterative cholangitis in neonates, but serologic evidence of reovirus III is absent in patients with PSC or PBC [37]. Acquired sclerosing cholangitis is associated with multiple types of immunodeficiencies, including familial, combined X-linked, angioimmunoblastic lymphadenopathy, hypogammaglobulinemia, and AIDS, presumably due to intermittent bacterial, viral, or parasitic infection. Cello [38] described 26 patients with AIDS who had right upper quadrant pain, fever, or increased alkaline phosphatase who underwent ERCP with ampullary biopsy. Twenty (77%) of these patients had abnormal cholangiograms. Seventy percent of the abnormal ERCP were compatible with sclerosing cholangitis, of which 10 had associated papillary stenosis and six had cytomegalovirus, cryptosporidium or *Mycobacterium avium intracellular* infection. A mechanism of biliary injury in these patients is suggested by the observation that *Cryptosporidium parvum* can induce apoptosis in biliary epithelial cells [39]. Sphincterotomy led to symptomatic relief but no improvement in progression of hepatobiliary disease. A similar irreversible progression of inflammation and secondary bacterial infection in inflamed and partially obstructed bile ducts may explain the lack of improvement of idiopathic PSC with immuno-suppressive therapy and the inexorable progression of inflammation and fibrosis [40–42].

Arthritis

There is no evidence of direct infection of synovial tissues in IBD-associated arthritis, but a reservoir of invasive enteric organisms seems to be necessary for postinfectious reactive arthritis. Patients with reactive arthritis secondary to *Yersinia* have prolonged fecal carriage and protracted serum immunoglobulin A (IgA) and secretory IgA responses to this organism. *Yersinia* and *Chlamydia* antigens and oligoclonal bacterial antigen-specific T cells have been recovered from synovial fluid of patients with reactive arthritis, but exhaustive cultures and polymerase chain reaction (PCR) studies demonstrate no viable bacteria in the joint [43–46]. Causative agents of reactive arthritis, including *Yersinia*, *Salmonella*, *Shigella*, and *Chla-mydia*, invade the mucosa and can proliferate within macrophages [47]. Enteric Gram-negative infections also can reactivate quiescent spondyloarthropathy [48]. However, antibiotics do not affect the course of reactive arthritis following enteric infections [10, 49].

Several rodent models of reactive arthritis conclusively link peripheral arthritis with intestinal enteric infections and commensal bacteria and provide insights into the pathogenesis of this disorder [46]. Adult Lewis rats inoculated intra-venously with *Y. enterocolitica* 0:8 strain develop arthritis 1 week after injection, which peaks at 3 weeks and persists for 6 weeks. Viable *Yersinia* are found in the spleen but not the joints of these rats [50]. In contrast, experimental animals with reactive arthritis induced by *Y. enterocolitica* 0:3 [51] or *S. enteritidis* [52] have transiently positive joint cultures, although persistently inflamed joints remain sterile after the first month. Inability to recover viable bacteria in human postinfectious and IBD-associated arthritis does not exclude transient early infection, as suggested by finding multiclonal *Salmonella*-reactive T cells in the synovium of a patient with postinfectious *Salmonella* arthritis [53]. The importance of commensal enteric bacteria is demonstrated by the lack of peripheral arthritis and colitis in germfree (sterile) HLA-B27 transgenic rats [54, 55]. Although these investigators did not culture

the inflamed joints, there is no evidence of sepsis in these rats.

Skin lesions

Erythema nodosum is commonly associated with tuberculosis, leprosy, histoplasmosis, and strepto-coccal, *Yersinia*, *Salmonella*, and *Shigella* infections, but the skin lesions are sterile. Refractory pyoderma gangrenosum resolves soon after selective elimina-tion of aerobic Gram-negative rods from the gastro-intestinal tract [56]. The skin pustules associated with bacterial overgrowth in patients with jejunoileal bypasses are sterile.

Iritis/uveitis

Patients with IBD who have anterior uveitis/iritis do not routinely undergo aqueous humor cultures, but responses to immunosuppressive therapy suggest an absence of invasive pathogens. However, Johnson *et al.* [57] found intracytoplasmic mollicute-like organisms, which are non-cultivatable, cell wall-deficient, intracellular bacterial pathogens, by electron microscopy, in three CD patients with acute flares of chronic recurrent ocular inflammation. Rifampin therapy improved the ocular and intestinal inflammation of these patients, and inoculation of mollicute-like organisms into mouse eyelids produced local and disseminated progressive granulomatous inflammation, which also involved the intestine. Sterile acute anterior uveitis is a frequent complication of Gram-negative enteric bacterial and *Chlamydia trachomatis* infections, which can be subclinical. For example, 43% of consecutive Australian patients with anterior uveitis but no gastrointestinal symptoms had serologic evidence of prior *Yersinia* infection [58].

Hematologic

Numerous chronic infections including tuberculosis, osteomyelitis, and subacute bacterial endocarditis produce anemia of chronic disease without direct infection of the bone marrow.

Conclusions

There is no consistent evidence of protracted infec-tion of target organs in extraintestinal inflammation associated with gut injury, although transient synovial infection after Gram-negative enteritis is suggested by animal models and antigen-specific T cells in reactive arthritis. *Helicobacter* species need to be further investigated in PSC. It is more likely that persistent enteric colonization and translocation of viable bacteria and bacterial components into the lymphatic and portal circulations serve as continuous sources of immunopathogenic antigens, as discussed below.

Immunologic mechanisms of injury

Immune mechanisms of extraintestinal inflammation are strongly suggested by the histologic appearance and response to immunosuppressive therapy. The critical questions to be addressed are primary vs secondary events and the origin of the antigen (absorbed vs host). Types of immunopathologic responses are individually discussed below.

Autoimmune events

Although UC and CD traditionally have been considered to have an autoimmune component based on the presence of circulating and tissue-bound Ig and lymphocytes which recognize epithelial cell and neutrophil epitopes these responses probably represent secondary rather than primary etiologic events [59, 60]. Crossreactivity of intestinal, biliary, synovial, dermal, and eye antigens is a plausible explanation for concurrent inflammation in these organs, particularly if molecular mimicry between organ-specific epitopes and highly conserved enteric bacterial antigens is considered.

Sclerosing cholangitis

PSC patients with IBD have an increased frequency of associated autoimmune disorders compared with IBD patients without liver disease (25% vs 9%, $p < 0.005$) [61], indicating an increased propensity for dysregulated immune responses. Serum anticolon antibodies from IBD patients were reported to react with proliferating bile ductules from obstructed livers [62]. Attempts to reproduce this observation demonstrated an increased frequency of anticolon antibodies in IBD patients with PSC, but these anticolon antibodies did not bind to biliary epithelium, although half of these patients had distinct serum antibodies that reacted with neutrophils [63, 64]. Approximately 70% of patients with UC have circulating IgG antineutrophil cytoplasmic antibodies with a characteristic perinuclear pattern (pANCA) [65, 66]. These antibodies are present in 65% of patients with PSC, regardless of associated UC, but in none of the patients with PBC and chronic active hepatitis or normal controls examined [67]. No correlation exists between ANCA titer and dis-

ease activity of PSC or UC, and these antibodies persist after colectomy. Unfortunately, from the diagnostic perspective, ANCA has been described in up to 39% of patients with PBC and the high frequency of pANCA in UC (60–70%) does not allow this assay to be used as a sensitive detector of PSC in IBD patients [68]. Thirty percent of rats developed pANCA following portal vein injections of trinitrobenzene sulfonic acid [69], further supporting the secondary nature of this antibody response. The majority of PSC patients (55%) displayed antibodies to neutrophil granule components, most notably bactericidal/permeability-increasing protein (46%), cathepsin G (23%), and lactoferrin (22%) with anti-lactoferrin antibody more frequent with associated UC [70]. Of note, Lindgren and co-workers reported only slightly lower frequencies of anti-neutrophil granule proteins in PBC patients (BPI 20%, lactoferrin 7%, cathepsin G 4%), hindering differentiation between these two cholestatic syndromes [68]. However, anti-catalase antibodies in 60% of PSC patients' sera vs 0% in UC [71], raises the possibility of a sensitive marker of PSC in UC patients. Moreover, crossreactivity of anticatalase antibodies with biliary epithelial cells suggests an autoimmune activity. The recent observation of reactivity of pANCA with nuclear histone H_1 as well as the common enteric commmensals *E. coli* and *Bacteroides* caccae suggests molecular mimicry as the genesis of this autoimmune response [72, 73]. 'Atypical' pANCA found in PSC and autoimmune hepatitis react to a 50 kDa nuclear envelope protein of neutrophils and myeloid cells [74].

Mieli-Vergani *et al.* [75] reported that antibodies to a liver membrane protein preparation and lymphocyte toxicity to autologous hepatocytes were present in the majority of patients with PSC and autoimmune chronic active hepatitis in children, although the biologic relevance of an autoimmune response to hepatocytes rather than to biliary epithelial cells in PSC is unclear. Inhibition of leukocyte migration by bile from patients with PSC raises the possibility of a reaction to biliary antigens, although similar changes in patients with PBC and chronic active hepatitis suggest this is a secondary event [76]. In a separate study 20 different autoantibodies were compared in 73 PSC patients and 75 healthy controls [77]. At least one autoantibody was positive in 97% of PSC patients and 81% had three or more positive autoantibodies in contrast to 24% of controls with at least one autoantibody. Antinuclear antibody (ANA), anticardiolipin, ANCA, rheumatoid factor, and antithyroperoxidase were positive significantly more often in PSC than in controls. The presence of IBD did not affect the rate of positivity. Anticardiolipin antibodies were the only markers that correlated with liver histology ($r = 0.30$, $p < 0.01$) and Mayo risk score ($r = 0.49$, $p < 0.001$).

Das *et al.* have reported crossreacting epitopes on colonic, biliary, ciliary body, and skin epithelial cells [78, 79]. IgG bound to UC tissue recognized a 40 kDa protein on colonic epithelial cells which has been identified as tropomyosin isoform 5, a component of the colonic epithelial cytoskeleton [80]. A monoclonal antibody raised to this partially purified protein also reacted with inflamed gallbladder, obstructed and inflamed extrahepatic bile ducts, and normal skin, but not with biliary epithelium in 10 liver biopsies. Five of eight patients with PSC with or without UC had circulating antibodies that competed with monoclonal antibody binding to extrahepatic biliary epithelium [81]. However, in previous studies [82] the same authors showed that IgG eluted from UC colons did not bind to homogenated normal human and rat livers. Additional conceptual problems include: (1) this epitope is distributed in all skin layers, which should lead to widespread exfoliative dermatitis rather than focal erythema nodosum and pyoderma gangrenosum; (2) skin inflammation is not linked to PSC, although both occur independently in patients with UC; (3) less than 10% of patients with UC develop skin or biliary inflammation, but colon-bound and serum IgG recognizing 40 kDa protein is found in 90% of ulcerative patients [82]; and (4) no complement deposition or IgG binding is found in PSC tissues by immunohistochemical studies.

In confirmatory studies, Sakamaki *et al.* [83] reported increased serum antibodies and antibody cell-mediated cytotoxicity (ADCC) to a nine amino acid peptide of tropomyosin in UC and PSC compared with CD and PBC patients. Moreover, this peptide can bind to HLA DPW9. Biancone *et al.* [84] found increased serum antibodies to tropomyosin isoform 1 in asymptomatic relatives of UC patients, suggesting that this antibody may precede inflammation, although antitropomyosin antibodies appear *after* the onset of experimental colitis in Gαi2$^{-/-}$ mice [85], indicating a secondary phenomenon. The lack of significant biliary inflammation in Gαi2-deficient and TCR$\alpha^{-/-}$ mice [85, 86] with colitis and serum and mucosal antitropomyosin antibodies argues against these autoantibodies mediating PSC in humans. Furthermore, Khoo *et al.* were unable to

detect IgA or IgG antibodies binding tropomyosin in mucosal washings of patients with UC with and without PSC [87].

Ueno and co-workers have developed a model in which rats immunized with purified autologous cholangiocytes in Freund's adjuvant developed non-suppurative cholangitis and small duct disease visualized by cholangiogram [88]. Inflammation was transferable by splenic lymphocytes and cholangiocyte-immunized splenocytes killed biliary epithelial cells *in vitro*. Because anticarbonic anhydrase II antibody was present in these immunized rats, these investigators created a murine model of cholangitis using injections of purified human carbonic anhydrase II that was transferable by T cells [89]. These studies suggest that PSC is caused by autoreactive T cells targeting cholangiocytes, perhaps after a nonspecific injury unveils previously hidden cholangiocyte antigens. Anticarbonic anhydrase II antibodies were not found in 12 PSC patients but were detected in five of six patients with autoimmune cholangitis [90]. The presence of a specific antigen is suggested by the finding of a predominant TCR V beta3 gene usage in liver tissues from patients with PSC [91]. These antigens are difficult to study due to heterogeneity among cholangiocytes [92].

The well-studied mouse model of graft-versus-host disease (GVHD) may also have implications for human PSC. Irradiated recipient BALB/c mice injected with spleen cells from mice minor histocompatibility complex differences develop non-suppurative destructive cholangitis with mononuclear cell infiltration. T cells responded to the minor histocompatibility antigen of cholangiocytes. No cholangiographic studies have been performed in this model but histologic evidence of periductal and duct wall fibroplasia occurs within 1 week and distinct extrahepatic and intrahepatic duct fibrosis develop after 2 months [93]. This model is T lymphocyte-dependent [94] and biliary epithelial injury is mediated in part by Fas-induced apoptosis [95], and tumor necrosis factor (TNF) [96], since hepatic GVHD is attenuated by T lymphocyte depletion, treatment with a Fas–Fc fusion protein or anti-TNF antibodies and transplantation in Fas-deficient lpr mice [97]. These studies demonstrate the potential for activated T cells responding to biliary epithelial cells to induce cholangitis. However, the relevance of these rodent studies is questioned by the observation that Fas and costimulatory molecules are expressed in only a small minority of biliary epithelial cells in

PSC tissues, in contrast to frequent expression in PBC [98].

Arthritis and ankylosing spondylitis

Shared epitopes between bacterial proteins and human HLA-B27 raise the possibility that molecular mimicry is the basis of the association of HLA-B27 with ankylosing spondylitis and reactive arthritis [99, 100]. Antibodies generated to either HLA-B27 lymphocytes or synthetic peptides crossreact with various Gram-negative enteric bacteria, especially *Klebsiella pneumoniae, Y. enterocolitica, Shigella flexneri, Salmonella typhimurium*, and *E. coli*. These findings are relevant because *Yersinia, S. flexneri*, and *Salmonella* are associated with reactive arthritis, and patients with ankylosing spondylitis have increased fecal isolation rates and serum antibodies to Klebsiella [101]. Sequence homology exists between HLA-B27 amino acids 72–77 and *K. pneumoniae* nitrogenase reductase amino acids 188–193 (Gln-Thr-Asp-ArgGlu-Asp) [99]. However, only 30% of patients with ankylosing spondylitis and 54% of those with Reiter's syndrome have circulating antibodies to HLA-B27, and there are no reports of synovial anti-HLA-B27 antibodies. Tsuchiya *et al.* [102] have demonstrated that a five amino acid peptide in a plasmid (pHS-2) isolated from four arthritogenic *S. flexneri* strains bears sequence homology with the same hypervariable segment in the B-27 molecule (amino acids 71–75). This epitope is expressed in synovial tissue of patients with ankylosing spondylitis who are B27-positive, but only 10.5% of patients with ankylosing spondylitis and 4.4% of those with Reiter's syndrome or reactive arthritis (4.1% of normal controls) had serum antibodies that reacted with pHS-2, and these sera displayed no cytotoxicity to HLA-B27 lymphocytes. Similar sequence homology applies to a four amino acid segment in a plasmid-coded outer membrane protein of *Yersinia*; 16.7% of men but no women with ankylosing spondylitis displayed increased anti-*Yersinia* peptide antibodies, but only one patient had crossreacting antibodies between *Yersinia* and HLA-B27 [103]. Although the molecular mimicry hypothesis is an appealing explanation of persistent inflammation induced by transient infection, only a minority of patients with ankylosing spondylitis and reactive arthritis have detectable crossreacting antibodies. Furthermore, molecular mimicry between HLA-B27 and bacteria does not explain tissue specificity of inflammation, why inflammation is confined to the axial skeleton, or the mechanism of inflammation in HLA-B27-negative patients, which comprise 30–40% of IBD patients with ankylosing spondylitis. Data from HLA-B27 transgenic mice suggest that experimental arthritis is mediated by antigen presentation by HLA-B27 rather than autoimmune responses to B27 peptides [104–106]. Confirmatory data are provided by susceptibility to arthritis in HLA-B27 transgenic rats transferred by bone marrow transplant, indicating that host antigens are not involved [107].

The strong homology between bacterial and mammalian heat-shock proteins (HSP) (stress proteins) also could lead to humoral and cell-mediated autoimmune responses. Serum antibodies to HSP 90 have been described in patients with ankylosing spondylitis, and lymphocyte clones from synovial fluid of patients with *Yersinia*-induced reactive arthritis proliferate upon exposure to *Yersinia* antigens and mycobacterial or human 65 kDa HSP [108]. Thiel *et al.* reported that HSP 60 is one of two dominant *Yersinia* antigens, inducing responses in 0.66% of synovial CD4$^+$ cells in patients with reactive arthritis [45]. HSP expression in human cells is increased by heat, viral infection, interferon gamma (IFN-γ), reactive oxygen metabolites, cytokines, and mitogens [109]. The expression of at least one 65 kDa HSP is increased in UC epithelial cells and goblet cells [110], although intraepithelial and peripheral blood lymphocytes from patients with CD do not display heightened reactivity to this protein [111]. T lymphocyte clones reactive to HSP 65 mediate experimental Freund's adjuvant-induced arthritis, whereas active immunization with HSP 65 prevents streptococcal cell wall and adjuvant-induced arthritis [112]. Monoclonal antibodies to HSP 65 react with rheumatoid arthritis synovium but not normal joints, raising the possibility that injured joint tissues express HSP on cell membranes. This hypothesis is given additional credence by the report that the HSP 90 family preferentially binds to HLA-B27 [113]. Three of the 11 peptides eluted from purified HLA-B27 molecules were HSP 89. However, a lack of arthritis accompanying small intestinal and hepatic inflammation induced in TCR$\beta^{-/-}$ mice by transfer of HSP 60-reactive CD8 T cells [114] suggests that autoreactive HSP responses cannot be induced without some preexisting injury to up-regulate HSP 60. Furthermore, Mertz *et al.* [115] demonstrated no crossreactivity of *Yersinia* HSP 60 T cell clones from a patient with post-*Yersinia* reactive arthritis with human HSP 60.

An immune response against matrix proteins is an additional means of perpetuating chronic ankylosing spondylitis. A cell-mediated response to cartilage proteoglycans in patients with ankylosing spondylitis and the development of progressive polyarthritis and ankylosing spondylitis in Balb/c mice immunized with fetal human proteoglycan depleted of chondroitin sulfate supports this hypothesis [116]. Moreover, evidence exists of crossreactive matrix protein and bacterial cell wall epitopes. Van den Broek *et al.* [117] demonstrated that synovial but not peripheral blood mononuclear cells from a patient with Crohn's colitis and arthritis proliferate in response to dermatan sulfate proteoglycan, chondroitin sulfate, and bacterial cell walls extracted from *Bacillus megaterium*, *E. coli*, and *Streptococcus pyogenes*. Murine T cells primed with cell wall polymers from group A streptococci or E. coli induce a humoral and cellular anticartilage response.

Thus, humoral and cellular immune responses to a variety of bacterial antigens crossreact with mammalian HLA-B27, HSP, and cartilage components, but the role of these epitopes as a primary event in the pathogenesis of arthritis is not yet clear. Tissue specificity is obvious for the cartilage components but less clear for HLA-B27 and HSP, which are present in all tissues. However, secondary autoimmune responses to cartilage matrix proteins and inducible HSP molecules may be one mechanism of perpetuating chronic spondyloarthropathy initiated by a transient infection or nonimmunologic injury.

Skin manifestations

Older studies describe circulating antibodies that recognize skin and colonic antigens [118], and monoclonal antibodies raised to the 40 kDa human colon epithelial antigen (tropomyosin) of Das *et al.* [78] crossreact diffusely with normal skin. Although deposition of Ig and complement could be interpreted as a primary humoral response to skin antigens rather than immune complex localization, very little direct evidence of autoimmune activity in common skin complications exists. However, 15 cases of epidermolysis bullosa acquisita, which is characterized by IgG autoantibodies against a 145–290 kDa protein of the dermaepidermal junction, have been described in patients with CD [119].

Uveitis

Although no direct evidence supports an autoimmune reaction in human disease, pANCA antibodies have been described in 29% of patients with anterior uveitis [120]. The well-characterized animal model of experimental allergic uveitis (EAU) raises the possibility of similar autoimmune cell responses in humans. Immunization with S protein, a watersoluble 45 kDa retinal protein with at least four active epitopes [121], interphotoreceptor retinoidbinding protein, or bovine melanin protein derived from uveal and retinal pigment epithelium [122] produces a chronic T lymphocyte-dependent posterior uveitis and retinitis [123].

Hematologic

Autoimmune Coomb's-positive hemolytic anemia and neutropenia unrelated to therapy are infrequently associated with IBD [124, 125], but their incidence in patients with IBD is not clearly increased over the general population. ANCA is found in 60% of patients with UC and 20% of those with CD [65], but these do not cause neutrophil lysis.

Conclusions

Supporting evidence of primary autoimmune mechanisms for hepatobiliary, skin, eye, and hematologic complications of intestinal inflammation is weak, but a humoral or cellular response to epitopes on HLA-B27, HSP, or cartilage matrix proteins that bear sequence homology to enteric bacteria, may play a role in reactive and spondyloarthropathies. Rodent models demonstrate the ability of T cells reactive to biliary epithelial antigens to induce experimental cholangitis, although evidence of autoimmune T lymphocyte responses in human PSC is not available.

Immune complex-mediated injury

Although controversial [126], findings of levels of circulating immune complexes in patients with UC and CD have been reported to correlate with disease activity [127]. Interestingly, serum immune complexes are associated with colonic involvement in CD (47% colon only, 28% ileocolitis, and 9% small intestinal only) but only weakly correlate with the extent of UC (33% substantial vs 26% distal). Circulating immune complexes are increased in patients with extraintestinal manifestations: 54 vs 22% of patients without extraintestinal disease [128]. In serum sickness circulating large immune complexes produce complement-mediated fever, leukopenia, arthritis, lymphadenopathy, urticaria, glomerulonephritis, and arteritis. However, as discussed by Soltis *et al.* [126], who failed to detect circulating immune complexes in patients with UC or CD, conventional methods are indirect and subject to false-positive results in the setting of low albumin, elevated globulin, and increased C reactive protein present in active IBD. Lack of activation of the classical complement pathway [129] supports the paucity of convincing evidence for pathogenic immune complexes in patients with IBD.

Sclerosing cholangitis

Serum immune complexes have been described in up to 80% of PSC patients with or without UC [130] and also have been found within bile [131]. Senaldi et al. [132] noted immune complexes in 88% of patients with PSC and provided evidence of classical complement activation but found no correlation between circulating immune complexes and complement or complement fragment concentrations. Hodgson et al. [128] found that 50% of IBD patients with pericholangitis and PSC, but 100% of patients with cirrhosis, had circulating, predominantly large immune complexes, consistent with an inability of diseased livers to clear these complexes. Defective clearance of IgG-opsonized red blood cells in patients with PSC compared with liver disease controls and normals raises the possibility of a similar defect in clearing immune complexes [133]. Immune complexes were found in these patients but in considerably lower frequency than disease controls 133]. The lack of specificity compared to disease controls of matched severity and the lack of correlation with disease activity and complement activation diminish the probability that immune complexes are involved in the pathogenesis of PSC.

Arthritis

Circulating antibody and cryoprotein complexes, some containing antibodies against E. coli and Bacteroides, were found in the majority of patients who develop arthritis following jejunoileal bypass [134]. A pathologic role of these complexes is suggested by complement activation in the serum, immune complexes in synovial fluid and Ig, and complement in dermal and synovial biopsy material [135, 136]. IgM complexes containing Yersinia antigens are present in the serum and sterile synovial fluid [137] of patients in the early phase of reactive arthritis after Yersinia enteritis. Immune complexes have not been described in synovial fluid of IBD patients with arthritis, although Hodgson et al. [128] reported that all 14 patients with acute arthritis, none of nine patients with chronic arthritis, and four of six patients with ankylosing spondylitis had circu-

lating small immune complexes. Serum IgA immune complexes were found in 75% of 40 patients with ankylosing spondylitis followed serially for 9 months [138]. Two patients with IBD and ankylosing spondylitis who developed nephropathy and leukocytoclastic vasculitis had circulating IgA immune complexes and perivascular IgA deposits in the skin and renal mesangium [139]. The association of IgA nephropathy with ankylosing spondylitis is well established, convincingly arguing for the pathogenic nature of circulating IgA immune complexes in this disorder. Drug-induced delayed-type hypersensitivity responses with arthritis, urticaria, and fever secondary to immune complexes develop in 25% of widely spread infliximab infusions [140].

Skin lesions

Data concerning immune complexes in human IBD-associated skin lesions are inconsistent and sparse, although the immunopathology of erythema nodosum and the association of this condition with infectious agents raises the possibility of immune complex involvement. In Hodgson's series the one IBD patient with erythema nodosum had immune complexes, whereas one patient with pyoderma gangrenosum did not [128]. Pyoderma gangrenosum occasionally responds to plasmapheresis, a treatment that could decrease the concentration of circulating immune complexes as well as autoantibodies, cytokines, and bacterial polymers.

Two IBD patients with skin necrosis described by Mayer et al. [141] had circulating cryoglobulins (one patient) and cryofibrinogen (one patient), but neither patient had circulating immune complexes, cutaneous vasculitis, or immunoglobulin or complement within skin biopsies. Patients with the arthritis–dermatitis syndrome associated with jejunoileal bypass have a neutrophilic vasculitis (Sweet's syndrome) or leukocytoclastic vasculitis with detectable IgG and complement on skin biopsy [3, 142, 143]. Granulomatous vasculitis without immune deposits is a prominent feature of dermal 'metastatic CD' [143]. The pathophysiology of these lesions may be relevant to the recently described granulomatous vasculitis in submucosal vessels draining areas of active CD [144] and perhaps Takayasu's arteritis occasionally associated with CD.

Iritis/uveitis

There is very little evidence that immune complexes play a role in iritis or uveitis complicating IBD. In Hodgson's series neither of two patients with uveitis had circulating immune complexes [128]. Immune complexes do not preferentially localize to the eye, and uveitis is not a common feature of serum sickness. Immune complexes are present in Behçet's disease, but they do not correlate with the course of uveitis and appear only during the healing phase of experimental autoimmune uveitis [145].

Conclusions

Circulating immune complexes or cryoproteins appear to be important in the pathogenesis of arthritis and cutaneous vasculitis associated with bacterial overgrowth in jejunoileal bypass, the rare dermal necrosis associated with IBD, and IgA nephropathy accompanying ankylosing spondylitis. Circulating immune complexes are present in postinfectious arthritis (best documented for *Yersinia*), in ankylosing spondylitis (IgA), and perhaps in acute arthritis of IBD, but their causal role in these syndromes has not yet been established. At present the role of immune complexes in the pathogenesis of systemic inflammation associated with IBD remains speculative.

Systemic absorption of toxic luminal contents

The distal intestine contains high concentrations of dietary antigens, digestive enzymes, and bacterial products capable of producing local and systemic inflammation if absorbed [146–148]. Increased intestinal permeability to inert markers in patients with CD, even during quiescent phases of inflammation [149], is well documented. Systemic absorption of bacterial lipopolysaccharide (LPS) [150] and increased serum antibodies to lipid A [151] occur in patients with active CD, whereas IBD patients with PSC have increased plasma concentrations of formylated oligopeptides (FMLP) [152]. Systemic absorption of FMLP [153, 154] and peptidoglycan-polysaccharide (PG-PS) [155] is dramatically increased in rats with acetic acid-induced colitis; both of these toxic bacterial products undergo biliary excretion. FMLP, LPS, PG-PS, and antigens produced by pathogenic as well as commensal bacteria inhabiting the distal intestine can induce inflammatory activities relevant to IBD and its systemic complications, including activation of immunoregulatory and effector immune cells, activation of the complement and kallikrein–kinin systems, and production of proinflammatory cytokines and eicosanoids [146, 156–158]. Circulating neutrophils from patients with active IBD have increased numbers of membrane FMLP receptors [159]. These bacterial

products have synergistic activities. For example, LPS can prime a cell to be triggered by low doses of FMLP or PG-PS, whereas low doses of PG-PS or LPS can reactivate arthritis in a joint previously injured by PG-PS [160]. A single intraperitoneal or intramural injection of PG-PS can induce systemic inflammation remarkably similar to the spectrum of extraintestinal manifestations of IBD (Table 4) [158]. Chronicity of experimental inflammation in this model depends on two factors: persistence of PG-PS polymers in tissue and genetically determined host susceptibility [158]. Easily biodegradable (derived from peptostreptococci or enterococci) or small PG-PS polymers induce only transient inflammation, whereas larger, lysozyme-resistant PG-PS complexes (derived from group A streptococci, certain eubacterial species, or mycobacteria) produce chronic, spontaneously relapsing granulomatous inflammation in susceptible inbred rat strains (Lewis and Sprague–Dawley). Although very few data are currently available for the role of intestinal bacterial products in systemic complications of IBD, the extensive experimental evidence of inflammation induced by these products is discussed below.

Hepatobiliary inflammation

Heat-killed non-pathogenic *E. coli*, either alone or opsonized with immune serum, injected into peripheral or portal veins of rabbits three times over 6 weeks caused acute periportal and focal parenchymal inflammation, which progressed to granulomatous periportal inflammation with fibrosis, proliferation of bile ducts and Kupffer cells [161]. Inflammation had resolved 1 month after the final injection, but marked circumductular fibrosis, portal vein sclerosis, and proliferation of small bile ducts persisted. No transaminase or alkaline phosphatase

Table 4. Systemic inflammation induced by peptidoglycan-polysaccharide

Single intraperitoneal or intestinal injection of purified PG-PS	Intestinal bacterial overgrowth with anaerobic bacteria
Peripheral arthritis	Hepatobiliary inflammation
Granulomatous hepatitis	Reactivation of arthritis*
Uveitis	Anemia*
Cutaneous vasculitis	
Anemia	
Leukocytosis	

*Correlated with experimental bacterial overgrowth, but mechanism of inflammation remains speculative.

alterations were found after 3 and 5 months. This experiment shows the injurious potential of non-viable normal flora bacteria and suggests that inflammatory molecules, cytokines, and growth factors that mediate fibrosis also induce bile duct proliferation. LPS up-regulates inducible nitric oxide synthase (iNOS) expression in biliary epithelial cells *in vivo* [162] and interleukin 6 (IL-6) *in vitro* [163] and stimulates proliferation of isolated biliary epithelial cells through an IL-6-mediated, p44/p42 MAP kinase-dependent pathway [163]. Luminal FMLP is absorbed following experimental gut inflammation [153] and macrophages are necessary for lymphocyte infiltration in a model of FMLP-induced cholangitis following acetic acid-induced colitis in rats [164].

Genetically susceptible rats challenged with experimental small intestinal bacterial overgrowth develop chronic hepatobiliary inflammation that resembles PSC [12]. A jejunal self-filling blind loop (SFBL) induces rapid proliferation of anaerobic bacteria and progressive hepatomegaly, spleno-megaly, elevation of aspartate aminotransferase (AST), and histologic evidence of hepatobiliary injury with a 50% mortality rate in Lewis rats. Bile duct inflammation is associated with periportal infiltration of mononuclear cells and scattered PMN (Fig. 1), periportal fibrosis, and bile duct injury with focal parenchymal inflammation and Kupffer cell hyperplasia. Differential genetic susceptibility is a unique feature of this model, with Lewis and Wistar rats developing hepatobiliary inflammation [12] but not Buffalo or Fischer F344 rats. The relevance of this model to human PSC is enhanced by the demonstration that susceptible rats have markedly thickened extrahepatic bile ducts due to epithelial hyperplasia and fibrosis and abnormal cholangio-grams with ectatic extrahepatic ducts and irregular, tortuous, and beaded intrahepatic bile ducts (Fig. 2) [165]. No evidence of extrahepatic biliary obstruc-tion was present, but intrahepatic bile duct strictures were demonstrated using cholangiography [165]. Anaerobic bacteria are important because hepato-biliary inflammation is prevented and treated by metronidazole and tetracycline but not by genta-micin or polymyxin B. The latter antibiotic binds lipopolysaccharide (LPS) in addition to providing Gram-negative aerobic coverage [166]. Preliminary studies suggest a role for *Bacteroides* species. The peritoneal cavity, bile, liver, and cardiac blood are consistently culture-negative.

PG-PS from luminal bacteria has been incrimi-nated in the pathogenesis of this inflammatory process. Plasma anti-PG IgA, IgM, and IgG are increased in all rat strains with small bowel bacterial overgrowth, indirectly indicating mucosal absorp-tion of PG-PS, but anti-PG antibodies do not correlate with hepatobiliary inflammation [167]. Increased concentrations of plasma and hepatic PG-PS in rats with SFBL after injection of PG-PS from group A streptococci into the proximal jejunum

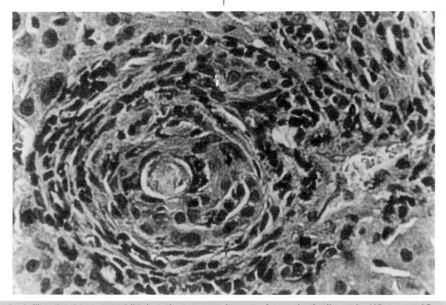

Figure 1. Periductular infiltration by neutrophils, lymphocytes, and macrophages in the liver of a Wistar rat 12 weeks after creation of jejunal self-filling blind loop. (Reprinted from ref. 12 with permission.)

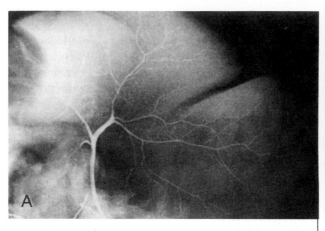 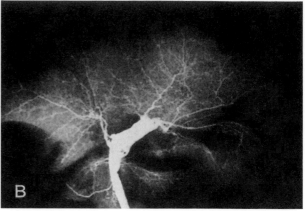

Figure 2. Cholangiograms using barium sulfate in Lewis rats 4 weeks after creation of a jejunal self-emptying blind loop (**A**) or self-filling blind loop (**B**). In the control rat (**A**) the intrahepatic ducts are smooth and gradually taper. After self-filling blind loop (**B**), the extrahepatic duct is ectatic, and intrahepatic ducts are tortuous and irregular with neoductularization. (Reprinted from ref. 165 with permission.)

provide direct evidence of luminal PG-PS absorption and systemic distribution. Intravenously injected PG-PS is detected in bile, suggesting an entero-hepatic circulation of this high-molecular weight polymer G-PS from endogenous luminal bacteria in this model is the observation that mutanolysin, a muralytic enzyme which splits the βI-4 polymer of PG-PS without direct antibiotic activity, prevents and treats the hepatobiliary inflammation [169]. The ability of PG-PS to cause hepatic inflammation is confirmed by the observation that purified PG-PS from group A streptococci injected into the perito-neal cavity or intestinal wall causes a T cell-mediated chronic granulomatous hepatitis with marked fibro-sis in inbred Lewis rats, but not Buffalo or Fischer rats [158, 170]. Moreover, PG-PS or LPS stimulate production of TNF, IL-1, and transforming growth factor β (TGF-β) by Kupffer cells and hepatic granuloma macrophages [169, 171]. A human correlate of this model is hepatic inflammation which develops in 20% of patients with anaerobic bacterial overgrowth following jejunoileal bypass performed for morbid obesity [142].

Accumulation of endotoxin in biliary epithelial cells has been documented in humans with PBC and PSC [172]. Although concentrations of peptido-glycan in PSC have not been investigated, serum antibodies to PG are increased in patients with PSC [173]. However, FMLP is detected in higher concen-trations in the plasma of patients with PSC [152] and LPS serum levels correlate with disease activity in IBD patients [150, 174], clearly demonstrating

enhanced uptake of bacterial products with intestinal inflammation. The role of luminal bacteria in hepatobiliary inflammation is further supported by decreased periportal inflammation in germfree IL-2 knockout mice compared with specific pathogen-free littermates [14].

Arthritis

Y. enterocolitica 0:3 LPS was detected by immuno-fluorescence within synovial fluid PMN in 10 of 15 patients with post-*Yersinia*-reactive arthritis, despite negative cultures [43]. Provocative but poorly controlled studies in patients with jejunoileal bowel bypass syndrome have demonstrated radiolabeled bacterial cell walls in circulating immune complexes [135], exacerbation of arthritis with skin testing with bacterial peptidoglycan [175], and *E. coli* antigen in dermal biopsies [135]. Similar studies in IBD-asso-ciated arthritis have not been performed, but serum anti-PG antibodies are elevated in patients with ankylosing spondylitis [176], and seronegative arthritis [177].

Commensal bacteria are involved in the patho-genesis of arthritis in HLA-B27 transgenic rats. Germfree B27 transgenic rats fail to develop arthritis, colitis, and gastritis, which are found in these rats raised under conventional conditions [54]. Aggressive disease was associated with increased cecal *E. coli* and *Enterococcus* species [178], and monoassociation studies in gnotobiotic B27 trans-genic rats indicate a selective role for *Bacteroides vulgatus* in the pathogenesis of colitis [179]. Similarly,

HLA-B27 transgenic/murine β_2-microglobulin-deficient mice develop arthritis only when transferred to conventional housing from specific pathogen-free conditions [180].

Bacterial cell wall polymers can induce and reactivate experimental peripheral arthritis in genetically susceptible rats. A single intraperitoneal injection of a sterile suspension of PG-PS from group A streptococci produces acute synovitis in ankle joints, which develops into chronic, spontaneously reactivating erosive polyarthritis in Sprague–Dawley and Lewis rats [181, 182]. PG-PS from bacterial species normally inhibiting the intestine, including *Enterococcus fecium*, *Lactobacillus casei*, and *Eubacterium contortum*, isolated from a patient with CD, can induce chronic arthritis, whereas transient non-erosive arthritis develops after intraperitoneal injection of PG-PS from a variety of Gram-positive normal enteric flora [183, 184]. Studies in *Eubacterium* species with different abilities to induce arthritis indicate that the chemical structure of PG is responsible for arthritogenicity [185]. Complement-mediated events are involved in the acute phase, whereas the chronic and reactivating phases of arthritis are T cell-dependent. Immune complexes are not involved. Once arthritis has been initiated by systemic or intra-articular injection of PG-PS, it can be reactivated by homologous or heterologous peptidoglycan polymers, LPS from normal enteric bacteria or pathogens (*S. typhimurium*), or superantigens in concentrations that do not cause inflammation in previously non-injured joints. Local or systemic injection of LPS into rats with joints not previously injured with PG-PS leads to mild, very transient arthritis [160]. Similarly, oral LPS can exacerbate collagen-induced arthritis [186]. Immunization with complete Freund's adjuvant, whose moiety is mycobacterial peptidoglycan, produces destructive arthritis and systemic inflammation.

We have extended these observations by showing that subserosal injection of group A streptococcal PG-PS into the distal intestine can produce chronic, erosive polyarthritis [158], and that experimental small intestinal anaerobic bacterial overgrowth can reactivate arthritis in genetically susceptible rats [13]. Reactivation of arthritis occurred within 3 days in Lewis rats with SFBL but not following control self-emptying blind loops or sham operations performed 7 days after intra-articular injection of PG-PS [13]. There was no evidence of systemic or joint infection. We hypothesize that systemic distribution of sterile bacterial cell wall polymers (PG-PS or LPS) derived from the intestine induced arthritis in a manner analogous to hepatobiliary inflammation accompanying experimental bacterial overgrowth [12]. The concept of systemic distribution of arthritogenic bacterial cell wall polymers is supported by the observation that transplanted livers from Lewis rats injected intraperitoneally with PG-PS reactivated quiescent arthritis in recipients, which accumulated PG-PS in the blood and spleen [187].

Skin inflammation

Poorly characterized epidermolytic substances have been extracted from stools of patients with pyoderma gangrenosum [188]. Guinea pigs systemically injected with PG-PS develop dermal necrosis secondary to vasculitis [189], but cutaneous lesions do not occur in rats. However, dermal injection of PG-PS leads to chronic spontaneously relapsing local granulomatous inflammation in rabbits [190].

Uveitis

Systemic injection of either heat-killed Gram-negative organisms, purified LPS [191], PG-PS [192] or lipoteichoic acid [193] induces an acute, transient uveitis in rats or mice, whereas more chronic uveitis is a feature of Freund's adjuvant-induced disease in Lewis rats [194]. A Lewis rat model of acute anterior uveitis induced by intravenous or oral injection of a *Salmonella enteritidis* or *Yersinia enterocolitica* 0:3 was not influenced by the presence of the HLA-B27 transgene [195]. Subcutaneous injection of LPS into C3H/HeN mice induces a biphasic acute uveitis, peaking at 1 and 5 days with an early infiltration of neutrophils and later influx of macrophages [196].

Hematologic

Chronic anemia, leukocytosis (increased PMN and monocytes), and thrombocytosis whose course closely parallels that of peripheral arthritis occurs after a single systemic or intramural intestinal injection of PG-PS in Lewis rats [197]. This experimental anemia resembles anemia of chronic disease as it is mild to moderate, red blood cell survival is decreased, red blood cells are slightly microcytic, serum iron and transferrin concentrations are decreased, reticuloendothelial iron stores are normal or increased, and no gastrointestinal blood loss occurs [197]. Chronic anemia also accompanies adjuvant arthritis in Lewis rats.

Conclusions

Experimental animal models convincingly indicate that bacterial products of intestinal origin can induce peripheral arthritis, hepatobiliary inflammation, uveitis, and hematologic abnormalities, and that systemic absorption of these luminal products is enhanced by mucosal inflammation. Only genetically susceptible hosts develop chronic inflammation, and inflammation which, once initiated, can be perpetuated and reactivated by very small amounts of a variety of bacterial products. To date only circumstantial evidence incriminates luminal antigens and bacterial polymers in the extraintestinal inflammation of IBD and gut injury, but this hypothesis merits further investigation.

Systemic distribution of inflammatory mediators

The intense inflammatory response of active UC and CD generates a complex array of immunologically active inflammatory mediators (see Chapters 7 to 12), including eicosanoids, cytokines, growth factors, complement products, kallikrein–kinin pathway components, reactive oxygen metabolites, and metalloproteinases. Although intestinal levels are much higher than circulating concentrations of these inflammatory products a number of cytokines have been detected in peripheral blood of patients with active IBD [59, 60], and plasma TNF concentrations are increased after experimental intestinal bacterial overgrowth [169]. Circulating cytokines could be produced by immunocytes within the inflamed intestine, reticuloendothelial system, or blood. Regardless of their origin, circulating inflammatory mediators can induce and reactivate inflammation in systemic organs. Interestingly, IL-1 [198] and TNF [199] production is greater in Crohn's colitis than ileitis, paralleling the incidence of extraintestinal manifestations.

Hepatobiliary inflammation

Inflammatory mediators produced by the inflamed colon and transported in relatively high concentrations through the portal vein could generate hepatobiliary injury. Systemic administration of TNF over 8 days produced hepatomegaly (almost twice that of pair-fed controls), bile duct proliferation, portal tract inflammation with an influx of predominantly mononuclear cells, and focal parenchymal necrosis in female Sprague–Dawley rats [200]. Continuous infusion of murine recombinant IL-1α into male Sprague–Dawley rats for 10 days increased transaminases [201]. Excessive TNF release was documented in rats with hepatobiliary injury caused by a SFBL [202]. Pentoxifylline prevented bacterial overgrowth-induced hepatobiliary injury in these rats [202], but did not affect liver enzymes in 20 PSC patients [203]. In the human study, however, antibodies to peptidoglycan did decrease in all patients taking pentoxifylline over a 1-year period [173]. Leukotrienes also have deleterious effects on the liver [204]. IL-1 and TGF-β have potent fibrogenic properties by virtue of direct and indirect effects on fibroblasts and matrix protein metabolism [205]. Development of PSC in a patient with a primary intestinal T cell lymphoma [206] raises the possibility that products of activated intestinal T cells can induce biliary lesions, although the number of IFN-γ-producing cells has been reported to be lower in the lamina propria of UC patients with PSC than in UC patients without liver disease [207], possibly related to disease activity at the time of tissue collection. No differences in colonic IL-2 or IL-4 were noted in this study [208], consistent with the lack of differences in serum IFN-γ and GM-CSF in patients with PSC, alcoholic liver disease, and controls [209]. However, soluble CD23, IL-8, and IL-10 were noted in the serum of PSC patients [209]. Thus inflammatory mediators probably produced in excess by inflamed colonic tissues have effects directly relevant to the inflammation, fibrosis, and bile duct proliferation of PSC.

Arthritis

Normally subarthropathic amounts of cytokines can reactivate arthritis in joints previously injured by PG-PS. IL-1, TNF, platelet-derived growth factor, IL-8, and substance P will reactivate arthritis, each with a characteristic time course [210, 211] (S.A. Stimpson, unpublished observations). Interestingly, IL-6 and C5a have no effect in this model. Repeated injections of IL-1 into a previously injured joint promotes chronic erosive synovitis [210]. Injection of IL-1 or TGF-β into normal rat joints will induce transient non-erosive arthritis; however, systemic injection of TGF-β diminishes both acute and chronic phases of polyarthritis induced by intraperitoneal PG-PS [212]. In addition to their immunoregulatory properties, IL-1 and TNF can cause joint destruction by inducing macrophages, fibroblasts, and synovial lining cells to secrete collagenase, elastase, proteoglycanase, plasminogen, and arachidonic acid metabolites [205]. Enhanced local and systemic production of TNF by deletion of adenine uracil (AU)-rich elements which destabilize mRNA results in peripheral arthritis and ileitis in TNF 'knock in' mice (TNF ARE$^{-/-}$)[16]. An important consequence of circulating proinflammatory cytokines such as IL-1β, TNF and IL-6 is bone loss through activation of osteoclasts and inhibition of osteoblasts [213], which may explain the propensity for osteoporosis in IBD patients, especially those with CD, even in the absence of steroid therapy [214]. Alveolar bone loss was noted in older HLA-B27 transgenic rats [215], presumably related to long-standing inflammation in the intestine and peripheral joints.

Skin inflammation

No known specific skin effects are noted after systemic injection of cytokines, but dermal injection of IL-1, TGF-β, and IL-8 causes an influx of inflammatory cells, whereas TGF-β induces fibroplasia.

Hematologic abnormalities

Chronic anemia with decreased red blood cell mass but no change in plasma volume began 4 days after systemic TNF administration in rats and progressed for 8 days [200]. Leukocytosis accompanies systemic administration of both IL-1 [201] and TNF [200]. TNF inhibits erythroid precursor cell proliferation *in vitro* while increasing production of GM-CSF and other cytokines that influence hematopoietic cell growth and differentiation.

Conclusions

Although speculative at this time, inflammatory mediators absorbed from the inflamed intestine, especially the colon, probably contribute to periportal hepatic injury, reactive hepatopathy, reactivation or exacerbation of systemic inflammation, suppression of bone marrow red blood cell production, and stimulation of an acute-phase response. This mechanism could help explain why certain extraintestinal inflammatory events are related to disease activity in the colon.

Immune activation in extraintestinal organs

Cytokines and other inflammatory mediators produced within inflamed systemic organs, perhaps stimulated by systemic distribution of absorbed bacterial products, are almost certainly involved in the pathogenesis of extraintestinal inflammation associated with gut injury. Cytokine and inflammatory mediator profiles in the joint and liver are remarkably similar to those in the inflamed gut and respond similarly to selective mediator inhibition, suggesting that the initiating agents (antigens, cell wall polymers, and autoimmune targets) and/or underlying host immunoregulatory defects which stimulate inflammation in the gut and systemic organs are similar, if not identical.

Hepatobiliary inflammation

Biliary injury appears to be immune-mediated, with infiltration of activated Th1 lymphocytes, macrophages, and, to a lesser extent, neutrophils and eosinophils which produce proinflammatory cytokines (Table 5). The biliary epithelium is clearly a target of these activated immune cells, with responses ranging from apoptosis, lysis, and increased permeability to hyperproliferation [216–218]. Progression of disease in PSC is related to fibrogenesis, stricture formation, and secondary bacterial infection. Biliary epithelial cells not only are a passive recipient of immune-mediated injury, but actively participate in the inflammatory process. Proinflammatory cytokines secreted by activated bone marrow-derived and parenchymal cells stimulate the expression of a variety of cytokines (IL-6, IL-8, MCP-1), class II MHC molecules, adhesion molecules (ICAM1) and enzymes (iNOS) in biliary epithelial cells (Table 6). These same molecules which are induced *in vitro* have increased expression *in vivo* (Table 5) in the inflamed ductal epithelium of PSC and PBC patients, with expression correlating with histologic stage of activity [162]. Enhanced expression of α$_4$β$_7$ integrins in PSC tissues provides a mechanism by which intestinal T cells could selectively home to the inflamed liver [219]. T lymphocyte-mediated injury in PSC is suggested by a predominant Th1 cytokine profile [220, 221].

The role of biliary epithelial cells as functional antigen-presenting cells which stimulate T lympho-

Table 5. Activation of biliary epithelial cells during *in vivo* inflammation

A. *Spontaneous expression*
    ↑ Epithelial IL-6, IL-6 receptor, TNF, TNF receptor, ICAM1, VCAM1, MHC II, and stem cell factor in PBC > PSC
    ↑ Bile IL-6, TNF in acute cholangitis
    ↑ Serum IL-8, IL-10 in PSC

B. *Inducible expression (systemic administration)*
    LPS↑iNOS
    IL-2↑MHC II (IFN-γ-dependent)

strains that do not develop arthritis, Lewis rats have prolonged and increased recovery of viable *Y. enterocolitica* 0:8 in their spleens after intravenous inoculation [50]. Similar results occur in HLA-B27 transgenic mice, which do not develop arthritis without parallel manipulations of β_2-microglobulin but have higher incidences of paraspinal abscesses and mortality rates than B27-negative controls after intravenous injection of *Y. enterocolitica* [263]. HLA-B27 transgenic Lewis rats that develop spontaneous enterocolitis and arthritis have no detectable pathogenic bacteria, but had increased cecal concentrations of *E. coli* and *Enterococcus* species [178]. Evidence of defective immune responses in these rats is provided by decreased anti-*Yersinia* cytotoxic T lymphocyte responses in transgenic vs wild-type rats infected with *Yersinia paratuberculosis*, which were not MHC restricted to HLA-B27 [264], and by defective dendritic cell function [265]. Finally, arthritis in HLA-B27 transgenic mice occurs only in the absence of endogenous murine β_2-microglobulin [180]. Recently, Kingsbury *et al.* demonstrated that mice deficient in β_2-microglobulin or transporter associated with antigen processing (TAP-1) develop arthritis even in the absence of human HLA-27, suggesting that defective class I MHC antigen presentation is the mechanism of arthritis in these mice [266]. This defect could potentially result in deficient production of CD8 regulatory (suppressive) T lymphocytes, thereby fostering unopposed aggressive CD4[+] T cell responses. Reactive arthritis can occur in patients with AIDS, but the relative contribution of enteric or pulmonary pathogens vs overgrowth of normal flora is unknown.

Conversely, joint injury could arise from a dysregulated, exaggerated immune response to ubiquitous antigens, as has been demonstrated in Lewis and HLA-B27 transgenic rats and HLA-B27 patients. Neutrophils of HLA-B27-positive patients with reactive arthritis and ankylosing spondylitis have increased PMN chemokinesis, whereas B27-positive patients with severe recurrent reactive arthritis have enhanced superoxide production [267]. LPS-stimulated monocytes from healthy B27-positive subjects produce more IL-1 and TNF than do B27-negative controls, although monocytes from both groups kill *Y. enterocolitica* equally [268]. In recent studies we have demonstrated a decreased IL-10/IL-12 ratio in mesenteric lymph node cells stimulated with cecal bacterial lysates from HLA-B27 transgenic rats compared with wild-type controls [269].

Skin inflammation

Pyoderma-like lesions occur in immunosuppressed patients, and inconsistent reports of depressed phagocytic cell (especially PMN) and lymphocyte activity in patients with pyoderma have been published, although their delayed-type hypersensitivity response was normal in the study of Powell *et al.* [270].

Conclusions

Abnormal immunoregulation in patients with IBD who have extraintestinal inflammation remains speculative but is an important area of investigation, based on well-documented abnormalities present in patients with post-infectious reactive arthritis and evidence in rodent strains prone to arthritis and hepatobiliary inflammation. It will be important to determine whether the immunosuppression seen in patients with reactive arthritis secondary to *Yersinia* is unique to that bacterium, which produces immunosuppressive proteins [262]. Either deficient antimicrobial responses to pathogens leading to protracted infections, or a loss of tolerance to commensal bacterial or ubiquitous self antigens could lead to systemic inflammation. Defective immunoregulation will most likely be the basis for genetic susceptibility to extraintestinal manifestations of IBD.

Genetic influences

Although multiply affected families with PSC, ankylosing spondylitis, or IBD with systemic inflammation [6] have been described, the clearest evidence of a genetic influence in extraintestinal disorders is the association of certain HLA haplotypes with ankylosing spondylitis, reactive arthritis, PSC, and anterior uveitis. Genetically determined host susceptibility is further implicated by differential susceptibility of inbred rodents to hepatobiliary, joint, and eye inflammation.

Sclerosing cholangitis

From 60% to 80% of patients with PSC have the HLA-B8 haplotype vs 17–25% of controls, and approximately 70% display HLA-DR3 [258]. These antigens are not increased in UC patients without liver disease but are associated with a variety of diseases of suspected autoimmune etiology, including insulin-dependent diabetes mellitus, myasthenia gravis, Graves' disease, lupoid chronic hepatitis, dermatitis herpetiformis, and celiac disease. Several studies have found an association of PSC with the extended HLA A1-B8-DR3 haplotype and with DRB3*0101–DRB1*0301–DQA1*0103–DQB1*0603 [271]. In five different European populations increased frequencies of the DRB1*03–DQA1*0501–DQB1*02 and DRB1*13–DQA1*0103–DQB1*0603 haplotypes were noted [272]. Polymorphism in the TNF gene, which is closely aligned with HLA class I and II loci, may account for some of these associations. Recently the TNF2 allele was found in 58% of PSC patients vs 29% of controls ($p < 0.0001$) and was linked to HLA-B8 and DRB3*0101 [273]. No specific association was found in PSC patients with five genetic markers of the IL-11 family, including markers for IL-1α, IL-1β and IL-1RA [252, 274]. These results raise the possibility that genetic markers could lead to detection of PSC at a preclinical stage that is more amenable to therapy.

The importance of host genetic susceptibility is illustrated by dramatically different phenotypes in inbred rat strains in the SFBL model of hepatobiliary inflammation. Lewis rats develop hepatobiliary injury within 2–3 weeks after creation of SFBL; Wistar rats develop similar lesions after 12 weeks, but inbred Buffalo and Fischer rats fail to develop clinical, biochemical, or histologic evidence of hepatobiliary injury even after 24 weeks of observation, even though all rat strains have essentially identical concentrations of bacteria within the SFBL [12].

Arthritis

The HLA-B27 haplotype is strongly correlated with idiopathic ankylosing spondylitis (90%) and post-infectious reactive arthritis (70%) but is found in only 60–70% of IBD patients with ankylosing spondylitis and is not increased over the control population (8–10%) in IBD patients with peripheral arthritis. HLA-B27 positivity is clearly a risk factor for ankylosing spondylitis in the population with IBD. Approximately 25% of B27-positive patients who have IBD will develop ankylosing spondylitis vs 1% of patients with IBD who are HLA-B27 negative. Conversely, IBD is a risk factor for ankylosing spondylitis, because only 2% of the general HLA-B27 population develop ankylosing spondylitis. Spontaneous development of gastrointestinal, joint, skin, and urogenital inflammation in B27 transgenic rats strongly supports the association of HLA-B27 with arthritis [275]. Interestingly, intestinal inflam-

mation routinely precedes systemic inflammation. It should be noted, however, that HLA-B27 transgenic mice do not develop arthritis, even when challenged with *Yersinia* [263], unless murine β$_2$-microglobulin is deleted [180]. However, arthritis develops in murine β$_2$-microglobulin-deficient mice even in the absence of HLA-B27 [266], suggesting that the defect in this model is at the level of class I MHC binding rather than expression of human HLA-B27 [266]. A single gene autosomal recessive mouse model of ankylosing spondylitis (ank/ank) was not affected by the association of HLA-B27 [276].

A number of innovative explanations have been advanced to explain the association of the HLA-B27 haplotype with axial and seronegative arthritis. The molecular mimicry, altered immunoreactivity, and HLA-B27 polymorphism, and epitope receptor hypotheses are currently in vogue [10, 277–279]. The first two theories have been discussed above. Class I MHC preferentially bind cytoplasmic oligopeptides of eight or nine amino acids. Initial binding occurs in the endoplasmic reticulum; then the complex is transported with β$_2$-microglobulin to the plasma membrane, where it is recognized preferentially by CD8$^+$ T lymphocytes. Binding of a particular oligopeptide depends on its fit within the antigenic groove of the MHC molecule, which is determined by binding to motifs unique to each MHC haplotype. Thus HLA-B27 could bind to a specific arthritogenic antigen not recognized by other class I haplotypes. This antigen could be of host joint- and eye-specific or infectious origin. For example, HLA-B27-cytotoxic T cell lines and transgenic mice preferentially recognize an influenza peptide [280], and HSP89 has been eluted from native HLA-B27 [113]. Evidence that peptides bound to HLA-B27 are involved in arthritis is provided by the demonstration that arthritis is inhibited in HLA-B27 transgenic rats by displacement of endogenous peptides by overexpression of an influenza nucleoprotein which binds to B27 with high affinity when targeted to the endoplasmic reticulum [104]. However, this theory does not explain why all HLA-B27 patients and transgenic rats or mice do not develop spontaneous spondyloarthritis and uveitis. One innovative suggestion is that a joint-derived oligopeptide binding to the cysteine at the 67 position of the HLA-B27 antigenic groove could cause a conformational change which generates an autoimmune response [277].

Recent studies by the Oxford group have demonstrated HLA genotype associations with IBD related peripheral arthritis phenotypes [281]. Type I peripheral arthritis (pauciarticular, asymmetrical) was associated with HLA-DRB1*0103 (relative risk 12.1), B35 and B27 (relative risk 4.0). In contrast, type II (symmetrical, small joint) arthritis was associated with HLA-B44. IBD-related ankylosing spondylitis is associated with HLA-B27 and DRB*0101. Reactive arthritis controls were associated with the same HLA markers as IBD arthritis type I, with a stronger HLA-B27 influence. It will be interesting to determine if type I IBD-related arthritis exhibits polymorphism of the IκB-like gene, an immunosuppressive protein associated with HLA-DRB1*0103 [282]. In addition, Schulte et al. [214] reported that bone loss in IBD patients was related to genetic variations in the IL-1RA and IL-6 alleles, consistent with the effects of these cytokines on bone resorption. The extent of bone loss was not correlated with disease activity or corticosteroid use in this study.

Differential susceptibility of inbred rodent strains to experimental arthritis provides additional evidence of a genetic influence in the pathogenesis of arthritis associated with intestinal bacterial products. Lewis rats develop peripheral arthritis after PG-PS, complete Freund's adjuvant (mycobacterial PG-PS), or *Y. enterocolitica* 0:8 injection, whereas Lewis-Brown Norway F_1 hybrids preferentially develop arthritis after *Salmonella* inoculation [46]. In striking contrast to the chronic, spontaneously relapsing T cell-mediated chronic peripheral arthritis which develops in Lewis rats injected with PG-PS, Buffalo and MHC identical Fischer F344 rats similarly injected display only transient, self-limited joint injury [158]. Susceptibility to chronic PG-PS-induced arthritis correlates with activation of the kallikrein–kinin system [158] and the hypothalamic/pituitary/adrenal axis [246]. Similarly, expression of arthritis in β_2-microglobulin-deficient mice on various inbred strains is dramatically influenced by genetic background, ranging from 30–50% incidence in mixed 129/C57 Bl6 mice to 10–15% in inbred C57/Bl6 or Balb/cJ mice [266].

Eye inflammation
HLA-B27 is associated with anterior uveitis in ankylosing spondylitis and reactive arthritis but is not clearly a feature of acute iritis/uveitis in IBD. Susceptibility of T lymphocyte-mediated experimental allergic uveitis is confined to certain inbred rodent strains such as Lewis rats and Hartley guinea pigs, and C3H/HeN mice preferentially develop recurrent LPS-induced uveitis [196].

Skin manifestations
Autosomal-dominant transmission of associated pyoderma gangrenosum, cystic acne, and aseptic arthritis in a three-generational kindred has been mapped to the long arm of chromosome 15 (LOD score 5.83), demonstrating the potential role of genes outside the MHC locus in inflammatory syndromes [283].

Conclusions
Although HLA haplotypes B27 and B8/DR3 are clearly associated with ankylosing spondylitis/reactive arthritis/anterior uveitis and PSC, respectively, clearly other modifying genes and environmental factors are also involved. Most HLA-B27- and DR3-positive patients do not develop inflammatory lesions, and although the risk for ankylosing spondylitis and PSC increases if a patient with one of these haplotypes develops IBD, still only a minority (about 25%) develop overt extraintestinal inflammation. Conversely, at least 30% of IBD patients with ankylosing spondylitis or PSC are HLA-B27- or DR3-negative. However, it is of considerable interest that the two extraintestinal inflammatory conditions that are strongly associated with specific HLA haplotypes (PSC and ankylosing spondylitis) pursue independent clinical courses from the associated IBD. IBD, ankylosing spondylitis, and PSC probably have fundamentally different perpetuating mechanisms, although the initiation of systemic inflammation is linked in some way to intestinal, especially colonic, injury.

Nonimmunologic factors
Although histopathologic evidence suggests at least a secondary role for immune-mediated events, nonimmunologic factors may explain why certain systemic complications of IBD localize in specific areas; for example, erythema nodosum to the anterior lower leg, and why certain conditions, such as PSC, do not respond to traditional immunosuppressive therapy.

Hepatobiliary inflammation
Enhanced colonic absorption of bacterially metabolized hepatotoxic bile acids could conceivably link colitis to PSC [37]. Lithocholic acid causes cholestasis, whereas chenodeoxycholic acid induces hepatocellular injury. Ursodeoxycholic acid reverses these injurious effects and ameliorates chronic active hepatitis and PBC, but has limited efficacy in PSC,

with decreased biochemical parameters but no change in histology or symptoms [284]. Although toxic bile acids are probably not major etiologic agents, they may contribute to the seemingly irreversible tissue damage of PSC. Similarly, partial ductular obstruction with or without secondary infection may perpetuate hepatobiliary injury of IBD in a manner similar to progressive liver damage associated with long-standing biliary obstruction and AIDS-associated sclerosing cholangitis. Balloon dilation of dominant strictures can delay progression of deteriorating liver function and improve symptoms of PSC. Vascular damage of diverse types causes bile duct injury resembling PSC [37]. The biliary tree is vascularized by a periductular vascular plexus supplied by the hepatic artery. Hepatic artery occlusion, particularly after hepatic transplant, can produce obliteration and fibrosis of intrahepatic bile ducts, mimicking PSC. Accumulation of copper in livers of patients with PSC is probably secondary to cholestasis rather than a primary event, because D-penicillamine has no benefit [285]. Finally, the potential of drug-induced biliary injury is emphasized by massive bile duct proliferation in response to α-naphthylisothiocyanate (ANIT), which causes Th1-mediated inflammation [220].

Arthritis

Localization of IBD-associated peripheral arthritis to the knees, hips, and shoulders could potentially be due to non-specific trauma of these weight-bearing joints, which by increasing vascular permeability could promote local deposition of circulating antigens or immune complexes. In the PG-PS reactivation model the previously injured joint is much more susceptible to reactivation by circulating bacterial polymers than the contralateral non-injured ankle [160]. Interestingly, recurrent bouts of peripheral arthritis in patients with IBD tend to localize to the same joints initially involved. The possibility of drug-induced arthritis is supported by descriptions of systemic lupus erythematosus in slow acetylators treated with sulfasalazine [286] and CD patients treated with infliximab [140], as well as immune complex disease in patients reinfused with infliximab more than 6 months after initial treatment [140].

Skin lesions

The predilection of erythema nodosum and pyoderma gangrenosum to the anterior lower leg suggests a role of trauma in the induction of these lesions, although only a minority of patients can recall specific traumatic events before developing inflammation.

Hematologic abnormalities

Patients with active UC and CD have multiple causes for anemia, including blood loss, iron deficiency, vitamin B_{12} and folic acid deficiencies, hemolytic anemia secondary to sulfasalazine, and bone marrow suppression secondary to immunosuppressive drugs.

Conclusions and unifying hypothesis

The previously outlined clinical clues for the pathogenesis of extraintestinal inflammation are now readdressed in light of the experimental data presented. The presence of extraintestinal inflammation in a minority of patients with intestinal injury can be explained by the requirement for permissive host susceptibility factors, most likely genetic in origin. The association of systemic inflammation with colonic involvement incriminates colonic bacterial species or their products, crossreactive epitopes unique to colonic epithelial cells, or increased colonic production and/or absorption of inflammatory mediators and cytokines by the inflamed colon. Systemic inflammation preferentially occurring with extensive, active intestinal disease implicates enhanced absorption of luminal antigens or viable bacteria through the inflamed gut, increased production or uptake of inflammatory mediators or effector cells by the diseased bowel, or shared mechanisms of intestinal and systemic inflammation. The non-random association of certain extraintestinal manifestations and their similar response to a single therapy suggests that activity-related manifestations (peripheral arthritis, erythema nodosum, and iritis) share common mechanisms. Finally it should be noted that IBD is only one of several stimuli, usually infectious, that can trigger reactive arthritis, ankylosing spondylitis, uveitis, erythema nodosum, and PSC.

A two-component hypothesis to reconcile these associations with the clinical and experimental observations discussed above is illustrated in Figs. 3 and 4. Intestinal inflammation with increased mucosal permeability and secondary bacterial invasion of crypt abscesses, ulcers, and fistulas leads to dramatically increased uptake of luminal constituents into portal and lymphatic circulations (Fig. 3). Bacterial products (FMLP, LPS, PG-PS, and superantigens) with intrinsic inflammatory properties, bacterial

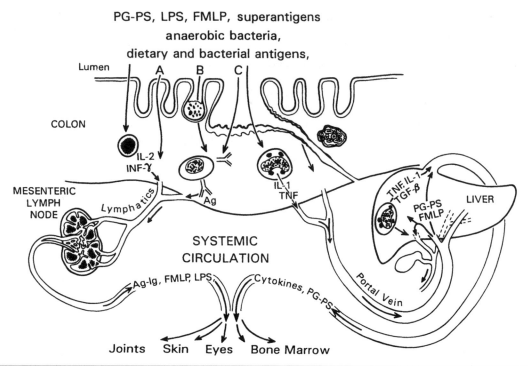

Figure 3. Systemic distribution of phlogistic mucosal products. Luminal bacterial and bacterial products cross the colonic mucosa in areas of enhanced permeability across leaky epithelia (**A**), crypt abscesses (**B**), or ulcers and fistulae (**C**). During transit through the lamina propria and submucosa antigens complex with immunoglobulin (Ig), and cell wall polymers stimulate macrophages and lymphocytes, which secrete cytokines. Bacterial products, cytokines, and immune complexes are transported through the mesenteric lymphatics or veins to regional lymph nodes or the liver, where further stimulation of immune cells occurs. In the liver PG-PS and FMLP can be excreted into the bile duct, activate Kupffer cells, or enter the hepatic vein. After entering the systemic circulation bacterial products, immune complexes, and inflammatory mediators are distributed to the joints, skin, eyes, and bone marrow, where local inflammation is incited in genetically susceptible hosts.

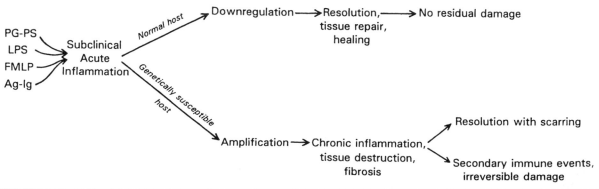

Figure 4. Genetically determined inflammatory response to luminal antigens and bacterial products. Systemically distributed bacterial polymers and immune complexes induce subclinical inflammation in all hosts. The normal response is appropriate down-regulation of inflammation with no residual damage (upper arm). However, genetically susceptible hosts (lower arm) amplify the inflammatory response leading to tissue injury, which either resolves when intestinal uptake or luminal antigens ceases (activity-related conditions) or pursues an independent, progressive course when secondary immune events become involved (activity-unrelated conditions).

antigens, activated T lymphocytes, inflammatory mediators, and immune complexes containing dietary or bacterial antigens are systemically distributed. These phlogistic materials induce local immune and inflammatory responses in joints, bile ducts, skin, the anterior chamber of the eye, and the reticuloendothelial systems of the bone marrow and liver. Organ specificity is dependent on tissue tropism of circulating bacterial polymers, cytokines, and immune complexes, selective migration of T lymphocytes recognizing randomly distributed antigens or localized vascular permeability caused by preexisting injury. Most patients develop only subclinical systemic inflammation, which quickly resolves through tightly regulated protective immune responses without residual tissue injury (Fig. 4). However, a genetically susceptible subset of patients with dysregulated immune responses develop systemic inflammation that progresses to clinical symptoms. The inflammatory stimuli inducing inflammation are not mutually exclusive and probably act synergistically such that inflammation initiated by bacterial cell wall polymers, antigens, or immune complexes can be reactivated and perpetuated by LPS, FMLP, superantigens, PG-PS, antigens, or cytokines derived from the colon.

This hypothesis predicts that extraintestinal inflammation should resolve when the intestinal injury abates, diminishing the systemic distribution of luminal antigens, activated T cells, bacterial polymers, or cytokines. The amount of residual damage depends upon the degree of tissue destruction. Activity-associated lesions fit easily into this paradigm, but additional factors must be invoked to explain the extraintestinal manifestations which do not correspond with underlying disease activity. Both PSC and ankylosing spondylitis are strongly associated (approximately 70% of patients with IBD) with HLA-B8/DR3 and HLA-B27, respectively. Under the influence of these stringent genetic factors independent inflammatory pathways may develop that are mechanistically distinct from those initiating tissue injury. Continued organ damage then proceeds independent of underlying intestinal injury (Fig. 4). For example, in ankylosing spondylitis an autoimmune response may be initiated against matrix constituents, heat-shock proteins, or crossreacting epitopes on the HLA-B27 molecule exposed during initial injury, whereas activated immune cells which respond to very low constitutive concentrations of PG-PS or FMLP in the bile, injured biliary epithelial cells, or to commensal

bacteria secondarily infecting obstructed ducts may perpetuate PSC. These events could then lead to progressive, irreversible fibrosis and destruction of the intra- and extrahepatic bile ducts or the joint–ligament–cartilage junction of the axial skeleton (entheseopathy). Critical components of this hypothesis are the interaction between genetic and environmental factors and the separate mechanisms for initiation and perpetuation of inflammation. Environmental and genetic factors are individually permissive, but spontaneous occurrence of inflammation with a single risk factor is a rare event. Confluence of both variables, however, results in a high frequency of disease. For example, clinically apparent ankylosing spondylitis develops in approximately 1% of HLA-B27-negative patients with IBD, 1–2% of the HLA-B27-positive population without IBD, but affects approximately 25% of the HLA-B27-positive IBD subpopulation. The incidence of ankylosing spondylitis in HLA-B27 patients with pancolitis is unknown but is presumably even higher. Similar incidence figures could be calculated for reactive arthritis with the concurrence of HLA-B27 and epidemic enteric infections [25]. As the immunogenetics of IBD are clarified (see Chapter 2) the mechanisms determining the association of extraintestinal inflammation with intestinal injury almost certainly will become more clearly delineated. Our hypothesis predicts that genetic susceptibility for UC and CD will be distinct from those genes which determine extraintestinal complications, particularly ankylosing spondylitis and PSC, which follow independent clinical courses from the underlying bowel disease.

Clinical evidence supporting this hypothesis in IBD patients with extraintestinal manifestations is limited and circumstantial, because definitive mechanistic studies are not available. However, reasonably firm experimental support exists for genetically determined defective immunoregulatory responses to bacteria and bacterial products in post-*Yersinia*-reactive arthritis patients, Lewis rats, and HLA-B27 transgenic rats. We suggest that extraintestinal inflammation is dependent on underlying intestinal injury as the source of luminal antigens or activated T lymphocytes which mediate the inflammatory events. Systemic distribution of enteric bacterial antigens has been documented in patients with reactive arthritis and the jejunoileal bypass syndrome. The spectrum of systemic inflammation induced by endogenous or exogenous bacterial cell wall polymers in Lewis rats is remarkably similar to the extraintestinal manifestations of human intestinal injury (see Table 4), although extrapolation of results from a rat model to humans is quite speculative. However, the Lewis rat model of PG-PS-induced arthritis clearly demonstrates that a variety of bacterial products and cytokines can initiate and reactivate immune-mediated inflammation. In addition, selected monoassociation studies in gnotobiotic HLA-B27 transgenic rats and IL-10-deficient mice indicate that different bacterial antigens stimulate similar inflammatory events in genetically distinct hosts. Concepts derived from these animal models and patients with postinfectious reactive arthritis or jejunoileal bypass syndrome [287] should help guide future investigations to identify the immunogenetic mechanisms and dominant bacterial or self antigens which cause extraintestinal inflammation associated with IBD.

References

1. Katz JP, Lichtenstein GR. Rheumatologic manifestations of gastrointestinal diseases. Gastroenterol Clin N Am 1998; 27: 533–62.
2. Leino R, Toivanen A. Arthritis associated with gastrointestinal disorders. In: Toivanen A, Toivanen P, eds. Reactive Arthritis. Boca Raton: CRC Press, 1988: 000
3. Jorizzo JL, Apisarnthanarax P, Subrt P et al. Bowel-bypass syndrome without bowel bypass. Arch Intern Med 1983; 143: 457–61.
4. Greenstein AJ, Janowitz HD, Sachar DB. The extraintestinal complications of Crohn's disease and ulcerative colitis: a study of 700 patients. Medicine 1976; 55: 401–12.
5. Rankin GB, Watts HD, Melnyk CS, Kelley ML Jr. National Cooperative Crohn's Disease Study: Extraintestinal manifestation and perianal complications. Gastroenterology 1979; 77: 914–20.
6. Monsen U, Sorstad J, Hellers G, Johansson C. Extracolonic diagnoses in ulcerative colitis: an epidemiological study. Am J Gastroenterol. 1990; 85: 711–16.
7. Jacobsen MB, Fausa O, Elgio K, Schrumpf E. Hepatic lesions in adult coeliac disease. Scand J Gastroenterol. 1990; 25: 656–62.
8. Bourne JT, Kumar P, Huskisson EC, Mageed R, Unsworth IJ, Wojtulewski JA. Arthritis and celiac disease. Ann Rheum Dis 1985; 44: 592–8.
9. Klein S, Mayer L, Present DH, Youner KD, Cerulli MA, Sachar DB. Extraintestinal manifestations in patients with diverticulitis. Ann Intern Med 1988; 108: 700–2.
10. Toivanen A, Toivanen P. Reactive arthritis. Curr Opin Rheumatol 2000; 12: 300–5.
11. Bocanegra TS, Espinoza LR, Bridgeford PH, Vasey FB, Germain BF. Reactive arthritis induced by parasitic infestation. Ann Intern Med 1981; 94: 207–9.
12. Lichtman SN, Sartor RB, Keku J, Schwab JH. Hepatic inflammation in rats with experimental small intestinal bacterial overgrowth. Gastroenterology 1990; 98: 414–23.
13. Lichtman SN, Wang J, Sartor RB et al. Reactivation of arthritis induced by small bowel bacterial overgrowth in rats: role of cytokines, bacteria, and bacterial polymers. Infect Immun 1995; 63: 2295–301.
14. Schultz M, Tonkonogy SL, Sellon RK et al. IL-2-deficient mice raised under germfree conditions develop delayed mild focal intestinal inflammation. Am J Physiol 1999; 276: G1461–72
15. Sartor RB, Bender DE, Holt LC. Susceptibility of inbred rat strains to intestinal and extraintestinal inflammation induced by indomethacin. Gastroenterology 1992; 102: A690 (abstract).
16. Kontoyiannis D, Pasparakis M, Pizarro TT, Cominelli F, Kollias G. Impaired on/off regulation of TNF biosynthesis in mice lacking TNF AU-rich elements: implications for joint and gut-associated immunopathologies. Immunity 1999; 10: 387–98.
17. Aadland E, Schrumpf E, Fausa O, Elgjo K, Heilo A. Primary sclerosing cholangitis: a long-term follow-up study. Scand J Gastroenterol 1987; 22: 655–64.
18. De Vos M, Cuvelier C, Mielants H, Veys E, Barbier F, Elewaut A. Ileocolonoscopy in seronegative spondylarthropathy. Gastroenterology 1989; 96: 339–44.
19. Rabinovitz M, Gavaler JS, Schade RR, Dindzans VJ, Chien MC, Van Thiel DH. Does primary sclerosing cholangitis occurring in association with inflammatory bowel disease differ from that occurring in the absence of inflammatory bowel disease? A study of sixty-six subjects. Hepatology 1990; 11: 7–11.
20. Suh CH, Lee CH, Lee et al. Arthritic manifestations of inflammatory bowel disease. J Korean Med Sci 1998; 13: 39–43.
21. Buskila D, Odes LR, Neumann L, Odes HS. Fibromyalgia in inflammatory bowel disease. J Rheumatol 1999; 26: 1167–171.
22. Wright V, Watkinson G. The arthritis of ulcerative colitis. Medicine 1959; 38: 243–59.
23. Olsson R, Danielsson A, Jarnerot G. Prevalence of primary sclerosing cholangitis in patients with ulcerative colitis. Gastroenterology 1991; 100: 1319–23.
24. Bardazzi G, Mannoni A, d'Albasio G et al. Spondyloarthritis in patients with ulcerative colitis. Italian J Gastroenterol Hepatol 1997; 29: 520–4.
25. Eastwood CJ Epidemic reactive arthritis. Ann Rheum Dis 1990; 49: 73–4.
26. Hermon-Taylor J, Bull TJ, Sheridan JM, Cheng J, Stellakis ML, Sumar N. Causation of Crohn's disease by *Mycobacterium avium* subspecies paratuberculosis. Can J Gastroenterol 2000; 14: 521–39.
27. Wakefield AJ, Montgomery SM, Pounder RE. Crohn's disease: the case for measles virus. Ital J Gastroenterol Hepatol 1999; 31: 247–54.
28. Ambrose NS, Johnson M, Burdon DW, Keighley MR. Incidence of pathogenic bacteria from mesenteric lymph nodes and ileal serosa during Crohn's disease surgery. Br J Surg 1984; 71: 623–5.
29. Brooke BN, Dykes PW, Walker FC. A study of liver disorder in ulcerative colitis. Postgrad Med J 1961; 37: 245–51.
30. Vinnik IE, Kern F, Struthers JE, Hill RB, Guzak S. Experimental chronic portal vein bacteremia. Proc Soc Exp Biol Med 1964; 15: 311–14.
31. Olsson R, Bjornsson E, Backman L et al. Bile duct bacterial isolates in primary sclerosing cholangitis: a study of explanted livers. J Hepatol 1998; 28: 426–32.
32. Cox KL, Coc KM. Oral vancomycin treatment of PSC in children with inflammatory bowel disease. J Pediatr Gastroenterol Nutr 1998; 27: 580–3.
33. Nilsson HO, Taneera J, Castedal M, Glatz E, Olsson R, Wadstrom T. Identification of *Helicobacter pylori* and other *Helicobacter* species by PCR, hybridization, and partial DNA sequencing in human liver samples from patients with primary sclerosing cholangitis or primary biliary cirrhosis. J Clin Microbiol 2000; 38: 1072–6.

34. Pearce CB, Duncan HD, Timmis L, Green JR. Assessment of the prevalence of infection with *Helicobacter pylori* in patients with inflammatory bowel disease. Eur J Gastroenterol Hepatol 2000; 12: 439–43.

35. Foltz CJ, Fox JG, Cahill R *et al.* Spontaneous inflammatory bowel disease in multiple mutant mouse lines: association with colonization by *Helicobacter hepaticus*. Helicobacter 1998; 3: 69–78.

36. Nilsson I, Lindgren S, Eriksson S, Wadstrom T. Serum antibodies to *Helicobacter hepaticus* and *Helicobacter pylori* in patients with chronic liver disease. Gut 2000; 46: 410–14.

37. Sherlock S. Pathogenesis of sclerosing cholangitis: the role of nonimmune factors. Semin Liver Dis 1991; 11: 5–10.

38. Cello JP. Acquired immunodeficiency syndrome cholangiopathy: spectrum of disease. Am J Med 1989; 86: 539–46.

39. Chen XM, Levine SA, Tietz P *et al. Cryptosporidium parvum* is cytopathic for cultured human biliary epithelia via an apoptotic mechanism. Hepatology 1998; 28: 906–13.

40. Narayanan Menon KV, Esner RH. Etiology and natural history of primary sclerosing cholangitis. J Hepato-Biliary-Pancreat Surg 1999; 6: 343–51.

41. Raj V, Lichtenstein DR. Hepatobiliary manifestations of inflammatory bowel disease. Gastroenterol Clin N Am 1999; 28: 491–513.

42. LaRusso NF. The Fifth Carlos E. Rubio Memorial Lecture. Sclerosing cholangitis: pathogenesis, pathology, and practice. PR Health Sci J 1999; 18: 11–17.

43. Granfors K, Jalkanen S, Essen RV. *Yersinia* antigens in synovial-fluid cells from patients with reactive arthritis. N Engl J Med 1989; 320: 216–21.

44. Wordsworth BP, Hughes RA, Allan L, Keat AC, Bell JI. Chlamydial DNA is absent from joints of patients with sexually acquired reactive arthritis. Br J Rheumatol 1990; 29: 208–10.

45. Thiel A, Wu P, Lauster R, Braun J, Radbruch A, Sieper J. Analysis of the antigen-specific T cell response in reactive arthritis by flow cytometry. Arthritis Rheum 2000; 43: 2834–42.

46. Yu DT. Pathogenesis of reactive arthritis. Intern Med 1999; 38: 97–101.

47. Wuorela M, Jal, Toivanen P, Granfors K. Intracellular pathogens and professional phagocytes in reactive arthritis. Pathobiology 1991; 59: 162–5.

48. Rynes RI, Volastro PS, Bartholomew LE. Exacerbation of B27 positive spondyloarthropathy by enteric infections. J Rheumatol 1984; 11: 96–7.

49. Wakefield D, McCluskey P, Verma M, Aziz K, Gatus B, Carr G. Ciprofloxacin treatment does not influence course or relapse rate of reactive arthritis and anterior uveitis. Arthritis Rheum 1999; 42: 1894–7.

50. Hill JL, Yu DTY. Development of an experimental animal model for reactive arthritis induced by *Yersinia enterocolitica* infection. Infect Immun 1987; 55: 721–6.

51. de los Toyos JR, Vazquez J, Sampedro A, Hardisson C. *Yersinia enterocolitica* serotype 0: 3 is arthritogenic for mice. Microb Pathogen 1990; 8: 370

52. Volkman A, Collins FM. Pathogenesis of *Salmonella*-associated arthritis in rats. Infect Immun 1975; 11: 222–30.

53. Hermann E, Mayet WJ, Poralla T, Meyer zum Buschenfelde KH. *Salmonella*-reactive synovial fluid T cell clones in a patient with post-infectious *Salmonella* arthritis. Scand J Rheumatol 1990; 19: 350–5.

54. Taurog JD, Richardson JA, Croft JT *et al.* The germfree state prevents development of gut and joint inflammatory disease in HLA-B27 transgenic rats. J Exp Med 1994; 180: 2359–64.

55. Rath HC, Herfarth HH, Ikeda JS *et al.* Normal luminal bacteria, especially *Bacteroides* species, mediate chronic colitis, gastritis, and arthritis in HLA-B27/human beta2

56. Driessen LHHM, van Saene HKF. A novel treatment of pyoderma gangrenosum by intestinal decontamination. Br J Dermatol 1983; 108: 108 (abstract).

57. Johnson LA, Wirostko E, Wirostko W. Parasitization of vitreous leukocytes by molliculte-like organisms. Am J Clin Pathol 1989; 91: 259–64.

58. Wakefield D, Stahlberg TH, Toivanen A, Granfors K, Tennant C. Serologic evidence of *Yersinia* infection in patients with anterior uveitis. Arch Ophthalmol 1990; 108: 219–21.

59. Sartor RB. Pathogenesis and immune mechanisms of chronic inflammatory bowel diseases. Am J Gastroenterol 1997; 92: 5S–11S.

60. Fiocchi C. Inflammatory bowel disease: etiology and pathogenesis. Gastroenterology 1998; 115: 182–205.

61. Saarinen S, Olerup O, Broom U. Increased frequency of autoimmune diseases in patients with primary sclerosing cholangitis. Am J Gastroenterol 2000; 95: 3195–9.

62. Koffler D, Minkowitz MD, Rothman W, Garlock J Immunocytochemical studies in ulcerative colitis and regional ileitis. J Exp Med 1962; 41: 733–41.

63. Chapman RW, Cottone M, Selby WS, Shepherd HA, Sherlock S, Jewell DP. Serum autoantibodies, ulcerative colitis and primary sclerosing cholangitis. Gut 1986; 27: 86–91.

64. Snook JA, Chapman RW, Fleming K, Jewell DP. Antineutrophil nuclear antibody in ulcerative colitis, Crohn's disease and primary sclerosing cholangitis. Clin Exp Immunol 1989; 76: 30–3.

65. Saxon A, Shanahan F, Landers C, Ganz T, Targan S. A distinct subset of antineutrophil cytoplasmic antibodies is associated with inflammatory bowel disease. J Allergy Clin Immunol 1990; 86: 202–10.

66. Roozendaal C, Kallenberg CG. Are anti-neutrophil cytoplasmic antibodies (ANCA) clinically useful in inflammatory bowel disease (IBD)? Clin Exp Immunol 1999; 116: 206–13.

67. Duerr RH, Targan SR, Landers CJ Neutrophil cytoplasmic antibodies: a link between primary sclerosing cholangitis and ulcerative colitis. Gastroenterology 1991; 100: 1385–91.

68. Lindgren S, Nilsson S, Nassberger L, Verbaan H, Wieslander J Anti-neutrophil cytoplasmic antibodies in patients with chronic liver diseases: prevalence, antigen specificity and predictive value for diagnosis of autoimmune liver disease. Swedish Internal Medicine Liver Club (SILK). J Gastroenterol Hepatol 2000; 15: 437–42.

69. Orth T, Neurath M, Schirmacher P, Treichel U, Meyer zum Buschenfelde KH, Mayet W. Anti-neutrophil cytoplasmic antibodies in a rat model of TNBS acid-induced liver injury. Eur J Clin Invest 1999; 29: 929–39.

70. Roozendaal C, van Milligen de Wit AW, Haagsma EB *et al.* Antineutrophil cytoplasmic antibodies in primary sclerosing cholangitis: defined specificities may be associated with distinct clinical features. Am J Med 1998; 105: 393–9.

71. Orth T, Kellner R, Diekmann O, Faust J, Meyer zum Buschenfelde BK, Mayet WJ Identification and characterization of autoantibodies against catalase and alpha-enolase in patients with primary sclerosing cholangitis. Clin Exp Immunol 1998; 112: 507–15.

72. Cohavy O, Bruckner D, Gordon LK *et al.* Colonic bacteria express an ulcerative colitis pANCA-related protein epitope. Infect Immun 2000; 68: 1542–8.

73. Eggena M, Cohavy O, Parseghian MH *et al.* Identification of histone H1 as a cognate antigen of the ulcerative colitis-associated marker antibody pANCA. J Autoimmun 2000; 14: 83–97.

microglobulin transgenic rats. J Clin Invest 1996; 98: 945–53.

74. Terjung B, Spengler U, Sauerbruch T, Worman HJ. 'Atypical p-ANCA' in IBD and hepatobiliary disorders react with a 50-kilodalton nuclear envelope protein of neutrophils and myeloid cell lines. Gastroenterology 2000; 119: 310–22.

75. Mieli-Vergani G, Lobo-Yeo A, McFarlane BM, McFarlane IG, Mowat AP, Vergani D. Different immune mechanisms leading to autoimmunity in primary sclerosing cholangitis and autoimmune chronic active hepatitis of childhood. Hepatology 1989; 9: 198–203.

76. McFarlane IG, Joycicka BM, Tsantoulas DC. Leukocyte migration inhibition in response to biliary antigens in primary biliary cirrhosis, sclerosing cholangitis and other chronic liver diseases. Gastroenterology 1979; 76: 1333–40.

77. Angulo P, Peter JB, Gershwin ME et al. Serum autoantibodies in patients with primary sclerosing cholangitis. J Hepatol 2000; 32: 182–7.

78. Das KM, Vecchi M, Sakamaki S. A shared and unique epitope(s) on human colon, skin and biliary epithelium detected by a monoclonal antibody. Gastroenterology 1990; 98: 464–9.

79. Bhagat S, Das KM. A shared and unique peptide in the human colon, eye, and joint detected by a monoclonal antibody. Gastroenterology 1994; 107: 103–8.

80. Geng X, Biancone L, Dai HH et al. Tropomyosin isoforms in intestinal mucosa: production of autoantibodies to tropomyosin isoforms in ulcerative colitis. Gastroenterology 1998; 114: 912–22.

81. Mandal A, Dasgupta A, Jeffers L et al. Autoantibodies in sclerosing cholangitis against a shared peptide in biliary and colon epithelium. Gastroenterology 1994; 106: 185–92.

82. Takahashi F, Das KM. Isolation and characterization of a colonic autoantigen specifically recognized by colon tissue-bound immunoglobulin G from idiopathic ulcerative colitis. Clin Invest 1985; 76: 311–18.

83. Sakamaki S, Takayanagi N, Yoshizaki N et al. Autoantibodies against the specific epitope of human tropomyosin(s) detected by a peptide based enzyme immunoassay in sera of patients with ulcerative colitis show antibody dependent cell mediated cytotoxicity against HLA-DPw9 transfected L cells. Gut 2000; 47: 236–41.

84. Biancone L, Monteleone G, Marasco R, Pallone F. Autoimmunity to tropomyosin isoforms in ulcerative colitis (UC) patients and unaffected relatives. Clin Exp Immunol 1998; 113: 198–205.

85. Ohman L, Franzen L, Rudolph U, Harriman GR, Hultgren HE. Immune activation in the intestinal mucosa before the onset of colitis in Galphai2-deficient mice. Scand J Immunol 2000; 52: 80–90.

86. Mizoguchi A, Mizoguchi E, Chiba C et al. Cytokine imbalance and autoantibody production in T cell receptor-alpha mutant mice with inflammatory bowel disease. J Exp Med 1996; 183: 847–56.

87. Khoo UY, Bjarnason I, Donaghy A, Williams R, Macpherson A. Antibodies to colonic epithelial cells from the serum and colonic mucosal washings in ulcerative colitis. Gut 1995; 37: 63–70.

88. Ueno Y, Phillips JO, Ludwig J, Lichtman SN, LaRusso NF. Development and characterization of a rodent model of immune-mediated cholangitis. Proc Natl Acad Sci USA 1996; 93: 216–20.

89. Ueno Y, Ishii M, Takahashi S, Igarashi T, Toyota T, LaRusso NF. Different susceptibility of mice to immune-mediated cholangitis induced by immunization with carbonic anhydrase. Lab Invest 1998; 78: 629–37.

90. Gordon SC, Quattrociocchi-Longe TM, Khan BA et al. Antibodies to carbonic anhydrase in patients with immune cholangiopathies. Gastroenterology 1995; 108: 1802–9.

91. Broome U, Grunewald J, Scheynius A, Olerup O, Hultcrantz R. Preferential V beta3 usage by hepatic T lympho-

cytes in patients with primary sclerosing cholangitis. J Hepatol 1997; 26: 527–34.

92. Alpini G, Galsser SS, Ueno Y et al. Heterogenicity of the proliferative capacity of rat cholangiocytes after bile duct ligation. Am J Physiol 1998; 274: G767–75.

93. Nonomura A, Kono N, Minato H, Nakanuma Y. Diffuse biliary tract involvement mimicking primary sclerosing cholangitis in an experimental model of chronic graft-versus-host disease in mice. Pathol Int 1998; 48: 421–7.

94. Howell CD, Yodre T, Claman HN, Vierling JM. Hepatic homing of mononuclear cells isolated during murine chronic graft-vs-host disease. J Immunol 1989; 143: 476–83.

95. Ueno Y, Ishii M, Yahagi K et al. Fas-mediated cholangiopathy in the murine model of graft versus host disease. Hepatology 2000; 31: 966–74.

96. Shalaby MR, Fendly B, Sheehan KC Schreiber RD, Ammann AJ Prevention of the graft-vs-host reaction in newborn mice by antibodies to tumor necrosis factor-alpha. Transplantation 1989; 47: 1057–61.

97. van der Brink MRM, Moore E, Horndasch KJ et al. Fas-deficient lpr mice are more susceptible to graft-vs-host disease. J Immunol 2000; 164: 469–80.

98. Dienes HP, Lohse AW, Gerken G et al. Bile duct epithelia as target cells in primary biliary cirrhosis and primary sclerosing cholangitis. Virchows Archiv 1997; 431: 119–24.

99. Yu DTY, Choo SY, Schaack T. Molecular mimicry in HLA-B27 related arthritis. Ann Intern Med 1989; 111: 581–91.

100. Lopez-Larrea C, Gonzalez S, Martinez-Borra J The role of HLA-B27 polymorphism and molecular mimicry in spondyloarthropathy. Mol Med Today 1998; 4: 540–9.

101. Chou CT, Uksila J, Toivanen P. Enterobacterial antibodies in Chinese patients with rheumatoid arthritis and ankylosing spondylitis. Clin Exp Rheumatol 1998; 16: 161–4.

102. Tsuchiya N, Husby G, Williams RC, Stieglitz H, Lipsky PE, Inman RD. Autoantibodies to the HLA B27 sequence crossreact with the hypothetical peptide from the arthritis associated *Shigella* plasmid. J Clin Invest 1990; 86: 1193–203.

103. Tsuchiya N, Husby G, Williams RC. Antibodies to the peptide from the plasmid coded *Yersinia* outer membrane protein (YOPI) in patients with ankylosing spondylitis. Clin Exp Immunol 1990; 82: 493–8.

104. Zhou M, Sayad A, Simmons WA et al. The specificity of peptides bound to human histocompatibility leukocyte antigen (HLA)-B27 influences the prevalence of arthritis in HLA-B27 transgenic rats. J Exp Med 1998; 188: 877–86.

105. Khare SD, Bull MJ, Hanson J, Luthra HS, David CS. Spontaneous inflammatory disease in HLA-B27 transgenic mice is independent of MHC class II molecules: a direct role for B27 heavy chains and not B27-derived peptides. J Immunol 1998; 160: 101–6.

106. Khare SD, Lee S, Bull MJ et al. Peptide binding alpha1 alpha2 domain of HLA-B27 contributes to the disease pathogenesis in transgenic mice. Hum Immunol 1999; 60: 116–26.

107. Breban M, Hammer RE, Richardson JA, Taurog JD. Transfer of the inflammatory disease of HLA-B27 transgenic rats by bone marrow engraftment. J Exp Med 1993; 178: 1607–16.

108. Hermann E, Lohse AW, van der Zee R. Synovial fluid-derived *Yersinia* reactive T cells responding to human 65 kDa heat shock protein and heat stressed antigen presenting cells. Eur J Immunol 1991; 21: 2139–43.

109. Kaufmann SH. Heat shock proteins and the immune response. Immunol Today 1990; 11: 129–36.

110. Winrow VR, Mojdehi GM, Ryder SD, Rhodes JM, Blake DR, Rampton DS. Stress proteins in colorectal mucosa. Enhanced expression in ulcerative colitis. Dig Dis Sci 1993; 38: 1994–2000.

111. Baca-Estrada ME, Gupta RS, Stead RH, Croitoru K. Intestinal expression and cellular immune responses to human heat-shock protein 60 in Crohn's disease. Dig Dis Sci 1994; 39: 498–506.

112. van den Broek MF, Hogervorst EJ, van Bruggen MC, Van Eden W, van der Zee R, van den Berg WB. Protection against streptococcal cell wall-induced arthritis by pretreatment with the 65-kD mycobacterial heat shock protein. J Exp Med 1989; 170: 449–66.

113. Jardetzky TS, Lane WS, Robinson RA, Madden DR, Wiley DC. Identification of self peptides bound to purified HLA-B27. Nature 1991; 353: 326–9.

114. Steinhoff U, Brinkmann V, Klemm U et al. Autoimmune intestinal pathology induced by hsp60-specific CD8 T cells. Immunity 1999; 11: 349–58.

115. Mertz AK, Wu P, Sturniolo T et al. Multispecific CD4+ T cell response to a single 12-mer epitope of the immunodominant heat-shock protein 60 of Yersinia enterocolitica in Yersinia-triggered reactive arthritis: overlap with the B27-restricted CD8 epitope, functional properties, and epitope presentation by multiple DR alleles. J Immunol 2000; 164: 1529–37.

116. Glant TT, Mikecz K. Antiproteoglycan antibodies in experimental spondyloarthritis. In: Kresina TF, ed. Monoclonal Antibodies, Cytokines, and Arthritis. New York: Marcel Dekker, 1991.

117. van den Broek MF, van de Putte LB, van den Berg WB. Crohn's disease associated with arthritis: a possible role for crossreactivity between gut bacteria and cartilage in the pathogenesis of arthritis. Arthritis Rheum 1988; 31: 1077–9.

118. Broberger O, Perlmann P. Autoantibodies in human ulcerative colitis. J Exp Med 1959; 110: 657–74.

119. Labeille B, Gineston JL, Denoeux JP, Capron JP. Epidermolysis bullosa acquisita and Crohn's disease. Arch Intern Med 1988; 148: 1457–9.

120. Gordon LK, Eggena M, Holland GN, Weisz JM, Braun J pANCA antibodies in patients with anterior uveitis: identification of a marker antibody usually associated with ulcerative colitis. J Clin Immunol 1998; 18: 264–71.

121. Singh VL, Donoso LA, Yamaki K, Shinohara T. Uveitopathogenic sites in bovines antigen. Autoimmunity 1989; 3: 177–87.

122. Li Q, Sun B, Dastgheib K, Chan CC. Suppressive effect of transforming growth factor beta1 on the recurrence of experimental melanin protein-induced uveitis: upregulation of ocular interleukin-10. Clin Immunol Immunopathol 1996; 81: 55–61.

123. Becker MD, Adamus G, Davey MP, Rosenbaum JT. The role of T cells in autoimmune uveitis. Ocular Immunol Inflamm 2000; 8: 93–100.

124. Altman AR, Maltz C, Janowitz HD. Autoimmune hemolytic anemia in ulcerative colitis. Dig Dis Sci 1979; 24: 282–5.

125. Stevens C, Peppercorn MA, Janowitz HD. Crohn's disease associated with autoimmune neutropenia. J Clin Gastroenterol 1991; 13: 328–30.

126. Soltis RD, Hasz D, Morris MJ, Wilson ID. Evidence against the presence of circulating immune complexes in chronic inflammatory bowel disease. Gastroenterology 1979; 76: 1380–5.

127. Lawley TJ, James SP, Jones EA. Circulating immune complexes: their detection and potential significance in some hepatobiliary and intestinal diseases. Gastroenterology 1980; 76: 626–41.

128. Hodgson HJ, Potter BJ, Jewell DP. Immune complexes in ulcerative colitis and Crohn's disease. Clin Exp Immunol 1977; 29: 187–96.

129. Lake AM, Stitzel AE, Urmson JR, Walker WA, Spitzer RE. Complement alterations in inflammatory bowel disease. Gastroenterology 1979; 76: 1374–9.

130. Bodenheimer HC, LaRusso NF, Thayer WR, Charland C, Staples PJ, Ludwig J Elevated circulating immune complexes in primary sclerosing cholangitis. Hepatology 1983; 3: 150–4.

131. Alberti-Flor JJ, Medina M, Jeffeers L, Schiff ER. Elevated immunoglobulins and immune complexes in the bile of patients with primary sclerosing cholangitis. Hepatology 1983; 3: 844 (abstract).

132. Senaldi G, Donaldson PT, Magrin S et al. Activation of the complement system in primary sclerosing cholangitis. Gastroenterology 1989; 97: 1430–4.

133. Minuk GY, Angus M, Brickman CM et al. Abnormal clearance of immune complexes from the circulation of patients with primary sclerosing cholangitis. Gastroenterology 1985; 88: 166–70.

134. Wands JR, LaMont JT, Mann E, Isselbacher KJ Arthritis associated with intestinal bypass procedure for morbid obesity. N Engl J Med 1976; 294: 121–4.

135. Utsinger PD. Systemic immune complex disease following intestinal bypass surgery: bypass disease. J Am Dermatol 1980; 2: 488–95.

136. Zapanta M, Aldo-Benson M, Madura J Clinical and immunological features in patients with postintestinal bypass arthritis. Arthritis Rheum 1978; 21: 599 (abstract).

137. Lahesmaa-Rantala R, Granfors K, Isomaki H, Toivanen A. Yersinia specific immune complexes in the synovial fluid of patients with Yersinia triggered reactive arthritis. Ann Rheum Dis 1987; 46: 510–14.

138. Peeters AJ, Warmold A, Van den Wall Bake L, Van Albada-Kuipers GA. IgA containing immune complexes and hematuria in ankylosing spondylitis. A prospective longitudinal study. J Rheumatol 1988; 15: 1662–7.

139. Peeters AJ, Van den Wall Bake AWL, Daha MR, Breedveld FC. Inflammatory bowel disease and ankylosing spondylitis associated with cutaneous vasculitis, glomerulonephritis, and circulating IgA immune complexes. Ann Rheum Dis 1990; 49: 638–40.

140. Sandborn WJ, Hanauer SB. Antitumor necrosis factor therapy for inflammatory bowel disease: a review of agents, pharmacology, clinical results, and safety. Inflam Bowel Dis 1999; 5: 119–33.

141. Mayer L, Meyers S, Janowitz HD. Cryoproteinemia in the cutaneous gangrene of Crohn's disease: a report of two cases. J Clin Gastroenterol 1981; 3: 17–21.

142. Stein HB, Otto LA, Schlappner WB, Gourlay RH, Reeve CE. The intestinal bypass arthritis dermatitis syndrome. Arthritis Rheum 1981; 24: 684–90.

143. Shum DT, Guenther L. Metastatic Crohn's disease. Arch Dermatol 1990; 126: 6455–8.

144. Wakefield AJ, Sankey EA, Dhillon AP, Sawyer AFM. Granulomatous vasculitis in Crohn's disease. Gastroenterology 1991; 100: 1279–87.

145. de Kozak Y. Antibody response in uveitis. Eye 1997; 11: 194–9.

146. Sartor RB. Microbial factors in the pathogenesis of Crohn's disease, ulcerative colitis and experimental intestinal inflammation. In: Kirsner JB, ed. Inflammatory Bowel Diseases: 5th edition. Philadelphia: W.B. Saunders, 1999: 153–78.

147. Sartor RB. Intestinal microflora in human and experimental inflammatory bowel disease. Curr Opin Gastroenterol 2001; 17 (In press).

148. Sartor RB, Veltkamp C. Interactions between enteric bacteria and the immune system which determine mucosal homeostasis vs chronic intestinal inflammation: Lessons from rodent models. In: Rogler G, Kullmann F, Rutgeerts P, Sartor RB, Scholmerich J, eds. IBD at the End of Its First Century. Dordrecht: Kluwer Academic Publishers, 2000: 30–41.

abound: stomach (chronic gastritis, atrophic gastritis, gastric carcinoma), pancreas (chronic pancreatitis, pancreatic carcinoma), liver (chronic hepatitis, cirrhosis, hepatocellular carcinoma).

Before embarking on gross and microscopic features of UC and CD some discussion on context is needed. The idiopathic IBD is separated from those conditions with established etiologies. Table 1 lists some inflammatory conditions of the alimentary tract that must always be in the mind of the physician evaluating a patient for IBD. Ischemic, iatrogenic, and infectious causes of injury with inflammation abound, and will run courses and have treatments distinct from IBD. Apart from those diseases with clear-cut etiology, non-UC and non-CD IBD exist [16–24]. They are not reviewed here except when necessary to distinguish them from UC and CD.

Importantly, nature does not provide a complete anatomic road map of every entity under the sun. Thus it cannot be overemphasized how much anatomic pathological overlap there can be among the different diseases. Realistically speaking, the best anatomical assessment is really only a constellation of weighted findings which may considerably narrow the differential diagnosis, but is not definitively diagnostic in its own right. The contribution of clinical input toward classifying a given patient's ailment is insurmountable [4, 24]; an example might be IBD presenting in the elderly [25]. Such a setting would require a thorough effort to exclude ischemic injury, drug-related injury, extraintestinal masses, diverticular disease, and of course not to overlook the likelihood of IBD itself. Clinical input at the time of pathologic assessment can greatly assist in rapid and precise diagnoses rather than purely descriptive ones that are less utilitarian, even if accurate.

Ulcerative colitis

Classic ulcerative colitis and general considerations

UC is more precisely an idiopathic chronic ulcerative colitis. UC is a chronic inflammatory disease of the colonic mucosa with an active component. Its diagnosis necessitates the exclusion of known pathogens and defined pathologic processes such as infections, vasculopathies, intoxications, and iatrogenic injury, as well as other idiopathic diseases. Anatomically it is truly localized to the colon, although there are systemic manifestations of the disease which are best described in several other chapters elsewhere in this text.

Table 1. Common inflammatory diseases of the alimentary tract

Acute self-limited enteritis/colitis
Infectious enteritis/ colitis
    Viral
    Bacterial
    Protozoal
Parasitic
Ischemic enteritis/colitis
Radiation enteritis/colitis
Drug related injury (e.g. non-steroidal anti-inflammatory drug (NSAID))
Microscopic colitis
Collagenous colitis
Food intolerance/hypersensitivity (e.g. gluten-sensitive enteropathy)
Crohn's disease
Ulcerative colitis
Indeterminate colitis
Acute appendicitis
Diverticulitis
Gastroesophageal reflux disease
Gastroduodenitis
    Peptic ulcer disease
    H. pylori infection
    Autoimmune gastritis

UC is most often described as an active chronic inflammatory disease of the colorectal mucosa that has a characteristic distribution. *Classic* UC is said to always involve the rectum; it can involve the colon but always in continuity with the rectum. Therefore it is a diffuse disease, its distal limit is always the rectum and it may extend proximally to any length of colon. It is believed to be most severe distally. Intrinsically, UC does not extend beyond the ileocecal valve. Ulcerative colitis does not skip areas within the colon. It always causes mucosal damage [3–10, 13]. The deep submucosa and muscularis propria are spared. Variations of the classic disease pattern are discussed later.

There are well-described peripheral features of UC that bear mentioning. They include 'backwash ileitis', which is an indirect injury causally related to bystander inflammatory change in the terminal ileum when UC involves the cecum. However, ulcerating injury is not found in the terminal ileum. UC will directly involve the appendix, and the appendiceal injury will parallel the affected colon. Severe mucosal activity, especially with ulceration, will cause some superficial submucosal damage in continuity with the overlying mucosal injury. Lastly, an exceptional but accepted variant is fulminant UC. This may be abrupt, and injure the full thickness of the colonic wall by a mechanism more akin to ischemia than the typical active chronic inflammatory mechanism. The most florid manifestation of fulminant UC is toxic megacolon.

At this point it is asserted that common practice observation and the literature support features of UC that deviate from the classic teaching. UC is a dynamic disease that frequently demonstrates a lack of diffuse changes and loss of continuity with the rectum over time [26–29]. It has a waxing and waning evolution that at one point in time may not adhere to what is taught to be classic. The most striking example of this is often referred to as *patchiness*. The term is meant to imply focality of disease or variations in activity or chronic injury that resemble skip lesions. The term 'skip lesion' is so entrenched in the lexicon of CD that it is avoided in the assessment of non-Crohn's IBD. In addition, patchiness does not always refer to unequivocally normal segments between diseased segments; but it does refer to variable disease impact rather than purely diffuse disease in continuity with the rectum. Nowadays, this non-uniform pattern is most frequently observed in (a) treated patients and (b) children at their first presentation. The distribution and severity of disease in the non-classic sense will be further described in the sections on anatomic pathology and non-classic UC.

Anatomic pathology of ulcerative colitis

The starting point of anatomic classification of UC is necessarily the classic and prototypically static pattern. At some time in the disease evolution there is a dominant morphology that has been determined to be the defining pathology for UC. The gross and microscopic pathology for classic UC is described below, and further illustrated in Table 2. Hints that the disease is more dynamic than the dogma indicates are present in the literature. Understandably, it is difficult to chronicle the course of UC for all patients. Indeed, who knows when the disease begins? Investigators have made efforts to describe the anatomic pathology of different points in the life of a colon so affected. These include early changes, chronic active changes, chronic inactive changes, quiescent colitis or colitis in remission, and fulminating colitis.

Gross pathology of ulcerative colitis

The anatomic pathology of UC that most reliably matches the classic description for UC can be found in a resection specimen from a patient in whom the clinical and radiographic data are supportive of the diagnosis. In practice the most commonly encountered resection specimen is the colectomy for intractable disease. Grossly, the colon is shortened. The reasons for shortening of the colon include contraction of the muscularis propria and are not related to significant mural fibrosis. Importantly, the serosa of the colon and the perirectal fat are soft, smooth, shiny, and lack fibrosis, creeping fat, and fistulas. The opened specimen has a variable appearance that reflects the degree of inflammatory activity and the extent of disease. The affected area includes the rectum and some length of colon proximal to it. The entire colonic mucosa may be involved. The gross mucosal disease is diffuse and may gradually appear less severe as one moves proximally, but the boundary to the residual normal proximal extent may be sharp. Gross mucosal pathology may reveal hemorrhage, congestion, and edema. Loss of haustral markings and the usual mucosal folds are evident. The mucosa may be granular, cobblestoned, pitted, and most importantly ulcerated. In cases with less activity the mucosa may appear more pale, tan, and atrophic. In cases with marked activity there may be inflammatory polyps. These polyps may appear as small knobs with a smooth surface, or in extreme cases they may form long processes with a filiform appearance. An inflammatory polyp rises above the level of the mucosa, and inflammatory pseudopolyp is an inflamed island of mucosa that is surrounded by ulceration and only appears raised. The cross-section of the bowel wall reveals mucosal disease, a normal loose submucosal interface between the mucosa and muscularis propria. The terminal ileum may have mild non-specific changes, but no significant gross pathology, and the appendix may have some mucosal disease but will not appear as an acute appendicitis with mural and serosal inflammation. The ulcers tend to be irregular (linear serpentine ulcers are more often seen in CD). Another finding is mucosal bridges; areas where there has been undermining ulceration of mucosa by inflammation and necrosis. The ulcer is partly roofed by mucosa with two attachments. Occasionally, a rim of squamous lined proximal anal canal will be attached at the distal end of the gross specimen. Squamous mucosa is pearly opaque white to pink, in contrast to the reddened

Table 2. Important pathologic features in typical IBD (i.e. classic, non-treated)

	Ulcerative colitis	Crohn disease
Gross pathology		
Involved organ	Colon	Any part of alimentary tract, commonly large and small bowel
Serositis	None	Frequent
Adenopathy	Common	Common
Creeping fat	None	Frequent
Strictures	None	Frequent
Fissures	None	Frequent
Distribution of disease	Diffuse, in continuity with rectum	Focal disease, segmental pattern with skip areas
Mucosal appearance	Granular, ulcerated	Cobblestoned
Aphthous lesions	None	Common
Inflammatory polyps	Common	Common
Perinanal disease	Rare	Common
Fistulas	None	Common
Other gross disease	Colonic shortening, non fibrotic	Adhesion to adjacent organs
Microscopic pathology		
Distribution of disease	Mucosal, diffuse even at microscopic level	Up to all layers of organ involved, can be focal at microscopic level
Mucosal architecture	Distorted	Distorted
Metaplasia	Paneth cell metaplasia	Pyloric gland metaplasia
Inflammatory cell infiltrate	Heavy mucosal lymphocytic and plasmacytic infiltrate, with neutrophils confined to crypt zones	Lymphoid aggregates and heavy lymphocytic and plasmacytic infiltrates with neutrophils
Crypt abscesses	Very common	Common
Granulomas	Rare, foreign-body type (usually associated with contents of ruptured crypt)	Frequent; non-caseating epithelioid histiocytes
Neuronal hyperplasia	None	Common
Dilated lymphatics	None	Common
Congestion, hemorrhage	Common	Rare
Fibrosis	Mucosal, minimal	Transmural

translucent glandular mucosa. Benign adenopathy is not uncommon [3–10].

Microscopic pathology of ulcerative colitis

Microscopically, the hallmark of ulcerative colitis is a diffuse mixed inflammatory cell infiltrate within the lamina propria and crypts in a background of architectural distortion. Like the gross specimen, this change diffusely involves the mucosa in the area sampled. The mixed infiltrate is partly dominated by lymphocytes and plasma cells that crowd the lamina propria. Neutrophilic activity is within the lamina propria predominantly confined to the pericrypt zone, within the crypt epithelial lining and filling the crypt lumens (crypt abscesses). Eosinophilic inflammation is variable, but may be quite prominent. Well-formed sarcoid like granulomas are not a feature of

UC. In areas of crypt injury, luminal contents and mucin may incite a foreign-body-type reaction with giant cells and loose collections of histiocytes that qualify as poorly formed granulomas [4, 5]. These are seen in the mucosa and can be surprising when there is no residual crypt present, but most often some kind of clue to the residual crypt is found on serial sections. The muscularis mucosa and superficial submucosa may show chronic inflammatory changes secondary to mucosal disease, but transmural disease or submucosal disease in isolation of overlying pathology are not features of UC.

The mucosal architecture provides important clues to classifying colitis as that of UC rather than an acute self-limited colitis. The usual colonic crypts run at 90 degrees to the muscularis mucosa, they are straight and have a single opening per crypt at the colonic lumen. With chronic inflammatory injury, erosion, and ulceration, the mucosa does not remodel normally. Crypts are seen to branch, with two or more irregular crypts with off-angle axes sharing a common orifice. Every possible permutation of crypt shape can occur; they are often cystically dilated, have buds, or run at odd angles relative to the muscularis mucosa. An important crypt feature that is regularly found in established UC is crypt shortening. Crypts fail to reach the muscularis mucosa. In some areas band-like infiltrates of lymphocytes and plasma cells or lymphoid aggregates resembling follicles separate the short crypts from the muscularis mucosa. The microscopist should be aware that a rare branched crypt can be found in normal colons, and in severe acute colitis (as with *Shigella* infection) some branching may be seen as the mucosa regenerates [4, 5]. Innominate glands, with a consistent branching pattern, are also found in normal mucosa [30]. The spectrum of atrophy, gland branching and shortening, minimal mucosal fibrosis, inflammatory polyps, etc. is referred to as architectural distortion. The architectural distortion, added to the heavy lymphocytic and plasmacytic infiltrates (apart from the physiologic lamina propria complement of mononuclear cells), comprise the diagnostic features of chronic colitis. The neutrophilic component and evidence of ongoing mucosal damage such as erosion, crypt regeneration, reactive epithelial and endothelial cytology comprise the activity of the disease. Paneth cell metaplasia in the left colon is another aspect of chronic injury.

Fulminant colitis and toxic megacolon in ulcertive colitis

Fulminant colitis is included for completeness [4, 5, 31]. This may occur with UC and a number of other causes of colitis such as infectious or ischemic colitis or even CD. It is a severe colitis with life-threatening complications such as hemorrhage and perforation (50% mortality if perforation occurs). It may be the primary presentation of UC, and in such cases the usually requisite signs of chronic injury will not be found.

Grossly, the colon often has disease seen on the external surface, and this may suggest an ischemic pathology with congestion imparting a dusky red hue. Other features resembling ischemia include a thin and friable wall. Microscopically one might find extensive and diffuse injury such that mucosal evaluation is difficult to impossible secondary to diffuse necrosis, ulceration, congestion, and hemorrhage. Contrary to what is usually seen in UC, this intense necrosis and congestion can extend into the deeper layers of the bowel wall and be seen in the muscularis propria. The fragile tissue may form cracks and force a consideration that the disease is fissuring CD. However, the cracks are not chronic fistulas, but are really due to lost cohesion in newly necrotic tissue. Even if there is not total mucosal necrosis findings such as architectural distortion, a band of chronic inflammatory cells along the mucosa, and crypt abscesses might not be found. Fulminant colitis may result in toxic megacolon, which is likely to result in colectomy. The bowel becomes dilated, there may be extensive intraluminal hemorrhage, and the wall is extremely thin and delicate. It is important to note that, in fulminant colitis, the anatomic pathological findings may not yield a 100% specific diagnostic etiology. The section on indeterminate colitis further addresses this.

Recognized variations in ulcerative colitis

Although traditional descriptions of UC abound, the length of the involved segment and the neutrophilic activity can be variable among patients and over time. The proximal extent of colitis is variable. Importantly, some people have only proctitis. Often the rectal involvement has greater lymphoid development. This appears as a chronic follicular proctitis. If the disease is truly limited to the rectum, and is diagnosed as ulcerative proctitis, the course of disease is distinct from UC. In ulcerative proctitis alone the important sequelae associated with extensive UC, such as a significantly increased risk of carcinoma, are not imparted. Reportedly, most of these patients do not go on to develop more proximal disease [4, 7, 8]. Other variations of involvement include left-sided disease, extensive disease, and pancolitis. However, what is the true extent or just a temporally assigned limit is disputed [29]. Histologically, the degree of acute inflammatory activity does not necessarily correlate with symptoms [4]. Acute inflammatory activity may abate, and some term these cases of UC 'quiescent' [7] or colitis in remission [32]. Usually, there are telltale signs of previous damage in the form of diffuse mucosal architectural distortion; these signs are referred to as 'footprints'. A quiescent pattern is one in which active inflammation with neutrophils, crypt damage and repair, and stromal vascular reactive changes are absent, but the more durable aspects of disease (mainly architectural distortion) persist. A resolved pattern is one in which the inflammatory infiltrate and remodeled mucosa appear normally, that a diagnosis of colitis cannot be made. Rarely, even the architecture may remodel well enough to make diagnosis impossible without relying on well-documented, well-sampled material from a time when the disease had more activity. Variations in UC pattern abound, including 'rectal sparing' [27, 33], cecal or right-sided flares [26], or appendiceal disease in left-sided colitis [34]. These phenomena, treatment effects, and the temporal dynamic nature are important considerations for the next section on non-classic UC.

Non-classic ulcerative colitis

The pattern of inflammatory injury in ulcerative colitis may deviate from the classic teachings [4, 26–29, 32–41]. The classic pattern of diffuse colitis, always in continuity with the rectum, and increasing severity distally is reiterated in teaching more often than is encountered in practice. The leading deviation encountered in practice is *patchy* inflammatory injury that often demonstrates proximal disease in excess of distal disease. 'Patchy' inflammatory injury is a description of variable inflammatory intensity or architectural distortion that may suggest a 'skip lesion', and is in direct opposition to 'diffuse disease in continuity with the rectum'. In practice, a pathologist may review more material from referred patients with long-standing and treated disease than from patients with disease at the primary presentation, and it has been suggested that treated UC with uneven healing may appear patchy in its distribution. It has also been said that children without prior treatment may present with a non-classic pattern of injury [39].

A successfully treated UC colon may have no residual inflammatory activity to be seen pathologically. More impressively, there may be extreme cases in which the architecture undergoes virtual reconstitution and would not be diagnostically different from normal colon. Most often, resolution is incomplete and inflammatory activity and architectural distortion persist to some degree. Often the resolution does not occur with the same bias as the classic distribution of UC. Witnessed pathologically are areas where there is diagnosable UC in the proximal colon, but not so in the distal colon. Nowhere is this seen more often than in a case of *rectal sparing* [26–28].

The dogma of (1) diffuse disease in continuity with the rectum and its corollary (2) rectal normalcy being an exclusion criterion for a diagnosis of UC, must be challenged carefully with example. A well-documented example is rectal sparing. A thorough description of this phenomenon was illustrated by Levine *et al.* [27], but alluded to by others [4, 25, 28]. The Levine study population had well-documented UC with rectal involvement. They found rare complete resolution in rectal biopsies of patients in remission. These workers found histopathologically borderline or normal biopsies that did not meet diagnostic criteria for UC in 46% of these patients. They studied both inflammatory activity and architectural distortion parameters. In addition, one patient developed severe clinical relapse without rectal disease, an appearance that would suggest CD if one adhered to dogma. Levine *et al.* also made the important observation that disease involvement in UC is dynamic, perhaps starting with a classic distribution, developing patchy resolution, but also suffering relapse. Thus, this example is illustrative of where the rectum is not always involved or is not the most severely involved segment in UC. Levine *et al.* were not alone in reporting this phenomenon; others have noted rectal sparing and often made the association with various treatments including 5-aminosalicylic acid and steroids [36–38]. Odze *et al.* [36] noted that rectal sparing occurred in placebo-treated patients, but significantly more often in topical 5-aminosalicylate treated patients. Importantly Levine *et al.* noted that rectal steroid treatment was not a factor in rectal sparing in their study. They also reported that rectal sparing was not a new observation but could be found in the literature going back decades. This gives credence to the assertion by Bernstein *et al.* [28] that the dogmatic message is so successful that practitioners do not acknowledge the important exceptions to the disease model despite their frequent occurrence. This has been firmly echoed by others [29]. Lastly, rectal sparing is not limited to long-standing treated UC but has also been reported in fulminant colitis [41].

The concept of patchiness is extended beyond rectal sparing by Bernstein *et al.* [28] and by Kleer and Appelman [29]. In their investigations patchiness can manifest as skip areas or segmental chronic colitis. Their study population all had well-documented UC, but deviated endoscopically and histologically over time. This gave the colon areas of pathologic chronic colitis without diffuse distribution. Areas of normal or near-normal mucosa could be found in the areas of chronic colitis. In addition, right-sided disease could be found to dominate over left-sided disease. The fraction of cases that developed patchiness in a way that might promote a pathologist to favor CD was significant at 30% [29]. Both groups of investigators support the consideration made by Levine *et al.* [27] that UC mucosal distribution is dynamic and does not necessarily adhere to the dogma of diffuse disease in continuity with the rectum. Rectal therapy was not a significant factor in developing patchiness. Patchiness in UC and its dynamic mucosal involvement were studied in populations with well-documented UC, necessarily. This provokes the notion that over time the disease changes but presents classically. However, Markowitz *et al.* [39] and Burnham *et al.* [35] have reported rectosigmoid pathology that did not support a diagnosis of UC, while the proximal colon did. These occurred in populations at primary presentation.

Understandably, one never knows the true time of primary onset of disease, only when it first comes to medical attention.

Another pattern of patchiness that can appear as segmental colitis or skip area occurs with appendiceal inflammation. Left-sided colitis can occur with a long normal right colonic segment. Somewhat paradoxically, this situation may be accompanied by an appendiceal involvement by UC. Biopsies at the appendiceal orifice might give the suggestion of cecal and left-sided chronic colitis and lead the pathologist to favor a diagnosis of Crohn's colitis [34].

In practice one encounters biopsies from patients with patchy disease distribution. In addition, severe ulcerating disease (lesions extending beyond the muscularis mucosa into the submucosa) may heal with fibrosis, sometimes obliterating the muscularis mucosa and superficial submucosa. It is not hard to imagine the scenario at biopsy where this might suggest CD, especially if crypt disruption has given rise to some foreign-body-type giant cells. It is for situations such as this that complete clinical data and all pertinent pathology be reviewed before one feels forced to change a diagnosis in a given patient. It should be stressed that the patchiness described above is not likely to have severe injury adjacent to normal mucosa like that seen in CD. Even, with excellent healing, one might still find tell-tale signs ('footprints') suggesting diffuse disease in areas that seem to be skip lesions. In some of these areas the healing is so good as to not be diagnostic of chronic colitis, but at the same time not entirely normal.

Neoplasia and ulcerative colitis

A major consequence of UC is the increased risk of colorectal adenocarcinoma. The risk of developing carcinoma in patients with extensive but unresected UC has been measured to be 3%, 5%, and 9% at 15, 20, and 25 years disease duration [42]. In this text Chapter 36 is devoted to cancer and dysplasia, and the reader is referred to that chapter for the broader issues covering neoplasia and UC. This section deals with the anatomic pathological concerns of dysplasia and carcinoma in UC. The various terms given to dysplastic lesions are covered. For the anatomic pathology to have any meaning its context in surveillance is discussed. Briefly, the main concern regarding UC and carcinoma is how to intervene such that colorectal carcinoma does not contribute to patient morbidity and mortality. In more practical terms, can surveillance programs and surgical intervention prevent an adverse outcome due to colorectal carcinoma in patients with UC? Exactly how and when to survey, and what surgical procedures to perform, are not the primary issues for the pathologist, but how tissue diagnoses affect management are. Removing carcinoma by way of colectomy at a stage where metastases have not yet occurred is the goal. Surveillance is directed toward the detection of dysplasia as well as carcinoma. This is because dysplasia is neoplastic and premalignant, parallels the carcinoma location, and is found in association with carcinoma in UC just as in non-IBD populations. Therefore, in surveillance, in the hope of catching early cancer we may overshoot and advise colectomy at precancer. This section will evaluate the anatomic pathology of dysplasia and carcinoma in UC, dysplasia not necessarily related to IBD and UC, and whether dysplasia not otherwise specified is a practical premalignant endpoint for intervention in UC.

For the sake of simplicity we will focus on the role of the pathologist in a surveillance program for dysplasia and carcinoma. Traditional management of UC maintains that a dysplasia diagnosis is an indication for colectomy. This has been reiterated throughout the literature [4, 5, 42–52] with notations of caution and various qualifications regarding grade, gross features, and second opinion. Simply put, those patients in a traditional surveillance protocol have a predetermined endpoint (a diagnosis of dysplasia) that would trigger a management decision to end in curative colectomy. Therefore, a diagnosis of a dysplastic lesion or carcinoma is an indication for colectomy. At our institution, low-grade dysplasia is sufficient indication in the appropriate candidate. Certainly other scenarios exist, such as finding dysplasia in a patient who is not in a surveillance protocol and refuses colectomy, but individualized considerations such as that would only confuse this section. The pathologist must identify dysplasia in biopsies taken from the colon at endoscopy and communicate this information prominently in the surgical pathology report. Surveillance is done at sufficiently close intervals so as to detect early neoplastic lesions that do not have life-threatening consequences for the patient.

Dysplasia must be defined as a term and a concept. First, dysplasia as it is discussed here is the unequivocal transformation of epithelial cells to a neoplastic state. Unless otherwise stated, dysplasia refers to a preinvasive epithelial neoplasm. It is believed that most colorectal adenocarcinomas arise from pre-existing dysplasia. Dysplastic lesions may gradually worsen and lead to carcinoma. This concept applies to UC just as it does to non-IBD-related colons. The particular issues of what makes dysplasia an indication for colectomy in UC but not non-IBD colons are discussed below. Dysplasia can be recognized via microscopic examination.

Dysplasia has characteristic gross and microscopic pathology and clear microscopic criteria [46, 53, 54]. The gross features include a lesion that may be polypoid (pedunculated or sessile), flat, or depressed. The surface is often papillary grossly and is distinct from inflammatory polyps (which appear smooth). It is the microscopy that specifically and definitively characterizes dysplasia. Microscopically the neoplastic glands are often tubular, or villous, occasionally serrated. The neoplastic glands are hyperchromatic; architecturally crowded, cytologically crowded, generally have immature cytoplasm; and demonstrate nuclear enlargement, lack of nuclear maturation, and increased mitotic activity. Variations occur and higher-grade lesions have more extreme deviations from normal. A low-grade lesion generally has simple gland shapes, pseudostratified epithelial cells, peg-shaped nuclei, and small dark nucleoli. High-grade lesions have complex gland shapes including cribriforming, true stratification of cells, and rounded nuclei with prominent somewhat amphophilic nucleoli. A high-grade lesion shares considerable overlap with early carcinoma.

There is currently a marked treatment difference between UC patients with a diagnosis of dysplasia versus non-IBD patients. In non-IBD the removal of a dysplastic lesion at endoscopy is adequate therapy and does not require colectomy. In UC it has been recommended that a dysplastic lesion found at endoscopy be followed by colectomy [52]. The very premise of surveillance is that most UC-related adenocarcinomas arise from preinvasive dysplastic lesions in a manner paralleling that for non-IBD [46]. In UC it is believed that a diagnosis of dysplasia is more ominous than in non-IBD. This implies that there is a significant risk of concomitant but unsampled carcinoma coincident with dysplasia. There are studies to support this [42, 45]. Anatomic pathologic assessment of colectomy specimens have found dysplasia in several forms (flat, polypoid, and sometimes associated with carcinoma). In addition neoplasia has been found to be multifocal [42, 45, 55, 56]. Carcinoma has been found at sites apart from dysplasia. Carcinoma has been found to be multifocal. So, unlike a non-IBD colon, there is a greater chance that the malignant potential of a UC colon is multifocal, and at sites either coordinate with a dysplasia diagnosis or away from identified dysplastic foci. Because of that risk, total colectomy is performed rather than segmental resection. A surveillance diagnosis of dysplasia can be seen as a marker of high malignant potential rather than the locator of the only worrisome focus. There may be a different biology to UC neoplasia than in non-IBD colons; interestingly a greater percentage of mucinous adenocarcinomas have been noted in UC [56].

With colectomy such a major surgical intervention, and missed carcinoma such a morbid state, the pitfalls in diagnosis need to be addressed. Traditional management of UC and dysplasia has found it difficult to distinguish different types of dysplasia, and has chosen to lump together all the dysplastic lesions in the affected colon and recommend colectomy for them all. Therefore the only issue remaining for traditional management is precision diagnoses. To this end the nuances of dysplasia diagnoses and observer agreement are addressed. However, in a subsequent section the concept of conservative management of dysplasia and IBD is discussed. When considering conservative management of UC patients in a surveillance protocol the following need to be addressed. Can a UC patient develop a dysplastic lesion akin to one in a non-IBD patient? Do UC patients have two separate pathogenic roads to colorectal carcinoma; one being UC related and one being just like that for non-IBD? If the last statement were true should we be able to distinguish between the UC-related dysplasia–carcinoma sequence and the sporadic adenoma–carcinoma sequence?

One pitfall in the diagnosis of dysplasia is sampling, and this was partly alluded to above. A visible lesion or a random sample of flat mucosa may be the gross target; but there is no guarantee that the highest-grade lesion has been adequately sampled, and therefore the true malignant potential of the UC colon may be underestimated.

Another major pitfall in the diagnosis of dysplasia lies in interpretation. The challenge can be seen in two ways: (1) the increased difficulty making the diagnosis in abnormal mucosa and (2) poor observer reproducibility. For a diagnosis of dysplasia there must be tissue obtained for microscopic examination. Clear-cut diagnostic criteria for the establishment of dysplasia exist. Regrettably, dysplasia is most easily diagnosed when the background is normal colonic mucosa; however, in UC the inflammatory milieu, regenerative atypia and architectural distortion increase the uncertainty in a diagnosis of dysplasia. This is because architecturally complex non-neoplastic glands can be found in UC as a result of distorted healing. In addition, cytologic atypia with nuclear enlargement and immature cytoplasm occur secondary to inflammation and regeneration. It has been well said that extreme caution should be exercised when evaluating dysplasia in the setting of active inflammation [3]. In addition, bona-fide dysplasia in IBD may not form the prototypical pedunculated polyp seen in textbooks, but may be superimposed onto the usual background of IBD (in fact this proposed difference may be what separates some non-IBD-related dysplasia from IBD-related dysplasia). Thus, non-dysplastic mucosa may mimic dysplasia, or it may obscure true dysplasia. 'Dysplasia' is usually descriptively modified and the terms used also highlight the uncertainty noted above. Accepted terminology for evaluating dysplasia include: indefinite for dysplasia, low-grade dysplasia, high-grade dysplasia [43, 46]. The indefinite category is not part of the spectrum of dysplasia in that it does not necessarily mean the low end of low-grade, but rather the combination of atypia and inflammation makes certainty unlikely and a diagnosis of dysplasia must be deferred until inflammation is removed from the equation.

Unfortunately, the uncertainty does not end with 'indefinite for dysplasia' but there is poor observer agreement when evaluating dysplasia in IBD [57]. When attempting to match a diagnosis grade for grade the agreement varied between 42% and 65%

between pathologists. Melville *et al.* [57] conceded that practice habits which include discussion with the referring gastroenterologist and review of previous material from a given patient might make the real agreement stronger than that found in a study set. In another study, using the standardized classification of dysplasia developed by Riddell *et al.* [46], observer variability was quite high. The standardized classification included negative for dysplasia (grade 0), indefinite for dysplasia (grade 0–1), low-grade dysplasia (grade 2), and high-grade dysplasia (grade 3). In addition there were subclassifications in the indefinite category. The intraobserver variability in that study was not insignificant, with the same pathologist averaging a 0.29 grade unit self disagreement. The interobserver disagreement was greater; 0.60 grade units. Fortunately there was greater agreement at the extremes (negative for dysplasia and high-grade dysplasia). However, the true measure of the grading system is partly based on the medical action taken. For instance, if the *grade* of dysplasia does not affect management, then a homogenization of the low and high-grade categories might allow for better agreement in terms of management. Both of the above studies note the additional difficulty of separating reactive changes on chronically injured mucosa and true dysplasia. Other investigations have verified the limits on pathological diagnostic reproducibility regarding dysplasia and UC [58].

At our institution surveillance is targeted for any grade of dysplasia, and carcinoma. A grade of indefinite directs the patient toward therapy to reduce inflammation and promote healing with subsequent rebiopsy. Any dysplasia results in a critical review of the endoscopic impression with the most likely recommendation being colectomy. We concur with the recommendations that diagnostically challenging biopsies should be reviewed by more than one experienced pathologist. If colectomy is not an option, then surveillance is not a logical part of management. Carcinoma has been reported to develop in patients with dysplasia but refusing colectomy, sometimes after many years [59].

The above section dealt with the realities and traditional role of surveillance in UC. Below, non-traditional management of IBD-related dysplasia is addressed. Various terms for dysplastic lesions as they occur in non-IBD colons and IBD colons are defined. It is possible that subsets of dysplastic lesions can be managed safely without colectomy. The scope of the possibility has not yet been clarified.

Non-traditional management of dysplasia

A controversial topic today revolves around the sporadic adenoma (for example a dysplastic lesion such as a tubular adenoma) and colitis-related dysplasia. In non-IBD a sporadic adenoma is usually a low-grade dysplastic lesion that is treated endoscopically and with follow-up. In surveyed UC patients IBD-related dysplasia is followed by colectomy. With significant improvements in treatment, more patients are living longer with manageable disease and are not requiring colectomies for intractable disease. As these patients reach the age of 50 years or more they acquire adenomatous lesions that are indistinguishable from those of non-IBD patients. Is it possible to make a diagnosis of sporadic adenoma in IBD and treat that patient just as one would a non-IBD patient? One example of this would be a typical tubular adenoma in the cecum found in a patient who had only left-sided colitis. It might be overkill to perform a colectomy, especially if the UC is well controlled symptomatically. But even this decision is easily mired in challenge since we know the disease to be dynamic (did the disease *ever* involve the cecum?) its true proximal extent is uncertain. What if the supposed adenoma were in an area of colitis? Also, what if the patient were 30 years old or younger, would we still believe it to be a sporadic adenoma?

Next needing defining are the various terms given to dysplastic lesions. Dysplastic lesions may be described as sporadic adenoma (SA), dysplastic lesion or mass (DALM), or flat dysplasia (also known as endoscopically invisible dysplasia) [45, 49]. For this section we are concerned with SA and DALM. A SA is the colonic epithelial lesion that is not uncommonly found in persons over 50 years of age at endoscopy (i.e. tubular adenoma or villous adenoma). A SA, like all adenomas in the GI tract, is a dysplastic lesion [54]. Because of its frequency and conservative management recent efforts have been made to separate SA from IBD-related dysplasia [43, 47, 49, 60–62]. It should be emphasized that there is near-total overlap in the criteria used to diagnose each, and this area is undergoing intensive and important work (discussed below). DALM was coined by Blackstone *et al.* in 1981 [45]. Their study demonstrated that an endoscopic biopsy of a visualized lesion in which only dysplasia was found (at biopsy) had a significant association with carcinoma (at resection). They had studied several lesions sufficiently suspicious for neoplasia to require biopsy, and found dysplasia alone in the biopsy sample in most cases. The dysplasia was frequently less than high-grade. However, at resection there was found to be carcinoma deep to the biopsy site. Their conclusion maintained that endoscopically worrisome lesions with histologic confirmation of dysplasia were so strongly linked to carcinoma that colectomy was warranted. The term DALM has clinical utility in that it alerts the medical team that the lesion may be more ominous than an adenoma. The term, however, suffers from definitional ambiguity. In the broadest sense, any visible lesion biopsied that is found to be dysplastic can be construed as a DALM, including a sporadic adenoma. This underscores the importance of separating SA from IBD-related dysplasia, if it is at all possible. Not so easily addressed is the potential for other foci of epithelial neoplasms of the colon are present once dysplasia has been found at one site. As was mentioned above, there are numerous reports of multifocal dysplasia, multifocal carcinoma, and carcinoma found at sites apart from the initial dysplastic site (this was another observation in the Blackstone paper [45]). It will be apparent from the discussion below that some investigators' estimates of occult malignancies of the colon (unselected dysplastic lesions) exceed those found by other investigators selecting for the least worrisome dysplastic lesions. Next, how does all the above affect the management of endoscopically invisible dysplasia picked up at a random biopsy site during surveillance? The last statement and question are largely under-addressed and unanswered.

Relatively recently some studies addressing the issue of IBD-related dysplasia versus SA diagnosis and management have appeared. In 1998 Torres *et al.* studied a highly selected group of raised dysplastic lesions in IBD (the study included a minority of CD patients) [60]. It is important to note that this study was not designed to fully evaluate the risk of carcinoma in colons with dysplasia and IBD, but to seek features that might help distinguish IBD-related dysplasia from SA. The selected lesions were those that would not be grossly distinguishable from a sporadic adenoma. As one would expect, the challenge of separating these lesions was high, particularly using anatomic pathology alone. In their design they incorporated a significant amount of clinical data to select their study set. Dysplastic lesions that had features suggesting carcinoma were excluded at the outset (for example, lesions associated with a stricture, or lesions with a broad-based mass underneath). Thus, selected out were cases that would likely increase the incidence of carcinoma at follow-up. Also, some lesions were assumed to be probably IBD-related if they occurred within a segment of colitis and had adjacent flat mucosa with dysplasia; in addition if follow-up biopsies of a dysplastic focus proved to have carcinoma or dysplasia then the lesion was thought to be IBD-related. This combination of a predetermined and retrospective classification underscores the difficulty in distinguishing the pathogenesis of a polyp at the time of biopsy. All the polyps were small enough to be removed endoscopically. At the completion of their study those polyps that were not in a region of colitis and were preassigned to the SA category were evaluated against those that were in the area of colitis. Among the latter, some polyps remained indeterminate in pathogenic origin, others were believed to be IBD-related. Those that were thought to be IBD-related were in a segment involved by IBD, occurred in younger patients, had active disease, had a longer disease duration, increased lamina propria inflammation, greater frequency of villous or tubulovillous architecture, admixed dysplastic epithelium, and non-dysplastic epithelium on the surface of the lesion. It is notable that there were as many clinical features as there were anatomic ones. The study was information-rich, and found multifocal dysplasia of polypoid and flat varieties. Mean follow-up was 13 months in 40 patients for whom additional material was available for pathologic study. In addition to recurrent polypoid dysplasia there was a 12.5% incidence of flat dysplasia and a 7.5% incidence of adenocarcinoma. Although statistically significant features were found to separate these selected polyps from SA it is important to note that the distinction was not entirely based in anatomic pathology. Also, with the exclusion of the most worrisome lesions at the outset and the relatively high incidence of recurrent dysplasia and carcinoma in the short follow-up, a dysplastic lesion appeared to be an ominous marker.

Additional work in this area has been illuminating, and has opened the door to colectomy sparing management in patients with IBD and dysplasia. Rubin et al. in 1999 reported conservative management in some cases of IBD-related dysplasia [47]. They noted that even the typical adenoma fit the definition of a DALM, and they acknowledged that a DALM lesion is an indication for colectomy. Their selection of dysplastic lesions that were amenable to excision by endoscopic polypectomy, allowed them to conservatively manage (by surveillance) 48

patients for a mean period of 4.1 years. Their selection process excluded patients in whom flat dysplasia had been found. They found no carcinomas at follow-up, even though at baseline some dysplastic lesions were high-grade and one carried adenocarcinoma. Recurrent polypoid dysplasia but not flat dysplasia was found. An extension of the work done by Torres et al. [60] was reported by Engelsgjerd et al. in 1999 [61]. In that study they contend that DALM are heterogeneous and broadly cover lesions which include carcinoma and nearly-inconsequential dysplasia akin to SA. In fact that work went to great lengths to select IBD-related dysplastic lesions that endoscopically and pathologically were so similar to SA as to make them indistinguishable (referred to as adenoma-like DALM). With that group of patients they found no carcinoma at follow-up (3.5 years) and found recurrent polypoid dysplasia at an incidence similar to non-IBD patients with a history of adenomatous polyps. In effect, they showed that the subset of DALM that had strong clinical and pathologic overlap with SA, behaved as SA. It is essential to reiterate that the decision to label a lesion as having a low probability of concern is based largely on the clinical (endoscopic) data, and not heavily on the microanatomic pathology.

The literature supports two truths about IBD-related dysplasia and carcinoma concerning patients for whom colectomy may be appropriate. First, taken as a whole, dysplastic lesions in IBD (especially DALM) are markers for carcinoma in a significant fraction of patients and serve as indications for colectomy. Second, polypectomized dysplastic lesions with endoscopic and pathologic features resembling those of SA behave like SA, as far out as 3–4 years, and may be managed conservatively. The paradox in these findings may not be easily resolved, but one thing does separate the two: the clinical endoscopic impression of the lesion. We cannot over-emphasize the magnitude of input required on the part of the endoscopist toward the latter statement (features such as size of lesion, overall morphology, surrounding mucosa, stricture association, colitis zone, etc.). On a related note, it is unclear whether the term DALM is having its intended impact, that is a diagnosis supporting colectomy. With studies referring to 'adenoma-like DALM' behaving as SA, some clinicians may no longer consider DALM as an indication for colectomy. A clearer description might be in order, if a lesion is clinically and endoscopically worrisome for malignancy and the pathologic assessment is dysplasia, a colectomy is likely the prudent course in the appropriate candidate. If a lesion has the endoscopic appearance of a sporadic adenoma and the pathologic assessment is exactly that for a SA (even in an area of active colitis) conservative management *may* be warranted. Lastly, still in question is the meaning of flat (or invisible) dysplasia, and the importance of recurrent or multifocal dysplasia.

Crohn's disease

Crohn's disease and general considerations

Some observers have found the gross appearance of CD striking, and some poetic gross descriptions such as 'An eel in a state of rigor mortis' have been made [9]. Multiorgan involvement, multifocality, transmural extension, and varied histopathology make CD anatomically more engaging than UC. The anatomic pathology of CD, with traditional attention to small bowel and colon in addition to the upper GI tract, is discussed in this section. Part of this anatomic pathological assessment will deal with dysplasia and carcinoma in CD. The histopathologic diagnostic assessment of CD is further discussed in Chapter 37, and further concerns regarding the cancer process are discussed in Chapter 36. This section is primarily concerned with Crohn's colitis and its distinction from UC (see Table 2), CD in the more proximal GI tract, and to some extent its emergence as a risk factor for carcinoma.

CD can involve any part of the alimentary tract. It has a predilection for the terminal ileum, but the colon and remaining small bowel are additional targets. It is a segmental process with areas of normal bowel intervening between diseased segments. The disease can involve all or part of the wall thickness, with subsequent involvement of adjacent structures through fissures and fistulas. A prototypical case might be a terminal ileitis with anal fissures and rectovaginal fistulas separated by a normal colon. The extent and distribution of the above example is contrary to UC. Because of the multiplicity of organ manifestations, variable histopathology and often limited anatomic pathologic sampling, a CD diagnosis must be made at the exclusion of other pathogenic etiologies such as ischemic, infectious, iatrogenic (radiation, NSAID), malignant, or diverticular (see Table 3). The etiology of CD remains idiopathic; the diagnosis requires strongly supportive clinical data and anatomic data for confirmation. The converse of making a diagnosis is also true; CD is difficult to exclude as a

Table 3. Potential mimics of Crohn's disease

Ischemic injury
Radiation injury
Granulomatous inflammation (*Mycobacteria, Salmonella, Yersinia, Chlamydia*)
Drug-related ulcers (NSAID, enteric coated potassium)
'Diaphragm disease' (NSAID-related)
Neuromuscular and vascular hamartoma
Behçet disease with enterocolonic involvement
Diverticular disease

potential diagnosis in many settings. For example, when evaluating a new patient for alimentary tract disease such as a small bowel stricture without clear etiology, CD may remain in the differential until a known cause of injury is identified [2–15, 63–70].

Gross pathology of Crohn's disease

The anatomic pathology of CD is typified by its small and large bowel involvement, but is generally applicable to other areas of the alimentary tract [9]. The gross pathology is known for its segmental distribution. If multifocal, the normal bowel between segments is referred to as a skip area. The small bowel is most frequently the primary organ involved (60%), followed by the colon (20%); the anus is a component of the disease in 75% of cases. The injury is what one might expect from any chronic inflammatory process, that is fibrosis and loss to the functional anatomy of the bowel layers. Thus inflammatory obliteration causes the serosa to no longer resist adhesion, the muscle coat and nerve plexes fail to allow for peristaltic movement, the submucosa loses its pliability, and the mucosal absorptive and barrier functions erode. Externally, the bowel is rigid, the serosa may be dull, the serosal fat adherent and firm. Fusion of the loop of bowel to adjacent structures, including other loops of bowel, non-alimentary organs or the body wall, may occur. The bowel wall may be edematous, especially at the mucosa and submucosa. The lymph nodes in the area are often reactively enlarged. Dissection of the diseased segment reveals transmural fibrosis with loss in distinctiveness of layers of muscle, submucosa, and mucosa. The mucosa may be ulcerated; the ulcers of CD are commonly aligned longitudinally (linear serpentine ulcers); the background mucosa can be a mixture of normal, atrophic, and granulating histology. Fissures through the wall forming sinus tracts or fistulas to other organs can be found. The thickened fibrotic bowel wall often narrows the lumen to form strictures.

Microscopic pathology of Crohn's disease

The microscopy of CD builds on the gross pathology. As the disease is focal grossly, it can also be so microscopically. The mucosa in a diseased segment can be normal in one part of the histologic section and next to a deep ulcer or sinus tract. This is a regular distinction from UC where focal disease is rarely seen; in CD the extremes of injury can be seen in the same section. The effects of chronic inflammation are present in the mucosa and mucosal architecture is distorted where there is disease. Thus, like UC, excess mononuclear cells in the lamina propria, branched and budded glands, and atrophy can be found in the mucosa. Ulcers, erosions, reactive and regenerative epithelium, and granulation tissue can all be found in the mucosa.

In our experience mucus gland metaplasia reminiscent of gastric pyloric glands is more easily found in CD than in UC. Strictly speaking there can be significant overlap between CD colitis mucosal disease and UC. Distinctions occur with microscopic skip areas and, of course, well-formed sarcoid-like granulomas, hallmarks of CD. Neutrophilic and eosinophilic infiltrates are variable. Edema and fibrosis may appear at any level of the bowel wall as a consequence of chronic active inflammation. The submucosa can also show hypertrophy of nerve trunks and demonstrate dilated lymphatic channels. Lymphoid aggregates, some with germinal centers, may decorate any layer of the wall. Deeper mural inflammation is not necessarily in continuity with overlying mucosal injury. Lymphoid aggregates, fibrosis, even collections of neutrophils can appear within the wall and are surrounded by uninvolved tissue.

CD is known for granulomatous inflammation and aphthoid lesions [3, 76, 77]. The granulomas are classically sarcoid-like and may be found in up to 60% of cases. In practice, granulomas are found in as few as 20% of patients with the diagnosis of CD. The granulomas of CD are often described as sarcoid-like, noncaseating and having multinucleated giant cells. Also common to CD are poorly formed granulomas resembling a collection of epithelioid histiocytes. The granulomas may be found anywhere in the bowel wall, even at the serosa, or even in the resected lymph node. Non-alimentary tract organs might be affected by granulomatous inflammation due to CD. In the mucosa, foreign body giant-cell granulomas may form due to crypt injury, with crypt mucin and intestinal contents leaking into the lamina propria. These granulomas can also be found in UC, reminding us that finding just any granuloma does not impart a diagnosis of CD. The aphthoid ulcer is a gross term that has had some microscopic characterization. In a mucosal site a tiny raised, reddened lesion with a whitish punctate center is aphthoid. The reported histologic equivalent is a subepithelial lymphoid aggregate with a tiny erosion where the epithelial cells and lymphoid cells meet. The erosion has a small amount of neutrophilic exudate. In practice, what is often described as 'aphthoid' endoscopically has no regularly defined histologic counterpart, but we have found the above-described histologic lesion on occasion. In CD, endoscopically normal or minimally abnormal mucosa had been found to contain tiny foci of epithelial necrosis, with or without any associated aphthoid lesions.

Fissures and sinus tracts also characterized CD. Kelly and Siu [73] described acute fissuring at the base of ulcers often in dilated segments. They also describe sinuses in a more chronic context with the lining being inflammatory cells and granulation tissue. Sinuses were most often found proximal to strictures. In both cases increased intraluminal pressure was hypothesized as part of the pathogenesis. Kelly and Preshaw [74] showed that fistulas arise from the sinus tracts, and were proximal to strictures at primary resection. However, they noted that at early recurrence of fistulas causing secondary resection, fistulas commonly arose from anastomotic sites. Thus, processes more complex than strictures probably induce fistulating disease in CD.

The lower GI tract in Crohn's disease

In practice the question of CD as it pertains to the anatomic pathologist often regards the distinction of Crohn's colitis from UC. If there is clinical or radiographic evidence of convincing small bowel disease, then UC is most likely excluded. Likewise, clear-cut segmental colitis with mural fibrosis, fissures, fistulas, and sarcoid-like granulomas will be Crohn's colitis and never UC. The real problems arise in the common occurrence of having only mucosal biopsies for review and no other clinical, radiographic or anatomic information. Granulomas become very helpful in these cases, but may be found in as few as

20% of cases (60% in resection specimens). Skip lesions and mucus gland metaplasia will also favor a Crohn's etiology over UC. It is understood from the section on UC that patchiness may masquerade as focal disease or skip lesions. However, even in patchiness there is often a residue of chronic disease rather than completely normal mucosa, and therefore not a true skip. Lastly, it must be stressed that, without maximal clinical and radiographic input, the mucosal biopsy anatomic pathology may be able to confirm chronic colitis, but not supply a definitive diagnosis of Crohn's colitis.

A fraction of chronic colitis cases will have no etiology, and in some settings a diagnosis is said to be 'indeterminate' [3, 75, 76]. Indeterminate colitis is further covered in its own section below. Examples of unusual diseases that may suggest a diagnosis of Crohn's colitis by virtue of segmental distribution or granulomatous inflammation are Behçet syndrome [19] and sarcoidosis [77], respectively. Crohn's colitis may have a fulminant course like that seen with UC or indeterminate colitis.

True segmental disease in the small bowel and colon should suggest CD [63–65]. One is obligated to exclude neoplasia such as a small bowel carcinoid tumor with multicentricity. Ischemic injury is also known to be segmental, and it can be chronic. Erosions and ulcers due to medications such as NSAID or enteric-coated potassium supplements might also give the impression of focal disease. Radiation injury will have atrophic, fibrotic, and chronic inflammatory changes mimicking CD. A pair of similar-appearing diseases, one termed 'diaphragm disease' and the other 'neuromuscular and vascular hamartoma' may form isolated or multifocal somewhat fibrotic and ulcerating lesions in the small bowel and colon. The diaphragm disease lesion is thought to be secondary to heavy NSAID use. Both can give the impression of CD, but have some distinctive gross and microscopic features [78–80].

The upper GI tract and Crohn's disease

The upper GI tract is involved by CD 15–25% of the time [4]. It should come as no surprise that the features of CD at the more distal small bowel and colon can be recapitulated in the esophagus, stomach, and duodenum. For that reason a reiteration of CD features is not necessary. The more common situation is one in which there has yet to be a definitive diagnosis of CD in the proximal GI tract

and the anatomic pathologic findings are an important component to guiding therapy. CD symptoms in the upper GI tract may be confused with gastro-esophageal reflux disease, *Helicobacter pylori* gastritis, peptic ulcer disease, or NSAID-type injury. CD in the upper GI tract should be part of the pathologic differential diagnosis in many situations. It has been gratifying to examine upper GI tract mucosal biopsies prior to incorporating all clinical data, and find that CD figures prominently in the differential diagnosis, and subsequently finding that CD is the best interpretation. Features such as focality, chronic inflammatory injury with altered mucosal architecture and fibrosis, and occasionally granulomas should alert the pathologist to a potential CD diagnosis. In real practice this has occurred, only to discover that the patient in question had typical lower GI tract CD.

Precise figures for unequivocal clinically significant upper GI involvement by CD are not known [69, 70]. Symptomatic involvement ranges from 0.5% to 13%, and histologic evidence may hover around 50%. Wright and Riddell [70] pointed out how rarely CD is described in the stomach and duodenum. Their study examined the gastro-duodenal anatomic pathology in patients with CD. Importantly, *H. pylori* infection is a major point in the differential. *H. pylori* is a major cause of chronic gastritis with neutrophilic activity and lymphoid aggregate formation. Wright and Riddell found that focal disease with neutrophilic activity was a characteristic of CD in the *H. pylori*-negative patient. This was true of the stomach and duodenum. Granulomas were rare (9%). They recommend adequate sampling to identify injury such as deep duodenal acute inflammation and focal active disease in the stomach and duodenum in a background of uninflamed mucosa. It should be noted that with *H. pylori* there is often diffuse superficial chronic active inflammation with deep lymphoid aggregates, and focality is not the common pattern. With resolved *H. pylori* infection all that might remain are the lymphoid aggregates, which might be difficult to separate from focal disease, but there should not be a neutrophilic component. In the study by Wright and Riddell, gastric lymphoid aggregates were a feature of H. pylori infection and not CD. Gastric metaplasia of the duodenum was not a frequent or specific finding. Wright and Riddell noted that NSAID-type erosions impart focal changes, NSAID injury often had very few inflammatory cell infiltrates (NSAID gastropathy).

In children the evaluation of gastritis and peptic ulcer disease requires a consideration of upper GI tract involvement by CD [81]. It would appear obvious that a granulomatous gastritis or duodenitis would prompt a diagnosis of CD, but so also should a focal non-*H. pylori* active gastritis. Signs of deep injury, chronic injury, and the exclusion of NSAID related injury would be supportive. Pure esophageal involvement by CD is anecdotally reported, and CD rarely but definitely may involve the esophagus [68]. We have encountered a patient with upper GI disease symptomatology who was found to have a granulomatous esophagitis; the additional work-up identified enterocolonic CD.

Neoplasia and Crohn's disease

For several decades the CD relationship to adenocarcinoma has been described [56, 82–89]. There is now believed to be an increased risk of colorectal adenocarcinoma and small bowel adenocarcinoma in segments involved by CD. Malignancies in the upper GI tract are anecdotally reported [83]. The major issue ripe for resolution is the issue of Crohn's colitis, and the magnitude of its risk for developing carcinoma. Even more importantly: is a surveillance protocol for detecting early cancer or dysplasia applicable to Crohn's colitis? CD and adenocarcinoma present challenges not seen with UC. With regard to the colon, diseased areas might not be as easily studied due to problems imposed by strictures. In regard to the disease in general, CD has greater variability of organ involvement than UC. Much of the non-colonic disease, such as small bowel, may be unsurveyable. However, small bowel adenocarcinoma is rare. Even with the added risk of CD, the number of CD patients in whom small bowel adenocarcinoma develops will probably be too few for what would be a huge technical surveillance challenge by today's methods. As has been stated, Chapter 36 has been devoted to these issues; presented here are the issues most appropriate to the anatomic pathologic concerns.

Segments of colon involved by Crohn's colitis are thought to be at increased risk for adenocarcinoma. The risk has been reported as 6.9–23.8-fold higher than the general population, although this has not always been uniformly the opinion [86]. In studies of colorectal carcinoma and Crohn's colitis, it has been shown that carcinoma occurs at a younger age than in non-IBD populations. The risk is proportional to duration and extent of disease, and in many ways

parallels that for UC [56, 88]. The histology of Crohn's colitis-related carcinoma is not distinctive. However, there are reports that the relative percent of unusual carcinoma phenotypes is altered, such that mucinous and poorly differentiated varieties are over-represented compared with non-IBD-related colorectal carcinoma [86, 89]. Dysplasia and CD is less well studied. It is likely that the diagnostic pitfalls and subtleties of sporadic adenoma and IBD-related dysplasia will closely parallel those for UC. Some studies on IBD and dysplasia include a minority of CD patients [60]. Mayer *et al.* [56] report a paucity of preoperative diagnoses of dysplasia and a concomitant lack of dysplasia associated with carcinoma in resection specimens in a series devoted to IBD-related colorectal carcinoma. Conversely, in a study of distinct design, Sigel *et al.* [89] were able to find dysplasia in resection specimens with Crohn's colitis-related colorectal adenocarcinoma 95% of the time. Eighty-six percent of the time dysplasia was in continuity with the carcinoma. In 41% of the cases dysplasia was found at a separate site (multifocal neoplasia). To date we are unaware of a study that shows surveillance to be protective against the mortality of colorectal carcinoma in Crohn's colitis. If surveillance were warranted, early cancer detection would be the most surgically conservative endpoint. Whether dysplasia is itself a significant risk factor warranting surgical intervention is not yet clear. As for UC, there will be diagnostic pitfalls in assessing dysplasia in inflamed and distorted mucosa. CD may impart new diagnostic challenges relating to early carcinoma or dysplasia appearing in strictures, bypassed segments, and fistulas.

Adenocarcinoma of the small bowel complicates Crohn enteritis. It has been associated with dysplasia [86, 89], and its frequency in bypassed segments suggested to Glotzer [86] that defunctionalized segments be removed rather than surgically bypassed. A large fraction (76%) of the carcinomas studied by Sigel *et al.* [89] were poorly differentiated.

Indeterminate colitis

When chronic colitis has no etiology, and no convincing morphologic distinction between CD and UC can be found, a diagnosis of indeterminate colitis may be rendered (some might prefer another term such as non-specific colitis). It is said that 10% of cases are indeterminate [3, 75, 76]. There are two main scenarios where this may occur. (1) The most prominent scenario is in fulminant colitis without antecedent definition of the underlying disease. As has been mentioned above, fulminant colitis with or without toxic megacolon may have such intense destruction, congestion, hemorrhage and comparatively little chronic inflammatory changes that the diagnostic features of UC or CD are absent or obscured. If fulminant colitis results in colectomy the patient may never again suffer from IBD, and no further data may appear to put the issue to rest. (2) The second scenario revolves around morphologic variants of classic UC, an unusual presentation of Crohn's colitis or an as-yet-undetermined cause of chronic active colitis. Examples might include UC, lacking the classic diffuse mucosal pattern and having multifocal deeper involvement. It is conceivable that Crohn's colitis might lack transmural disease, granulomas, edema, or fibrosis, and involve a more superficial area of the distal colon. It would be nearly impossible to consistently resolve the overlap without additional information. This raises the question regarding indeterminate colitis; that is when can one make the diagnosis in the absence of colectomy for full pathologic examination? This should be given great consideration. Often, in the work-up of chronic colitis, only limited anatomic pathologic data are available. Few or many endoscopic biopsies give only mucosal information, and the vast majority of the colon is unsampled. The pathologist may feel pressure to commit to a diagnosis of UC or CD based on an incomplete picture. This is a mistake. Apart from fulminant colitis, a diagnosis of indeterminate colitis should be made only after exhaustive clinical, radiographic, and anatomic pathologic assessment has guaranteed that no new information will be forthcoming and no decisive distinction between UC and CD can be made. In cases in which a distinction between UC and CD cannot be made, but the setting is premature for concluding the investigation, a diagnosis of 'IBD, precise classification yet to be determined' might be more prudent. In reflection there are likely other idiopathic causes of IBD that are not CD or UC, namely (a) infection (50% of cases have no detectable organisms) or (b) drug injury. Considering that IBD is thought to be of composite etiology having interplay between genetic susceptibility, immunologic repertoire, and environmental influences, we should be relatively gratified that there are not dozens of clinically mandatory alternative diagnoses. Unusual but distinct diseases may confound discovery of the best diagnostic category for a chronic colitis.

Systemic disease with colonic involvement may be the culprit (sarcoidosis. tuberculosis, Behçet disease, vasculopathy).

Conclusion

The traditional anatomic pathology of IBD and its relationship to diagnosis and management has been well described. In recent work it is recognized how UC is a dynamic disease. Deviations from classic morphology occur with time, disease remission or treatment, or even primary presentation. Still it is recalled that the nearly singular dogmatic description of UC accurately described a majority of cases, but neglected a significant fraction of others. A colloquial term 'patchiness' has been used to describe the main deviation from dogma, and is useful as a way to alert for a non-classic distribution without implying segmental colitis. Recognition of patchy distribution of disease, especially when all other factors indicate UC over CD, is one way to avoid a diagnostic pitfall.

The anatomic pathology of CD is fairly unchanged, but it has remained as a cause of distal enterocolitis in almost everyone's mind; it is important to emphasize its potential role in upper GI disease. Features suggesting upper GI involvement include all the usual findings of lower GI disease, but also an alertness for focal, active gastroduodenal inflammatory injury when *H. pylori* and NSAID-related injuries are excluded.

Dysplasia and carcinoma in IBD remain hotly investigated issues. The molecular pathology of these processes is beyond the scope of this chapter, but those studies in addition to advanced epidemiology are where most of our answers will come. Strictly speaking, the anatomic pathology of dysplasia, adenoma, and carcinoma is not new, and not in need of review. What does require attention are the concepts in *diagnosis* and *management* of alimentary tract epithelial neoplasia in IBD. The colon is the only organ that is even remotely well addressed. In the colon there are a few strongly supported concepts. First, unqualified dysplasia is a significant marker for carcinoma and multifocal dysplasia. Second, there is no reason not to expect that older IBD patients will develop sporadic adenomas in the segment of colon with or without IBD, and that these adenomas may not impart morbidity and mortality of IBD-related dysplasia. In the case of an endoscopically removed sporadic adenoma, no further treatment may be needed. Thirdly, the diagnosis of dysplasia and the distinction of sporadic adenomas from IBD-related dysplasia is fraught with difficulty. The distinction is heavily dependent on clinical input such as the lesion appearance, the state of the adjacent bowel, age of the patient, etc. There is no role for the surgical pathologist to make the distinction between SA and IBD-related dysplasia without superior input by the endoscopist, and probably not without the opinion of a pathologist with experience in the area. Fourth, Crohn's colitis likely imparts a risk of colorectal adenocarcinoma similar to that seen with UC. The pitfalls in diagnosis are likely at least as hazardous as those in UC. The role of surveillance and the target pathology of surveillance in CD are unsettled.

Acknowledgements

The authors gratefully acknowledge Dr Stephen Geller who penned the corresponding chapter in this text's prior edition. It provided a superior scaffold for critical anatomic pathologic assessment in IBD.

References

1. Wilks S, Moxon W. Lecture on Pathological Anatomy, 2nd ed. London: Churchill, 1875; 408, 672.
2. Crohn BB, Ginzburg L, Oppenheimer GD. Regional ileitis: a pathologic and clinical entity. J Am Med Assoc 1932; 99: 1323–9.
3. Geller SA. Pathology of inflammatory bowel disease: a critical appraisal in diagnosis and management. In: Targan SR, Shanahan, F eds. Inflammatory Bowel Disease: From Bench to Bedside. Baltimore: Williams and Wilkins, 1994: 336–51.
4. Lewin KJ, Riddell RH, Weinstein WM. Gastrointestinal Pathology and Its Clinical Implications. New York: Igaku-Shoin, 1992: 812 989.
5. Goldman H. Ulcerative colitis and Crohn's disease. In: Ming SC, Goldman H, eds. Pathology of the Gastrointestinal Tract, 2nd edn. Baltimore: Williams & Wilkins, 1998: 675–718.
6. Morson BC, Dawson IMP. Gastrointestinal Pathology, 2nd edn. Oxford: Blackwell Scientific Publications, 1979: 272–336.
7. Mottet NK. Histologic Spectrum of Regional Enteritis and Ulcerative Colitis. Philadelphia: WB Saunders, 1971: 63–176.
8. Hamilton SR. Diagnosis and comparison of ulcerative colitis and Crohn's disease involving the colon. In: Norris HT, ed. Pathology of the Colon, Small Intestine, and Anus. New York: Churchill Livingstone, 1983: 1–20.
9. Price AB, Morson BC. Inflammatory bowel disease: the surgical pathology of Crohn's disease and ulcerative colitis. Human Pathol 1975; 6: 7–29.
10. Lockhart-Mummery HE, Morson BC. Crohn's disease (regional enteritis) of the large intestine and its distinction from ulcerative colitis. Gut 1960; 1: 87–105.
11. Greenstein AJ, Gellar, SA, Dreiling, DA, Aufses AH. Crohn's disease of the colon: IV. Clinical features of Crohn's (ileo) colitis. Am J Gastroenterol 1975; 64: 191–9.
12. Lockhart-Mummery HE, Morson BC. Crohn's disease of the large intestine. Gut 1964; 5: 493–509.
13. Haggit RC. The differential diagnosis of idiopathic inflammatory bowel disease. In: Norris HT, edr. Pathology of the Colon, Small Intestine, and Anus. New York: Churchill Livingstone, 1983: 21–60.
14. Lewin KJ, Riddell RH, Weinstein WM. Gastrointestinal pathology and its clinical implications. New York: Igaku-Shoin, 1992: 401–39, 506–69, 701–1151.
15. Goldman H. Infectious disorders of the intestines. In: Ming SC, Goldman H, eds. Pathology of the Gastrointestinal Tract, 2nd edn. Baltimore: Williams & Wilkins, 1998: 651–72.
16. Veress B, Lofberg R, Bergman L. Microscopic colitis syndrome. Gut 1995; 36: 880–6.
17. Offner FA, Jao RV, Lewin KJ, Havelec L, Weinstein WM. Collagenous colitis: a study of the distribution of the morphological abnormalities and their histologic detection. Human Pathol 1999; 30: 451–7.
18. Jawhari A, Talbot IC. Microscopic, lymphocytic and collagenous colitis. Histopathology 1996; 29: 101–10.
19. Lee RG. The colitis of Behçet's syndrome. Am J Surg Pathol 1986; 10: 888–93.
20. Dumot JA, Adal K, Petras RE, Lashner BA. Sarcoidosis presenting as granulomatous colitis. Am J Gastroenterology 1998; 93: 1949–51.
21. Price AB. Overlap in the spectrum of non-specific inflammatory bowel disease – 'colitis indeterminate'. J Clin Pathol 1978; 31: 567–77.
22. Isaacson PG. Gastrointestinal lymphomas of T- and B-cell types. Mod Pathol 1999; 12: 151–8.
23. Roberts PF, Stebbings WS, Kennedy HJ. Granulomatous visceral neuropathy of the colon with non-small cell lung carcinoma. Histopathology 1997; 30: 588–91.
24. Carpenter HA, Talley NJ. The importance of clinicopathologic correlation in the diagnosis of inflammatory conditions of the colon: histological patterns with clinical implications. Am J Gastroenterol 2000; 95: 878–96.
25. Linder AE. Inflammatory bowel disease in the elderly. Gastroenterology 1999; 15: 487–97.
26. Bernstein CN, Shanahan F, Anton PA. Patchiness of mucosal inflammation in treated ulcerative colitis: a prospective study. Gastrointest Endosc 1995; 42: 232–7.
27. Levine TS, Tzardi M, Mitchell S, Sowter C, Price AB. Diagnostic difficulty arising from rectal recovery in ulcerative colitis. J Clin Pathol 1996; 49: 319–23.
28. Bernstein CN, Shanahan F, Weinstein WM. Histological patchiness and sparing of the rectum in ulcerative colitis: refuting the dogma. J Clin Pathol 1997; 50: 354–5.
29. Kleer CG, Appelman HD. Ulcerative colitis: patterns of involvement in colorectal biopsies and changes with time. Am J Surg Pathol 1998; 22: 983–989.
30. Levine DS, Haggit RC. Colon. In: Sternberg SS, ed. Histology for Pathologists. New York: Raven Press, 1992: 573–92.
31. Swan NC, Geoghegan JG, O'Donoghue DP, Hyland JMP, Sheahan K. Fulminant colitis in inflammatory bowel disease. Dis Colon Rectum 1998; 41: 1511–15.
32. Sachar DB. Maintenance therapy in ulcerative colits. J Clin Gastroenterol 1995; 20: 117–22.
33. Oshitani N, Kitano A, Nakamura S *et al*. Clinical and prognostic features of rectal sparing in ulcerative colitis. Digestion 1989; 42: 39–43.
34. Davison AM, Dixon MF. The appendix as a 'skip lesion' in ulcerative colitis. Histopathology 1990; 16: 93–5.

35. Burnham WR, Ansell ID, Langman MJS. Normal sigmoidoscopic findings in severe ulcerative colitis: an important common occurrence. Gut 1980; 21: A460.

36. Odze R, Antonioli D, Peppercorn M, Goldman H. Effect of topical 5-aminosalicylic acid (5-ASA) therapy on rectal mucosal biopsy morphology in chronic ulcerative colitis. Am J Surg Pathol 1993; 17: 869–75.

37. Zaitoun AM, Cobden I, Al Mardini H, Record CO. Morphometric studies in biopsy specimens from patients with ulcerative colitis: effect of oral 5 amino salicylic acid and rectal prednisolone treatment. Gut 1991; 32: 183-7

38. Danielsson A, Hellers G, Lyrenas E. et al. A controlled randomized trial of budesonide versus prednisolone retention enemas in active distal ulcerative colitis. Scand J Gastroenterol 1987; 22: 987–92.

39. Markowitz J, Kahn E, Grancher K, Hyams J, Treem W, Daum F. Atypical rectosigmoid histology in children with newly diagnosed ulcerative colitis. Am J Gastroenterol 1993; 88: 2034–7.

40. Spiliadis CA, Lennard-Jones JE. Ulcerative colitis with relative rectal sparing of the rectum. Clinical features, histology, and prognosis. Dis Colon Rectum 1987; 30: 334–6.

41. Lennard-Jones JE, Vivian AB. Fulminating ulcerative colitis. Recent experience and management. Br J Med 1960; 2: 96.

42. Lennard-Jones JE, Melville DM, Morson BC, Ritchie JK, Williams CB. Precancer and cancer in extensive ulcerative colitis: findings among 401 patients over 22 years. Gut 1990; 31: 800–6.

43. Riddell RH. Dysplasia in inflammatory bowel disease. In: Norris HT, ed. Pathology of the Colon, Small Intestine, and Anus. New York: Churchill Livingstone, 1983: 77–108.

44. Nugent FW, Haggitt RC, Colcher H, Kutteruf GC. Malignant potential of chronic ulcerative colitis. Gastroenterology 1979; 76: 1–5.

45. Blackstone MO, Riddel RH, Gerald Rogers BH, Levin B. Dysplasia-associated lesion or mass (DALM) detected by colonoscopy in long-standing ulcerative colitis: and indication for colectomy. Gastroenterology 1981; 80: 366–74.

46. Riddell RH, Goldman H, Ransohoff DF et al. Dysplasia in inflammatory bowel disease: standardized classification with provisional clinical applications. Human Pathol 1983; 14: 931–66.

47. Rubin PJ, Friedman S, Harpaz N et al. Colonscopic polypectomy in chronic colitis: conservative management after endoscopic resection of dysplastic polyps. Gastroenterology 1999; 117: 1295-1300.

48. Bernstein CN. ALMs versus DALMs in ulcerative colitis: polypectomy or colectomy? Gastroenterology 1999; 117: 1488–91.

49. Odze RD. Adenomas and adenoma-like DALMs in chronic ulcerative colitis: a clinical, pathological, and molecular review. Am J Gastroenterol 1999; 94: 1746–50.

50. Geboes K, Rutgeerts P. Dysplasia in inflammatory bowel diseases: definition and clinical impact. Can J Gastroenterol 1999; 13: 671–8.

51. Levin B. Inflammatory bowel disease: role of endoscopic surveillance. American Society for Gastrointestinal Endoscopy Clinical Update; 2000 Jan; 7(3): 1–4.

52. Bernstein CN, Shanahan F, Weinstein WM. Are we telling the truth about surveillance colonoscopy in ulcerative colitis. Lancet 1994; 343: 71–4.

53. Kent TH, Mitros FA. Polyps of the colon and small bowel, polyp syndromes, and the polyp-carcinoma sequence. In: Norris HT, ed. Pathology of the Colon, Small Intestine, and Anus. New York: Churchill Livingstone, 1983: 167–200.

54. Lewin, KJ. Nomenclature problems of gastrointestinal epithelial neoplasia. Am J Surg Pathol 1998; 22: 1043–8.

55. Mottet NK. Histologic Spectrum of Regional Enteritis and Ulcerative Colitis. Philadelphia: WB Saunders, 1971: 217–35.

56. Mayer R, Wong DW, Rothenberger DA, Goldberg SM, Madoff RD. Colorectal cancer in inflammatory bowel disease. Dis Colon Rectum 1999; 42: 343–7.

57. Melville DM, Jass JR, Morson BC, et al. Observer study in the grading of dysplasia in ulcerative colitis: comparison with clinical outcome. Human Pathol 1989; 20: 1008–14.

58. Dixon MF, Brown LJR, Gilmour HM et al. Observer variation in the assessment of dysplasia in ulcerative colitis. Histopathology 1988; 13: 385–7.

59. Lindberg JO, Steinling RB, Rutegard JN. Eighteen-year surveillance of dysplasia associated lesion in ulcerative colitis. Endoscopy 2000; 32: 359–60.

60. Torres C, Antonioli D, Odze RD. Polypoid dysplasia and adenomas in inflammatory bowel disease. A clinical, pathologic, and follow-up study of 89 polyps from 59 patients. Am J Surg Pathol 1998; 22: 275–84.

61. Engelsgjerd M, Farraye FA, Odze RD. Polypectomy may be adequate treatment for adenoma-like dysplastic lesions in chronic ulcerative colitis. Gastroenterology 1999; 117: 1288–94.

62. Fogt F, Urbanski, SJ, Sanders ME et al. Distinction between dysplasia associated lesion or mass (DALM) and adenoma in patients with ulcerative colitis. Human Pathol 2000; 31: 288–91.

63. Rickert RR. The important 'imposters' in the differential diagnosis of inflammatory bowel disease. J Clin Gastroenterol 1984; 6: 153–63.

64. Tanaka M, Riddell RH. The pathological diagnosis and differential diagnosis of Crohn's disease. Hepatogastroenterology 1990; 37: 18–31.

65. Shepherd, NA. Pathological mimics of chronic inflammatory bowel disease. J Clin Pathol 1991; 449: 726–33.

66. Marteau P. Inflammatory bowel disease. Endoscopy 2000; 32: 131–7.

67. Goldstein NS, Leon-Armin C, Mani A. Crohn's colitis-like changes in sigmoid diverticulitis specimens is usually an idiosyncratic inflammatory response to the diverticulosis rather than Crohn's colitis. Am J Surg Pathol 2000; 24: 668–75.

68. Geboes K, Janssens J, Rutgeerts P, Vantrappen G. Crohn's disease of the esophagus. J Clin Gastroenterol 1986; 8: 31–7.

69. Wagtmans MJ, Verspaget HW, Lamers CB, van Hogezand RA. Clinical aspects of Crohn's disease of the upper gastrointestinal tract: a comparison with distal Crohn's disease. Am J Gastroenterol 1997; 92: 1467–71.

70. Wright CL, Riddell RH. Histology of the stomach and duodenum in Crohn's disease. Am J Surg Pathol 1998; 22: 383–90.

71. Dourmashkin RR, Davies H, Wells C et al. Epithelial patchy necrosis in Crohn's disease. Human Pathol 1983; 14: 643–8.

72. Rotterdam H, Korelitz BI, Sommers SC. Microgranulomas in grossly normal rectal mucosa in Crohn's disease. Am J Clin Pathol 1977; 67: 550–4.

73. Kelly JK, Siu TO. The strictures, sinuses, and fissures of Crohn's disease. J Clin Gastroenterol 1986; 8: 594–8.

74. Kelly JK, Preshaw RM. Origin of fistulas in Crohn's disease. J Clin Gastroenterol 1989; 11: 193–6.

75. Price A B. Overlap in the spectrum of non-specific inflammatory bowel disease – 'colitis indeterminate'. J Clin Pathol 1978; 31: 567–77.

76. Lee KS, Medline A, Shockey S. Indeterminate colitis in the spectrum of inflammatory bowel disease. Arch Pathol Lab Med 1979; 103: 173–6.

77. Dumot JA, Adal K, Petras RE, Lashner BA. Sarcoidosis presenting as granulomatous colitis. Am J Gastroenterol 1998; 93: 1949–51.
78. Lang J, Price AB, Levi AJ, Burke M, Gumpel JM, Bjarnason I. Diaphragm disease: pathology of disease of the small intestine induced by non-steroidal anti-inflammatory drugs. J Clin Pathol 1988; 41: 516–26.
79. Fernando SS, McGovern VJ. Neuromuscular and vascular hamartoma of small bowel. Gut 1982; 23: 1008–12.
80. Cortina G, Wren S, Armstrong B, Lewin K, Fajardo L. Clinical and pathologic overlap in nonsteroidal anti-inflammatory drug-related small bowel diaphragm disease and the neuromuscular and vascular hamartoma of the small bowel. Am J Surg Pathol 1999; 23: 1414–17.
81. Blecker U, Gold BD. Gastritis and peptic ulcer disease in childhood. Eur J Pediatr 1999; 158: 541–6.
82. Ginsburg L, Schnieder KM, Dreizin DH, Levinson C. Carcinoma of the jejunum occuring in a case of regional enteritis. Surgery 1956; 39: 347–51.
83. Patel M, Banerjee B, Block JG, Marshall JB. Gastric Crohn's disease complicated by adenocarcinoma of the stomach: case report and review of the literature. Am J Gastroenterol 1997; 92: 1368–71.
84. Weedon DD, Shorter RG, Ilstrup DM, Huizenga KA, Taylor WF. Crohn's disease and cancer. N Engl J Med 1973; 289: 1099–103.
85. Perrett AD, Truelove SC, Massarella GR. Crohn's disease and carcinoma of colon. Br Med J 1968; 2: 466–8.
86. Glotzer DJ. The risk of cancer in Crohn's disease. Gastroenterology, 1985; 89: 438–41.
87. Gillen CD, Walmsley RS, Prior P, Andrews HA, Allan RN. Ulcerative colitis and Crohn's disease: a comparison of the colorectal cancer risk in extensive colitis. Gut, 1994; 35: 1590–2.
88. Ribeiro MB, Greenstein AJ, Sachar DB *et al.* Colorectal adenocarcinoma in Crohn's disease. Ann Surg 1996; 223: 186–93.
89. Sigel JE, Petras RE, Lashner BA, Fazio VW, Goldblum JR. Intestinal adenocarcinoma in Crohn's disease: a report of 30 cases with a focus on coexisting dysplasia. Am J Surg Pathol 1999; 23: 651–5.

18 | An endoscopic and histologic perspective of diagnosis: when, where, and what to do

CHARLES N. BERNSTEIN AND ROBERT H. RIDDELL

Introduction

Endoscopy and biopsy of the colon is an important diagnostic tool in the investigation of the inflammatory bowel diseases (IBD). There are a number of scenarios in which colon biopsies are of particular importance:

1. Biopsies in the patient with undiagnosed diarrhea: (a) biopsies in the patient with normal colonoscopy, (b) biopsies in the patient with colitis endoscopically.

2. Distinguishing different forms of IBD.

3. Assessing disease extent and disease activity.

4. Differential diagnosis of IBD and diagnosing other disorders superimposed on IBD.

5. Neoplasia in patients with IBD.

We will discuss the utility of (a) colonoscopy, with colon biopsies for each of these scenarios, (b) ileoscopy plus biopsy and (c) esophagogastroduodenoscopy plus biopsy.

Colonoscopy plus biopsy

Biopsies in the patient with undiagnosed diarrhea

Is 'mild' colitis early or minimally active IBD or is it an overcall by the pathologist?

In the evaluation of patients with diarrhea, once infection has been excluded as far as possible with stool studies, endoscopic examination and biopsies have become routine [1–6]. Particularly for patients with chronic diarrhea, the possibility of IBD always heads the differential diagnosis list. Most gastroenterologists pursue either sigmoidoscopy or colonoscopy plus biopsies. Table 1 lists a differential diagnosis of diarrhea in the setting of either normal or abnormal lower endoscopy.

Few studies have proven the utility of endoscopy plus biopsies on the care of patients with chronic diarrhea. Recently a study from a tertiary-care university-affiliated endoscopy facility revealed that the diagnostic yield from lower endoscopy plus biopsy in chronic, painless non-bloody diarrhea was 18% [7]. Painless diarrhea was chosen to minimize enrollment of patients with irritable bowel syndrome. The specific diagnoses found in the group with abnormal endoscopy or abnormal biopsies are listed in Table 2. IBD accounted for 22% of positive diagnoses and lymphocytic and collagenous colitis accounted for 14%. There were nine patients with normal endoscopy but abnormal biopsies who were categorized as having biopsy findings inconsistent with the final diagnosis. The majority of these patients' biopsy results described only 'minimal' or 'mild' histologic changes. Of all cases with normal endoscopies and abnormal biopsies, histologic ulcers or crypt abscesses were never seen in this group. The point here is that findings of ulcers or crypt abscesses should minimize any confusion as to whether an inflammatory cause of diarrhea exists. Cryptitis, increased inflammatory cells, and edema were not discriminating for clinical diagnosis.

Definite collagenous and lymphocytic colitis that remained as persistent clinical problems were uncommon in this study. Two cases were labeled by the original pathologists as lymphocytic colitis and confirmed as such on blinded review by the gastrointestinal pathologist coinvestigator. That these cases have been clinically described as acute self-limited diarrhea may reflect as much the natural history of this entity rather than an overcall by the pathologist [8]] That is, these two cases were likely bona-fide lymphocytic colitis; however, the patients became asymptomatic and remained so at the time of review by their clinicians.

Stephan R. Targan, Fergus Shanahan and Loren C. Karp (eds.), Inflammatory Bowel Disease: From Bench to Bedside, 2nd Edition, 357–370.
© 2003 *Kluwer Academic Publishers. Printed in Great Britain*

Table 1. Differential diagnosis of diarrhea in the setting of normal and abnormal lower endoscopy

Normal lower endoscopy

(i) Abnormal biopsies
   Microscopic colitis: collagenous colitis, lymphocytic colitis, quiescent IBD
   Amyloidosis
   Melanosis coli
   Acute self limited diarrhea

(ii) Normal biopsies
   Irritable bowel syndrome
   Small bowel diseases, including celiac disease, Crohn's disease, giardiasis
   Drug-induced
   Non-absorbable carbohydrate-induced
   Bacterial overgrowth
   Diabetes mellitus
   Thyrotoxicosis
   Addison's disease
   Bile salt-induced
   Other disorders: including gastric hypersecretory disorders, intestinal lymphoma and other malabsorption states, pancreatic disease, neuroendocrine tumors

Abnormal lower endoscopy

(i) Colitis
   IBD (ulcerative colitis or Crohn's disease)
   Infectious colitis (Enterobacteriaciae, *Clostridium difficile*, cytomegalovirus, herpes simplex virus, *Mycobacterium tuberculosis*, fungal, *Entamoeba histolytica*, *Dientamoeba fragilis*, *Treponema pallidum*, acute self-limited colitis (organism not defined)
   Ischemic
   Radiation-induced
   Drug-induced
   Granulomatous diseases (Melkersson–Rosenthal syndrome, sarcoidosis, Behçet's)

(ii) No colitis, but abnormal endoscopy
   Large villous adenoma
   Ileocecal valve and ileal and/or segmental colonic resection
   Gastrocolic or enterocolic fistula
   Colonic lymphoma or neuroendocrine tumor
   Endometriosis

Table 2. Specific diagnoses of the patients with abnormal biopsies in the study of 205 patients with chronic painless non-bloody diarrhea

(a) Abnormal endoscopy/abnormal biopsy group ($n = 24$): specific diagnoses made in 24 cases

Specific diagnoses	No. of cases
Pseudomembranous colitis	7
Ulcerative colitis	4
Crohn's disease	2
Villous adenoma >5 cm	3
Indeterminate colitis	2
Melanosis coli	2
Ischemic colitis	1
Rectal prolapse	1
Collagenous colitis	1
Peridiverticulitis	1
Total	24

(b) Normal endoscopy/abnormal biopsy group ($n = 21$): specific diagnoses made in 12 cases

Specific diagnoses	No. of cases
Acute self-limited colitis	5
Microscopic colitis	4
Melanosis coli	3
Total	12

Adapted from: Patel Y, Pettigrew NP, Grahame GR, Bernstein CN. The outcome of endocopy plus biopsy in the evaluation of patients with chronic diarrhea. Gastrointest Endosc 1997; 46: 338–43, with permission.

It is unknown as to how long the symptoms or microscopic changes of acute self-limited colitis last; however, microscopic changes that persist beyond 6 months should no longer be viewed as part of an acute self-limited process. The labeling of otherwise normal biopsies as inflamed with some bland descriptor as 'minimal', or 'non-specific' may lead the unwary clinician to a final diagnosis of IBD. This may create a dilemma for both patient and physician who become unnecessarily caught up in chronic anti-inflammatory therapy regimens.

There are at least three problems regarding the histologic interpretation of inflammation in the colon. One undefined issue pertains to the quantification of the normal amount of inflammation in the normal colon. Data are lacking to definitively answer this question. This clearly has a subjective component but also the implication that pathologists call only abnormal when it is unequivocally abnormal, and not when equivocal changes are present. Some pathologists appear to be unwilling to call anything normal or without abnormality. Furthermore, in the colon, most inflammation is non-specific so that the use of the word 'non-specific' is superfluous. It is the pattern and distribution both within the bowel and within the mucosa specifically that fall into reasonably well defined clinicopathological entities.

The second issue pertains to how much additional inflammation is needed to cause symptoms? There are no criteria on where 'colitis' starts and normality finishes. Hence the whole problem of what constitutes microscopic colitis is in the 'unequivocal increase' in (chronic) inflammatory cells in the lamina propria plus or minus an intraepithelial lymphocytosis (lymphocytic colitis). Symptoms may be indistinguishable among patients who have only an increase in intraepithelial lymphocytes (Brainerd-type diarrhea) versus patients who fulfill the criteria of lymphocytic colitis and also have increased lamina propria lymphocytes. It also seems that some chronic diarrheas with microscopic abnormalities have the histologic appearance of acute infectious-type colitides.

Third, the distribution of inflammation is also likely important. The suspicion is that while microscopic/lymphocytic/collagenous colitis usually involves most of the large bowel, focal inflammation is much more difficult to deal with. Microscopic proctitis is much more likely to be symptomatic than the same change limited to part of the right colon, or even localized sigmoiditis, e.g. as seen accompanying diverticular disease.

It may be warranted to begin a standardized approach to the description of colonic biopsies (analogous to that for liver biopsies) so as to move away from descriptions such as 'mild', 'minimal', or 'non-specific' colitis, and thereby limit any clinical confusion. This should also help to avoid incorrectly labeling a patient with the diagnosis of colitis and the stigma and implications associated with it. Nonetheless, regarding the issue of 'mild' colitis, it is important that endoscopists and their pathologists have an open dialog as to the threshold for labeling a patient's biopsy as being truly inflamed [9].

Biopsies in the patient with normal colonoscopy

Where do the microscopic colitides fit within the spectrum of IBD?

The main diagnostic possibilities in patients with diarrhea, normal endoscopies, and abnormal biopsies include amyloidosis, melanosis coli, and the microscopic (including collagenous and lymphocytic) colitides [8, 10–13]. Histologic criteria have been developed for diagnosing microscopic colitis [13], but they are not universally agreed upon. The acceptance of the uniqueness of collagenous and lymphocytic colitis has sharpened our focus on pathology reports that identify mild inflammation. A frequent problem for clinicians is in deciding whether to ignore these reports (and thereby potentially miss some true cases of microscopic colitis) or

to accept all these diagnoses and overtreat a large number of patients whose mild histologic inflammation is really a variant of normal. The issue of pathologists using labels such as 'mild' or 'non-specific' colitis has been alluded to above.

It is unclear how many biopsies should be obtained in the work-up of diarrhea in the endoscopically normal colon and from how many and which sites. There are no data to guide us on this. In the Patel study, which was retrospective, there were nearly two sites of biopsies and nearly five biopsies on average taken per endoscopy [7]. It is unknown whether more biopsies and more sites would increase the yield. Endoscopists should also be aware of cecal 'inflammation' in health [14]. We recommend a minimum of two biopsies from the descending colon, sigmoid, and rectum at flexible sigmoidoscopy [15] or at total colonoscopy, including those sites plus the transverse colon, ascending colon, and cecum. A rigorous protocol of multiple biopsy sites would require a prospective study of patients with chronic diarrhea. Such a study would help delineate the true extent of patchiness of conditions such as microscopic colitis, which may predominate in the proximal colon in some patients [15].

Although the Patel study has proven the utility of endoscopy plus biopsy in the investigation of painless non-bloody diarrhea there are differing opinions on the need for a biopsy in endoscopically normal-appearing mucosa [16–19]. One study supported the findings by Patel *et al.* with a 22% rate of making specific histologic diagnoses in patients with normal endoscopy [16]. The indications for the colonoscopies were not stated in this report. One study found no cases of confirmed microscopic colitis [18]. One study found no histologic abnormalities on rectal biopsies of 89 patients with apparent irritable bowel syndrome [19]. This study did not evaluate whether biopsies proximal to the rectum would be of value. The work-up of typical irritable bowel syndrome should not be the same as other undiagnosed diarrheal states, especially as the rectum has the lowest yield in biopsies taken for microscopic, lymphocytic, or collagenous colitis [13, 15]. Making a specific diagnosis of microscopic colitis, melanosis coli, or even acute infectious-type colitis may have important implications for patient management, and may prevent any further unnecessary investigations or inappropriate medical therapy. Thus, biopsies of the normal colon are essential in the evaluation of patients undergoing endoscopy for diarrhea.

counterpart of aphthoid ulcers) or markedly focal acute inflammation may be evident and these findings should not prejudice the surgical approach.

In a prospective series of 39 patients with longstanding known UC 33% were found to have histologic patchiness, including two patients who had absolute rectal sparing. Both of these cases had rectal involvement at diagnosis, and at the time of the study did not even have evidence of quiescent colitis [53]. Fig. 1 shows a rectal biopsy from a patient who had 10 years of UC. The patient ultimately came to colectomy and had UC confirmed. The biopsy revealed patchiness within the biopsy specimen. Endoscopic or histologic patchiness in this study was not related to the use of rectal therapy. In a 5-ASA enema treatment trial one group showed that 64% of patients had histologic evidence of patchiness within the rectum, but they did not compare the rectum with more proximal sites [51]. Two groups have suggested that patients with first presentations of UC can present with endoscopic rectal sparing [26, 52]; therefore this phenomenon may not simply be one associated with long-standing or treated disease.

One group of pathologists has reported that up to 46% of rectal biopsies from patients with longstanding UC have lost the typical features of UC, in fact two of their 24 cases reverted to completely normal histology [54]. The implication is that UC can never be excluded on rectal biopsies alone. Kleer and Appelman have reported that 30% of biopsy sites from 41 patients with UC had focal inflammation implying that not all pieces from a single site were involved [55]. Thirty-six percent of cases had histologic rectal sparing at some time in the course of their disease. These authors also reported that histologically inflamed mucosa at some colonic site reverted to normal mucosa at a later time in the disease in over 50% of cases. In a prospective sequential endoscopy plus biopsy study of patients with UC, Appelman's group reported that patients may have patchiness histologically at different points in time through the course of their disease [56].

If the endoscopist does not recognize patchy inflammation, and does not biopsy, for instance, colorectal areas of differential endoscopic inflammation, then the reporting pathologist may not have the opportunity to recognize that patchiness in UC exists. If the endoscopist recognizes definite skip areas at endoscopy, it is critical that the non-inflamed areas be biopsied. It may very well be that, histologically, these areas are inflamed and are not truly skip

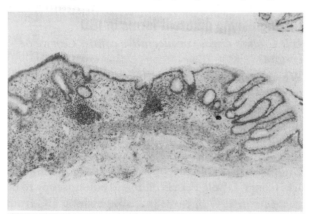

Figure 1. Example of histologic patchiness in the rectum of a patient with longstanding ulcerative colitis. Rectal biopsy from a patient with 10 years of ulcerative colitis at a time of active disease. The patient at the time of this endoscopy plus biopsy was using azathioprine, 5-ASA orally and by enema, and oral prednisone. At endoscopy there was one area in the rectum that was patchy, however, the rest of the rectum and colon were diffusely actively inflamed. Within 1 month after this endoscopy the patient underwent successful total colectomy with ileoanal pouch procedure. His colon pathology was consistent with ulcerative colitis. On the left side of the biopsy is moderately severe inflammation with gland loss, and shortening, loss of goblet cells, increased subcryptal space, and increased inflammatory cell infiltrate. On the right side of the biopsy there is quiescent colitis. There is gland branching; however, the goblet cells are preserved and the glands reach the muscularis mucosae. There is minimal inflammatory cell infiltrate.

areas, making inferences toward CD much less certain [57].

Some years ago [58] and more recently [47, 48] investigators found evidence of periappendiceal inflammation in cases of long-standing typical UC. Perhaps their finding has nothing to do with UC, and is only associated with a large burst into the cecum of lavage solution. Nonetheless, periappendiceal inflammation is not typically noted in colonoscopy of the non-inflamed colon. A study of 152 colectomy specimens reported eight cases with 'islands typical of ulceration in areas of mucosa which were otherwise normal' [59]. They reported that most of these skip lesions occurred in the cecum, including a lesion at the base of the appendix. The implications of periappendiceal inflammation are unknown at present, particularly in light of the data suggesting that UC patients have a lower than expected past history of appendectomies [60]. Does smoldering inflammation in an intact appendix in some way predispose to left-sided colitis or does the appendix

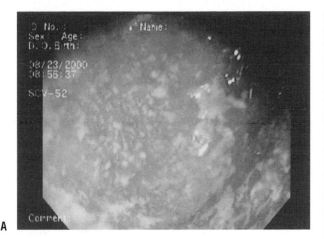

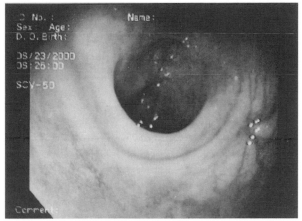

Figure 2. Colonoscopic findings in a patient with ulcerative proctitis. **A**: Exudate, friability and loss of vascular pattern in the rectum. This endoscopic picture could be found in any of ulcerative colitis, ulcerative proctitis, Crohn's colitis, or infectious colitis. **B**: View at 10 cm showing demarcation between abnormal rectal mucosa to the lower right (at 7 o'clock) and normal mucosa with intact vascular pattern beyond. Only histologic biopsies at 15–18 cm could confirm or refute whether this case is in fact one of ulcerative proctitis or ulcerative colitis.

share common antigenic determinants with the distal large bowel?

When standard endoscopic and histologic landmarks fail to clearly distinguish Crohn's colitis from UC, novel methods may soon be available to better classify what may otherwise be labeled as indeterminate colitis. This includes serologic testing for a variety of antibodies, and may soon include assessing colon biopsy specimens by magnetic resonance spectroscopy [61].

Distinguishing ulcerative proctitis from procto-sigmoiditis (or UC) depends upon biopsies taken above 15–18 cm in instances where endoscopic inflammation is limited to the rectum (see Fig. 2).

Assessing disease extent and disease activity

Appreciating the dynamic changes including regression over time

While traditionally UC tends to extend proximally during relapses, when quiescent for long periods of time, healing can occur, in that both endoscopically and histologically, the mucosa can return to a condition where it is indistinguishable from normal. Indeed it is surprising how many apparently normal biopsies are encountered in patients undergoing surveillance colonoscopy. Furthermore, some exacerbations may involve only part of the mucosa. Usually this takes the form of architectural changes proximally but with no active disease while distally active disease may be present.

Kleer and Appelman reported that 32 of 41 cases of UC followed with repeat colonoscopy with biopsies over a median of 7 years had changes over time in the extent of their disease, including recession of proximal disease extent in several cases [55]. A Scandinavian study reported that 68% of 384 UC patients had changes in disease extent either proximally or distally 1 year after initial diagnosis [62]. For some clinicians the extent of disease will alter their cancer surveillance practice (with earlier surveillance initiated in cases of pancolitis). For others it may alter their approach to therapy, reserving rectal therapy only for those with limited disease.

Clinicians typically decide therapy based on patients' symptoms more than on their endoscopy or histology results. Few data have been available to instruct as to the prognostic abilities of histologic outcomes. In one study Riley *et al.* reported on the rectal biopsies in 82 patients with UC in remission and with chronic quiescent colitis on biopsy [63]. At 1 year 33% had relapsed. The features that significantly predicted relapse included acute inflammatory cell infiltrate, crypt abscesses, mucin depletion, and breaches in the surface epithelium when patients were in remission clinically. Chronic inflammatory cell infiltrate and crypt architecture distortion were not predictive of relapse. This type of data may encourage clinicians either to alter their practice in terms of biopsying patients in remission as a means of deciding who requires ongoing or to step up maintenance therapy. It certainly provides a ratio-

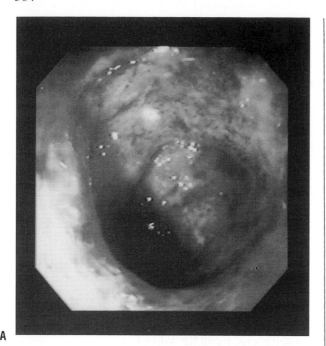

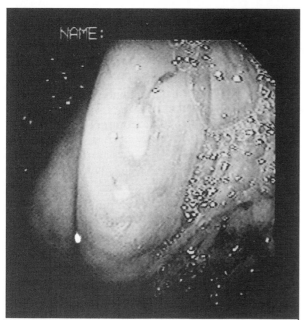

Figure 3. Examples of colonic injury that could be indistinguishable endoscopically from IBD. **A**: Friable hemorrhagic rectal mucosa in a patient with diversion proctitis who underwent descending colostomy and a Hartmann's pouch procedure for acute diverticulitis. **B**: Ulcers with surrounding erythema on the ileocecal valve. This injury was caused by shock wave lithotrypsy for renal lithiasis [84].

nale for conducting studies on the rational use of long-term maintenance 5-ASA in certain patient subtypes (e.g comparing the value of maintenance of 5-ASA in those with active histologic disease versus those with quiescent disease histologically).

Differential diagnosis of IBD and diagnosing other disorders superimposed on IBD

The clues to other diagnoses when IBD is and is not present

In newly diagnosed colitis a variety of disorders must be ruled out. These include radiation injury and drug-induced injury (see Fig. 3), both of which should have specific histories if carefully sought. Ischemic colitis typically presents in older patients; however, so can IBD. Ischemic colitis has features of epithelial sloughing into empty ghost tubules. Mucosal and submucosal microthrombi and fibrosis may be present [64]. More long-standing disease is characterized by dense fibrosis of the lamina propria which may be much less extensive than the endoscopic disease. The solitary rectal ulcer syndrome which may be associated with straining at stools and rectal prolapse has histologic features of fibromuscular replacement of the lamina propria with the muscle fibers running parallel to the crypts, villous surface with superficial erosions, and occasional misplacement of mucus-filled glands into the submucosa [65, 66]. Enterocolonic endometriosis is uncommon, but a cyclic history and the presence of endometrial glands should be evident in those patients in whom the mucosa or superficial submucosa is involved, which is rare. Thickened serosa with an endometrioma can be mistaken for adenocarcinoma and architectural distortion and crypt abscesses may lead to confusion with IBD [67, 68]. Chronic diverticulitis can be confused with left-sided CD [69]. This distinction can be particularly difficult in older patients, since CD in the elderly often presents as left-sided colitis [70]. One troubling feature of a series of chronic diverticulitis cases, recently reported, was the presence of granulomas histologically [69]. Granulomas in diverticultis are most usually a reaction to foreign material extruded following local perforation. Perhaps only a localized resection without recurrence will ultimately define that CD is not present in the setting of possible chronic diverticulitis. Diverticulitis can also be associated with mucosal inflammation that may extend distally and present a scenario that is indistinguishable from UC [71].

Some disorders of host neutrophil response can be associated with enterocolitides that may mimic CD. These include Hermansky–Pudlak syndrome (oculocutaneous albinism), glycogen storage disease type 1b, and autoimmune neutropenia [72–74]. Other granulomatous diseases can be patchy and mimic CD, such as Melkersson–Rosenthal syndrome (labial and vulvar granulomatous inflammation associated with facial nerve and autonomic neuropathy, and patchy enterocolonic disease), sarcoidosis and Behçet's disease [75–77]. These diseases require a constellation of extraintestinal findings to clinch their diagnoses.

In newly diagnosed colitis infections must be ruled out. This is usually done through microbiology studies of stool and occasionally of mucosal biopsies. However, when typical acute infectious colitis is present histologically only about one-half of all patients will have an identifiable pathogen. Failure to find such a pathogen does not mean that the disease was not infectious in origin. Most enteropathic *Escherichia coli* associated with verotoxin production are detected on routine cultures. When crypt architecture distortion is present this indicates prior mucosal or crypt destruction, and is mostly frequently seen as part of chronic (non-infectious) IBD. However, one study of patients from India with shigellosis suggested that some of these patients' biopsies showed evidence of crypt architecture changes [78]. Similar changes can be present whenever a pathogen causes ulceration of the mucosa, but this invariably occurs only with culturable pathogens – including *Clostridium difficile* on occasions. In cases with known IBD it is important to review drug and travel histories when patients present with a flare of disease. Mucosal biopsies may not be helpful to uncover superimposed drug or infectious injuries. Pseudomembranes may be present in IBD. However, superficial injury with volcano lesions should lead the clinician to reconsider whether a *C. difficile*-associated pseudomembranous colitis is present, which would lead to very specific therapy.

Mycobacterium tuberculosis should be considered in the initial differential diagnosis of enterocolitis in the appropriate patient setting. It may be associated with caseating granulomas and positive acid-fast staining (or auramine rhodamine which is fluorescent but far more sensitive), and if necessary tissue can be taken from paraffin for polymerase chain reaction. There has also been an increasing apprecia-tion for other bacterial colonic infections that can have predilections for the right colon and masquerade as CD, such as *Yersinia* or *E. coli* 0-157 [79]. The presence of eosinophilia in an acute colitis should lead one to consider *Dientamoeba fragilis* [80]. There have been several reports [81–83] of cytomegalovirus (CMV) infection being evident either at the time of exacerbation of known IBD or at the time of presentation of newly diagnosed IBD. In some cases therapy directed at CMV was beneficial. Trauma is an uncommon cause of colitis but recently extracorporeal shockwave lithotripsy for urinary calculi has been reported to cause an acute self-limited colitis [84]. Finally, there are iatrogenic effects of oral Fleet's phosphosoda producing focal active colitis histologically and aphthoid ulcers endoscopically [85].

Neoplasia in patients with IBD

The ultimate fear, the lack of good predictors, the complicated chase

Both Crohn's colitis and UC are associated with an increased risk of developing colorectal cancer. Endoscopists pursue dysplasia utilizing surveillance colonoscopy, usually beginning at 8 years of disease when the cancer risk starts to increase. Dysplasia is an unequivocal neoplastic change limited to the mucosa. It was hoped that establishing a standardized grading system would help facilitate dysplasia surveillance endoscopy [86]. The distinction of low-grade and high-grade dysplasia was established with the presumption that low-grade changes are early and less associated with imminent cancer [86]. The data from dysplasia surveillance programs have shown that high-grade dysplasia is more likely to be associated with concurrent cancer or with progression over time to cancer [87–89]. However, low-grade dysplasia is associated with concurrent cancer in up to 20% of cases and has a rate of progression to high-grade dysplasia or cancer of 35–50% [87–89]. One large series of cancers in UC reported that as many as approximately 50% were associated with low-grade dysplasia as the highest grade of synchronous dysplasia [90].

Therefore, there appears to be no good reason to follow patients with low-grade dysplasia, Increasingly the position taken is that when the patient is free from dysplasia, then the chances that an invasive carcinoma will be present are low (but not zero). However, other than for adenomas, proctocolectomy should be considered when dysplasia is found. Further, as dysplasia tends to be very focal, it is not uncommon for repeat colonoscopy 'to confirm the diagnosis' to be negative, resulting in a suspicion that dysplasia 'comes and goes'. Despite the establishment of standardized criteria for dysplasia diagnosis, its diagnosis is often problematic and requires an experienced pathologist. Pathologist interagreement in dysplasia diagnosis studies is at least 70% for high-grade dysplasia but can be as low as 40–50% for low-grade or epithelium indefinite dysplasia [88, 91]. The latter is diagnosed when the answer to both questions 'Is the epithelium unequivocally not dysplastic?' and 'Is the epithelium unequivocally dysplastic?' is No.

Despite the flaws associated with dysplasia surveillance, it is currently widely practiced and remains the foremost screening tool for dysplasia, and sometimes carcinoma, in UC. There is a wide variation in how dysplasia surveillance is performed. Endoscopists may take anywhere from two to six biopsies per site and biopsy at anywhere from six to ten sites in the colon [92]. This variability is also evident in published dysplasia surveillance series, although mostly an approach of two biopsies every 10 cm is used [93]. Rubin *et al.* published a detailed histology assessment of patients with UC who underwent colectomy [94]. They reported that 33 biopsies were required to have a 95% sensitivity that any dysplasia was present, but up to 64 biopsies were required to find the highest degree. If the endoscopist and patient are willing to pursue colectomy for any degree of definite dysplasia, it may be reasonable to aim for at least 30 biopsies. Since there is an increased risk of rectosigmoid cancer in UC [90] an increased number of biopsies should be obtained from these sites. A recent series of dysplasia surveillance in Crohn's colitis has been reported, and substantiates the approach that patients with long-standing Crohn's colitis should be screened similarly to patients with UC [95].

Another important issue in surveillance is the approach to mass lesions. When dysplastic mass lesions are large or associated with strictures then there is little doubt that surgery is required. When dysplastic lesions are irregular and large, and do not resemble typical inflammatory polyps or adenomas, they may be termed a dysplasia-associated lesion or mass (DALM). This lesion induces fear in gastroenterologists and most pursue colectomy in this setting [90]. When dysplastic mass lesions look like typical adenomas (that would occur in a non-UC colon) and occur within colitic mucosa, and there is no synchronous dysplasia in flat mucosa, there is evidence that it is safe to simply perform polypectomy and further endoscopic surveillance [96, 97]. The caveat is that it needs to be demonstrated that the lesion has been completely removed endoscopically, by examination of a stalk if present, or by taking multiple biopsies around the base of the lesion to ensure that dysplastic mucosa has not extended into the adjacent mucosa, when polypectomy would not be curative. The evidence does not yet include sufficient numbers of patients who have been followed out to 5 years; however, the evidence is sufficient to allow this approach to be incorporated in post-dysplasia surveillance discussions with patients. It certainly may be worth pursuing polypectomy in older patients who might otherwise be at risk for developing sporadic adenomas, while it may be more prudent to recommend colectomy to a patient who has not yet reached the usual adenoma-bearing age range (e.g. < 40 years of age) who presents with an adenoma-like mass and who has many years of risk mucosa ahead. For polyps on stalks, and for polyps presenting in normal mucosa distant from any microscopic evidence of colitis, it is reasonable to pursue polypectomy and further surveillance, but again long-term data in these settings are lacking [98].

Ileoscopy plus biopsy

Intubation of the terminal ileum at the time of colonoscopy has become commonplace with success rates of greater than 80%. The value of this technique in the evaluation of patients with undiagnosed diarrheal disorders has been debated. We feel that there is no debate in the setting of a high suspicion for IBD or when colitis is present. In a recent report of colonoscopies in patients with undiagnosed diarrheal disorders, endoscopic ileal lesions were found in 123 of 257 patients [99]. Ileal disease in the absence of colonic disease was present in 44 patients. In 88 cases a diagnosis of CD was made. In all, ileal biopsies were essential for a final diagnosis in 15 and contributive in 53.

In the event that the ileocecal valve cannot be fully intubated then the biopsy forceps can usually be passed through the valve and blind biopsies obtained. One potential confounding issue for the pathologist may arise if the endoscopist has blindly biopsied over a lymphoid follicle and the pathologist reports a large influx of chronic inflammatory cells.

In the absence of cecitis the presence of acute ileal inflammation indicates discontinuous disease in the ileum, which is strongly suggestive of CD. The differential diagnosis is that of other acute inflammatory conditions in the terminal ileum, that are most commonly drugs such as NSAID and some infections such as *Salmonella*. Rarely, ileal biopsies are utilized to rule out *Mycobacterium tuberculosis*, lymphoma, or superimposed adenocarcinoma. In the presence of cecitis, which is part of a pancolitis, ileal inflammation will make the diagnosis of CD rather than UC more likely.

Esophagogastroduodenoscopy plus biopsy

Esophageal CD is rare, but biopsies of isolated ulcers in the esophagus or stomach can rule out cytomegalovirus or herpes simplex virus ulceration when routine histopathology, immunohistochemistry, and viral culture are utilized. *Helicobacter pylori* is less frequent than expected in patients with CD, and *H. pylori*-associated disease such as peptic ulcer disease is similarly less frequent [100–103]. Nonetheless, patients with any form of IBD may develop routine peptic ulcer disease, or NSAID-induced ulcers, but they can also develop ulcers as a manifestation of upper gastrointestinal CD. The presence of ulcers in patients with CD warrants multiple biopsies from affected and non-affected areas. In the case of gastroduodenal ulcers, biopsies of prepyloric antrum and mid-body greater curve are necessary to assess for *H. pylori*. There has been an emerging literature on the histologic findings in the gastric antrum of patients with CD. These changes may be present whether or not ulcers or erosions are present, or even if the mucosa appears completely normal. Focally enhanced gastritis in *H. pylori*-negative mucosa has been reported [100–103] (see Fig. 4). This includes a focal infiltration of CD3+ lymphocytes, CD68+ histiocytes, granulocytes, and in some cases granulomas. The findings were twice as likely to be present in the antrum than in the body, and in total occurred in 76% of CD patients negative for *H. pylori* [101]. Focally active gastritis was rarely seen in a series of 200 control patients without CD. Recently focal gastritis had an 84% specificity for CD and a 71% positive predictive value in a comparative study of 141 consecutive patients with CD, 71 with UC, and 141 controls [103].

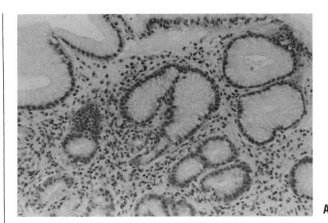

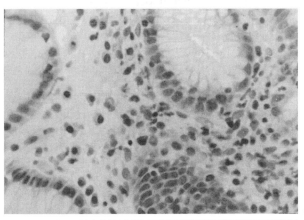

Figure 4. Biopsy of focal active gastritis in a patient with endoscopically normal stomach and ileal Crohn's disease. **A**: Overview of gastric antral mucosa with superficial focus of chronic inflammation. **B**: Detailed view of focal collection of lymphocytes. The biopsies were *Helicobacter pylori*-negative.

Finding these histologic changes on gastric biopsies may help discern the diagnosis in cases of indeterminate colitis. Duodenal biopsies may be abnormal in CD even in the absence of overt endoscopic pathology. The presence of partial villous atrophy on duodenal biopsies of patients with CD should not necessarily prompt a search for any other diagnosis unless clinically indicated. In a comparative study of 22 cases of CD and 23 cases of UC it was recently reported that the presence of microaggregates of immunostained macrophages and/or granulomas within non-inflamed gastroduodenal mucosa were found only in CD and not in UC [104]. The sensitivity was only 55% but the specificity was 100%, which suggests these histologic features of a normal-appearing stomach and/or duodenum may prove to be a valuable tool in differentiating indeterminate colitis.

Summary

Colon biopsies are critical in helping to diagnose diarrhea, to distinguish different forms of colitis, to determine the extent of disease, and to determine if neoplasia has arisen in the setting of chronic colitis. Colon biopsies in some instances can be definitive, but this usually requires the appropriate clinical scenario. For instance, to appreciate that segmental granulomatous colitis is CD and not the much rarer colonic sarcoidosis requires ancillary clinical information. Often colon biopsies may definitively reveal an abnormality, but the findings may be non-specific in regard to a definitive diagnosis. Thus, to utilize colon biopsies most appropriately in patient management usually requires frequent clinician–pathologist interaction, often repeat endoscopy with biopsies at a different time, and the assessment of any prior biopsies or resections. Once a patient has a firm diagnosis of CD he/she rarely converts to a disease that is indistinguishable from UC, and typically continue to behave like CD. Conversely, it is not too uncommon for patients with UC to develop features that strongly suggest that CD is the real underlying disease. These patients also tend to behave like those with CD. The ileum should be intubated whenever possible in cases of undiagnosed diarrhea and in cases of colitis to help distinguish if CD might be present. Gastric biopsies may reveal a pattern of focally active gastritis and this may serve as a clue for CD when the diagnosis is unknown or in doubt.

References

1. Fine KD, Krejs GJ, Fordtran JS. Diarrhea. In: Sleisenger MH, Fordtran JS, eds. Gastrointestinal Disease: Pathophysiology, Diagnosis, Management, 5th edn, vol. 2. Philadelphia: W.B. Saunders, 1993: 1043–72.
2. Powell DW. Approach to the patient with diarrhea. In: Yamada T, ed. Textbook of Gastroenterology. Philadelphia: J.B. Lippincott, 1991: 732–78.
3. Afzalpurkar R, Schiller L, Little K, Santangelo W, Fordtran J. Self-limited nature of chronic idiopathic diarrhea. N Engl J Med 1992; 327: 1849–52.
4. Donowitz M, Kokke FT, Saidi R. Evaluation of patients with chronic diarrhea. N Engl J Med 1995; 332: 725–9.
5. Greenberger NJ. Diagnostic approach to the patient with chronic diarrheal disorder. Dis Month 1990; 36: 139–79.
6. Fine KD, Schiller LR. AGA technical review on the evaluation and management of chronic diarrhea. Gastroenterology 1999; 116: 1464–86.
7. Patel Y, Pettigrew NP, Grahame GR, Bernstein CN. The outcome of endocopy plus biopsy in the evaluation of patients with chronic diarrhea. Gastrointest Endosc 1997; 46: 338–43.
8. Kingham JGC. Microscopic colitis. Gut 1991; 32: 234–5.
9. Lewin DN, Lewin KJ, Weinstein WM. Pathologist–gastroenterologist interaction. Am J Clin Pathol 1995; 103(Suppl. 1): S9–S12.
10. Kingham JGC, Levison DA, Morson BC, Dawson AM. Collagenous colitis. Gut 1986; 27: 570–7.
11. Zeroogian J, Chopra Sanjiv. Collagenous colitis and lymphocytic colitis. Annu Rev Med 1994; 45: 105–18.
12. Veress B, Lofberg R, Bergman L. Microscopic colitis syndrome. Gut 1995; 36: 880–6.
13. Lazenby AJ, Yardley JH, Giardello FM, Jessurun J, Bayless TM. Lymphocytic ('microscopic') colitis: a comparative histopathologic study with particular reference to collagenous colitis. Human Pathol 1989; 20: 18–27.
14. Ang ST, Bernstein CN, Robert ME, Weinstein WM. Cecal inflammation (infl) occurs in health and may result in false diagnoses of pancolitis: a prospective study. Gastroenterology 1993: 104; A1028.
15. Tanaka M, Mazzoleni G, Riddell RH. Distribution of collagenous colitis: utility of flexible sigmoidoscopy. Gut 1992; 22: 65–70.
16. Prior A, Lessells AM, Whorwell PJ. Is biopsy necessary if colonoscopy is normal? Dig Dis Sci 1987; 32: 673–6.
17. Bertomeu A, Ros E, Barragan V, Sachje L, Navarro S. Chronic diarrhea with normal stool and colonic examination: organic of functional? J Clin Gastroenterol 1991; 13: 531–6.
18. Marshall JB, Singh R, Diaz-Arias AA. Chronic, unexplained diarrhea: are biopsies necessary if colonoscopy is normal? Am J Gastroenterol 1995; 90: 372–6.
19. MacIntosh DG, Thompson WG, Patel DG, Barr R, Guindi M. Is rectal biopsy necessary in irritable bowel syndrome? Am J Gastroenterol 1992; 87: 1407–9.
20. Baert F, Wouters K, D'haens G et al. Lymphocytic colitis: A distinct clinical entity? A clinicopathological confrontation of lymphocytic and collagenous colitis. Gut 1999; 45: 375–81.
21. Mullhaupt B, Guller U, Anibitarte M, Guller R, Fried M. Lymphocytic colitis: clinical presentation and long term course. Gut 1998; 43: 629–33.
22. Surawicz CM, Haggitt RC, Husseman M, McFarland LV. Mucosal biopsy diagnosis of colitis: acute self-limited colitis and idiopathic inflammatory bowel disease. Gastroenterology 1994; 107: 755–63.
23. Allison MC, Hamilton-Dutoit SJ, Dhillon AP, Pounder RE. The value of rectal biopsy in distinguishing self-limited colitis from early inflammatory bowel disease. Q J Med 1987; 248: 985–95.
24. Schumacher G, Kollberg B, Sandstedt B. A prospective study of first attacks of inflammatory bowel disease and infectious colitis. Histologic course during the first year after presentation. Scand J Gastroenterol 1994; 29: 318–32.
25. Surawicz CM, Belic L. Rectal biopsy helps to distinguish acute self-limited colitis from idiopathic inflammatory bowel disease. Gastroenterology 1984; 86: 104–13.
26. Odze R, Antonioli D, Peppercorn MA, Goldman H. Effect of topical 5-aminosalicylic acid (5-ASA) enema therapy on mucosal biopsy morphology in chronic ulcerative colitis. Am J Surg Pathol 1993; 17: 869–75.
27. Tanaka M, Riddell RH, Saito H, Soma Y, Hidaka H, Kudo H. Morphologic criteria applicable to biopsy specimens for effective distinction of inflammatory bowel disease from other forms of colitis and of CD from ulcerative colitis. Scand J Gastroenterol 1999; 34: 55–67.
28. Bernstein CN, Surawicz CM, Bronner M, Weinstein WM. Is follicular proctitis a distinct form of ulcerative proctitis? Gastroenterology 1994; 106; A652.
29. Jenkins D, Goodall A, Scott BB. Ulcerative colitis; one disease or two? Gut 1990; 31: 426–30.

30. Blanche M, Rossini FP, Ferrari A, Roatta L, Gilli E, Cirillo R. The role of coloscopy in the differential diagnosis between idiopathic ulcerative colitis and Crohn's disease of the colon. Am J Gastroenterol 1975; 65: 539–45.

31. Pera A, Bellando P, Caldera D *et al.* Colonoscopy in inflammatory bowel disease. Diagnostic accuracy and proposal of an endoscopic score. Gastroenterology 1987; 92: 181–5.

32. Palnaes Hansen C, Hegnhoj J, Moller A, Brauer C, Hage E, Jarnum S. Ulcerative colitis and Crohn's disease of the colon. Is there a macroscopic difference? Ann Chir Gynecol 1990; 79: 78–81.

33. Tanaka M, Riddell RH. The pathological diagnosis and differential diagnosis of Crohn's disease. Hepatogastroenterology 1990; 37: 18–31.

34. Jenkins D, Balsitis M, Gallivan S *et al.* Guidelines for the initial biopsy diagnosis of suspected chronic inflammatory bowel disease. The British Society of Gastroenterology Initiative. J Clin Pathol 1997; 50: 93–105.

35. Seldenrijk CA, Morson BC, Meuwissen SGM, Schipper NW, Lindeman J, Meijer CJLM. Histopathological evaluation of colonic mucosal biopsy specimens in chronic inflammatory bowel disease: diagnostic implications. Gut 1991; 32: 1514–20.

36. Chambers TJ, Morson BC. The granuloma and Crohn's disease. Gut 1979; 20: 269 74.

37. Price AB, Morson BC. Inflammatory bowel disease: The surgical pathology of Crohn's disease and ulcerative colitis. Human Pathol 1975; 6: 7–29.

38. Surawicz CM, Meisel JL, Ylvisaker T, Saunders DR, Rubin CE. Rectal biopsy in the diagnosis of Crohn's disease: value of multiple biopsies and serial sectioning. Gastroenterology 1981; 81: 66–71.

39. Theodossi A, Spiegelhalter DJ, Jass J *et al.* Observer variation and discriminatory values of biopsy features in inflammatory bowel disease. Gut 1994; 35: 961–8.

40. Petras RE. Non-neoplastic intestinal disease. In: SS Sternberg, ed. Diagnostic Surgical Pathology. Raven Press; New York 1989: 967–1014.

41. Haggitt RC. Ulcerative colitis. In: Goldman H, Appelman HD, Kaufman N, eds. Gastrointestinal Pathology. Baltimore: Williams & Wilkins; USA 1990: 325–55.

42. Hodgson HJF. Non-specific inflammatory bowel disease: one disease or two? In: Allan RN, Keighley MRB, Alexander-Williams J, Hawkins C, eds. Inflammatory Bowel Disease. New York: Churchill Livingston, 1990: 121 6.

43. Hamilton SR, Morson BC. Ulcerative colitis. Pathology. In: Bockus HL, Berk JE, eds. Bockus Gastroenterology. Philadelphia: WB Saunders, 1985: 2139–53.

44. Modigliani R, Bitoun A. Endoscopic assessment of inflammatory bowel disease. In: Anagnostides AA, Hodgson HJF, Kirsner JB, eds. Inflammatory Bowel Disease. London: Chapman Hill, 1991: 108–21.

45. Farmer RG. Ulcerative colitis. Clinical features. In: Bockus HL, Berk JE, eds. Bockus Gastroenterology. Philadelphia: WB Saunders, 1985: 2153–7.

46. Waye JD. Endoscopy in inflammatory bowel disease. In: Kirsner JB, Shorter RG, eds. Inflammatory Bowel Disease, 4th edn. Baltimore: Williams & Wilkins, 1995: 555–82.

47. D'Haens G, Geboes K, Peeters M, Baert F, Ectors N, Rutgeerts P. Patchy inflammation associated with distal ulcerative colitis: a prospective endoscopic study. Am J Gastroenterol 1997; 92: 1275–9.

48. Okawa K, Aoki T, Sano K, Harihara S, Kitano A, Kuroki T. Ulcerative colitis with skip lesions at the mouth of the appendix: a clinical study. Am J Gastroenterol 1998; 93: 2405–10.

49. Goligher JC, deDombal FT, Watts JM, Watkinson G. Ulcerative Colitis. London: Bailliere Tindall & Cassell, 1968: 66–7.

50. Burnham WR, Ansell ID, Langman MJS. Normal sigmoidoscopic findings in severe ulcerative colitis: an important and common occurrence. Gut 1980; 21 : A460.

51. Whitehead R, Ulcerative colitis. In: Whitehead R, ed. Gastrointestinal and Oesophageal Pathology. Edinburgh: Churchill Livingston, 1989: 522–31.

52. Markowitz J, Kahn E, Grancher K, Hyams J, Treem W, Daum F. Atypical rectosigmoid histology in children with newly diagnosed ulcerative colitis. Am J Gastroenterol 1993; 88: 2034–7.

53. Bernstein CN, Shanahan F, Anton PA, Weinstein WM. Patchiness of mucosal inflammation in treated ulcerative colitis: a prospective study. Gastrointest Endosc 1995; 42: 232–7.

54. Levine TS, Tzardi M, Mitchell S, Sowter C, Price AB. Diagnostic difficulty arising from rectal recovery in ulcerative colitis. J Clin Pathol 1996; 49: 319–23.

55. Kleer CG, Appelman HD. Ulcerative colitis: patterns of involvement in colorectal biopsies and changes with time. Am J Surg Pathol 1998; 22: 983–9.

56. Kim B, Barnett JL, Kleer CG, Appelman HD. Endoscopic and histological patchiness in treated ulcerative colitis. Am J Gastroenterol 1999; 94: 3258 62.

57. Riddell RH. Pathology of idiopathic indflammatory bowel disease. In: Kirsner JB, Shorter RG, eds. Inflammatory Bowel Disease, 3rd edn. Philadelphia: Lea and Febiger, 1988: 329–50.

58. Davison AM, Dixon MF. The appendix as a 'skip lesion' in ulcerative colitis. Histopathology 1989; 16: 93–4.

59. Lumb G, Prothroe RHB. Ulcerative colitis. Gastroenterology 1958; 34: 381–407.

60. Rutgeerts P, D'Haens G, Hiele M, Geboes K, Vantrappen G. Appendectomy protects against ulcerative colitis. Gastroenterology 1994; 106: 1251–3.

61. Bezabeh T, Somorjai RL, Smith IC, Nikulin AE, Dolenko B, Bernstein CN. The use of ^{1}H magnetic resonance spectroscopy in inflammatory bowel diseases: distinguishing ulcerative colitis from Crohn's disease. Am J Gastroenterol 2001; 96: 442–8.

62. Moum B, Ekbom A, Vatn MH, Elgjo K. Change in the extent of colonoscopic and histological involvement in ulcerative colitis over time. Am J Gastroenterol 1999; 94: 1564–8.

63. Riley SA, Mani V, Goodman MJ, Dutt S, Herd ME. Microscopic activity in ulcerative colitis: what does it mean? Gut 1991; 32: 174–8.

64. Dignan H, Greenson J. Can ischemic colitis be differentiated from *C. difficile* colitis on biopsy specimens? Am J Surg Pathol 1997; 21:706–10.

65. Madigan MR, Morson BC. Solitary ulcer of the rectum. Gut 1969; 10: 871–81.

66. Rutter KRP, Riddell RH. The solitary rectal ulcer syndrome of the rectum. Clin Gastroenterol 1975; 4: 505–30.

67. Rowland R, Langman J. Endometriosis of the large bowel. Pathology 1989; 21: 259–65,

68. Parr NJ, Murphy C, Holt S, Zakhour H, Crosbie RB. Endometriosis and the gut. Gut 1988; 29: 1112–15.

69. Gledhill A, Dixon MF. Crohn's-like reaction in diverticular disease. Gut 1998; 42: 392–5.

70. Carr N, Schofield PF. Inflammatory bowel disease in the older patient. Br J Surg 1982; 69: 223–5.

71. Makapugay LM, Dean PJ. Diverticular associated chronic colitis. Am J Surg Pathol 1996; 20: 94–102.

72. Gahl WA, Brantly M, Kaiser-Kupfer MI *et al.* Genetic defects and clinical characteristics of patients with a form

of oculocutaneous albinism (Hermansky–Pudlak syndrome). N Engl J Med 1998; 338: 1258–64.

73. Roe TF, Thomas DW, Gilsanz V, Isaacs H Jr, Atkinson JB. Inflammatory bowel disease in glycogen storage disease type 1B. J Pediar 1987; 110: 166.

74. Stevens C, Peppercorn MA, Grand RJ. Crohn's disease associated with autoimmune neutropenia. J Clin Gastroenterol 1991; 13: 328–30.

75. Ilnyckyj A, Aldor TAM, Warrington R, Bernstein CN. Crohn's disease and the Melkersson–Rosenthal syndrome. Can J Gastroenterol 1999; 13: 152–4.

76. Bulger K, O'Riordan M, Purdy S, O'Brien M, Lennon J. Gastrointestinal sarcoidosis resembling Crohn's disease. Am J Gastroenterol 1988: 83; 1415–17.

77. O'Connell DJ, Courtney JV, Riddell RH. Colitis of Behçet's syndrome: radiologic and pathologic features. Gastrointest Radiol 1980; 5: 173–9.

78. Anand BS, Malhotra V, Bhattacharya SK *et al*. Rectal histology in acute bacillary dysentery. Gastroenterology 1986; 90: 654–60.

79. Ilnyckyj A, Greenberg H, Bernstein CN. *Escherichia coli* 0157:H7 infection mimicking Crohn's disease. Gastroenterology 1997; 112: 995–9.

80. Cuffari C, Oligny L, Seidman EG. *Dientamoeba fragilis* masquerading as allergic colitis. J Pediatr Gastroenterol Nutr 1998; 26: 16–20.

81. Berk T, Gordon SJ, Choi HY, Cooper HS. Cytomegalovirus infection of the colon: a possible role in exacerbation of inflammatory bowel disease. Am J Gastroenterol 1985; 80: 355–60.

82. Orvar K, Murray J, Carmen G, Conklin J. Cytomegalovirus infection associated with onset of inflammatory bowel disease. Dig Dis Sci 1993; 38: 2307–10.

83. Vega R, Bertran X, Menacho M *et al*. Cytomegalovirus infection in patients with inflammatory bowel disease. Am J Gastroenterol 1999; 94: 1053–6.

84. Inyckyj A, Hosking DH, Pettigrew NM, Bernstein CN. Extracorporeal shock wave lithotripsy causing colonic injury: first case report. Dig Dis Sci 1999; 44: 2485–8.

85. Driman DK, Preiksaitis HG. Colorectal inflammation and increased cell proliferation associated with oral sodium phosphate bowel preparation solution. Human Pathol 1998; 29: 972–8.

86. Riddell RH, Goldman H, Ransohoff DF *et al*. Dysplasia in inflammatory bowel disease: standardized classification with provisional clinical applications. Human Pathol 1983; 14: 931–68.

87. Bernstein CN, Shanahan F, Weinstein WM. Are we telling patients the truth about surveillance colonoscopy in ulcerative colitis? Lancet 1994; 343: 71–4.

88. Connell WR, Lennard-Jones JE, Williams CB, Talbot IC, Price AB, Wilkinson KH. Factors affecting the outcome of endoscopic surveillance for cancer in ulcerative colitis. Gastroenterology 1994; 107: 934–44.

89. Lindberg B, Persson B, Veress B, Ingelman-Sundberg H, Granqvist S. Twenty years' colonoscopic surveillance of patients with ulcerative colitis. Detection of dysplastic and malignant transformation. Scand J Gastroenterol 1996; 31: 1195–204.

90. Connell WR, Talbot IC, Harpaz N *et al*. Clinicopathological characteristics of carcinoma complicating ulcerative colitis. Gut 1994; 35: 1419–23.

91. Melville DM, Jass JR, Morson BC *et al*. Observer study of the grading of dysplasia in ulcerative colitis: comparison with clinical outcome. Human Pathol 1989; 20: 1008–14.

92. Bernstein, CN, Weinstein WM, Levine DS, Shanahan F. Physicians' perceptions of dysplasia and approaches to surveillance colonoscopy in ulcerative colitis. Am J Gastroenterol 1995: 90; 2106–14.

93. Bernstein CN. Challenges in designing a randomized trial of surveillance colonoscopy in IBD. Inflamm Bowel Dis 1998; 4: 132–41.

94. Rubin CE, Haggitt RC, Burmer GC *et al*. DNA aneuploidy in colonic biopsies predicts future development of dysplasia in ulcerative colitis. Gastroenterology 1992; 103: 1611–20.

95. Friedman S, Rubin PH, Goldstein E, Harpaz N, Bodian C, Present DH. The efficacy of a 10 year surveillance study in 260 chronic Crohn's colitis (CC) patients. Gastroenterology 1999; 116: A487.

96. Engelsgjerd M, Torres C, Odze RD. Adenoma-like polypoid dysplasia in chronic ulcerative colitis: a follow up study of 23 cases. Gastroenterology 1999; 117:1288–94.

97. Rubin PH, Friedman S, Harpaz N *et al*. Colonoscopic polypectomy in chronic colitis: are we removing adenomas or 'DALMs'. Gastroenterology 1999; 117: 1295–300.

98. Bernstein CN. ALMs versus DALMs in ulcerative colitis: polypectomy or colectomy? Gastroenterology 1999; 117: 1488–91.

99. Geboes K, Ectors N, D'Haens G, Rutgeerts P. Is ileoscopy plus biopsy worthwhile in patients presenting with symptoms of inflammatory bowel disease? Am J Gastroenterol 1998; 93: 201–6.

100. Halme L, Karkkainen P, Rautelin H, Kosunen TU, Sipponen P. High frequency of *Helicobacter*-negative gastritis in patients with Crohn's disease. Gut 1996; 38: 379–83.

101. Oberhuber G, Puspok A, Oesterreicher C *et al*. Focally enhanced gastritis: a frequent type of gastritis in patients with Crohn's disease. Gastroenterology 1997; 112: 698–706.

102. Wright CL, Riddell RH. Histology of the stomach and duodenum in Crohn's disease. Am J Surg Pathol 1998; 22: 383–90.

103. Parente F, Cucino C, Bollani S *et al*. Focal gastric inflammatory infiltrates in inflammatory bowel diseases: prevalence, immunohistochemical characteristics, and diagnostic role. Am J Gastroenterol 2000; 95: 705–11.

104. Yao K, Yao T, Iwashita A, Matsui T, Kamachi S. Microaggregate of immunostained macrophages in noninflamed gastroduodenal mucosa: a new useful histological marker for differentiating Crohn's colitis from ulcerative colitis. Am J Gastroenterol 2000: 95: 1967–73.

19 | Radiologic (radiographic) and imaging features of ulcerative colitis and Crohn's disease

EDWARD FITZGERALD

Introduction

Since the previous edition of this book several advances have occurred in the radiologic evaluation of both ulcerative colitis (UC) and Crohn's disease (CD). The most important of these is the definition of the place of computed tomography (CT) in the evaluation and management of these conditions. Other imaging techniques such as magnetic resonance imaging (MRI), radionuclide imaging (NM) and ultrasonography (US) have also become more important in evaluation of both UC and CD.

Imaging studies are used in all phases of these conditions: (1) in the initial evaluation of the patient to allow a diagnosis to be established; (2) in the preoperative patient to determine the full extent of disease; (3) in the postoperative patient to evaluate complications of treatment and the presence of recurrent disease; (4) during clinical exacerbations to determine if complications are present; (5) to demonstrate extraluminal and extra-abdominal manifestations; and (6) to allow imaging-guided interventional procedures to be undertaken in patients with complicated inflammatory bowel disease (IBD).

Imaging techniques

Plain abdominal radiographs

This is the least expensive and least sophisticated imaging modality; it is often very useful [1, 2]. Air is an excellent contrast medium for outlining the bowel lumen on plain films (Fig. 1A,B). IBD may be diagnosed based on the loss of haustration of the air-filled colon. Nodularity of the luminal margin may suggest pseudopolyps or mucosal ulceration. Marked dilation of the large bowel may mean that the patient has developed fulminant colitis or toxic megacolon (see Fig. 32A,B).

Dilated small bowel may be secondary to a distal stenotic lesion of CD. Evidence of an unsuspected perforation or abscess may be present on plain abdominal radiographs. Some of the extraintestinal manifestations of IBD, such as renal stones, gallstones and arthritis, may also be demonstrated on plain abdominal films.

Barium techniques
Double-contrast barium examinations

These are currently the most accurate imaging method for evaluating bowel mucosa to detect the early changes of IBD [3–10]. Studies of the esophagus, stomach and colon are performed using high-density barium to coat the mucosa and with air to distend the lumen. In double-contrast examination of the complete gastrointestinal tract it is important that the gut be as clean as possible before the examination.

No preparation is necessary for an esophagram. The only preparation necessary for barium examination of the stomach and small bowel is that the patient has nothing by mouth for at least 8 h before the examination. For colonic studies, irritating laxatives are contraindicated in the patient with acute IBD. A clear liquid diet for approximately 48 hours before the examination is usually adequate preparation. In someone with fulminant colitis or when developing toxic megacolon is suspected, barium or other contrast medium examination of the colon is contraindicated, and plain film radiology is suggested instead [11–14]. For these patients CT is the ideal technique, providing both an accurate diagnosis and demonstrating the complications associated with all of IBD [15]. CT has replaced the older antegrade barium examinations that were occasionally performed in the past.

Stephan R. Targan, Fergus Shanahan and Loren C. Karp (eds.), Inflammatory Bowel Disease: From Bench to Bedside, 2nd Edition, 371–407.
© 2003 *Kluwer Academic Publishers. Printed in Great Britain*

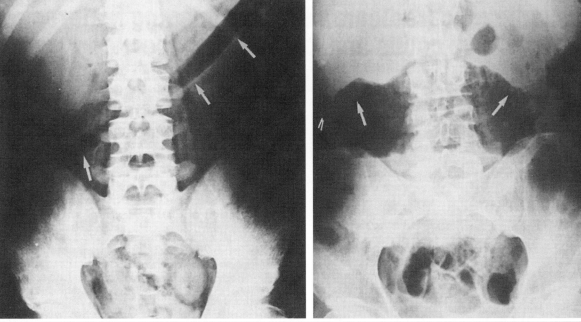

Figure 1. Plain abdominal radiograph in inflammatory bowel disease. **A**. Chronic ulcerative colitis with air column outlining a tubular ahaustral transverse colon (arrows). **B**. Crohn's colitis. The air column shows the colon to be dilated and have a nodular mucosal margin (arrows) in a patient with disease recurring in the colon after ileo-ascending colostomy.

Small bowel studies

The small intestine can be examined by a conventional small bowel meal, in which the patient is given at least 500 ml (450 g) of barium by mouth. Radiographs and compression spot films of the small bowel are taken at regular intervals until the barium reaches the colon. This is quite an accurate examination [16]. An alternative technique is enteroclysis (small bowel enema) [16–19] (Fig. 2A,B,C). For this procedure it is necessary for the radiologist to intubate the patient and position the tube with its tip beyond the ligament of Treitz. This can be a challenge for both the patient and radiologist. Mild sedation, such as 100 µg of Sublimaze is useful. A high-density barium is injected through the tube followed by methylcellulose (or water) as the double-contrast agent. The barium coats the wall of the bowel and the methylcellulose distends the lumen, giving the small bowel a translucency that allows a clear view of the mucosa. Another advantage is that the entire small bowel is filled at the same time. The distension of the bowel may demonstrate small strictures. Radiographs are obtained and suspicious areas can be compressed. Problems with

this procedure are the discomfort of a nasojejunal tube for the patient, and the time and radiation exposure need to place the tube [18]. This examination is particularly useful in preoperative assessment of stricture site and number in known IBD.

If, using conventional studies, there is difficulty in demonstrating the pelvic loops and terminal ileal region, a pneumocolon should be performed [20, 21]. To perform the pneumocolon a small enema catheter is placed in the rectum with the patient in the left lateral decubitus position. CO_2 or air is insufflated as the patient turns prone. The fluoroscopic table is first elevated and then returned to the horizontal position to aid distribution of gas throughout the colon. If reflux does not occur spontaneously, a muscle relaxant such as hyoscine butylbromide 20 mg (Buscopan) or glucagons 0.5 mg can be used [21] (Fig 3).

Sinography

When a bowel fistula has developed a cutaneous communication, a catheter can be threaded into the opening and iodinated contrast medium injected under fluoroscopic control. Contrast medium can

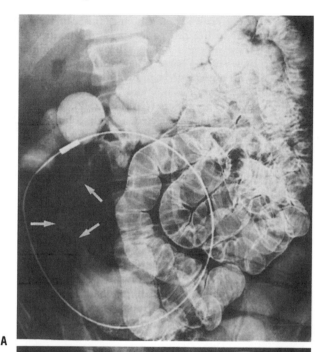

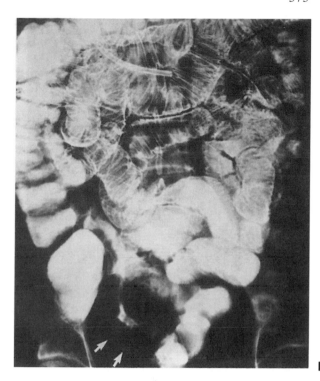

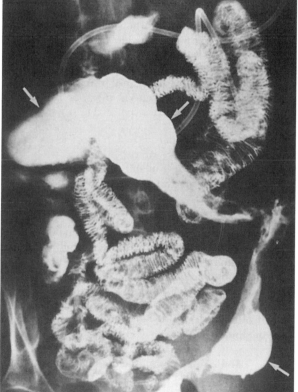

Figure 2. Enteroclysis studies. **A**: Distal ileal Crohn's disease. Arrows outline a narrowed segment with no mucosal folds (string sign). There is distension immediately proximal to the diseased segment and normal bowel proximal to this. **B**. Distal ileal Crohn's disease. Arrows indicate a sinus tract arising from an involved segment of distal ileum. **C**. Delayed radiograph shows Crohn's colitis with skip areas of disease in the transverse, descending, and sigmoid colons (arrows).

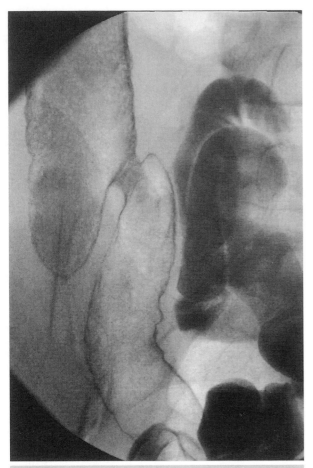

Figure 3. Pneumocolon outlining Crohn's disease of terminal ileum and caecum.

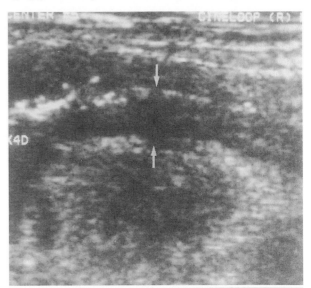

Figure 4. Ultrasound of Crohn's disease of the distal ileum. Arrows outline thickened wall of longitudinally scanned segment.

also be injected into a catheter placed after abscess drainage to determine if a bowel fistula is present (see Fig. 31B). A sinogram should always be performed prior to removal of such drainage catheters.

Abdominal computed tomography

This technique is now often the only one needed in patients with IBD. Particularly for acutely ill patients CT is often the only study required for accurate diagnosis and management of the many complications associated with IBD [15]. Complete opacification of a well-distended gut is needed for accurate CT examination. This can be achieved with 1000 ml of 2% barium solution (Readi-CAT2, E-ZM, Westbury, NY) followed by 200–300 ml immediately prior to the scan.

The entire thickness of the bowel wall, rather than just the mucosal surface, can be visualized. The surrounding structures such as mesentery and lymph nodes can clearly be seen. Complications such as bowel wall thickening, phlegmon, abscess, obstruction, carcinoma and fistulas are all shown on CT. Extraintestinal manifestations of IBD which occur in one-third to one-quarter of patients with these diseases are clearly seen. The liver, gallbladder, kidneys, ureters, sacroiliac joints and bones all need to be carefully evaluated on CT scan in patients with all forms of IBD [22–30] (Fig. 16).

Ultrasound

Ultrasound is often the first imaging examination performed on the patient with abdominal symptoms who does not yet have a diagnosis. Bowel wall thickening, in a segment involved by IBD, may be seen, as can evidence of complications of IBD such as abscesses or distended bowel due to obstruction (Figs. 4 and 5). Extraintestinal manifestations of IBD in the liver, gallbladder or kidney may also be diagnosed by ultrasound examination [31, 32]. Transrectal ultrasonography is useful for demonstration of perirectal abscesses and fistulas, especially in CD (Fig. 5).

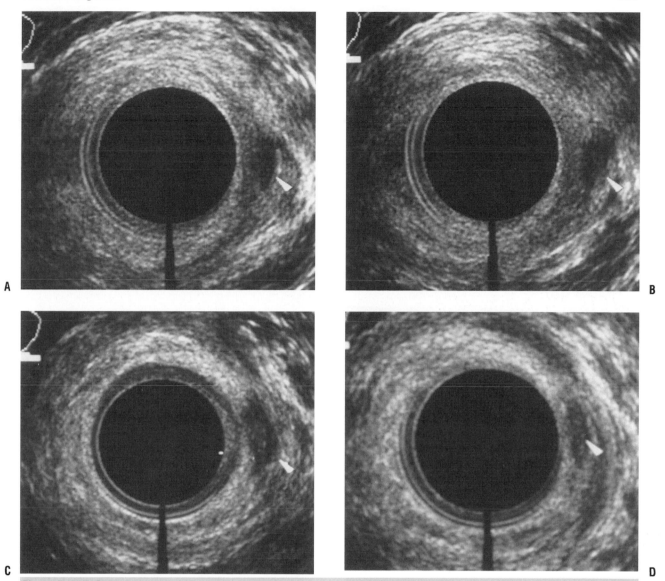

Figure 5 (A, B, C, D). Endoluminal ultrasound showing caudal extension of transphincteric fistula (arrowed).

Nuclear medicine

NM techniques offer a non-invasive method that may help identify and monitor disease activity and sites of bowel involvement. Radionuclides used in clinically available methods include gallium-67 citrate, indium-111 and technetium-99m-labeled leukocytes [32–36]. Leukocytes labeled with radio-isotopes migrate to segments of bowel that are acutely inflamed. Delayed images show accumulation of tracer in these areas (Fig. 6). Severity of inflammation may also be inferred from the quantity of labeled leukocytes recovered in stool samples. Positron emission tomography (PET) scanning with fluorodioxyglucose has also been used in diagnosis and follow-up of CD (Fig. 7).

Patients with ischaemic bowel, pseudomembranous colitis and active bleeding may also have positive labeled leukocyte studies because of accumulation of white blood cells in their bowel lumen.

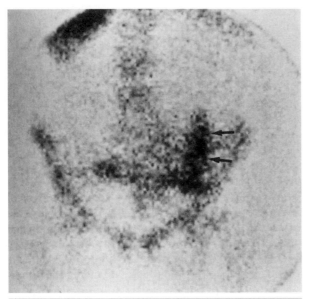

Figure 6. Indium-111-labeled leukocyte study. A zone of increased tracer activity is present in the left lower quadrant in a segment of bowel involved by recurrent Crohn's disease (arrows).

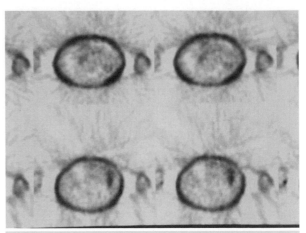

Figure 7. Transaxial PET scan showing increased uptake in left-sided Crohn's colitis.

Magnetic resonance imaging

MRI is now the method of choice for evaluation of the perianal complications of CD such as perianal abscesses and fistulas. Imaging with surface coils is sufficient to show the anal anatomy and to reliably describe perianal abscesses and fistulas according to surgical terminology [37] (see Fig. 30).

Magnetic resonance enteroclysis is now performed in many units. Its advantages include soft-tissue contrast, direct multiplanar capacity and lack of ionizing radiation. These give it the potential to become the ideal diagnostic method for imaging the small bowel [38, 39].

Crohn's disease

CD can involve any portion of the gastrointestinal tract, from mouth to anus. It most frequently involves the terminal ileum. UC is usually diagnosed without delay, because most cases present with bloody diarrhea, leading to early colonoscopy. In CD the delay between onset of symptoms and diagnosis varies between 2 and 4 years [40].

For assessment and diagnosis of CD the current diagnostic and imaging techniques used include radiography of the small and large bowel, ileocolonscopy, ultrasonography and CT. MRI is of particular use in evaluation of perineal fistulas and sinuses [41].

Esophageal Crohn's disease

This is usually diagnosed on endoscopy at the present time. It may be diagnosed on barium studies. CD involving the esophagus rarely occurs in isolation. The radiographic findings are not pathognomonic for CD. As in the remainder of the gastrointestinal tract, appearances vary in early disease and subtle mucosal lesions such as aphthous ulcers are found [42–46] (Fig. 8). With more advanced disease ulcers may be numerous, the ulcers may be deep, and thickened mucosal folds may be present. Deep ulcers may progress into sinus tracts or fistulize into the bronchial tree, mediastinum or stomach. In advanced cases strictures can occur, as they do in the rest of the bowel.

Stomach and duodenum

When the stomach is affected the disease occurs most frequently in the distal portion. Aphthous ulcers (discrete, small ulcerations seen as a collection of barium surrounded by edema) are found on double-contrast barium studies (Fig. 9). It can be impossible to differentiate aphthous ulcers from gastric erosions due to other causes. With progression of the disease scarring of the antrum can occur. On barium studies this may look like a linitis plastica [47]. Gastrocolic

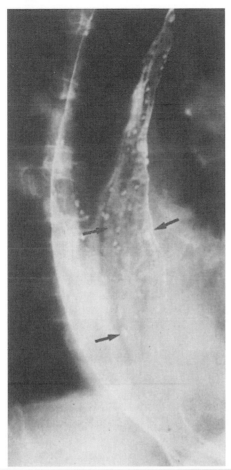

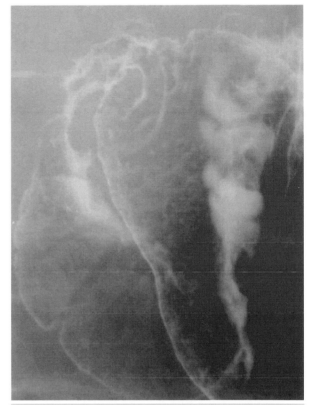

Figure 9. Gastroduodenal Crohn's disease.

Figure 8. Crohn's disease of the esophagus. Extensive aphthous lesions of the esophagus are present (arrows). This patient also had ileal involvement by Crohn's disease.

fistulas have been reported, but these are more usually due to disease of the transverse colon invading the stomach [48].

CD of the duodenum is usually seen in conjunction with gastric involvement (Fig. 9). Once again the earliest radiographic finding is the aphthous ulcer (Fig. 9). Then larger ulcers occur in a bulbar or post-bulbar location [42, 43, 45]. With more severe disease a cobblestone pattern develops because of a cross-hatchet distribution of linear ulceration. If fibrosis occurs strictures may be seen. These are commonest in the post-bulbar duodenum (Fig. 10A). With asymmetric fibrosis (as occurs anywhere in the bowel) uninvolved segments may distend in an area of fixed disease, giving this normal area the appearance of a diverticulum. These are referred to as pseudodiverticulae [49].

As in other segments of both large and small bowel, skip areas can occur. Stenotic areas can cause obstruction of stomach and duodenum. Fistulas are rare. If present they usually occur between transverse colon and the third part of the duodenum. These are usually secondary to colonic disease and are most likely to be shown on colonic barium studies. Occasionally fistulas into the biliary tree can be seen (Fig. 10B).

Small bowel Crohn's disease

Jejunal involvement by CD occurs in between 4% and 10% of patients with this disease [45]. Thickened mucosal folds may be the earliest finding (Fig. 11A). These may be in skip lesions, which appear as short strictures. A cobblestone pattern may occur in patients with longitudinal and transverse ulceration (Fig. 11B). Separation of bowel loops is frequently present and is due to thickening of the bowel wall and fibrofatty changes in the mesentery [42, 45, 49].

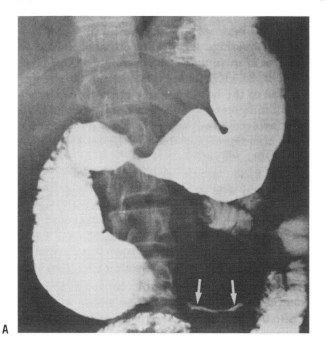

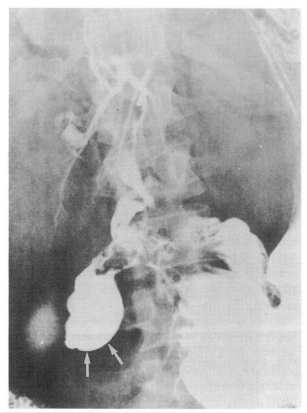

Figure 10. Gastroduodenal Crohn's disease. **A**: Distal duodenal involvement with a string sign (arrows). **B**: Nodular mucosal pattern of the distal antrum and marked irregular duodenal narrowing. Arrows indicate a spared segment (pseudodiverticulum). A fistula from the duodenum to the biliary tree is present with barium filling the intrahepatic bile ducts.

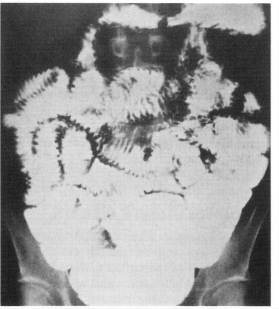

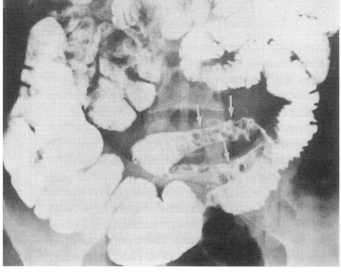

Figure 11. Crohn's disease the jejunum. **A**: Thickening of the jejunal mucosal folds represents early changes. **B**: Multiple involved narrowed segments (arrows) with dilated spared segments between them.

Almost all patients with CD have involvement of the terminal ileum either as the sole site or as one of multiple sites in the small and large bowel [42, 47, 49–51] (Fig. 12A). It is the only site of involvement in 14–30% of patients and, along with colonic disease, is involved in 55–75% of reported patients. The terminal ileum is spared in only 3–5% of cases. The extent of diseased bowel may be from 10 to 30 cm proximal to the ileocecal valve, and milder changes may be present 10–20 cm proximal to the more clearly involved area.

The earliest detectable radiographic findings are aphthous ulcers. When these are the sole abnormality differentiation from infectious processes such as *Yersinia*, *Salmonella*, tuberculosis or *Candida* cannot be made with confidence. Mucosal folds may be thickened (Fig. 12A). The bowel lumen is often narrowed, frequently markedly so; and this has led to the term 'string sign' [50] (Fig. 12E). Longitudinal and transverse ulceration may give the mucosal surface a cobblestone appearance (Fig. 12C). In some patients severe ulceration and edema may give the appearance of a bowel segment that is devoid of mucosa. Contrast-filled bowel loops may be separated because of thickening of involved bowel wall and fibrofatty proliferation of the mesentery [51] (Figs. 12B,D,E, see Fig. 21A,B). With transmural disease tracts may occur into the wall of the bowel (Fig. 13). These may progress to fistulas between loops of bowel or between bowel and skin, bladder, ureters, prostate, vagina or skin, frequently in the perineal area (Fig. 14A,B,C). The commonest fistulous communication is between diseased ileum and cecum or ascending colon (Fig. 13). Skip areas of disease are frequent as in asymmetric involvement of the bowel. There is a tendency for the mesenteric side of the bowel to show greater involvement than the antimesenteric side [52, 53].

Pseudodiverticulae occur when uninvolved bowel segments distend in otherwise restricted asymmetrically diseased bowel loops (Fig. 10B).

When fibrosis occurs, stenotic segments may lead to obstruction. Plain radiographs may show markedly distended bowel loops proximal to chronically obstructed segments (see Fig. 20A,B). In a patient with long-standing chronic obstructions the distension is more likely to be in bowel loops near the obstructed segment. The degree of proximal chronic distension may be so great as to be confused with colonic dilation on plain radiographs (Fig. 15). Occasionally, enteroliths are seen in bowel proximal

to an obstructing lesion or in a pseudodiverticulum [46, 48–50] (see Fig. 53C).

Perforation of the bowel has been reported, but is an unusual complication of CD (Fig. 16A,B).

Ultrasound may show the thickened wall of involved bowel segments (Fig. 4). These may have a target appearance if the segment is scanned transversely, with the center of the target being the narrowed lumen. Distended fluid-filled bowel may be seen proximal to a stricture. Irregular fluid-filled collections can be seen when abscesses are present [29]. Ultrasound may also identify fistulas, 20 out of 23 in one series [55].

CT gives a unique diagnostic perspective in both small and large bowel CD. It can depict abnormalities in the bowel wall as well as extraluminal complications [56]. Findings on CT include thickening of the wall of diseased segments, often with a target appearance (Fig. 17A,B). Bowel loops can be separated due to fibrofatty proliferations of the mesentery and to lymphadenopathy (Fig. 18). Fistulous tracts may be seen. Sometimes small amounts of air or contrast present in the bladder or other abnormal location may be the first sign of a sinus tract or fistula [54, 57] (Fig. 19). Such evidence is often seen on CT in the presence of normal conventional plain film or contrast radiography. Bladder wall thickening is sometimes seen due to direct extension of inflammation from adjacent involved bowel loops. Abscesses can appear as a well-defined zone of low attenuation with a thick wall (Fig. 20). Frequently it may not be as well defined but may contain extraluminal air bubbles. CT can be used to guide aspiration or catheter drainage of such fluid collections and abscesses.

Once the disease is established in the small bowel it may become more severe and stenotic in the involved areas. It is unusual for it to spread, either proximally or distally, in the absence of surgery (Fig. 21A,B; Fig. 22A,B) [50]. Regression of the radiographic changes of CDe in the upper gastrointestinal tract and small bowel is rare [58, 59]. It is important to note that, particularly in chronic disease, the findings on imaging studies often correlate poorly with the clinical status of the patient. Therefore, once the diagnosis is established, unless a complication such as obstruction, perforation, abscess or fistula (Fig. 23A,B) is suggested by the patient's clinical condition, frequent routine follow-up radiographic examinations of the patient are usually not necessary.

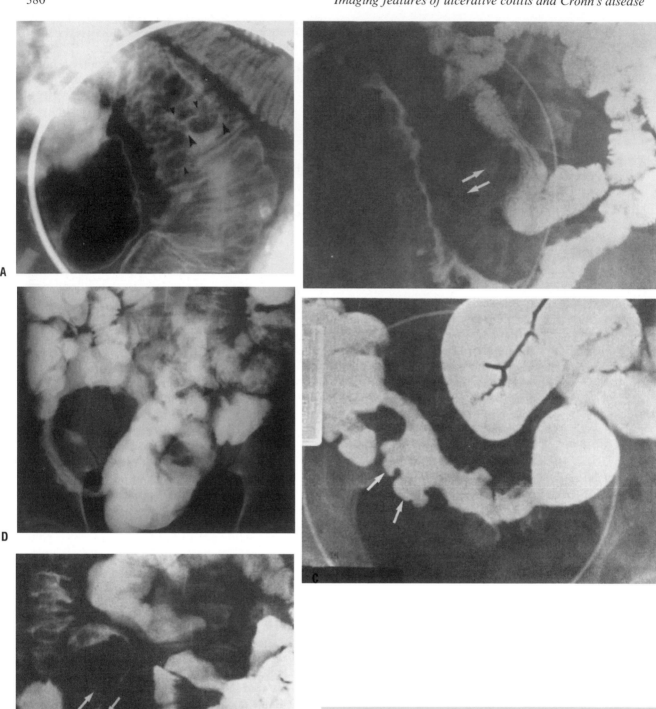

Figure 12. A: Pneumocolon showing early involvement of terminal ileum by Crohn's disease with mucosal thickening. **B**: Marked nodularity of terminal ileal mucosal folds, luminal narrowing, and separation of bowel loops (arrows). **C**: Loss of normal distal ileal mucosal pattern, sinus tracts into the wall of the bowel, and diverticular outpouchings (arrows) which are spared segments. **D**: Separation of loops due to bowel wall thickening and abscess with fistula in right iliac fossa. **E**: Marked narrowing of the terminal ileum (strong sign) with multiple sinus tracts arising from the diseased segment (arrows).

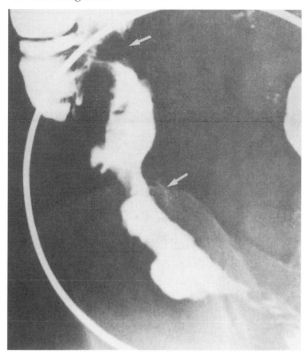

Figure 13. Crohn's disease with ileocecal fistulae. Sinus tract into the bowel wall and fistula from the terminal ileum to the ascending colon are indicated by arrows.

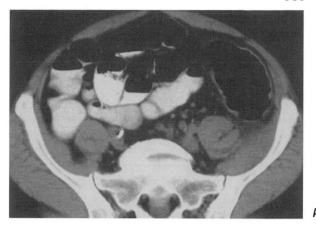

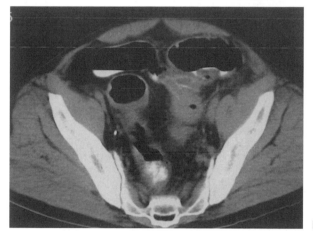

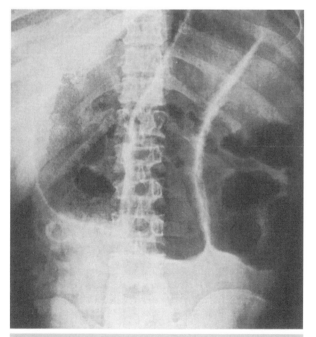

Figure 15. Marked bowel distension on plain radiograph (proven to be small bowel on subsequent studies) due to obstruction by small bowel Crohn's disease.

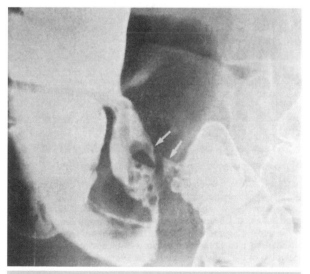

Figure 14. **A**: CT with colo-jejunal fistula. **B**: CT with colovesical fistula with 3 tracts from colon to left wall of bladder. **C**: Crohn's disease with ileosigmoid fistulae. A fistulous tract passes from the terminal ileum to the sigmoid and causes tenting of the secondarily involved colon.

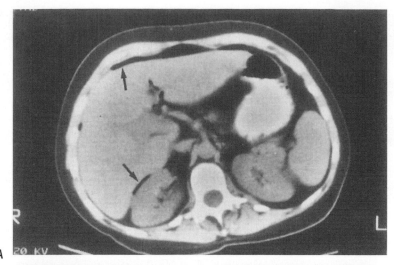

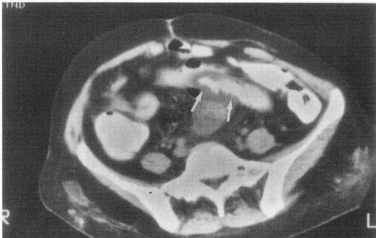

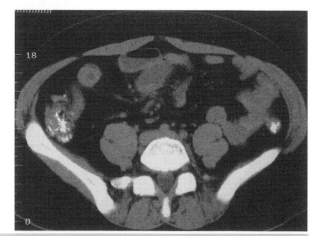

Figure 16. **A**: Arrows indicate free air in Morrison's pouch, and the perihepatic region in another patient with bowel perforation. **B**: Thick-walled segment of jejunum involved by Crohn's disease (arrows) which was found to be perforated at the time of surgery.

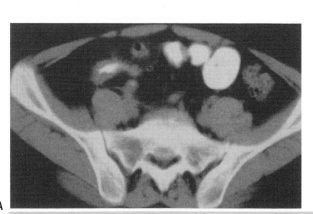

Figure 17. **A**: Thickening of terminal ileum in early Crohn's disease. **B**. Target sign of terminal ileum in Crohn's disease.

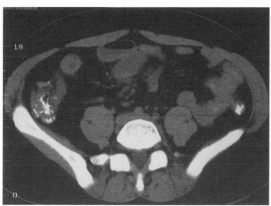

Figure 18. CT with creeping fat due to Crohn's disease.

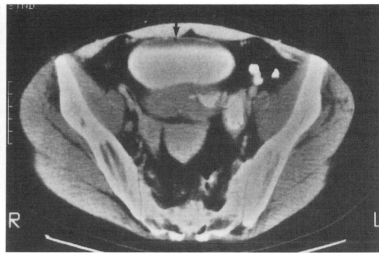

Figure 19. Crohn's disease with ileovesicle fistula. An inflammatory mass posterior to the bladder surrounds a fistula which communicates from the ileum to the bladder. A single air bubble is present in the bladder (arrows).

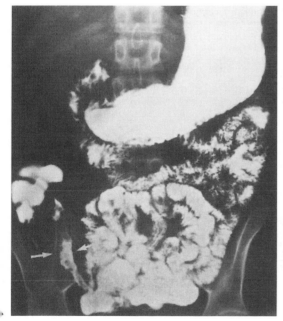

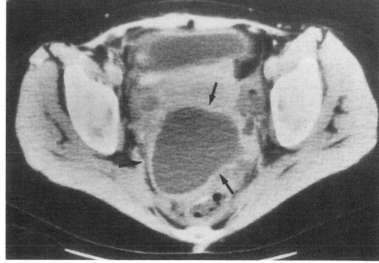

Figure 20. Crohn's disease with large pelvic abscess (CT findings). **A**: Terminal ileal involvement with nodular mucosal pattern and separation of bowel loops in the right lower quadrant (arrows). **B**: CT shows thickened bowel wall in areas of diseased segments (arrows). **C**: Arrows indicate large thick-walled pelvic abscess in same patient.

B

C

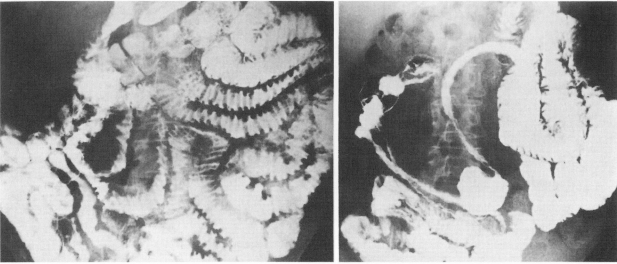

A   B

Figure 21. Crohn's disease of the jejunum and ileum with rapid progression from non stenotic to stenotic phases of disease. **A**: Thickened but preserved mucosal folds and separation of bowel loops due to thickened walls. **B**: Loss of mucosal folds, stenosis, and marked separation of bowel segments in same patient 3 years later.

Postoperative recurrence

Postoperative recurrence and subsequent progression of disease is a well-known complication. It is said to occur with an incidence as high as 80% (Fig. 22). It usually recurs at anastomosis; more frequently on the ileal side of an ileocolonic anastomosis, but it can be seen on the colonic side (Fig. 22A). The first radiographic features which suggest recurrence include aphthous ulceration and mucosal fold thickening [50, 51, 60]. Recurrent disease may progress, and all the previously mentioned complications may occur within the areas of recurrence (Fig. 23A,B).

Crohn's colitis

This disease was first recognized as a distinct entity in 1959, when the pathologic findings were described by Lockart-Mummery and Morson and the radiographic features by Marshak and Wolf [61, 62]. Prior to this, most patients with Crohn's colitis carried the diagnosis of UC.

Partial colonic involvement by CD is more common than pancolitis. Disease of the colon and terminal ileum with sparing of the rectum and sigmoid is the most usual distribution [62–64].

Radiographically the subtlest mucosal changes are best demonstrated using double-contrast barium enema techniques. The earliest find is the aphthous ulcer (as seen elsewhere in this disease); this, as already described, appears as a shallow ulcer surrounded by normal mucosa (Fig. 24A).

Small irregular nodules may occur along the contour of the bowel with thickening of the haustra or asymmetric loss of haustra in areas of disease. There may be a concavity of the medial wall of the cecum, with normal-appearing cecal mucosa. This is most likely due to inflammation of the terminal ileum and mesentery causing an extrinsic pressure defect on the cecum.

With progression, ulcers may appear which are large and deep, and which undermine the mucosa [65] (Fig. 24A,B; Fig. 25). If they occur in a longitudinal and transverse orientation they give the bowel a cross-hatched or cobblestone appearance (Fig. 25). These tracts may parallel the bowel wall or may extend into adjacent bowel or other organs to produce fistulas (Fig. 26A,B).

As in the small bowel, discontinuous or skip areas of disease and asymmetric involvement of the bowel are frequent (Fig. 27A), but symmetrical and continuous involvement can occur (Fig. 27B). Pseudo-diverticula of localized distensible uninvolved

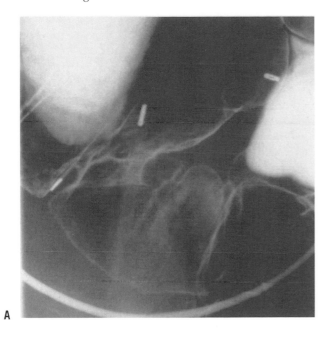

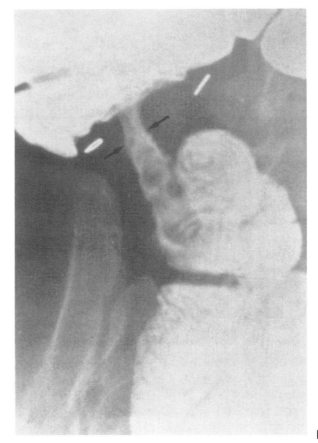

Figure 22. A: Recurrent Crohn's disease with aphthous ulcers at anastomosis on small bowel pneumocolon study. B: Short narrowed segment of recurrent disease (arrows).

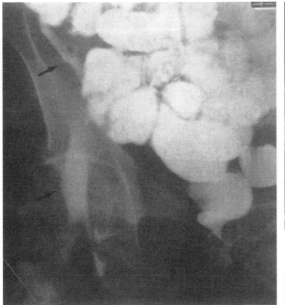

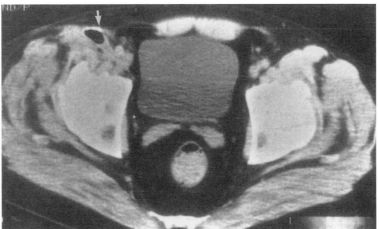

Figure 23. Recurrent ileal Crohn's disease with sinus tract. A: The tract is seen to pass inferiorly and into the right hip and thigh. B: CT scan.

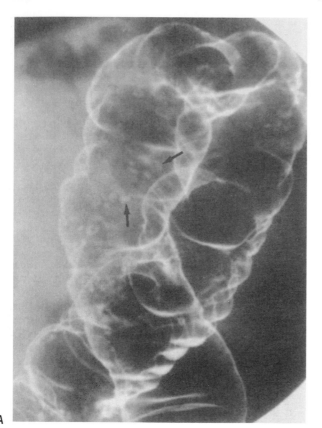

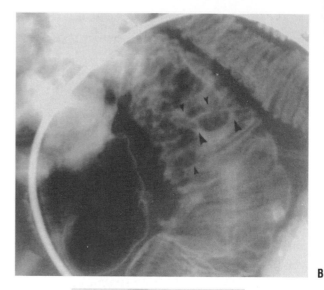

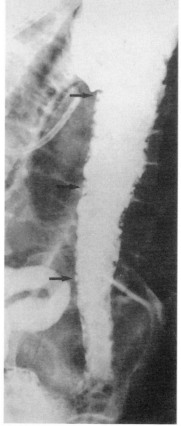

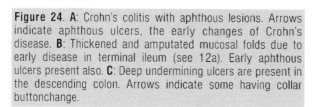

Figure 24. A: Crohn's colitis with aphthous lesions. Arrows indicate aphthous ulcers, the early changes of Crohn's disease. **B:** Thickened and amputated mucosal folds due to early disease in terminal ileum (see 12a). Early aphthous ulcers present also. **C:** Deep undermining ulcers are present in the descending colon. Arrows indicate some having collar buttonchange.

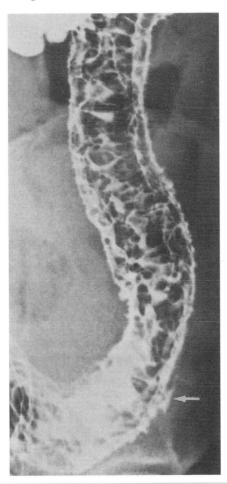

Figure 25. Crohn's colitis with cobblestone mucosal pattern. Cobblestoned mucosa of the descending colon. Arrow indicates deep ulceration into bowel wall.

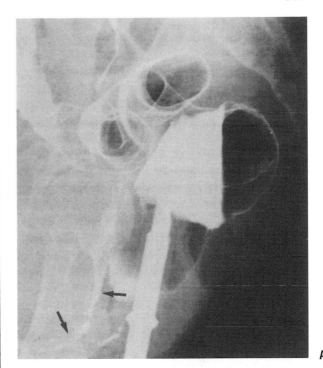

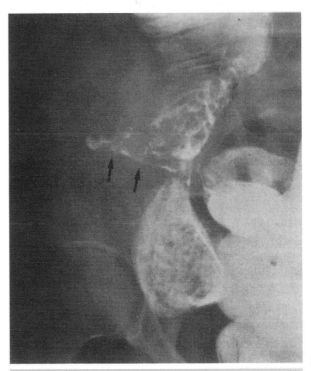

Figure 26. Crohn's colitis with fistulas. **A**: Rectovaginal fistula (arrows). **B**: Fistulous tract into R hip (arrows).

segments may be present (Fig. 28A,B). These need to be differentiated from the pseudosacculations seen in the colon in scleroderma, where the abnormal bowel segment balloons because of muscle atrophy.

The stenotic phase of the disease is characterized by bowel strictures which can be variable in length and configuration. Occasionally an asymmetric stricture, caused by pronounced transmural disease, may be difficult to differentiate radiologically from a colon cancer (Fig. 29). Obstruction secondary to colonic CD is unusual, and is more likely to occur with ileocolonic disease.

Filling defects may project into the lumen and the terms pseudopolyps, inflammatory polyps and post-inflammatory polyps have been used to describe them [66, 67]. Inflammatory polyps are not known

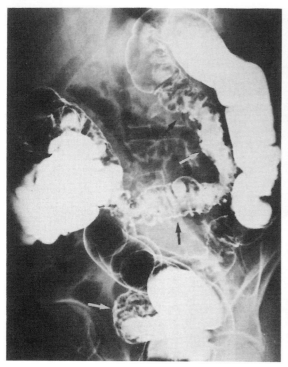

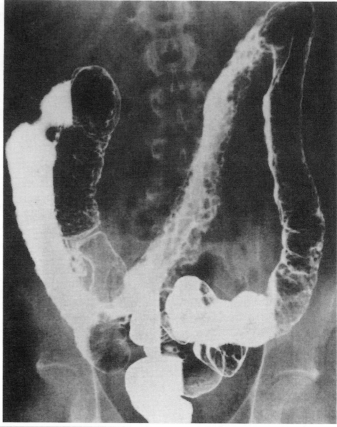

Figure 27. A: Asymmetric diseased segments are present in the sigmoid and transverse colon (arrows). **B**: Crohn's disease with uniform and symmetric bowel involvement, sparing only the rectum and distal sigmoid colon.

to have malignant potential. Adenomatous polyps, which are true neoplasms, are unusual in patients with CD. Perirectal disease is very common in patients with CD (Fig. 30). MRI is the method of choice for imaging such fistulas [68], and will show whether a fistulous tract or abscess is located above or below the levator ani muscle. It will also show whether it involves the rectal sphincters or ischioanal space. An abscess or fistula which crosses the levator ani muscle will often have two components. If surgery is required both will need to be drained.

As with CD of the small bowel, the radiographic picture often correlates poorly with the clinical status of the patient. There has been some evidence in the radiology literature that regression may be seen in patients with mild disease. Healing of aphthous ulcers and fissures after steroid treatment has been noted; unfortunately, follow-up suggests that such regressions are temporary. Radiographic resolution in more advanced cases has not been reported [69].

Complications

Fistulas

As with CD of the small bowel, colonic Crohn's may be complicated by fistulas to other bowel loops, to bladder, skin, vagina or urethra (Fig. 14A,B; Fig. 30). However, enterovesical fistulas are commoner with ileocolonic than pure colonic disease. Abscesses may also occur (Fig. 31).

Toxic megacolon

Toxic dilations or toxic megacolon is an acute life-threatening complication which may occur with Crohn's colitis [1, 12, 14, 70] (Fig. 32A,B). It is more likely to occur with pancolitis than with limited colonic involvement. Dilation of the mid-transverse colon above 6.5 cm can be seen on supine radiographs. The haustral pattern may be diminished and soft-tissue filling defects, caused by pseudopolyps, may protrude into the distended lumen. The mucosal margin may be irregular due to ulceration. Toxic

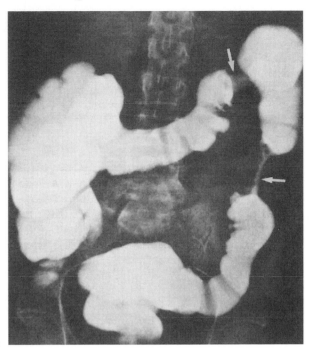

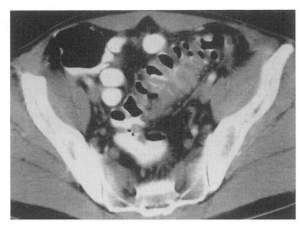

Figure 28. A: Skip areas of stenotic bowel involved by Crohn's disease (arrows). The asymmetric involvement of the superior aspect of the transverse colon has produced pseudo-diverticulae on the inferior aspect. **B**: Pseudosacculation of large bowel due to Crohn's disease.

megacolon was previously thought to occur only with UC, but it is now a well-recognized complication of Crohn's colitis. It may also occur in association with pseudomembranous colitis, typhoid fever, cholera, amebiasis, ischemia and Behçet's disease.

Serial plain films should be taken to evaluate changes in dilation and to look for sings of perforation. Contrast enemas should be avoided [11, 13]. The normal width of the transverse colon is 6 cm. In patients with toxic megacolon the width ranges from 6 to 15 cm, with a mean of 8 cm. Some people with fulminant disease may not have the capacity to dilate significantly due to thickening of the bowel wall. Therefore, progression or otherwise of dilation, rather than the absolute diameter, is the important factor to measure. This disease process is not limited to the transverse colon. When the patient is supine the transverse colon is anterior and the air column rises to this area. Decubitus views or CT will demonstrate distension of the remainder of the colon.

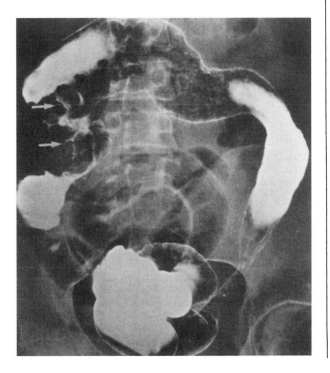

Figure 29. Crohn's colitis with strictures and pseudopolyps simulating carcinoma. Irregular narrowed segment with large pseudopolyps in the ascending colon (arrows) in a patient with Crohn's colitis sparing only the rectum. Lesion was benign on pathological examination.

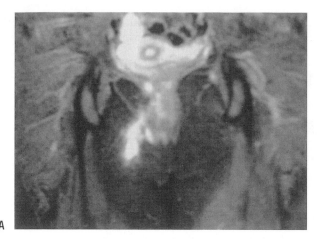

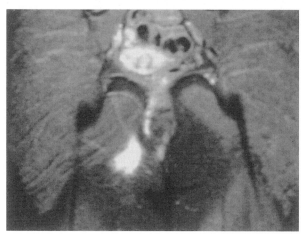

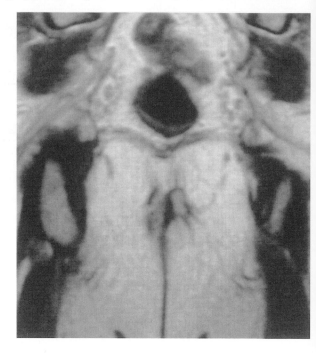

Figure 30. **A**: More posterior coronal STIR MRI scan showing right-sided transphincteric fistula in Crohn's disease. **B**: Coronal STIR MRI scan showing right-sided transphincteric fistula in Crohn's disease. **C**: Coronal T1 MRI scan showing left-sided extrasphincteric fistula in Crohn's disease.

Carcinoma

Carcinoma is a complication of Crohn's disease [71, 72]. It is most commonly seen in bypassed segments of bowel and in fistulous tracts. There is also an increased incidence of carcinoma around the anal canal in patients with Crohn's disease. As these areas are difficult to image, preoperative diagnosis is unusual. CT and MRI may be more helpful than contrast bowel studies in detecting these lesions. Carcinoma usually occurs in patients with long-standing disease, but may be discovered on first presentation. The appearance of carcinoma in the bowel with CD is more likely to be that of an infiltrative lesion rather than the more usual abrupt annular-type tumor seen in non-colitic patients (Fig. 33A,B).

Extraintestinal manifestations

Extraintestinal complications develop in a quarter to a third of patients with inflammatory bowel disease. These complications can be divided into three categories: (1) those intimately related to the activity or extent of disease such as arthritis or iritis; (2) those independent of the severity of diseas, such as sclerosing cholangitis or ankylosing spondylitis; and (3) those that result from inadequate or disordered intestinal function such as cholelithiasis or nephrolithiasis (Fig. 34).

Multiple imaging modalities may be necessary to show the full extent of the extraintestinal manifestations of CD. CT will show the majority of these manifestations. Asymptomatic sacroiliitis is shown on CT in 32% of patients [15]. In the hepatobiliary system, fatty liver is found on biopsy in 20–50% of patients and 30–50% of patients with CD develop gallstones which may be seen on ultrasound or CT.

About 1–2% of patients with CD will develop pancreatitis, and CD complications now account for 73% of all pyogenic psoas abscesses [15].

Genitourinary complications include calculus disease (Fig. 34), ureteral obstruction due to inflammatory masses involving the bladder (Fig. 35) [73, 74].

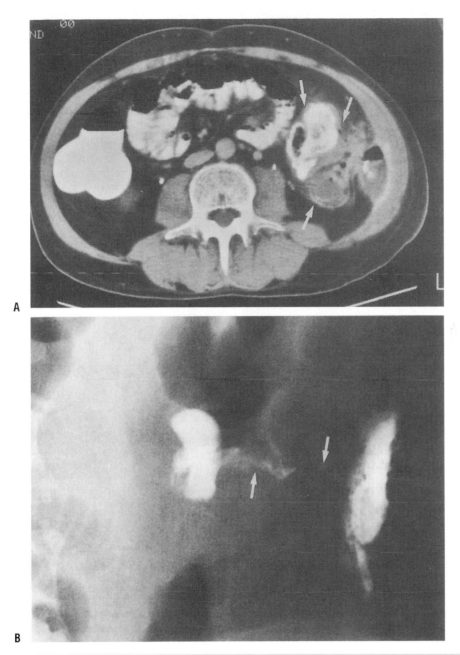

Figure 31. Crohn's colitis with abscess (CT findings). **A**: On CT a phlegmonous mass surrounding the descending colon is present (arrows). An air-fluid level and a small amount of contrast material is present in an abscess formed as a result of a sinus tract from the involved colon segment. **B**: The abscess was drained percutaneously and sinogram performed through drainage catheter shows fistulous communication to the colon (arrows).

The earliest mucosal changes, which are due to edema, are seen as a fine granularity as compared to the relatively featureless appearance of normal bowel (Fig. 37). Small superficial erosions may cause a more coarsely granular effect (Fig. 38). With progression discrete ulceration occurs. These ulcers may be deep and sometimes 'collar button' in configuration (Fig. 39), this effect is due to submucosal undermining.

The disease almost always involves the rectum and extends proximally for varying distances, or it may involve the entire colon (pancolitis). If only the rectum is involved (which occurs commonly) the disease may be referred to as ulcerative proctitis [79]. The rectum may be narrowed, and there is often an increase in the retrorectal space (Fig. 40). (This space usually measures less than 1 cm; it may also be increased in obesity, Cushing's disease, other IBD, radiation fibrosis, pelvic lipomatosis and in pelvic carcinomatosis).

UC involves the bowel in continuity and in a symmetrical manner (Fig. 41). There are no spared areas or pseudodiverticulae within the involved area (Fig. 42). The terminal ileum is spared, except in some cases of total colonic involvement (pancolitis) when the terminal ileum may be dilated, smooth or have multiple small ulcers (Fig. 43). In these patients the ileocecal valve is often patulous; these changes are commonly referred to as 'backwash ileitis' (Fig. 43).

Pseudopolyps, representing either edematous mounds of non-ulcerated tissue or overgrowth of regenerating mucosa, may be in the form of filiform polyps, mucosal bridges or sessile filling defects [66, 67, 83] (Fig. 44). Occasionally, large masses of coalescent polyps can be present and may simulate a neoplasm [84, 85]. Adenomatous polyps occur rarely (Fig. 45).

Loss of haustration and narrowing of bowel lumen may occur in acute recent-onset disease or may be seen in long-standing chronic colitis (Figs. 41 and 42). The colon in chronic UC becomes shortened with depressed flexures, it lacks distensibility and is tubular in appearance (Fig. 42B).

Unlike Crohn's colitis, radiographic remission of findings may correlate with clinical remission. In early disease the ahaustral, ulcerated, non-distensible portion of involved bowel may revert to a normal X-ray appearance when the patients are in remission [86–90]. If the original episode of colitis was severe, postinflammatory pseudopolyps may persist as the

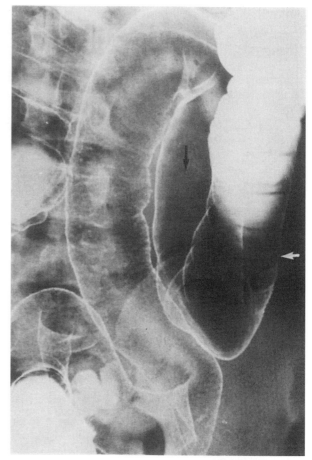

A

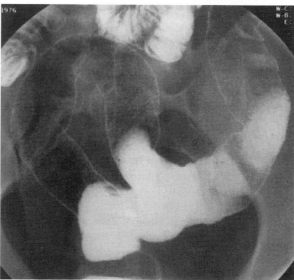

B

Figure 37. Ulcerative colitis with fine granular mucosal pattern. **A:** Rather than the normal featureless mucosa of the distal descending and proximal colon (arrows), the rectum and distal sigmoid show the granular pattern of ulcerative colitis. **B:** Early ulcerative colitis with granular mucosa.

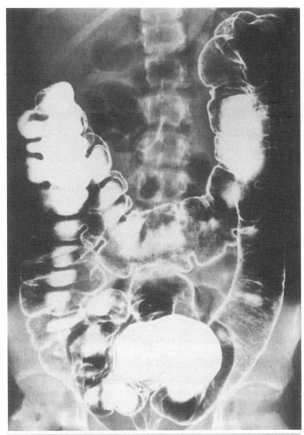

Figure 38. Pancolitis with preservation of haustral pattern.

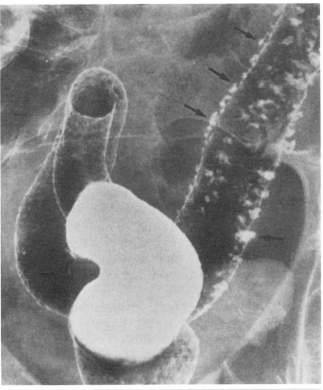

Figure 39. Ulcerative colitis with discrete ulceration. Arrows indicate deep ulcerations, some of which are undermined and collar button in configuration. Note the coarsely granular background mucosa and the symmetry and continuity of involvement.

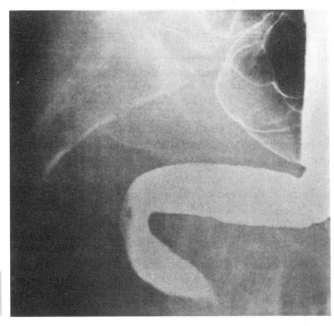

Figure 40. Ulcerative proctitis. Narrowing of the rectum, pseudopolyps along the posterior rectal wall, and marked increase in the retrorectal space.

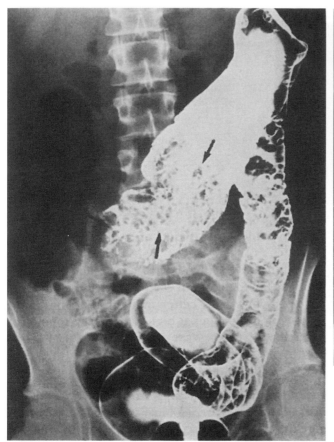

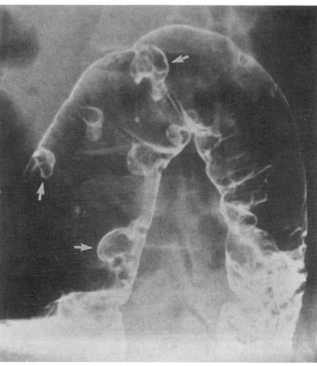

A

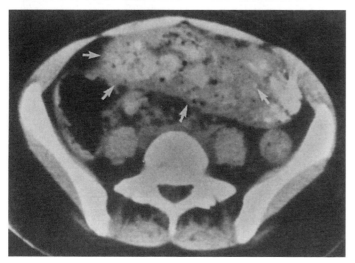

B

Figure 45. Ulcerative colitis in remission, with masses of pseudopolyps causing partial obstruction. **A**: Ulcerative colitis in remission with obstruction to the retrograde flow of barium due to giant pseudopolyposis of the colon (arrows). **B**: CT in the region of the transverse colon shows mass of pseudopolyps with a small amount of contrast passing between them (arrows). **C**: Arrows show sessile pseudopolyps in this same patient in the splenic flexure. There is no mucosal ulceration and the haustral pattern is normal as the colitis is in remission.

only radiographic abnormality during a remission phase (Fig. 45).

CT is not recommended as a primary means of diagnosing acute UC because of its low diagnostic sensitivity for early disease [15]. In chronic UC the muscularis mucosa becomes markedly hypertrophied and the submucosa becomes thickened because of the deposition of fat [15] (Fig. 46). The increase in the presacral space can be appreciated as due to a combination of fat proliferation and rectal contraction [86] (Fig. 46B). Carcinoma, if present, may be seen as irregular thickening of bowel wall with infiltration of the pericolic fat. The mesenteric and retroperitoneal fat abnormalities seen in patients with CD do not occur in UC.

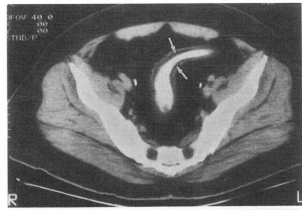

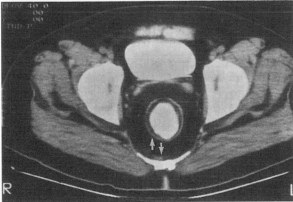

Figure 46. Ulcerative colitis-CT appearance. **A**: The bowel is ahaustral with a thickened wall which contains a zone of fat density (arrows). **B**: The rectum also has a thickened wall including an area of fat. There is a large amount of fat surrounding the rectum which causes an increase in the retrorectal space (arrows).

Toxic megacolon

Toxic megacolon is seen more frequently with UC than with other IBD. It may be the first manifestation of UC or may occur with long-standing disease. Follow-up with plain films is adequate [12, 14]. The transverse colon appears dilated on supine views, but ascending and descending portions of bowel wall also appear dilated if decubitus views are obtained (Fig. 47). When the transverse colon is dilated to greater than 6 cm haustration may be absent, and the margin of the bowel may be irregular due to pseudopolyps or ulceration; linear streaks or air in the bowel wall should alert the radiologist to impending perforations. Care should be taken to look for subtle signs of free air, which indicate that colonic perforation has already occurred (Fig. 47B).

Carcinoma

Carcinoma of the colon is a well-known complication of UC [72, 91]. The reported incidence in the radiology literature covers a wide range. It is accepted, however, that long-standing disease (morer than 10 years) and disease involving a long segment of colon (usually pancolitis) increase the risk for development of colonic cancer. Occasional patients may develop carcinoma after only 7–10 years of disease. Studies indicate that approximately 3–4% of all patients with UC develop carcinoma. This number rises to over 13% when considering people with pancolitis [72].

Diagnosis of colon cancer in people with UC is often difficult radiologically. Cancer in this group may have the appearance of a stricture and can be multicentric (Fig. 48). These cancers may also be flat and infiltrating, better seen on colonoscopy than on radiology. Dysplastic lesions may appear as a solitary nodule or a group of nodules with a radiographic appearance identical to pseudopolyps [92, 93].

Even the best double-contrast examinations of the colon may fail to detect an early cancer. Colonoscopy with biopsy is the better method for follow-up in UC patients at high risk for developing colonic carcinoma.

Extraintestinal manifestations

Extraintestinal manifestations of UC include a long list of hepatobiliary abnormalities. These range in severity from fatty infiltration of liver to cholangio-

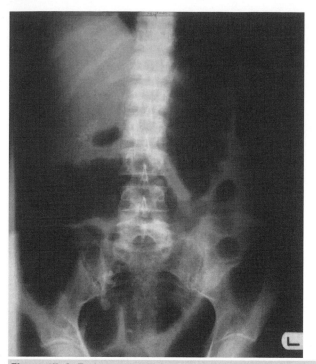

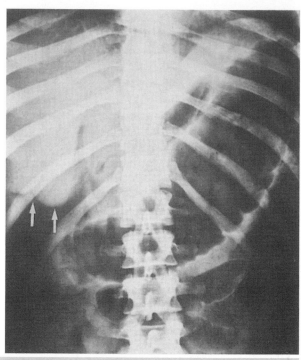

A   B

Figure 47. A: Toxic megacolon with ulcerative colitis (note presence of gallstones). **B:** Ulcerative colitis with toxic megacolon and colonic perforation. Arrows indicate subhepatic air clearly outlining the gallbladder and liver margin as a result of large bowel perforation.

carcinoma [72, 73, 75]. Primary sclerosing cholangitis is seen in approximately 5.5% of patients with substantive UC; 65–75% of patients with sclerosing cholangitis have UC. Hepatic dysfunction may either precede the diagnosis of UC or may present years after colectomy for UC. If abnormal liver function tests suggest cholangitis, the biliary tree can be imaged with ERCP (endoscopic retrograde cholangiopancreatography) or transhepatic cholangiography (PTC) [94]. Magnetic resonance cholangiopancreatography (MRCP) is beginning to replace both these techniques: On these techniques short multifocal strictures give the biliary tree a beaded appearance (Fig. 49). Fine mural irregularities cause the duct margin to have a blurred appearance. In most instances (80%) the extrahepatic as well as the intrahepatic biliary tree is involved. CT may show focal intrahepatic biliary dilation which is discontinuous with thickening of the walls of the extrahepatic bile ducts (Fig. 50).

Interventional radiologic procedures such as biliary drainage with stent placement and stricture dilation may be need in patients with advanced changes of sclerosing cholangitis.

Bile duct carcinoma may develop in patients with UC and sclerosing cholangitis, or it may develop without preceding cholangitis (Fig. 51). In patients who have developed cholangiocarcinoma the biliary tree may show changes which are often difficult to differentiate from those of sclerosing cholangitis alone. These changes are: (1) an annular constricting lesion with proximal dilation, (2) diffuse infiltration of the biliary tree, or (3) an intraluminal polypoid mass lesion. These findings are best seen on MRCP or ERCP. These tumors are often infiltrating, but not bulky, which means they are often inapparent on CT.

The arthritides seen in patients with UC are similar to those seen with CD.

Pulmonary abnormalities associated with both UC and CD can present years after the onset of the disease and they can involve any part of the lung. In one series 13/14 showed high-resolution CT (HRCT) changes like those of bronchiectasis; one patient had changes with peripheral reticular change similar to cryptogenic fibrosing alveolitis [95]. Early recognition of pulmonary change is important as these changes can be strikingly steroid-responsive.

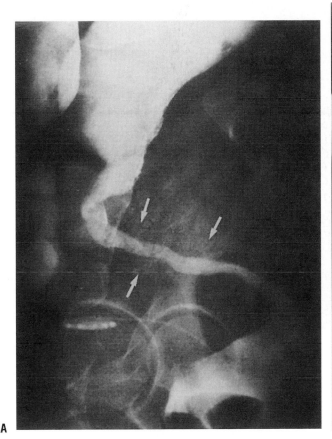

A

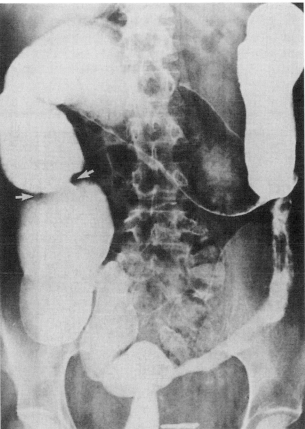

B

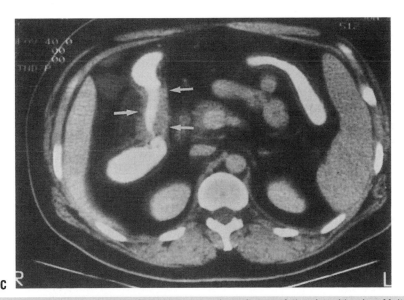

C

Figure 48. Ulcerative colitis with colon carcinoma. **A**: Long strictured carcinoma of the sigmoid colon. Multiple calcifications are present in this mucinous tumor (arrows). **B**: Supine radiograph on same patient as in A shows benign stricture of ascending colon (arrows). Also note backwash ileitis and patulous ileocecal valve. **C**: CT shows infiltration of the wall of the ascending colon (arrows) due to carcinoma in patient with ulcerative colitis. Note smooth ahaustral splenic flexure.

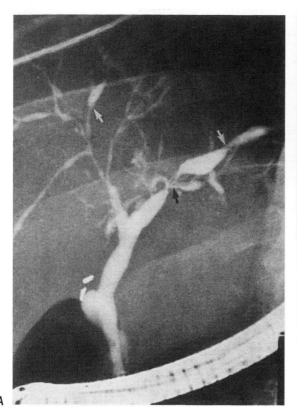

A

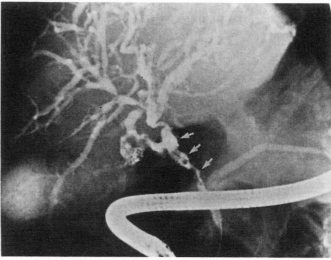

B

Figure 49. Ulcerative colitis with sclerosing cholangitis (ERCP). **A**: Diffuse involvement of the intrahepatic biliary tree with alternating segments of ductal stenosis and dilation (arrows). **B**: Mural irregularities of the extrahepatic biliary tree with diverticula-like outpouchings.

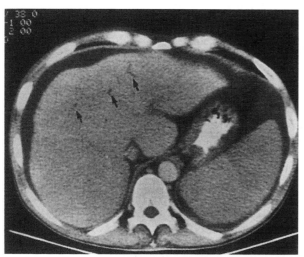

Figure 50. Ulcerative colitis with sclerosing cholangitis (CT). Arrows indicate discontinuous ductal dilatation due to sclerosing cholangitis. Ascites and splenomegaly are present due to cirrhosis and portal hypertension.

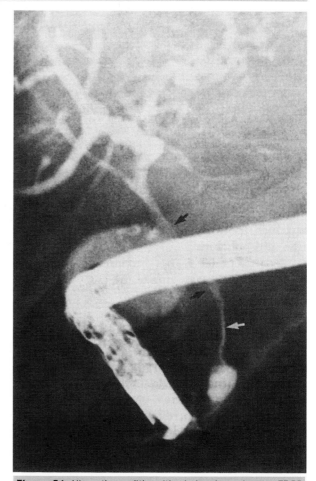

Figure 51. Ulcerative colitis with cholangiocarcinoma. ERCP shows long, irregularly narrowed common bile duct (arrows) due to infiltrating cholangiocarcinoma.

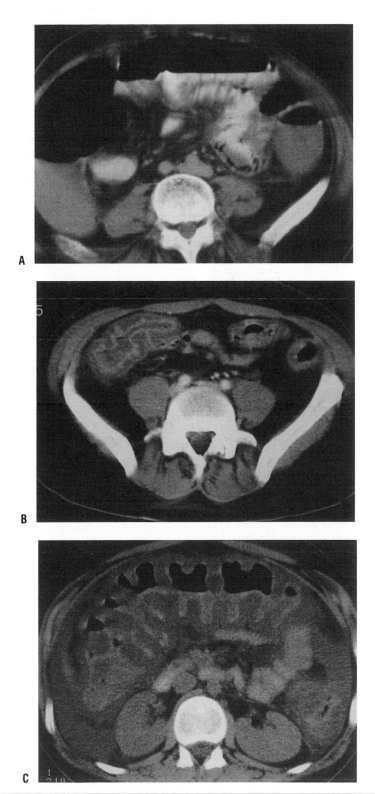

Figure 52. **A**: CT with ischemic colitis and jejunitis. **B**: Pseudomembranous colitis with accordion sign. **C**: Typhilitis in an immunocompromized patient causing marked thickening of bowel wall.

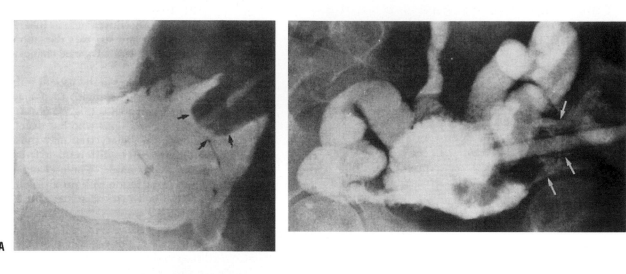

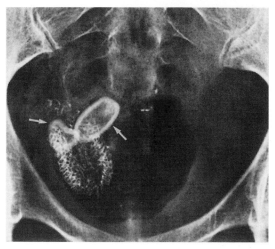

Figure 53. Koch pouch. **A**: The pouch is created of ileal segments. The nipple valve is indicated by arrows. The shaggy luminal margin suggests pouchitis may be present. **B**: Leakage of contrast from the pouch (arrows) indicates incompetence of the nipple valve. **C**: Two large calcified enteroliths (arrows) have formed in the gas-filled Koch pouch probably as a result of stasis.

Differential diagnosis

CT gives a unique diagnostic perspective in IBD. It is frequently the first imaging test used, especially in acute disease. There are several features on CT which may help to differentiate different types of inflammatory disease. In CD the mean colonic wall thickness is significantly greater than in UC [56]. Fibrofatty proliferation (Fig. 19A) is seen exclusively in CD. Small bowel involvement isC most frequent in CD but may occur in up to 36% of patients with infectious disease.

Ten of 13 patients with ischemic colitis had disease limited to the left side of colon [56] (Fig. 52A). CT findings can be highly suggestive for pseudomembranous colitis (PMC). Classically these show marked mucosal thickening with average width 15 mm (Fig. 52B). The mucosal thickening is low attenuation, and strips of contrast medium trapped between the swollen haustra produce the so-called accordion sign [96]. The colonic wall thickening is approximately twice that of UC, ischemic or infectious colitis.

Typhilitis (Fig. 52C) classically occurs in neutrapenic patients. In UC the bowel wall may have a heterogeneous appearance due to fatty infiltration (Fig. 46).

Imaging of surgically-treated patients

Total proctocolectomy is the definitive treatment for patients with UC who are refractory to conservative management or who have developed complications such as progressive toxic megacolon or carcinoma.

Koch was among the first to describe an operation to create a continent ileostomy [97]. With the Koch pouch a reservoir is created from distal ileal loops. An inverted nipple valve is fashioned to aid continence and the patient intubates the pouch at intervals to empty it (Fig. 53). Complications include incontinence due to leaking through and around the nipple, internal fistulas and inflammation of the mucosa of the pouch, 'pouchitis'. This procedure is not recommended for patients with CD because of the likelihood of recurrent disease in the small bowel. Radiographic examination of the pouch is possible by intubating it, injecting contrast and air to obtain double-contrast radiographs (Fig. 53). CT can also be used to assess these pouches after filling them with air or dilute contrast medium [98–100].

More recently the ileoanal reservoir has become a more frequently used method for creating a continent ileostomy [101–103]. This method eliminates the need for a permanent stoma and preserves anal sphincter function. Several different surgical procedures are described using the same type of staged procedure (J-pouch, S-pouch). The pouch can be imaged using a contrast enema, by CT or by nuclear medicine technique. Immediate complications of this technique include anastomotic leak, obstruction, abscesses or pouchitis. Late complications which may be seen are obstruction and pouchitis.

Again this pouch is not recommended for patients with CD due to the risk of recurrent disease.

References

1. Rice RP. Plain abdominal film roentgenographic diagnosis of ulcerative diseases of the colon. Am J Roentgenol 1968; 104: 544–50.
2. Prantera C, Lorenzetti R, Cerro P, Davoli M, Brancato G, Fanucci A. The plain abdominal film accurately estimates extent of active ulcerative colitis. J Clin Gastroenterol 1991; 13: 231–4.
3. Laufer I. The radiologic demonstration of early changes in ulcerative colitis by double contrast technique. Can Assoc Radiol J 1975; 26: 116–21.
4. Laufer I, Hamilton J. The radiological differentiation between ulcerative and granulomatous colitis by double contrast radiology. Am J Gastroenterol 1976; 66: 259–69.
5. Brahme F, Fork F-T. Roentgenology of the colon in Crohn's disease. Radiologe 1976; 16: 489–96.
6. Laufer I. Air contrast studies of the colon in inflammatory bowel disease. Crit Rev Diagn Imaging 1977; 8: 421–47.
7. Kelvin FM, Oddson TA, Rice RP, Garbutt JT, Bradenham BP. Double contrast barium enema in Crohn's disease and ulcerative colitis. Am J Roentgenol 1978; 131: 207–13.
8. Williams HJ Jr, Stephens DH, Carlson HC. Double-contrast radiography: colonic inflammatory disease. Am J Roentgenol 1981; 137: 315–22.
9. Winthrop JD, Balfe DM, Shackelford GD, McAlister WH, Rosenblum JL, Siegel MJ. Ulcerative and granulomatous colitis in children. Radiology 1985; 154: 657–60.
10. Freeny PC. Crohn's disease and ulcerative colitis. Postgrad Med 1986; 80: 139–54.
11. Wruble LD, Bronstein MW. Toxic dilatation of the colon following barium enema examination during the quiescent stage of chronic ulcerative colitis. Am J Dig Dis 1968; 13: 918–24.
12. Diner WC, Barnhard, HJ. Toxic megacolon. Semin Roentgenol 1973; 8: 433–4.
13. Goldberg HI. The barium enema and toxic megacolon: cause–effect relationship? (Letter). Gastroenterology 1975; 68: 617–18.
14. Halpert RD. Toxic dilatation of the colon. Radiol Clin N Am 1987;25: 147–55.
15. Gore RM, Balthazar EJ, Ghahremani GG, Miller FH. CT features of ulcerative colitis and Crohn's disease. Am J Roentgenol 1996; 187: 3–15.
16. Cohen AJ, Rowen SJ, Pelod D, Dana ER. The role of antegrade barium studies in the evaluation of colitis. Am J Gastroenterol 1986; 81: 656–61.

17. Ekberg O, Lindstrom C. Superficial lesions in Crohn's disease of the small bowel. Gastrointest Radiol 1979; 4: 389–93.
18. Herlinger H. The small bowel enema and the diagnosis of Crohn's disease. Radiol Clin N Am 1982; 20: 721–42.
19. Ott DJ, Chen YM, Gelfand DW, Van Swearingen F, Munitz HA. Detailed per-oral small bowel examination vs. enteroclysis. Radiology 1985; 155: 29–34.
20. Deignan RW, Malone DE, Taylor S et al. Improving visualisation of distal and terminal ileum during the small bowel meal: an evaluation of fluoroscopic manoeuvres. Clin Radiol 1995; 50: 548–52.
21. Fitzgerald EJ, Thompson GT, Somers SS, Franic SF. Pneumocolon as an aid in small-bowel studies. Clin Radiol 1985; 36: 633–7.
22. Gore RM, Marn CS, Kirby DF, Vogelzang RL, Neiman HL. CT findings in ulcerative, granulomatous and indeterminate colitis. Am J Roentgenol 1984; 143: 279–84.
23. Riddlesburger MM Jr. CT of complicated inflammatory bowel disease in children. Pediatr Radiol 1985; 15: 384–7.
24. Gore RM, Cohen MI, Vogelzang RL, Neiman HL, Tsang T-K. Value of computed tomography in the detection of complications of Crohn's disease. Dig Dis Sci 1985; 30: 701–9.
25. Gore RM. Cross-sectional imaging of inflammatory bowel disease. Radiol Clin N Am 1987; 25: 115–31.
26. Fishman EK, Wolf JJ, Jones B, Bayless TM, Siegelman SS. CT evaluation of Crohn's disease: effect on patient management. Am J Roentgenol 1987; 148: 537–40.
27. Orel SG, Rubesin SE, Jones B, Fishman EK, Bayless TM, Siegelman SS. Computed tomography vs barium studies in an acutely symptomatic patient with Crohn's disease. J Comput Assist Tomogr 1987; 11: 1009–16.
28. Jabra AA, Fishman EK, Taylor GA. Crohn disease in the paediatric patient: CT evaluation. Radiology 1991; 179: 495–8.
29. Yeh H-C, Rabinowitz JG. Granulomatous enterocolitis: findings by ultrasonography and computed tomography. Radiology 1983; 149: 253–9.
30. Goldberg HI, Gord RM, Margulis AR, Moss AA, Baker EL. Computed tomography in the evaluation of Crohn disease. Am J Roentgenol 1983; 140: 277–82.
31. Kaftori JK, Pery M, Kleinhaus U. Ultrasonography in Crohn's disease. Gastrointest Radiol 1984; 9: 137–42.
32. Buxton-Thomas MS, Dickinson RJ, Maltby P, Hunter JO, Wright EP. Evaluation of indium scintigraphy in patients with active inflammatory bowel disease. Gut 1984; 25: 1372–5.
33. Fotherby KJ, Wriaight EP, Garforth H, Hunter O. Indium-111 leucocyte scintigraphy in the investigation and management of inflammatory bowel disease. Postgrad Med J 1986; 62: 457–62.
34. Froelich JW. Nuclear medicine imaging of inflammatory bowel disease. Radiol Clin N Am 1987; 25: 133–41.
35. Park RHR, McKillop JH, Duncan A, MacKenzie JF, Russell RI. Can 111 indium autologous mixed leucocyte scanning accurately assess disease extent and activity in Crohn's disease? Gut 1988; 29: 821–5.
36. Scholmerich J, Schmidt E, Schumichen C, Billmann P, Schmidt H, Gerok W. Scintigraphic assessment of bowel involvement and disease activity in Crohn's disease using technique 99m-hexamethyl propylene amine oxine as leukocyte label. Gastroenterology 1988; 95: 1287–93.
37. Laniado M, Makowiec F, Dammann F, Jehle EC, Claussen CD, Starlinger M. Perianal complications of Crohn disease: MR imaging findings. Eur Radiol 1997; 7: 1035–42.
38. Maglinte DT, Siegelman ES, Kelvin FM. MR Enteroclysis: the future of small bowel imaging? Radiology 2000; 215: 639–41.
39. Umshaden HW, Szolar D, Gasser J, Umschaden M, Haselback H. Small bowel disease: comparison of MR enteroclysis images with conventional enteroclysis and surgical findings. Radiology 2000; 215: 717–25
40. Maccioni F, Viscido A, Broglia L et al. Evaluation of Crohn disease activity with magnetic resonance imaging. Abdom Imaging 2000; 25: 219–28.
41. Carroll K. Crohn's disease: new imaging techniques. Baillieres Clin Gastroenterol 1998; 12: 35–72.
42. Harper RAK. The radiological spectrum of Crohn's disease. Proc R Soc Med 1971; 64: 43–8.
43. Bagby RJ, Rogers JV Jr, Hobbs C. Crohn's disease of the esophagus, stomach and duodenum: a review with emphasis on the radiographic findings. South Med J 1972; 65: 515–23.
44. Cynn W-S, Chon H, Gureghian PA, Levin BL. Crohn's disease of the esophagus. Am J Roentgenol Rad Ther Nucl Med 1975; 125: 359–64.
45. Levine MS. Crohn's disease of the upper gastrointestinal tract. Radiol Clin N Am 1987; 25: 79–91.
46. Javors BR, Wecksell A, Fagelman D. Crohn's disease: less common radiographic manifestations. Radiographics 1988; 8: 259–75.
47. Farman J, Faegenburg D, Dallemand S, Chen C-K. Crohn's disease of the stomach: the 'rams's horn' sign. Am J Roentgenol Rad Ther Nucl Med 1975; 123: 242–51.
48. Kokal W, Pickleman J, Steinburg M, Jameson P, Banich FE. Gastrocolic fistula in Crohn's disease. Surg Gynecol Obstet 1978; 146: 701–4.
49. Nelson SW. Some interesting and unusual manifestations of Crohn's disease ('regional enteritis') of the stomach, duodenum and small intestine. Am J Roentgenol Rad Ther Nucl Med 1969; 107: 86–101.
50. Marshak RH. Granulomatous disease of the intestinal tract (Crohn's disease). Radiology 1975; 114: 3–22.
51. Glick SN. Crohn's disease of the small intestine. Radiol Clin N Am 1987; 25: 25–45.
52. Glass RE, Ritchie JK, Lennard-Jones JE, Hawley PR, Todd IP. Internal fistulas in Crohn's disease. Dis Colon Rectum 1985; 28: 557–61.
53. Katz I, Fischer RM. Enteroliths complicating regional enteritis. A report of two cases. Am J Roentgenol Rad Ther Nucl Med 1957; 78: 653–61.
54. Brettner A, Euphrat EJ. Radiological significance of primary enterolithiasis. Radiology 1970; 94: 283–8.
55. Gast P, Belaiche J. Rectal endosonography in inflammatory bowel disease: differential diagnosis and prediction of remission. Endoscopy 1999; 31: 158–66.
56. Philpotts LE, Heiken JP, Westcott MA, Gore RM. Colitis: use of CT findings in differential diagnosis. Radiology 1994; 190: 445–9.
57. Goldman SM, Fishman EK, Gatewood OMB, Jones B, Siegelmann SS. CT in the diagnosis of enterovesical fistulae. Am J Roentgenol 1985; 144: 1229–33.
58. Gossios KJ, Tsianos EV. Crohn disease: CT findings after treatment. Abdom Imaging 1997; 22: 160–3.
59. Goldberg HI, Caruthers SB Jr, Nelson JA, Singleton JW. Radiographic findings of the national cooperative Crohn's disease study. Gastroenterology 1979; 77: 925–37.
60. Ekberg O, Fork F-T, Hildell J. Predictive value of small bowel radiography for recurrent Crohn disease Am J Roentgenol 1980; 135: 1051–5.
61. Lockhart-Mummery HE, Morson BC. Crohn's disease (regional enteritis) of the large intestine and its distinction from ulcerative colitis.Gut 1960; 1: 87–105
62. Marshak RH, Wolf BS, Eliasoph J. Segmental colitis. Radiology 1959; 73: 707–16.
63. Joffe N, Antonioli DA, Bettmann MA, Goldman H. Focal granulomatous (Crohn's) colitis: radiologic–pathologic correlation. Gastrointest Radiol 1978; 3: 73–80.

64. Marshak RH, Lindner AE, Maklansky D. Granulomatous colitis. Mt Sinai J Med 1979; 46: 431–54.
65. Goldberg HI. Focal ulcerations of colon in granulomatous colitis. Am J Roentgenol Rad Ther Nucl Med 1967; 101: 296–300.
66. Blum JC, Kelvin FM. Radiologic spectrum of polypoid lesions in ulcerative colitis and Crohn's disease. South Med J 1981; 74: 850–5.
67. Lichtenstein JE. Radiologic–pathologic correlation of inflammatory bowel disease. Radiol Clin N Am 1987; 25: 3–24.
68. O'Donovan AN, Somers S, Farrow R, Mernagh JR, Sridhar S. MR imaging of anorectal Crohn disease: a pictorial essay. Radiographics 1997; 17: 101–7.
69. Brahme F, Fork F-T. Dynamic aspects of colonic Crohn's disease. Radiologe 1975; 15: 463–8.
70. Siskind BN, Burrell MI, Klein MI, Princenthal RA. Toxic dilatation in Crohn disease with CT correlation. J. Comput Assist Tomogr 1985; 9: 193–5.
71. Miller TL, Skucas J, Gudex D, Listinsky C. Bowel cancer characteristics in patients with regional enteritis. Gastrointest Radiol 1987; 12: 45–52.
72. Feczko PJ. Malignancy complicating inflammatory bowel disease. Radiol Clin N Am 1987; 25: 157–74.
73. Williams SM, Harned RK. Hepatobiliary complications of inflammatory bowel disease. Radiol Clin N Am 1987; 25: 175–88.
74. Banner MP. Genitourinary complications of inflammatory bowel disease. Radiol Clin N Am 1987; 25: 199–209.
75. Feczko PJ. Intestinal and extraintestinal complications of inflammatory bowel disease. Radiol Clin N Am 1987; 25: 145–6.
76. Bjorkengren AG, Resnick D, Sartoris DJ. Enteropathic arthropathies. Radiol Clin N Am 1987; 25: 189–98.
77. Rioux M, Gagnon J. Imaging modalities in the puzzling world of inflammatory bowel disease. Abdom Imaging 1997; 22: 173–4.
78. Fennessy J, Sparberg M, Kirsner JB. Early roentgen manifestations of mild ulcerative colitis and proctitis. Radiology 1966; 87: 848–58.
79. Sparberg M, Fennessy J, Kirsner JB. Ulcerative proctitis and mild ulcerative colitis: a study of 220 patients. Medicine 1966; 45: 391–412.
80. Bartram CI. Radiology in the current assessment of ulcerative colitis. Gastrointest Radiol 1977; 1: 383–92.
81. Bartram CI, Walmsley K. A radiological and pathological correlation of the mucosal changes in ulcerative colitis. Clin Radiol 1978; 29: 323–8.
82. Zeman R, Burrell M, Gold JA. Ulcerative colitis in the elderly. Am J Roentgenol 1980; 135: 164–6.
83. Goldberger LE, Neely HR, Stammer JL. Large mucosal bridges. An unusual roentgenographic manifestation of ulcerative colitis. Gastrointest Radiol 1978; 3: 81–3.
84. Keating JW Jr, Mindell HJ. Localized giant pseudopolyposis in ulcerative colitis. Am J Roentgenol 1976; 126: 1178–80.
85. Lesher DT, Phillips JC, Rabinowitz JG. Pseudopolyposis as the only manifestation of ulcerative colitis. Am J Gastroenterol 1978; 70: 670–2.
86. Gore RM. Colonic contour changes in chronic ulcerative colitis: reappraisal of some old concepts. Am J Roentgenol 1992; 158: 59–61.
87. Kolodny M. Reversible right colonic strictures in chronic ulcerative colitis. Radiology 1970; 97: 83–4.
88. Keeley F, Gohel VK, Hodes PJ. A roentgenologic remission in ulcerative colitis. Am J Roentgenol Rad Ther Nucl Med 1961; 86: 906–10.
89. Goldberg HI, Carbone JV, Margulis AR. Roentgenographic reversibility of ulcerative colitis in children treated with steroid enemas. Am J Roentgenol Rad Ther Nucl Med 1968; 103: 365–79.
90. Lennard-Jones JE. Reversibility of some radiological abnormalities in inflammatory disease of the colon. Proc R Soc Med 1970; 63: 66–8.
91. James EM, Carlson HC. Chronic ulcerative colitis and colon cancer: can radiographic appearance predict survival patterns? Am J Roentgenol 1978; 130: 825–30.
92. Frank PH, Riddell RH, Feczko PJ, Levin B. Radiological detection of colonic dysplasia (precarcinoma) in chronic ulcerative colitis. Gatrointest Radiol 1978; 3: 209–19.
93. Hooyman JR, MacCarty RL, Carpenter HA, Schroeder KW, Carlson HC. Radiographic appearance of mucosal dysplasia associated with ulcerative colitis. Am J Roentgenol 1987; 149: 47–51.
94. Kolmannskog F, Aakhus T, Fausa O et al. Cholangiographic findings in ulcerative colitis. Acta Radiol Diagn 1981; 22: 151–7.
95. Mahadeva R, Walsh G, Flower CD, Shneerson JM. Clinical and radiological characteristics of lung disease in inflammatory bowel disease. Eur Resp J 2000; 15: 41–8.
96. Ros PR, Buetow PC, Pantograg-Brown L, Forsmark CE, Sobin LH. Pseudomembranous colitis. Radiology 1996; 198: 1–9.
97. Stephens DH, Mantell BE, Kelly KA. Radiology of the continent ileostomy. Am J Roentgenol 1979; 132: 717–21.
98. Hillard AE, Mann FE, Becker JM, Nelson JA. The ileoanal J pouch: radiographic evaluation. Radiology 1985; 155: 591–4.
99. Kremers PW, Scholz FJ, Schoetz DJ Jr, Veidenheimer MC, Coller JA. Radiology of the ileoanal reservoir. Am J Roentgenol 1985; 145: 559–67.
100. Thoeni RF, Fell SC, Engelstad B, Schrock TB. Ileoanal pouches: comparison of CT, scintigraphy, and contrast enemas for diagnosing postsurgical complications. Am J Roentgenol 1990; 154: 73–8.

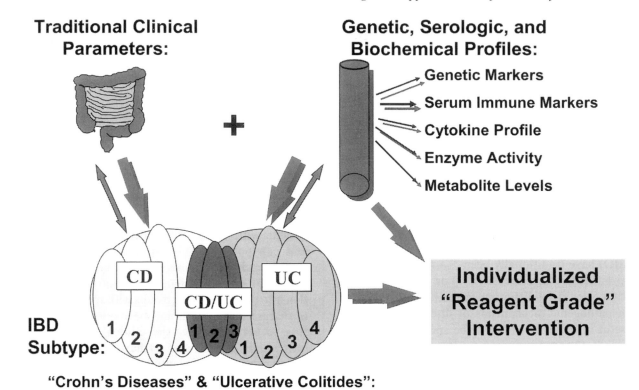

Figure 1. 'Reagent-grade' therapeutic intervention. In the near future it is foreseeable that when patients present to the clinician their traditional clinical parameters will be combined with their specific genetic (i.e. HLA, TNF microsatellite, TPMT genotype), serologic (i.e. immune markers), and biochemical (i.e. TPMT activity, drug metabolite) profiles. Based on the composite profile, the specific subtype of CD and UC could be determined and the most appropriate individualized treatment intervention selected (Modified from ref. 97).

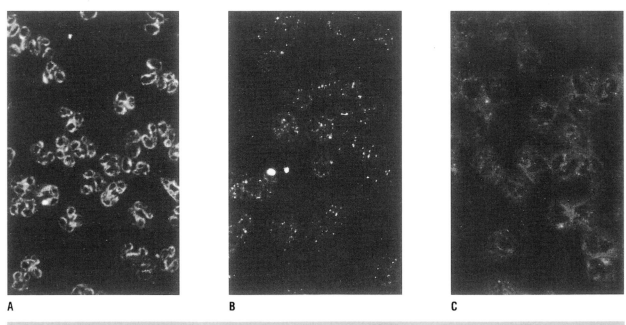

Figure 2. Immunofluorescence staining patterns of sera from patients with IBD. Three subtypes of serum ANCA expression have been characterized in patients with IBD based on the predominant immunofluorescent (IIF) microscopy staining patterns of neutrophils. **A**: The characteristic perinuclear highlighting of pANCA. **B**: Cytoplasmic highlighting of cANCA. **C**: The newly-described diffuse 'speckled' staining pattern over the entire neutrophil of sANCA.

Serum ANCA determination and ANCA subtype characterization in IBD

While the incidence of ANCA detection in IBD has varied greatly, the reported prevalence in most series ranges between 50% and 80% in UC and 10–50% in CD [10, 12, 17–44]. Differences in patient populations including ethnicity and referral center bias may account for some discrepancies between studies. Methodologic differences, however, are most likely the greatest contributor to the variation in results, as the techniques used to identify serum ANCA are numerous and varied, as are criteria used to define a positive result. This point is best highlighted by the results of a recent study undertaken at the Mayo Clinic in which serum blood samples from the same 296 patients from a population-based cohort with confirmed IBD were sent to six different US and foreign laboratories to assess the prevalence of pANCA and ASCA (Table 1) [42]. Most commercial and even many research laboratories use techniques and criteria originally designed to identify the ANCA found in patients with *vasculitis*. The ANCA assays of most clinical laboratories are validated to *vasculitides*, such as Wegener's granulomatosis rather than IBD, and are optimized to detect cANCA. In many reports ANCA expression in IBD is determined by IIF alone. Other clinical and research laboratories use specific enzyme-linked immunosorbent assays (ELISA) to detect the specific, well-characterized *vasculitis-associated* ANCA antigens, such as elastase, lactoferrin, myeloperoxidase, proteinase 3, and cathepsin G. Numerous investigators have shown that the previously characterized granule proteins of neutrophils mentioned above are *not* recognized by the majority of IBD-associated pANCA [17–19, 21, 22, 30, 43, 45].

The most sensitive and specific method for detecting IBD-associated ANCA is a three-step method that first screens for the presence of serum ANCA using a fixed neutrophil ELISA developed to specifically expose the IBD-specific ANCA antigen(s) at a high dilution of 1:100 [10, 18, 42]. Screening by this ELISA technique detects all forms of ANCA expressed in patients with IBD. Serum samples positive for ANCA by ELISA are subsequently examined by IIF to determine the predominant staining pattern. While a diffuse cytoplasmic (cANCA) or speckled (sANCA) staining pattern may be observed, the majority of IBD-associated ANCA exhibit the more typical perinuclear neutrophil highlighting pattern (pANCA). Serum samples that are pANCA-positive by IIF are subsequently treated with DNase. The pANCA of IBD is DNase-sensitive, losing the characteristic perinuclear staining pattern when neutrophils are pretreated with DNase [46, 10, 39, 47]. This method of detecting pANCA is very specific for IBD, such that <5% of individuals who do not have IBD, including inflammatory controls, express pANCA. sANCA is characterized by a positive ANCA ELISA value, the presence of a diffuse to overtly speckled staining pattern displayed over the entire neutrophil on both the untreated and DNAse-treated IIF slides, rather than the distinct perinuclear (pANCA) or cytoplasmic (cANCA) staining patterns previously described [44].

It is now recognized that the pANCA characteristic of patients with IBD is unique amongst ANCA. UC-associated pANCA differ from vasculitis-associated ANCA in that the pANCA in UC are mainly composed of the IgG1 and IgG3 antibody subclasses but lack the IgG4 antibodies that are expressed in relatively high IgG4 titers in patients with vasculitis

Table 1. Inter-laboratory comparison for determining prevalence of pANCA, ASCA, and APA in IBD patients (percentages)

Assay	Type IBD	Prometheus	CHRU de Lisle	Oxford	Wurzburg	Mayo	Smith Kline Beecham
pANCA	UC	63	–	39	32	48	0
	CD	25	–	22	14	19	1
ASCA	UC	13	13	–	–	–	–
	CD	44	39	–	–	–	–
APA	UC	–	–	–	0	–	–
	CD	–	–	–	15	–	–

pANCA, perinuclear anti-neutrophil cytoplasmic antibody; ASCA, anti-*Saccharomyces cerevisiae* antibody; APA, anti-pancreatic antibody.

–, Test not available

Adapted from Sandborn *et al.* [42].

[48]. Unlike the ANCA of patients with *vasculitides,* when pANCA-containing sera from patients with UC are incubated with neutrophils the vast majority of pANCA localize to the *inner side* of the nuclear membrane periphery, as demonstrated on confocal microscopy (Fig. 3) [49]. Evaluation with immuno-electron microscopy has also shown that pANCA from patients with UC reacts to antigen located within the inner nuclear membrane periphery, co-localizing with nuclear heterochromatin DNA. Candidate autoantigens for the IBD-specific pANCA include histone H1 [50]. pANCA has also been found to crossreact with an autoantigen that is expressed in colonic mucosa, more specifically in mast cells, *mast cell cytoplasmic antibody* within the colonic lining [51]. Crossreactivity with protein epitopes expressed by colonic bacteria has also been suggested [52].

Serum pANCA in IBD reflects mucosal pANCA production. The intestinal mucosa has been demonstrated to be the site of antigenic B cell priming and pANCA production in patients with UC, suggesting that recognition of mucosal antigen(s) leads to local production of pANCA [53]. While the antigen to which pANCA(s) in IBD react(s) has not been definitively determined, it has been well characterized and several lines of evidence support the concept that the pANCA of CD is the same as pANCA of UC. The proportion of DNase-sensitive pANCA CD sera converting from P→Ø and from P→C is similar to that seen in the pANCA⁺ UC population (70%

and 30%) [10, 46]. The CD subpopulation expressing pANCA is clinically distinct, having a 'UC-like' behavioral phenotype, with clinical features of left-sided colitis and endoscopic and/or histopathologic features typical of UC [10, 37]. Furthermore, the serum immunoglobulin G (IgG) subclass profile of pANCA⁺ 'UC-like CD' is similar to that of UC [54]. This clinical and immunologic/serologic commonality suggests that the presence of serum pANCA reflects a specific type of mucosal inflammation that may be common to the subgroups, both UC and CD expressing pANCA. sANCA has been detected in approximately 14–20% of patients with CD; the incidence in UC has not been reported [44, 55, 56]. ELISA levels of sANCA in CD tend to be very low [56].

ASCA

Overview

Anti-*Saccharomyces cerevisiae* antibodies (ASCA) are present in the majority of sera of patients with CD and a smaller proportion of patients with UC [10, 15, 38–40, 42, 57–60]. ASCA is rarely expressed in individuals who do not have IBD. Sendid *et al.* demonstrated that yeast cell wall phosphopeptido-mannans are the epitopes responsible for the antigenic reactivity in ASCA⁺ CD sera [59]. *S. cerevisiae* is the species of yeast commonly used in baking and brewing. The presence of serum ASCA in patients

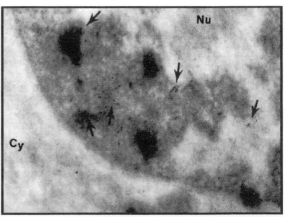

A
B

Figure 3. IBD-Associated pANCA. IBD-associated pANCA is unique amongst ANCA antigens, for unlike the ANCAs associated with vasculitides, the majority of IBD-associated pANCA do *not* recognize the proteins in the granules of neutrophils. **A**: IBD-associated pANCA exhibits peri-nuclear highlighting with immunofluorescence staining. **B**: Confocal microscopy demonstrates that the vast majority of IBD-associated pANCA localize to the *inner side* of the nuclear membrane periphery. (Adapted from refs. 49 and 107).

with IBD is not simply a matter of increased permeability, as elevated levels of antibodies to *Candida albicans*, another common yeast, and to other common antigens such as gliadin, ovalbumin, and beta-lactoglobulin, have *not* been observed in CD [61]. While ASCA is not believed to be a true auto-antibody, evidence suggests that, as with pANCA, expression of this marker antibody is not an epiphenomenon of intestinal insult, but rather a reflection of a specific mucosal immune-mediated response [10, 62–64]. It has been suggested that ASCA production may reflect antigenic cross-reactivity to epitopes coincidentally shared with a true etiologic agent of the disease. The target antigen for ASCA is likely a luminal bacterial antigen that crossreacts with *Saccharomyces*. Mannans are believed to be the major antigenic component of yeast cell walls and are an important antigenic constituent of mycobacteria and other micro-organisms [57]. Soluble preparations of *S. cerevisiae* have been demonstrated to induce a lymphoproliferative response *in vitro*, similar to that of known recall antigens [62, 63]. As with ANCA, familial associations have been observed in patients with ASC [15, 16, 65]. Taylor *et al.* described the association of ASCA with the TNF microsatellite haplotype a11b4c1d3e3 in patients with IBD [64]. Yang *et al.* demonstrated that, in addition to CD, the expression of ASCA as a quantitative trait is also linked to the MHC region, suggesting the MHC-determined susceptibility to CD may be related to reactivity to certain antigens reflected in ASCA expression. These findings suggest that a gene related to ASCA expression resides on chromosome 6 within the MHC, in the vicinity of this haplotype [66]. A mutation located on the haplotype may be contributing to ASCA expression. In combination, these findings suggest that ASCA expression, like pANCA, reflects specific mucosal immune mechanisms.

Serum ASCA determination and characterization

The reported prevalence of ASCA expression in most series ranges between 5% and 70% in CD and from 6% to14% in UC [10, 39, 42, 67]. In addition to methodologic differences, differences in the age of disease onset contribute to the variation in results [10, 38, 42]. The most sensitive and specific method detects serum ASCA using a purified antigen preparation and a fixed ELISA assay optimized for detection of serum IgG and IgA antibodies to *S. cerevisiae* [10, 42]. Microtiter plates are coated with

a purified antigen preparation of phosphopeptido-mannans obtained from yeast *S. uvarum*. Sera exhibiting ASCA reactivity (IgG and/or IgA) exceeding the normal reference range were termed 'ASCA positive' (ASCA$^+$).

Serologic markers to bacterial antigens

Loss of tolerance to normal commensal bacteria has been implicated as an initial step in the inflammatory cascade in some IBD patients [68]. Serologic responses to bacterial antigens have been studied in IBD patients (see Chapter 10) and may represent another family of serologic markers that may be associated with specific subgroups of IBD patients. These bacterial antigens may be crossreactive with other already identified serologic markers of IBD such as pANCA. For example, the precise antigen for pANCA may not be a single antigen, but may represent homologous protein sequences shared among a number of different bacterial antigens. Outer membrane proteins (OmpC) and histone proteins (HupB) are two bacterial antigens that may represent the target antigen for pANCA [52, 69]. The presence of a combination of serologic markers directed against these bacterial antigens and pANCA may identify a subgroup of IBD patients that are particularly immunologically reactive to intestinal bacteria, and most likely to respond to treatments that alter gut bacteria populations.

Escherichia coli OmpC and HupB

The outer cell wall membrane of *E. coli* and other *Enterobacteriacae* is responsible for controlling the flow of nutrients, metabolites, and small hydrophilic antibiotics both in and out of the cell. This function is predominantly controlled by outer membrane proteins called porins [70]. Different organisms manufacture various different porins located on their outer membrane (OmpC, OmpF, PhoE, NmpC). These porins may have surface antigenic determinants that are species-dependent, but contain shared protein sequences between organisms [71, 72]. HU proteins are histone-like DNA-binding proteins, which are involved in the maintenance of DNA tertiary structure. HU proteins are composed of two subunits (HupA and HupB), and participate in various DNA replication and repair process [50].

In a recent study by Cohavy *et al.* libraries of colonic bacteria and clonal isolates were evaluated for crossreactivity with pANCA monoclonal antibody. pANCA identified two major species of proteins that were immunoreactive to pANCA: an *E coli* OmpC, and a *B. caccae* HupB. In addition, human sera from UC patients and healthy controls were evaluated for immunoglobulins crossreactive with these antigens. Patients with UC showed increased IgG to OmpC compared to controls, suggesting that these antibodies may detect a recurrent antigenic protein sequence or epitope expressed by colonic bacteria [52]. Since it is hypothesized that normal gut bacteria are immunogenic in the IBD patient, detection of a combination of pANCA and anti-OmpC may be important in identifying patients who have lost their tolerance to their own bacterial flora, and may be most likely to respond to antibiotic therapy. This hypothesis is currently being studied in a number of ongoing clinical trials.

pANCA antibodies also identify an epitope on the COOH-terminal region of the human histone H1 protein [50]. In mycobacterial species a novel 32 kDa, 214 amino-acid HupB protein has also been shown to have homologous sequences shared with the human histone-1, and has confirmed cross-reactivity to pANCA [69]. When serum IgG activity was measured in UC patients compared to controls, there was no significant correlation between anti-HupB binding activity, anti-H1 activity, the presence of pANCA, nor the diagnosis of UC. This suggests that, although HupB and H1 may share homologous protein sequences that may be recognized by a pANCA monclonal antibody, in clinical UC the antigenic determinants of pANCA and H1 are not crossreactive with HupB, illustrating the complexity of immune responses in IBD. However, when serum IgA activity was measured in a subgroup of IBD patients, anti-HupB IgA was strongly associated with CD [69]. Anti-HupB IgA may simply reflect the presence of mycobacterial species in the intestinal microenvironment of CD patients, but may also be potentially useful in identifying subgroups of CD patients. Thus, the utilization of pANCA, along with serologic evidence of response to bacterial antigens such as OmpC and/or HupB, may be useful in characterizing some subgroups of IBD patients.

I2 Peptide

Sutton *et al.* recently-described a novel RNA-derived immunologically associated bacterial sequence, the I2 peptide, which exhibits seroreactivity and specific lesional abundance in CD. I2 was initially isolated by subtractive cloning in lamina propria mononuclear cells from colonic mucosa histologically involved with CD [73].

Using quantitative competitive polymerase chain reaction (PCR) analysis they detected I2 DNA in 43% of involved CD colonic mucosa, but in only 9% of UC and 5% of non-IBD colonic controls. Serum antibodies to an I2-encoded peptide were also observed to be disease-associated. ELISA analysis with a recombinant I2 glutathione-*S*-transferase fusion protein demonstrated that while the majority of CD patients expressed IgA binding (54%), sero-reactivity was less common in patients with UC (10%), other enteric inflammatory controls (19%), or normals (4%). The mean serum anti-I2 absorbance for patients with CD was similarly elevated compared with UC, non-IBD disease controls, who were not significantly different from normals. As an I2 sequence was commonly detectable in the ileum of non-IBD controls, I2 seroreactivity did not necessarily reflect the mucosal presence of I2.

The I2 protein was undetectable by PCR in most human tissues, and when detected it was quantitated at $<0.1\%$ of the genomic single copy rate. The I2 sequence is thus not of human origin: The seroreactivity to the I2 peptide may represent crossreactivity or secondary microbial exposure. The infrequent detection of I2 in inflamed colonic specimens from patients with UC and other non-IBD acute and chronic colitides, including ischemic colitis, argues against non-specific entry of I2 at sites of mucosal disruption secondary to inflammation. The observation that I2 was present in most ileal specimens, regardless of patient disease status or histologic evidence of inflammation, suggests that the putative I2-expressing organism is a normal resident of the ileal mucosa. Isolation of the I2 sequence from lamina propria mononuclear cells, and failure to grow the putative organism under diverse axenic culture conditions, suggest that it may undergo intracellular growth, consistent with elicitation of granulomatous inflammation, a cardinal feature of mucosal damage in CD. The I2 sequence was not detected from seven mycobacterial isolates, including a CD isolate of *M. paratuberculosis*. Sutton *et al.* suggested that it is possible that the I2 sequence is derived from a novel bacterium, or perhaps a well-known enteric bacterium not yet characterized for this gene segment.

Preliminary evidence suggests that I2 induces both humoral and T cell responses in patients with CD [74].

Heat shock proteins

Other bacterial antigens that may induce an immunologic response in IBD patients are heat-shock proteins (HSP-60), which are intracellular molecules that are induced by proinflammatory cytokines [75]. IgA antibodies to heat-shock proteins were found to be elevated in patients with CD compared to healthy and infectious diarrhea controls. IgA HSP-60 levels were independent of disease activity. In UC the median level of IgA HSP-60 was not significantly different compared to control. However, after substratification for disease activity, HSP-60 IgA was significantly elevated in UC patients with active disease compared to inactive UC or controls. The pathogenesis of heat-shock protein antibodies may be related to increased mucosal permeability with subsequent increased exposure to bacterial antigens [75]. However, since anti-HS proteins were not elevated in infectious diarrhea controls who also have damaged epithelium, immune reactivity to these bacterial antigens may be more complex than increased exposure due to leaky epithelium, and may involve dysfunctional immune responses and regulation.

Cathepsin G

pANCA has been shown to be elevated in primary sclerosing cholangitis (PSC), as well as UC and some patients with CD. Halbwachs *et al.* report that pANCA reacts to an azurophilic granule component of the polymorphonuclear neutrophil (PMN) which is distinct from other reported autoantigens of pANCA (proteinase 3, elastase, and myeloperoxidase). This antigenic target has been identified as cathepsin G, which has been associated with the presence of UC, PSC, and CD, suggesting a similar pathogenic mechanism for these diseases [76]. Furthermore, Mayet *et al.* report that IgG antibodies to cathepsin G were detected in 38% of a cohort of CD patients, and 74% of these patients had colonic disease. In this report cathepsin G antibodies were not significantly present in UC. This suggests that cathepsin G may be another target antigen for antibodies detected in a subgroup of IBD patients with colonic CDe [77].

Other novel disease markers of ulcerative colitis or Crohn's disease

Anti-pancreatic antibodies (PAB) and anti-goblet cell antibodies (GAB)

Antibodies to pancreatic juice (PAB) have been reported to be increased in patients with IBD. The PAB antigen has been partially characterized and is a large >800 kDa macromolecular trypsin-sensitive protein, but not part of a panel of defined pancreatic exocrine proteins [78]. Seibold *et al.* studied 222 CD and 51 UC patients for PAB and found that 31% and 4% of CD and UC patients respectively were positive for PAB, which was statistically significant [79]. PAB were not found in other inflammatory controls, and were not associated with disease severity or location. Of the seven patients with concurrent CD and pancreatic disease, four were positive for PAB. A subsequent study by Seibold *et al.* confirmed these observations. They reported that 40% of CD patients in their study population were positive for PAB. Furthermore, pancreatic insufficiency was detected in seven of 26 PAB-positive patients but in only three of 38 negative patients [80]. These observations support PAB as a specific marker for CD and possibly for associated pancreatic insufficiency.

While PAB were found to be associated with CD, anti-goblet cell antibodies (GAB) have been associated with the diagnosis of UC. GAB were found in 13 of 51 patients with UC (29%) and in none of the CD patients or inflammatory controls. However, neither antibody was associated with disease behavior, nor suggested an antigen in the etiopathogenesis of IBD [79]. When the presence of PAB and pANCA was examined in first-degree relatives with UC and CD, neither marker wsd elevated, suggesting that they do not represent genetic markers of disease [81, 82].

IL-1/IL-1ra ratio

IL-1 is a proinflammatory cytokine that is inhibited by its naturally occurring receptor (IL-1ra). In IBD, it has been hypothesized that an imbalance in the production of IL-1 and IL-1ra exists in the gut mucosa as a result of a dysregulated immune system. The quantitative level of IL-1ra detected in peripheral blood from patients with UC, CD, and inflammatory controls has been observed to be significantly elevated in active CD and UC compared to control. These levels were also higher in active CD versus active UC [83]. When the ratio of IL-1ra to IL-1 (IL-1ra/IL-1) was examined, the ratio was significantly decreased in the mucosa of UC and CD patients, compared to healthy controls or patients with self-limited colitis [84]. The decreased IL-1ra/IL-1 ratio also correlated with disease severity. These data suggest that the measurement of IL-1ra or the IL1ra/IL-1 ratio may be a useful diagnostic test and indicator of disease activity.

The polymorphism on intron 2 of the IL-1ra gene has been previously characterized [85]. Carriage of allele 2 of this gene has been associated with 60–70% of patients with UC. Tountas *et al.* also showed that a decreased level of IL-1ra production in PBMC was correlated with the carriage of allele 2 (IL-1RN*2) [86]. In this study, when patients were stratified according to ethnicity, carriage of allele 2 of the IL-1ra polymorphism was significantly increased in the Hispanic and Jewish subgroups, but not in the subgroup of patients of Italian descent [86]. Similar studies in other ethnic subgroups have also not been able to confirm the increased carriage of allele 2 of the IL-1ra polymorphism in their UC populations from England, Spain, and Germany [87–89]. However, Roussomoustakaki *et al.* did confirm that, in their UC subgroup from England, extensive disease was significantly associated with increased carriage of allele 2 of the IL-1ra gene [87]. Heresbach *et al.* also showed that, in severe UC patients who required colectomy, there was a higher carriage of the IL-1ra allele 1–2 than non-operated UC patients. Furthermore, non-surgically treated UC patients had a significantly lower frequency of IL-1ra allele 2 compared to surgically treated UC patients or controls [90]. These observations suggest that the genetic polymorphism for the IL-1ra gene in UC may be associated with genetic heterogeneity among different ethnic groups, accounting for the variable carriage rates in different populations. The carriage of allele 2 of the IL-1ra gene may also be associated with more extensive and severe disease in UC.

The IL-1β gene polymorphism was studied in a group of Dutch UC and CD patients, but did not show any significant associations. However, when carriage of the IL-1β polymorphism and allele 2 of the IL-1ra gene polymorphism were combined, UC as well as CD patients showed an increased carriage of IL-1ra allele 2, but a decreased frequency of the IL-1β polymorphism. These observations provide genetic support for the hypothesis that an imbalance in the IL-1ra/ IL-1 ratio may be important in the pathogenesis of IBD [91]. However, in a similar study by Hacker *et al.*, neither the IL-1β gene polymorphism nor the combination with the IL-1ra gene polymorphism showed any associations within this population of IBD patients. Neither could any association between the allele 2 polymorphism and UC patients be identified or associated with severity of disease. These disparate results may again reflect the genetic heterogeneity between various ethnic subgroups within UC patients [89].

Papo and co-workers studied a subgroup of Spanish UC patients for ANCA and allelic frequencies of IL-1ra gene polymorphism, and polymorphisms of TNFα and TNF-β. Overall there was no association between these polymorphisms in UC patients. However, when this study population was stratified according to ANCA status, pANCA-positive patients had a significantly higher frequency of the allele 1-2 of the IL-ra polymorphism. This suggests that pANCA and allele 2 of the IL-1ra gene may also identify a distinct genetic subgroup of UC patients [88].

The frequency of other polymorphisms in the genes for IL-1 and IL-1ra have been studied (Mwo1, MspAI1, Alu1, Taq1, BsoF1), but have not been shown to be associated with UC or CD compared to controls [92].

Other genetic markers as novel markers of IBD

Genetic markers have been associated with the presence of ANCA in IBD, and may further identify distinct subgroups of IBD patients in combination with ANCA serology. In a cohort of 53 IBD patients, Hirv *et al.* reported a significantly higher frequency of the HLA-DRB1*15 allele in UC, and a significantly lower frequency of this allele in CD. When UC patients were substratified according to ANCA status the increased HLA-DRB1*15 association was due to a significantly increased frequency of the allelic subtype HLA-DRB1*1501 in the ANCA-positive subgroup compared to controls [93]. Although larger populations of IBD patients need to be studied, this observation supports the role of ANCA in combination with genetic markers in identifying more homogeneous IBD subgroups.

Other genetic markers have been observed to be associated with the severity and prognosis of IBD. For example, in a study population of UC patients the presence of HLA-DR2 was associated with poor prognosis and medically resistant disease [94]. HLADRB1*15 and HLA-DRB1*0103 alleles have also been reported to be associated with more extensive and severe disease in ulcerative colitis [95]. In CD HLA-DRB1*03 was found to be significantly less frequent in a selected population of fistulizing CD patients compared to control [96]. Taken together, these data suggest that a combination of genetic and serologic markers may identify specific phenotypic subgroups characterized by common patterns in disease severity and prognosis.

Clinical applications

Serum immune and genetic markers can potentially be utilized at several levels including: diagnosis (IBD vs non-IBD), differentiation (UC vs CD), stratification (phenotyping), or prognostication, as well as potential therapeutic and research implications.

Diagnostic utility: differentiation of IBD from non-IBD

Early recognition of IBD may allow for therapeutic interventions at an earlier point in the inflammatory process, thereby potentially avoiding or minimizing subsequent disease- and therapy-related complications. The current gold standard for the diagnosis of IBD is based on a combination of established clinical, endoscopic, histopathologic, radiologic, and serologic criteria [1]. The sensitivity and specificity of these combined tests enable clinicians to differentiate IBD for other disease processes. Establishing a definitive diagnosis of IBD, and knowing in whom and to what extent to pursue more extensive diagnostic evaluations, can be challenging. The presenting symptoms of IBD, in particular CD, can be subtle and non-specific. Initial symptoms may be non-gastrointestinal in nature and may include: arthritis, arthralgias, menstrual irregularities, unexplained fevers, anorexia, or fatigue. Indeed, once a diagnosis of IBD has been established, it is not uncommon for patients and family members to relate how, in retrospect, symptoms associated with unrecognized IBD predated the definitive diagnosis by months or years, having been attributed to 'irritable bowel syndrome', 'chronic recurrent abdominal pain', or other conditions [97, 98]. Despite exhibiting minimal or no gastrointestinal symptoms, predominant manifestations of IBD in children and adolescents may include

delayed pubertal maturation or failure to gain weight and height appropriately [97, 99, 100]. Under these circumstances IBD may go unrecognized, or the degree of involvement may go under-appreciated for an extended period of time. Underscoring this point is that growth retardation is already present in 30–50% of pediatric CD patients, including prepubertal children, at the time of presentation, with decreased height velocity preceding the onset of gastrointestinal symptoms by as much as 11 years [101–103]. Failure to recognize and address 'silent' active inflammatory disease in a timely fashion ultimately manifests permanent deficits and adult height [97, 104, 105]. Thus for pediatric patients in particular, early diagnosis, adequate nutrition, and successful control of disease activity set the stage for optimizing appropriate linear growth, normal sexual maturation, and restoration of well-being.

Delays in diagnosis are common and may in part be related to patient or parental resistance and anxiety due to the invasive nature of the work-up. Radiographic and endoscopic procedures require cooperation and are unpleasant and invasive, especially from the perspective of the child or the young adolescent. Less invasive traditional blood tests are non-specific, primarily looking for evidence of inflammation, including: elevated white blood cells with a left shift and elevated band counts, thrombocytosis, elevated sedimentation rate and/or C-reactive protein, decreased serum albumin levels, and decreased iron stores. Stool markers, such as stool α_1-antitrypsin, have also been used as diagnostic aids [97].

Of the described IBD-specific serum immune markers, pANCA and ASCA are clinically the best characterized and studied. As previously described, these serum immune markers are present in the majority of UC and CD patients, respectively, and are infrequently present in non-IBD controls, including patients with irritable bowel syndrome (IBS). These tests are thus specific for IBD and the false-positive rate is low for each. Non-invasive and less expensive diagnostic screening in the form of an 'IBD serum immune marker panel' could thus provide the evidence to direct further appropriate evaluation, a strategy similar to that currently applied in patients with suspected systemic lupus erythematosus [106].

Ideally patients identified with UC and CD should have the appropriate traditional work-up to characterize their disease, and expensive and invasive testing to rule out disease should be avoided in patients who do not have IBD despite symptoms compatible with these disorders. Such a strategy was recently tested in a pediatric population presenting with non-specific symptoms suggestive of IBD, yet a normal physical examination [60]. For the purposes of testing the assays as a screening tool, an ELISA-based modification of the pANCA and ASCA assays without immunofluorescence or DNase pANCA confirmation was used. Cut-off values were recalculated for the purpose of optimizing diagnostic sensitivity (understanding that this also lowers specificity). In this study all patients underwent simultaneous invasive and non-invasive modified serodiagnostic testing. Applying this strategy the authors found that 95% of non-IBD patients were accurately identified by way of the modified pANCA and ASCA panel, demonstrating that had this 'IBD serum immune marker panel' been the only diagnostic tool utilized, these non-IBD patients could have avoided an unnecessary invasive evaluation. On the other hand, the third of patients with non-specific symptoms whose diagnosis would have been delayed with this approach would likely have returned with persistent or progressive symptoms more suggestive of IBD, which would have then mandated the needed further work-up.

The addition of OmpC, I2 and other serum immune markers to such an 'IBD panel' could further improve sensitivity and specificity. In the appropriate clinical setting, a negative 'IBD panel' can provide reassurance and avoid unnecessarily extensive work-up, unneeded discomfort, or anxiety [60, 107]. On the other hand, a positive test may provide the evidence to pursue further appropriate evaluation. It must be emphasized, however, that the absence of serum pANCA or ASCA expression does not rule out IBD. The IBD panel is an excellent non-invasive adjunct to a good history, and clinical, endoscopic, radiologic, and histopathologic findings.

Differentiation of ulcerative colitis from Crohn's disease

Both pharmacologic and surgical management decisions are often heavily influenced by whether the patient has a diagnosis of CD or UC. Serum immune markers have been used in an attempt to differentiate UC from CD. While there is a strong tendency for patients who express ASCA or OmpC to have CD and pANCA to have UC, it is not surprising that overlap is seen in serum immune marker expression, just as an overlap between CD

and UC has been demonstrated at multiple levels including: clinical, endoscopic, radiographic, histopathologic, epidemiologic, genetic, immunopathologic, and response therapies [9, 13, 64, 108–115]. In general up to 30% of CD patients are pANCA$^+$ and up to 14% of UC patients are ASCA$^+$. Selective marker antibody expression combining ASCA and pANCA improves the ability to differentiate between CD and UC [10, 38]. In addition to the absolute presence or absence of immune marker expression, the clinical relevance of taking into account the level of marker antibodies has recently been demonstrated [10]. An inverse relationship between ANCA and ASCA levels within CD has been observed (i.e. the higher the ASCA level, the lower the ANCA level and vice-versa) [10]. A similar inverse relationship is seen in UC (personal observations). This inverse relationship suggests that the presence and levels of a specific marker antibody could reflect distinct immunologic reactivity that leads to differences in clinical expression among CD patients. The vast majority of patients who are positive for both IgA and IgG ASCA, and/or express very high levels of either ASCA subtype, have CD (personal observations). Expression of both IgG and IgA ASCA subtypes is unusual in UC, and levels of ASCA tend to be low. Interestingly, ASCA is coexpressed in only about half of pANCA$^+$ CD patients, generally at low levels [10]. Of further clinical relevance is that many patients with indeterminate colitis are not surprisingly pANCA$^+$, which is consistent with their 'UC-like' presentation, and as such the ANCA and ASCA profiles are of limited usefulness in determining whether these patients will truly manifest as UC or CD [116]. I2 is detected more commonly in CD than UC and non-inflammatory controls (51–54%, 10%, and 4%, respectively) [73, 117]. Interestingly, I2 is present in 44% of pANCA$^+$ CD patients and additionally was detected in a third of those CD patients negative for ASCA and pANCA [117]. OmpC is present in nearly half of CD patients lacking the above two markers. The value of collective serum marker profiles, combined with the presence of specific genetic markers, may ultimately prove to be the most beneficial strategy.

Stratification

Overview

Serum immune and genetic markers may serve as subclinical indicators of specific patterns of disease expression. Numerous attempts have been made to characterize CD and UC patients into uniform subgroups to better understand and predict clinical courses and responses to medical and surgical interventions. Most stratification analyses of CD, particularly in therapeutic trials, continue to focus predominantly on anatomic location of inflammation. Behavior characteristics of inflammation, aggressiveness of disease, and responsiveness to medical interventions also need to be considered [1, 5]. Patients with UC are generally characterized by location of disease as having either proctitis, proctosigmoiditis, left-sided colitis, or pancolitis. While this description of extent of disease may guide initial approaches to treatment and future dysplasia screening recommendations, it is important to realize that this does not correlate with or predict aggressiveness of disease. Such classifications have generally been descriptive and not reflective of specific pathogenic mechanisms.

Inflammatory bowel diseases can now be further stratified into distinct subgroups by pairing clinical features with the *presence* and *levels* of serum antibody markers [10, 41, 67]. Serum immune marker expression in IBD permits stratification at the mucosal, clinical, immunologic, genetic, and therapeutic levels. To date these associations have been best characterized with pANCA and ASCA. In IBD, pANCA and ASCA production appear to reflect distinct and divergent mucosal inflammatory processes and thereby are reflective of immunologically distinct subpopulations. Both have been associated with distinct disease subgroups [10, 31, 35, 37, 41, 44, 118–120].

Ulcerative colitides

In UC pANCA has been associated with the clinical features of: (1) treatment-resistant left-sided disease [119]; (2) aggressive disease course [31, 120]; (3) surgery early in the disease course [35]; and (4) development of pouchitis following ileal pouch–anal anastomosis (IPAA) [41, 118, 121]. While many studies have found no association of pANCA expression with disease activity [18, 21, 22, 24–27, 31], and persistence of pANCA positivity after coletomy [19, 21, 24, 33, 34, 87, 122] others have observed higher levels of antibody expression in patients with more active disease [20, 28, 29, 123] and lower or absent levels in patients following colectomy with active disease [32, 39, 123, 124]. Some studies have shown an increased incidence of ANCA expression in

family members of ANCA$^+$ UC patients [12, 14, 34]. Genetic studies have suggested that subpopulations of UC can be defined by ANCA expression in association with specific HLA markers [13, 14, 87, 115, 125, 126] and it has recently been suggested that certain genotypes may be associated with clinical phenotypes, such as disease behavior or an increased likelihood of developing chronic pouchitis [67, 87, 127, 128].

Crohn's diseases

The *presence* of the immunologic markers ASCA and pANCA expression in CD have been found to correlate with different disease locations [14, 26, 30, 37–39, 61, 129]. Most studies evaluating ASCA expression in CD have found an association with small bowel involvement. Giaffer *et al.* observed that patients with isolated small bowel involvement had significantly higher ASCA IgG titers against two strains of *S. cerevisiae* than those with colonic disease [129]. In a study examining ASCA expression in monozygotic twins, Lindberg *et al.* found higher IgG ASCA levels (to whole yeast) in patients with CD limited to the small bowel compared to those with both small bowel and colonic involvement [61]. Vasiliauskas *et al.* also observed that the presence of ASCA was associated with small bowel involvement (alone or in combination with colonic disease), noting minimal ileal involvement in all [10]. In contrast, several investigators have maintained that in CD pANCA expression is related to colonic involvement disease, which at minimum is left-sided and 'UC-like' [10, 14, 25, 26, 37, 39, 130]. 'UC-like' behavioral attributes are the predominant behavior pattern common to the subgroup of CD patients expressing serum pANCA, providing additional evidence that pANCA is a marker of a distinct mucosal inflammatory process. In addition to features of 'classic CD' (such as fistula, fibrostenosis, and anal or small bowel involvement) pANCA$^+$ CD patients have at some point in the course of their disease a minimal left-side colitis with endoscopic and/or histopathologic features of UC [37]. Review of the clinical histories of pANCA$^+$ CD patients reveals that nearly a third are initially diagnosed as having UC, prior to the development of characteristics diagnostic of CD (i.e. small bowel fibrostenosing or penetrating disease, multiple fistulas, or the finding of granuloma, which by definition convert the diagnosis to CD (unpublished personal observations). Using the same methods of pANCA detection this association of

Table 2. Clinical features in Crohn's disease: results of multivariate analysis

	Disease location	Fibrostenosing disease	Internal penetrating disease	Perianal penetrating disease	UC-like features
ASCA level					
β	–	0.33	0.32	–	−0.29
R^2	–	0.13	0.03	–	0.02
p-Value	n.s.	0.0001	0.022	n.s.	0.063
ANCA level					
β	–	–	–	–	0.67
R^2	–	–	–	–	0.15
p-Value	n.s.	n.s.	n.s.	n.s.	0.0001

β, regression coefficient; R^2, proportion of the total variation of a dependent variable which can be explained by the variation of each independent variable

Modified from ref. 10.

'UC-like' features has been confirmed in several CD populations by investigators in England and Canada [14, 39, 130].

It has recently been suggested that not only the type, but also the magnitude of the immune marker expression (as measured by level of host marker antibody production) reflects divergent immune responses, that manifest as specific disease behaviors (phenotypes) in IBD. A recent study by Vasiliauskas *et al.* demonstrated that the associations with behavioral manifestations in CD become more evident at higher levels of both ASCA and pANCA expression (particularly if they expressed one, but not the other, immune marker) [10]. Higher levels of ASCA and pANCA expression identify CD subgroups which are immunologically and clinically progressively more homogeneous, with distinct and divergent clinical characteristics, suggesting that ASCA and pANCA are serum markers for different mucosal inflammatory mechanisms that influence disease expression [10]. Higher levels of ASCA are independently associated with earlier age of onset of CD and a tendency toward developing 'classic' fibrostenosing and internal penetrating small bowel complications, and less often UC-like features (Table 2) [10]. In contrast, higher levels of pANCA in CD are associated with later age of onset and with a 'UC-like' inflammatory response, as well as a relative lack of fibrostenosis and penetrating disease (Table 2).

The combination of selective pANCA or ASCA expression with the added variable of the magnitude of expression (those expressing high levels of a single marker antibody and lacking the other) further defines subgroups of CD patients into more

immunologically and clinically homogeneous subgroups, including a group with a more aggressive disease course [10]. While fibrostenosing and internal penetrating behaviors have been considered by some to be indicators of a more aggressive form of small bowel CD, the need for small bowel surgery or recurrent surgeries has been suggested as a further measure of disease severity. In the study by Vasiliauskas *et al.* the subgroup of CD patients expressing high levels of IgG and IgA ASCA and lacking pANCA were characterized by the universal occurrence of fibrostenosis and the frequent development of internal penetrating complications (Fig. 4) [10]. Small bowel surgery was not only required by a larger percentage of CD patients expressing very high levels of ASCA and not pANCA (Fig. 5A), but the mean number of small bowel surgeries per patient with small bowel disease was also higher (Fig. 5B). Similarly, the incidence of 'UC-like' behavior is greatest at higher ELISA levels of pANCA expression and by exclusion of ASCA expression. The frequency of UC-like features in low-level expression of pANCA is no different from that in the overall population, stressing the importance of taking into account the magnitude of the immune response. These data strengthen the assertion that CD and UC pANCA subgroups share a similar mucosal immune response. The associations and findings seen in the subgroup of CD patients expressing high levels of ASCA and pANCA are provocative, and suggest that the presence of serum immune markers (in this case ASCA and pANCA), and the magnitude of the host immune response (level of serum immune marker expression), correlate with

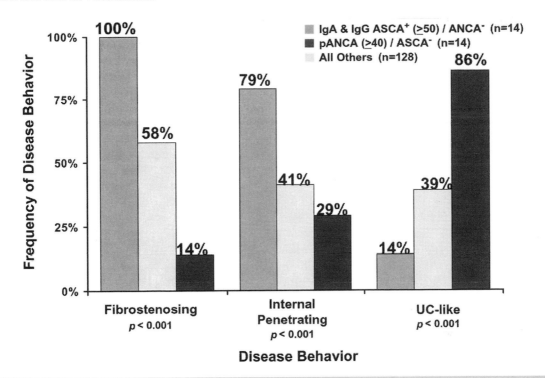

Figure 4. Substratification of Crohn's disease using selected expression of immune markers. Disease behavior characteristics were examined in more immunologically homogeneous CD subgroups (those expressing high levels of a single marker antibody) and compared to all other CD study patients. Overall differences in proportions were evaluated using the χ^2 test for trend ($p < 0.001$ for each of the disease behavior characteristics). Higher ASCA levels are associated with both fibrostenosing and internal penetrating disease behaviors. In contrast, higher ANCA levels are associated with an 'UC-like' inflammatory response (Modified from ref. 10).

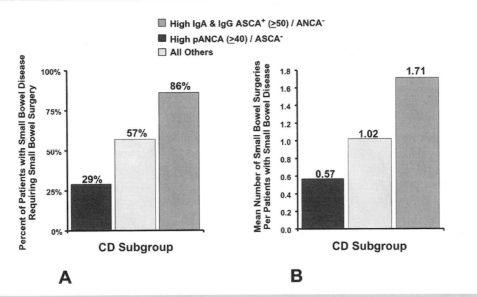

Figure 5. Surgery as a measure of disease aggressiveness in Crohn's disease. Substratification of the subset of patients with small bowel disease (CD involving the small bowel alone or in combination with the colon) using selective immune marker expression: **A**: percentage of patients requiring small bowel surgery and **B**: total number of small bowel surgeries per patient with small bowel involvement. Overall differences in proportions were evaluated using the χ^2 test for trend. (**A**: $p < 0.0001$; **B**: $p < 0.005$). Small bowel surgery was not only required by a larger percentage of CD patients expressing very high levels of ASCA and not pANCA, but the mean number of small bowel surgeries per patient with small bowel disease was higher as well, suggesting that very high levels of ASCA without ANCA may reflect more aggressive small intestinal disease (Modified from ref. 10).

distinct, and indeed divergent, clinical characteristics, suggesting that ASCA and pANCA are serum markers for different mucosal inflammatory mechanisms that influence disease expression.

These marker antibodies have also provided insight into the perforating behaviors characteristic of CD, as manifested by abscess or fistula formation or perforation. While internal penetrating disease is positively correlated with high levels of ASCA expression, and negatively correlated with high levels of ANCA expression, no significant correlation was seen with these markers and perianal fistulizing disease (Table 2) [10]. This suggests that these two penetrating forms of CD involve different immunologic mechanisms, and might be considered not only clinically, but also immunologically, distinct. Of note is that, while perforating and non-perforating behaviors are clinically (and likely in some ways immunologically) distinct also, the observation that higher levels of ASCA expression are associated with both of these traditional 'classic' fibrostenosing and internal penetrating features of CD, suggests an overlapping mucosal mechanism, rather than solely distinct mechanisms [10].

The association of ANCA and ASCA expression with age of onset of CD is intriguing. The relationship between age of disease onset and both disease behavior and anatomic location has long been appreciated. The majority of epidemiologic studies examining age of presentation suggest a bimodal age distribution in CD [131–134]. It has been observed that childhood-onset CD is characterized by a greater prevalence of small bowel disease and stricturing/penetrating complications, compared to late-onset CD which is associated with more colonic disease and 'UC-like' features and a lower incidence of fibrostenosis or internal perforating complications [10, 135, 136]. Some studies suggest that childhood-onset CD has a more aggressive course [136–138], while older-onset CD is associated with a comparatively favorable prognosis, better response to medical therapies, and lower risk of recurrence in the minority requiring surgery [134, 135, 139, 140 140]. Clinical differences between childhood- and adult-onset CD in disease distribution and clinical course may be associated with different immune responses [135–142]. The relationship between age of onset of CD and expression of ASCA and pANCA has been examined. ASCA+ CD patients have been shown to experience onset of IBD symptoms earlier in life than patients not expressing ASCA [10, 38]. The study by Vasiliauskas *et al*, compared patients

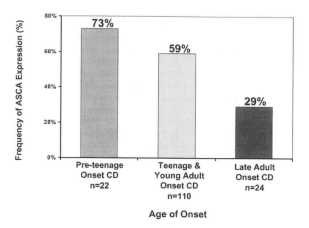

Figure 6. ASCA expression varies with age of onset of Crohn's disease. ASCA expression was more common in patients with pre-teenage onset of CD than those with later onset of disease ($p_{\chi2 \text{ for trend}} < 0.003$) (Adapted from ref. 10).

with pre-teenage onset of CD to patients with onset between 13 and 40 years, and patients with disease onset after age 40 years (age > 40 has been described as the start of the second age peak for onset of CD) [10, 131–134]. As depicted in Fig. 6, 73% (16/22) of patients with pre-teenage onset of CD were ASCA+, compared to 59% (65/110) of patients with onset between 13 and 40 years, and only 29% (7/24) of patients with disease onset after age 40 years. In this same study age of onset was further shown to be independently associated with *levels* of both IgG and IgA ASCA. A negative correlation between IgG and IgA ASCA levels and age of onset of CD was suggested as further evidence for the association of this immune response with younger age of onset. Although the percent of CD patients expressing pANCA did not vary significantly with age of onset, there was a tendency toward higher levels of ANCA expression with increasing age of onset. These findings suggest that early- and late-onset CD may have distinct immunologic responses. These differences in disease location and behavior pattern tendencies imply that pediatric and later adult-onset CD represent pathogenetically distinct forms of this disease [143]. The underlying pathogenetic mechanisms for these clinical differences observed between adult- versus childhood-onset CD remain unclear. Although familial clustering supports the role of genetic factors in the pathogenesis of pediatric and adult-onset CD, additional factors must also be involved to account for the observed differences

[113, 144–148]. It has been hypothesized that young children may be more immunologically reactive than older children or adults [149–151]. Age-dependent immune influences have been described in other immune-mediated disorders [106, 152–156]. The results of this study provide evidence that age of onset associated with host-dependent immune responses may influence intestinal location, phenotypic expression, and CD behavior.

While neither sANCA nor I2 has been associated with a unique clinical phenotype based on traditional descriptive parameters of disease behavior or location, it has been suggested that expression of sANCA in CD is associated with a clinically relevant therapeutic phenotype characterized by enhanced responsiveness to intervention with the anti-TNF monoclonal antibody infliximab [44, 55]. Of interest is that I2 positivity has been highly associated with ASCA positivity, not pANCA, and level of serum I2 reactivity also correlated significantly with ASCA levels [117].

The serologic and distinct clinical commonality seen in IBD patients expressing high levels of these serum immune markers suggests that patients with IBD may be stratified based on types of mucosal inflammation into immunologically and clinically more uniform subgroups.

Potential prognostic implications

Stratification of ulcerative colitides and Crohn's diseases into more uniform subgroups with genetic and immune markers may ultimately permit better clinical characterization and prediction of natural history. This information could potentially allow for earlier and more aggressive treatment in order to avoid predictable complications in selected patients, without unnecessarily exposing others to potential adverse side-effects of overaggressive therapeutic regimens. For example, given the aggressive nature of the small bowel disease in the subgroup of patients with high levels of both IgG and IgA subtypes of ASCA and the correlation with small bowel stricturing and penetrating disease and need for surgery, earlier and more aggressive intervention may prove to be prudent to thwart these complications. Analysis of a prospective population of UC patients undergoing colectomy and IPAA revealed that very high preoperative pANCA is associated with subsequent development of chronic pouchitis, while the risk for those with lower levels of pANCA was similar to those who lacked this marker [41]. Thus UC patients

with proven identifiable preoperative risk factors for subsequent chronic pouchitis development (i.e. PSC, oral ulcerations, certain genotypes, and specific immune marker profiles) may need to be appropriately counseled regarding this risk, and strategies aimed at pouchitis prophylaxis may be entertained.

Identification of therapeutic subgroups

Overview

A further important clinical application is the identification of therapeutically relevant subgroups. Both CD and UC exhibit immunologic and genetic heterogeneity, suggesting that underlying pathogenic mechanisms and therefore potential therapeutic targets vary within different disease subgroups [157]. Stratification of IBD with serum immune and genetic markers may thus ultimately allow for identification of those individuals most likely to benefit from specific therapeutic interventions [44, 55, 97]. By combining clinical findings with genetic and serologic profiles the most appropriate individualized treatment intervention can then be selected based on the composite subprofile (Fig. 1). The following examples illustrate how, though still in its infancy, pharmacogenetics has begun to provide the tools necessary to further individualize and optimize therapeutic regimens.

Cytokine-specific interventions

Responses to newer cytokine-specific therapies are likely related to the nature of the underlying mucosal inflammatory process (Fig. 7). The specificity of specific cytokine-directed interventions provides a unique opportunity to evaluate clinical responses with relation to immunologically or genetically determined patient subgroups. Subanalysis of the patients in the multicenter, placebo-controlled anti-TNF monoclonal antibody (infliximab) trial reported by Targan *et al.* [158] and subsequent open-label experiences have demonstrated that the subgroup of CD patients that are pANCA$^+$ (a subgroup that has been correlated with the UC-like phenotype) have a poorer response to cytokine-specific anti-TNF chimeric monoclonal antibody therapy than those who lacked this marker [44, 55]. Additionally, it has been our experience that, when treated with infliximab, pANCA$^+$ CD patients tend not to respond as quickly or as dramatically as patients

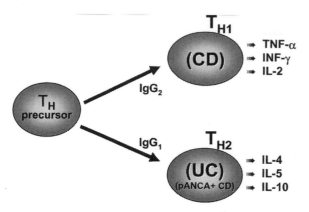

Figure 7. Fundamental concept: IBD = mucosal inflammation. Responses to the newer cytokine-specific interventions may be related to the nature of the mucosal inflammatory process. It has been suggested that the T helper cell type 1 (Th1) and Th2 balance is divergent in IBD, each being characterized by different cytokine profiles. Generalizations regarding the immune mechanisms characterize CD as Th1-dominant, while UC and pANCA+ 'UC-like' CD have been suggested to be predominantly Th2-mediated. Preliminary clinical experience with anti-TNF-α monoclonal antibodies support this, in that while the majority of CD patients improve with this form of therapy, those with UC or pANCA+ CD respond less well to this same intervention (Adapted from ref. 97).

who lack this serum immune marker, and the clinical effect frequently is of shorter duration [55] (personal observations). CD patients expressing the newly described sANCA, however, tend to be more responsive to this same intervention [44, 55]. This preliminary evidence suggests serum immune marker expression correlates with response to specific cytokine-directed therapy and thus may indeed be helpful in guiding decisions with respect to which patients might best benefit from specific interventions. Such substratification may allow for enhanced selection/identification of appropriate patient subgroups for specific appropriate therapeutic interventions, and may allow for more meaningful interpretation of study results with specific therapies.

Thiopurine therapy

The clinical availability of thiopurine methyltransferase (TPMT) genotyping and thiopurine metabolite level testing has shed new insight on the use of these medications, and should be helpful in optimizing this cornerstone of IBD therapy. TPMT, the key enzyme involved in the metabolism of 6-mercaptopurine (6-MP)/azathioprine (AZA) is subject to significant genetic variability [159]. Indivi-

duals with very low TPMT activity are at risk for severe toxicity, even death, from an inability to metabolize these drugs [160]. Thus it is of clinical relevance that determination of the TPMT genotype prior to initiation of 6-MP/AZA allows for identification of these at-risk patients. Furthermore, patients with intermediate enzyme activity generally achieve 6-thioguanine nucleotide (6-TGN) levels in the therapeutic range at lower drug doses. AZA is non-enzymatically converted to 6-MP, which in turn is intracellularly converted to the thiopurine metabolites, 6-TGN and 6-methylmercaptopurine ribonucleotides (6-MMPR). Erythrocyte 6-TGN levels over $230-235$ pmol$/8 \times 10^8$ red blood cells are significantly associated with therapeutic response to 6-MP/AZA in IBD [160, 161]. 6-MMPR production is TPMT-dependent and very high 6-MMPR levels are associated with hepatotoxicity and/or leukopenia [160, 162]. It should be noted that dose escalation does not always result in the attainment of therapeutic 6-TGN levels and clinical response in patients failing 6-MP/AZA therapy; in fact, an important unique subgroup of IBD patients resistant to 6-MP/AZA therapy has recently been identified based on patterns 6-MP/AZA of metabolite profiles [162]. This subgroup of patients is biochemically characterized by preferential shunting of the 6-MP substrate toward the overproduction of potentially toxic 6-MMPR levels upon dose escalation, while negligible to absent rises in the desired beneficial 6-TGN levels are observed. Thus, this identifiable metabolic pattern explains the majority of dose-related 6-MP hepatotoxic and/or bone marrow-suppressive adverse events limiting the usefulness of 6-MP/AZA in this subset of patients. The strategies of blocking the TPMT enzyme with sulfasalazine or olsalazine, and splitting the daily dose of 6-MP/AZA are being evaluated as potential ways of diminishing 6-MMP production. Importantly, alternate or additional pharmacologic approaches will ultimately be required by the majority of patients in this phenotypically distinct subgroup of IBD patients in whom traditional thiopurine therapy alone tends not to adequately suppress disease activity.

Pouchitis prophylaxis

Given that in the future UC patients with certain serum immune marker profiles (i.e. very high preoperative pANCA levels) and certain genotypes may be identified as being at higher risk for subsequent development of chronic pouchitis following IPAA, strategies aimed at prophylaxis against subsequent development of pouchitis in select UC patients could potentially be undertaken [41, 127, 128].

Genetic research implications

Expression and level of expression of serum immune markers may also allow for stratification of IBD at the genetic level. In order to understand the complex genetic influences predisposing to clinical phenotype expression it is crucial that patients with IBD be stratified into more appropriate pathogenically homogeneous disease subgroups. Most attempts at stratification of IBD to date have been descriptive, focusing on stratifying patients with IBD based on traditional approaches: the anatomic distribution of inflammation and on characteristic fibrostenosing and perforating/fistulizing behavior patterns, rather than on suspected etiology of pathogenic mechanisms of disease. The immunologic responses in IBD, as measured by type and level of marker antibody production, may well reflect different host genetic profiles. Thus stratification based on serum immune marker expression may filter out the 'background noise' inherent in studies of a heterogeneous group of diseases with some similar characteristics, and may facilitate the identification of pathogenically more homogeneous subsets of patients, and perhaps identify 'at-risk individuals' in a group of diseases with complex genetic influences, including reduced penetrance or variable expressivity of disease. Preliminary genetic analyses stratifying on type and level of immune marker expression suggest that this approach may be indeed fruitful [66, 163].

Summary

To approach the underlying mechanisms involved in the various forms of Crohn's diseases and ulcerative colitides, clinical and genetic studies of IBD must rely upon homogeneous patient subgroups [5, 10]. Current stratification strategies which focus on the clinical characteristics of anatomic distribution of inflammation and disease behavior patterns do not reflect specific pathogenic mechanisms. The immunologic responses in IBD, as measured by marker antibody production, may well reflect different host genetic profiles. The use of ASCA and pANCA, and potentially other serum and genetic markers, allows for identification of more homogeneous subgroups of patients with common subclinical and clinical characteristics, based on immune mechanisms of disease.

References

1. Lennard-Jones JE. Classification of inflammatory bowel disease. Scand J Gastroenterol 1989; 24(Suppl.): 2–6.
2. Allchin WH. Ulcerative colitis. Proc Roy Soc Med 1909; 2: 59–75.
3. Dalziel Tk. Chronic interstitial enteritis. Br Med J 1913; 2: 1068–70.
4. Crohn BB, Ginzburg L, Oppenheimer GD. Regional ileitis. J Am Med Assoc 1932; 99: 1323–9.
5. Sachar DB, Andrews HA, Farmer RG et al. Proposed classification of patients subgroups in Crohn's disease. Gastroenterol Int 1992; 5: 141–54.
6. Targan S, Murphy LK. Serologic and mucosal markers of ulcerative colitis and Crohn's disease: implications of pathophysiology for diagnosis. In: Scholmerich J, Kruis W, Goebell H et al, eds. Inflammatory Bowel Diseases – Pathophysiology as a Basis of Treatment. Dordrecht: Kluwer Academic Publishers, 1993: 283–6.
7. Rotter JI, Yang H. Delineating the major aetiological risk factors for IBD: the genetic susceptibilities. In: Scholmerich J, Kruis W, Goebell H et al, eds. Inflammatory Bowel Diseases – Pathophysiology as a Basis of Treatment. Dordrecht: Kluwer Academic Publishers, 1993: 9–18.
8. Yang H, Rotter JI. The genetics of inflammatory bowel disease: genetic predispositions, disease markers, and genetic heterogeneity. In: Targan SR, Shanahan F, eds. Inflammatory Bowel Disease: From Bench to Bedside. Baltimore: Williams & Wilkins, 1994: 32–64.
9. Satsangi J, Jewell DP, Rosenberg WMC, Bell JI. Genetics of inflammatory bowel disease. Gut 1994; 35: 696–700.
10. Vasiliauskas EA, Kam LY, Karp LC, Gaiennie J, Yang HY, Targan SR. Marker antibody expression stratifies Crohn's disease into immunologically homogeneous subgroups with distinct clinical characteristics. Gut 2000; 47: 487–96.
11. Duerr RH, Targan SR, Landers CJ, Sutherland LR, Shanahan F. Anti-neutrophil cytoplasmic antibodies in ulcerative colitis: comparison with other colitides/diarrheal illnesses. Gastroenterology 1991; 100: 1590–6.
12. Shanahan F, Duerr RH, Rotter JI et al. Neutrophil autoantibodies in ulcerative colitis: familial aggregation and genetic heterogeneity. Gastroenterology 1992; 103: 456–61.
13. Yang HY, Rotter JI, Toyoda H et al. Ulcerative colitis: a genetically heterogeneous disorder defined by genetic (HLA class II) and subclinical (antineutrophil cytoplasmic antibodies) markers. J Clin Invest 1993; 92: 1080–4.
14. Satsangi J, Landers CJ, Welsh KI, Koss K, Targan S, Jewell DP. The presence of anti-neutrophil antibodies reflects clinical and genetic heterogeneity within inflammatory bowel disease. Inflam Bowel Dis 1998; 4: 18–26.
15. Sendid B, Quinton JF, Charrier G, Goulet O, Cortot A, Grandbastien B, Poulain D, Colombel JF. Anti-Saccharomyces cerevisiae mannan antibodies in familial Crohn's disease. Am J Gastroenterol 1998; 93: 1306–10.
16. Sutton CL, Yang H, Li Z, Rotter JI, Targan SR, Braun J. Familial expression of anti-Saccharomyces cerevisiae mannan antibodies in affected and unaffected relatives of patients with Crohn's disease. Gut 2000; 46: 58–63.
17. Jennette JC, Hogan S, Wilkman AS, Tuttle R, Jones D, Falk RJ. Anti-neutrophil cytoplasmic autoantibody (ANCA) disease associations. Scand J Gastroenterol 1989; 24 (Suppl. 158): 206–7 (A39).
18. Saxon A, Shanahan F, Landers C, Ganz T, Targan S. A distinct subset of antineutrophil cytoplasmic antibodies is associated with inflammatory bowel disease. J Allergy Clin Immunol 1990; 86: 202–10.
19. Duerr RH, Targan SR, Landers CJ et al. Neutrophil cytoplasmic antibodies: a link between primary sclerosing cho-

langitis and ulcerative colitis. Gastroenterology 1991; 100: 1385–91.

20. Seibold F, Weber P, Klein R, Berg PA, Wiedmann KH. Clinical significance of antibodies against neutrophils in patients with inflammatory bowel disease and primary sclerosing cholangitis. Gut 1992; 33: 657–62.

21. Colombel JF, Reumaux D, Duthilleul P et al.Antineutrophil cytoplasmic autoantibodies in inflammatory bowel diseases. Gastroenterol Clin Biol 1992; 16: 656–60.

22. Cambridge G, Rampton DS, Stevens TRJ, McCarthy DA, Kamm M, Leaker B. Anti-neutrophil antibodies in inflammatory bowel disease: prevalence and diagnostic role. Gut 1992; 33: 668–74.

23. Lo SK, Fleming KA, Chapman RW. Prevalence of anti-neutrophil antibody in primary sclerosing cholangitis and ulcerative colitis using an alkaline phosphatase technique. Gut 1992; 33: 1370–3.

24. Oudkerk Pool M, Ellerbroek PM, Ridwan BU et al. Serum antineutrophil cytoplasmic autoantibodies in inflammatory bowel disease are mainly associated with ulcerative colitis. A correlation study between perinuclear antineutrophil cytoplasmic autoantibodies and clinical parameters, medical, and surgical treatment. Gut 1993; 34: 46–50.

25. Hardarson S, Labrecque DR, Mitros FA, Neil GA, Goeken JA. Antineutrophil cytoplasmic antibody in inflammatory bowel and hepatobiliary diseases. Am J Clin Pathol 1993; 99: 277–81.

26. Proujansky R, Fawcett PT, Gibney KM, Treem WR, Hyams JS. Examination of anti-neutrophil cytoplasmic antibodies in childhood inflammatory bowel disease. J Pediatr Gastroenterol Nutr 1993; 17: 193–7.

27. Reumaux D, Colombel JF, Delecourt L, Noel LH, Cortot A, Duthilleul P. Anti-neutrophil cytoplasmic auto-antibodies (ANCA) in patients with ulcerative colitis (UC): influence of disease activity and familial study. Adv Exp Med Biol 1993; 336: 515–18.

28. Broekroelofs J, Mulder AH, Nelis GF, Esterveld BD, Ervaert JWC, Allenberg CGM. Anti-neutrophil cytoplasmic antibodies (ANCA) in sera from patients with inflammatory bowel disease (IBD): relation to disease pattern and disease activity. Dig Dis Sci 1994; 39: 545–9.

29. Mulder AHL, Broekroelofs J, Horst G, Limburg PC, Nelis GF, Kallenberg CGM. Anti-neutrophil cytoplasmic antibodies (ANCA) in inflammatory bowel disease: characterization and clinical correlates. Clin Exp Immunol 1994; 95: 490–7.

30. Sung JY, Chan FKL, Lawton J et al. Anti-neutrophil cytoplasmic antibodies (ANCA) and inflammatory bowel diseases in Chinese. Dig Dis Sci 1994; 39: 886–92.

31. Vecchi M, Bianchi MB, Sinico RA et al. Antibodies to neutrophil cytoplasm in Italian patients with ulcerative colitis: sensitivity, specificity and recognition of putative antigens. Digestion 1994; 55: 34–9.

32. Winter HS, Landers CJ, Winkelstein A, Vidrich A, Targan SR. Anti-neutrophil cytoplasmic antibodies in children with ulcerative colitis. J Pediatr 1994; 125: 707–11.

33. Patel RT, Stokes R, Birch D, Ibbotson J, Keighley MRB. Influence of total colectomy on serum antineutrophil cytoplasmic antibodies in inflammatory bowel disease. Br J Surg 1994; 81: 724–6.

34. Seibold F, Slametschka D, Gregor M, Weber P. Neutrophil autoantibodies: a genetic marker in primary sclerosing cholangitis and ulcerative colitis. Gastroenterology 1994; 107: 532–6.

35. Boerr LA, Sambuelli AM, Katz S et al. Clinical heterogeneity of ulcerative colitis in relation to frequency of pANCA reactivity. Gastroenterology 1995; 108: A785.

36. Lee JCW, Lennard-Jones JE, Cambridge G. Antineutrophil antibodies in familial inflammatory bowel disease. Gastroenterology 1995; 108: 428–33.

37. Vasiliauskas EA, Plevy SE, Landers CJ et al. Perinuclear antineutrophil cytoplasmic antibodies in patients with Crohn's disease define a clinical subgroup. Gastroenterology 1996; 110: 1810–19.

38. Quinton J-F, Sendid B, Reumaux D et al. Anti- Saccharomyces cerevisiae mannan antibodies combined with antineutrophil cytoplasmic autoantibodies in inflammatory bowel disease: prevalence and diagnostic role. Gut 1998; 42: 788–91.

39. Ruemmele FM, Targan SR, Levy G, Dubinsky M, Braun J, Seidman EG. Diagnostic accuracy of serological assays in pediatric inflammatory bowel disease. Gastroenterology 1998; 115: 822–9.

40. Hoffenberg EJ, Fidanza S, Sauaia A. Serologic testing for inflammatory bowel disease. J Pediatr 1999; 134: 447–52.

41. Fleshner PR, Vasiliauskas EA, Kam LY et al. High level perinuclear antineutrophil cytoplasmic antibody (pANCA) in ulcerative colitis patients before colectomy predicts the development of chronic pouchitis after ileal pouch–anal anastomosis. Gut 2001 49: 671–7.

42. Sandborn WJ, Loftus EV, Colombel JF et al. Utility of perinuclear anti-neutrophil cytoplasmic antibodies (pANCA), anti-Saccharomyces cerevisiae (ASCA), and anti-pancreatic antibody (APA) as serologic markers in a population based cohort of patients with Crohn's disease (CD) and ulcerative colitis (UC). Gastroenterology 2000; 118: A106 (no. 696) .

43. Deusch K, Oberstadt K, Schaedel W, Weber M, Classen M. p-ANCA as a diagnostic marker in ulcerative colitis. Adv Exp Med Biol 1993; 336: 527–31.

44. Taylor K, Plevy SE, Yang H et al. ANCA pattern and LTA haplotype relationship to clinical responses to anti-TNF antibody treatment in Crohn's disease. Gastroenterology 2001; 120: 1347–55.

45. Vasiliauskas E, Targan SR. Do pANCA define a clinical subgroup in patients with Crohn's disease? Gastroenterology 1997; 112: 316–17.

46. Vidrich A, Lee J, James E, Cobb L, Targan S. Segregation of pANCA antigenic recognition by DNase treatment of neutrophils: ulcerative colitis, type 1 autoimmune hepatitis, and primary sclerosing cholangitis. J Clin Immunol 1995; 15: 293–9.

47. Vasiliauskas EA, Kam LY, Abreu-Martin MT et al. An open-label pilot study of low-dose thalidomide in chronically-active, steroid-dependent Crohn's disease. Gastroenterology 1999; 117: 1278–87.

48. Ellerbroek PM, Oudkerk Pool M, Ridwan BU et al. Neutrophil cytoplasmic antibodies (p-ANCA) in ulcerative colitis. J Clin Pathol 1994; 47: 257–62.

49. Billing P, Tahir S, Calfin B et al. Nuclear localization of the antigen detected by ulcerative colitis-associated perinuclear antineutrophil cytoplasmic antibodies. Am J Pathol 1995; 147: 979–87.

50. Eggena M, Cohavy O, Parseghian MH, et al. Identification of histone H1 as a cognate antigen of the ulcerative colitis-associated marker antibody pANCA. J Autoimmun 2000; 14: 83–97.

51. Gordon LK, Eggena M, Targan SR, Braun J. Mast cell and neuroendocrine cytoplasmic autoantigen(s) detected by monoclonal pANCA antibodies. Clin Immunol 2000; 94: 42–50.

52. Cohavy O, Bruckner D, Gordon LK et al. Colonic bacteria express an ulcerative colitis pANCA-related protein epitope. Infect Immun 2000; 68: 1542–8.

53. Targan SR, Landers CJ, Cobb L, MacDermott RP, Vidrich A. Perinuclear anti-neutrophil cytoplasmic antibodies are

spontaneously produced by mucosal B cells of ulcerative colitis patients. J Immunol 1995; 155: 3262–7.

54. Plevy SE, Landers CJ, Vasiliauskas EA, Targan SR, Vidrich A. Alterations in serum immunoglobulin (Ig) G subclasses provide evidence for distinct immune responses in pANCA positive Crohn's disease patients. Gastroenterology 1996; 110: A993 .

55. Kam LY, Vasiliauskas EA, Landers CJ, Targan SR. Magnitude of response to Remicade™ correlates with marker antibody expression. Gastroenterology 1999; 116: A744 (G3232).

56. Vasiliauskas EA, Plevy SE, Targan SR. Stratification of Crohn's disease by antineutrophil cytoplasmic antibodies (ANCA) & anti-*Saccharomyces cerevisiae* antibody (ASCA) distinguishes phenotypic subgroups. Gastroenterology 1997; 112: A1112.

57. McKenzie H, Main J, Pennington CR, Parratt D. Antibody to selected strains of *Saccharomyces cerevisiae* (baker's and brewer's yeast) and *Candida albicans* in Crohn's disease. Gut 1990; 31: 536–8.

58. Barclay GR, McKenzie H, Pennington J, Parratt D, Pennington CR. The effect of dietary yeast on the activity of stable chronic Crohn's disease. Scand J Gastroenterol 1992; 27(Suppl.): 196–200.

59. Sendid B, Colombel JF, Jacquinot PM et al. Specific antibody response to oligomannosidic epitopes in Crohn's disease. Clin Diagn Lab Immunol 1996; 3: 219–26.

60. Dubinsky MC, Ofman JJ, Urman M, Targan SR, Seidman EG. Clinical utility of serodiagnostic testing in suspected pediatric inflammatory bowel disease. Am J Gastroenterol 2001; 96: 758–65.

61. Lindberg E, Magnusson KE, Tysk C, Järnerot G. Antibody (IgG, IgA, and IgM) to baker's yeast (*Saccharomyces cerevisiae*), yeast mannan, gliadin, ovalbumin and betalactoglobulin in monozygotic twins with inflammatory bowel disease. Gut 1992; 33: 909–13.

62. Darroch CJ, Christmas SE, Barnes RMR. In vitro human lymphocyte proliferative responses to a glycoprotein of the yeast *Saccharomyces cerevisiae* . Immunology 1994; 81: 247–52.

63. Young CA, Sonnenberg A, Burns EA. Lymphocyte proliferation response to baker's yeast in Crohn's disease. Digestion 1994; 55: 40–3.

64. Taylor KD, Li Z, Barry M et al. Tumor necrosis factor microsatellite haplotype a11b4c1d3e3 is associated with anti-*Saccharomyces cerevisiae* antibody (ASCA) across clinical forms of inflammatory bowel disease. Gastroenterology 1998; 114: A1098 (G4492).

65. Lubinski SM, LaBuda MC, Cho JH, Hanauer SB, Bayless TM, Brant SR. Anti-*Saccharomyces* Antibodies (ASCA) are highly positive in familial Crohn's disease (CD). Gastroenterology 1999; 116: A766 (G3323).

66. Yang H, Taylor K, Lin YC, Targan SR, Rotter JI. Magnitude of anti-*Saccharomyces cerevisiae* antibody (ASCA) expression is linked, in Crohn's disease, families to the major histocompatibility complex (MHC) region. Gastroenterology 2000; 118: A339 (no. 1833).

67. Plevy SE, Vasiliauskas EA, Taylor K et al. The Crohn's disease associated tumor necrosis factor (TNF) microsatellite a2b1c2d4e1 haplotype and anti-*Saccharomyces cerevisiae* antibody (ASCA)define medically resistant forms of ulcerative colitis. Gastroenterology 1997; 112: A1062.

68. Duchmann R, Kaiser I, Hermann E et al. Tolerance exists towards resident intestinal flora but is broken in active inflammatory bowel disease (IBD). Clin Exp Immunol 1995; 102: 448–55.

69. Cohavy O, Harth G, Horwitz M et al. Identification of a novel mycobacterial histone H1 homologue (HupB) as an antigenic target of pANCA monoclonal antibody and serum immunoglobulin A from patients with Crohn's disease. Infect Immun 1999; 67: 6510–17.

70. Murry PR, Rosenthal KS, Kobayashi GS, Pfaller MA. Medical Microbiology, 4th edn. St Louis, Missouri: Mosby-Yearbook Inc, 2002: 11–24.

71. Singh SP, Upshaw Y, Abdullah T, Singh SR , Klebba PE. Structural relatedness of enteric bacterial porins assessed with monoclonal antibodies to *Salmonella typhimurium* OmpD and OmpC. J Bacteriol 1992; 174: 1965–73.

72. Painbeni E, Caroff M, Rouviere-Yaniv J. Alternations of the outer membrane composition in *Escherichia* lacking the histone-like protein HU. Proc Natl Acad Sci 1997; 94: 6712–17.

73. Sutton CL, Kim J, Yamane A et al. Identification of a novel bacterial sequence associated with Crohn's disease. Gastroenterology 2000; 119: 23–31.

74. Landers CJ, Braun J, Targan SR. I2, a mucosal Crohn's disease (CD) associated bacterial antigen, induces both humoral *and* T-cell responses in CD patients: I2 induced interferon-Γ (INF-Γ) production is associated with higher levels of serum IgA reactivity. Gastroenterology 2000; 118: A347 (no. 1870).

75. Stevens TR, Winrow VR, Blake DR, Rampton DS. Circulating antibodies to heat–shock protein 60 in Crohn's disease and ulcerative colitis. Clin Exp Immunol 1992; 90: 271–4.

76. Halbwachs-Mecarelli L, Nusbaum P, Noël LH et al. Antineutrophil cytoplasmic antibodies (ANCA) directed against cathepsin G in ulcerative colitis, Crohn's disease and primary sclerosing cholangitis. Clin Exp Immunol 1992; 90: 79–84.

77. Mayet WJ, Hermann E, Finsterwalder J et al. Antibodies to cathepsin G in Crohn's disease. Eur J Clin Invest 1992; 22: 427–33.

78. Fricke H, Birkhofer A, Folwaczny C, Meister W, Scriba PC. Characterization of antigens from the human exocrine pancreatic tissue (Pag) relevant as target antigens for autoantibodies in Crohn's disease [See comments]. Eur J Clin Invest 1999; 29: 41–5.

79. Seibold F, Weber P, Jenss H, Wiedmann KH. Antibodies to a trypsin sensitive pancreatic antigen in chronic inflammatory bowel disease: specific markers for a subgroup of patients with Crohn's disease. Gut 1991; 32: 1192–7.

80. Seibold F, Scheurlen M, Muller A, Jenss H, Weber P. Impaired pancreatic function in patients with Crohn's disease with and without pancreatic autoantibodies. J Clin Gastroenterol 1996; 22: 202–6.

81. Seibold F, Mork H, Tanza S et al. Pancreatic autoantibodies in Crohn's disease: a family study. Gut 1997; 40: 481–4.

82. Folwaczny C, Noehl N, Endres SP, Loeschke K, Fricke H. Antineutrophil and pancreatic autoantibodies in first-degree relatives of patients with inflammatory bowel disease. Scand J Gastroenterol 1998; 33: 523–8.

83. Propst A, Propst T, Herold M, Vogel W, Judmaier G. Interleukin-1 receptor antagonist in differential diagnosis of inflammatory bowel diseases. Eur J Gastroenterol Hepatol 1995; 7: 1031–6.

84. Cassini-Raggi V, Kam L, Chong YT, Fiocchi C, Pizarro TT, Cominelli F. Mucosal imbalance of IL-1 and IL-1 receptor antagonist in inflammatory bowel disease. J Immunol 1995; 154: 2434–40.

85. Mansfield JC, Holden H, Tarlow JK et al. Novel genetic association between ulcerative colitis and the anti-inflammatory cytokine interleukin-1 receptor antagonist. Gastroenterology 1994; 106: 637–42.

86. Tountas NA, Casini-Raggi V, Yang H et al.. Functional and ethnic association of allele 2 of the interleukin-1 receptor antagonist gene in ulcerative colitis. Gastroenterology 1999; 117: 806–13.

21 | Differential diagnosis of colitis

SUE C. ENG AND CHRISTINA M. SURAWICZ

Introduction

The classic symptoms of colitis are diarrhea (which may be bloody) and abdominal pain. They may be accompanied by fever, cramps, or other symptoms such as malaise, vomiting, chills, myalgias, and nausea. When symptoms of colitis begin suddenly, the usual differential is between an infectious colitis and a first attack of idiopathic inflammatory bowel disease (IBD). However, there are many other causes of colitis (Table 1). Diagnostic clues can be obtained by history and physical examination, as well as laboratory tests and stool cultures. Examination of the colonic mucosa via sigmoidoscopy or colonoscopy and by biopsy is often required for a definitive diagnosis. This chapter will describe differentiation of IBD from infectious colitis. Pathogens that cause acute self-limiting colitis are described; these differ from those which cause sexually transmitted colitis and from those which cause colitis in persons who are immunosuppressed. Finally, differential diagnosis of ulcerative colitis (UC) from Crohn's disease (CD) will be defined, as well as colitis of other etiologies.

Distinguishing acute self-limiting colitis from idiopathic IBD

History and physical examination

The initial differential of acute diarrhea is often between an infectious type of colitis, i.e. acute self-limited colitis, and a first episode of IBD. By definition, acute self-limiting colitis is a colitis that resolves in less than 4 weeks. Although an infectious etiology is often suspected, stool cultures yield a pathogen in only 55% of cases. By contrast, IBD is a chronic illness. In a prospective study of first attacks of colitis, historical clues favoring infectious colitis included acute onset in 81%, fever within the first week after onset of disease in 75%, and at least 10

bowel movements in a 24-h period in 76%. In contrast, in patients eventually diagnosed with IBD, the onset was insidious in 56%, there was no fever or fever more than 1 week after the onset of disease in 83%, and no more than six bowel movements in a 24-h period in 85% [1]. Physical examination is rarely helpful because left lower quadrant tenderness over the area of the descending and sigmoid colon is non-specific. However, a right lower quadrant mass should suggest Crohn's ileocolitis.

Laboratory evaluation

Laboratory evaluation may be helpful but is never diagnostic. For example, an elevated white blood cell count can be seen with either acute self-limiting colitis or IBD. Anemia, especially iron-deficiency anemia, suggests IBD, as the usual course in acute self-limiting colitis is too short for significant blood loss. Anemia in IBD may be due to iron lack from blood loss, or due to vitamin B_{12} deficiency in CD with malabsorption due to small intestinal disease. Anemia may also be due to marrow suppression. A study of clinical and laboratory parameters in 239 adults, 212 of whom had infective diarrhea and 27 who proved to have IBD, revealed that the clinical features which predicted IBD were long-standing diarrhea, fecal blood, anemia, leukocytosis, thrombocytosis, and a decrease in serum albumin [2]. Interestingly, the most helpful differentiating feature was the platelet count which was greater than 450×10^9/liter in 59% of patients with IBD compared to only 1.6% of patients with infective diarrhea. Fecal leukocytes are insensitive in distinguishing IBD from infectious colitis because they can be seen in both [3].

Routine stool cultures will identify a pathogen only about 55% of the time. Of presumed infectious diarrhea, cultures obtained early in the course will have a higher yield. In hospitalized patients, if the stool specimens were obtained within 3 days of

Stephan R. Targan, Fergus Shanahan and Loren C. Karp (eds.), *Inflammatory Bowel Disease: From Bench to Bedside, 2nd Edition*, 431–455.
© 2003 Kluwer Academic Publishers. Printed in Great Britain

Table 1. Differential diagnosis of colitis

I.   Idiopathic
     A.   Inflammatory bowel disease
          1.   Crohn's disease
          2.   Ulcerative colitis
          3.   Indeterminate colitis
     B.   Diversion colitis
     C.   Collagenous colitis
     D.   Microscopic (lymphocytic) colitis

II. Infections
     A.   Bacteria
     B.   Parasites
     C.   Viruses
     D.   Fungi
     E.   *C. difficile* (antibiotic-associated pseudomembranous
          colitis)

III. Ischemia
     A.   Mesenteric ischemia or thrombosis
     B.   Drug-induced (cocaine, oral contraceptives)
     C.   Proximal to mechanical obstruction

IV. Physical agents
     A.   Radiation
     B.   Solitary rectal ulcer syndrome (prolapse)
     C.   Glutaraldehyde or hydrogen peroxide (endoscopic cleaning
          solutions)
     D.   Drug-induced
          1.   Gold
          2.   Isotretinoin
          3.   Laxatives
          4.   Allopurinol
          5.   Non-*C. difficile* antibiotic-induced i.e. ampicillin (usually
               right-sided colitis)
          6.   Chemotherapeutics (5-fluorouracil)
          7.   Non-steroidal anti-inflammatory drugs

Immunologic
     A.   Allergic proctitis
     B.   Eosinophilic colitis
     C.   Graft-versus-host disease
     D.   Immunodeficiency syndromes

Associated with systemic disease
     A.   Vasculitis
     B.   Behçet's disease
     C.   Sarcoidosis

Miscellaneous
     A.   Diverticulitis
     B.   Colon cancer

Adapted with permission from Surawicz CM. Diagnosing colitis. Contemp Intern Med 1991; 3: 17.

admission, cultures were positive for *Salmonella, Shigella,* or *Campylobacter* species in 12.6% (compared to 1.4% if obtained after 3 days of admission). Cytotoxin for *C. difficile* was detectable in 12.8% and rotavirus was detected in 12.5% from specimens obtained within 3 days versus 9.8% and 11.8% if the stools were obtained after 3 days of hospitalization [4]. If stool cultures were not sent, or are negative, intraluminal fluid obtained during colonoscopy can be sent for culture [5], but biopsy cultures add little to the diagnosis of infectious colitis. In industrialized countries the most common pathogens are *Campylobacter jejuni/Escherichia coli* spp. [6], followed by *Salmonella* spp. (Table 2). In travelers to underdeveloped countries, *E. coli* spp., *Shigella* spp., and *Campylobacter* spp., are the most frequent pathogens [7]. 'New' organisms that cause colitis continue to be discovered. In addition, multifocal colitis has been detected in two separate epidemics of chronic diarrhea from which no pathogens were ever identified, the Brainerd diarrhea and the Henderson County outbreak [8, 9].

Routine stool cultures for enteric pathogens can identify *Shigella, Salmonella, Campylobacter,* and *E. coli* O157:H7 in about 55% of cases. The presence of *Aeromonas, Plesiomonas,* and *Vibrio* can also be detected on routine cultures, but their identities

Table 2. Infectious colitis in immunocompetent individuals

Bacteria
   Campylobacter spp.
   Salmonella spp.
   Shigella spp.
   C. difficile
   Vibrio/non-cholera spp.
   Y. enterocolitica
   Tuberculosis

Fungi
   Histoplasmosis
   South American blastomycosis
   ? Candida

Parasites
   E. histolytica
   Schistosomiasis
   B. hominis

Viruses
   Herpes simplex virus type II
   Cytomegalovirus

require further work-up by the laboratory in order to identify them further. Specific requests are needed if *Yersinia* or *Clostridium difficile* is suspected.

Evaluating the colonic mucosa

When a specific diagnosis is necessary it may be important and necessary to look at the colonic mucosa, both grossly and microscopically. It is best to perform sigmoidoscopy without a harsh laxative or enema preparation, as these can cause mucosal damage which may be mistaken for colitis. If stool obscures the lumen, a tapwater or saline enema can be given. The visual appearance of UC is typical, with almost uniform rectal involvement, edematous and erythematous mucosa with loss of vascular pattern and friability. Discrete ulcers are rare. CD, in contrast, is focal and transmural. Its early lesions are isolated aphthous ulcers; later there are linear ulcers in normal surrounding mucosa, although areas of diffuse colitis can also be seen.

The appearance of the mucosa which suggests an infectious colitis is patchy petechial hemorrhage, with focal edema and erythema [3]. However, this does not differentiate between one infection and another, nor does it preclude another diagnosis such as UC, or a superinfection such as shigellosis. Pseudomembranous colitis due to *C. difficile* has a characteristic appearance, with creamy yellow–white plaques that bleed when they are removed.

Mucosal biopsy can be very helpful in distinguishing between IBD, especially UC, and acute self-limiting colitis, because crypt distortion, which is a hallmark of the former, is rare in infectious colitis [10–12]. The mucosa in UC shows branched or forked crypts, present even with an early presentation, suggesting that crypt changes may precede the development of symptoms. In addition to branched glands, distortion of architecture can include a villous surface and crypt atrophy (sparse crypts that are shortened and do not reach the muscularis mucosae). In contrast, in acute self-limiting colitis, crypt architecture remains normal, both during the disease and after healing has occurred (Figs. 1 and 2). There may be some exceptions to this general rule. For instance, in an epidemic of shigellosis in India, which involved 78 000 cases and 2200 deaths, mucosal biopsies showed frequent crypt architectural distortion [13]. However, it may be that this was due to differences in the patient population or due to that especially virulent pathogen.

Other histologic clues that help distinguish acute self-limiting colitis from IBD include the nature of the lamina propria inflammation, the presence or absence of granulomas, and the location of isolated giant cells [11].

The inflammatory infiltrate in acute self-limiting colitis is predominantly acute, i.e. polymorphonuclear cells, and may be most prominent in the upper half of the mucosa. In contrast, in IBD the inflammation consists of both acute and chronic inflammatory cells (polymorphonuclear cells as well as plasma cells and lymphocytes). It should be noted that the normal lamina propria cells include plasma cells and lymphocytes but not polymorphonuclear cells; thus an increase in polymorphonuclear cells is easy to detect, but an increase in 'chronic cells' should only be called abnormal if their numbers are clearly increased. Some have noted an increase in plasma cells near the crypt bases, described as 'basilar plasmacytosis' [12]. Focal or diffuse basal plasmacytosis is seen in 69% of patients with IBD and only in 3% of infectious colitis [14]. This is an area where plasma cells are normally sparse so that an increase can be detected easily. Basilar lymphoid aggregates are increased in UC (two or more per average-sized biopsy is abnormal). Crypt abscesses are a non-specific indication of inflammation and do not indicate a specific diagnosis. Similarly, goblet cell mucin depletion is probably a response to intense inflammation rather than a specific diagnostic clue for UC.

Interestingly, isolated giant cells are also a non-specific inflammatory response. However, in IBD they occur more frequently at the bases of crypts, and in infectious colitis they are more frequent superficially, in the upper third of the mucosa. Granulomas, however, strongly suggest CD, although they can occur in rare cases of infectious colitis due to lymphogranuloma venereum (LGV) strains of *Chlamydia trachomatis* or syphilis [15]. Some have found the presence of basal giant cells, granulomas, and epithelial surface erosions to be the most reliable histologic features in early diagnosis of IBD [16]. Focal inflammation may be seen in resolving acute self-limiting colitis as well as in CD [12]. Thus, the clinical setting and follow-up are important to avoid misdiagnoses [17].

It is usually not possible to diagnose specific infections by biopsy, although some biopsy features are specific (Table 3). Viral inclusions suggest cytomegalovirus or herpes simplex virus type II, and granulomas are seen in tuberculosis, *Mycobacterium*

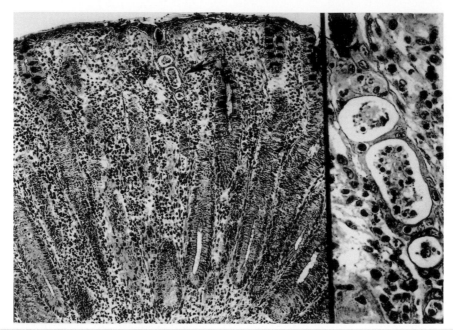

Figure 1. Rectal biopsy from a patient with *Campylobacter* colitis. Note normal architecture, predominantly acute inflammatory cells in the lamina propria, and crypt abscesses (arrow). Right: string of pearls crypt abscess (higher power).

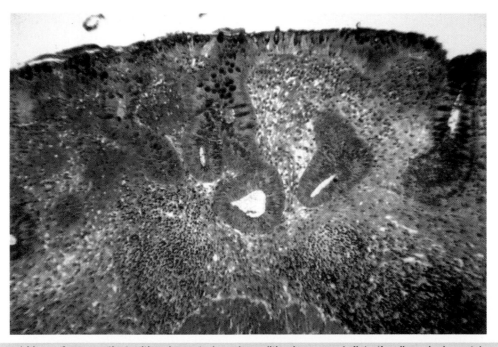

Figure 2. Rectal biopsy from a patient with quiescent ulcerative colitis shows crypt distortion (branched crypts), crypts atrophy (crypts are sparse and shortened), and basal lymphoid aggregates above the muscularis mucosa. (Reprinted with permission from Surawicz CM, Belic L. Rectal biopsy helps to distinguish acute self-limited colitis from idiopathic inflammatory bowel disease. Gastroenterology 1984; 86: 106.)

avium-intracellulare infection (in AIDS), syphilis, or *C. trachomatis* infection (in sexually transmitted proctitis). The histologic findings of pseudomembranous colitis are characteristic, with preservation of crypt architecture and a pseudomembrane composed of fibrin, polys, and debris which emanates from the surface epithelium in a 'volcanic' fashion, called a 'summit' lesion (Fig. 3). The histology of *E. coli* O157:H7, an infectious colitis, can suggest ischemic injury with superficial necrosis, and occasionally an inflammatory pseudomembrane [18] (Fig. 4).

Table 3. Histology of infectious colitis

Non-specific features	
Preservation of normal architecture	
Acute inflammation	
Crypt abscesses	
Suggestive specific features	
Pseudomembranes	*C. difficile*
	E. coli O157:H7
Viral inclusions	
Intranuclear and/or	
Intracytoplasmic	Cytomegalovirus
Intranuclear	Herpes simplex virus type II
Parasites	
Diagnostic organism on	*E. histolytica*
surface of biopsy	*Cryptosporidium*
Granuloma around organism	Shistosomiasis
Granulomas	*C. trachomatis*
	Syphilis
	Tuberculosis
Microgranulomas	Non-specific can be seen with *Campylobacter* or *Yersinia* colitis, for example

Specific infections in immunocompetent individuals

Gastrointestinal infections can mimic IBD, making it imperative to be able to differentiate the two; they can also aggravate IBD. The bloody diarrhea that is a classic presenting sign of UC is mimicked by the infectious agents that cause dysentery. These include *Campylobacter*, *Shigella*, *Salmonella*, and *E. coli* O157:H7. Other pathogens are *Aeromonas*, *Plesiomonas*, *Yersinia*, *Entameba histolytica*, severe *C. difficile*, and *Chlamydia trachomatis*.

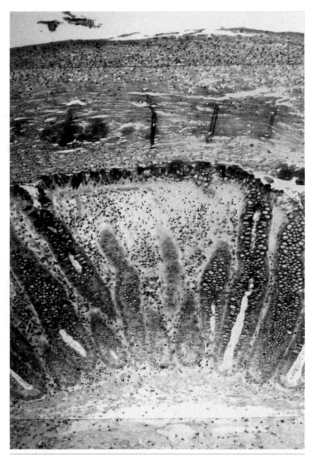

Figure 3. Rectal biopsy from a woman with pseudomembranous colitis; note the pseudomembrane, composed of fibrin, polymorphonuclear cells, and debris, erupting from the surface in a 'volcanic' manner.

Bacteria

Shigellosis

Shigella spp. cause colitis by invading the colonic epithelium and by producing an enterotoxin. Rectal involvement is frequent, but pancolitis can occur. The organism usually causes a dysenteric syndrome with passage of bloody diarrhea or bloody mucus and fever. The course is usually less than a week. Stool cultures are usually diagnostic; bacteremia can occur. A recent paper reviews the epidemiology and clinical and laboratory features [19].

Campylobacter

Campylobacter jejuni has been recognized as a significant cause of dysentery since the late 1970s, and in many areas of the United States it is the

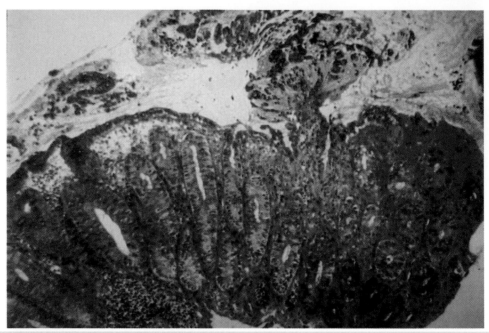

Figure 4 Rectal biopsy from a young woman with *E. coli* O157:H7 colitis who developed hemolytic uremic syndrome. Crypt architecture is normal; there is superficial necrosis, and a pseudomembrane. Histolocially, these features can suggest ischemia or pseudomembranous colitis.

pathogen most frequently isolated from diarrheal stool samples. It accounts for 5–11% of infectious diarrhea [20]. *Campylobacter* is acquired from an animal source, often from undercooked chicken, unpasteurized milk, or pets. In the vast majority of cases this is a limited illness; however, a fulminant *C. jejuni* colitis with toxic megacolon complicated by perforation was recently reported [21]. This case illustrates the difficulty in differentiating IBD from infectious colitis, as the patient was simultaneously treated with corticosteroids which may have exacerbated the infectious colitis.

E. coli

E. coli can cause diarrhea by several mechanisms. Enterotoxigenic *E. coli* (which elaborate a toxin) and enteropathogenic *E. coli* cause diarrhea but usually affect the small intestine rather than the colon. Enteroinvasive *E. coli* causes dysentery and colitis. Other organisms which cause a similar illness include *C. jejuni*, *Shigella*, *Y. enterocolitica*, *Vibrio parahemolyticus*, and *Salmonella*. Enterohemorrhagic *E. coli* results in gross blood per rectum; one-third of cases have neither fecal leukocytes nor fever.

In 1982 the toxigenic *E. coli* O157:H7 was found to cause colitis, including hemorrhagic colitis and hemolytic uremic syndrome [22]. This organism is usually acquired in an epidemic setting; but sporadic cases occur. Outbreaks have been traced to unpasteurized milk and apple juice, undercooked ground beef [23] but also venison, swimming-pool water, and basil pesto, among other vehicles. The young and the elderly are most likely to be seriously ill, and fatalities can occur. One epidemic in a nursing home involved several elderly people who presented with colitis [24]. Given its predilection for the right colon and rectal sparing, it needs to be differentiated not only from ischemic colitis, but also from CD. In two recent cases, radiologic and endoscopic findings on abdominal computerized tomography (CT) and colonoscopy were consistent with CD; only when stool specimens were positive for *E. coli* O157:H7 was the correct diagnosis made and antibiotics and steroids discontinued [25]. In children this infection may cause an illness which presents as suspected IBD or intussusception. Prompt recognition of an epidemic setting and appropriate cultures using special media will allow proper diagnosis. Although the organism is susceptible to most antibiotics, it remains unclear whether antibiotic therapy has any effect on the course of the disease. The organism may be more common than previously suspected. When all diarrheal stools were appropriately cultured, it was found to be the fourth most common bacterial stool pathogen (following *Campylobacter*, *Salmonella*, and *Aeromonas* spp.) at the Mayo Clinic [26].

C. difficile

C. difficile is the most common nosocomially acquired cause of infectious diarrhea. This Gram-positive anaerobic bacillus was recognized in 1979 as the cause of pseudomembranous colitis [27]. Antibiotics perturb the bowel flora and allow for overgrowth of *C. difficile*, which causes disease by producing its toxins. There are two toxins: an enterotoxin, toxin A, which causes mucosal damage and a cytotoxin, toxin B, which can be detected in the stool. The clinical spectrum of disease ranges from diarrhea due to antibiotics (antibiotic-associated diarrhea), in which one-third of patients will have a significant overgrowth of *C. difficile*, to the more serious pseudomembranous colitis, where all patients will have *C. difficile* and toxin in their stools. This illness can range from mild diarrhea to severe colitis with a toxic colon or even megacolon [28]. Any antibiotic can lead to pseudomembranous colitis, although broad-spectrum antibiotics that destroy the protective Gram-negative fecal flora are the usual culprits. Pseudomembranous colitis occurs more frequently after oral than after intravenous antibiotics. There are even a few cases that have occurred after single-dose cephalosporins given as a preoperative antibiotic [29]. Other factors that predispose to pseudomembranous colitis include prolonged hospitalization, surgery, elderly age, and female sex. However, many patients who have received antibiotics and develop diarrhea do not have *C. difficile* in their stools. In addition, some patients with *C. difficile* in their stools but without toxin have diarrhea and are classified as *C. difficile*-positive, toxin-negative diarrhea [30].

Although the most specific test for *C. difficile* is the cell cytotoxin assay and the most sensitive test is the stool culture, both are expensive, and rapid results are not possible. Rapid enzyme immunoassays for the detection of toxin A and B have reasonable sensitivity and specificity and are used in many hospitals [31]. However, a negative test should not exclude the diagnosis if clinical indicators suggest it.

Antibiotics should be discontinued if possible or an antibiotic with a narrower spectrum should be chosen. If the patient is quite ill empiric treatment with metronidazole 500 mg three times a day can be started until results from stool studies are available. Flexible sigmoidoscopy can be performed to look for diagnostic pseudomembranes. Rarely will full colonoscopy be necessary as isolated right-sided pseudomembranous colitis occurs in less than 10% of cases [32].

Yersinia

Y. enterocolitica and *Y. pseudotuberculosis* are pathogens that can cause acute or chronic colitis. When they cause an acute terminal ileitis with mesenteric adenitis, this can be misdiagnosed as acute appendicitis or CD. From a large Dutch study, of 261 patients with *Yersinia* enterocolitis, 8.9% were complicated by arthritis and nearly 25% had chronic symptoms lasting from several months to 1 year [33]. Coupled with its predilection for the terminal ileum, a diagnosis of CD could mistakenly be made if stool cultures are not sent. The colonoscopic features include aphthoid ulcers, in the left or right colon; terminal ileoscopy reveals edema, ulcers, and round or oval elevations of the mucosa [34]. As mentioned, a request to specifically test for *Yersinia* must be made as a special cold-enrichment technique is required [35]. Cultures of lymph nodes, blood, or peritoneal fluid may also be positive, but it may take weeks for the organism to grow. Serology with elevated antibody titers in a typical clinical setting may be useful to make the diagnosis.

Salmonella

Salmonella spp. infection causes diarrhea, usually as a result of involvement of the small intestine. Less frequently it causes colitis and a dysenteric syndrome. A recent paper reviews the epidemiology, clinical features, and diagnostic techniques [19].

Aeromonas

Aeromonas spp. are Gram-negative vibrios that are not part of the normal fecal flora and are recognized as pathogens. Heavy growths have been found in patients with diarrhea [36]. Aeromonas-associated colitis is rare, but there have been reports of chronic colitis due to *Aeromonas* infection which can mimic UC [37–39] or ischemic colitis [40].

Plesiomonas

Plesiomonas is a freshwater organism that is associated with diarrheal illnesses. In one study from Bangladesh it was the fourth most common organism isolated in cases of bacterial gastroenteritis [41]. Although abdominal pain or cramping is the most common symptom, bloody stools can be the presenting symptom in 36% [42].

Tuberculosis

Intestinal tuberculosis frequently involves the ileo-cecal area, as does CD. In primary tuberculosis of the gastrointestinal tract the lungs will be involved in only about 20% of cases, while in primary pulmonary tuberculosis the gastrointestinal tract is involved in 25% of cases [43, 44]. A recent case report illustrates the difficulty in differentiating intestinal tuberculosis from CD. Despite the absence of acid-fast bacilli and histologic findings on colonic biospy consistent with Crohn's, the correct diagnosis of tuberculosis was only made several months after the patient had been started on corticosteroids [45].

Parasites

Amebiasis

The protozoan *Entamoeba histolytica* invades the colon, causing ulcers, typically 'flask-shaped' ulcers in normal surrounding mucosa. Presenting symptoms include abdominal pain, fever, non-bloody diarrhea, or dysentery. Asymptomatic carriage is common. The diagnosis is made by identifying the parasite in fresh stool specimens (90% will be positive for trophozoites) or in biopsy specimens. Because amebic colitis can be chronic it may be mistaken for IBD, either UC or CD. For this reason it is important to exclude amebiasis in such patients, and serology can be quite helpful.

Blastocystis hominis/Balantidium coli

B. hominis is a large protozoan formerly classified as a yeast. Sporadic cases report an associated colitis that responds to therapy [46–49], but other studies show no correlation of the organism's presence in stools of patients with gastrointestinal symptoms [50]. It may be a more significant pathogen in immunosuppressed patients. Rare cases of chronic colitis associated with the parasite *B. coli* have been described, with resolution after tetracycline therapy [51, 52].

Strongyloidiasis

Although *Strongyloides* usually affects the small intestine, it can rarely involve the colon and should be considered in the differential diagnosis of colitis, especially in endemic areas of the US. The diagnosis is made on colonic biopsy when *Strongyloides* larvae are identified, usually near eosinophilic infiltrates in the lamina propria [53].

Fungi

Most fungal infections occur in immunosuppressed patients, with the exception of histoplasmosis, which can involve the colon and small intestine when it disseminates, as well as other areas of the gastrointestinal tract. Perianal ulcers have been previously described and can lead to an incorrect diagnosis of CD [54]. In South America paracoccidiomycosis (South American blastomycosis) can cause a granulomatous inflammation that resembles CD. In both of these infections, organisms can be recognized in biopsy specimens. *Candida* occurs ubiquitously but can invade in immunosuppressed patients in whom the infection may be diagnosed at autopsy, with detection of colonic ulcers.

Gastrointestinal manifestations of sexually transmitted colitis and human immunodeficiency virus

Sexually transmitted colitis

With the advent of the acquired immune deficiency syndrome epidemic in the 1980s, sexual practices in the homosexual male population have changed. With 'safer sex' practices that prevent transmission of human immunodeficiency virus (HIV), there has been a decline in reported cases of sexually transmitted diseases in the US. A recent paper reviews the epidemiology, etiology, and clinical syndromes of sexually acquired proctitis and proctocolitis [55].

Clinical syndromes

Sexually transmitted colitis was recognized in the 1970s, in homosexually active men who presented with frequent gastrointestinal symptoms, including anorectal pain and discharge, diarrhea, and abdominal pain [56] (Table 4). The possible infectious causes, including gonorrhea and syphilis, were recognized early but the landmark study of Quinn *et al.* provided additional significant insight as to pathogens and clinical syndromes [57]. This prospective study of homosexual men with gastrointestinal symptoms presenting to a sexually transmitted disease clinic included comprehensive microbiologic evaluation as well as sigmoidoscopy and biopsy.

Eighty percent of symptomatic and 40% of asymptomatic homosexual men had intestinal pathogens, and multiple infections were common. In addition, it was clear that certain pathogens were associated with the specific clinical syndromes of proctitis, proctocolitis, and enteritis. For example, proctitis, an inflammation limited to the distal rectum, which could mimic ulcerative proctitis, was due to herpes simplex virus type II, syphilis, *N. gonorrhoeae, C. trachomatis*, or ameba.

Proctocolitis presents as bloody diarrhea and abdominal pain due to inflammation extending beyond the rectum, and thus can mimic UC and CD. Specific infectious causes include *Campylobacter* and *Shigella*. Stool cultures were usually diagnostic. Finally, enteritis (abdominal pain and bloating) usually was due to *Giardia lamblia* infection, which can be detected by stool ova and parasite examination. When this is negative, organisms can be detected in duodenal fluid obtained by a string test (Entero-test) or small bowel biopsy. Occasionally, a therapeutic trial of metronidazole can be tried.

Specific infections

Neisseria gonorrhoeae

Gonorrhea is usually accompanied by a mucopurulent discharge and very distal inflammation (5–10 cm above the dentate line) [58, 59]. A smear of the anal mucus is usually diagnostic with intracellular Gram-negative diplococci. Cultures of anal swabs can be innoculated directly onto ThayerMartin media. Biopsies of rectal mucosa are non-specific but may show mild inflammation [60].

Table 4. Common enteric pathogens in homosexual men with sexually-transmitted colitis and patients with AIDS

Clinical syndrome	Sexually transmitted colitis	AIDS
Proctitis	Herpes simplex virus type II Syphilis *C. trachomatis* Gonorrhea Amebiasis	Herpes simples virus type II
Colitis	*Campylobacter* *Shigella*	Cytomegalovirus *Campylobacter* Rare causes include: adenovirus, *H. capsulatum,* and B. *hominis,* among others
Enteritis	*G. lamblia*	Mycobacterium avium- intracellulare Cryptosporidia *I. belli* Microsporidia Cytomegalovirus HIV *Salmonella*

Herpes simplex virus type II

Herpes simplex virus type II also involves the very distal rectum, since it infects squamous epithelium. The gross appearance and symptoms that suggest herpes simplex virus type II include severe anal pain, often associated with constipation, urinary hesitancy, or retention (possibly due to neural involvement), and ulcerative lesions with vesicles [61, 62]. Diagnosis can be made by anal culture or less often by recognizing diagnostic intracellular inclusions in biopsy specimens.

C. trachomatis

The non-LGV strains of *C. trachomatis* can cause an ulcerative proctitis [63, 64]. The LGV strains can also cause a proctocolitis which may be mistaken for CD, because biopsies show epithelioid granulomas such as those seen in CD [65]. Other clinical manifestations include rectal strictures and fistula formation or abscesses [66]. Many patients are asymptomatic. Diagnosis may be difficult but the organism can be isolated in cultures. Direct immunofluorescent staining and enzyme immunosorbent assays can detect the presence of *C. trachomatis*. The lesions heal with antibiotic therapy (doxycycline).

Syphilis

Syphilitic infection of the anorectal area is uncommon but can present with proctitis [67], an anal mass, or an ulcer [68]. Diagnosis is best made by dark-field examination of a swab taken from the lesion, or by serology.

E. histolytica

Most (90%) homosexual men infected with *E. histolytica* are asymptomatic or have vague abdominal complaints. It is likely that these organisms are less virulent than those types that cause invasive amebiasis. Rectal biopsy is often normal.

Diagnostic approach

Determine whether the patient has proctitis, proctocolitis, or enteritis by history. If anoscopy shows pus, culture for *N. gonorrhoeae*. If anoscopy is normal, or symptoms suggest proctitis or proctocolitis, culture for herpes simplex virus type II, *C. trachomatis*, and enteric pathogens, and look for ova and parasites. Empiric therapy has a role; in men with evidence of acute proctitis or proctocolitis, a single dose of ceftriaxone 125 mg intramuscularly and doxycycline 100 mg per os twice a day for 7 days will cure gonorrhea, *Chlamydia* and incubating syphilis [55]. Sigmoidoscopy can be performed when no specific diagnosis can be made with culture and anoscopy or when symptoms do not respond to treatment of a pathogen.

Diarrhea in acquired immune deficiency syndrome (AIDS)

Immunosuppression with HIV is associated with frequent gastrointestinal symptoms, due to involvement of the esophagus, small bowel, and/or colon. Diarrhea is a frequent symptom and may occur in up to 80% of persons infected with HIV. There are many infectious causes. Microbiologic examination will reveal a pathogen in 50–80% of cases, and histology will detect even more pathogens, such as cytomegalovirus [69, 70]. Interestingly, there is very little overlap with the pathogens which cause gay

bowel syndrome (see Table 4). Combination antiretroviral therapy for HIV has resulted in a decrease in gastrointestinal opportunistic infection [71].

Enteric bacteria

Enteric infections such as *Shigella* and *Campylobacter* can cause colitis, as in immunocompetent individuals. But in persons with HIV infection, stool cultures can occasionally be negative although the organism can be detected by blood culture [69]. Another difference compared with immunocompetent individuals is occasional lack of response of the infection to antibiotic therapy, or frequent relapse after antibiotics are stopped, necessitating longer courses of therapy [72–74]. The oral quinolone antibiotics may be especially useful in this setting [75].

Parasites

Parasitic infections such as *Isospora belli* and *Cryptosporidium* can cause a self-limited diarrhea in immunocompetent individuals [76], but in immunosuppressed individuals the diarrhea may be profuse and unrelenting [77]. While these organisms are harbored in the small intestine, cryptosporidial infection of the stomach (40%) and colon (74%) can be appreciated on biopsy as evident by mucosal injury [78].

Microsporidia can be found in small intestinal mucosa of persons with HIV infection and is a significant cause of diarrhea [79]. In a recent retrospective analysis of diarrhea in HIV positive patients, yearly positive rates for microsporidia in stool specimens collected over a 4-year period ranged from 2.9% to 9.7% [80]. Microsporidia can be diagnosed by direct visualization in stool specimens with modified trichrome stain, in intestinal biopsy by light or electron microscopy, or by PCR amplification of stool [81]. Treatment for cryptosporidiosis is limited to combination azithromycin and paromomycin [82]. There are two species of microsporidia: *Enterocytozoon bieneusi* and *Encepalitozoon intestinalis*. The former may respond to albendazole [82] or thalidomide [83]. Invasive amebiasis causes colitis in HIV infection [84].

Viruses

Herpes simplex virus type II infection can cause extensive perianal ulceration as well as distal proctitis, and it may not always respond well to acyclovir. Cytomegalovirus (CMV) is the most common pathogen of the gastrointestinal tract in AIDS; it is especially common in the colon, where it causes an endothelial vasculitis [85]. The symptoms of CMV colitis (diarrhea, bleeding, weight loss, and fever) are similar to those of IBD. Its protean manifestations include mucosal ulceration, diffuse or segmental colitis, and ileocolitis which can mimic CD when detected by barium enema or by sigmoidoscopy or colonoscopy [86]. CMV can cause a toxic megacolon, fulminant colitis, or ulcers that can bleed or perforate. Barium enema X-ray findings include diffuse mucosal ulcers, or linear or aphthous ulcers [87, 88]. The diagnosis of CMV colitis is best made by culture and histology [89] (Fig. 5) as the colonoscopic and X-ray manifestations are not specific. Therapy with ganciclovir or foscarnet can improve the symptoms, although relapse is common when therapy is discontinued.

Adenovirus infection may be a cause of diarrhea as it has been rarely identified in colonic mucosa of HIV-positive men with diarrhea. This may be secondary to underdiagnosis because of lack of familiarity by pathologists. At a single institution, 62% of cases were not diagnosed on the original pathology report as adenovirus [90].

Other

Intestinal infection with *M. avium-intracellulare* can mimic Whipple's disease when it occurs in the proximal small intestine, because bacteria-filled macrophages fill the lamina propria [91]. However, the correct diagnosis is obvious when an acid-fast stain of the biopsy is done, which can even reveal individual microorganisms. When this infection involves the distal small intestine, it can cause terminal ileal stenoses which can be mistaken for CD [92]. The organism may be present in the stool, but it is not known at this time whether this has any clinical significance. Although optimal therapy has yet to be defined, the combination regimen of clarithromycin, ethambutol, and ciprofloxacin has led to improved survival compared to clarithromycin and ethambutol alone [93].

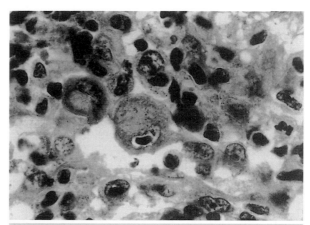

Figure 5. Cytomegalovirus inclusion in an endothelial cell in a colonic biopsy from a woman with a self-limited colitis due to cytomegalovirus. Note the typical cytomegalovirus intranuclear inclusion surrounded by a clear halo; the cytoplasm is also enlarged. This cell is diagnostic of cytomegalovirus. (Reprinted with permission from Surawicz CM. Histopathology of infectious colitis. Can J Gastroenterol 1989; 3: 168.)

Colitis due to *Histoplasma capsulatum* has also been reported in one man with AIDS [94].

Some patients without pathogens may have small intestinal disease causing their diarrhea; mild changes in villous architecture have been seen [95–97].

In addition to intestinal infections, tumors of the gastrointestinal tract may be present, including Kaposi's sarcoma and lymphoma. These may present with obstruction or bleeding, and surgery may be required for definitive diagnosis and/or therapy.

Diagnostic approach to diarrhea with HIV

Initial evaluation should include stool culture for enteric pathogens (including *C. difficile*) and three ova and parasite examinations and a blood culture. If these are negative, flexible sigmoidoscopy with biopsy is sufficient endoscopic evaluation for detecting specific pathogens [98], although some feel a complete evaluation requires colonoscopy and esophagogastroduodenoscopy (EGD). Alternatively, empiric therapy with antidiarrheals can be given, or a trial of an empiric antibiotic such as metronidazole or a quinolone.

Differentiating ulcerative colitis from Crohn's disease

History and physical examination

Bloody diarrhea is more common with UC but can occur in CD. Tenesmus is more often seen in UC because of the uniform rectal involvement.

Historical clues that suggest CD include any evidence of fat malabsorption, such as easy bruisability from vitamin K malabsorption, night-blindness (vitamin A malabsorption), and hypocalcemia with tetany (vitamin D malabsorption).

Physical examination clues that suggest CD include a right lower quadrant mass (due to terminal ileal and cecal involvement), typical perianal disease, i.e. violaceous undermined indolent anal ulcers or multiple perianal fistulas, or non-rectal fistulation. Fissures and perirectal abscesses are non-specific and can be seen with either UC or CD.

Laboratory evaluation

Serum tests

Laboratory tests which have been used in evaluation of IBD include erythrocyte sedimentation rate, orosomucoid, and C-reactive protein. None of these is specific, however, as they merely indicate the presence of inflammation.

However, it is now well recognized that perinuclear antineutrophil cytoplasmic autoantibodies (pANCA) and antibodies to the oligomannosidic epitopes of the yeast *Saccharomyces cerevisiae* (ASCA) are very specific for UC and CD respectively in both adults and children. When both tests are used in conjunction, the specificity and positive predictive value of a positive pANCA and a negative ASCA for UC is 97% and 92.5% respectively in adults, while the specificity of a positive pANCA in children is 92%. For a negative pANCA and a positive ASCA the specificity and positive predictive value for CD in adults is 97% and 96% respectively, while in children the specificity of a positive ASCA is 95% [99,100].

Stool cultures

Chronic UC can be exacerbated by superinfection with enteric organisms such as *Salmonella* [101], *Listeria monocytogenes* [102], and even *Legionella* [103]. *C. difficile* and its cytotoxin may be present [104]; its overgrowth is probably due to antibiotics or sulfasalazine. Occasionally this may contribute to relapse, although there is no consensus on this [105]. Aside from stool cultures and empiric therapy there is no good way to detect bacterial superinfections in IBD.

Ameba serology

It is important to remember that *E. histolytica* infection can mimic IBD, and serology should be performed because stool examination is unreliable [106]. As mentioned previously, every patient with suspected IBD should have tests done to exclude amebiasis [107].

CMV

Not only can CMV mimic IBD but it more frequently complicates UC than CD. In a retrospective review of a 12-year period at a single institution, 172 patients who underwent colectomy for UC had a prevalence of CMV colitis of 4.6%. During the same time period 376 patients with CD had intestinal resections and, of these, 0.8% had CMV colitis or enteritis [108].

X-ray and ultrasound/computerized tomographic scanning

The different imaging modalities useful in the diagnosis and management of IBD have recently been reviewed and are briefly discussed below [109].

Contrast radiography

Radiographic differentiation of IBD follows its pathologic distinctions. Double-contrast barium enema is the main radiologic procedure in patients with subacute or quiescent IBD. It should not be performed in patients with suspected perforation or toxic colon. In these situations, if an X-ray is necessary, water-soluble contrast should be used. In general it is best to wait until the colitis subsides, if possible. Bowel preparation should be gentle, and modification of the standard preparation may be wise in patients with UC, to avoid exacerbating their disease with harsh laxatives.

Characteristic changes of UC include fine diffuse granularity, thickened irregular mucosal detail, continuous disease, uniform rectal involvement, and a normal terminal ileum, although a patulous terminal ileum ('backwash ileitis') can be seen in some. When strictures occur, carcinoma must be excluded. Characteristic changes of CD are aphthous ulcers, non-continuous disease with skip areas, and asymmetry. Deeper ulcers can occur, as can strictures, fistulas, abscesses, and inflammatory masses [110].

Pseudopolyps and strictures can be seen in either disease. Because patients with both diseases can develop dysplasia, and adenocarcinoma, differentiation of these lesions from dysplasia and cancer is important, but may be difficult.

Ultrasound

Ultrasound is an indirect test that is useful in evaluating IBD. Bowel wall thickening can be seen in both UC and CD, but it is usually more marked in CD. There is right lower quadrant involvement in CD which contrasts with left lower quadrant involvement in UC [111].

Ultrasound is also useful in differentiating mesenteric adenitis and acute terminal ileitis from appendicitis [112].

Scanning

Contrast radiography, i.e. upper gastrointestinal series with small bowel follow-through and barium enema, is superior to abdominal CT scan in evaluating patients with IBD [113]. However, imaging by CT scans may help detect complications, such as abscesses and fistulas. In general these are more common with CD.

Radionuclide scanning

Radionuclide scanning is an adjunct to X-ray and endoscopy in the evaluation of IBD, and may be especially helpful in detecting terminal ileal disease or abscesses. The technique involves selective labeling of autologous granulocytes with radioactive isotopes, such as indium-111, technetium-99m (^{99m}Tc) stannous colloid, or ^{99m}Tc-hexamethyl propylene amine oxine (HM-PAO) [114, 115]. These scans may be useful when other modalities are too invasive, such as in critically ill patients who cannot undergo endoscopy. While the role of radionuclide scans is still evolving, it is likely they will continue to be used as adjunctive tests [115, 116]. The obvious drawbacks are the radiation dose and the fact that these scans are not available in many centers.

Colonoscopy

Colonoscopy during severe attacks of IBD is usually contraindicated; however, when diagnosis is necessary, it can be performed safely [117], and the information obtained may guide therapy and provide information which may postpone emergent surgery [118]. Both a skilled endoscopist and a mild bowel preparation are recommended. When CD is suspected, colonoscopy with ileoscopy and biopsy are helpful [119].

In a large prospective study of 357 patients with an endoscopic diagnosis of UC, CD, or indeterminate colitis, who were followed for about 22 months, a final endoscopy-independent diagnosis was made in 71% based on autopsy, surgery, or histology. Endoscopic diagnosis was correct in 89%. The most discriminating signs at endoscopy for CD are anal lesions, cobblestoning, discontinuous and discrete distribution of lesions, and rectal sparing; in UC the signs are erosions, granularity, continuous and symmetrical distribution of lesions, and rectal involvement [120]. However, two recent studies challenge this traditional teaching of continuous mucosal lesions in UC [121, 122]. While rectal sparing and patchy inflammation have been considered hallmarks of CD, one center reported that in over half of their UC patients these findings were present at some time on endoscopy [122].

It is important to remember that double-contrast barium examination of the colon and endoscopy (colonoscopy) can be complementary procedures [123].

Histology

Mucosal biopsy is an important adjunct to visual examination of the colon in diagnosing colitis. It is important to biopsy abnormal as well as normal-appearing mucosa. There are several reasons to biopsy normal-appearing colonic mucosa: to detect occult CD, where granulomas may be present in 18% of patients with CD elsewhere [124, 125]; to diagnose collagenous or microscopic colitis; and to detect other changes which may or may not be clinically relevant, such as intestinal spirochetosis [126] or changes due to laxatives.

Pathologically there are some similarities between UC and CD, but it is more important to emphasize the differences (see Table 5). UC is a diffuse mucosal inflammation which almost always involves the rectum and variable continuous lengths of colon, from left colon (left-sided colitis) to the entire colon (pancolitis). Histologic criteria for UC and CD have been described by many, including classic descriptions by Morson and Dawson [127] and Yardley and Donowitz [128]. Involvement is limited to the colon, although occasionally a dilated terminal ileum ('backwash ileitis') can be detected by small bowel X-rays. In contrast, CD is focal or segmental, can have transmural involvement which can lead to stricture and fistula formation, and can involve any part of the gastrointestinal tract from the mouth to the anus.

In general, useful pathologic criteria are discontinuous inflammation in CD and crypt distortion in UC. Morphometric studies, used to distinguish between UC and CD, showed no useful criteria except granulomas because of the wide overlap. Discontinuous inflammation can be found in resolving UC and infectious colitis.

Microscopically, inflammation in UC is characterized by increased lamina propria inflammatory cells, both acute and chronic, as well as crypt abscesses. Paneth cell metaplasia is frequent, especially at crypt bases. Distortion of crypt architecture is diffuse, with branched or forked crypts, crypt atrophy (a sparsity and shortening of crypts), and a villiform surface (Fig. 6). Changes can range from mild to severe. Isolated giant cells are a non-specific indicator of inflammation. Any of these changes can also be seen in CD; one difference is that inflammation may involve the submucosa, and that granulomas can be present in up to 28% of biopsies if searched for, i.e. serial sections [129, 130] (Fig. 7).

Although findings on histology contribute greatly to the diagnosis of the different colitides, there are limitations that clinicians should be aware of. In a retrospective review of 280 colorectal biopsies from 100 consecutive patients at a single institution over a 6-week period, the original diagnosis was compared to the reviewer's evaluation. Fifty-six percent of cases

originally diagnosed as inflamed were found by the reviewers to be normal or showing non-specific changes. Of the cases in whom a specific diagnosis was made, 59% were originally diagnosed only with a descriptive terminology [131]. This places clinicians in the quandary of making their own diagnosis based on histologic descriptions, and emphasizes the importance of dialog between clinician and pathologist.

In 10% of cases it is impossible to distinguish UC from Crohn's, usually in patients who present with fulminant colitis. Indeterminate colitis occurs in 5–10% of surgical specimens, and can be IBD or infectious. Rectal sparing can occur, as can patchy involvement, aphthous ulcers, and abnormal architecture [132].

The presence of extraintestinal symptoms does not differentiate, although pyoderma gangrenosum and sclerosing cholangitis are more frequent complications of UC.

Colitis with other causes
Ischemic colitis

Ischemic colitis is usually a disease of the elderly, who are susceptible to a decrease in blood flow, but young people can also develop significant ischemia. Certain clinical settings are classical, such as after aortic aneurysm repair or after hypotension for whatever cause (congestive heart failure, sepsis, etc.). Ischemic colitis has been reported in women who take pseudoephedrine [133] and oral contraceptive pills [134]. Colonoscopic features include rectal sparing and

Table 5. Differentiation of ulcerative colitis from Crohn's disease

	Ulcerative Colitis	Crohn's Disease
Site of disease	Colon only	Any part of GI tract
Distribution	Diffuse	Focal (segmental)- skip areas
	Mucosal	Transmural
Colonoscopic appearance	Diffuse friability	Focal/aphthous ulcers
	Cobblestoning	
	Linear ulcers with normal surrounding mucosa	
Histopathology		
Crypt architecture	Distorted	Normal or focally distorted
Inflammation	Acute or chronic	Normal or acute/chronic
Epithelioid granulomas	Never	Yes
Complications	Fistulae/abscess never or rarely occur	Fistulae/abscess can occur
Strictures	Uncommon	Common
Cancer risk after long-standing disease	+ + + +	+ +

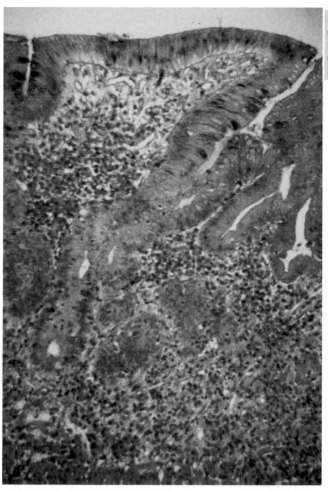

Figure 6. Rectal biopsy from a patient with active ulcerative colitis shows distorted crypt architecture and diffuse lamina propria inflammation with acute and chronic inflammatory cells. (Reprinted with permission from Surawicz CM. Diagnosing colitis. Contemp Intern Med 1991; 3: 19.)

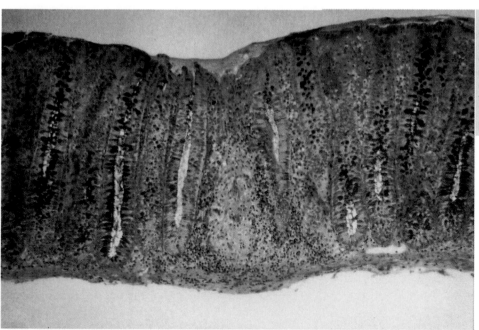

Figure 7. Rectal biopsy from a patient with Crohn's disease shows a typical epithelioid granuloma in otherwise normal mucosa. (Reprinted with permission from Surawicz CM. Diagnosing colitis. Contemp Intern Med 1991; 3: 20.)

discrete ulcers which can suggest CD [135]. Some of the colitis that develops in long-distance or marathon runners may be ischemic [136]. The most frequent clinical presentation is lower abdominal pain with bloody diarrhea or hematochezia. There may be slight fever and leukocytosis. X-ray films may show thumbprinting of the mucosa, which is due to submucosal hemorrhage. Because IBD often has a second peak of incidence in the elderly, ischemia may be in the differential. Only 3–5% of Crohn's patients present after 65 years, and 75% of non-infectious colitis in persons more than 60 years old is probably ischemic.

Classically, colonic involvement occurs in 'watershed' areas between overlapping blood supplies, such as the splenic flexure which is frequently involved. The rectum, with its abundant dual blood supply, is rarely involved; thus rectal sparing is characteristic but not uniform. The diagnosis can be quickly made by flexible sigmoidoscopy, where dusky blue/purple mucosa can be seen. The examination should be performed carefully by an experienced endoscopist, and it is best not to use excessive air insufflation. Histology shows that crypt architecture remains, often with 'ghosts of crypts', minimal inflammatory infiltrate, and superficial necrosis (Fig. 8). There are no good noninvasive tests to diagnose intestinal ischemia. Ischemia either heals or causes chronic colitis with submucosal fibrosis, strictures, or obstruction.

Radiation colitis

Up to 50% of patients treated with pelvic radiation will develop acute radiation colitis, usually within 2 weeks of initiation of therapy. Signs will generally include abdominal cramping, tenesmus, diarrhea, and rectal bleeding. Chronic radiation colitis can occur 6 months to decades after radiation therapy and occurs in only about 5% of patients. The most common symptoms are rectal bleeding, rectal ulcers, and diarrhea. These occur due to a progressive vasculitis leading to small vessel thrombosis [137]. The histology resembles ischemia, with superficial necrosis and hyalinized blood vessel walls. The most important risk factor for chronic radiation colitis is the total dose of radiation.

Solitary rectal ulcer syndrome

The incidence is thought to be about 1 in 100 000 per year. Typical features include blood and mucus per rectum with associated straining and a sense of incomplete evacuation accompanied by rectal prolapse. The endoscopic appearance can range from rectal erythema to ulceration to polypoid lesions. Histology shows hyperplastic, elongated, and distorted crypts; an edematous lamina propria with excess collagen deposits; and engorgement of superficial capillaries. The differential diagnosis includes IBD and ischemic colitis. The diagnosis is made by or with a combination of clinical signs and symptoms, endoscopic appearances, and histology [138] (Fig. 9).

Microscopic colitis

Microscopic colitis is characterized by chronic watery diarrhea with normal endoscopic and radiologic studies but histologic abnormalities of inflammatory changes in the lamina propria. It encompasses collagenous colitis and lymphocytic colitis. In addition to the inflammatory infiltrate, both entities require an increase in intraepithelial lymphocytes, damage to the surface epithelium, and minimal crypt distortion [139]. A recent population-based study found a mean annual incidence 1.1 per 100 000 for collagenous colitis and 3.1 per 100 000 for lymphocytic colitis [139]. While some believe that collagenous and lymphocytic colitis may represent a spectrum [140], others believe that they are two distinct clinical syndromes [141]. These entities are clearly distinct from IBD, and patients do not develop it later.

Collagenous colitis

This entity was first described in 1976 by Lindstrom, and the first case remains a typical example [142]. The illness occurs in middle-aged women (4:1). Because the colonic mucosa looks normal grossly, it is unlikely to be confused with UC. Typically, these patients have chronic watery diarrhea, and an evaluation is normal. Biopsy is necessary to make the diagnosis. The histology is diagnostic, with a thickened subepithelial band of collagen that measures 10 μm at least [143]. Normally this layer is 0.4–4.6 μm thick. Various therapies exist, but it is not clear which are more efficacious as the studies have been small open-label studies. Bile acid binders [144], sulfasalazine [145], mesalamine, budesonide [146],

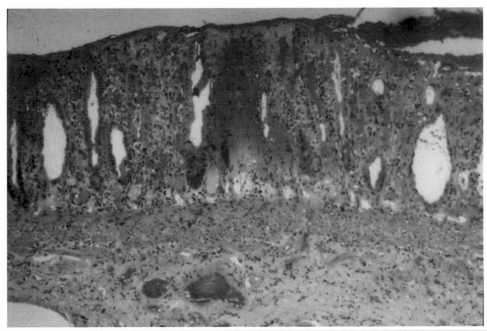

Figure 8. Colorectal biopsy from a patient with ischemic colitis shows superficial necrosis and 'erased' crypts without an inflammatory response. (With permission from Dr Cyrus E. Rubin, University of Washington, Seattle, WA.)

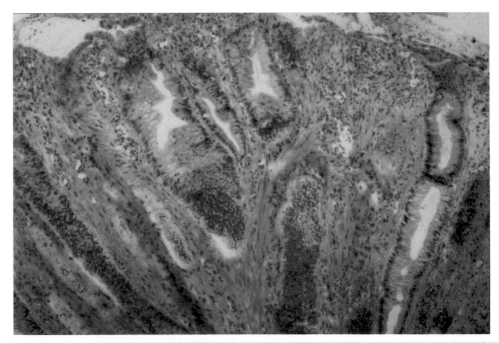

Figure 9. Rectal biopsy from a patient with solitary rectal ulcer syndrome shows classic pathological findings of hyperplasic crypts and mucosal fibrosis. The excess diffuse mucosal collagen in the lamina propria is easily seen when stained yellow with saffron. (With permission by Dr Douglas Levine, Seattle, WA.)

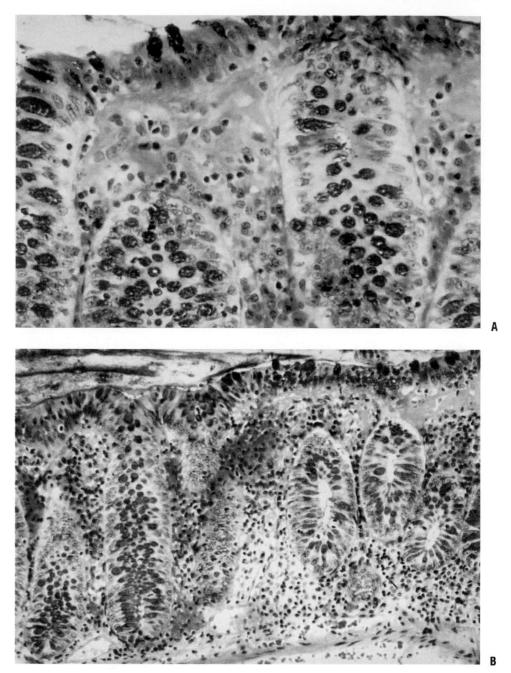

Figure 10. **A:** Two biopsies from a patient with collagenous colitis show the thickened subepithelial band of collagen (here stained yellow with saffron). **B:** Note that the collagen band is focal; thus multiple biopsies should be taken to exclude the diagnosis.

and bismuth subsalicylate [147] have all shown good efficacy in these small studies (Fig. 10A,B).

Lymphocytic colitis

This entity was first described in 1982 in a small number of patients with chronic watery diarrhea in whom mild histologic changes in colonic biopsies from normal-appearing mucosa were noted [148]. To diagnose lymphocytic colitis more than 20 intraepithelial lymphocytes per 100 epithelial cells are required without the presence of a collagen band [141]. As in collagenous colitis, other evaluation is negative and biopsy is necessary for diagnosis. Basically, the histology is the same as collagenous colitis, minus the diagnostic thickened collagen band. Colonic absorption is decreased [149].

Diversion colitis

This is an inflammatory reaction that occurs in surgically defunctionalized segments of colon [150] and resolves when bowel continuity is restored. The endoscopic changes of friable mucosa, with ulcers in some cases, can mimic UC or CD. Histology shows chronic lymphoplasmacytic inflammatory infiltrates, with crypt abscesses, mucin granulomas, and lymphoid follicular hyperplasia [151,152]. Despite these inflammatory changes, patients can be clinically asymptomatic or have symptoms of abdominal pain with bloody mucus discharge. The spectrum of histologic changes that can been seen in diversion colitis is dependent upon the nature of the presurgical intestinal mucosa [153]. In patients with normal bowel the inflammation seen in diversion colitis is limited to the mucosa and there is minimal crypt distortion. In patients with underlying UC the histology may also display vertical fissuring and transmural lymphoid aggregates which can be confused with CD. In contrast, patients with underlying CD will have more quiescent disease clinically and histologically after a diversion procedure [153]. Resolution of histologic abnormalities with short-chain fatty acid irrigation suggests that the inflammation may be due to a luminal nutritional deficiency [154].

Colitis with systemic disease (vasculitis)

Any systemic vasculitis can affect the colon and cause colitis, including polyarteritis nodosa and systemic lupus erythematosus. Colonoscopic pete-

chial lesions in the colon have been described in patients with Henoch–Schönlein purpura [155]. These lesions resemble the skin lesions. Vasculitis has been demonstrated by biopsy.

Churg–Strauss syndrome is a rare entity with asthma, hypereosinophilia, necrotizing vasculitis, and extravascular granulomas [156]. Colonic involvement is rare, but multiple colonic ulcers can occur [157]. There are a few cases published describing colitis in patients with Wegener's granulomatosis with endoscopic findings of ulcerating mucosa but histology demonstrating non-specific findings for IBD [158].

Granulomatous colitis
Sarcoidosis

Gastrointestinal sarcoidosis can clinically present like IBD with endoscopic and histologic appearances of CD in biopsies demonstrating chronic inflammatory infiltrates, crypt abscesses, and non-necrotizing granulomas. The correct diagnosis of sarcoidosis can usually be made when the usual extraintestinal signs of sarcoid are manifest [159]. Unlike CD there is no transmural inflammation, and no lymphoid aggregates or strictures [160].

Diverticulosis

A small series of patients with sigmoid diverticulitis who underwent sigmoid colectomy had histologic findings of epithelioid granulomas, crypt abscesses, lymphoid aggregates, and chronic mucosal inflammation which are indistinguishable from CD. After a median follow-up of 51 months, none of the patients developed any clinical signs of CD [161].

Behçet's syndrome

Behçet's syndrome consists of uveitis and oral and genital ulcers. There can also be gastrointestinal involvement in the form of deep flask-shaped ulcers in the background of chronic inflammation that may demonstrate granulomas, thus raising the possibility of CD. Some feel that Behçet's is indistinguishable from CD [162]. The prevalence of Behçet's syndrome varies significantly not only with geography, but also with the presence of gastrointestinal involvement. In Japan the prevalence is 1:10 000 while in North America it is 1:500 000. In a large study from Turkey involving 1000 patients with Behçet's, none had colitis [163].

Drugs

Many drugs can cause colitis including Aldomet (methyldopa), penicillamine, oral potassium supplements, and 5-fluorouracil. Another chemotherapy agent, irinotecan, or Campostar, which is used for colon, prostate, ovarian, and esophageal cancer, has been associated with hemorrhagic colitis [164]; a good review is available [165]. Proctosigmoiditis in a teenager was associated with isotretinoin (Accutane); it resolved with removal of the drug but recurred after challenge [166]. Colitis also occurs with gold therapy, but this is rare. The endoscopic appearance is similar to UC; pseudomembranes have been reported [167]. The illness usually resolves after gold is discontinued. Chronic non-steroidal anti-inflammatory drug (NSAID) therapy can cause both small bowel and colonic lesions that can mimic CD or infectious colitis. These include patchy colitis, lymphoplasmacytic infiltrates, ulcerations, crypt disarray, and diaphragm-like strictures of the colon [168–170]. An acute self-limited colitis can occur after colonoscopy which is thought to be secondary to the contamination of the instrument by the glutaraldehyde used for disinfection of the colonoscopes [171]. Another iatrogenic cause of colitis is the rare inflammatory reaction of the colonic mucosa to the carbon particles in India ink used for endoscopic tattooing. The inflammatory reaction can result in the histologic appearance of ulcerative colits [172].

Neutropenic colitis (necrotizing enterocolitis in cancer patients)

This is a complication of cytotoxic drug therapy often for leukemia or lymphoma. It is usually due to clostridial infection (*Clostridium septicum*, *C. perfringens*, or *C. paraperfringes*) whose toxins cause hemorrhagic necrosis. This diagnosis needs to be considered in any neutropenic patient with fever, abdominal pain, and diarrhea, which can be bloody. It can progress to peritonitis, septicemia, shock, and death. Endoscopically the bowel is edematous with ulceration and hemorrhages. Histologically there is submucosal edema, hemorrhage, necrosis, and very few inflammatory infiltrates. Perforation can occur in 5–10%, and in this case series the mortality rate was 28% [173].

Graft-versus-host disease

Graft-versus-host disease occurs in the setting of bone marrow transplant. Both the skin and intestinal mucosa are targets for this syndrome. A diagnosis of graft-versus-host disease of the gastrointestinal tract may be made by rectal biopsy which reveals focal proctitis, isolated injury to crypts, and apoptosis [174], but it is routinely diagnosed via gastric biopsy [175, 176] currently.

Eosinophilic colitis

Eosinophilic infiltration of the mucosa of the gastrointestinal tract can involve the stomach, small intestine, or colon. When ileocecal involvement occurs it may mimic CD [177, 178]. Symptoms are nonspecific but include abdominal pain and cramps, diarrhea, and rectal bleeding. Biopsies show intense eosinophilic infiltration, more marked than the increase in lamina propria eosinophils which can be seen in IBD. Peripheral blood eosinophilia is quite marked.

NSAID enteropathy

NSAID use is very common. There are three ways NSAIDs are relevant to IBD – they can mimic IBD; they can cause relapses of IBD; and their use is associated with collagenous colitis, a diarrheal illness often included in the differential diagnosis of IBD. NSAIDs are the most frequently prescribed class of drug in the US. Their adverse effects on the stomach, including gastritis and ulcers, are well known. Over the past decade there has been increasing recognition of the effects of NSAIDs on the small bowel and colonic mucosa. Mucosal injury is more common in the stomach than in the small intestine, and less frequent in the colon. The pathogenesis of injury appears to be related to the inhibition of prostaglandin synthesis. Symptoms of small bowel injury include diarrhea, bleeding, and protein loss. Discrete ulcers can occur in the colon.

Small intestine

Small intestinal damage was first indicated by epidemiologic studies of Langman *et al.*, who found that chronic NSAID use was more common in patients with small and large bowel perforation and bleeding [179]. Recent estimates suggest that 40–70% of long-term NSAID users have inflammatory changes in the small intestine [180]. Small intestinal diaphragm lesions have been found, sometimes requiring surgery to relieve symptoms of obstruction. These lesions appear to be specific for NSAID injury [181]. Ulcers and other mucosal lesions can cause bleeding and protein loss with resulting iron-deficiency anemia and/or hypoalbuminemia. Discrete ulcers can also perforate. The term 'NSAID enteropathy' has been used to describe this low-grade inflammation with blood and protein loss [182]. The differential diagnosis can include small bowel CD. Diagnosis can be made by enteroscopy, though this technique is not widely used. Indirect measures of protein or blood loss can also suggest mucosal injury.

Colon

Colonic lesions are less common than gastric and small intestinal lesions. Symptoms include diarrhea, chronic blood loss, and iron-deficiency anemia. Lesions are most frequently detected at colonoscopy – ulcers, usually sharply demarcated and clean-based, either single or multiple, are typical [183]. While lesions can occur throughout the colon, the ileocecal area and ascending colon appear most commonly affected [184] (Fig. 11). Rectal ulcers are often associated with suppository use [185]. Diaphragm lesions and strictures of the colon can occur [186]. These signs and symptoms can mimic IBD [182]. Lesions typically heal upon withdrawal of NSAIDs, usually within a few weeks. Concurrent upper gastrointestinal tract damage can occur – it was present in four of 14 with colon lesions in one recent study [184].

Treatment

Withdrawal of NSAIDs is usually recommended, if feasible. Concurrent treatment with misoprostil is another option. The newer selective Cox-2 NSAIDs have less gastrointestinal tract toxicity, but lesions can still occur [180].

Summary

NSAID injury can mimic IBD, can exacerbate IBD, and NSAID use may also be more common in the diarrheal syndrome of collagenous colitis, though there is no clear role in pathogenesis.

References

1. Schumacher G, Sandstedt B, Kolleberg B. A prospective study of first attacks of inflammatory bowel disease and infectious colitis. Clinical findings and early diagnosis. Scand J Gastrenterol 1994; 29: 265–74.

2. Harris RD, Beeching NJ, Rogerson SJ, Nye FJ. The platelet count as a simple measure to distinguish inflammatory bowel disease from infective diarrhoea. J Infect 1991; 22: 247–50.

3. Tedesco FJ, Hardin RD, Harper RN, Edwards BH. Infectious colitis endoscopically simulating inflammatory bowel disease: a prospective evaluation. Gastrointest Endosc 1983; 29: 195–7.

4. Rohner P, Pittet D, Pepey B, Thompson N, Auckenthaler R. Etiologic agents of infectious diarrhea: implications for request for microbial culture. J Clin Microbiol 1997; 35: 1427–32.

5. Barbut F, Beaugerie, Delas N et al. Comparative value of colonic biopsy and intraluminal fluid culture for diagnosis of bacterial acute colitis in immunocompetent patients. Clin Infect Dis 1999; 29: 356–60.

6. Rautelin HI, Renkonen OV, Von Bonsdorff CH et al. Prospective study of the etiology of diarrhea in adult outpatients. Scand J Gastroenterol 1989; 24: 329–33.

7. Taylor DN, Houston R, Shlim DR et al. Etiology of diarrhea among travelers and foreign residents in Nepal. J Am Med Assoc 1988; 260: 1245–8.

8. Osterholm, MT, MacDonald KL, White KE et al. An outbreak of a newly recognized chronic diarrhea syndrome associated with raw milk consumption. J Am Med Assoc 1986; 256: 484–90.

9. Janda RC, Conklin JL, Mitros FA, Parsonnet J. Multifocal colitis associated with an epidemic of chronic diarrhea. Gastroenterology 1991; 100: 458–64.

10. Kumar NB, Nostrant TT, Appelman HD. The histopathologic spectrum of acute self-limited colitis (acute infectious-type colitis). Am J Surg Pathol 1982; 6: 523–9.

11. Surawicz CM, Haggitt RC, Husseman M, McFarland LV. Mucosal biopsy diagnosis of colitis: acute self-limited colitis and idiopathic inflammatory bowel disease Gastroenterology 1994; 107: 755–63.

12. Nostrant TT, Kumar NB, Appelman HD. Histopathology differentiates acute self-limited colitis from ulcerative colitis. Gastroenterology 1987; 92: 318–28.

13. Anand BS, Malhotra V, Bhattacharya SK et al. Rectal histology in acute bacillary dysentery. Gastroenterology 1986; 90: 654–60.

14. Schumacher G, Kollberg B, Sandstedt B. A prospective study of first attacks of inflammatory bowel disease and infectious colitis. Histologic course during the first year after presentation. Scand J Gastroenterol 1994; 29: 318–32.

15. Surawicz CM, Goodell SE, Whinn TC et al. Spectrum of rectal biopsy abnormalities in homosexual men with intestinal symptoms. Gastroenterology 1986; 91: 651–9.

16. Allison MC, Hamilton-Dutoit SJ, Dhillon AP, Pounder RE. The value of rectal biopsy in distinguishing self-limited colitis from early inflammatory bowel disease. Q J Med 1987; 65: 985–95.

17. Therkildsen MD, Jensen BN, Teglbjaerg P, Rasmussen S. The final outcome of patients presenting with their first episode of acute diarrhea and an inflamed rectal mucosa crypt architecture. A clinopathologic study. Scand J Gastroenterol 1989; 24: 158–64.

18. Griffin PM, Olmstead LC, Petras RE. *Escherichia coli* O157: H7-associated colitis. Gastroenterology 1990; 99: 142–9.

19. Edwards BH. *Salmonella* and *Shigella*. Clin Lab Med 1999; 19: 469–87.

20. Mishu A, Blaser MJ. *Campylobacter jejuni* and the expanding spectrum of related infections. Clin Infect Dis 1995; 20: 1092–9.

21. Jackson TL, Young RL, Thompson J, McCashland TM. Toxic megacolon associated with *Campylobacter jejuni* colitis. Am J Gastroenterol 1999; 94: 280–2.

110. Caroline DR, Evers K. Colitis: radiographic features and differentiation of idiopathic inflammatory bowel disease. Radiol Clin N Am 1987; 25: 47–66.

111. Worlicek H, Lutz H, Heyder N, Matek W. Ultrasound findings in Crohn's disease and ulcerative colitis: a prospective study. J Clin Ultrasound 1987; 15: 153–63.

112. Puylaert JB. Mesenteric adenitis and acute terminal ileitis: US evaluation using graded compression. Radiology 1986; 16: 691–5.

113. Lubat E. Bathazar EJ. The current role of computerized tomography in inflammatory disease of the bowel. Am J Gastroenterol 1988; 83: 107–13.

114. Cucchiara S, Celentano L, de Magistris TM et al. Colonoscopy and technetium-99m white cell scan in children with suspected inflammatory bowel disease. J Pediatr 1999; 135: 727–32.

115. Weldon MJ, Lowwe C, Joseph AE, Maxwell JD. Review article: quantitative leukocyte scanning in the assessment of inflammatory bowel disease activity and its response to therapy. Aliment Pharmacol Ther 1996; 2: 123–32.

116. Giaffer MH, Tindale WB, Holdworth D. Value of technetium-99m HMPAO-labelled leucocyte scintigraphy as an initial screening test in patients suspected of having inflammatory bowel disease. Eur J Gastroenterol Hepatol 1996; 8: 1195–200.

117. Waye JD, Endoscopy in inflammatory bowel disease: indications and differential diagnosis. Med Clin N Am 1990; 74: 51–65.

118. Alemayehu G, Jarnerot G. Colonoscopy during an attack of severe ulcerative colitis is a safe procedure and of great value in clinical decision making. Am J Gastroenterol 1991; 86: 187–90.

119. Coremans G, Rutgeerts P, Geboes K, Van den Oord J, Ponette E, Vantrappen G. The value of ileoscopy with biopsy in the diagnosis of intestinal Crohn's disease. Gastrointest Endosc 1984; 30: 167–72.

120. Pera A, Bellando P, Caldera D et al. Colonoscopy in inflammatory bowel disease. Diagnostic accuracy and proposal of an endoscopic score. Gastroenterology 1987; 92: 181–5.

121. D'Haens G, Geboes K, Peeters M et al. Patchy cecal inflammation associated with distal ulcerative colitis: a prospective endoscopic study. Am J Gastroenterol 1997; 92: 1275–9.

122. Byungki K, Barnett J, Kleer C et al. Endoscopic and histological patchiness in treated ulcerative colitis. Am J Gastroenterol 1999; 94: 3258–62.

123. Freeny PC. Crohn's disease and ulcerative colitis. Evaluation with double-contrast barium examination and endoscopy. Postgrad Med 1986; 80: 139–56.

124. Korelitz BI, Sommers SC. Rectal biopsy in patients with Crohn's disease. J Am Med Assoc 1977; 237: 2741–4.

125. Korelitz BI. Inclusion of rectal biopsies at colonsocopy. Dig Dis Sci 1988; 533: 1048–9.

126. Surawicz CM, Roberts PL, Rompalo A et al. Intestinal spirochetosis in homosexual men. Am J Med 1987; 82: 587–92.

127. Morson BC, Dawson IMP. Gastrointestinal Pathology. Oxford: Blackwell Scientific Publications, 1974.

128. Yardley JH, Donowitz M. Colorectal biopsy in inflammatory bowel disease. In: Yardley JH, Morson BC, Abell MR, eds. The Gastrointestinal Tract. International Academy of Pathology Monograph No. 18. Baltimore: Williams & Wilkins, 1977: 50–94.

129. Surawicz CM, Meisel JL, Ylvisaker T et al. Rectal biopsy in the diagnosis of Crohn's disease: value of multiple biopsies and serial sectioning. Gastroenterology 1981; 81: 66–71.

130. Surawicz CM. Serial sectioning of a portion of a rectal biopsy detects more focal abnormalities. A prospective study of patients with inflammatory bowel disease. Dig Dis Sci 1982; 27: 434–6.

131. Tsang P, Rotterdam H. Biopsy diagnosis of colitis. Possibilities and pitfalls. Am J Surg Pathol 1999; 23: 423–30.

132. Tanka M, Riddell RH. The pathological diagnosis and differentiatial diagnosis of Crohn's disease. Hepato-gastroenterology 1990; 37: 18–31.

133. Dowd J, Bailey D, Moussa K et al. Ischemic colitis associated with pseudoephedrine: four cases. Am J Gastroenterol 1999; 94: 2430–4.

134. Cotton PB, Thomas ML. Ischemic colitis and the contraceptive pill. Br Med J 1971; 2: 27–8.

135. Tedesco FJ, Volpicelli NA, Moore FS et al. Estrogen-and progesterone-associated colitis: a disorder with clinical and endoscopic features mimicking Crohn's colitis. Gastrointest Endosc 1982; 28: 247–9.

136. Lucas W, Schroy P. Reversible ischemic colitis in a high endurance athlete. Am J Gastroenterol 1998; 93: 2231–4.

137. Donner C. Pathophysiology and therapy of chronic radiation-induced injury to the colon. Dig Dis 1998; 16: 253–61.

138. Vaizey CJ, van der Bogaerde JB, Emmanuel AV et al. Solitary rectal ulcer syndrome. Br J Surg 1998; 85: 1617–23.

139. Fernandez-Banares F, Salas A, Forne M et al. Incidence of collagenous and lymphocytic colitis: a 5 year population-based study. Am J Gastroenterol 1999; 94: 418–23.

140. Zins BJ, Sandborn WJ, Tremaine WJ. Collagenous and lymphocytic colitis: subject review and therapeutic alternatives. Am J Gastroenterol 1995; 90: 1394–400.

141. Baert F, Wouters K, D'Haens G. Lymphocytic colitis: a distinct clinical entity? A clinicopathologic confrontation of lymphocytic and collagenous colitis. Gut 1999; 45: 375–81.

142. Lindstrom CG. 'Collagenous colitis' with watery diarrhea – a new entity? Pathol Eur 1987; 11: 87–9.

143. Wang HW, Owings DV, Antonioli DA et al. Increased subepithelial collagen deposition is not specific for collagenous colitis. Mod Pathol 1988; 1: 329–35.

144. Ung KA, Gillberg R, Kilander A, Abrahamssen H. Role of bile acids and bile acid binding agents in patients with collagenous colitis. Gut 2000; 46: 170–5.

145. Bohar, J Tysk C, Erriksson S et al. Collagenous colitis: a retrospective study of clinical presentation and treatment in 163 patients. Gut 1996; 39: 846–51.

146. Tromm A, Gringa T, Mollmann HW et al. Budenoside for treatment of collagenous colitis: first results of a pilot trial. Am J Gastroenterol 1999; 94: 1871–5.

147. Fine RD, Lee EL. Efficacy of open-label bismuth subsalicylate for treatment of microscopic colitis. Gastroenterology 1998; 114: 29–36.

148. Kingham JGC, Levinson DA, Ball JA et al: Microscopic colitis – a cause of chronic watery diarrhea. Br Med J 1982; 285: 1601–4.

149. Bo-Linn GW, Vendrell DD, Lee E et al. An evaluation of the significance of microscopic colitis in patients with chronic diarrhea. J Clin Invest 1985; 75: 1559–69.

150. Glotzer DJ, Glick ME, Goldman H. Proctitis and colitis following diversion of the fecal stream. Gastroenterology 1981; 80: 438–41.

151. Murray FE, O'Brien MJ, Birkett DE et al. Diversion colitis: pathologic findings in a resected sigmoid colon and rectum. Gastroenterology 1987; 93: 1404–8.

152. Komorowski RA. Histologic spectrum of diversion colitis. Am J Surg Pathol 1990; 14: 548–54.

153. Edwards CM, Geroge B, Warren B. Diversion colitis – new light through old windows. Histopathology 1999; 34: 1–5.

154. Harig JM, Soergel KH, Komorowski RA et al. Treatment of diversion colitis with short-chain fatty acid irrigation. N Engl J Med 1989: 320: 213–28.

155. Cappell MS, Gupta AM. Colonic lesions associated with Henoch–Schonlein purpura. Am J Gastroenterol 1990; 85: 1186–8.

156. Churg J, Strauss L. Allergic granulomatosis, allergic angiitis, and periarteritis nodosa. Am J Pathol 1951; 27: 277–301.

157. Shimamoto C, Hirata I, Ohshiba S et al. Churg–Strauss syndrome (allergic granulomatous angiitis) with peculiar multiple colonic ulcers. Am J Gastroenterol 1990; 85: 316–19.

158. Schneider A, Menzel J, Gaubitz M et al. Colitis as the initial presentation of Wegener's granulomatosis. J Intern Med 1997; 242: 513–17.

159. Dumot JA, Adal K, Petras RE, Lashner BA. Sarcoidosis presenting as granulomatosis colitis. Am J Gastroenterol 1998; 93: 1949–51.

160. Bulger K, O'Riordan M, Purdy S et al. Gastrointestinal sarcoidosis resembling Crohn's disease. Am J Gastroenterol 1988; 83: 1415–17.

161. Burroughs SH, Bowrey DJ, Morris-Stiff GJ, Williams GT. Granulomatous inflammation in sigmoid diverticulitis: two diseases or one? Histopathology 1998; 33: 349–53.

162. Lee RG. The colitis of Behçet's syndrome. Am J Surg Pathol 1986; 101: 888–93.

163. Yurdakul S, Tuzuner N, Yurdakul I et al. Gastrointestinal involvement in Behçet's syndrome: a controlled study. Ann Rheum Dis 1996; 55: 208–10.

164. Sears S, McNally P, Bachinski MSZ, Avery R. Irinotecan (CPT-11) induced colitis: report of a case and review of Food and Drug Administration MEDWATCH reporting. Gastroint Endosc 1999; 50: 841–4.

165. Cappell MS, Simon T. Colonic toxicity of administered medications and chemicals. Am J Gastroenterol 1993; 88: 1684–99.

166. Martin P, Manley PN, Depew WT et al. Isotretinoin-associated proctosigmoiditis. Gastroenterology 1987; 93: 606–9.

167. Reinhart WH, Kappeler M, Hlater F. Severe pseudomembranous and ulcerative colitis during gold therapy. Endoscopy 1984; 30: 120.

168. Goldstein NS, Cinenza AN. The histopathology of nonsteroidal anti-inflammatory drug-associated colitis. Am J Clin Pathol 1998; 110: 622–8.

169. Buchmen AL, Schwartz MR. Colonic ulceration associated with systemic use of nonsteroidal anti-inflammatory medication. J Clin Gastroenterol 1996; 22: 224–6.

170. Hooker GD, Gregor JC, Ponich TP et al. Diaphragm-like strictures of right colon due to indomethacin suppositories: evidence of systemic effect. Gastrointest Endosc 1996; 44: 199–202.

171. Caprilli R, Viscido A, Frieri G, Latella G. Acute colitis following colonoscopy. Endoscopy 1998; 30: 428–31.

172. Gopal D, Morava-Protzner I, Miller H, Hemphill D. Idiopathic inflammatory bowel disease associated with colonic tattooing with India ink preparation – case report and review of literature. Gastrointest Endosc 1999; 49: 636–9.

173. Gomez L, Martino R, Rolston KV. Neutropenic enterocolitis: spectrum of the disease and comparison of definite and possible cases. Clin Infect Dis 1998; 27: 695–9.

174. Epstein RJ, McDonald GB, Sale GE et al. The diagnostic accuracy of the rectal biopsy in acute graft-versus-host disease: a prospective study of thirteen patients. Gastroenterology 1980; 78: 764–71.

175. Ponec RJ, Hackman RC, McDonald GB. Endoscopic and histologic diagnosis of intestinal graft-versus-host disease after marrow transplantation. Gastrointest Endosc 1999; 49: 1–9.

176. Washington K, Bentley R, Green A et al. Gastric graft-versus-host disease: a blinded histologic study. Am J Surg Pathol 1997; 21: 1037–46.

177. Haberkern CM, Christie DL, Haas JE. Eosinophilic gastroenteritis presenting as ileocolitis. Gastroenterology 1978; 74: 896–9.

178. Tedesco FJ, Huckaby CB, Hamyr AM et al. Eosinophilic ileocolitis: expanding spectrum of eosinophilic gastroenteritis. Dig Dis Sci 1981; 26: 943–8.

179. Langman MJ, Morgan L, Worrail A. Use of anti-inflammatory drugs by patients admitted with small or large bowel perforations and haemorrhage. Br Med J 1985; 290: 347–9.

180. Davies NM, Saleh JY, Skjodt NM. Detection and prevention of NSAID-induced enteropathy. J Pharm Pharmaceut Sci 2000; 3: 137–55.

181. Kwo PY, Tremaine WJ. Nonsteroidal anti-inflammatory drug-induced enteropathy: case discussion and review of the literature. Mayo Clin Proc 1995; 70: 55–61.

182. Bjarnason I, Hayllar J, MacPherson AJ, Russell AS. Side effects of nonsteroidal anti-inflammatory drugs on the small and large intestine in humans. Gastroenterology 1993; 104: 1832–47.

183. Davies NM. Toxicity of nonsteroidal anti-inflammatory drugs in the large intestine. Dis Colon Rectum 1995; 38: 1311–21.

184. Puspok A, Kiener H-P, Oberhuber B. NSAID Colitis – resolving a diagnostic dilemma? Dis Colon Rectum 2000; 43: 685–91.

185. Kurahara K, Matsumotos T, Iida M, Honda K, Yao T, Fujishima M. Clinical and endoscopic features of nonsteroidal anti-inflammatory drug-induced colonic ulcerations. Am J Gastroenterol 2000; 96: 473–80.

186. Smith JA, Pineau BC. Endoscopic therapy of NSAID-induced colonic diaphragm disease: two cases and a review of published reports. Gastrointest Endosc 2000; 52: 120–5.

care spending (ranging from ~8.8% in the US to 16.8% in France), and the data on prescription drug use were relatively easy to identify. Other problems associated with drug use also added to the total expense of health care, the resolution of which would lower the costs. These problems included prescription errors [4], complications of drug therapy [5], and non-utilized drugs once prescribed [6]. The most common prescription errors were lack of knowledge of the drug, lack of information about possible drug interactions or allergies, and incomplete or poorly legible prescriptions [7]. The largest expense by far related to drug complications in the US was from hospital admissions [8]. Similar figures for levels of error have been reported from Australia, Israel, and the United Kingdom [9]. In Sweden the average difference in cost between prescribed and dispensed medications was about 20% [10].

To address these issues, and to save money, PBM companies were created to manage the reimbursement of pharmaceutical products, normally including only prescription drugs (a 'carve-out' model). A prerequisite for an effective PBM is a well-established network of pharmacies and an infrastructure enabling interventions at the point of service. These companies were very successful in driving down the costs by negotiating with pharmaceutical manufacturers for price discounts, by providing services to payers such as drug utilization review (DUR), formulary management, prior authorization, and physician profiling [11]. Many of these features improved care as well as controlling costs.

PBM could address a broad spectrum of problems, and their economic value became apparent early. The DM strategy started later, and focused on common chronic illnesses that accounted for a majority of the hospitalized care, the major expense in any health-care system. Initially the idea was to deliver 'comprehensive' DM for these disorders. Because the illnesses were chronic, and because they were many, demonstrating economic value for DM has been more difficult to demonstrate across an entire health-care system. DM aimed to assist in identifying and monitoring long-term care of patients with chronic diseases at high risk for hospitalization (e.g. diabetes, coronary artery disease, congestive heart failure, osteoporosis, depression, asthma, cancer, benign prostatic hypertrophy, osteoarthritis, and peptic ulcer disease) [12]. Although some companies have attempted to take over management of such patients (another example of a 'carve-out' model), most programs have aimed at providing assistance to

the physician, based on evidence-based algorithms and/or on nationally accepted guidelines for management of specific disorders. Up to this point there was little direct involvement with physicians, who were not themselves at financial risk from the changes that were introduced.

However, the legislative climate is changing rapidly. The Balanced Budget Act of 1997 in the US includes a possible change in reimbursement to providers who do not follow standards of care. Medicare may be called on to enforce these standards and withhold payment when they are not followed [13]. In the UK the white paper on the National Health Service (NHS) created primary care groups who would be responsible for accepting some of the financial risk, in that they would be cash limited, but able to move money from one service to another [14, 15]. These groups will be responsible for commissioning secondary care, and tackling the variations in quality of care [16]. However, the health authorities, the regional organization responsible for the performance of general practice, face many barriers to implementing the new NHS. Among these barriers are the poor quality of the data, the unclear roles and responsibilities of physicians and managers, and the fact that doctors and health authority managers do not work sufficiently closely together to improve the quality of practice [17]. In the US group-model and staff-model health maintenance organizations, such as Group Health Cooperative of Puget Sound and Kaiser Health Plan, have developed in house programs of DM (the 'primary care-based' model) [3]. This model provides electronic information systems that allow viewing of an information spreadsheet for specific diseases, e.g. diabetes.

Clearly the time has come for physicians to be better informed about the solutions being proposed for health care, the reasons behind those solutions, and the role that they can play in improving their practice before changes are imposed upon them. The rest of this chapter will cover these areas based on published information relating to primary-care physicians, the group most often targeted for DM programs. Because of the magnitude of the problems, the most practical and successful approaches have been very focused. 'Comprehensive' DM, if it becomes a reality, will be composed of a group of smaller, more focused, and successful programs that all deal with a given disease entity.

What was the disease management solution originally proposed?

The concept of managed health care, of which DM was a component, developed in the 1980s as an adaptation of the reorganization of industrial management skills (also called total quality management, business process design, etc.). In this paradigm businesses committed to placing customers' needs first, decentralizing responsibility, placing reliance on well-defined economic/statistical tools, and to quality teamwork and measurement of results. The first programs 'borrowed' from industry in the early 1990s were designed to cut cost by using physician oversight, including gatekeepers, second opinions, and utilization review. As the concepts of DM took hold, the experience in the managed health care industry regarding the concepts of total quality management was applied in part to the components of managed care. In the latter part of the decade, as more quality tools were developed, so also were clinical pathways, algorithms, guidelines, automated prompts, and financial incentives. None of these programs by themselves, however, are equated with DM, although most are included in it.

DM is medical decision-making driven by data. The data must be captured and transformed into actionable information for use by providers to improve efficiency and effectiveness of health-care delivery. In its comprehensive form it involves an integrated, systematic approach to patient care, based on identifying at-risk patients, capturing clinical data, intervening in the course of the illness, and improving outcomes. Implicit in such a program is that the information and analysis of decision-making will help to change the behavior of patients, providers, and payers. Although DM was meant to be comprehensive, its goals were so broad that all programs have been composed of fragments of overall disease care. These components are listed in Table 1.

For DM to work requires the collection and management of large volumes of patient data. Because many elements of this information-based system are foreign to providers, development of such programs must include education of and support from providers for successful implementation. This will lead to sophisticated analysis, tracking, and measurement systems to provide useful interventions and outcomes data. The provider, therefore, is a crucial element in the planning and administration of DM programs. Reluctance to change or participate is a danger that the medical profession must

Table 1. General components of disease management

- Identify patients
- Provide treatment guidelines to physicians
- Educate patients
- Deliver interventions and support services to patients
- Measure clinical and financial outcomes

overcome, if the promise of information-based decision-making is to be achieved.

Why were economic evaluations an important driver to the development of disease management?

DM concepts developed at the same time as did the search for alternative methods of health resource allocation. Thus, it was originally thought that DM would save money. For this reason DM programs were developed initially by companies who would profit from such activities. One fear commonly expressed was that the profit motive would interfere with the delivery of quality health care. These fears have been mollified by the need for physician groups to control health-care costs, as reimbursement decreases and expenses increase. As DM programs have been developed with physicians, however, their involvement focuses naturally on the health-care aspects. 'Reduction in the costs of care is often a beneficial product of such programs, but it is a secondary goal and, importantly, not always achieved' [18]. Because economic forces continue to be important drivers of health-care policies and of managed care programs, it is useful for the physician to understand some aspects of medical economics [19, 20]. What follows is not meant to be comprehensive, but to take aspects of this large field that apply to DM concepts, explain some of the methods used, and put them into perspective for the physician.

The concept of DM was relevant to care needed by a population with a given disease, instead of focusing on individually taken decisions during multiple physician–patient interactions. Thus, health was considered a commodity, and DM principles (as managed health care principles) were adopted from the business world. However, health differs from money. One cannot trade health across time or individuals, and it is not stable, but affected by illness benefit analyses address only the absolute costs, but not whether the benefits are worth the cost. Neither takes into account cost shifting, nor variations in the delivery of health care. Finally, the power of the studies is often too low.

A few of these points are worth mentioning in a bit more detail. The outcome measures used have ranged from randomized controlled trials (RCT) to guesses by experts [35], but most involve RCT. Thus, their conclusions may not be applicable to a wider patient population. Cost shifting has been well demonstrated when comparing population costs of smokers versus non-smokers [36]. Although cost savings were estimated for the age group 45–70, most of these costs would probably be shifted to the surviving patients over age 70. The power of a study becomes important when one realizes that there is no absolute cut-off to determine what degree of cost savings is clinically meaningful. There is no *a-priori* reason for assuming that the 10–15% differences usually applied to clinical problems will be reasonable economically, or to suppose that such a cost difference would be worth a change in clinical practice [37]. Moreover, to achieve a 10–15% difference in costs often requires a very large sample, because cost data are likely to have large variances, to be highly skewed, and to require log transformation [38]. Thus, the sample size to achieve a meaningful cost difference may be much greater than that needed to find a clinically important difference. Thus, more care needs to be taken in prospectively deciding what size of cost difference would be worth achieving, and what study power would be needed to achieve such a difference, based on estimates of the variance in the cost projections. Finally, even when cost-effectiveness data are available, e.g. on drug usage, these data are often not applied, because they cannot be properly evaluated or do not seem to apply to the setting in which they might be helpful [39].

Why is disease management important for physicians, and vice-versa?

Despite the problems linking economic benefit to health care, the concepts behind DM are still valid, and should be pursued, regardless of whether or not they lead to tangible economic benefit. The economic issue will only factor into the decision to fund such programs. The major reason behind the need for

implementing DM is the variation in physician practice. There is so much information to be used, but even the relatively small number of evidence-based decisions that can be made are not necessarily widely or uniformly applied [40]. When physician variation is quantified, as for example by indices related to total medical expenses, a wide scatter with a range of $\pm 30\%$ was found [21]. Lack of knowledge of the drug was the major reason in prescription errors by physicians [7]. Even diagnostic precision should be improved, as reflected by the fact that the ability of clinicians to achieve consensus on a diagnosis from a given data set is limited [41]. Even using similar historical criteria, the probability of a given diagnosis may vary greatly depending on the clinical setting [42]. Thus, any system that improved such variability in a decision-making area should be welcome.

The reasons for practice variation are multiple [43]. There are first and foremost variations in the characteristics of the patients. The variability of the physician/provider includes not only how the physician responds to these characteristics, but what differences there are locally in availability and/or access to services, and what local differences there are in thresholds for actions. These provider-related issues involve processes that could be made more efficient by computer assistance, although the acceptance of such assistance by physicians depends heavily on the ease of use of the interface [44]. The need for local modification of these processes, however, is easily forgotten when introduction of DM programs is widely offered [45].

DM is best suited to decision nodes that are supported by evidence-based medicine [46]. However, doctors do not make most decisions based on 'hard' scientific evidence. They also retain a moral commitment to intervene on behalf of their individual patient, and not in response to a population-focused best-case scenario. Finally, personal intuition and physician expertise is encouraged for its advantages in professional esteem and market place advantage. After all, if all physicians looked and performed the same, what would there be to choose between them? 'The model of the clinician ... encourage[s] individual deviation from codified knowledge on the basis of personal, first-hand observation of concrete cases. This deviation is called "judgement" or even "wisdom"' [47]. The health-care system needs to change, in part due to increased inefficiency, but also due to increased cost, and information overload. The problem has been stated clearly, but it is unclear how this is to be accomplished. 'For the organization to break even they have to somehow control what the individual doctor does. The real trick is, can those entities ... find collegial methods to sort of control utilization [of medical resources] without the rancour?' [48]. 'Managed care firms have enormous incentives to promulgate rules that may rationalize medical practice economically, but may not give doctors and patients the flexibility they need to deal with the limitless variables of real life' [49].

Does disease management work?

The process of DM consists of four main steps: (1) identification of the target patient group, (2) intervention to introduce preventive or curative treatment according to validated therapeutic guidelines and/or best-evidence, (3) education to improve physician performance and patient compliance, and (4) measure outcomes to ensure that the result is beneficial. Typically guidelines are established nationally or internationally by medical experts, but as local practice may vary in many ways (including those that do not alter the medical decision), these guidelines must be locally adapted and adopted. There are many studies showing that the application of clinical guidelines does improve the process of clinical practice. Because the concept of DM was meant to affect populations of patients, the majority of the studies and the examples discussed here will be confined to general practice sites and issues [50]. When outcomes are examined these usually also improve, although the data are not so numerous nor so robust [51]. This survey is meant not to be comprehensive, but to represent what might come closest to situations that reflect general clinical practice. The 'bottom line' to be extracted from these studies is that DM *can* work in office practice, and that when it does physicians appreciate the results [52].

The studies shown in Table 3 have been selected from the meta-analyses of Grimshaw and Russell [50], and from a Medline search, if they combined the application of guidelines to assessment of both physician compliance and patient outcome, if they were randomized controlled studies, and if they were carried out in a general medical or primary-care setting. In only a few studies has the economic impact of an altered outcome been studied at the same time [53, 54]. Some studies have dealt with acute hospital-based care. One study tested the effects of incorporating adherence to essential criteria of medical care into concurrent quality control [55]. The criteria were simply placed in the hospital with no attempt at education of physicians or patients, and it was a multicenter study involving 24 study and 26 control hospitals. Nonetheless, there was a small increase in physician compliance with guidelines, and poorer outcomes associated with lack of compliance to guidelines for treatment of bacterial pneumonia and acute myocardial infarction. An algorithm was developed for resuscitation of patients with hypotension in a surgical emergency room, combined with physician education, and it was found that physicians will use an algorithm even under stress [56]. The use of the guidelines prevented delays in resuscitation with less mortality and morbidity (the percentage of patients leaving emergency on ventilators declined from 33% to 14%). A highly structured continuing education program to impart guidelines regarding management of burns in the emergency room was employed, and demonstrated a benefit among patients admitted to hospital in decreased early complications (30% vs 45% among patients whose physicians were not instructed) [57]. This was a large study involving 298 physicians and over 2500 patients.

Hypertension and diabetes mellitus are conditions with well-publicized guidelines and fairly standard outcomes measures, and should be ideal for DM [58]. An automated surveillance system with a computer-based medical record system was used to improve the follow-up of patients with newly diagnosed hypertension [59]. Physicians who received reminders improved the frequency of follow-up blood pressure checks in 6 months, and this led to adequate control of pressure in 70%, compared to patients whose physicians did not receive a reminder (52%). Sixty physicians were provided not only with computer reminders, but on-line information on treatment protocols and their patients' blood pressure percentile [60]. In this study of over 3000 patients such reminders led to diastolic pressure of <90 mmHg for more days out of the year (323 vs. 255 for controls). In the diabetes studies improvement in physician compliance was marked, and led to a decrease in hospitalization using only computer-based reminders [61] and improved glycemic control using extensive education programs for physicians and patients [62].

Preventive medicine is another area in which guidelines should produce non-controversial applications and improved results. Computer-based reminders to 115 physicians (12 467 patients) led to

Table 3. Changes in clinical outcome using specific guidelines

Patient group [ref no.]	Guideline used	Results	
		Physician compliance	Patient outcome
Acute hospital			
Various [55]	External, national Placed in records	2% more (all MDs)	Better for MI and bacterial pneumonia if guideline compliant
Shock [56]	External, personal instruction	37% more (45→82%) (ER MDs)	19% fewer patients on ventilators (33→14%)
Burns [57]	National, seminars	5% more (90→95%) (ER MDs)	15% fewer complications (45→30%)
Hypertension			
Ambulatory [9]	External, patient-specific computer prompts	52% more follow-up (46→98%) (GPs)	18% more diastolic BP <100 (52→70%)
Ambulatory [60]	Provincial, patient-specific computer prompts	Patients followed longer (GPs)	19% more days with diastolic BP <90 (255→323)
Preventive			
Various [63]	External, computer prompts	20% more (29→49%) (GPs)	Fewer hospitalizations or ER visits in vaccinated patients
Smokers [66]	External, trained	64% more(12→76%) (GPs)	4% more not smoking after 1 year (4.4→8.8%)
Smokers [64]	National, chart reminders	32% more (23→55%) (GPs)	8% more not smoking after 1 year (2.7→11.1%)
Smokers [65]	External, trained, patient prompts	12% more (10→22%) (internists)	1% more not smoking after 1 year
Diabetes mellitus			
Ambulatory [84]	External, computer reminders	13% more (37→50%) (GPs)	Fewer days in hospital for 2/3 of group
Ambulatory [62]	ADA, MD and patient education	Nearly complete (medical HOs)	Lower fasting glucose HbA1c, body weight
Self-limited conditions			
Outpatients [10]	Internal, mailed to MDs	8% more for five conditions (GPs.	Fewer days/month SOB (4.2→1.7 days)
Diarrhea, URI [53]	WHO guidelines local courses	More use of ORS, less use of antibiotics (GPs)	Higher benefit/cost ratios
Depression			
Island of Gotland [54]	Internal, courses	33% more antidepressants (GPs)	48% fewer suicides (39→20% predicted)
Island of Gotland [69]	No courses during follow up	More inpatient care (GPs, academic)	Higher suicide rate
Older patients [70]	Patient-specific recommendations	More diagnosis and use of antidepressants	No significant effect
Depressed patients [71]	AHCPR guide-lines	Complete (GPs)	50% more complete recovery (20→70%)

ADA, American Diabetic Association; AHCPR, Agency for Health Care Policy and Research; BP, blood pressure; ER, emergency room; GP, general practitioner; MI, myocardial infarction; ORS, oral rehydration solution; SOB, shortness of breath; URI, upper respiratory infection; WHO, World Health Organisation better compliance in providing occult blood testing and mammography for cancer screening, weight reduction diets and programs, and influenza and pneumococcal vaccines, compared with controls [63]. Moreover, hospitalizations and emergency room visits were decreased among the vaccinated patients. Three studies on smoking cessation used short courses to physicians to improve delivery of information to the patient [64–66]. In all studies it was clear that continuing educational programs substantially changed the way physicians counseled smokers. As a result there was a small improvement in long-term abstinence, especially among patients who wanted to quit.

Although DM is considered usually only for chronic conditions, programs have been applied successfully to medically self-limited conditions. The North of England Study is unique in that the general practitioners in the study developed their own guidelines, which were mailed to all physicians, but only the study group had educational programs related to them [67]. Although the control group that received guidelines may also have improved its performance, there was still improved compliance in the study group, and in one condition (recurrent wheezing) there was clear improvement in outcome. The study from Mexico involved a large number of patients and rather limited formal physician education [53]. Guidelines were developed in a small research project as proof of concept, and the guidelines were provided to a health district and then to the state level where one physician oversaw the education of over 100 other physicians. Drug use in acute diarrhea was dramatically decreased and use of oral rehydration solution dramatically increased over the 2 years of the study ($>52\,000$ district patients and $>126\,000$ state patients), with demonstrated cost-effectiveness.

Depression is a disorder also amenable to disease management, as it is underdiagnosed and treated [68]. After establishing baseline data the Swedish Committee for Prevention and Treatment of Depression launched an educational program for the diagnosis and treatment of depression for all general practitioners on the island of Gotland, and the immediate effects were evaluated after 2 years. The direct benefits were fewer days in hospital and reduced (by half) rate of suicides [54]. The amount of money saved depended on the value placed on a life, but however calculated, the indirect benefits of the program corresponded to a significant portion ($>10\%$) of the total health expenditure. A follow-up study from the same group documented that, 3 years after cessation of the educational program for general practitioners, the use of antidepressants (intervention) and the suicide rate (outcome) had returned to pre-study levels [69]. Thus, it would appear that educational programs will have lasting effects only if they are repeated and/or continued.

More recent studies on depression confirmed that, after a brief educational program, primary-care physicians improved recognition and treatment of late-life depression, and demonstrated improved symptomatic control [70]. When the diagnosis was confirmed before the intervention was applied, the value of standardized pharmacotherapy or psychotherapy was dramatic in 8 months, with complete recovery of 70% in the study group, versus 20% in controls [71].

None of these studies is perfect, but then none of the studies attempted a comprehensive approach to the clinical problem. If the modest results reported above were multiplied by the number of interventions needed to manage an entire disease, the results would be impressive. In such a setting it would be less important whether all such interventions worked. In such a world of the future the successful interventions could be selected and the others dropped. However, even the ones that did not change disease outcome might very well be valued for their ability to save time or simply manage record-keeping better. Although DM is difficult to develop and implement, the underlying concepts are sound and supported by the available evidence.

How can disease management be implemented?

The most difficult task in DM programs involves implementation. As is evident from Table 3, multiple methods and interventions have been used, even in a single study. A meta-analysis of multifaceted interventions in general practice (61 controlled studies) revealed that multifaceted interventions were most effective (Table 4). Information linked to performance (feedback, physician and patient reminders) was the most effective single intervention [72]. When three or four interventions were used together the strategy was nearly always successful.

It is worth stressing at the outset of this section that computer methods are enablers of DM concepts, but are not essential to the concepts themselves. However, many of the studies in DM

Table 4. Effectiveness of strategies for implementing changes in primary care

Strategy used	Strategy components	Effectiveness (no. of 61 best-evidence studies)		
		Complete	Partial	None
Information transfer (I)	Reading materials. Group, patient education	2	6	9
Information linked to performance (II)	Feedback, physician and patient reminders	10	4	1
Learning through social influence (III)	Individual instruction, Peer review, patient reports	2	3	2
Management support (IV)	Resources, incentives, rules, obligations, patient incentives	1	2	–
I + III		4	4	12
I + IV		3	3	1
II + III		1	2	–
3 or 4 interventions		5	–	1

Modified from ref. 77.

have used electronic media to provide either information or reminders. A few have even used the computer to compile or calculate patient data that are then fed back to the physician or provider. Such computer-based clinical decision support systems (CDSS in current jargon) are increasing in frequency [73]. A review of such studies in 1994 found 28 controlled trials [74], while a similar review in 1998 found 65 [75]. One must keep in mind, however, that the use of computers does not ensure a better outcome. In fact, in one study where blood pressure was lowered by use of guidelines and computer-prompts, there was no statistically significant effect of the reminders for follow-up blood pressure measurements themselves on lowered pressure [59]. This may be related to the fact that there is a wide range of factors that affect changes in clinical practice, and none was dominant [76]. The most frequent reasons for change were organizational (e.g. hospital management, staffing, improved services), education, contact with professionals, availability of technology, and clinical experience. The use of computers could be considered either as a new technology or as an organizational change. Other reasons for change, such as education and contact with professionals and patients, can also be delivered through the computer. Thus, the computer has the greatest potential for changing practice.

Information provided by computer is more accessible, more thoroughly indexed, potentially more up-to-date, more linked to related data sources, and can be incorporated into a local decision support system that includes decision-making advice and warnings. Thus, it is good at identifying patients, at intervening by providing pathways and reminders, at educating patients and physicians to maintain the program, and at measuring outcomes: all the key features required for a DM program. As with all DM programs such a system would not dictate decisions, but would provide the basis for making more consistent and logical decisions. The electronic medical record (EMR) is not an essential part of a computer-based program, but it can make the practice of medicine more efficient. The fully implemented EMR can be interfaced with the laboratory, enabling transfer of reports directly to the record. Prescriptions can be transmitted directly to the pharmacy at the time of the patient's visit, and the pharmacist can confirm that the prescription was filled and picked up. Referral letters can be generated automatically, based on the data from the most recent patient encounter. The record can be programmed to note potential drug interactions, and can produce patient recall letters for preventive services. Patient educational information can be provided automatically at the end of the patient visit. And the potential of this EMR can increase markedly once patients also come on line, and the confidentiality concerns are overcome.

Table 5. Computerized decision support systems can improve clinical performance and patient outcome (1982–1992)

Strategy used	Results of 29 PRCTs	
	Improvement	No improvement
Computer-assisted diagnosis	1	4
Computer-assisted drug dosing	3	1
Preventive-care reminders	4	2
Computer-aided active medical care	7	2
Fewer errors in test ordering	3	0
Response rate to clinical events	3	0
Adherence to hypertension protocol	1	2
Effect on patient outcome	2	3

Modified from ref. 74.

Even without an EMR there is strong evidence that CDSS can improve physician performance, as shown in Table 5 [74]. It is difficult to judge these results by themselves, however, as doctors change behavior most when multiple interventions are performed [77]. Thus, it might appear from Table 5 that computers cannot help in diagnosis. However, it is known that education can do this very nicely. Thus, if education were delivered electronically in easy and usable form, that result might change. More recent studies have utilized the computer outside the doctor's office, a setting in which its use is much more familiar. For example, the pharmacy can track antibiotics during acute hospitalization, and produce reduction in overdose, allergies, mismatches, and adverse events [78]. Anticoagulation is another area of drug control in which nurses can provide excellent follow-up via computer, leading to a longer time in the therapeutic range [79]. In the primary-care setting regulation of anticoagulation using a CDSS has been remarkable, with acceptable INR control from 23% of the time to 86% [80].

Applying evidence from these clinical trials to the care of individual patients is a very large challenge [49]. Knowing when results obtained from the process of 'evidence-based medicine' apply to a given patient still requires a great deal of skill and experience, and must be individualized. Thus, guidelines for deciding how and when this should be done can only be process-driven, with or without computer assistance. This is true even in a system such as the NHS in the UK where such implementation is now a national priority. Evidence-based indicators linked to interventions that improve outcomes have been suggested [81] as an adjunct to primary-care practices to help them find a way to succeed. Physicians must become involved with these systems, and most likely computer-based decision systems, as guidelines and drug information become more widely distributed and constitute the standard of care [82]. The delivery of such systems for implementation via the Internet is a sign of the direction in which the physician must go. One such aid is the System for Interactive Electronic Guidelines with Feedback and Resources for Intructional and Educational Development (SIEGFRIED), designed to present clinical practice guidelines interactively to providers at a point of care, by means of a series of questions that apply to a specific patient [83]. It is clear that these developments will take time to implement and to learn. Even writing inpatient orders through computer workstations required more physician time than did paper charts [84]. Moreover, no immediate gain, related either to outcomes or cost, may be realized by physicians during the initial learning phase using decision support systems. However, the longer the profession waits to enter the field of electronic medicine, the more they will have to catch up with consumers, laboratories, and other groups who will be consistent and expectant users of computers.

What is the evidence for disease management programs in IBD?

The number of patients involved and their use of drugs, the most easily monitored aspect of medical costs, is relatively small, so that no organization has felt compelled yet to turn its attention to DM for IBD. The process of establishing a meaningful DM protocol takes considerable commitment and energy [85]. In addition, the complexity of the disease has left most patients cared for by specialists who, because of their better education in dealing with fewer diseases, may feel less need for such programs. Furthermore, drugs account for only about 6% of the total cost of care in Crohn's disease [12]. Indirect costs due to sick leave and early retirement account for 71% of the cost, but these are harder to measure, and do not add to the annual outlay for medical care. Another review of all IBD patients, however, suggests that surgery and hospitalization account for about 50% of all costs. If this is really the case, HMOs or other payers may become interested in programs to decrease health-care costs in IBD.

Cost-effectiveness studies are beginning to be performed for difficult decision areas in IBD, such as the surveillance of patients with ulcerative colitis [86]. A cost analysis of the role of colonoscopy vs sigmoidoscopy for initial evaluation of ulcerative colitis has shown that, based on the physician preference for knowing disease location, colonoscopy is most cost-effective [87]. However, the real question of how important it is to know precise disease location was not addressed. One must be alert always to ask if the outcome will really be affected by the intervention [88]. The same is true for the study analyzing lifetime cost-utility for patients with inactive Crohn's disease [89]. A small incremental benefit for mesalamine was found using QALY as the utility measure, but also a small incremental cost. The conclusion was that long-term maintenance should not be discouraged on a cost-utility basis. More correctly the authors pointed out that the real question is the long-term prognosis of such patients. After all, if mesalamine has no long-term benefit, or if only patients with clinically active disease are benefited, then a population-based study will not be helpful. The same kind of careful clinical questions have been raised in a study of the cost of endoscopic screening for intestinal precancerous conditions [90]. The variabilities in the clinical questions (incidence of tumors, effectiveness of timely diagnosis, sensitivity of endoscopy, etc.) produce sufficiently large margins of error that a DM program could not really be constructed at this time.

These studies point out that DM should be used when the evidence is convincing to assist in decision-making. However, all physicians should be acquainting themselves with the concepts and methodologies involved and, most importantly, advancing to greater use of the computer, so that when the clinical evidence is available, programs helpful to the physician and patient can be rapidly introduced [91]. It is already clear that some patients with ulcerative colitis (about 30%) are willing to provide their medical information over the World Wide Web [92]. One could wonder if that high a percentage of physicians would be willing to access a computer-based program. To leave such programs to forces imposed during economic crisis by payers, employers, or insurers is to abdicate an important aspect of the physician as the advocate of the patient and good-quality delivery of health care.

Acknowledgement

This work was supported in part by Diversified Health Systems, Ltd, a division of SmithKline Beecham plc.

References

1. Bodger AU, Daly MJ, Heatley RV. 1997. Clinical economics review: *Helicobacter pylori*-associated peptic ulcer disease. Aliment Pharmacol Ther 11: 273–82.
2. Hadorn D. The Oregon priority-setting exercise: cost-effectiveness and the rule of rescue, revisited. Med Decis Making 1996; 16: 117–19.
3. Bodenheimer T. 1999. Disease management – promises and pitfalls. N Engl J Med 340:1202–5.
4. Lesar TS, Briceland LL, Delcoure K, Parmalee JC, Masta-Gornic V, Pohl H. Medication prescribing errors in a teaching hospital. J Am Med Assoc 1990; 263: 2329–33.
5. Bates DW, Cullen DJ, Laird N et al. Incidence of adverse drug events and potential adverse drug events. Implications for prevention. J Am Med Assoc 1995; 274: 29–34.
6. Beardon PH, McGilchrist MM, McKendrick AD, McDevitt DG, MacDonald TM. Primary non-compliance with prescribed medication in primary care. Br Med J 1994; 307:846–48.
7. Leape LL, Bates DW, Cullen DJ et al. Systems analysis of adverse drug events. J Am Med Assoc 1995; 274: 35–43.
8. Johnston JA, Bootman JL. Drug-related morbidity and mortality: a cost-of-illness model. Arch Intern Med 1995; 155: 1949–56.
9. Berwick DM, Leape LL. Reducing errors in medicine: it's time to take this more seriously. Br Med J 1999; 319: 136–7.
10. Nilsson JLG, Johansson H, Wennberg M. Large differences between prescribed and dispensed medicines could indicate undertreatment. Drug Inform J 1995; 29: 1243–6.
11. Schumock GT, Meek PD, Ploetz PA, Vermeulen LC. Economic evaluations of clinical pharmacy services – 1988–1995. The Publications Committee of the American College of Clinical Pharmacy. Pharmacotherapy 1996; 16: 1188–208.
12. Ekbom A, Blomqvist P. Costs to society in Crohn's disease. Res Clin Forums 1998; 20: 33–9.
13. Epstein RS, Sherwood LM. From outcomes research to disease management: a guide for the perplexed. Ann Intern Med 1996; 124: 832–7.
14. Butler T, Roland M. How will primary care groups work? Br Med J 1998; 316: 214.
15. Department of Health. The New NHS. London: Stationery Office, 1997.
16. Gilley J. Meeting the information and budgetary requirements of primary care groups. Br Med J 1999; 318: 168–70.
17. Marshal MN. Improving quality in general practice: qualitative case study of barriers faced by health authorities. Br Med J 1999; 319: 164–7.
18. Mark DB. Economics of treating heart failure. Am J Cardiol 1997; 80: 33H–8H.
19. Sloan FA (editor). Valuing Health Care: Costs, Benefits, and Effectiveness of Pharmaceuticals and Other Medical Technologies. New York: Cambridge University Press, 1996.
20. Sloan FA, Conover CJ. The use of cost-effectiveness/cost-benefit analysis in actual decision making: current status and prospects. In: Sloan FA, ed. Valuing Health Care. New York: Cambridge University Press, 1996: 207–22.

21. Phelps CE. Good technologies gone bad: how and why the cost-effectiveness of a medical intervention changes for different populations. Med Decis Making 1997; 17: 107–17.

22. Rich MW, Beckham V, Wittenberg C, Leven CL, Freedland KE, Carney RM. A multidisciplinary intervention to prevent the readmission of elderly patients with congestive heart failure. N Engl J Med 1995; 333: 1190–5.

23. Rich MW, Nease RF. Cost-effectiveness analysis in clinical practice: the case of heart failure. Arch Intern Med 1999; 159: 1690–700.

24. DaSilva RV. A disease management case study on asthma. Clin Ther 1996; 18: 1374–82.

25. Neumann PJ, Zinner DE, Wright JC. Are methods for estimating QALYs in cost-effectiveness analyses improving? Med Decis Making 1997; 17: 402–8.

26. Guyatt GH, Feeny DH, Patrick DL. Measuring health-related quality of life. Ann Intern Med 1993; 118: 622–9.

27. Bergner M, Bobbitt RA, Carter WB et al. The sickness impact profile: development and final revision of a health status measure. Med Care 1981; 19: 787–805.

28. Stewart AL, Greenfield S, Hays RD et al. Functional status and well-being of patients with chronic conditions: Results from the medical outcomes study. J Am Med Assoc 1989; 262: 907–13.

29. Deverill M, Brazier J, Green C, Booth A. The use of QALY and non-QALY measures of health-related quality of life. Assessing the state of the art. Pharmacoeconomics 1998; 13: 411–20.

30. Detsky AS, McLaughlin JR, Abrams HB et al. Quality of life of patients on long-term total parenteral nutrition at home. J Gen Intern Med 1986; 1: 26–33.

31. Russell LB, Gold MR, Siegel JE, Daniels N, Weinstein MC, for the Panel on Cost-Effectiveness in Health and Medicine. The role of cost-effectiveness analysis in health and medicine. J Am Med Assoc 1996; 276: 1172–7.

32. Weinstein MC, Siegel JE, Gold MR, Kamlet MS, Russell LB, for the Panel on Cost-Effectiveness in Health and Medicine. Recommendations of the panel on cost-effectiveness in health and medicine. J Am Med Assoc 1996; 276: 1253–8.

33. Goldman L, Weinstein MC, Goldman PA, Williams LW. Cost-effectiveness of HMG-CoA reductase inhibition for primary and secondary prevention of coronary artery disease (CAD). J Am Med Assoc 1991; 265: 1145–51.

34. Oster G, Borok GM. Menzin J et al. Cholesterol reduction intervention study (CRIS): a randomized trial to assess effectiveness and costs in clinical practice. Arch Intern Med 1996; 156: 731–9.

35. Detsky AS. Evidence of effectiveness: evaluating its quality. In: Sloan FA, ed. Valuing Health Care. New York: Cambridge University Press, 1996: 5–29.

36. Barendregt JJ, Bonneux L, van der Maas PJ. The health care costs of smoking. N Engl J Med 1997; 337:1052–7.

37. Drummond M, O'Brien B. Clinical importance, statistical significance and the assessment of economic and quality-of-life outcomes. Health Econ 1993; 2: 205–12.

38. Gray AM, Marshall M, Lockwood A, Morris J. Problems in conducting economic evaluations alongside clinical trials: Lessons from a study of case management for people with mental disorders. Br J Psychiatry 1997; 170: 47–52.

39. Sloan FA, Whetten-Goldstein K, Wilson A. Hospital pharmacy decisions, cost containment, and the use of cost-effectiveness analysis. Soc Sci Med 1997; 45: 523–33.

40. Gill P, Dowell AC, Neal RD, Smith N, Heywood P, Wilson AE. Evidence based general practice: a retrospective study of interventions in one training practice. Br Med J 1996; 312: 819–21.

41. Dolan JG, Bordley DR, Mushlin AI. An evaluation of clinicians' subjective prior probability estimates. Med Decis Making 1986; 6: 216–23.

42. Sox HC Jr, Hickam DH, Marton KI et al. Using the patient's history to estimate the probability of coronary artery disease: a comparison of primary care and referral practices. Am J Med 1990; 89: 7–14.

43. van Miltenburg-van Zijl AJ, Bossuyt PM, Nette RW, Simoons ML, Taylor TR. Cardiologists' use of clinical information for management decisions for patients with unstable angina: a policy analysis. Med Decis Making 1997; 17: 292–7.

44. Kopelman PG, Sanderson AJ. Application of database systems in diabetes care. Med Inform (Lond) 1996; 21: 259–71.

45. Sullivan F, Mitchell E. Has general practitioner computing made a difference to patient care? A systematic review of published reports. Br Med J 1995; 311: 848–52.

46. Sackett DL. Evidence Based Medicine: How to Practice and Teach EBM. New York: Churchill Livingstone, 1997.

47. Friedson E. Profession of Medicine: A Study of the Sociology of Applied Knowledge. New York: Dodd, Mead, 1970, p. 347.

48. Reinhardt U. Quoted in Hilzenrath DS. Can doctors heal themselves? The Washington Post National Weekly Edition. 22–9 Dec 1997: 30 1.

49. Reed SE. Miss Treatment. New Republic 217 (29 Dec 1997): 20–2.

50. Grimshaw JM, Russell IT. The effect of clinical guidelines on medical practice: a systematic review of rigorous evaluations. Lancet 1993; 352: 1317–22.

51. Grimshaw JM, Russell IT. Achieving health gain through clinical guidelines. II: Ensuring guidelines change medical practice. Qual Health Care 1994; 3: 45–52.

52. Grol R, Dalhuijsen J, Thomas S, Veld Ci, Rutten G, Mokkink H. Attributes of clinical guidelines that influence use of guidelines in general practice: observational study. Br Med J 1998; 317: 858–61.

53. Guiscafre H, Martinez H, Reyes H et al. From research to public health interventions. I. Impact of an educational strategy for physicians to improve treatment practices of common diseases. Arch Med Res 1995; 26 (Suppl.) S31–9.

54. Rutz W, Carlsson P, von Knorring L, Walinder J. Cost-benefit analysis of an educational program for general practitioners by the Swedish Committee for the Prevention and Treatment of Depression. Acta Psychiatr Scand 1992; 85: 457–64.

55. Sanazaro PF, Worth RM. Concurrent quality assurance in hospital care. Report of a study by private initiative in PSRO. N Engl J Med 1978; 298: 1171–7.

56. Hopkins JA, Shoemaker WC, Greenfield S, Chang PC, McAuliffe T, Sproat RW. Treatment of surgical emergencies with and without an algorithm. Arch Surg 1980; 115: 745–50.

57. Linn BS. Continuing medical education. Impact on emergency room burn care. J Am Med Assoc 1980; 244:565–70.

58. Grundel BL, White GL Jr, Eichold BH. Diabetes in the managed care setting: a prospective plan. South Med J 1999; 92: 459–64.

59. Barnett GO, Winickoff RN, Morgan MM, Zielstorff RD. A computer-based monitoring system for follow-up of elevated blood pressure. Med Care. 1983; 21: 400–9.

60. McAlister NH, Covvey HD, Tong C, Lee A, Wigle ED. Randomised controlled trial of computer assisted management of hypertension in primary care. Br Med J 1986; 293: 670–4.

61. Thomas JC, Moore A, Qualls PE. The effect on cost of medical care for patients treated with an automated clinical audit system. J Med Syst 1983; 7: 307–13.

62. Vinicor F, Cohen SJ, Mazzuca SA et al. DIABEDS: a randomized trial of the effects of physician and/or patient education on diabetes patient outcomes. J Chronic Dis 1987; 40: 345–56.

63. McDonald CJ, Hui SL, Smith DM et al. Reminders to physicians from an introspective computer medical record. A two-year randomized trial. Ann Intern Med 1984; 100: 130–8.

64. Cohen SJ, Christen AG, Katz BP et al. Counselling medical and dental patients about cigarette smoking: the impact of nicotine gum and chart reminders. Am J Public Health 1987; 77: 313–16.

65. Cummings SR, Coates TJ, Richard RJ et al. Training physicians in counselling about smoking cessation. A randomized trial of the "Quit for Life" program. Ann Intern Med 1989; 110: 640–7.

66. Wilson DM, Taylor DW, Gilbert JR et al. A randomized trial of a family physician intervention for smoking cessation. J Am Med Assoc 1988; 260: 1570–4.

67. North of England Study of Standards and Performance in General Practice. II: Effects on health of patients with common childhood conditions. Br Med J 1992; 304: 1484–7.

68. Santiago JM. Commentary: The costs of treating depression. J Clin Psychiatry 1993; 54: 425–6.

69. Rutz W, von Knorring L, Walinder J. Long-term effects of an educational program for general practitioners given by the Swedish Committee for the Prevention and Treatment of Depression. Acta Psychiatr Scand 1992b; 85: 83–8.

70. Callahan CM, Hendrie HC, Dittus RS, Brater DC, Hui SL, Tierney WM. Improving treatment of late life depression in primary care: a randomized clinical trial. J Am Geriatr Soc 1994; 42: 839–46.

71. Schulberg HC, Block MR, Madonia MJ et al. Treating major depression in primary care practice. Eight-month clinical outcomes. Arch Gen Psychiatry 1996; 53: 913–19.

72. Wensing M, Grol R. Single and combined strategies for implementing changes in primary care: A literature review. Int J Quality Health Care 1994; 6: 115–32.

73. Classen DC. Clinical decision support systems to improve clinical practice and quality of life (Editorial). J Am Med Assoc 1998; 280: 1360–1.

74. Johnston ME, Langton KB, Haynes RB, Mathieu A. Effects of computer-based clinical decision support systems on clinician performance and patient outcome: a critical appraisal of research. Ann Intern Med 1994; 120: 135–42.

75. Hunt DL, Haynes RB, Hanna SE, Smith K. Effects of computer-based decision support systems on physician performance and patient outcomes. A systematic review. J Am Med Assoc 1998; 280: 1339–46.

76. Allery LA, Owen PA, Robling MR. Why general practitioners and consultants change their clinical practice: a critical incident study. Br Med J 1997; 314: 870–4.

77. Wensing M, van der Weijden T, Grol R. Implementing guidelines and innovations in general practice: which interventions are effective? Br J Gen Pract 1998; 48: 991–7.

78. Evans RS, Pestotnik SL, Classen DC et al. A computer-assisted management program for antibiotics and other anti-infective agents. N Engl J Med 1998; 338: 232–8.

79. Vadher BD, Patterson DL, Leaning M. Comparison of oral anticoagulant control by a nurse-practitioner using a computer decision-support system with that by clinicians. Clin Lab Haematol 1997; 19: 203–7.

80. Fitzmaurice DA, Hobbs FD, Murray ET, Bradley CP, Holder R. Evaluation of computerized decision support for oral anticoagulation management based in primary care. Br J Gen Pract 1996; 46: 533–5.

81. McColl A, Roderick P, Gabbay J, Smith H, Moore M. Performance indicators for primary care groups: an evidence based approach. Br Med J 1998; 317: 1354–60.

82. Meyer LC. Why centers of excellence are gaining momentum. J Health Care Benefits 1994; 3: 52–6.

83. Lobach DF, Underwood HR. Computer-based decision support systems for implementing clinical practice guidelines. Drug Benefit Trends 1998; 10: 48–53.

84. Tierney WM, Miller ME, Overhage JM, McDonald CJ. Physician inpatient order writing on microcomputer workstations: effects on resource utilization. J Am Med Assoc 1993; 269: 379–83.

85. Rall CJN, Munshi AD, Stasior DS. Disease management strategies and the gastroenterologist. Gastroenterol Clin N Am 1997; 26: 873–94.

86. Ward FM, Bodger K, Daly MJ, Heatley RV. Clinical economics review: medical management of inflammatory bowel disease. Aliment Pharmacol Ther 1999; 13: 15–25.

87. Deutsch DE, Olson AD. Colonoscopy or sigmoidoscopy as the initial evaluation of pediatric patients with colitis: a survey of physician behaviour and a cost analysis. J Pediatr Gastroenterol Nutr 1997; 25: 26–31.

88. Provenzale D, Wong JB, Onden JE, Lipscomb J. Performing a cost-effectiveness analysis: surveillance of patients with ulcerative colitis. Am J Gastroenterol 1998; 93: 872–80.

89. Trallori G, Messori A. Drug treatments for maintaining remission in Crohn's disease. A lifetime cost-utility analysis. Pharmacoeconomics 1997; 11: 444–53.

90. Sonnenberg A, El-Serag HB. Economic aspects of endoscopic screening for intestinal precancerous conditions. Gastrointest Endosc Clin N Am 1997; 7: 165–84.

91. McKee M, Britton A. Conducting a literature review on the effectiveness of health care interventions. Health Policy Plan 1997; 12: 262–7.

92. Soetikno RM, Provencale D, Lenert LA. Studying ulcerative colitis over the World Wide Web. Am J Gastroenterol 1997; 92: 457–60.

23 | Pharmacoeconomics and inflammatory bowel disease

BRIAN G. FEAGAN

Introduction

The past decade has seen an unprecedented increase in our understanding of the biology of chronic inflammation. The pharmaceutical industry has harnessed this new knowledge to produce important new treatments for such chronic debilitating diseases as multiple sclerosis, rheumatoid arthritis, and inflammatory bowel disease (IBD). Unfortunately, monoclonal antibodies and recombinant human cytokines are expensive; annual treatment costs of greater than US$10 000 are common. In the near future many additional biopharmaceuticals will become available. However, since health-care resources are limited, sound decisions must be made regarding the appropriate allocation of resources for these products. Is society obtaining good value for expenditures on drugs? How can we provide the best care at the lowest cost? Which new treatments should be funded? These are some of the questions which are addressed by pharmacoeconomic analyses.

IBD has a large economic impact on society for several reasons. First, drug treatments to ameliorate symptoms of abdominal pain, diarrhea, and bleeding are expensive. Although many individuals require surgery to alleviate symptoms, surgery itself may also cause considerable morbidity and, rarely, death. Second, patients with IBD are typically young [1] and life-long treatment is often required [2]. Third, although conventional medical treatments such as glucocorticoids and immunomodulatory drugs are moderately effective, they also cause adverse effects. Thus both the symptoms of IBD and treatment negatively influence patients' health-related quality of life (HRQL) [3]. Since the cost of IBD is high in both humanistic and monetary terms it is vital to understand the economic consequences of new treatments. This chapter reviews the fundamental concepts of pharmacoeconomic analysis, and examines cost and quality-of-life assessments in IBD.

Classification of pharmacoeconomic analyses

Four fundamental procedures can be performed: cost-minimization, cost-benefit, cost-effectiveness, and cost-utility analyses [4, 5]. All of these analyses relate expenditures, expressed in dollars, to specific outcomes. The key distinction is the choice of outcome to which costs are related.

The most basic technique, cost-minimization analysis [6], is utilized when *equivalent* clinical outcomes result from two competing treatments. Logically, the least expensive treatment is preferred given that no difference in efficacy exists. However, this approach is overly simplistic since the usual situation is that a new drug is likely to be both more expensive and more effective than a standard therapy. Even in the rare instance when equivalent clinical efficacy for two treatment alternatives has been demonstrated other differences usually exist, such as convenience of administration or side-effect profile, which make this form of analysis inappropriate. Thus more sophisticated types of pharmacoeconomic comparisons are usually required.

The most commonly employed method, cost-effectiveness analysis [7], relates costs to a discrete, clinically meaningful outcome. The incremental cost of a new therapy in comparison to a standard treatment is then expressed in terms of dollars expended per beneficial outcome attained or negative outcome prevented. This approach is useful for disorders such as cardiovascular disease in which robust clinical endpoints occur frequently (i.e. death or myocardial infarction). Since these events have a distinct meaning to both health-care providers and patients, the concept of expressing the cost of a new treatment in terms of dollars expended per adverse outcome avoided is easily understood. However, this type of analysis has some important limitations. Most importantly cost-effectiveness analysis does

Stephan R. Targan, Fergus Shanahan and Loren C. Karp (eds.), Inflammatory Bowel Disease: From Bench to Bedside, 2nd Edition, 471–480.
© 2003 *Kluwer Academic Publishers. Printed in Great Britain*

Table 2. Comparison of costs of inflammatory bowel disease in United States (1990)

Medical services	Crohn's disease		Ulcerative colitis	
	Annual cost (US$)	Percentage (%)	Annual cost (US$)	Percentage (%)
Diagnostic work-up	98	1.5	116	7.6
Outpatient services	192	2.9	105	7.1
Medications	671	10.2	125	8.4
Surgery	3032	46.2	233	15.6
Other inpatient services	2209	33.7	469	31.5
Treatment of long-term complications	358	5.5	439	29.5
Total	6561	100	1488	100

Sums are not exact because of rounding.

Reprinted with permission from ref. 13.

$1.0–1.2 billion annually compared with $0.4–0.6 billion for UC. The indirect cost of these diseases, based exclusively on economic loss in the workplace, was estimated to be $0.4–0.8 billion. Based on these data the total (direct plus indirect) economic burden for UC and CD was estimated at $1.8–2.6 billion per year (Table 2).

A recently reported cost-of-illness study evaluated reimbursement charges from patients enrolled in a health benefit claims program serving 50 of the largest US employers [16]. Eligible patients were enrolled in their health plan for a minimum of 3 years and had at least one CD-related claim during 1994–1995. Patients were retrospectively classified into three mutually exclusive health states: *mild disease* – patients who were in remission or those with disease requiring less than 6 months of active treatment over the period of observation; *moderate disease* – patients who required chronic treatment (>6 months) with prednisone or antimetabolites as outpatients, and *severe disease* – those patients who required admission to hospital for treatment. A total of 607 eligible patients generated average charges of $12417 per patient. Charges for the mild, moderate, and severe disease groups were $6277, $10033 and $37135, respectively. Twenty-five percent of the patients generated 80% of the total charges; 57% of the charges occurred as a consequence of caring for inpatients.

Finally, Bernstein and colleagues [17] estimated the direct costs of hospitalization for patients with CD and UC admitted to a tertiary-care hospital in Manitoba, Canada, during 1994 and 1995. Based on a sample of 275 admissions the mean cost of CD was $3149 compared with $3726 for UC. Surgery accounted for 49.8% of all admissions and 60.5% of the total inpatient costs.

What conclusions can be drawn from these three studies?

First, two of the studies show that the direct cost of care for CD, in the setting of a US HMO during the first half of the 1990s, was approximately $6600–8800 per annum (The first estimate is from Hay and Hay [13]; the latter is calculated from Feagan *et al.* [16] following adjustment for: (1) a cost-to-charge ratio of 0.65 and (2) an annual rate of inflation of 3%). Second, the studies demonstrate that provision of inpatient care to a minority of patients – 20–25% – is responsible for the majority of costs. Third the data of Hay and Hay indicate that UC likely has less overall economic impact than CD. Finally, the relatively low cost estimates obtained by the Manitoba study underscore the importance of obtaining jurisdiction-specific cost estimates.

Although all three of these studies provide valuable information they also suffer from an important limitation. Since only highly selected individuals who sought medical treatment were assessed, it is likely that the cost of treatment was overestimated. Ideally, cost data should be obtained from a defined cohort of patients (1) who are residents of a region where health care is readily accessible and (2) where an administrative database exists which has the capacity to reliably measure the total costs of care. Two such studies have been reported; one from Minnesota, the other from Sweden. The former study concentrated on the direct cost of CD whereas the latter provides us with the only published information regarding indirect costs for both disorders.

Poulation-based cost estimates

Olmstead County

Silverstein *et al.* [18] performed a retrospective evaluation of the direct costs of CD based on a cohort of Olmstead County Minnesota residents who were diagnosed between 1970 and 1993. Patients were classified into one of eight unique health states. A Markov model estimated the duration of time spent in each health state over the follow-up period for the entire cohort of patients. The transition probabilities between each of these states were estimated based on 2-month periods. The direct costs of CD were assigned to the specific health states using 1987–1996 charge data from the Olmstead County Utilization and Expediture Database. Charges were converted to cost estimates in 1995 US dollars using the Medical Price Index. The average lifetime cost of CD was estimated at $125 404 per patient. Expressed on an annual basis this translates into a cost of $4308 per patient per year. Surgery accounted for 44% of the total costs, treatment with 5-aminosalicyclic acid (5-ASA) accounted for 29% of all costs.

Sweden

A second population-based study, performed in Sweden, provides unique indirect cost data. Blomquist and Ekbom [19] identified all cases of CD in Sweden during 1994. Because access to health care is universal in Sweden this study is a comprehensive, cross-sectional evaluation of the direct and indirect economic burden of the disease. However, the latter analysis was restricted to economic loss due to disease-related absence from work. The total direct cost of CD, expressed in 1994 US dollars, was estimated to be $27.5 million. Admission to hospital was responsible for 58% of the cost. The estimate of indirect costs was even greater at $58.4 million total. These large indirect costs were attributable to: (1) a small group of patients who were permanently disabled and (2) a significant rate of absenteeism due to illness (the average sick leave was greater than 40 days).

Taken collectively these population-based studies suggest that the average cost estimates derived from HMO data likely overstate the true direct costs of CD. This discordance probably reflects an overrepresentation of more severely ill patients in the claims-based HMO data sets. The Swedish study also underscores the large potential effects of the disease on indirect costs. These costs are important from a societal perspective and should be considered when decisions are made regarding payment for new drugs. However, it should be emphasized that social programs differ greatly among countries. Thus further indirect costs studies from a broad sample of jurisdictions should be performed.

Although these population-based studies may not reflect more recent trends in therapy which include: (1) the use of newer, more expensive forms of medical treatments (aminosalicylates, antibiotics, 6-mercaptopurine, azathioprine, methotrexate, infliximab); (2) increased reliance on outpatient care; and (3) increased surgery rates for patients with CD, a consistent message is identifiable. Treatments which reduce the need for admission to hospital, surgery, or absenteeism may result in important direct and indirect cost saving

Measuring outcomes: quality of life

As described previously, pharmacoeconomic analyses assess the incremented cost required to achieve clinically meaningful improvement in outcomes such as disease activity, hospitalization, surgery, complications, death, or HRQL. In patients with CD, HRQL is perhaps the most relevant outcome because: (1) hospitalization, surgery, disease-related complications, and death occur infrequently; and (2) the burden of symptoms and social and psychological morbidity are lifelong.

HRQL is not simply the absence of disease, but comprises four major components: physical function, emotional and social well-being, ability to work productively, and freedom from disease-related symptoms [20, 21]. Although physical complaints of pain, diarrhoea, and fatigue are important to patients with IBD, other components of HRQL, such as the presence of disease-related emotional stress, are also relevant [22].

Patients with CD and UC have lower HRQL than healthy individuals. The greatest impact on HRQL occurs during disease exacerbations, but patients are also affected while in remission. In a Danish study [23], a majority of patients reported that IBD had a negative influence on their lives. This may be related to concerns about disease recurrence, the need for surgery, and the effect of chronic illness on family or professional relationships.

In an attempt to measure the relative importance of the factors which affect quality of life, HRQL instruments have been developed. The two major forms of HRQL assessments are psychometric questionnaires and utility measures.

Psychometric questionnaires

HRQL questionnaires range widely in complexity – from asking the patient to rate pain on a 10-point scale to completing a computerized instrument containing more than 100 individual questions.

Quality-of-life instruments are either generic or disease-specific. Generic instruments evaluate most aspects of physical, mental, and social health, and are especially useful comparing differences in health status between diseases. Many such instruments exist, including the Sickness Impact Profile [24], the Short Form-36 [25], and the McMaster Health Status Questionnaire [26]. Disease-specific HRQL instruments address only the problems commonly encountered by individuals with a given disease, and generally respond better than generic instruments to small changes in the well-being of patients.

The IBD questionnaire

The IBD questionnaire (IBDQ) [27] is a disease-specific measurement of quality of life which measures four dimensional scores, namely bowel function (e.g. loose stool, abdominal pain), systemic function (e.g. fatigue, altered sleep pattern), social function (e.g. work attendance, need to cancel social events), and emotional function (e.g. anger, depression, irritability). Each item is scored on a seven-point Likert scale where a score of 1 indicates a very severe problem, while a score of 7 denotes no problem at all. Thus, the aggregate score ranges from 32 (very poor HRQL) to 224 (very good HRQL).

The IBDQ has been validated [28, 29] and has excellent reliability and responsiveness.

Utility analysis

Valid and reliable HRQL questionnaires may help the clinician to assess the psychological and social needs of the patient and improve patient management [29]. Unfortunately, these scores are unsuitable for use in a cost-effectiveness analyses, i.e. analysing the marginal cost per unit of IBDQ score gained is not a meaningful metric.

An alternative method of evaluating HRQL is utility analysis [9, 30]. Utility refers to the value placed on a given health state by an individual or society. The concept of utility analysis incorporates the evaluation of preference. For example, given a choice, most individuals would prefer to have mild myopia (high utility) than to be blind (low utility).

Estimating utility

Three generally accepted methods exist for estimating utility: the Standard Gamble, the Time Trade-off, and the Visual Analogue Scale (VAS) [31].

The gold standard for utility estimation is the Standard Gamble. This procedure asks patients to consider their current state of health, and then choose between two alternatives: Choice A – to remain in that health state; or Choice B – to opt for a hypothetical gamble with two possible outcomes. The possible outcomes with Choice B are: (1) a probability (P) of returning to perfect health or; (2) a complementary probability ($1 - P$) of immediate death. In a simplified theoretical situation, if a patient with chronically active CD was offered a 99% chance of returning to perfect health with an associated 1% risk of immediate death, most patients would accept the gamble. Conversely, most people in this situation would not choose to gamble based on the complementary probability of a 99% chance of sudden death against a 1% risk of returning to health. As the probability P is varied the patient should reach a point at which it is difficult to decide whether or not to gamble. At this point of equipoise the utility score is identified. In the Time Trade-off method an individual identifies the number of years of life in his/her current health state that he/she would be willing to trade in exchange for perfect health. The number of years is varied until the patient is ambivalent about the trade. The utility score is calculated by expressing the number of years traded as a proportion of the patient's calculated life expectancy (estimated from an actuarial table). For example, if a 40-year-old malet with chronically active CD is willing to trade 6 of his estimated 38 years of life expectancy, the utility score is $38 - 6/38 = 0.84$.

In the visual analog scale (VAS) method, the subject chooses a point on a 100-mm visual aid that best expresses the current health state where 0 signifies death and 1.0 means perfect health. Utility measures assess patient preference.

Although the use of methods such as the Standard Gamble have been criticized as abstract it can be pointed out that clinical medicine routinely requires doctors and patients to make choices under uncertainty. Usually these choices are associated with quantifiable risks to the patient.

Utility in IBD

Few studies have measured utility scores in patients with IBD. A 1997 publication [32] collected data from 180 patients with CD using the three accepted measures for utility estimation (Standard Gamble, Time Trade-off, and VAS). Patients were stratified into one of four health states (Table 3).

Utility scores were demonstrated to be valid and reliable measures of HRQL. However, utility determination was less responsive to changes in disease severity than the CD Activity Index (CDAI).

This observation indicates that utilities may be less useful than other measurements for detecting small, but clinically important, differences in HRQL. Validity was demonstrated by: (1) the observation that all three measures of utility ordered the hypothetical health states according to an *a-priori* prediction (patients with more severe disease scored poorer than those whose disease was in remission and (2) that the Time Trade-off and Standard Gamble scores correlated with two other widely accepted measures of disease severity: the IBDQ, which assesses HRQL, and the CDAI, which assesses disease activity. Reliability (reproducibility) was also demonstrated since utility scores in stable patients were remarkably similar at the first visit and 8 weeks thereafter.

Table 3. Evaluation of utility measurement in Crohn's disease [32]

Health State	Definition
Chronically active therapy-responsive disease	CDAI score <150 with continuous prednisone therapy ($\geq$10 mg/day) and/or continuous treatment with methotrexate or purine antimetabolites for >6 months
Chronically active therapy-resistant disease	CDAI score $\geq$150 despite continuous prednisone therapy ($\geq$10 mg/day) and/or continuous treatment with methotrexate or purine antimetabolites for >6 months
Acute disease exacerbation	A recent flare of disease (CDAI $\geq$150) and no steroid or immunosuppressive therapy in the 12 weeks preceding the initiation of current course of treatment
Remission	Inactive Crohn's disease defined by presence of CDAI score <150 for a minimum of 6 months in the absence of steroid or immunosuppressive therapy

CDAI = Crohn's Disease Activity Index.

Reprinted with permission from ref. 32.

Table 4. Mean utility scores (95% confidence interval) for the three hypothetical disease-severity states [32]

| Model | Mild disease | | Moderate disease | | Severe disease | |
	Visit 1	Visit 2	Visit 1	Visit 2	Visit 1	Visit 2
Time Trade-off	0.95 (0.94–0.97)	0.96 (0.95–0.97)	0.88 (0.87–0.91)	0.88 (0.86–0.91)	0.73 (0.69–0.76)	0.71 (0.68–0.75)
Standard Gamble	0.81 (0.79–0.83)	0.82 (0.80–0.85)	0.72 (0.69–0.75)	0.73 (0.71–0.77)	0.50 (0.46–0.54)	0.54 (0.50–0.59)
Visual Analogue Scale	0.80 (0.78–0.82)	0.82 (0.80–0.84)	0.57 (0.55–0.59)	0.61 (0.58–0.63)	0.27 (0.23–0.30)	0.31 (0.28–0.33)
Estimated CDAI	134 (122–164)		266 (215–318)		483 (404–562)	
Estimated IBDQ	174 (167–180)		154 (140–169)		117 (107–128)	

Reprinted with permission from ref. 32.

Additional analyses of these data showed that utility estimates are highly dependent upon methodology (Table 4). The VAS yielded the lowest utility estimates. This result was attributed to the well-recognized phenomenon of 'response-spreading', a bias associated with visual scales which systematically lowers scores. Time Trade-off estimates were significantly higher than the Standard Gamble scores since approximately one-third of respondents refused to trade life expectancy. This finding was observed consistently irrespective of the health state of the patient. For these reasons the Standard Gamble was considered a more accurate reflection of utility than the other two measures.

Application of utility measurements

Utility scores can compare the HRQL of patients with chronic diseases. In a study of symptomatic patients with angina a utility score of approximately 0.9 was reported [33]. In contrast patients with chronic renal failure have a utility of 0.4 – meaning very poor quality of life. In the previously described study a Standard Gamble utility score of 0.82 was shown in patients with mild CD. This suggests that the HRQL of patients with CD is substantially worse than those with heart disease. In summary, these utility data demonstrate that CD has a profoundly negative effect on the well-being of patients. How then can this information be used? One application is in cost-utility analysis.

Cost-utility analysis

In a cost-utility analysis, treatment alternative regimens are compared in terms of the incremental cost per QALY [34]. As noted previously, society is generally willing to pay for health-care interventions that cost less than US$50 000 per QALY [11].

Cost-utility analyses are suitable for evaluating new treatments for the following reasons: (1) therapy now focuses on improving patient well-being rather than changing life expectancy; (2) a single measurement can assess both the positive and negative aspects of a treatment; and (3) society must make critical decisions regarding reimbursement for effective yet relatively costly new treatments

Cost-utility models in Crohn's disease

Only two cost-utility analyses have been described in IBD. Trallori and Messori [35] evaluated the incremental cost utility of 5-ASA maintenance therapy in comparison to a strategy of no-maintenance therapy. This model evaluated two hypothetical groups of 100 patients. The natural history of the disease was estimated using data from a large-scale survey of Italian gastroenterologists [36]. The efficacy of 5-ASA maintenance therapy was derived from a meta-analysis performed by one of the authors [37]. Cost estimates were based on the Hay and Hay data [13] using a 5% annual discount rate. Both lifetime and 2-year time horizons were evaluated. Utility estimates were derived from 10 expert gastroenterologists who assigned a utility score to five health states (remission in non-operated patients, remission in operated patients, relapse not requiring hospitalization, relapse requiring hospitalization without surgical intervention, and relapse requiring hospitalization and surgical intervention).

The lifetime cost per QALY of maintenance therapy was estimated to be US$5015. The authors concluded that chronic therapy with 5-ASA was associated with a small incremental benefit and costs. Sensitivity analyses indicated that the result was insensitive to differences in utility estimates but highly sensitive to variances in the cost of illness. If the cost of CD was decreased by 20% the cost per QALY gained was increased to US$26 436. The effect of varying efficacy estimates for 5-ASA was not examined in this study.

This landmark study is the first attempt to examine economic and quality-of-life outcomes for CD. It should be emphasized that the authors were limited by the quality of the available data at the time of publication. Since this time, additional information suggests that the marginal cost-utility estimate obtained in this study likely overstates the value of 5-ASA maintenance therapy. First, the efficacy of maintenance therapy is probably less than the 12% annual absolute risk reduction used in the model. A subsequent meta-analysis by Camma *et al.* [38] could not identify a statistically significant effect of maintenance therapy following a medically induced remission. A modest benefit (9% absolute risk reduction per year) was observed following surgery. The authors also assumed that 5-ASA therapy prevented surgery and hospitalization. No data are available to support these assumptions. Second, as noted previously, the cost estimates of Hay and Hay likely overestimate the economic burden of CD in the population. Since this model is highly sensitive to cost these inputs favor maintenance therapy. Two-way sensitivity analyses, which simultaneously examine the consequences of varying costs and efficacy estimates, might have provided useful information. Finally the utility and natural history estimates used by Trallori and Messori were derived by expert opinion and are almost certainly weighted towards a tertiary-care hospital experience. Again this bias would favor 5-ASA treatment. Notwithstanding these criticisms this study is an important contribution to the literature which illustrates the potential value of cost-utility models.

The second cost-utility model, by Wong and colleagues [39], examined the role of infliximab therapy for the treatment of refractory CD. Data from a randomized controlled trial were used to estimate the efficacy of infliximab. The Olmstead County Markov model served as the basis for natural history and cost estimates. Utility estimates were adapted from the study of Gregor and colleagues [32]. A marginal cost-effectiveness ratio of $14 200–40 000 per QALY gained was estimated for infliximab therapy: and the investigators concluded that infliximab therapy is likely cost-effective depending on the durability of the treatment benefit. Since these data have been published only as an abstract it is difficult to critique the assumptions used in the model. However, a significant limitation of this analysis is the lack of long-term data regarding the efficacy of infliximab therapy.

Conclusion

Over the past decade preliminary data regarding the pharmacoeconomics of inflammatory bowel disease have emerged. The synthesis of this information has culminated in the first models which evaluate the marginal cost-utility of competing therapies. Since the validity of these comparisons is critically dependent upon accurate efficacy, natural history, cost and utility inputs investigators must identify areas where important data are lacking. Through this process, more sophisticated and valid models will be developed.

Highly effective, yet costly, new treatments for IBD will soon be in widespread use. Because societal resources are limited, health-care providers must make intelligent choices regarding the introduction of new technologies. Consideration of data from cost-utility models is likely to become an important part of the decision-making process.

References

1. Andres PG, Friedman LS. Epidemiology and the natural course of inflammatory bowel disease. Gastroenterol Clin N Am 1999; 28: 255–75.
2. Hanauer SB, Meyers S. Management of Crohn's disease in adults. Am J Gastroenterol 1997; 92: 559–66.
3. Binder V. Prognosis and quality of life in patients with ulcerative colitis and Crohn's disease. Int Disabil Stud 1988; 10: 172–4.
4. Torrance GW. Preferences for health outcomes and cost-utility analysis. Am J Manag Care 1997; 3: S8–S20.
5. Spilker B. Quality of life and pharmacoeconomics in clinical trials, 2nd edn. Philadelphia: Lippencott-Raven, 1996.
6. Marra FO, Frighetto LO, Marra CA *et al.* Cost-minimization analysis of piperacillin/tazobactam versus imipenem/cilastatin for the treatment of serious infections: a Canadian hospital perspective. Ann Pharmacother 1999; 33: 156–62.
7. Teutsch SM, Murray JF. Dissecting cost-effectiveness analysis for preventive interventions: a guide for decision makers. Am J Manag Care 1999; 5: 301–5.
8. Jimenez FJ, Guallar-Castillon P, Rubio TC, Guallar E. Cost-benefit analysis of *Haemophilus Iifluenzae* type B vaccination in children in Spain. PharmacoEconomics 1999; 15: 75–83.
9. Gerard K, Smoker I, Seymour J. Raising the quality of cost-utility analyses: lessons learnt and still to learn. Health Policy 1999; 46: 217–38.
10. Weinstein MC, Stason WB. Foundations of cost-effectiveness analysis for health and medical practices. N Engl J Med 1977; 296: 716–21.
11. Laupacis A, Feeny D, Detsky AS, Tugwell PX. How attractive does a new technology have to be to warrant adoption and utilization? Tentative guidelines for using clinical and economic evaluations. Can Med Assoc J 1992; 146: 473–81.
12. Brooten D. Methodological issues linking costs and outcomes. Med Care 1997; 35: 87–95.
13. Hay JW, Hay AR. Inflammatory bowel disease: cost-of-illness. J Clin Gastroenterol 1992; 14: 309–17.
14. Schulman KA, Ohishi A, Park J, Glick HA, Eisenberg JM. Clinical economics in clinical trials: the measurement of cost and outcomes in the assessment of clinical services through clinical trials. Keio J Med 1999; 48: 1–11.
15. Jacobs P, Fassbender K. The measurement of indirect costs in the health economics evaluation literature. A review. Int J Technol Assess Health Care 1998; 14: 799–808.
16. Feagan BG, Vreeland MG, Larson LR, Bala MV. Annual cost of care for Crohn's disease patients. A claims-based cost of illness evaluation. Am J Gastroenterol 2000; 95: 1955–60.
17. Bernstein CN, Papineau N, Zajaczkowski J, Rawsthorne P, Okrusko G, Blanchard JF. Direct hospital costs for patients with inflammatory bowel disease in a Canadian tertiary care university hospital. Am J Gastroenterol 2000; 95: 677–83.
18. Silverstein MD, Loftus EV, Sandborn WJ *et al.* Clinical course and costs of care for Crohn's disease: Markov model analysis of a population-based cohort. Gastroenterology 1999; 117: 49–57.
19. Blomqvist P, Ekbom A. Inflammatory bowel disease: health care and costs in Sweden in 1994. Scand J Gastroenterol 1997; 32: 1134-9.

20. Fitzpatrick R. Quality of life measures in health care. Br Med J 1992; 305: 74–7 (Abstract).
21. Turnbull GK, Vallis TM. Quality of life in inflammatory bowel disease: the interaction of disease activity with psychosocial function. Am J Gastroenterol 1995; 90: 1450–4.
22. Mitchell A, Guyatt G, Singer J *et al.* Quality of life in patients with IBD. J Clin Gastroenterol 1988; 10: 306–10.
23. Munkholm P, Langholz E, Davidsen M, Binder V. Disease activity courses in a regional cohort of Crohn's disease patients. Scand J Gastroenterol 1995; 30: 699–706.
24. Bergner M, Bobbitt RA, Carter WB, Gilson BS. The Sickness Impact Profile: development and final revision of a health status measure. Med Care 1981; 19: 787–805.
25. Ware JE, Jr., Sherbourne CD. The MOS 36-item short-form health survey (SF-36). I. Conceptual framework and item selection. Med Care 1992; 30: 473–83.
26. Chambers LW, MacDonald LA, Tugwell P, Buchanan WW, Kraag G. The McMaster Health Index Questionnaire as a measure of quality of life for patients with rheumatoid disease. J Rheumatol 1982; 9: 780–4.
27. Guyatt G, Mitchell A, Irvine EJ *et al.* A new measure of health status for clinical trials in inflammatorybowel disease. Gastroenterology 1989; 96: 804–10.
28. Irvine EJ, Feagan B, Rochon J *et al.* Quality of life: a valid and reliable measure of therapeutic efficacy in the treatment of inflammatory bowel disease. Gastroenterology 1994; 106: 287–96.
29. Irvine EJ. Quality of life – measurement of inflammatory bowel disease. Scand J Gastroenterol 1993; 199: 36–9.
30. Hellinger FJ. Expected utility theory – a risky choice with health outcomes. Med Care 1989; 27: 273–9.
31. Read JL, Quinn RJ, Berwick DM, Fineberg HV, Weinstein MC. Preferences for health outcomes. Comparison of assessment methods. Med Decis Making 1984; 4: 315–29.
32. Gregor JC, McDonald JWD, Klar N *et al.* An evaluation of the utility measurement in Crohn's disease. Inflam Bowel Dis 1997; 3: 265–76.
33. Nease RF, Kneeland T, O'Connor GT *et al.* Variations in patient utilities for outcomes of the management of chronic stable angina. J Am Med Assoc 1995; 273: 1185–90.
34. Drummond MF, Heyse J, Cook J, McGuire A. Selection of end points in economic evaluations of coronary-heart-disease interventions. Med Decis Making 1993; 13: 184–90.
35. Trallori G, Messori A. Drug Treatments for maintaining remission in Crohn's disease. A lifetime cost-utility analysis. PharmacoEconomics 1997; 11: 444–53.
36. Pera A, Rocca B. Le malattie infiammatorie croniche intestinali: profili di diagnosi e terapia. EDRA srl 1995;
37. Messori A, Brignola C, Trallori G *et al.* Effectiveness of 5-aminosalicylic acid for maintaining remission in patients with Crohn's disease: a meta-analysis. Am J Gastroenterol 1994; 89: 692–8.
38. Camma C, Giunta M, Rosselli M, Cottone M. Mesalamine in the maintenance treatment of Crohn's disease: a meta-analysis adjusted for confounding variables. Gastroenterology 1997; 113: 1465–73.
39. Wong JB, Loftus EV, Sandborn J, Feagan BG. Estimating the cost-effectiveness of infliximab for Crohn's disease. Gastroenterology 1999; 116: G0451 (Abstract).
40. Hay AR, Hay JW. Inflammatory bowel disease: medical cost algorithms. J Clin Gastroenterol 1992; 14: 318–27.

24 Measuring quality of life in inflammatory bowel disease

E. Jan Irvine

Introduction

Most patients with inflammatory bowel disease (IBD) are not significantly at risk of dying from their disease [1]. However, other serious outcomes, such as hospitalization and the need for surgery, are clearly related to disease severity [2] In contrast, daily functioning, health perception, life satisfaction, and ambulatory health-care use correlate best with health-related quality of life (HRQL) status. Thus, clinicians and researchers must assess both disease severity and HRQL, using well-validated instruments. These applications allow increased patient participation in disease management, fuller assessment of the disease impact, and the ability to implement the most cost-effective therapies [3–7]. The HRQL instruments, which appear to play a critical role in IBD assessment, will be discussed in this chapter.

Disease activity measurement

Traditionally, disease severity has been quantified in IBD by assessing symptoms, endoscopic or radiologic bowel appearance, and tissue or serum markers that reflect the degree of inflammation. These features have been assessed with three major objectives: (1) to stratify patients for optimal management; (2) to predict disease outcome; and (3) to measure response to therapy.

Several activity indices are available and their pros and cons are discussed in the previous chapter. In general there are sufficient differences in the clinical manifestations and pathophysiology of Crohn's disease (CD) and ulcerative colitis (UC) to justify the development and application of distinct severity indices. These differences are, however, less important when assessing HRQL. Although there may be good reasons to use a unique instrument to answer a particular research question, there is a strong correlation ($r > 0.5$) between disease severity and the physical domain of HRQL and considerable overlap in the psychosocial HRQL features of CD and UC. Generally, HRQL instruments developed for use in IBD research have been applied in both diseases.

Defining HRQL

HRQL measurement assesses both function and attitude in three broad categories: physical, social, and emotional domains, as they relate to health or chronic illness. HRQL encompasses physical symptoms, mobility, body image, pain and discomfort, ability to engage in recreation or leisure activities, social and family relationships, sexual function, enjoyment of food and drink, satisfaction in and performance of work or school activities, and emotional function [3–6]. In chronic illnesses such as IBD, HRQL scores are partly predicted by disease severity, but are also influenced by psychological and social factors. These include such features as the patient's cognitive function, knowledge concerning the disease, socioeconomic status, educational level, personality, appropriate use of coping strategies, social support network, culture, beliefs, and other less clear determinants [7]. These predictors of HRQL may help explain why no two IBD patients are exactly alike, even in the face of comparable disease severity. For example, one patient might be fully employed with a spouse and children, while another is socially withdrawn, depressed, and receiving long-term disability. HRQL features can also help explain why different patients choose different treatment pathways. For example, one patient with refractory UC might consider temporary cyclosporine therapy, to delay surgery for work or family reasons, while another might opt for immediate surgery. Other potential applications of HRQL mea-

Stephan R. Targan, Fergus Shanahan and Loren C. Karp (eds.), Inflammatory Bowel Disease: From Bench to Bedside, 2nd Edition, 481–494.

surement include assessing an individual patient's needs, monitoring health-care delivery, assessing or predicting disease outcome or efficacy of treatments, and evaluating the cost-utility of different treatment interventions [4, 6].

Measuring HRQL

In most studies which have adequately assessed HRQL, standardized questionnaires are administered to obtain data from different populations, while providing useful information for patient treatment. The three kinds of HRQL instruments that are used include the global assessment, generic instrument, and disease-specific instrument [8, 9]. Advantages and disadvantages of each type of questionnaire are shown in Table 1 and are briefly discussed here, but are well reviewed in the literature [2–4, 6–9].

The global assessment provides a summary of HRQL, often using a graded scale such as good, fair, or poor or a percent score based on a 10-cm visual analog scale (VAS). Such scores permit rapid comparisons with other conditions but cannot identify the determinants of a particular health state. Generic instruments are derived in and for general populations and consist of multi-item problem lists that are meant to be gender-, age-, and disease-independent. Items can be clustered in subscores, using statistical techniques to describe a series of domains, such as 'physical function', 'somatic sensation', or 'mental health', or may also be collapsed into summary scores to compare different populations or diseases.

Generic instruments are the most likely to detect unexpected factors affecting HRQL. Examples of these include the Sickness Impact Profile [10], the Short Form-36 [11], or the EuroQoL [12]. Disease-specific instruments are also multidimensional inventories, that have been derived in and for patients with a single condition [8, 9]. Such instruments are used to detect important treatment effects or change over time. To optimize HRQL assessment, most studies now combine generic and disease-specific instruments. Some of the questionnaires that have been applied in IBD HRQL research are shown in Table 2.

Factors affecting the portrayal of HRQL

Traditionally, HRQL assessment has been assessed from the patient's viewpoint and is supported by data in IBD and other conditions showing that spouses, family members, and physicians impose biases that underestimate the impact of IBD on HRQL [2, 13]. Clinicians and researchers selecting a HRQL instrument must consider the strength of the psychometric properties validity, reliability, and responsiveness of the instrument [8, 9]. *Validity* is a comparison of the new index score against a reference score (convergent validity) or a construct of what the new index is measuring, such as a prediction that patients with less severe disease will have better HRQL scores (construct validity). *Reliability* is a statistical summary trait describing the degree of measurement

Table 1. HRQL assessment in IBD

Advantages	Disadvantages
Global assessment	
Simple summary	Specific domains of dysfunction difficult to discern
Easily administered	May not detect small but important changes
Easily scored	
Generic instrument	
Permits comparisons among groups or populations	Complex administration and scoring
Can detect unanticipated effects	Insensitive to important clinical changes
Disease-specific instrument	
Reflects most important problems to a specific population	Complex administration and scoring
Can detect important clinical changes with time or treatment	May miss unexpected effects
Utility	
Necessary for economic analysis	Insensitive to detect changes over time

Table 2. HRQL instruments used in inflammatory bowel disease

Global assessments
Visual analog scale (10-cm line)
Graded scale (excellent, very good, good, poor, extremely poor)
Utilities (Standard Gamble or Time Trade-off; 0.0 death to 1.0 perfect health)

Generic instruments
1. Sickness Impact Profile (136 items, 12 subscores; higher score = worse HRQL)
2. Short Form-36 (36 items, 8 subscores; score 0, worst–100, best)
3. Grogono and Woodgate (20 items, 10 subscales)
4. Psychological General Well-being (22 items; 6 subscales (anxiety, depression, well-being, self-control, health, vitality); reliability 0.61–0.89; score 22–132, lower score better)
5. Cleveland Clinic Questionnaire (47 items, 4 subscores)
6. Euro-QL (5 items – utility)

Disease-specific instruments
1. Inflammatory Bowel Disease Questionnaire (IBDQ; 32 items, 4 subscores: 32–224)
2. Rating Form of IBD Patient Concerns (RFIPC) (25 items, subscores, 0–100)
3. Cleveland Clinic Questionnaire (18 items, 4 subscores; 0–100)
4. Pentasa Study instrument (7 items 0–100)

error, as in test–retest reliability, or the correlations among individual items or subscores [14]. *Responsiveness* provides an estimate of the signal-to-noise ratio of an instrument and allows the user to understand the degree of change that is considered to be clinically important [15]. Psychometric properties of some disease-specific instruments are illustrated in Table 3. The application of non-validated instruments and unsanctioned modification of well-validated instruments by investigators who have not followed rigorous questionnaire development methods are among the most common problems facing HRQL research. Investigators not familiar with questionnaire development methods must understand the pitfalls of inappropriate and unjustified alteration of questionnaires. Selecting an instrument for a particular study should also be based upon the research question, population to be assessed, study design, type of response options needed, questionnaire length, whether it is interviewer-administered, and how it is scored and interpreted.

Historical descriptive studies

One of the earliest studies assessing HRQL was a British study, employing a global assessment to describe the 'good' outcome for IBD patients. Sixty-nine percent of a cohort of 501 Oxford patients who had survived their UC were described as having 'normal function' (requiring some ambulatory visits)

while 19.3% had 'essentially normal function' (with frequent visits) [16]. In examining the predictors of HRQL in American adolescents with UC, Michener *et al.* observed that better HRQL occurred when the time to diagnosis was short [17]. In a series of adults with CD, postsurgical patients were less likely to describe their HRQL as 'good' compared to those who had been treated only medically (40% versus 53%; $p = 0.01$), suggesting that more severe disease was associated with poorer HRQL [18]. Another series of patients with CD unanimously recalled poor function preoperatively, with 37–84% describing an impact on symptoms, personal relations, school and employment, recreation, sexuality, or body image [19]. At postoperative follow up, 6 29% reported dysfunction and dissatisfaction with their outcome, particularly in the presence of an ileostomy. These studies collectively suggested that more severe disease was associated with poorer HRQL and that most aspects of a person's life were affected by IBD. However, further work was needed to identify more specific problems.

Mallett *et al.* interviewed 84 British UC patients and observed a limited social life in 25% and reduced earning capacity in 21%, even when disease was well controlled [20]. Almost 75% described impaired domestic or sex lives, while approximately 30% claimed to have better family relations as a result of their disease. In a similar study of 85 ambulatory patients with CD, 11% felt their marriage had

Table 3. Disease-specific HRQL instruments

IBDQ (Inflammatory Bowel Disease Questionnaire)
32 items, total score; 4 subscores (bowel, systemic, emotional, social)
Total score 32–224; some users report average score per item (1 to 7)
Higher score connotesbetter HRQL
Face validity: obtained from literature review, patients, caregivers
Discriminative validity: poorer scores with more severe disease
Convergent validity: correlates with CDAI, global assessments, Rand
Test–retest reliability: ICC = 0.90; Cronbach alpha: 0.83
Clinical change over time: within patients: 0.5–1.0 per item (16–32 total score)
Several modifications of IBDQ published based on face validity only

Short IBDQ
10 items, 1–7
Discriminative validity and sensitivity to change over time shown
Reliability, internal consistency, responsiveness similar to IBDQ

RFIPC
25 items, 4 factors (impact of disease, sexual intimacy, complications of disease, body stigma), score 0–100; test–retest reliability
Individual item score 10 cm VAS
Higher score = more worries and concerns
Discriminative validity, more worries and concerns in hospitalized or anxious patients, Crohn's disease after surgery, or stoma
Test–retest reliability: ICC = 0 .87
Responsiveness to change: surgical patients

Cleveland Clinic Questionnaire
18 items, 4 subscales (functional/economic, social/recreational, affect/life in general, medical)
Items score 1–5 – strongly agree to strongly disagree
Reliability: Spearman r = 0.75–0.95
Higher score, poorer HRQL
Responsiveness not demonstrated

suffered due to their disease, 33% reported less frequent sexual intercourse, and 14% had completely stopped all sexual activity [21]. Thirty-three percent had received treatment for depression, and many with impaired well-being had signs of neurosis. Joachim *et al.* in a similar study, reported 42% of 80 IBD patients had decreased overall life satisfaction [22].

In studies from McMaster University, Mitchell *et al.* identified 150 potential problems described by IBD patients and their caregivers [23]. Bowel symptoms such as frequent or loose stools and abdominal pain, feeling unwell or seriously fatigued, were the commonest and most severe symptoms. Emotional difficulties such as frustration and depression also played an important role, while social problems, such as canceling or missing social events, were somewhat less important. Surprisingly, emotional and social problems were elicited only after prompting subjects with a list of problems, suggesting that these problems were overlooked or underrated by patients,

families, or health-care givers. On average, patients had each experienced up to 50 of the problems listed. In a more recent study in children, the impact of IBD on physical and emotional domains was also greater than social impairment ($p < 0.01$), and physical symptoms had a more profound effect than reduced physical activities ($p < 0.01$) [24]. These children also described some positive outcomes, which had an even greater mean impact than the negative factors, such as more support from parents. Drossman *et al.* described a series of worries and concerns in their IBD patients and noted that a fear of cancer, having a stoma, needing surgery, and worries about the future or when the next flare would strike were among their most prominent concerns [25, 26]. Many problems were common to both UC and CD, although the fear of developing cancer was a greater worry in UC, and the uncertain nature of the disease and when the next flare would occur were greater worries in CD. Hospitalized patients had more worries and concerns than ambulatory patients. However, the severity of concerns correlated with their psychological well-being and daily function. Table 4 provides a list of items that have been included in generic or disease-specific HRQL instruments. More recent studies have begun to examine homogeneous patient subgroups, by diagnosis or disease pattern as well as control groups, to focus on problems of IBD patients compared to normal populations or groups with other conditions. The ability to quantify the impact of these problems is necessary if researchers hope to address patients' concerns or intervene with counseling or education for maladaptive coping behaviors.

Comparative studies in IBD

Several comparative studies have assessed HRQL using generic instruments. The Sickness Impact Profile (SIP), a well-known generic instrument, measures sickness-related dysfunction using 136 questions and 12 subscores [10]. The scores can then be aggregated into physical and psychosocial dimensional scores, and an overall score with independent categories of work, eating, sleep and rest, home management, and recreation and pastimes. Drossman *et al.* and Farmer *et al.* suggested that IBD patients functioned relatively well compared to those

Table 4. Problems and issues in HRQL instruments

Bowel	*Well-being*
Frequent stool passage	Energy
Loose stools	Fatigue
Excess gas	Sleep
Excess bloating	Self-control
Rectal bleeding	
Urgency	*Leisure and recreation*
Tenesmus	Travel
Mucus	Food/drink
Incontinence	Visit friend's homes
Borborygmi	Vacation
	Nearness to toilet facilities
Relationships	Hobbies and sports
Intimacy and sexual function	
Body image	*Emotional*
Understanding from others	Anger
Coping and support	Embarrassment
Relations with children and extended family	Anxiety
Friendships	Irritability
	Happiness
Treatment	Worries or fears
Efficacy	Ability to relax
Adverse effects	Frustration
	Depression/sadness
Pain and discomfort	Satisfaction
Abdominal pain	
Abdominal cramps	*Job – education*
Abdominal discomfort	Attendance
Joint pain	Concentration
Back pain	Task completion
Headaches	Achievement/promotion
	Financial reward
Mobility and self-care	Satisfaction
Walking	
Running	
Climbing	
Grooming	
Eating	
Physical endurance	

with other conditions such as chronic back pain or rheumatoid arthritis, but fared worse than adults enrolled in a group health plan [25, 27]. They described psychosocial function to be more impaired than physical function, perhaps reflecting the emphasis on mobility and activities of daily living of the SIP physical domain (rather than on loose stools, abdominal pain, or urgency) or the frustration of having a disease that is difficult to discuss with others. They further observed that patients with UC had better HRQL than those with CD, but the patients who required surgery were worse than those who had only received medical therapy. Later studies suggested this had been due to both a greater disease severity and psychological dysfunction in the CD group [26]. Using Grogono and Woodgate's health status [28] (Score range 0, poor, to 1.0, excellent) which assesses work, hobby and recreation, physical health, mental health, communication, sleep, dependency on others, feeding, excretion, and sexual function, 120 Dutch patients with CD described their mean health index at 0.70 ± 0.3 (versus 0.90 ± 0.1 in healthy controls, $p < 0.00001$). They could then be ranked between patients with a benign fistula-in-ano (score 0.75) and others with stomach cancer (score 0.65) [29]. However, only 6% were completely satisfied with their health compared to 51% of healthy controls. Hobbies and recreation were not significantly affected, but even when disease was in remission, 73% had major complaints. Interestingly, the perceived benefits of surgery were greatest prior to the first operation and declined for many afterwards, while those for medical therapy increased [29]. This example demonstrates the role of perception in quality-of-life assessment.

In contrast to the previously described results no significant differences were noted in two early Danish studies between patients with UC [30] or CD [31] and hospitalized controls, in marital status, sexual activity, family problems, previous psychiatric problems, social activity, or employment status. However, 54% with CD perceived a strain on their professional or family life during exacerbations, 23% had experienced a reduced work capacity in the previous year, and 21% felt that their leisure activities had been adversely affected. A more recent study by Guassora et al., involving only Crohn's patients, suggested they had poorer HRQL than age- and sex-matched buddy controls, but that patients in remission had better quality of life than those in relapse [32]. Two studies examining the full Danish cohorts of UC and CD observed that almost 90% of patients, were fully or partially able to work with limited absenteeism by 5 years after diagnosis [33, 34]. Sonnenberg estimated that 10% of German IBD patients annually underwent work rehabilitation, and that 3% obtained a disability pension because of IBD [35]. Female gender, and those with white-collar occupations, were particularly at risk. A survey in Wales of educational and work experience in 58 CD patients and community controls showed that significantly more patients than controls had missed school due to hospitalization (42% vs 4%, $p < 0.001$) [36]. In addition, patients felt that CD had restricted their education (14%) or career prospects (24%), yet rates of postsecondary education and employment were similar between groups. Despite this, 30% actively concealed the disease from employers, fearing recrimination. These results suggested the importance of assessing control subjects for comparison to eliminate perception bias.

Eckardt et al. compared HRQL, health-care use, and work disability in 106 outpatients with CD and in 83 spouses [37]. No significant difference was found between the respective groups when asked (yes or no) if their illness had affected their partnership (20% vs 8%), compromised their professional career (17% vs 11%), or affected their overall quality of life (28% vs 10%). However, when response options were changed to a visual analog scale (range 1 (worst) to 9 (best)), patients reported a significantly greater impact of illness than their spouses in these areas. In a follow-up study examining a British cohort of children hospitalized for IBD, perhaps the sickest of children, only three patients (8.5%) were unemployed due to their disease and all had CD [38]. These studies suggested that IBD affects many aspects of patients' lives and that the disease, its severity, and methods of measuring HRQL can all affect HRQL outcomes.

Medical vs surgical therapy

Most studies suggest that, irrespective of the type of surgery, there is substantial improvement in HRQL after surgery, although subtle differences become detectable only when large numbers of patients are studied and specific domains of function are carefully assessed. Few surgical series have fully assessed subjective HRQL and even fewer have avoided major methodologic flaws. Sagar et al. compared medically treated patients with UC to those who had undergone colectomy and pelvic pouch construction [39].

Significantly more medically treated patients described urgency, the need for topical steroids or antidiarrheals, and restricted social activities than did patients with a pelvic pouch. The latter, however, also had significantly more daytime and nocturnal stools. In an Italian study Martin *et al.* observed, that J-pouch patients, approximately 4 years after surgery, had mean HRQL scores similar to patients with mild disease, significantly better than those with moderate or severe disease, but worse than control non-IBD subjects [40]. Cohen *et al.* in Chicago [41], compared two groups 3 years after treatment, who had received either intravenous cyclosporine ($n = 18$) or colectomy ($n = 46$) for severe UC. Ten patients who were initially treated with cyclosporine later underwent surgery, accounting for the larger surgical treatment group. Using the IBDQ, a disease-specific questionnaire, there was no significant difference between groups in overall quality of life, bowel symptoms, fatigue, ability to sleep, social function, or emotional function, possibly reflecting an inadequate sample size. Nevertheless, using a visual analog scale (10 cm line), the cyclosporine patients reported significantly ($p < 0.01$) better stool consistency, ability to sleep through the night, somewhat less abdominal or rectal pain, and fewer trips to the toilet. They did, however, need more medications than their surgical counterparts. While the authors seemed to imply that HRQL was better after cyclosporine than after surgery, disease severity and willingness to try cyclosporine were important selection biases in the study.

Postsurgical HRQL

Additional data regarding the impact of surgery have come from cross-sectional and observational series of surgical patients. In a series from the Mayo Clinic with UC or familial polyposis, who had undergone colectomy, functional and performance activities were assessed in 406 Brooke ileostomates, 313 patients with a Kock pouch, and 298 patients with an ileal J-pouch–anal anastomosis (IPAA) [42]. Most patients (97% Brooke, 96% Kock, and 95% IPAA) reported satisfaction with their diet, and nearly two-thirds of each group noted an improved attitude following surgery. Very few (5%, 4%, and 4%, respectively) felt their attitude had deteriorated. Social activities, recreation, housework, and family relationships were similar among groups. However, patients with IPAA performed better in sports and

sexual activities than those with a Kock pouch ($p < 0.05$) while the latter had better sports and sexual performance than those with a Brooke ileostomy, but more restrictions in travel ($p = 0.05$). In a small study, patients with familial polyposis were somewhat less satisfied than patients with UC after colectomy and IPAA, suggesting that prior experience of health (poor for IBD and good for polyposis) also had an impact on satisfaction [43].

Other studies comparing different pouch procedures in patients with UC have suggested that women may experience greater sexual dysfunction than men after surgery, due to dyspareunia and vaginal discharge, and that this may also be more prevalent following a stapled than with a hand-sewn anastomosis [44–46]. In general, however, the majority of patients describe improved sexual function after surgery.

Several HRQL instruments have demonstrated the ability to discriminate among patient groups, based on disease severity. Using the Short Form-36 (SF-36) [11] from the Medical Outcomes Survey, which assesses eight subscales (physical function, role-physical, bodily pain, general health, vitality, social functioning, role-emotional and mental health), Colombel *et al.* observed significantly lower scores in UC or CD for all eight subscales compared to age- and sex-matched controls [47]. In addition, patients with active disease had significantly worse scores than did those with disease in remission. Richards and Irving, who also used the SF-36, observed that 35 patients with CD who were on home parenteral nutrition (HPN) scored significantly worse than population norms in six of the eight subscales, except in role-emotional and mental health scores [48]. Older patients scored worse than younger patients and, when compared to other disease populations, Crohn's patients scored between those with type II diabetes (better than CD) and congestive heart failure (worse than CD). Using the EuroQL, a utility instrument, which assesses HRQL on a continuum between 0 (death) and 100 (best possible health) in domains of mobility, self-care, activity, pain, and mental well-being, 51 HPN subjects scored a mean of 53.3 compared to 84.0 in the normal population ($p = 0.05$) [48]. Other studies confirmed that HPN improved HRQL over pre-HPN status and that patients with CD did relatively well compared to subjects with other causes of short bowel [49–51].

A retrospective series from Israel comparing patients who had undergone surgery for impaired

HRQL with a different group who had surgery for a disease complication, demonstrated a better outcome in the HRQL group [52]. While this could merely represent a lead-time bias due to less severe illness, it is worth further investigation. Two small studies [53, 54] in patients who had undergone colectomy for severe UC observed that generic HRQL scores (SIP, Time Trade-off utility, SF-36) were similar to those of a normal population and that a significant improvement occurred between preoperative and postoperative scores (mean SIP improved from 11.9 to 4.3; TTO increased from 0.58 to 0.98, both $p < 0.05$). However, none of these instruments could detect differences according to the type of surgery [54]. Only one small study, using a non-validated questionnaire in 71 patients who had surgery for UC, has suggested an advantage in body image for IPAA that was discounted by a disadvantage in bowel emptying [55]. In an 8-year follow-up of 68 Finnish subjects after IPAA, a modified Short Form-36 [56], demonstrated that problems postoperatively differed slightly from those experienced preoperatively. Sixty-five percent were fully continent, 28% had disturbed sleep, 25% could not discriminate gas from stool, and 71% had anal itching, although this was chronic in only 15%. Most J-pouch patients had similar HRQL scores to the normal Finnish population, although in a small group there was a strong relationship between poor bowel function (if > 10/day), chronic pouchitis, anal incontinence, and poor HRQL. Table 5 demonstrates the relative rankings of HRQL among different diseases and strata of inflammatory bowel disease.

Disease-specific HRQL

Three disease-specific HRQL instruments have been developed for IBD applications. They are shown in Table 3 together with some of their psychometric properties. The Inflammatory Bowel Disease Questionnaire (IBDQ) was developed as an outcome to assess treatment efficacy in clinical trials [57]. The Rating Form of IBD Patient Concerns was derived to discriminate IBD patients from those with other intestinal disorders and to predict health outcome [25], and the Cleveland Clinic Questionnaire was also derived to discriminate among different disease groups [27]. Other questionnaires, often described as *new*, have combined older generic instruments, changed scaling, or slightly modified some questionnaires. As previously emphasized, such application is inappropriate without rigorous revalidation.

Table 5. Relative HRQL of IBD patients groups

Healthy volunteers
Normal population
Health maintenance organization attendees

Cured ulcerative colitis
    Pelvic pouch
    Koch pouch
    Brook ileostomy

Remission ulcerative colitis
Remission Crohn's disease
Angina
Ambulatory but active ulcerative colitis
Crohn's disease
    Ambulatory – medical treatment only
    Prior surgery
    Active disease with mood disorder
    Steroid-dependent
    Narcotic-dependent
    Depressed
    Home parenteral nutrition
        Younger
        Older patients
Ulcerative colitis – hospitalized (severe)
Crohn's disease – hospitalized

Rheumatoid arthritis
Stomach cancer

The IBDQ was able to clearly discriminate statistically between healthy hospital workers and ambulatory UC or CD patients (possible range: 1, worst to 7, best; healthy mean 6.66 versus IBD mean 5.47; $p < 0.01$) [58]. The latter result was similar to that of a Crohn's and Colitis Foundation membership postal survey (mean modified IBDQ score 5.14) [59] and a subgroup of Danish patients with CD who had poorer HRQL than age- and sex-matched buddy controls [32]. In each of these studies significantly worse HRQL scores occurred in IBD patients in all domains (bowel, systemic, social, emotional) ($p < 0.01$) compared to healthy controls and in active versus quiescent disease [58–61]. Similar IBDQ scores were observed for medical and surgical remission [61]. When the IBDQ was assessed in patients with non-intestinal chronic diseases, only social function was impaired compared to healthy controls (7.0 versus 6.40), supporting its disease specificity [58]. Mean IBDQ scores were similar in ambulatory patients with IBD or irritable bowel syndrome, highlighting the overlap in problems of both groups, including psychosocial problems. In a large study (2000 patients) IBDQ scores were significantly worse

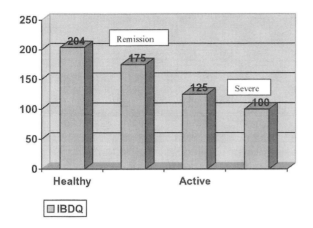

Figure 1. Mean IBDQ scores in patient groups with IBD by disease severity.

in CD than in UC, and could be explained by differences in disease severity [62]. In a later Canadian study, using the short IBDQ, significant impairment in mean HRQL was strongly predicted by depression, active disease, and low socioeconomic status [63]. Fig. 1 shows typical mean IBDQ scores in patients by disease severity.

The RFIPC [25], which was developed to discriminate IBD from other intestinal diseases and to predict outcomes, showed no difference between active and inactive CD or UC in French ambulatory patients [47]. Correlations of the SIP and the RFIPC subscores were moderate ($r = 0.4$), suggesting that they provided complementary information. A Swedish study had similar findings, and after performing a cluster analysis, a ceiling effect was noted for the SIP as well as inconsistent psychosocial function in groups with more severe disease [64]. Moser *et al.* also observed a low correlation between concerns and disease severity in ambulatory patients [65]. They also found that increased worries and concerns occurred in patients who perceived a lack of disease information. However, a recent trial of intense short-term education, while improving psychological status, did not change disease clinical course [66].

Maunder *et al.* assessed RFIPC scores in patients who were referred or had sought counseling versus those who did not seek psychiatric counseling [67]. A higher rate of interpersonal and emotional concerns was seen in the patients who had sought counseling. Postoperative RFIPC scores in 22 patients who had undergone colectomy and IPAA for UC were significantly better (median 16.6) than Crohn's and Colitis Foundation of America surveyed patients

(median 38.3), $p < 0.01$ [68]. In a similar small study in Vienna, 16 patients with CD showed significant improvement compared to preoperative scores for up to 24 months postoperatively, provided they did not experience a relapse [69].

All of these studies, using generic and disease-specific questionnaires, support the theory that poorer HRQL occurs in patients with more severe disease and that medical and surgical treatments seem to improve HRQL. Further, there are some subgroups of patients in whom there are discrepancies between perception and performance. Those who perceive lack of information, who are depressed or require counseling also experience impaired HRQL. Tailored interventions for those in need might well improve their health status.

Clinical trials

Several clinical trials, using generic instruments, have shown significant improvement in HRQL following effective treatments. Two trials of mesalamine (Pentasa) showed significant improvement for both UC and CD in a dose-responsive manner of seven domains measured by a 10-cm VAS (work activities, hobbies and social activities, outdoor activities, indoor activities, sexual function, sleep, energy) [70, 71]. Most benefit was demonstrated from 4 g/day. Gasche *et al.* noted significantly improved HRQL (mood, well-being, physical and social activities) in patients treated with erythropoietin plus intravenous iron for severe anemia associated with CD compared to those who received iron alone [72]. Recently, Thomsen *et al.* [73] reported significantly improved Psychological General Well Being scores [74] in patients with active ileal or ileocecal CD who were treated with budesonide 9 mg/day compared with mesalamine 3 g/day.

A number of trials have shown markedly improved mean IBDQ scores in CD, after effective therapy with prednisone (40 mg/day tapering protocol) [75], controlled ileal release budesonide (9 mg/day) in active ileocolitis [76], after methotrexate (25 mg, intramuscularly once weekly) in steroid-dependent patients [77], and with single or multiple infusions of infliximab in steroid-refractory patients [78, 79]. In these studies it appeared that going from active disease to remission resulted in a score improvement (increase) of between 16 and 32 points, or between 0.5 and 1.0 point per question. In the Canadian cyclosporine trial, which demonstrated no significant benefit from active treatment, patients who required surgery for active CD had significantly poorer social subscores than those who improved with medical therapy, suggesting that it might be useful in predicting patients who require surgery [57, 80].

The IBDQ, which was originally interviewer-assessed, was later revalidated as a self-administered questionnaire [81]. After one administration, even patients who had not previously completed the IBDQ could do so with good reliability ($r > 0.90$). A short version, the SIBDQ, consisting of 10 of the original 32 questions, explained over 90% of the variance of the IBDQ in both UC and CD [82]. The SIBDQ was able to discriminate between groups with inactive versus active disease ($p = 0.0006$) and an average score deterioration of 0.93 ± 0.55 ($p = 0.001$) occurred in patients at the time of relapse. Han *et al.* [83] in testing for differences between UC and CD, further validated the SIBDQ in over 300 British UC patients. They confirmed the excellent reliability (>0.95) of the SIBDQ and convergent validity of the instrument and saw no advantage in adopting separate instruments for UC and CD. This questionnaire, which can be completed in 3 minutes, may therefore be useful in clinical trials or in clinical practice to identify patients who are coping poorly and who would benefit from adjuvant counseling or more aggressive therapy.

Psychological disturbance in IBD

North *et al.* undertook two overviews examining psychological relationships and noted that early studies which reported psychological abnormalities were methodologically more flawed than those with negative findings [84, 85]. Studies in UC failed to find a direct association, while in CD there was an increased incidence of psychopathology, although less than that observed in irritable bowel syndrome. The most prevalent findings were those of anxiety and depression, and the degree of disturbance appeared to correlate with disease severity. Turnbull and Vallis noted that both psychological function and disease severity were needed to predict HRQL scores [86]. In 150 outpatients Kinash *et al.* found that younger patients ($\leqslant 35$ years), females, those with a depressive mood or affective coping style (prayer, substance abuse) had the worst HRQL. Patients who used problem-solving techniques to reduce stress tended to do better [87]. Drossman *et al.* also noted that higher rates of concern about

Table 6. Factors associated with poor HRQL in IBD	
Disease	
Severe	
Extensive	
Treatment	
Medical	More medication
Surgical	Differing problems such as incontinence
Surgery	
Koch pouch	For selected patients
Brook ileostomy	For older/elderly patients
Ileorectal anastomosis	
For selected patients	
Complicated (abscess or leak)	
Handsewn anastomosis	
Elderly	
Female	

surgery, being treated as different and feeling out of control, occurred in patients who used unconventional therapies [2, 25]. It is possible that these subjects perceived stress more than others and that this might play a role in depression and illness behavior. Levenstein *et al.* described seven of 29 patients who had no symptoms but did have endoscopic evidence of rectal inflammation, their perceived stress levels were higher than in patients who had no rectal inflammation [88]. A later study by the same group suggested that patients with quiescent UC, who scored in the upper tertile of the Perceived Stress Questionnaire, had a significantly higher risk of exacerbation over long-term follow-up than those with lower scores [89]. This may have been related to poorer sleep pattern, shorter remission, persistent histological inflammation, or the use of drugs that might trigger exacerbation. However, no studies have adequately shown a temporal relationship between depression or anxiety and disease occurrence. Katon summarized the impact of major depression on chronic medical illness as leading to increased visits and medical costs, increased functional impairment and decreased HRQL, increased somatization, difficulty adhering to self-care regimens (medication compliance, diet or quitting smoking), and increased mortality [90].

Other factors affecting HRQL

Demographic and lifestyle factors also appear to have an effect on HRQL. A list of factors predicting poor HRQL is shown in Table 6. These include gender, age, and smoking status. Several studies have observed poorer HRQL in women than in men [2, 8, 22]. In a Dutch study smoking was associated with poorer HRQL in females with CD, particularly young females, while males with UC who smoked moderately fared better than non-smoking UC patients [91]. However, no adjustment was made for disease severity, which explains approximately 40% of the IBDQ variance [62]. In patients taking HPN for CD, older patients seemed to do more poorly, likely due to the presence of comorbid disease [48]. Two surveys using the RFIPC and SF-36, respectively, observed that African-American patients had a significantly poorer quality of life ($p < 0.002$) [92] and greater disease burden than non-African-Americans, with more frequent and longer hospitalizations, more work loss, and a greater likelihood of having a stoma than non-African-Americans, despite a similar clinical course [93]. However, an adjusted analysis suggested that differences were due to social and economic factors rather than disease features [94]. Thus, age, gender, socioeconomic status, and lifestyle practices may impact on HRQL. Clearly further work is needed to elicit the specific reasons for these differences.

Does HRQL really matter?

HRQL is what matters most to patients with IBD. While the majority of patients have reasonable functional status and HRQL, some with particularly aggressive disease, depression or anxiety, a poor understanding of the disease, or maladaptive coping strategies tend to do less well. Appropriate tools can be used to identify these patients, to optimize management.

Most clinicians do elicit data regarding symptoms; social and emotional issues; support network; family interactions; and ability to carry on with education, domestic, or job activities. Responses are then used to develop clear objectives, tailored to the individual, with patient involvement in decision-making (perhaps selecting a less efficacious drug with fewer adverse effects). Already, many patients self-medicate and appreciate the ability to do so. This is in keeping with an observed improvement in HRQL of UC patients who used a patient-developed guidebook for self-management [95].

The use of alternative medicines in IBD often occurs due to frustration with lack of efficacy of conventional treatments. As a new generation of immunologicals is being tested, we must still be prepared to advise and address individual worries and concerns. This includes providing letters of documentation for patients when disability arises or the need for retraining occurs. Membership in local societies should be encouraged for some patients, particularly early in the disease course.

Future directions in HRQL assessment could consider the use of modular questionnaires and will need to further address crosscultural translation and validation. This is already occurring with instruments such as SIP, SF-36, PGWB, RFIPC, and IBDQ but further refinement of instruments will still be needed for broader applications. More efficient data collection and analysis techniques are also needed, a problem which might be addressed by the use of computerized questionnaires [96]. Finally, cost-effectiveness and cost-utility assessments are beginning to appear in the literature. However, some of these are premature, while others are assessing outdated or ineffective treatments. These will likely be the most important applications when a wider array of effective treatment options is available.

References

1. Travis SPL. Review article: insurance risks for patients with ulcerative colitis or Crohn's disease. Aliment Pharmacol Ther 1997; 11: 51–9.
2. Drossman DA, Patrick DL, Mitchell CM et al. Health-related quality of life in inflammatory bowel disease: functional status and patient worries and concerns. Dig Dis Sci 1989; 34: 1379–86.
3. Irvine EJ. Activity scores and quality of life indices in inflammatory bowel disease. Curr Opin Gastroenterol 1995; 11: 331–6.
4. Irvine EJ. Quality of life – rationale and methods for developing a disease-specific instrument for inflammatory bowel disease. Scand J Gastroenterol 1993; 28(Suppl. 199): 22–7.
5. Maunder RG, Cohen Z, McLeod RS et al. Effect of intervention in inflammatory bowel disease on health-related quality of life: a critical review. Dis Colon Rectum 1995; 38: 1147–61.
6. Fitzpatrick R, Fletcher A, Gore S et al. Quality of life measures in health care. I: Applications and issues in assessment. Br Med J 1992; 305: 1074–7.
7. Garrett JW, Drossman DA. Health status in inflammatory bowel disease: biological and behavioral considerations. Gastroenterology 1990; 99: 90-6.
8. Guyatt GH, Feeny DH, Patrick DL. Measuring health related quality of life in chronic disease. Ann Intern Med 1993; 118: 622–9.
9. Patrick DL, Deyo RA. Generic and disease-specific measures in assessing health status and quality of life. Med Care 1989; 27(Suppl.): S217–32.
10. Bergner M, Bobbitt RA, Carter WB et al. The Sickness Impact Profile: development and final revision of a health status measure. Med Care 1981; 19: 787–805.

11. Ware JE, Sherbourne CD. The MOS 36 item Short Form Health Survey (SF-36). Conceptual framework and item selection. Med Care 1992: 30: 473–83.

12. The EuroQol Group. EuroQol – a new facility for the measurement of health-related quality of life. Health Policy 1990; 16: 199–208.

13. Guyatt GH, Mitchell A, Irvine EJ et al. A new measure of health status for clinical trials in IBD. Gastroenterology 1989; 96: 804–10.

14. Deyo RA, Diehr P, Patrick DL. Reproducability and responsiveness of health status measures: statistics and strategies for evaluation. Control Clin Trials 1991; 12: 142–58S.

15. Guyatt GH, Walter S, Norman G. Measuring change over time: assessing the usefulness of evaluative instruments. J Chron Dis 1987; 40: 171–8.

16. Edwards FC, Truelove SC. The course and prognosis of ulcerative colitis. Gut 1963; 4: 299–315.

17. Michener WM, Farmer RG, Mortimer EA. Long-term prognosis of ulcerative colitis with onset in childhood or adolescence. J Clin Gastroenterol 1979; 1: 301–5.

18. Farmer RG, Whelan G, Fazio VW. Long-term follow-up of patients with Crohn's disease. Gastroenterology 1985; 88: 1818–25.

19. Meyers S, Walfish JS, Sachar DB, Greenstein AJ, Hill AG, Janowitz HD. Quality of life after surgery for Crohn's disease: a psychological survey. Gastroenterology 1980; 78: 1–6.

20. Mallett SJ, Lennard-Jones JE, Bingley J, Gilon E. Colitis. Lancet 1978; 2: 619–21.

21. Gazzard BG, Price HL, Libby GW, Dawson AM. The social toll of Crohn's disease. Br Med J 1978; 2: 117–19.

22. Joachim G, Milne B. The effects of inflammatory bowel disease on lifestyle. Can Nurse 1985; 81: 39–40.

23. Mitchell A, Guyatt G, Singer J et al. Quality of life in patients with IBD. J Clin Gastroenterol 1988; 10: 306–10.

24. Forget S, Issenman RM, Gold N, Irvine EJ. Assessment of functional status in children and adolescents with inflammatory bowel disease. Gastroenterology 1997; 112: A974.

25. Drossman DA, Leserman J, Li Z et al. The rating form of IBD patient concerns: a new measure of health status. Psychosom Med 1991; 53: 701–12.

26. Drossman DA, Leserman J, Mitchell CM et al. Health status and health care use in persons with inflammatory bowel disease: a national sample. Dig Dis Sci 1991; 36: 1746–55.

27. Farmer RG, Easley KA, Farmer JM. Quality of life assessment of patients with inflammatory bowel disease. Cleve Clin J Med 1992; 59: 35–42.

28. Grogono AW, Woodgate DJ. Index for measuring health. Lancet 1971; 1: 1024–6.

29. Shivananda S, van Blankenstein M, Schouten WR, Themans B, vsDoes E. Quality of life in Crohn's disease: results of a case–control study. Eur J Gastroenterol Hepatol 1993; 5: 919–25.

30. Hendriksen C, Kreiner S, Binder V. Long term prognosis in ulcerative colitis – based on results from a regional patient group from the county of Copenhagen. Gut 1985; 26: 158–63.

31. Sorensen VZ, Olsen BG, Binder V. Life prospects and quality of life in patients with Crohn's disease. Gut 1987; 28: 382–5.

32. Guassora AD, Kruuse C, Thomsen OO, Binder V. Quality of life study in a regional group of patients with Crohn's disease. Scand J Gastroenterol 2000; 35: 1068–74.

33. Munkholm P, Langholz E, Davidsen M et al. Disease activity courses in a regional cohort of Crohn's disease patients. Scand J Gastroenterol 1995; 30: 699–706.

34. Langholz E, Munkholm P, Davidsen M, Binder V. Course of ulcerative colitis. Analysis of changes in disease activity over years. Gastroenterology 1994; 107: 3–11.

35. Sonnenberg A. Disability and need for rehabilitation among patients with inflammatory bowel disease. Digestion 1992; 51: 168–78.

36. Mayberry MK, Probert C, Srivastava E, Rhodes J, Mayberry AJF. Perceived discrimination in education and employment by people with Crohn's disease: a case control study of educational achievement and employment. Gut 1992; 33: 312–14.

37. Eckardt VF, Lesshafft C, Kanzler G et al. Disability and health care use in patients with Crohn's disease: A spouse control study. Am J Gastroenterol 1994; 89: 2157–62.

38. Ferguson A, Sedgwick DM, Drummond J. Morbidity of juvenile onset inflammatory bowel disease: effects on education and employment in early adult life. Gut 1994; 35: 665-8.

39. Sagar PM, Lewis W, Holdsworth PJ et al. Quality of life after restorative proctocolectomy with a pelvic ileal reservoir compares favorably with that of patients with medically treated colitis. Dis Colon Rectum 1993; 36: 584-92.

40. Martin A, Dinca M, Leone L et al. Quality of life after proctocolectomy and ileo-anal anastomosis for severe ulcerative colitis. Am J Gastroenterol. 1998 Feb; 93: 166–9.

41. Cohen RD, Brodsky AL, Hanauer SB. A comparison of the quality of life in patients with severe ulcerative colitis after total colectomy versus medical treatment with intravenous cyclosporin. Inflam Bowel Dis 1999; 5: 1–10.

42. Köhler LW, Pemberton JH, Zinsmeister AR et al. Quality of life after proctocolectomy. A comparison of Brooke ileostomy, Kock pouch, and ileal pouch–anal anastomosis. Gastroenterology 1991; 101: 679–84.

43. Tjandra JJ, Fazio VW, Church JM, Oakley JR, Milsom JW, Lavery IC. Similar functional results after restorative proctocolectomy in patients with familial adenomatous polyposis and ulcerative colitis. Am J Surg 1993; 165: 322–5.

44. Scaglia M, Bronsino E, Canino V et al. Impatto della proctocolectomia convenzionale sulla funzione sessuale (Influence of conventional proctocolectomy on sexual function). Minerva Chir 1993; 48: 903–10.

45. Moody G, Probert CS, Srivastava EM, Rhodes J, Mayberry JF. Sexual dysfunction amongst women with Crohn's disease: a hidden problem. Digestion 1992; 52: 179–83.

46. Moody GA, Mayberry JF. Perceived sexual dysfunction amongst patients with inflammatory bowel disease. Digestion 1993; 54: 256–60.

47. Colombel JF, Yazdanpanah Y, Laurent F, Houcke P, Delas N, Marquis P. Qualite de vie dans les maladies inflammatoires chroniques de l'intestin. Gastroenterol Clin Biol 1996; 20: 10771–77.

48. Richards DM, Irving, MH. Assessing the quality of life of patients with intestinal failure on home parenteral nutrition. Gut 1997; 40: 218–22.

49. Mughal M, Irving M. Home parenteral nutrition in the United Kingdom and Ireland. Lancet 1986; 2: 383–7.

50. Galandiuk S, O'Neill M, McDonald P, Fazio VW, Steiger E. A century of home parenteral nutrition for Crohn's disease. Am J Surg 1990; 159: 540–4; discussion 544–5.

51. Detsky AS, McLaughlin JR, Abrams HB et al. Quality of life of patients on long-term total parenteral nutrition at home. J Gen Intern Med 1986; 1: 26–33.

52. Nissan A, Zamir O, Spira R, Seror D, Alweiss T et al. A more liberal approach to the surgical treatment of Crohn's disease. Am J Surg 1997; 174: 339–41.

53. McLeod RS, Churchill DN, Lock AN, Vanderburgh S, Cohen Z. Quality of life with ulcerative colitis preoperatively and postoperatively. Gastroenterology 1991; 101: 1307–13.

54. Provenzale D, Phillips-Bute B, Shearin M *et al.* Clinical predictors of post-colectomy health status in patients with a history of ulcerative colitis. Gastroenterology 1995; 108: A30 (Abstract).

55. O'Bichere A, Wilkinson K, Rumbles S *et al.* Functional outcome after restorative Panproctocolectomy for ulcerative colitis decreases an otherwise enhances quality of life. Br J Surg 2000; 87: 8802–7.

56. Tiainen J, Matikainen M. Functional outcome of conversion of ileorectal anastomosis to ileal pouch anal anastomosis in patients with familial adenomatous polyposis and ulcerative colitis. Scand J Gastroenterol 1999; 34: 601–5.

57. Irvine EJ, Feagan B, Rochon J *et al.* Quality of life: a valid and reliable measure of outcome for clinical trials in inflammatory bowel disease. Gastroenterology 1994; 106: 287–96.

58. Irvine EJ, Donnelly M. Quality of life is comparably impaired in patients with ulcerative colitis and irritable bowel syndrome. Gastroenterology 1994; 106: A517.

59. Love JR, Irvine EJ, Fedorak RN. Quality of life in inflammatory bowel disease. J Clin Gastroenterol 1992; 14: 15–19.

60. Martin A, Naccarato R, Fries W, Leone L. Quality of life in inflammatory bowel disease. Ital J Gastroenterol 1995; 27: 450–4.

61. Casellas F, Lopez-Vivancos J, Badia X, Vilaseca J, Malagelada JR. Impact of surgery for Crohn's disease on health-related quality of life. Am J Gastroenterol 2000; 95: 177–82.

62. Irvine EJ, Bolin T, Grace E *et al.* and the International Quality of Life Study Group. Geographic differences in health related quality of life in inflammatory bowel disease. Gastroenterology 1997; 112: A1003.

63. Farrokhyar F, Marshall JK, Cawdron R, Irvine EJ. Mood disorders worsen health-related quality of life in inflammatory bowel disease. Gastroenterology 2001; 119A (In press).

64. Almeida RT, Hjortsway H, Strom M, Almer S, Persson J. Technology assessment using the association between outcome measures and patterns of illness severity. Med Biol Eng Comput 1997; 35: 386–90.

65. Moser G, Tillinger W, Sachs G *et al.* Disease-related worries and concerns: a study on out-patients with inflammatory bowel disease. Eur J Gastroenterol Hepatol 1995; 7: 853-8.

66. Lange A, Haslbeck E, Bregenzer N, Gross V, Scholmerich J, Lamparter-Lang R. Ambulatory education of Crohn's disease/ulcerative colitis. Z Gastroenterol 1996; 34: 411–15.

67. Maunder RG, de Rooey EC, Toner BB *et al.* Health-related concerns of people who receive psychological support for inflammatory bowel disease. Can J Gastroenterol 1997; 11: 681–5.

68. Provenzale D, Shearin M, Phillips-Bute BG *et al.* Health related quality of life after ileoanal pull-through: evaluation and assessment of new health status measures. Gastroenterology 1997; 113: 7–14.

69. Tillinger W, Mittermaier C, Lochs H, Moser G. Health-related quality of life in patients with Crohn's disease. Influence of surgical operation-a prospective trial. Dig Dis Sci 1999; 44: 932–8.

70. Robinson M, Hanauer S, Hoop R *et al.* Mesalamine capsules enhance the quality of life for patients with ulcerative colitis. Aliment Pharmacol Ther 1994; 8: 27–34.

71. Singleton JW, Hanauer S, Robinson M. Quality of life results of a double-blind placebo controlled trial of mesalamine in patients with Crohn's disease. Dig Dis Sci 1995; 40: 931–5.

72. Gasche C, Dejaco C, Waldhoer T *et al.* Intravenous iron and erythropoietin for anemia associated with Crohn's disease. Ann Intern Med 1997; 126: 782–7.

73. Thomsen OO, Cortot A, Jewell D *et al.* A comparison of budesonide and mesalamine for active Crohn's disease. N Engl J Med. 1998; 339: 370–4.

74. Dupuy HJ. The Psychological General Well-Being (PGWB) Index. In: Wenger NK, Masson ME, Furberg CD, Elinson J, eds. Assessment of Quality of Life in Clinical Trials of Cardiovascular Therapies. New York: Le Lacq, 1984: 170–83.

75. Martin F, Sutherland L, Beck IT *et al.* Oral 5ASA versus prednisone in short term treatment of Crohn's disease: a multicentre controlled trial. Can J Gastroenterol 1990; 4: 452–58.

76. Greenberg GR, Feagan BG, Martin FM *et al.* Oral budesonide for active Crohn's disease. N Engl J Med 1994; 331: 836–41.

77. Feagan BG, Rochon J, Fedorak RN *et al.* Methotrexate for the treatment of Crohn's disease. N Engl J Med 1995; 332: 292–7.

78. Targan S, Hanauer SB, Van Deventer SJH *et al.* A short-term study of chimeric monoclonal antibody cA2 to tumor necrosis factor α for Crohn's disease. N Engl J Med 1997; 337: 1029–35.

79. Rutgeerts P, D'Haens G, Targan S *et al.* Efficacy and safety of retreatment with anti-tumour necrosis factor antibody (infliximab) to maintain remission in Crohn's disease. Gastroenterology 1999; 117: 761–9.

80. Feagan B, McDonald JWD, Rochon J *et al.* Chronic low dose cyclosporine in the treatment of Crohn's disease. N Engl J Med 1994: 330: 1846–51.

81. Irvine EJ, Feagan B, Wong C. Does self-administration of a quality of life instrument change the results? J Clin Epidemiol 1996; 49: 1177-85.

82. Irvine EJ, Zhou Q, Thompson A and the CCRPT Investigators. The short IBDQ: a quality of life instrument for community physicians managing inflammatory bowel disease. Am J Gastroenterol 1996; 91: 1571–8.

83. Han SW, Gregory W, Nylander D *et al.* The SIBDQ: Further validation in ulcerative colitis patients. Am J Gastroenterol 2000; 95: 145–51.

84. North CS, Alpers DH. A review of studies of psychiatric factors in Crohn's disease. Ann Clin Psychiatry 1994; 6: 117–24.

85. North CS, Clouse RE, Spitznagel EL, Alpers DH. The relation of ulcerative colitis to psychiatric factors: a review of findings and methods. Am J Psychiatry 1990; 147: 974–8.

86. Turnbull GK, Vallis TM. Quality of life in inflammatory bowel disease: the interaction of disease activity with psychosocial function. Am J Gatroenterol 1995; 90: 1450–4.

87. Kinash RG, Fischer DG, Lukie BE, Carr TL. Inflammatory bowel disease impact and patient characteristics. Gastroenterol Nurs 1993; Feb: 147–55.

88. Levenstein S, Prantera C, Varvo V *et al.* Psychological stress and disease activity in ulcerative colitis: a multidimensional cross-sectional study. Am J Gastroenterol 1994; 89: 1219–25.

89. Levenstein S, Prantera C, Varvo V *et al.* Stress and exacerbation in ulcerative colitis: a prospective study of patients enrolled in remission. Am J Gastroenterol 2000; 95: 1213–20.

90. Katon W. Editorial: The impact of major depression on chronic medical illness. Gen Hosp Psychiatry 1996; 18: 215–19.

91. Russel MG, Nieman FH, Bergers JM, Stockbrugger RW. Cigarette smoking and quality of life in patients with inflammatory bowel disease. Eur J Gastroenterol Hepatol 1996; 8: 1075–81.

92. Eisen GM, Straus WL, Sandler RS *et al.* Health status in Crohn's disease: comparison of the rating form of IBD patient concerns in African and non-African Americans. Gastroenterology 1996; 110: A15.

93. Straus WL, Eisen GM, Sandler RS *et al.* Race and Crohn's disease: clinical and therapeutic comparison of African

Americans and non-African Americans. Report of a multi-center survey. Gastroenterology 1996; 110: A1021

94. Straus WL, Eisen GM, Sandler RS, Murray SC, Sessions JT. Crohn's disease: does race matter? Am J Gastroenterol 2000; 95: 479–83.

95. Drummond HE, Ghosh S, Ferguson A, Brackenridge D, Tiplady B. Electronic quality of life questionnaires: a comparison of pen-based electronic questionnaires with conventional paper in a gastrointestinal study. Qual Life Res 1995; 4: 21–6.

96. Kennedy AP, Thompson DG, Robinson AJ, Wilkin D. Randomized controlled trial of a patient-centred guidebook; effect on quality of life in ulcerative colitis. Gastroenterology 2000; 118(Suppl. 2): A213.

25 | Clinical pharmacology in inflammatory bowel disease: optimizing current medical therapy

LAURENCE J. EGAN AND WILLIAM J. SANDBORN

Introduction

Effective therapy of inflammatory bowel disease (IBD) often requires the implementation of diverse pharmacologic strategies (Fig. 1). Unlike, for example, the treatment of an acid-peptic disease where blockade of the proton pump, a specific target enzyme, is highly effective in inhibiting the pathogenic process, investigators have been unable to identify a specific unifying etiologic or pathogenic factor in IBD to pharmacologically target. For this reason, current therapy of ulcerative colitis (UC), Crohn's disease (CD) and pouchitis often requires the use of more than one drug that belong to different therapeutic classes, and that are non-specific in action.

In this chapter the clinical pharmacology of drugs that are effective in IBD is reviewed. The pharmacokinetics and mechanisms of action of these agents are discussed, with particular reference to their use in IBD patients. Although the list of medicines available to treat IBD is expanding, none is universally effective or safe. Therefore, we also explore various strategies to individualize and optimize drug therapy in IBD, including therapeutic drug monitoring and the potential use of pharmacogenetic data to guide therapeutic decision-making. Several agents recently introduced for use in IBD, such as mycophenolate mofetil, interleukin (IL)-10 and thalidomide are not discussed because of a paucity of information on their use.

Aminosalicylates

Chemistry

Drugs that contain 5-aminosalicylic acid (5-ASA) have been used successfully in the treatment of IBD for decades. The aminosalicylates have evolved to become a cornerstone of modern IBD therapy since the observation that the 5-ASA-containing agent sulfasalazine, designed to provide both anti-inflammatory and antibacterial activities for rheumatoid arthritis therapy, produced symptomatic improvement of bowel disease in patients with coexisting colitis [1]. Sulfasalazine consists of one molecule of 5-ASA azo-bound to a molecule of the sulfa antibiotic sulfapyridine. A number of studies have suggested that the therapeutic action of sulfasalazine in IBD resides with the 5-ASA moiety, rather than with sulfapyridine [2–4]. Olsalazine is an azo-conjugated dimer of 5-ASA, and balsalazide consists of a molecule of 5-ASA azo-bound to 4-aminobenzoylalanine, an inert carrier (Fig. 2).

Mechanisms of action

5-ASA differs from salicylic acid only by the addition of an amino group at the 5 (meta) position. However, this change produces a chemical entity with pharmacologic properties different from conventional salicylates, and appears to be necessary for activity in IBD. The primary anti-inflammatory, antipyretic and analgesic actions of salicylates such as aspirin are due to blockade of prostaglandin

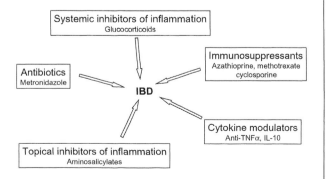

Figure 1. Effective therapy of IBD often requires a combination of diverse pharmacological approaches.

Stephan R. Targan, Fergus Shanahan and Loren C. Karp (eds.), Inflammatory Bowel Disease: From Bench to Bedside, 2nd Edition, 495–521.
© 2003 *Kluwer Academic Publishers. Printed in Great Britain*

of Pentasa allows 5-ASA to dissolve and diffuse into the gut lumen over several hours.

Three azo-conjugated preparations of 5-ASA are available: sulfasalazine, balsalazide and olsalazine. Compared to free 5-ASA, oral administration of azo-conjugated 5-ASA results in greatly reduced systemic absorption of the active drug, and therefore greater delivery of drug to the site of presumed pharmacologic activity [30–38]. Intestinal bacteria contain azo-reductase activity, and are most abundant in the terminal ileum and colon. Azo-conjugated aminosalicylates reach the distal bowel largely unabsorbed, and there are effectively metabolized to yield free 5-ASA and the carrier molecule. In the case of olsalazine, two molecules of 5-ASA are released. These preparations thus deliver high concentrations of active drug to the terminal ileum and colon. Compared to the delayed-release preparations, azo-conjugated aminosalicylates are less subject to absorption in the small bowel and consequently, less drug is delivered systemically (Table 1).

A number of factors may affect the delivery of orally administered 5-ASA to the site of disease in IBD patients. For example, rapid intestinal transit may decrease exposure of the small intestine to delayed-release preparations of 5-ASA, and alterations in bacterial flora due to antibiotic use or small bowel bacterial overgrowth could affect liberation of 5-ASA from the azo-bound aminosalicylates. Clinically significant differences between the available oral 5-ASA preparations have been difficult to detect and, compared to sulfasalazine, the newer products have not been shown to have superior clinical efficacy. However, aminosalicylates lacking sulfapyridine are tolerated better than sulfasalazine [39]. Comparisons between doses of azo-bound aminosalicylates and free aminosalicylates should be made on the basis of molar content of 5-ASA; thus, 1 g of sulfasalazine contains approximately 0.4 g of 5-ASA.

Rectal administration of 5-ASA as a suppository or enema provides a high concentration of drug at the site of disease in distal UC. Suppositories deliver 5-ASA to the rectum only. Enemas contain an aqueous suspension of 5-ASA that gradually dissolves into the luminal free water to deliver active drug to the rectum and left colon [40]. The effectiveness and absorption of rectally administered 5-ASA depend on the patient's ability to retain the drug, which can be difficult for individuals with active proctitis. The absorption of rectal 5-ASA averages around 20% of the administered dose.

Adverse effects

Aminosalicylates are well tolerated, especially the newer drugs lacking the sulfapyridine moiety of sulfasalazine [39, 41]. Sulfasalazine, but not 5-ASA, has been associated with oligospermia [42] and folate deficiency [43]. Adverse reactions to 5-ASA are generally mild and reversible. In most of the efficacy trials the frequency of drug reactions sufficient to warrant discontinuation was not significantly greater in the active treatment group (3–4%) than in the placebo group. The most frequently reported side effects of 5-ASA include dizziness, fever, headache, abdominal pain, nausea and rash [44–46].

Certain rare and potentially serious adverse events are occasionally associated with 5-ASA use. These include pneumonitis and pericarditis [47, 48], aplastic anemia [49], pancreatitis [50] and rarely, exacerbation of existing colitis [51].

High doses of aminosalicylates that are associated with higher salicylate blood levels have generated concern about potential nephrotoxicity [52, 53]. Careful studies of renal function and urinary sediment have documented subtle changes indicative of tubular epithelial cell damage in IBD patients receiving high doses of 5-ASA drugs [54]. However, despite this concern, clinically significant renal dysfunction appears to occur very infrequently in IBD patients treated with 5-ASA drugs.

Optimizing therapy

The effectiveness of aminosalicylate therapy of IBD depends on getting a high concentration of the drug to the site of disease. The different preparations of 5-ASA listed in Table 1 offer unique characteristics that can theoretically be exploited to deliver the greatest amount of drug to the site of disease in individual patients. Thus, many clinicians use 5-ASA suppositories and enemas in patients with proctitis or proctosigmoiditis. Indeed, even in the presence of pancolitis, the use of rectal 5-ASA may be very useful to control distal disease, the source of the most troublesome symptoms. In more extensive UC, both the azo-conjugated and delayed-release formulations of oral 5-ASA are suitable. No individual preparation has been conclusively shown to have an efficacy advantage over another in UC. For the treatment of small bowel CD, the timed-release Pentasa preparation has the theoretical, but not clinically proven, advantage over the other oral aminosalicylates.

Table 2. Comparison of the potency, bioavailability and common doses of oral and rectal glucocorticoid preparations for use in IBD

Drug	Anti-inflammatory potency	Bioavailability	Usual maximum dose, mg/day
Hydrocortisone	1	Oral: > 50%; rectal: 16–30%	100–200
Prednisone	4	Oral: > 50%	40–80
Prednisolone	4	Oral: > 50%; rectal, as metasulfobenzoate: < 10%	40–80
Budesonide, controlled-ileal-release	200	Oral : 10%; rectal: 16%	9–15

A consistent theme to emerge from clinical trials of aminosalicylates in IBD is that more is better. For active UC, doses of 5-ASA in the 2.4–4.8 g per range were more efficacious than 1.6 g or placebo [44, 46]. Similarly, in the treatment of active CD, 5-ASA doses of 3–4 g per day [55] are more effective than 1–2 g per day [56, 57]. For maintenance of medically or surgically induced remission in CD, 5-ASA doses of 2.4 g or greater are effective, but lower doses are not [58–60]. Furthermore, in studies which have compared oral and rectal 5-ASA for distal UC, combination therapy seems to be superior to either alone. Higher doses of 5-ASA produce higher mucosal drug levels [61], and the occurrence of ileal relapse after resection in CD patients on prophylactic 5-ASA, 2.4 g per day, was found to be associated with lower ileal mucosa drug levels [62]. Taken together, these data support the concept that the optimum use of aminosalicylates in active IBD demands the highest tolerated dose. In quiescent disease, lower doses may be more tolerable to the patient and are less costly.

5-ASA is primarily metabolized by *N*-acetylation to a product that does not appear to possess significant anti-inflammatory activity. Of the two *N*-acetyltransferase isoenzymes, *N*-acetyltransferase-1 has much greater affinity for aminosalicylates than *N*-acetyltransferase-2 [63]. *N*-acetyltransferase-1 is highly expressed in the epithelium of the small bowel and colon [64]. The *NAT1* gene is polymorphic, and inactivating mutations are associated with a phenotype of decreased enzymatic activity [65]. Conversion of 5-ASA to acetyl-5-ASA by *N*-acetyltransferase-1 takes place in the gut epithelium [66, 67] and in the liver, where phase II conjugation with glucuronic acid also takes place. After oral or rectal administration of an aminosalicylate, acetyl-5-ASA is the chief species present in the serum and urine [32, 33, 68] and in the intestine [36].

One study has examined the potential role of *NAT1* polymorphisms and *N*-acetyltransferase-1 activity in colonic mucosa as a determinant of clinical response to 5-ASA [69]. In this study IBD patients classified on clinical grounds as normal or poor responders to 5-ASA were compared with respect to *NAT1* polymorphisms and colonic *N*-acetyltransferase-1 activity. Interestingly, poor responders had a lower rate of 5-ASA acetylation than normal responders, and three out of five poor responders, but none of the normal responders, were heterozygous for *NAT1* polymorphisms. These intriguing but preliminary data run contrary to the notion that acetylation inactivates 5-ASA, but require confirmation.

Glucocorticoids

Chemistry

The glucocorticoids that are useful in the therapy of IBD are synthetic molecules that bear a number of modifications or substitutions of the naturally occurring steroid, cortisol (hydrocortisone). These alterations to the steroid molecule result in dramatic differences in its absorption, transport, metabolism and molecular actions. The synthetic analogs of cortisol have been developed with the primary goal of maximizing glucocorticoid activity while minimizing mineralocorticoid effects, and decreasing the protean adverse effects of high quantities of systemically active glucocorticoid. Prednisone and prednisolone are the steroids most commonly used to treat IBD, and have an intermediate duration of action that allows once-daily dosing. A variety of high glucocorticoid potency, low-bioavailability synthetic molecules have been developed. Delayed-release oral preparations of these molecules, for example controlled-ileal-release budesonide, allow topical delivery of the drug to the site of disease in IBD (Table 2).

Mechanisms of action

Glucocorticoids exert a diverse range of effects on most tissues of the body. When present at supraphysiological amounts after exogenous administration, the glucocorticoids have pronounced anti-inflammatory and immunosuppressive actions. The majority of the physiologic and pharmacologic effects of glucocorticoids are dependent on diffusion of the steroid across the cell membrane to the cytoplasm where they bind to the glucocorticoid receptor, a member of the superfamily of steroid hormone receptors (Fig. 3). The glucocorticoid receptor exists in the cytosol bound to the 90 kDa heat-shock proteins that act as chaperone molecules and prevent nuclear translocation. After steroid binding, the glucocorticoid–glucocorticoid receptor–heat-shock protein complex undergoes conformational changes that allow dissociation of the steroid and its receptor from the heat-shock proteins. The steroid–receptor complex is then transported to the nucleus where it can interact via its zinc finger domains with glucocorticoid response elements that are found in the 5′ promotor regions of up to 100 genes. Binding of the steroid–receptor complex to glucocorticoid response elements changes the rate of transcription of target genes. In some situations this favors the assembly of the transcription initiation complex and up-regulates the rate of gene transcription. In contrast, when the steroid–receptor complex binds to negatively acting glucocorticoid response elements, repression of gene transcription results. In addition to these direct effects on the rate of gene transcription, activated glucocorticoid receptors also physically associate with other transcription factors in the nucleus via leucine zipper interactions, and reciprocally modulate each others' activities. One important example of this mechanism is the inhibition of NF-κB and activator protein-1 binding to DNA by activated glucocorticoid receptors [70, 71]. Glucocorticoids also inhibit the activity of NF-κB by inducing transcription of its natural inhibitor, IκBα [72, 73].

These direct effects, and numerous indirect effects resulting from the modulation of gene expression,

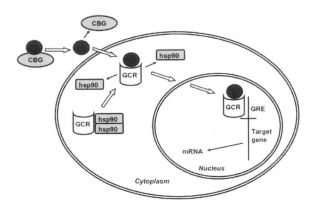

Figure 3. Mechanism of action of glucocorticoids (GC). After dissociation from corticosteroid-binding globulin (CBG), GC diffuse across the plasma membrane. In the cytoplasm the steroid binds to the glucocorticoid receptor (GCR), inducing conformational changes that cause dissociation of two chaperone molecules, heat-shock protein-90 (hsp90). The GC–GCR complex migrates to the nucleus and binds to glucocorticoid response elements (GRE) in the promoter regions of various target genes, regulating the rate of gene transcription. In addition, the GC–GCR complex interacts with important peptide transcription factors in the nucleus such as NF-κB, and can regulate their activity (not illustrated).

are the major molecular mechanisms of action of glucocorticoids. The dramatic capacity of glucocorticoids to inhibit inflammation relates to the potent inhibitory actions that these drugs exert on molecules that promote the activity of immune and inflammatory processes (Table 3). Effects of glucocorticoids that are well documented include inhibition of the production of proinflammatory cytokines such as TNF-α and IL-1, and chemokines such as IL-8; repression of the transcription of the genes for certain enzymes such as inducible nitric oxide synthase, phospholipase A_2 and cyclo-oxygenase II; and blockade of adhesion molecule expression. These molecular actions of glucocorticoids result in a blockade of leukocyte migration and function, and inhibit the effects of numerous important peptide- and lipid-derived mediators of inflammation.

A number of studies have examined the anti-inflammatory or immune-modulating effects of glucocorticoids in patients with IBD. Nitric oxide is found in elevated quantity in the inflamed mucosa in IBD [79], where it is produced by the inducible form of nitric oxide synthase. Glucocorticoids inhibited *in-vitro* production of nitric oxide by cultured mucosal biopsy specimens, but glucocorticoid treatment of severe UC was not shown to down-regulate immunoreactive nitric oxide synthase [80]. In

Table 3. Gene targets of glucocorticoids that are important in mediating their anti-inflammatory actions

Target substance	Effect of glucocorticoid	Target cell	Mechanism [ref.]	Result
Cytokines and chemokines				
IL-1, TNFα, IL-8	Decrease	Many	Inhibition of NF-κB [15]	Decreased inflammatory signaling
IL-2	Decrease	Lymphocytes	Inhibition of AP-1 [74]	Decreased lymphocyte activation
Enzymes				
Inducible nitric oxide synthase	Decrease	Epithelial and endothelial	Inhibition of NF-κB [15]	Decreased vascular permeability
Phospholipase A$_2$	Decrease	Many	Inhibition of NF-κB, induction of lipocortin gene expression [75]	Decreased eicosanoid production
Cyclo-oxygenase II	Decrease	Many	Inhibition of NF-κB [15]	Decreased prostaglandin production
Receptors				
IL-1 receptor type II	Increase	Many	Direct induction of gene expression [76]	Decreased availability of IL-1 for biological activity
Adhesion molecules				
E-selectin	Decrease	Endothelial	Inhibition of NF-κB [77]	Decreased leukocyte extravasation
Intracellular adhesion molecule-1	Decrease	Epithelial, monocytic	Inhibition of NF-κB [78]	Decreased leukocyte migration

patients with active CD prednisolone, but not budesonide, has been demonstrated to inhibit neutrophil and peripheral blood lymphocyte expression of activation markers and the proinflammatory cytokines, IL-1 and TNF-α [81]. Similarly, expression of the adhesion molecules intracellular adhesion molecule-3 and β_2-integrin by peripheral blood lymphocytes in CD and UC was lower in patients receiving prednisone [82]. At the level of the inflamed mucosa in UC, prednisolone enemas and oral tablets have been shown to decrease the luminal concentrations of the arachidonic acid metabolites prostaglandin-E$_2$ and leukotriene-B$_4$ [22]. At the mechanistic level prednisolone therapy inhibits the activation of NF-κB in the gut mucosa [11, 14], supporting an important role for this transcription factor in mediating the beneficial effects of glucocorticoids in IBD. Overall, these human studies provide evidence that the effects of glucocorticoids on expression of the genes listed in Table 3 underlie the *in-vivo* anti-inflammatory effects of these drugs in IBD.

Pharmaceutics and pharmacokinetics

The conventional synthetic corticosteroids prednisone and prednisolone are the drugs of this class most commonly used in IBD. Prednisone is a prodrug that requires metabolic activation in the liver to prednisolone. There is some evidence that chronic liver disease may impair this process [83], and for this reason prednisolone may be preferable in patients with advanced liver disease. Both of these drugs are well absorbed after oral administration and bioavailability is high, averaging over 70%. There is some evidence suggesting decreased absorption of prednisolone in patients with CD of the small bowel [84, 85], but it is not clear if this difference is clinically significant. After absorption, glucocorticoids circulate in the plasma partially bound to corticosteroid-binding globulin and albumin, but it is only the free form that is available for biologic activity. The affinity of different corticosteroids for these carrier proteins varies considerably and in part determines anti-inflammatory potency. Although various physiologic and pathologic conditions alter the plasma concentration of the steroid-binding proteins, the resulting changes that occur in the concentration of free glucocorticoid are transient and are not likely to be significant.

There has been a considerable effort to develop glucocorticoids for delivery to the site of disease in IBD, with the goal of providing high disease–tissue drug concentrations, with less systemic absorption than conventional steroids. One approach is rectal administration of the drug. Hydrocortisone enemas are used in ulcerative proctosigmoiditis to provide topical delivery of glucocorticoid directly to the diseased tissue, with good clinical results. Absorption of hydrocortisone enemas is less than after oral administration; nevertheless, bioavailability ranges from about 15% to 30% [86, 87], sufficient to suppress adrenal steroid production. A derivative of prednisolone with a metasulfobenzoate substitution is also used rectally in distal UC. Compared to prednisolone this agent is less well absorbed and should therefore provide a therapeutic advantage by acting locally and causing less systemic exposure to glucocorticoid activity [88, 89]. However, careful studies of adrenal function and bone turnover demonstrate that prednisolone metasulfobenzoate enemas do result in significant systemic glucocorticoid activity when used to treat distal UC [90, 91].

Budesonide is a synthetic analog of prednisolone that has proved to be therapeutically effective as oral delayed-release capsules in CD of the ileum and right colon, and as an enema in distal UC. This drug has high affinity for the glucocorticoid receptor resulting in very high potency, and is subject to rapid inactivation in the liver leading to low systemic bioavailability [92, 93]. A controlled-ileal-release formulation of budesonide is used orally, in which the drug is formulated as capsules containing microgranules of budesonide coated with Eudragit L100-55, an acrylic resin that dissolves above pH 5.5 to release the drug in the distal ileum. The systemic bioavailability of oral budesonide capsules is approximately 10% [94], and the majority of absorption appears to occur in the distal small bowel. However, even this degree of systemic exposure is sufficient to suppress adrenal steroid production, but is less than occurs with equivalent doses of prednisolone [95–97]. For rectal delivery, budesonide is formulated as a suspension enema. The bioavailability of budesonide administered by this route, mean 16%, is greater than found with the oral controlled-ileal-release formulation, probably reflecting absorption into the distal rectal veins that drain directly into the systemic venous system [98]. Rectal administration of budesonide

produces dose-dependent suppression of adrenal function [99]. Thus, with both the oral and rectal formulations of budesonide, some degree of adrenal suppression occurs, but this appears it to be less than seen with conventional steroids.

A number of other high glucocorticoid potency, low systemic bioavailability corticosteroids have been developed and tested for use in IBD. Tixocortol pivalate is a potent, well-absorbed and rapidly metabolized steroid molecule that has been used as an enema for distal UC. Fluticasone is a high potency fluorinated corticosteroid that is poorly absorbed from the intestine and undergoes extensive first-pass inactivation, leading to systemic bioavailability of less than 1%. Fluticasone has been evaluated for oral use in CD and UC, but in preliminary studies was not found to be efficacious [100, 101]. Beclomethasone is a highly potent glucocorticoid with low systemic bioavailability. Preliminary studies of beclomethasone enemas in active distal UC have revealed efficacy and little adrenal suppression, but further studies are needed [102–104].

Adverse effects

The use of glucocorticoids for prolonged periods in IBD patients is associated with serious side-effects. These are not different from those that occur when these drugs are given chronically for other indications. In the National Cooperative Crohn's Disease Study, adverse drug effects that occurred more frequently in prednisone-treated patients than in those receiving placebo were petechiae and bruising of skin, striae, moon face, acne, hypertension and infection [105]. About 30% of prednisone-treated patients in this study experienced a side-effect of this therapy, and the likelihood of occurrence of most of the reported adverse events increased with duration of exposure to the drug.

Physicians who care for IBD patients requiring frequent use of glucocorticoids also recognize that the full gamut of steroid-induced problems develop with prolonged consumption of these drugs. Certain adverse effects of glucocorticoids are of particular relevance in IBD. Hyperglycemia and non-alcoholic steatohepatitis are frequent metabolic complications of chronic glucocorticoid therapy. Abnormal liver chemistry test results in IBD patients can also be due to primary sclerosing cholangitis, or short-bowel syndrome, so one must consider steroid-induced steatohepatitis in the differential diagnosis of abnormal liver tests in IBD. Individuals with IBD are at greatly increased risk for the development of osteoporosis [106–108]. The use of glucocorticoids may increase this risk, as in one study 58% of steroid-treated patients had lumbar spine osteopenia, compared to 28% of steroid non-users [108]. In these studies the use of glucocorticoids may simply be a marker of more active disease, itself a risk factor for osteoporosis. However, in diseases other than IBD that are not strongly associated with osteoporosis, glucocorticoid use induces bone loss and fractures [109]. Aseptic necrosis of the hip is an unpredictable, devastating complication of glucocorticoid use. The newer high-potency, low-bioavailability steroids such as budesonide may be associated with less risk of inducing bone disease. Options for treating and preventing bone disease due to glucocorticoids include calcium and vitamin D, estrogen for post-menopausal women, and bisphosphonates. IBD patients who have been treated with glucocorticoids within 1 year should receive a short course of steroids perioperatively to protect against an inadequate adrenal response to the stress of surgery [110].

Optimizing therapy

It is paradoxical that glucocorticoids, the first therapy proven effective for IBD [111, 112] have not been as carefully studied as most other classes of drugs. The optimum doses of glucocorticoids to induce remission in active UC and CD are not known. Few studies have addressed the question of the optimum rate at which to taper the dose of steroids after a patient responds, so individual clinical judgement and experience, rather than data, direct practice.

Nevertheless, there are some well-established principles to guide the effective and safe use of glucocorticoids in IBD. Almost all IBD patients with moderately to severely active disease should be treated with a corticosteroid, as these drugs are highly efficacious for induction of remission and are probably responsible for reducing the high death rate first reported for severe UC [111]. Although oral steroids are well absorbed, most authorities recommend intravenous administration in the sickest patients, because alterations in gut motility and mucosal function may compromise absorption [84, 85]. However, after a patient responds, the dose should be tapered gradually to minimize development of corticosteroid-related side-effects. A typical rate of withdrawal for oral prednisone is by 5 mg per day each week, but this is only a guideline. Medications other than glucocorticoids, such as aminosalicylates and immunosuppressives, should be used to maintain remission because of superior efficacy and toxicity profiles. Rectally administered steroids have lower systemic absorption than oral, and therefore may provide a therapeutic advantage by acting locally in distal UC. Similarly, in CD of the terminal ileum and right colon, controlled-ileal-release budesonide appears to be almost as effective as prednisolone, but has significantly less systemic effect [97].

Intravenous, oral and rectal steroids are highly efficacious in most patients with IBD. However, up to 20% of the IBD population do not respond clinically to oral prednisolone after 30 days [113], and on clinical grounds are resistant to steroids. The molecular basis for resistance to the anti-inflammatory effects of glucocorticoids is an important issue in IBD therapy. A syndrome of familial steroid resistance has been described not only for glucocorticoids, but also for sex hormones, mineralocorticoids and vitamin D [114]. Familial glucocorticoid resistance is a rare disorder that appears to be due to a mutation in the glucocorticoid receptor. More common is isolated resistance to the anti-inflammatory effects of glucocorticoids, which has been best described in asthma [115]. In asthma, steroid resistance is associated with defects in the suppression of peripheral blood mononuclear cell function by glucocorticoids [116]. This may be related to alterations in the number of glucocorticoid receptors, and to altered affinity for ligand in target cells [117–119]. The molecular basis for these abnormalities has been linked to increased expression of the transcription factor c-fos in the peripheral blood mononuclear cells of glucocorticoid-resistant asthmatics [120]. In CD, peripheral blood leukocytes have reduced sensitivity to the inhibitory effects of dexamethasone on cytokine secretion after *ex-vivo* stimulation, compared to controls [121]. Among a group of patients with severely active UC, a therapeutic response to intravenous hydrocortisone was significantly more likely in those with the greatest sensitivity of peripheral T cells to dexamethasone-induced inhibition of proliferation after *ex-vivo* stimulation [122]. In IBD, more study is clearly needed to delineate the molecular mechanisms that underlie sensitivity and resistance to glucocorticoids.

Azathioprine and 6-mercaptopurine

Chemistry

Azathioprine and 6-mercaptopurine are purine anti-metabolite drugs that were found to have immune-suppressing properties when used for cancer chemotherapy, leading to their investigation and ultimate use as immunosuppressive drugs in a variety of clinical settings. Azathioprine is a pro-drug that is rapidly converted to 6-mercaptopurine in a non-enzymatic reaction by sulfhydryl-containing substances such as glutathione. These two drugs possess identical actions with respect to their use in IBD. Considering mass (azathioprine is 55% 6-mercaptopurine by weight) and the efficiency of conversion of azathioprine to 6-mercaptopurine (88%), one must administer approximately twice as much azathioprine as 6-mercaptopurine to achieve similar amounts of bioavailable active drug. 6-Mercaptopurine can enter three known metabolic pathways (Fig. 4). Two of these routes, leading to the inactive metabolites 6-methylmercaptopurine and 6-thiouric acid, are catalyzed by thiopurine methyltransferase and xanthine oxidase, respectively. The action of hypoxanthine phosphoribosyl transferase commits 6-mercaptopurine to conversion to the 6-thioguanine nucleotides, the putative active metabolites [123].

Mechanism of action

After administration of azathioprine or 6-mercaptopurine, the 6-thioguanine nucleotides accumulate intracellularly, and are believed to mediate the biologic actions of these drugs. Despite over 50 years of investigation the precise molecular basis for the therapeutic effects of the purine analogs is not known. However, intracellular accumulation of 6-thioguanine nucleotides causes inhibition of the pathways of purine nucleotide metabolism and DNA synthesis and repair, resulting in inhibition of cell division and proliferation. It is plausible, but not proven, that antiproliferative or functionally inhibitory actions on cells of the immune system, such as lymphocytes, underlie the immunosuppressive actions of azathioprine and 6-mercaptopurine.

Pharmacokinetics and pharmacogenetics

The bioavailability of azathioprine, estimated as 6-mercaptopurine, ranges from 27% to 83%, and of 6-

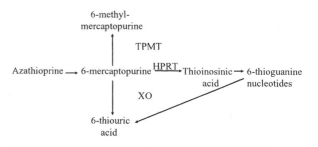

Figure 4. Metabolic pathways of azathioprine and 6-mercaptopurine. TPMT, thiopurine methyltransferase; HPRT, hypoxanthine phosphoribosyltransferase; XO, xanthine oxidase. Reproduced with permission from Chan GL *et al.*, J Clin Pharmacol 1990; 30: 358–63.

mercaptopurine ranges from 5% to 37%. An oral preparation of azathioprine coated with Eudragit-S, designed for release above pH 7 in the distal ileum, had a mean bioavailability of 7%. Rectal administration of azathioprine in hydrophilic or hydrophobic enemas consistently resulted in less than 10% systemic bioavailability [124]. At present there are no data on the clinical efficacy or toxicity of rectal or delayed-release oral azathioprine in IBD.

Many studies have examined the kinetics of the active metabolites of azathioprine and 6-mercaptopurine, the 6-thioguanine nucleotides. Although azathioprine and 6-mercaptopurine are rapidly cleared from plasma, 6-thioguanine nucleotides are concentrated in cells resulting in a half-life of elimination of many days [125]. In patients with CD and other conditions, erythrocyte 6-thioguanine nucleotide concentration gradually rises to a plateau after 2–4 weeks of oral azathioprine [126–128] (Fig. 5). The rather delayed time to reach steady-state 6-thioguanine nucleotide kinetics parallels the slow onset of therapeutic benefit of oral azathioprine or 6-mercaptopurine therapy in IBD, which has been estimated to average 17 weeks [129]. This observation prompted a pilot study [130], followed by a placebo-controlled trial of an intravenous loading-dose of azathioprine to hasten the onset of clinical benefit in CD [126]. In this study, despite initially higher erythrocyte 6-thioguanine nucleotide concentration in those who received active intravenous drug, a clinical response was seen no sooner than in placebo-treated patients. However, the median time to steady-state erythrocyte 6-thioguanine nucleotide concentration and first clinical improvement was only 4 weeks, suggesting that azathioprine may act more quickly than had previously been realized.

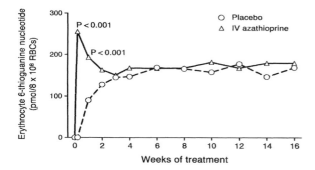

Figure 5. Mean erythrocyte 6-thioguanine nucleotide concentration in Crohn's disease patients after beginning azathioprine 2 mg/kg per day by mouth. △, received an intravenous loading dose of azathioprine; ○, received a placebo intravenous loading dose. Reproduced with permission from Sandborn WJ *et al.*, Gastroenterology 1999; 117: 527–35.

One of the pathways of biotransformation that is available to 6-mercaptopurine is metabolized by a polymorphically expressed enzyme, thiopurine methyltransferase [131]. Erythrocyte thiopurine methyltransferase activity correlates well with the enzyme's activity in other cells and tissues. The majority of the Caucasian population, ~90%, have an erythrocyte thiopurine methyltransferase activity of about 14–25 U/ml erythrocytes, and these individuals are homozygous for two wild-type *TPMT* alleles. Approximately 10% of this population have an enzyme activity that is detectable but below 14 U/ml erythrocytes, and are heterozygous for one active and one inactive copy of *TMPT*. One percent or less of individuals have no detectable thiopurine methyltransferase activity and have 2 inactive *TPMT* alleles [131, 132]. The erythrocyte 6-thioguanine nucleotide concentration varies considerably among patients being treated with azathioprine or 6-mercaptopurine, and appears to be dependent on the individuals' inherent, genetically determined thiopurine methyltransferase activity [132, 133]. Thus, patients with low thiopurine methyltransferase activity have greater 6-thioguanine nucleotide concentrations, presumably because more 6-mercaptopurine is shunted into the hypoxanthine phosphoribosyl transferase pathway.

Adverse effects

Two categories of adverse effects to azathioprine and 6-mercaptopurine have been described: allergic, occurring early during treatment; and dose-related, generally occurring later. Allergy to these drugs can manifest as pancreatitis, fever, rash, nausea, diarrhea, and hepatitis. Approximately 5% of the IBD population beginning treatment with azathioprine or 6-mercaptopurine will experience an allergic reaction to the drug [134], which can be confirmed by rechallenge if necessary. Dose-related toxicities of azathioprine or 6-mercaptopurine include bone marrow depression leading to leukopenia, anemia or thrombocytopenia. If severe, leukopenia can potentially cause profound immune suppression, and thus predispose to opportunistic infections or neoplasms. Cytopenias have been reported to develop from 2 weeks to 11 years after beginning therapy, at a cumulative frequency of about 10% [126, 135, 136]. Although the numbers are insufficient for statistical analysis, there are enough reports of fatal or life-threatening opportunistic infections in leukopenic IBD patients treated with azathioprine or 6-mercaptopurine to dispel any tendency towards complacency [134, 135]. If leukopenia and a serious infection develop in a patient receiving azathioprine or 6-mercaptopurine, reversal of bone marrow suppression is usually possible with granulocyte colony-stimulating factor.

It is not completely clear if azathioprine or 6-mercaptopurine therapy confers an excess risk of malignancy. In the New York series, a wide spectrum of malignant neoplasms developed in IBD patients who had at some point received 6-mercaptopurine, but the overall rate of 3.1% was low and probably not greater than the general population [134]. In the British series, of 755 patients treated with azathioprine for a median duration of 12.5 years at a dose of 2 mg/kg per day, 31 developed a cancer compared to 24.3 expected cases [137]. The difference was significant only when considering colorectal adenocarcinomas, a recognized complication of IBD. Thus, the data are quite reassuring, but isolated and anecdotal reports of unusual lymphomas arising in IBD patients during or after azathioprine or 6-mercaptopurine therapy continue to generate some concern [136, 138]. Nevertheless, if there is an increased cancer risk attributable to these drugs, the magnitude of the increased risk is small.

Optimizing therapy

In some studies of patients being treated with azathioprine or 6-mercaptopurine for diseases other than IBD, low thiopurine methyltransferase activity, resulting in greater 6-thioguanine nucleotide concentration, has been associated with the development of leukopenia [123, 139]. Conversely, patients with higher thiopurine methyltransferase activity may be undertreated with standard doses of azathioprine or 6-mercaptopurine. For example, in childhood acute leukemia the risk of relapse during therapy with 6-mercaptopurine is greatest in those patients with the highest erythrocyte thiopurine methyltransferase activity, because they inactivate the drug more efficiently and have lower concentrations of active 6-thioguanine nucleotides [140, 141].

In IBD patients it is currently uncertain if significant associations exist between azathioprine or 6-mercaptopurine metabolism and the occurrence of clinical response or toxicity. A number of studies that were performed in CD patients selected without regard to thiopurine methyltransferase activity have suggested that 6-mercaptopurine pharmacogenetics may in fact be clinically relevant. In a group of pediatric CD patients receiving 6-mercaptopurine therapy, one study found that disease severity was least in those with the highest erythrocyte 6-thioguanine nucleotide concentration [142]. Another found that 65% of patients with inactive disease had 6-thioguanine nucleotide levels greater than 230 pmol/8×10^8 erythrocytes, compared to 28% of patients with active CD [143]. Similar studies in adults with CD and UC have documented a greater mean 6-thioguanine nucleotide concentration among responders to azathioprine or 6-mercaptopurine than among patients with persistent active disease [144, 145].

In contrast, two prospective studies of azathioprine in CD arrived at different conclusions. These clinical trials examined the relationships between thiopurine methyltransferase activity and erythrocyte 6-thioguanine nucleotide concentration, and the clinical outcomes of leukocyte count and efficacy [126, 130]. To minimize the potential for toxicity in these studies, individuals were excluded if thiopurine methyltransferase activity was in the heterozygous or homozygous low range (approximately 20% of the screened population, unpublished observation, W.J. Sandborn). No significant correlations were found between thiopurine methyltransferase activity or erythrocyte 6-thioguanine nucleotide concentration, and leukocyte count or clinical efficacy. The exclusion of individuals with intermediate or low thiopurine methyltransferase activity probably decreased the power of these studies to detect pharmacogenetic differences. Furthermore, a cross-sectional study of

IBD patients that included individuals with intermediate-range thiopurine methyltransferase activity who were receiving azathioprine or 6-mercaptopurine also found no significant associations between thiopurine methyltransferase activity or erythrocyte 6-thioguanine nucleotide concentration and disease severity [146].

Based on these data the benefit of monitoring erythrocyte 6-thioguanine nucleotide levels during azathioprine or 6-mercaptopurine therapy of IBD remains uncertain. Prospective studies that examine if a clinical benefit derives from using erythrocyte 6-thioguanine nucleotide concentrations to guide therapy in IBD are needed. It is our practice to measure thiopurine methyltransferase activity before beginning therapy with one of these drugs, to exclude the rare patient that is completely deficient in this enzyme. Individuals who have intermediate thiopurine methyltransferase activity can probably be treated safely with azathioprine or 6-mercaptopurine, but at half the standard dose. We currently do not routinely use erythrocyte 6-thioguanine nucleotide concentration for therapeutic drug monitoring, but this practice is commonplace at some centers.

Therapeutic trials have demonstrated that azathioprine should be given at a dose of 2–2.5 mg/kg per day, and 6-mercaptopurine at 1.5 mg/kg per day. There is no role for an intravenous loading dose to hasten the onset of clinical response. We counsel patients about the risk of leukopenia, and check a complete blood count every month during therapy. The results of one retrospective study suggested that the development of mild leukopenia, an indicator of intensity of treatment with 6-mercaptopurine, identified CD patients with a greater likelihood of a favorable response [147]. Based on this observation, one group of investigators has tried dose escalation in CD patients refractory to standard-dose azathioprine. In this uncontrolled study, after increasing the dose of azathioprine from a mean of 2 mg/kg per day to 2.7 mg/kg per day, 14 of 18 patients improved and were able to discontinue steroids [148]. Although no significant leukopenia was observed, two patients developed serious cytomegalovirus infection. Other studies that have examined the relationship between leukocyte count and clinical response during azathioprine and 6-mercaptopurine therapy of IBD have not supported the concept that leukopenia is associated with efficacy [126, 146]. For these reasons we do not recommend use of greater than standard doses of these agents.

Methotrexate

Chemistry and metabolism

Methotrexate is an antimetabolite anticancer drug that, like azathioprine, has been found to have beneficial effects in a number of chronic inflammatory diseases. Structurally, methotrexate is the 4-amino, N-10 methyl analog of folic acid. Like folic acid, methotrexate is a substrate for intracellular enzyme folylpolyglutamate synthase, which adds up to five glutamic acid residues to these compounds [149]. This modification promotes intracellular retention of methotrexate and increases the drug's affinity for a number of target enzymes [150, 151]. Over 90% of a dose of parenteral methotrexate is excreted unchanged in the urine [152]. In the liver a minor metabolic pathway of methotrexate produces small quantities of the 7-hydroxy derivative.

Mechanism of action

The principal biochemical action of methotrexate, and the mechanism that is believed to be responsible for the drug's cytotoxic activity, is inhibition of dihydrofolate reductase. This enzyme is critical for regenerating the fully reduced folate co-factors that are required for reactions involving transfer of one-carbon fragments, such as the production of thymidylate and purines. Methotrexate acts as a reversible, competitive inhibitor of dihydrofolate reductase. The polyglutamated metabolites of methotrexate are important not only because they are retained intracellularly, but also because they are potent inhibitors of enzymes that lie downstream of dihydrofolate reductase in the metabolic pathway of folic acid [151, 153]. Inhibition of these enzymes, including thymidylate synthase and 5-aminoimidazole-4-carboxamide ribotide transformylase, further impairs folate-dependent synthetic reactions.

At the high doses used in cancer chemotherapy, methotrexate blocks de-novo synthesis of DNA precursors leading to inhibition of cellular proliferation and cytotoxicity. Although methotrexate is beneficial in a number of chronic inflammatory diseases, cytotoxic or antiproliferative effects of folic acid analog therapy are difficult to invoke as the anti-inflammatory mechanism of action because clinically efficacious doses of methotrexate do not decrease circulating neutrophil, lymphocyte or platelet numbers [154, 155]. The occurrence of cytopenias or mucositis, clinical evidence of cytotoxicity, are in fact indications to lower the dose of methotrexate in chronic inflammatory diseases. Also, administration of folic acid ameliorates some of the toxicities of methotrexate that are attributable to its antiproliferative effects, without impairing its anti-inflammatory action [156].

In efforts to identify the mechanism of action of methotrexate in inflammatory diseases the effects of this drug on a number of mediators of inflammation have been examined, principally in patients with rheumatoid arthritis. Methotrexate has been found to decrease neutrophil production of leukotriene B_4 [157], to decrease IL-1 concentration in synovial fluid [158] and to lower plasma IL-6 and soluble IL-2 receptor concentrations [159]. However, other agents such as glucocorticoids produce similar effects, so these changes may reflect general improvement rather than methotrexate-specific phenomena.

It has alternatively been proposed that the anti-inflammatory action of methotrexate may be mediated by increased release of the endogenous anti-inflammatory autocoid, adenosine. Experiments in tissue culture and animal models of acute inflammation have demonstrated that methotrexate can promote extracellular release of adenosine, which inhibits neutrophil adherence to endothelial cells and accumulation at sites of inflammation [160, 161]. In animal experiments, methotrexate has also been shown to decrease leukocyte–endothelial cell interactions through release of adenosine and occupancy of adenosine A_2 receptors [162].

To determine if the methotrexate-induced elevations of extracellular adenosine concentration that were demonstrated in tissue culture and animal models of acute inflammation were relevant to the use of this drug in humans with IBD, the effect of methotrexate on rectal and plasma adenosine was studied. In 10 IBD patients with varying degrees of rectal involvement, adenosine was measured in the rectal lumen using in-vivo rectal dialysis [163]. The concentration of adenosine in the rectum tended to correlate with the severity of proctitis. After a subcutaneous injection of methotrexate 15 or 25 mg the mean rectal adenosine concentration did not change. Furthermore, the plasma adenosine concentration did not differ significantly from baseline at any time during the 24 h after the methotrexate injection. These data suggest that the in-vivo anti-inflammatory actions of methotrexate are not related to alterations of adenosine metabolism.

Activated T lymphocytes form an important part of the inflammatory infiltrate in IBD, and the major contribution of T lymphocytes in the pathogenesis of mucosal inflammation is highlighted by the many animal models of IBD that occur with various perturbations of T lymphocyte function [164]. The effect of methotrexate on T lymphocyte survival has been studied [165]. Methotrexate-treated T lymphocytes were found to be primed to die by apoptosis when stimulated with mitogens, by a Fas-independent mechanism. Furthermore, the inhibitory effect of methotrexate was confined to cells that were activated at the time of drug exposure. This process was inhibited by fully reduced folate and thymidine, indicating that methotrexate-induced lymphocyte apoptosis was dependent on inhibition of dihydrofolate reductase and thymidylate synthase. These results demonstrate that methotrexate inhibits the activation of T lymphocytes, a process that is likely to be important to this drug's *in-vivo* anti-inflammatory actions.

Pharmacokinetics

For the treatment of chronic inflammatory diseases, such as psoriasis and rheumatoid arthritis, methotrexate has traditionally been given once weekly, because the incidence of hepatotoxicity appeared to be less with this approach than with daily administration [166]. The doses that have been used range from 7.5 to 25 mg per week, usually given orally or by intramuscular injection. When methotrexate was first tried for IBD, this therapeutic regime was empirically adopted [167].

The bioavailability of oral methotrexate is dose-dependent, because the pathways of absorption are saturable, and at higher doses methotrexate induces malabsorption through its antiproliferative effects on epithelia [168]. Reported oral bioavailability at the low doses used in chronic inflammatory diseases range from 50% to 90% [169–171]. Intramuscular and subcutaneous methotrexate exhibit near-complete bioavailability [152, 172]; thus, considering ease of administration, the subcutaneous route is preferred.

After administration, methotrexate is widely distributed and rapidly cleared, mostly in unchanged form by the kidney. However, a small fraction of the drug is concentrated in many cell types as polyglutamated methotrexate. In IBD patients receiving weekly injections of methotrexate, the drug has been shown to gradually accumulate in erythrocytes, reaching a plateau after about 8 weeks (Fig. 6) [173]. Methotrexate also accumulates in many other

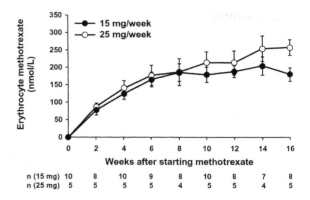

Figure 6. Mean erythrocyte methotrexate concentrations after starting methotrexate 15 mg/week (●) or 25 mg/week (○) by subcutaneous injection. Reproduced with permission from Egan LJ *et al.*, Aliment Pharmacol Ther 1999; 13: 1597–604.

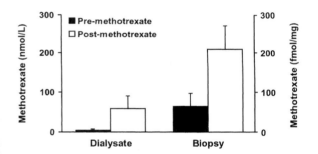

Figure 7. In IBD patients receiving weekly injections of methotrexate the drug can be detected in the rectal lumen and mucosa 7 days after the last dose. The concentration is higher in biopsy material than in dialysate, indicating intracellular concentration of methotrexate. Reproduced with permission from Egan LJ *et al.*, Clin Pharmacol Ther 1999; 65: 29–39.

tissues, including the intestinal mucosa. Methotrexate was easily identified in rectal dialysate and biopsies 7 days after a dose, at a time when plasma methotrexate was barely detectable (Fig. 7). Comparison of rectal lumen and rectal mucosa methotrexate concentrations reveals that the drug is also concentrated intracellularly at this site. The trough rectal mucosa methotrexate concentration was found to be sufficient to exert pharmacologic activity, and this observation thus provides a potential explanation for the continuous activity of methotrexate throughout a 7-day dosing interval [152].

Adverse effects

The long-term use of methotrexate for chronic inflammatory diseases has the potential for serious toxicity. In reported series of IBD patients treated with methotrexate about 10% have discontinued the drug because of suspected drug-induced toxicity [167, 173–179]. The adverse effects of methotrexate can be considered in three categories: predictable dose-related anti-proliferative effects on bone marrow, gut epithelia and hair follicles; idiosyncratic allergic/hypersensitive-type reactions; and hepatic damage due to the cumulative effects of chronic exposure.

Methotrexate inhibits cellular proliferation in a dose-dependent manner, by depleting cells of the fully reduced folate co-factors needed for thymidylate and purine biosynthesis. At the high doses used for cancer chemotherapy, bone marrow depression, gastrointestinal ulceration and stomatitis, and alopecia predictably occur, necessitating 'rescue' with tetrahydrofolate. For effective therapy of chronic inflammatory diseases with methotrexate, it is not clear that overt inhibition of cellular proliferation is required. Consequently, most clinicians regard the occurrence of cytopenias, intestinal distress or alopecia as indicators of unacceptable toxicity, and reduce the dose of methotrexate or co-administer folic acid [156].

Idiosyncratic allergic-type reactions to methotrexate include rash and pneumonitis. Methotrexate-induced lung damage is important, because in the rheumatologic literature this is reported to occur in 3–11% of patients, and has occasionally been fatal [180]. Clinically, methotrexate-induced pneumonitis is characterized by cough, dyspnea, fever, hypoxemia, a restrictive ventilatory defect with impaired gas exchange, and a radiographic picture of a diffuse alveolar/interstitial process. Discontinuation of methotrexate usually results in resolution.

Long-term use of weekly methotrexate is associated with abnormal serum transaminase activity in up to 30% of patients [177, 181]. However, hypertransaminasemia does not correlate well with histologic liver damage. The spectrum of histologic lesions attributed to chronic methotrexate use includes macrovesicular steatosis, hepatocyte necrosis and portal inflammation, progressing to fibrosis and cirrhosis [182]. It has been difficult to determine the true incidence of significant methotrexate-induced liver disease. In studies of psoriasis patients treated with methotrexate, progressive histologic liver damage has been well documented [183, 184].

In one study of 364 liver biopsies from 168 patients with psoriasis, only 50% of patients were without hepatic fibrosis after a cumulative dose of 3 g methotrexate [185]. However, in rheumatoid arthritis, the risk of cirrhosis over 5 years of methotrexate therapy appears to be only 1 in 1000 [186, 187]. Thus, there may be a disease-specific risk for methotrexate liver damage. In addition to the cumulative dose of methotrexate, other identified risk factors for liver damage include heavy alcohol ingestion, obesity and diabetes [185].

Optimizing therapy

The effective and safe use of methotrexate in IBD demands a trade-off between efficacy and toxicity, both of which may be dose-dependent. Studies in rheumatoid arthritis have demonstrated that higher doses of methotrexate are clinically more effective than lower doses [188], and some forms of methotrexate-induced toxicity are clearly dose-dependent. In patients with refractory IBD a 16-week comparison of methotrexate 15 or 25 mg per week did not reveal different rates of efficacy or toxicity between the two doses [173]. Until more data become available the clinical approach is necessarily somewhat empiric. Typically, patients are started on methotrexate 15 or 25 mg per week by subcutaneous injection. Once a satisfactory clinical response occurs the dose is reduced to 15 mg per week. Our proposed guidelines for liver monitoring in methotrexate-treated IBD patients are outlined in Table 4. We advise patients to refrain from alcohol consumption during methotrexate therapy.

Erythrocyte methotrexate concentration reflects intensity of exposure to the drug (Fig. 6). To determine if an association exists between the occurrence of clinical response or drug toxicity and circulating methotrexate concentrations, the mean trough concentrations of erythrocyte and plasma methotrexate, and plasma 7-hydroxymethotrexate were compared in IBD patients who responded or did not respond to weekly methotrexate injections [173]. No significant differences were found, suggesting that this approach to therapeutic drug monitoring of methotrexate in IBD is not helpful.

In cancer chemotherapy, poor outcomes are associated with the development of resistance to methotrexate. Two primary mechanisms have been identified: increased expression of the main target enzyme, dihydrofolate reductase, and increased drug efflux from cells, mediated by expression of the multi-

Table 4. Guidelines for preventing and monitoring hepatotoxicity in IBD patients receiving long-term methotrexate

Baseline		Withhold methotrexate
Liver tests	AST, ALT, ALP, bilirubin Hepatitis B and C tests	If > 2 × normal If actively infected
Liver biopsy	If abnormal AST, ALT, ALP, bilirubin; if clinical suspicion of liver disease	If hepatitis, fibrosis or cirrhosis is present
During treatment		*Stop or reduce methotrexate*
AST	Every 6 weeks	If > 2 × baseline
Liver biopsy	Every cumulative 1.5 g methotrexate; if progressive elevation of AST; if > 50% of AST tests are high	If hepatitis, fibrosis or cirrhosis is present

AST, aspartate aminotransferase; ALT alanine aminotransferase, ALP alkaline phosphatase.

drug resistance pump, p-glycoprotein [189]. It is not known if either of these mechanisms operates in IBD patients who do not respond to methotrexate.

Monoclonal antibody anti-TNF-α therapy

Several observations suggest that TNF-α is an important factor in the pathogenesis of mucosal inflammation [190]. This cytokine is capable of triggering intracellular signaling cascades, such as the NF-κB pathway, that result in an inflammatory phenotype in epithelial cells and cells of the lamina propria. Stool and mucosal levels of TNF-α are elevated in IBD [9, 191–193]. Recently, specific monoclonal antibody therapies to antagonize TNF-α have demonstrated clinical efficacy in CD [194–196].

Structure of monoclonal antibodies and fusion proteins against TNF-α

There are three currently available synthetic anti-TNF-α molecules: two monoclonal antibodies and one fusion protein (Fig. 8). These molecules have been developed with the goal of binding free and membrane-bound TNF-α and thereby preventing the cytokine from binding to its cell-surface receptor and exerting biologic activity. Linkage of the TNF-α binding portions of these molecules to immunoglobulin-like structures slows their clearance from plasma and allows for a variety of effector functions related to the immunoglobulin constant regions,

such as complement fixation and antibody-mediated cellular cytotoxicity.

Infliximab (cA2) is a chimeric mouse–human monoclonal antibody to human TNF-α. This molecule consists of human IgG_1 constant regions, human kappa light chains and transplanted monoclonal murine variable regions that recognize TNF-α with very high affinity [197]. CDP571 is a 'humanized' monoclonal antibody to TNF-α. This molecule consists of human IgG_4 constant regions, human kappa light chains and transplanted complementarity determining regions from a murine monoclonal antibody that recognizes TNF-α, also with very high affinity [198]. Etanercept is a fusion protein that is generated by linking the human p75 TNF-α receptor to the Fc portion of IgG_1 [199].

Pharmacokinetics

Infliximab and CDP571 are administered as intravenous infusions, and etanercept is given by subcutaneous injections. Pharmacokinetic studies of infliximab and CDP571 demonstrate that the plasma concentrations of these monoclonal antibodies are linearly proportional to dose, and that their elimination follows first-order kinetics [198, 200, 201]. At therapeutic doses of 5–10 mg/kg the half-lives of infliximab and CDP571 are in the range of 8–10 days. This results in plasma disappearance of these antibodies after approximately 8–12 weeks. In contrast, the receptor fusion protein etanercept has a shorter plasma existence. After subcutaneous injections of 25 mg etanercept, the median half-life of elimination was approximately 5 days [202].

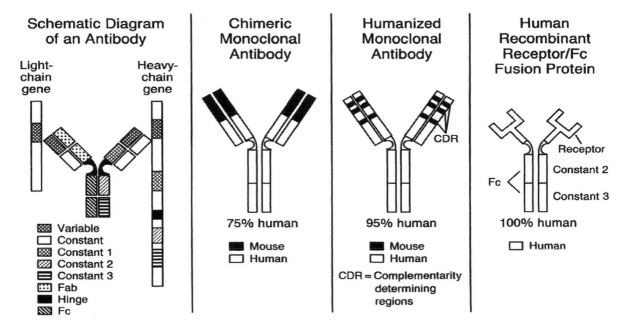

Figure 8. Schematic comparison of the available anti-TNF-α monoclonal antibodies infliximab and CDP571, and the TNF-α receptor–Fc fusion protein, etanercept. Reproduced with permission from Sandborn WJ *et al*, Inflam Bowel Dis 1999; 5: 119–33.

Mechanism of action

The biologic activity of TNF-α is mediated by the binding of soluble trimers of the cytokine, or membrane-bound trimers, to the cell-surface TNF-α receptors, types I and II. Infliximab, CDP571 and etanercept all bind to soluble TNF-α trimers with high affinity (Table 5). As a result serum TNF-α concentrations may actually increase because binding to the long-residing TNF-α antagonist molecules slows clearance [200, 202]. However, the binding of circulating TNF-α by the antagonist molecules prevents the cytokine from binding to its receptors, and thus the biologic activity of TNF-α is effectively neutralized [197, 199, 203, 204].

Membrane-bound TNF-α also exhibits biologic activity. Infliximab, CDP571 and etanercept can bind to this form of TNF-α and probably neutralize its activity. Immunoglobulin isotype is an important determinant of antibody function. For example, antibodies of the IgG_1, but not the IgG_4 isotype, can stimulate secondary effector mechanisms mediated by the Fc portion of the molecule. Fc receptor binding can result in complement activation and antibody-mediated cellular cytotoxicity [205]. In this regard infliximab but not CDP571 or etanercept can generate Fc receptor-dependent effector functions

Table 5. Comparison of the anti-TNF-α activities of infliximab, CDP571 and etanercept

	Binding to soluble TNF-α	Binding to membrane-bound TNF-α	Lysis of cells expressing membrane-bound TNF-α
Infliximab	Yes	Yes	Yes
CDP571	Yes	Probably	No
Etanercept	Yes	Yes	No

resulting in cytotoxicity [206]. This function may in part underlie the effects of infliximab *in vivo*, and thus may represent an important difference from CDP571 and etanercept, which do not appear to cause complement-mediated or antibody-mediated cytotoxicity [202, 205].

In vivo, treatment with infliximab has been demonstrated to down-regulate Th-1 type cytokine production in CD mucosa [10], to decrease the activity of pathways of coagulation and fibrinolysis [207], and to decrease circulating levels of phospholipase A_2. Further, in rheumatoid arthritis patients, infliximab has been shown to decrease circulating IL-1, IL-6, E-selectin, intracellular adhesion molecule-1 and matrix metalloproteinases [208-210]. CDP571 has been shown to decrease IL-1 production in an animal model [211]. Etanercept has been shown to decrease levels of IL-1, IL-6, E-selectin, intracellular adhesion molecule-1 and matrix metalloproteinases [202].

Adverse effects

The most important adverse effects of anti-TNF-α monoclonal antibody and fusion protein therapies are the development of infusion reactions, and induction of treatment-related antibodies. Initial infusions of infliximab have resulted in adverse reactions in approximately 17% of patients, but in only 2% was the reaction severe enough to warrant discontinuation of the infusion [201]. Four percent of patients experienced fever or chills, 1% experienced pruritis or urticaria and 1% experienced cardiopulmonary symptoms such as chest pain, dyspnea or hemodynamic instability. Infusion reactions are more common with the second or subsequent infusions, than with the first. In CD patients who were retreated with infliximab after a break of 2–4 years, 25% experienced adverse reaction that occurred 3–12 days after the infusion. These reactions consisted of myalgia; arthralgia; fever; rash; urticaria; and facial, hand and lip edema. In all cases of infusion reactions to infliximab, symptomatic treatment with antihistamines or corticosteroids resulted in resolution. The development of a reaction to infliximab was more common in CD patients who subsequently had detectable circulating anti-infliximab antibodies (36%) than in those without the antibodies (see below). The incidence of adverse reactions to infusions of CDP571 or to injections of etanercept appears to be less than occurs with infliximab. Thus, the risk of adverse infusion reactions seems to be proportional to the amount of murine protein in the antibody.

Administration of a foreign protein can stimulate development of an immune response directed at exogenous peptide antigens. Thus, it is not surprising that human antibodies that recognize epitopes on the foreign protein have been reported to develop in patients treated with infliximab, CDP571 and etanercept. Anti-infliximab antibodies developed in 10% of CD patients who were receiving concomitant immunosuppressive therapy with azathioprine or 6-mercaptopurine, and in 23% of those who were not [201]. A similar trend was seen in rheumatoid arthritis patients, suggesting that the development of a detectable acquired immune response to infliximab can be retarded by immune suppression. Higher doses of infliximab have been associated with lower rates of development of anti-infliximab antibodies [212]. Antibodies to CDP571 were detected in 35% of CD patients after an infusion [196]. Anti-etanercept antibodies developed in 16% of rheumatoid arthritis patients after receiving this drug. It is presently unclear if these antibodies are clinically significant.

The development of autoantibodies has been reported to occur after treatment with infliximab [201] and etanercept [202]. There are currently no data available on autoantibodies in CDP571-treated patients. After treatment with infliximab, 34% of CD patients developed antinuclear antibodies, and 9% developed antidouble-stranded DNA antibodies. A small minority of these patients developed a lupus-like syndrome that resolved gradually.

A variety of malignant neoplasms have developed in patients who were treated with the anti-TNF-α agents, infliximab and etanercept. However, the numbers have been too small to determine if the risk of cancer is greater than in appropriate control groups.

Optimizing therapy

Currently, infliximab is the preferred anti-TNF-α agent for use in CD. Further studies of CDP571 and etanercept in IBD are awaited. For induction of remission in active inflammatory or fistulizing CD, an initial dose of infliximab, 5 mg/kg is indicated [194, 195]. Because favorable clinical responses to infliximab tend to last only 2–4 months it is our practice to initiate immunosuppressive therapy with azathioprine or 6-mercaptopurine at this time, to act as a long-acting maintenance drug. Methotrexate is probably a good alternative for patients not tolerating azathioprine or 6-mercaptopurine. It is reasonable to retreat patients who do not respond to an initial dose of infliximab after about 4 weeks, because in the fistula study some patients responded only after the second or third dose [195]. Long-term retreatment with infliximab should be reserved for patients who relapse despite concomitant use of a long-acting immunosuppressive agent. The optimum dose and frequency of infliximab infusions for maintenance of remission in CD are not known. However, a recent study of every 8 week doses of infliximab suggested that retreatment may be a reasonable approach in patients who have failed other options.

Cyclosporine and tacrolimus (FK 506)

Chemistry and mechanism of action

Cyclosporine is a cyclic polypeptide of fungal origin, and tacrolimus is a macrolide antibiotic. Although these entities are chemically unrelated their mechanisms of immunosuppression are very similar. Both drugs bind to cytoplasmic proteins; cyclosporine to cyclophilin, and tacrolimus to FK-binding protein. These drug–protein complexes inhibit the cytoplasmic phosphatase calcineurin, an enzyme essential for activation of the T lymphocyte-specific nuclear factor of activated T cells. This transcription factor regulates the rate of transcription of cytokines important in T lymphocyte activation, notably IL-2 and IFN-γ [213]. Through this mechanism cyclosporine and tacrolimus act as powerful and specific inhibitors of T lymphocyte activation.

Pharmacokinetics

Standard cyclosporine is poorly and erratically absorbed, with oral bioavailability of only 20–50%. In patients with small bowel CD absorption may be even lower [214, 215]. The newer microemulsion formulation of cyclosporine is better absorbed by a factor of about two [216]. Tacrolimus is much more potent than cyclosporine. Although oral tacrolimus is also not highly available systemically, it is less dependent than cyclosporine on the presence of bile for absorption.

Adverse effects

Both cyclosporine and tacrolimus have low therapeutic indices. With chronic use of either agent, toxicity is likely to develop. The most frequently reported adverse effects of cyclosporine in IBD patients are paresthesias (26%), hypertrichosis (13%), hypertension (11%), tremor (7%), reversible decline of renal function (6%), headache (5%), and nausea (6%) [217]. The experience with tacrolimus in IBD is much more limited than with cyclosporine, but in addition to the side-effects reported with cyclosporine, hyperglycemia can occur. Rare but potentially life-threatening adverse effects of cyclosporine and tacrolimus include opportunistic infections and malignancies [218, 219].

Optimizing therapy

Optimum use of these powerful immunosuppressives requires a careful consideration of the risk to benefit ratio. There is a significant risk of long-term toxicity with cyclosporine and tacrolimus, and most clinical trials with oral cyclosporine in CD have been negative [220–222]. However, the short-term use of intravenous cyclosporine and tacrolimus has been highly effective in very sick IBD patients [223–226]. For these reasons we rarely initiate cyclosporine or tacrolimus in IBD patients with the anticipation of long-term use.

The key principles to effective and safe cyclosporine and tacrolimus therapy of IBD are use only in highly selected patients, concomitant initiation of safer forms of long-term immune suppression, the use of blood levels to guide dosing, and careful toxicity monitoring. Intravenous cyclosporine has a role in the management of patients with severely active UC who have failed to respond to high-dose intravenous steroids, who do not have colonic dilation or impending perforation, and who are not immediate surgical candidates [223]. In CD patients there are several potential situations in which cyclosporine or tacrolimus may be beneficial. Severely active inflammatory or fistulizing disease without a stricture, that cannot be controlled with intravenous steroids or infliximab, may respond to intravenous cyclosporine or tacrolimus [224, 225]. There is no role for oral cyclosporine or tacrolimus in the long-term management of UC or CD. The use of these rapidly acting drugs should be considered a 'bridge' to the onset of action of a safer, slow-acting immunosuppressive such as azathioprine, 6-mercaptopurine or methotrexate. It is our practice to start one of these agents along with cyclosporine or tacrolimus, and to overlap them for a sufficient duration to allow the slow-acting drug to work.

Monitoring of blood levels is essential during cyclosporine and tacrolimus therapy, because of inter- and intra-individual variation in absorption and metabolism. During intravenous therapy the drug blood levels should be checked daily, at least until a stable dose is achieved. During oral therapy the levels should be checked twice weekly initially and once every 1–2 weeks after a stable dose is achieved. Target blood levels of cyclosporine that correlate with clinical efficacy range from 150 to 300 ng/ml (high-pressure liquid chromatography assay) [217, 224]. Effective tacrolimus concentrations range from 3 to 8 ng/ml [225, 226]. Both cyclosporine and tacrolimus are metabolized by the 3A4 isoform of cytochrome P450. This enzyme is inhibited by grape-fruit juice, so patients should be cautioned against drinking this juice, unless they consume a constant amount on a regular basis, when its use may allow a lower dose of drug to be effective [227]. Toxicity to cyclosporine and tacrolimus often occur at these levels, and dose adjustment may be necessary. Hypo-cholesterolemia should be excluded before initiating cyclosporine [228]. Blood pressure should be checked twice weekly, and serum creatinine, potassium and glucose should be monitored every 1–2 weeks.

Nicotine

Chemistry and mechanism of action

Nicotine is a naturally occurring drug that is an agonist at ganglionic cholinergic receptors. This drug evokes a wide range of pharmacologic effects mediated by binding to receptors in autonomic ganglia, the adrenal medulla, the neuromuscular junction and in the central nervous system. In the gut, nicotine stimulates parasympathetic ganglia to cause increased cholinergic outflow, resulting in elevated smooth muscle tone and motor activity. In UC the therapeutic mechanism of action of nicotine is not known. This drug undoubtedly has profound effects of gastrointestinal motility that may be relevant to its action in UC. However, endoscopic inflammation is reduced by nicotine [229], suggesting an anti-inflammatory effect. In patients with UC, cigarette smoking is associated with decreased colonic production of IL-1, IL-8 and TNF-α [230]. One study has found that colon mucosal expression of IL-8 decreases in UC patients who respond to nicotine patches, but not in those who fail to respond, or who were treated with placebo [231]. Based on our current level of knowledge no firm conclusions can be drawn about the mechanism of nicotine's beneficial action in UC, and more study is needed.

Pharmacokinetics

The systemic bioavailability of nicotine from inhalation and transdermal patch is high, ranging from 75% to 90% [232, 233]. For use with therapeutic intent in UC, high blood levels of nicotine are not desirable because of side-effects. One study has evaluated the bioavailability of nicotine after oral and rectal administration [234]. Both oral and various rectal formulations of nicotine were found to have approximately 20% systemic bioavailability.

A delayed-release formulation of nicotine had a mean oral bioavailability of 40% [235].

Adverse effects

In therapeutic trials for UC, transdermal nicotine has caused considerable side effects [229, 236, 237]. Adverse events occurring more frequently with nicotine than with placebo included dermatitis, dizziness and nausea. The occurrence of side-effects appears to be dose-related, but significant associations with plasma nicotine levels have not been found [229, 234, 236].

Optimizing therapy

Nicotine therapy of UC is hampered by only modest efficacy in the face of considerable dose-limiting toxicity. Ex-smokers seem to be somewhat resistant to the nausea and light-headedness caused by nicotine [236]. Patients who develop UC for the first time, or who experience a disease flare after quitting smoking, may therefore represent a subpopulation that would be more likely to benefit from nicotine. When nicotine patches are prescribed for UC it is wise to start with a low dose, such as 7 mg/day, and gradually titrate the dose upwards according to response. Nicotine doses in the 22–25 mg/day range appear to be most effective. Nicotine is metabolized by the polymorphic cytochrome P450 2A6 enzyme. Individuals with decreased activity of this enzyme metabolize nicotine more slowly than normal, are less likely to become smokers, and when they do smoke they consume less cigarettes [238]. It is not known if nicotine metabolizer status is predictive of clinical outcome in the therapy of UC, but serum nicotine levels did not correlate with response [229]. Thus, there is no role for therapeutic drug monitoring of nicotine in IBD at present.

References

1. Svartz N. Salazopyrine, a new sulfanilamide preparation. Acta Med Scand 1942; 110: 577.
2. Azad Khan AK, Piris J, Truelove SC. An experiment to determine the active therapeutic moiety of sulfasalazine. Lancet 1977; 2: 892–5.
3. van Hees PA, Bakker JH, van Tongeren JH. Effect of sulphapyridine, 5-aminosalicylic acid, and placebo in patients with idiopathic proctitis: a study to determine the active therapeutic moiety of sulphasalazine. Gut 1980; 21: 632–5.
4. Klotz U, Maier K, Fischer C, Heinkel K. Therapeutic efficacy of sulfasalazine and its metabolites in patients with

ulcerative colitis and Crohn's disease. N Engl J Med 1980; 303: 1499–502.

5. Sharon P, Ligumsky M, Rachmilewitz D, Zor U. Role of prostaglandins in ulcerative colitis. Enhanced production during active disease and inhibition by sulfasalazine. Gastroenterology 1978; 75: 638–40.

6. Ligumsky M, Karmeli F, Sharon P, Zor U, Cohen F, Rachmilewitz D. Enhanced thromboxane A2 and prostacyclin production by cultured rectal mucosa in ulcerative colitis and its inhibition by steroids and sulfasalazine. Gastroenterology 1981; 81: 444–9.

7. Punchard NA, Boswell DJ, Greenfield SM, Thompson RP. The effects of sulphasalazine and its metabolites on prostaglandin production by human mononuclear cells. Biochem Pharmacol 1992; 43: 2369–76.

8. Hawkey CJ, Broughton-Smith NK, Whittle BJR. Modulation of human colonic arachadonic acid metabolism by sulphasalazine. Dig Dis Sci 1985; 30: 1161–5.

9. Isaacs KL, Sartor RB, Haskill S. Cytokine messenger RNA profiles in inflammatory bowel disease mucosa detected by polymerase chain reaction amplification. Gastroenterology 1992; 103: 1587–95.

10. Plevy SE, Landers CJ, Prehn J et al. A role for TNF-alpha and mucosal T helper-1 cytokines in the pathogenesis of Crohn's disease. J Immunol 1997; 159: 6276–82.

11. Schreiber S, Nikolaus S, Hampe J. Activation of nuclear factor kappa B inflammatory bowel disease. Gut 1998; 42: 477–84.

12. Rogler G, Brand K, Vogl D et al. Nuclear factor kappa B is activated in macrophages and epithelial cells of inflamed intestinal mucosa. Gastroenterology 1998; 115: 357–69.

13. Neurath MF, Pettersson S, Meyer zum Buschenfelde KH, Strober W. Local administration of antisense phosphorothioate oligonucleotides to the p65 subunit of NF-kappa B abrogates established experimental colitis in mice. Nat Med 1996; 2: 998–1004.

14. Thiele K, Bierhaus A, Autschbach F et al. Cell specific effects of glucocorticoid treatment on the NF-kappaBp65/IkappaBalpha system in patients with Crohn's disease. Gut 1999; 45: 693–704.

15. Barnes PJ, Karin M. Nuclear factor kappa B – a pivotal transcription factor in chronic inflammatory diseases. N Engl J Med 1997; 336: 1066–71.

16. Kopp E, Ghosh S. Inhibition of NF-kB by sodium salicylate and aspirin. Science 1994; 265: 956–8.

17. Wahl C, Liptay S, Adler G, Schmid RM. Sulfasalazine: a potent and specific inhibitor of nuclear factor kappa B. J Clin Invest 1998; 101: 1163–74.

18. Egan LJ, Mays DC, Huntoon CJ et al. Inhibition of interleukin-1-stimulated NF-kappaB RelA/p65 phosphorylation by mesalamine is accompanied by decreased transcriptional activity. J Biol Chem 1999; 274: 26448–53.

19. Kaiser GC, Yan F, Polk DB. Mesalamine blocks tumor necrosis factor growth inhibition and nuclear factor kappaB activation in mouse colonocytes. Gastroenterology 1999; 116: 602–9.

20. Shanahan F, Niederlehner A, Carramanzana N, Anton P. Sulfasalazine inhibits the binding of TNF alpha to its receptor. Immunopharmacology 1990; 20: 217–24.

21. Crotty B, Rosenberg WM, Aronson JK, Jewell DP. Inhibition of binding of interferon-gamma to its receptor by salicylates used in inflammatory bowel disease. Gut 1992; 33: 1353–7.

22. Lauritsen K, Laursen LS, Bukhave K, Rask-Madsen J. Effects of topical 5-aminosalicylic acid and prednisolone on prostaglandin E2 and leukotriene B4 levels determined by equilibrium *in vivo* dialysis of rectum in relapsing ulcerative colitis. Gastroenterology 1986; 91: 837–44.

23. Roberts WG, Simon TJ, Berlin RG et al. Leukotrienes in ulcerative colitis: results of a multicenter trial of a leukotriene biosynthesis inhibitor, MK-591. Gastroenterology 1997; 112: 725–32.

24. Dallegri F, Ottonello L, Ballestrero A, Bogliolo F, Ferrando F, Patrone F. Cytoprotection against neutrophil derived hypochlorous acid: a potential mechanism for the therapeutic action of 5-aminosalicylic acid in ulcerative colitis. Gut 1990; 31: 184–6.

25. Sandoval M, Liu X, Mannick EE, Clark DA, Miller MJ. Peroxynitrite-induced apoptosis in human intestinal epithelial cells is attenuated by mesalamine. Gastroenterology 1997; 113: 1480–8.

26. Burress GC, Musch MW, Jurivich DA, Welk J, Chang EB. Effects of mesalamine on the hsp72 stress response in rat IEC-18 intestinal epithelial cells. Gastroenterology 1997; 113: 1474–9.

27. Yu DK, Elvin AT, Morrill B et al. Effect of food coadministration on 5-aminosalicylic acid oral suspension bioavailability. Clin Pharmacol Ther 1990; 48: 26–33.

28. Almer S, Norlander B, Strom M, Osterwald H. Steady-state pharmacokinetics of a new 4-g 5-aminosalicylic acid retention enema in patients with ulcerative colitis in remission. Scand J Gastroenterol 1991; 26: 327–35.

29. Klotz U. Clinical pharmacokinetics of sulphasalazine, its metabolites and other prodrugs of 5-aminosalicylic acid. Clin Pharmacokinet 1985; 10: 285–302.

30. Staerk Laursen L, Stokholm M, Bukhave K, Rask-Madsen J, Lauritsen K. Disposition of 5-aminosalicylic acid by olsalazine and three mesalazine preparations in patients with ulcerative colitis: comparison of intraluminal colonic concentrations, serum values, and urinary excretion. Gut 1990; 31: 1271–6.

31. Stretch GL, Campbell BJ, Dwarakanath AD et al. 5-Amino salicylic acid absorption and metabolism in ulcerative colitis patients receiving maintenance sulphasalazine, olsalazine or mesalazine. Aliment Pharmacol Ther 1996; 10: 941–7.

32. Gionchetti P, Campieri M, Venturi A et al. Systemic availability of 5-aminosalicylic acid: comparison of delayed release and an azo-bond preparation. Aliment Pharmacol Ther 1996; 10: 601–5.

33. Goebell H, Klotz U, Nehlsen B, Layer P. Oroileal transit of slow release 5-aminosalicylic acid. Gut 1993; 34: 669–75.

34. Norlander B, Gotthard R, Strom M. Pharmacokinetics of a 5-aminosalicylic acid enteric-coated tablet in patients with Crohn's disease or ulcerative colitis and in healthy volunteers. Aliment Pharmacol Ther 1990; 4: 497–505.

35. Layer PH, Goebell H, Keller J, Dignass A, Klotz U. Delivery and fate of oral mesalamine microgranules within the human small intestine. Gastroenterology 1995; 108: 1427–33.

36. Yu DK, Morrill B, Eichmeier LS et al. Pharmacokinetics of 5-aminosalicylic acid from controlled-release capsules in man. Eur J Clin Pharmacol 1995; 48: 273–7.

37. Lauritsen K, Hansen J, Ryde M, Rask-Madsen J. Colonic azodisalicylate metabolism determined by *in vivo* dialysis in healthy volunteers and patients with ulcerative colitis. Gastroenterology 1984; 86: 1496–500.

38. Dew MJ, Ebden P, Kidwai NS, Lee G, Evans BK, Rhodes J. Comparison of the absorption and metabolism of sulphasalazine and acrylic-coated 5-amino salicylic acid in normal subjects and patients with colitis. Br J Clin Pharmacol 1984; 17: 474–6.

39. Sutherland SR, May GR, Schaffer GA. Sulfasalazine revisited: a meta-analysis of 5-aminosalicylic acid in the treatment of ulcerative colitis. Ann Intern Med 1993; 118: 540.

40. Gionchetti P, Venturi A, Rizzello F et al. Retrograde colonic spread of a new mesalazine rectal enema in patients with

119. Corrigan CJ, Brown PH, Barnes NC, Tsai JJ, Frew AJ, Kay AB. Glucocorticoid resistance in chronic asthma. Peripheral blood T lymphocyte activation and comparison of the T lymphocyte inhibitory effects of glucocorticoids and cyclosporin A. Am Rev Respir Dis 1991; 144: 1026–32.

120. Lane SJ, Adcock IM, Richards D, Hawrylowicz C, Barnes PJ, Lee TH. Corticosteroid resistant bronchial asthma is associated with increased *c-fos* expression in monocutes and T lymphocytes. J Clin Invest 1998; 102: 2156–64.

121. Franchimont D, Louis E, Dupont P et al. Decreased corticosensitivity in quiescent Crohn's disease: an *ex vivo* study using whole blood cell cultures. Dig Dis Sci 1999; 44: 1208–15.

122. Hearing SD, Norman M, Probert CS, Haslam N, Dayan CM. Predicting therapeutic outcome in severe ulcerative colitis by measuring *in vitro* steroid sensitivity of proliferating peripheral blood lymphocytes. Gut 1999; 45: 382–8.

123. Lennard L. The clinical pharmacology of 6-mercaptopurine. Eur J Clin Pharmacol 1992; 43: 329–39.

124. Van Os EC, Zins BJ, Sandborn WJ et al. Azathioprine pharmacokinetics after intravenous, oral, delayed release oral and rectal foam administration. Gut 1996; 39: 63–8.

125. Lennard L, Brown CB, Fox M, Maddocks JL. Azathioprine metabolism in kidney transplant recipients. Br J Clin Pharmacol 1984; 18: 693–700.

126. Sandborn WJ, Tremaine WJ, Wolf DC et al. Lack of effect of intravenous administration on time to respond to azathioprine for steroid-treated Crohn's disease. North American Azathioprine Study Group. Gastroenterology 1999; 117: 527–35.

127. Lennard L. Clinical implications of thiopurine methyltransferase – optimization of drug dosage and potential drug interactions. Ther Drug Monit 1998; 20: 527–31.

128. Bergan S, Rugstad HE, Bentdal O, Stokke O. Monitoring of azathioprine treatment by determination of 6-thioguanine nucleotide concentrations in erythrocytes. Transplantation 1994; 58: 803–8.

129. Pearson DC, May GR, Fick GH, Sutherland LR. Azathioprine and 6-mercaptopurine in Crohn disease. A meta-analysis. Ann Intern Med 1995; 122: 132–42.

130. Sandborn WJ, Van O, EC, Zins BJ, Tremaine WJ, Mays DC, Lipsky JJ. An intravenous loading dose of azathioprine decreases the time to response in patients with Crohn's disease. Gastroenterology 1995; 109: 1808–17.

131. Weinshilboum RM, Sladek SL. Mercaptopurine pharmacogenetics: monogenic inheritance of erythrocyte thiopurine methyltransferase activity. Am J Hum Genet 1980; 32: 651–62.

132. Weinshilboum R. Methyltransferase pharmacogenetics. Pharmacol Ther 1989; 43: 77–90.

133. Lennard L, Van Loon JA, Lilleyman JS, Weinshilboum RM. Thiopurine pharmacogenetics in leukemia: correlation of erythrocyte thiopurine methyltransferase activity and 6-thioguanine nucleotide concentrations. Clin Pharmacol Ther 1987; 41: 18–25.

134. Present DH, Meltzer SJ, Krumholz MP, Wolke A, Korelitz BI. 6-Mercaptopurine in the management of inflammatory bowel disease: short- and long-term toxicity. Ann Intern Med 1989; 111: 641–9.

135. Connell WR, Kamm MA, Ritchie JK, Lennard-Jones JE. Bone marrow toxicity caused by azathioprine in inflammatory bowel disease: 27 years of experience. Gut 1993; 34: 1081–5.

136. Bouhnik Y, Lemann M, Mary JY et al. Long-term follow-up of patients with Crohn's disease treated with azathioprine or 6-mercaptopurine. Lancet 1996; 347: 215–19.

137. Connell WR, Kamm MA, Dickson M, Balkwill AM, Ritchie JK, Lennard-Jones JE. Long-term neoplasia risk after azathioprine treatment in inflammatory bowel disease. Lancet 1994; 343: 1249–52.

138. Larvol L, Soule JC, Tourneau AL. Reversible lymphoma in the setting of azathioprine therapy for Crohn's disease. N Engl J Med 1994; 331: 883–4.

139. Krynetski EY, Tai HL, Yates CR et al. Genetic polymorphism of thiopurine *S*-methyltransferase: clinical importance and molecular mechanisms. Pharmacogenetics 1996; 6: 279–90.

140. Lennard L, Lilleyman JS, Van Loon J, Weinshilboum RM. Genetic variation in response to 6-mercaptopurine for childhood acute lymphoblastic leukaemia. Lancet 1990; 336: 225–9.

141. Lilleyman JS, Lennard L. Mercaptopurine metabolism and risk of relapse in childhood lymphoblastic leukaemia. Lancet 1994; 343: 1188–90.

142. Cuffari C, Theoret Y, Latour S, Seidman G. 6-Mercaptopurine metabolism in Crohn's disease: correlation with efficacy and toxicity. Gut 1996; 39: 401–6.

143. Dubinsky MC, Lamothe S, Yang HY et al. Optimizing and individualizing 6-MP therapy in IBD: the role of 6-MP metabolite levels and TPMT genotyping. Gastroenterology 1999; 116: A702.

144. Dubinsky M, Hassard P, Yang HY et al. 6-MP metabolite levels correlate with clinical response and drug toxicity in adult IBD. Am J Gastroenterol 1999; 94: 2641.

145. Cuffari C, Sharma S. 6-Mercaptopurine metabolite levels tailored to achieve clinical responsiveness in pediatric Crohn's disease. Gastroenterology 1999; 116: A694.

146. Lowry PW, Franklin CL, Weaver AL et al. Measurement of thiopurine methyltransferase activity and azathioprine metabolites in patients with inflammatory bowel disease. Gut 2001; 49: 665–70.

147. Colonna T, Korelitz BI. The role of leukopenia in the 6-mercaptopurine-induced remission of refractory Crohn's disease. Am J Gastroenterol 1994; 89: 362–6.

148. Barbe L, Matyeau P, Lemann M et al. Dose raising of azathioprine beyond 2.5 mg/kg/day in Crohn's disease patients who fail to improve with a standard dose. Gastroenterology 1998; 114: A925.

149. Jolivet J, Schilsky RL, Bailey BD, Drake JC, Chabner BA. Synthesis, retention, and biological activity of methotrexate polyglutamates in cultured human breast cancer cells. J Clin Invest 1982; 70: 351–60.

150. Allegra CJ, Drake JC, Jolivet J, Chabner BA. Inhibition of phosphoribosylaminoimidazolecarboxamide transformylase by methotrexate and dihydrofolic acid polyglutamates. Proc Natl Acad Sci USA 1985; 82: 4881–5.

151. Baggott JE, Vaughn WH, Hudson BB. Inhibition of 5-aminoimidazole-4-carboxamide ribotide transformylase, adenosine deaminase and 5′-adenylate deaminase by polyglutamates of methotrexate and oxidized folates and by 5-aminoimidazole-4-carboxamide riboside and ribotide. Biochem J 1986; 236: 193–200.

152. Egan LJ, Sandborn WJ, Mays DC, Tremaine WJ, Fauq AH, Lipsky JJ. Systemic and intestinal pharmacokinetics of methotrexate in patients with inflammatory bowel disease. Clin Pharmacol Ther 1999; 65: 29–39.

153. Jolivet J, Chabner BA. Intracellular pharmacokinetics of methotrexate polyglutamates in human breast cancer cells. Selective retention and less dissociable binding of 4-NH2-10-CH3-pteroylglutamate4 and 4-NH2- 10-CH3-pteroylglutamate5 to dihydrofolate reductase. J Clin Invest 1983; 72: 773–8.

154. Weinstein GD, Jeffes E, McCullough JL. Cytotoxic and immunologic effects of methotrexate in psoriasis. J Invest Dermatol 1990; 95: 49–52S.

155. Olsen NJ, Murray LM. Antiproliferative effects of methotrexate on peripheral blood mononuclear cells. Arthritis Rheum 1989; 32: 378–85.

156. Morgan SL, Baggott JE, Vaughn WH *et al.* Supplementation with folic acid during methotrexate therapy for rheumatoid arthritis. A double-blind, placebo-controlled trial. Ann Intern Med 1994; 121: 833–41.

157. Sperling RI, Benincaso AI, Anderson RJ, Coblyn JS, Austen KF, Weinblatt ME. Acute and chronic suppression of leukotriene B4 synthesis *ex vivo* in neutrophils from patients with rheumatoid arthritis beginning treatment with methotrexate. Arthritis Rheum 1992; 35: 376–84.

158. Thomas R, Carroll GJ. Reduction of leukocyte and interleukin-1 beta concentrations in the synovial fluid of rheumatoid arthritis patients treated with methotrexate. Arthritis Rheum 1993; 36: 1244–52.

159. Crilly A, McInness IB, McDonald AG, Watson J, Capell HA, Madhok R. Interleukin 6 (IL-6) and soluble IL-2 receptor levels in patients with rheumatoid arthritis treated with low dose oral methotrexate. J Rheumatol 1995; 22: 224–6.

160. Cronstein BN, Eberle MA, Gruber HE, Levin RI. Methotrexate inhibits neutrophil function by stimulating adenosine release from connective tissue cells. Proc Natl Acad Sci USA 1991; 88: 2441–5.

161. Cronstein BN, Naime D, Ostad E. The antiinflammatory mechanism of methotrexate. Increased adenosine release at inflamed sites diminishes leukocyte accumulation in an in vivo model of inflammation. J Clin Invest 1993; 92: 2675–82.

162. Asako II, Wolf RE, Granger DN. Leukocyte adherence in rat mesenteric venules: effects of adenosine and methotrexate. Gastroenterology 1993; 104: 31–7.

163. Egan LJ, Sandborn WJ, Mays DC, Tremaine WJ, Lipsky JJ. Plasma and rectal adenosine in inflammatory bowel disease: effect of methotrexate. Inflam Bowel Dis 1999; 5: 167–73.

164. Elson CO, Sartor RB, Tennyson GS, Riddell RH. Experimental models of inflammatory bowel disease. Gastroenterology 1995; 109: 1344–67.

165. Genestier L, Paillot R, Fournel S, Ferraro C, Miossec P, Revillard J-P. Immunosuppressive properties of methotrexate: apoptosis and clonal deletion of activated peripheral T cells. J Clin Invest 1998; 102: 322–8.

166. Dahl MGG, Gregory MM, Scheurer PJ. Methotrexate hepatotoxicity in psoriasis. Comparison of different dose regimens. Br Med J 1972: 654–56.

167. Kozarek RA, Patterson DJ, Gelfand MD, Botoman VA, Ball TJ, Wilske KR. Methotrexate induces clinical and histologic remission in patients with refractory inflammatory bowel disease. Ann Intern Med 1989; 110: 353–6.

168. Phelan MJ, Taylor W, van Heyningen C, Williams E, Thompson RN. Intestinal absorption in patients with rheumatoid arthritis treated with methotrexate. Clin Rheumatol 1993; 12: 223–5.

169. Teresi ME, Crom WR, Choi KE, Mirro J, Evans WE. Methotrexate bioavailability after oral and intramuscular administration in children. J Pediatr 1987; 110: 788–92.

170. Jundt JW, Browne BA, Fiocco GP, Steele AD, Mock D. A comparison of low dose methotrexate bioavailability: oral solution, oral tablet, subcutaneous and intramuscular dosing. J Rheumatol 1993; 20: 1845–9.

171. Oguey D, Kolliker F, Gerber NJ, Reichen J. Effect of food on the bioavailability of low-dose methotrexate in patients with rheumatoid arthritis. Arthritis Rheum 1992; 35: 611–14.

172. Seideman P, Beck O, Eksborg S, Wennberg M. The pharmacokinetics of methotrexate and its 7-hydroxy metabolite in patients with rheumatoid arthritis. Br J Clin Pharmacol 1993; 35: 409–12.

173. Egan LJ, Sandborn WJ, Tremaine WJ *et al.* A randomized dose-response and pharmacokinetic study of methotrexate for refractory inflammatory Crohn's disease and ulcerative colitis. Aliment Pharmacol Ther 1999; 13: 1597–604.

174. Baron TH, Truss CD, Elson CO. Low-dose oral methotrexate in refractory inflammatory bowel disease. Dig Dis Sci 1993; 38: 1851–6.

175. Lemann M, Chamiot-Prieur C, Mesnard B *et al.* Methotrexate for the treatment of refractory Crohn's disease. Aliment Pharmacol Ther 1996; 10: 309–14.

176. Arora S, Katkov WN, Cooley J *et al.* A double-blind, randomized, placebo-controlled trial of methotrexate in Crohn's disease. Gastroenterology 1992; 102: A591.

177. Feagan BG, Rochon J, Fedorak RN *et al.* Methotrexate for the treatment of Crohn's disease. The North American Crohn's Study Group Investigators. N Engl J Med 1995; 332: 292–7.

178. Oren R, Arber N, Odes S *et al.* Methotrexate for chronic ulcerative colitis: a double-blind, randomized, Israeli multicenter trial. Gastroenterology 1996; 110: 1416–21.

179. Oren R, Moshkowitz M, Odes S *et al.* Methotrexate in chronic active Crohn's disease: a double-blind, randomized, Israeli multicenter trial. Am J Gastroenterol 1997; 92: 2203–9.

180. Goodman TA, Polisson RP. Methotrexate: adverse reactions and major toxicities.. Rheum Dis Clin N Am 1994; 20: 513–28.

181. Kremer JM, Alarcon GS, Lightfoot RW, Jr. *et al.* Methotrexate for rheumatoid arthritis. Suggested guidelines for monitoring liver toxicity. American College of Rheumatology. Arthritis Rheum 1994; 37: 316–28.

182. Podurgiel BJ, McGill DB, Ludwig J, Taylor WF, Muller SA. Liver injury associated with methotrexate therapy for psoriasis. Mayo Clin Proc 1973; 48: 787–92.

183. Zachariae H, Kragballe K, Thestrup-Pedersen K, Kissmeyer-Nielsen F. HLA antigens in methotrexate-induced liver cirrhosis. Acta Dermato-Venereol 1980; 60: 165–6.

184. Nyfors A, Poulsen H. Liver biopsies from psoriatics related to methotrexate therapy. 2. Findings before and after methotexate therapy in 88 patients. A blind study. Acta Pathol Microbiol Scand Pathol 1976; 84: 262–70.

185. Newman M, Auerbach R, Feiner H *et al.* The role of liver biopsies in psoriatic patients receiving long-term methotrexate treatment. Improvement in liver abnormalities after cessation of treatment. Arch Dermatol 1989; 125: 1218–24.

186. Lewis JH, Schiff E. Methotrexate-induced chronic liver injury: guidelines for detection and prevention. The ACG Committee on FDA-related matters. American College of Gastroenterology. Am J Gastroenterol 1988; 83: 1337–45.

187. Walker AM, Funch D, Dreyer NA *et al.* Determinants of serious liver disease among patients receiving low-dose methotrexate for rheumatoid arthritis. Arthritis Rheum 1993; 36: 329–35.

188. Seideman P. Methotrexate – the relationship between dose and clinical effect. Br J Rheumatol 1993; 32: 751–3.

189. Gorlick R, Goker E, Trippett T, Waltham M, Banerjee D, Bertino JR. Intrinsic and acquired resistance to methotrexate in acute leukemia. N Engl J Med 1996; 335: 1041–8.

190. Van Deventer SJ. Tumour necrosis factor and Crohn's disease. Gut 1997; 40: 443–8.

191. Braegger CP, Nicholls S, Murch SH, Stephens S, MacDonald TT. Tumour necrosis factor alpha in stool as a marker of intestinal inflammation. Lancet 1992; 339: 89–91.

192. Nicholls S, Stephens S, Braegger CP, Walker-Smith JA, MacDonald TT. Cytokines in stools of children with inflammatory bowel disease or infective diarrhoea. J Clin Pathol 1993; 46: 757–60.

193. Cappello M, Keshav S, Prince C, Jewell DP, Gordon S. Detection of mRNAs for macrophage products in inflam-

26 | Multi-site therapeutic modalities for inflammatory bowel diseases – mechanisms of action

GERHARD ROGLER

Introduction

Genetic susceptibilities such as the recently identified polymorphisms in the *NOD2* gene, as well as environmental factors such as certain bacteria, play a role in the etiology of inflammatory bowel diseases (IBD). Over the years many factors have been identified that contribute to the pathogenesis and the process of inflammation in Crohn's disease (CD) and ulcerative colitis (UC), leading to new therapeutic concepts. Among these contributing factors are cytokines and chemokines, as well as adhesion molecules, which are relevant for the emigration of immune cells into the intestinal mucosa. Mucosal *and* systemic concentrations of many proinflammatory cytokines are elevated in IBD. An inadequate, and/or prolonged activation of the intestinal immune system plays an important role in the pathophysiology of chronic mucosal inflammation. An 'imbalance' between proinflammatory and anti-inflammatory cytokines has been described in the inflamed mucosa of patients with CD and UC.

Many, if not all, of the involved cytokine-mediated pathways have back-up systems. Therefore a therapeutic intervention at a particular, singular, very specific point in the complex network of cytokine and chemokine interactions with each other or their receptors is frequently less likely to be successful than a multi-site targeted anti-inflammatory strategy [1].

Even when the etiology of IBD is completely elucidated a causative therapy might not be possible, and the multi-site anti-inflammatory strategy could still be favorable. Therefore the improvement of 'classic' multi-site targeted anti-inflammatory therapies, as well as the development of new concepts for this approach, is of great importance for the future management of patients with IBD. The improvement of 'classic' concepts and therapies is necessary, as so far no therapeutic strategy has proved successful in all patients. Clinically we observe a 'resistance' of a certain percentage of patients to any particular therapy. An important goal for the future must be a better understanding of mechanisms leading to a relative resistance to classic multi-site anti-inflammatory strategies. This would allow the early identification of patients who are not likely to respond to a treatment modality, would avoid frustrating treatments for the patient and the physician, and could allow more specific concepts for the individual patient. To understand the mechanisms of resistance to a particular multi-site targeted anti-inflammatory therapy we first have to understand the molecular and cellular mechanisms involved in an effective therapy. Important insights into a number of those mechanisms of drug action have been made in the last two decades.

A classic example for a multi-site targeting anti-inflammatory treatment is therapy with glucocorticoids. Therefore the principles of glucocorticoid therapy, the structure of the effect-mediating receptor, the molecular mechanisms of action and the effects on the cellular levels will be highlighted first in this chapter. The glucocorticoid receptor (GR) is a member of a family of receptors, the so-called nuclear receptor superfamily, which shares structural and functional similarities. Other members of this family are the peroxisome proliferation-activated receptors (PPAR). Ligands to PPARγ have recently been shown to be effective in animal models of IBD whereas potential ligands of PPAR-α were beneficial in a clinical study in active IBD. The inhibition of the proinflammatory transcription factor nuclear factor kappa B (NF-κB) is likely to be the most important target of glucocorticoid therapy as well as PPAR-mediated effects. Therefore, finally the mechanisms and pathways of NF-κB activation, as well as the consequences of NF-κB inhibition, will be explained.

Stephan R. Targan, Fergus Shanahan and Loren C. Karp (eds.), Inflammatory Bowel Disease: From Bench to Bedside, 2nd Edition, 523–551.
© 2003 *Kluwer Academic Publishers. Printed in Great Britain*

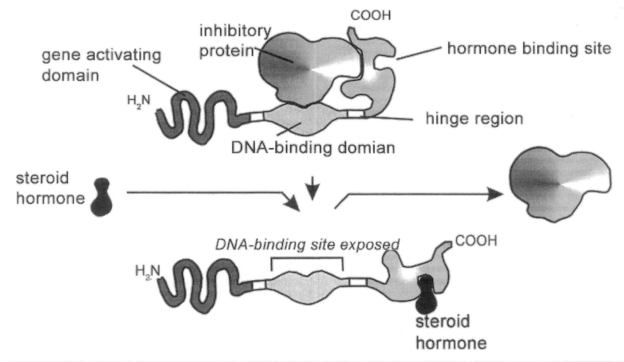

Figure 2. Molecular structure of the glucocorticoid receptor. The N-terminal part of GR contains a *trans*-activation domain that plays an important role in gene regulation. The DNA binding site (DBD) consists of two zinc-finger domains and contains an invariant pattern of eight cysteins arranged in two groups of four. Between the DBD and the carboxyl-terminal ligand binding domain (LBD) is a so-called 'hinge region'. This region of the GR protein contains a nuclear localization signal, a binding region for heat-shock protein 90 (hsp90) and a second *trans*-activating domain. The C-terminal LBD not only represents the specific binding sites for glucocorticoids but also serves as a homodimerization domain. Additionally it interacts with other proteins regulating GR activity. The inactivated GR is bound to a protein complex of approximately 300 kDa including two molecules of hsp90. The hsp90 proteins cover the nuclear localization site preventing the unliganded GR from localizing to the nuclear compartment. After binding of the specific ligand to the LBD the tertiary structure of the molecule changes, followed by a release of hsp90 from the complex.

Molecular mechanisms of glucocorticoid receptor action

Activated and nuclear-translocated GR can act in two principal ways. It can mediate *trans*-activation of gene transcription leading to an increased mRNA expression or *trans*-repression followed by a down-regulation of shut-off of a certain gene product.

Transactivation

In the nucleus GR can bind to classical GRE to activate transcription of the response gene [61–63] (Fig. 3A). The GRE has a palindromic motif (consensus sequence: **GGT ACA** NNN **TGT TCT**). Usually GR binds this or similar DNA sequences cooperatively as a homodimer (Fig. 3A). For homo-dimerization interaction of a group of five AA known as the dimerization or D loop is needed. They are located within the DBD of the GR molecule and are essential for dimerization and transcriptional activation.

A direct *trans*-activation of gene transcription by GR has been described for *IL-1 type II receptor* that binds IL-1 without induction of signal transduction, thus preventing cells from activation and inflammatory reaction [64–67] (Fig. 3A). Another important protein whose transcription is *trans*-activated by GR is IκBα, the inhibitory protein for the proinflammatory transcription factor NF-κB (see below).

For other genes such as *serine protease inhibitor 3* or *arginase* a cooperative *trans*-activation involving GR and another transcription factor such as C/EBP or AP-1 has been described (Fig. 3B). This means that binding of activated and translocated GR is necessary but not sufficient for the increased transcription of these genes. However, as soon as both, GR and the cooperating transcription factor (C/EBP or AP-1) are bound to the promoter, increased gene-transcription takes place.

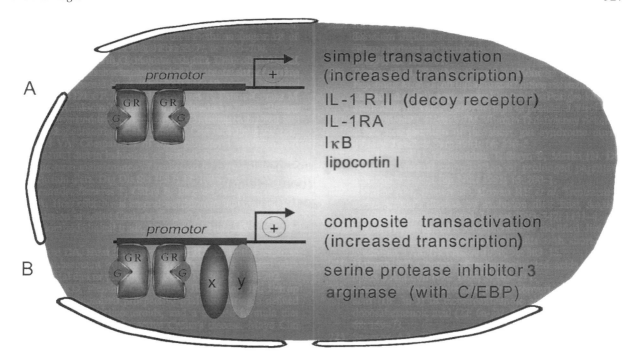

Figure 3. *Trans*-activation of gene transcription by glucocorticoid receptor. **A**: GR binds as a homodimer to classical GRE to activate transcription of response genes. The GRE has a palindromic motif (consensus sequence: **GGT ACA** NNN **TGT TCT**). A direct *trans*-activation of gene transcription by GR has been described for IL-1 type II, IκB, IL-1 RA or lipocortin I. **B**: For other genes such as serine protease inhibitor 3 or arginase a cooperative *trans*-activation involving GR and other transcription factors like C/EBP has been described.

GR-mediated *trans*-activation of genes is also involved in the induction of apoptosis in T cells by dexamethasone [68–78]. The detailed mechanisms mediating the induction of apoptosis are not yet elucidated.

In addition to these *trans*-activating actions described, which usually take several hours, GR have more rapid *trans*-repressing activities.

Trans-repression via DNA binding

After characterization of positive transcriptional regulating GRE the existence of negative GRE sites (nGRE) mediating a negative regulation of transcription (*trans*-repression) via glucocorticoids was postulated [63]. However, the concept of a nGRE site is still a matter of discussion, as the consensus binding site is variable and described for only a few genes [13]. A binding to a promoter sequence and subsequent *trans*-repression by GR has been shown for the *pro-opiomelanocortin (POMC)* gene, an ACTH precursor allowing a negative feedback circle [79, 80] (Fig. 4A). Another promoter containing a negative GR binding site (at –278 to –249 of the

promoter) is the *corticotropin-releasing hormone* (CRH) promoter [81, 82]. Thus it seems that direct *trans*-repression activity is reserved for the negative feedback circle in the hypothalamic–pituitary–adrenal axis.

GR and *trans*-activating transcription factors may also compete for binding sites in promoters [83]. In this case the presence of GR blocks *trans*-activation by another factor and does not actively *trans*-repress transcription itself (Fig. 4B). In the *osteocalcin* promoter GR overlaps the TATA box. Activation and nuclear translocation of GR can therefore prevent the binding of the basal transcription factor, TATA-binding protein (TBP), which is necessary for the recruitment of RNA polymerase II and initiation of transcription [84]. This may be one of the reasons for the occurrence of osteoporosis during long-term glucocorticoid therapy.

Trans-repression without DNA binding

Besides the competition for binding sites in promoters a *trans*-repression mechanism for GR has been described that does not involve DNA binding (Fig.

Regulation of glucocorticoid receptor in IBD

The regulation of GR action and the mechanisms involved in its function are complex. Investigations on possible mechanisms of steroid-refractory IBD are still at early stages. The few studies raise more questions than they answer. Hsp90 has some features of an inhibitory protein of GR and is bound to its inactive form (see above). The expression of human hsp90 in patients with CD and UC was studied; however, no differences between patients and controls were found, making a role of hsp90 in glucocorticoid-refractory IBD unlikely [134].

The number and dissociation constant (K_d) of GR in peripheral blood mononuclear cells of six non-responders of glucocorticoid treatment with UC, five responders and 10 healthy controls was determined in another study [135]. A significant increase in the number of binding sites and the dissociation constant in non-responders compared to responders was found. Surprisingly the number of binding sites was highest in non-responders.

When GR levels were determined via dexamethasone binding only in the cytosolic fraction to ensure that only free receptor and not already steroid-associated, translocated receptor molecules could bind [^{3}H]dexamethasone, the situation seemed to be different. The dexamethasone binding in cytosol isolated from peripheral blood mononuclear cells (PBMNC) of corticosteroid-treated IBD patients was significantly lower compared to controls and IBD patients not treated with glucocorticoid [136]. Systemic GR levels in untreated IBD patients did not differ significantly from controls [136]. There was no difference in the binding affinity of patients and control, with an obvious lower binding maximum indicating a reduced receptor number in the steroid-treated patients group, which is in contrast to the results reported by Shimada *et al.* In contrast to the findings in PBMNC mucosal GR levels of IBD patients were significantly decreased in both steroid-treated and untreated patients compared to controls [136].

The reduced binding of [^{3}H]dexamethasone in cytosol from steroid-treated IBD patients is most likely due to a feedback regulation of GR in the cells by the ligand. This assumption is supported by a number of studies [137–139]. The data indicate that, in contrast to patients with rheumatoid arthritis or other connective tissue diseases in IBD, there is no difference in systemic GR levels between patients not treated with glucocorticoids and controls. This could mean that a localized inflammation in the intestinal mucosa is not followed by a systemic depression of GR levels in leukocytes.

Honda and co-workers studied the expression of GRα and GRβ in PBMNC of patients with UC and controls [140]. They found expression of GRβ in only 9.1% of patients with steroid-sensitive disease whereas it was present in 83.3% of steroid-resistant patients as detected by polymerase chain reaction (PCR). The authors conclude that the determination of GRβ expression could provide a tool to predict steroid responsiveness of UC patients [140]. However, other laboratories have reported that GRβ transcripts could be amplified from all control patients investigated, making a role of GRβ for glucocorticoid refractivity unlikely (personal communication).

Despite these studies most of the questions regarding the mechanisms of steroid-refractory disease are still unanswered [141]. It is not clear why some patients express GRβ and others do not. It is not clear whether changes in glucocorticoid binding are just an epiphenomenon or a cause of different disease courses. It is not clear whether GRβ expression or decreased GRα levels are really crucial for treatment success.

Future studies on GR expression in IBD need to answer several important questions: are GR levels at the onset of the disease predictive for the success of glucocorticoid therapy? Are low levels correlated with the development of a steroid-refractory disease? The question of whether measurement of GR in the mucosa can be predictive for therapy success needs to be answered for the future management of patients with IBD. Patients with low GR levels could then be primarily treated with other drugs such as azathioprine. Prospective studies investigating GRα and GRβ transcripts, as well as glucocorticoid binding in PMNC and in the mucosa at the onset of disease before any treatment, will need to be performed to clarify whether both mechanisms are related to steroid-refractory IBD.

Cellular mechanisms of glucocorticoid action in IBD

Glucocorticoid receptors that can be activated by ligand binding mediate glucocorticoid action and induce *trans*-activation or *trans*-repression of genes as well as an inhibition of proinflammatory transcription factors such as NF-κB and AP-1. The question arises as to which effects the ligand-induced

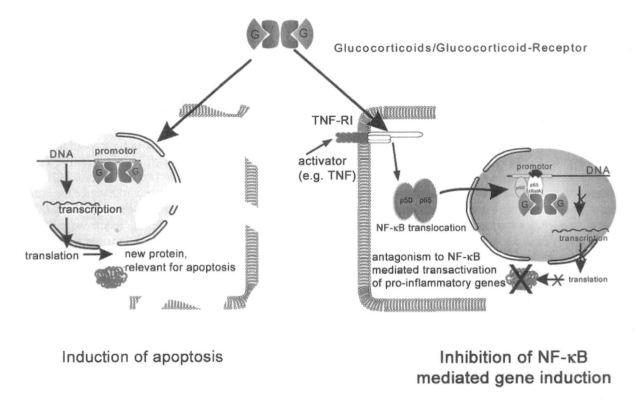

Induction of apoptosis

**Inhibition of NF-κB
mediated gene induction**

Figure 5. Glucocorticoid-induced anti-inflammatory mechanisms. Two major principles mediate the anti-inflammatory effect of glucocorticoids. After penetrating the cell membrane and binding to the GR nuclear translocation occurs. The complex can then *trans*-activate genes that are involved in the induction of apoptosis. The induction of apoptosis in activated lymphocytes, eosinophils, basophils and other cell types reduces the overall amount of circulating cytokines and inflammatory mediators and allows reconstitution of the intestinal mucosa. On the other hand the heterodimer of GR interacts with translocated NF-κB and prevents transcriptional activation by this proinflammatory transcription factor. As NF-κB activation has anti-apoptotic effects in a number of cell types antagonism to its action also has pro-apoptotic effects, indicating the interconnection of both mechanisms of glucocorticoid action.

activation of GR have at the cellular level, or more precisely which effects can be observed in different cell types? A simplified view could focus on two major principles (Fig. 5):

1. The cellular effects induced by a down-regulation of proinflammatory transcription factors. As mentioned this is facilitated by an incompletely understood antagonism to transcription factors such as NF-κB and AP-1 (Fig.5).

2. The induction of apoptosis of activated immune cells, which limits the immune response and as a consequence is also followed by reduced levels of circulating proinflammatory factors (Fig. 5).

In this chapter only a few of the effects on some of the relevant cell populations in the intestinal immune system can be highlighted.

Lymphocytes

Glucocorticoids affect the growth, differentiation and function of lymphocytes, the distribution of cellular subsets, and the production of cytokines [142]. In the chronic inflamed mucosa the number of lymphocytes is greatly increased. Most of these cells are activated T-helper cells.

Glucocorticoids reduce lymphocyte proliferation and induce apoptosis in these cells [143–146]. Studies indicate that mainly transcriptional *trans*-activation functions are required for this glucocorticoid-mediated apoptosis [147]. Interestingly intestinal intraepithelial lymphocytes (IEL) may be resistant to steroid-induced apoptosis, which could be due to the expression of high levels of the anti-apoptotic protein Bcl-2 and Bcl-x [148].

Recent data indicate that glucocorticoid-mediated inhibition of cytokine secretion in inflammatory diseases may be mediated not only by direct action on lymphocyte and monocyte/macrophage NF-κB but in addition indirectly through promotion of a T-helper cell type 2 (Th2) induction [143] with increased levels of Th2 cytokine (IL-4) and reduced levels of Th1 cytokine (IL-12) secretion [149]. In addition dexamethasone can inhibit IL-12-induced phosphorylation of STAT-4 without altering IL-4-induced STAT-6 phosphorylation [149]. Both would result in a blockade of proinflammatory T-helper cell type 1 (Th1) cytokine expression.

A further example of the multi-site mechanisms involved in glucocorticoid action is given by another monocyte/macrophage–lymphocyte interaction. Glucocorticoids have been shown to down-regulate T-cell co-stimulatory molecules B7-1 and B7-2 on macrophages which are essential for clonal T-cell expansion in reaction to antigen-presenting cells [150]. On the other hand co-stimulatory molecules can prevent cells from glucocorticoid-induced apoptosis [151]. It is interesting to note in this context that normal intestinal macrophages express no co-stimulatory molecules, whereas there is a clear up-regulation in IBD [152, 153].

Macrophages

Macrophages are known to play an important role during inflammation in many different tissues [154]. Intestinal macrophages represent one of the largest compartments of the mononuclear phagocyte system in the body [155]. They are localized preferentially in the subepithelial region and constitute 10–20% of mononuclear cells in the intestinal lamina propria [156]. Macrophages are able to secrete proinflammatory cytokines which are known to be regulated by NF-κB such as IL-1β, TNF-α, IL-6, IL-8, MCP-1.

In normal mucosa only very few macrophages express activation-associated markers such as CD14, CD16, HLA-DR, CD11b, and CD11c [152, 153, 157], supporting a concept of anergy in the normal mucosa. Several findings indicate a phenotypic change of the intestinal macrophage population in IBD. Mahida *et al.* demonstrated the presence of CD16 (FcγIII receptor) in IBD by immuno-histochemical methods and in isolated cells [158]. CD54 (ICAM1) expression increased from 7% to 70% in UC and to 46% in CD [159]. Inflammation-

associated intestinal macrophages express LPS receptors, Fc receptors and co-stimulatory molecules [152, 153, 157], which enable them to stimulate T cells and partially prevent them from gluco-corticoid-induced apoptosis (see above).

The number of macrophages is clearly increased in both CD and UC mucosa [160–162]. The activated macrophage population secretes a multitude of inflammatory mediators such as prostaglandins; leukotrienes; cytokines such as TNF, IL-1, IL-12; chemokines such as MCP-1 or IL-8 as well as tissue-damaging reactive radicals and tissue-degrading enzymes [163–176]. The transcription, translation and secretion of almost all molecules mentioned above can be reduced or inhibited by the administration of glucocorticoids. In the promoters of most of those gene NF-κB binding sites can be found [177–187], indicating that the glucocorticoid-mediated inhibition of NF-κB activation may be the most important mechanism for their anti-inflammatory potential.

Intestinal epithelial cells

Intestinal epithelial cells (IEC) play an active role in the intestinal immune system [188–190]. After stimulation with IFN-γ they express MHC molecules [191–195]. In addition there is evidence that epithelial cells are able to respond to damage or bacterial invasion by secreting cytokines and chemokines [196–205]. Among the cytokines secreted by intestinal epithelial cells are inflammatory mediators such as IL-6 and IL-8.

As already discussed for the other cell types, it could be shown that, for example, the induction of IL-6 production in human intestinal epithelial cells following stimulation with IL-1β was associated with activation of the transcription factor NF-κB [206]. Jobin and co-workers demonstrated that adeno-virus-mediated transfection of HT-29 and Caco-2 cells with a NF-κB superrepressor caused a reduced induction of inducible nitric oxide synthase (iNOS), IL-1β and IL-8 by IL-1 or TNF, indicating involvement of the NF-κB system in regulation of these genes [207]. In the inflamed mucosa activation of NF-κB has been demonstrated in intestinal epithelial cells, whereas activation was absent in non-inflamed mucosa [208, 209].

Glucocorticoids down-regulate the expression of IL-6, IL-8, iNOS and class II molecules in intestinal epithelial cells and restore epithelial cell physiology [210, 211]. This is again likely to be mediated by the inhibition of NF-κB activation.

Other cell types

As GR are expressed in most if not all cell types, effects of glucocorticoid therapy on all cell types involved in intestinal inflammation have been found. During the course of IBD increased numbers of eosinophils and mast cells are present in the intestinal mucosa [212–216]. These cells are activated and secrete different tissue-damaging proteins as well as cytokines and chemokines [217–224]. Again NF-κB has been found to be a major factor in activation of eosinophils [225], and glucocorticoids have been shown to down-regulate the production and secretion of the proinflammatory proteins [226, 227]. In addition the number of mucosal and circulating eosinophils is decreased by glucocorticoids. This is probably mediated by an induction of apoptosis in these cells [228–233].

As well as the number of eosinophils and mast cells, the number of basophils is increased in IBD mucosa [212]. Glucocorticoids reduce the number of basophils similar to the reduction described for eosinophils.

Neutrophils are a major component in active lesions in UC and to a lesser extent in CD [234–240]. They are recruited under the influence of the neutrophil chemoattractant IL-8 [237]. An important feature of these neutrophils is their ability to induce the so-called 'oxidative burst' reaction involving the NADPH oxidase system leading to a secretion of oxygen radicals that not only kill surrounding bacteria but also damage surrounding tissue [238]. Glucocorticoids act in different ways in neutrophils. They down-regulate the oxidative burst reaction and reduce IL-8 secretion, leading to a reduced immigration of neutrophils into the mucosa. On the other hand an increased release from the bone marrow, followed by a leukocytosis, is induced [241].

Another important feature of the treatment with glucocorticoids is down-regulation of the expression of adhesion molecules on endothelial cells, mononuclear cells and epithelial cells [89, 241–247], which again may be mainly mediated by antagonistic effects to NF-κB.

Glucocorticoid therapy in combination with other anti-inflammatory drugs in IBD

Due to this multitude of desired effects the standard therapy for acute flares of IBD is still the systemic application of glucocorticoids. The effectiveness of a glucocorticoid regimen has been shown in numerous multicenter trials [23, 248]. Initial remission rates in patients with acute flares of CD under a standard therapy vary from 60% to 80%, which is higher than under treatment with sulfasalazine or 5-aminosalicylic acid (40–50%). The combination of glucocorticoids and anti-inflammatory drugs, e.g. sulfasalazine, shows no additive effect and no higher remission rates than therapy with prednisolone alone [23]. This may indicate that glucocorticoids and drugs such as sulfasalazine may both act in a common signal transduction cascade. Recently evidence has been found that some of the anti-inflammatory effects of 5-ASA and sulfasalazine in IBD patients may be mediated by the inhibition of the proinflammatory transcription factor NF-κB. Acetylsalicylic acid, 5-ASA and sodium salicylate inhibit activation of NF-κB by blocking IκB-kinases (IKK), which are key factors in NF-κB activation [249–251]. Similar results were found for sulfasalazine [252, 253]. The inhibition of both IKKα and IKKβ has been shown [254].

The lack of additional effects of a combination of glucocorticoid and salicylate therapy indicates that the glucocorticoid effect on NF-κB inhibition may be superior. However, long-term studies show that, despite the high initial response rates, only 44% of patients initially treated with glucocorticoids show long-term remission; 25–35% of patients become 'steroid dependent', indicating that steroid treatment cannot be completely tapered and omitted. About 20% of glucocorticoid-treated patients prove to be primarily 'glucocorticoid resistant' [255, 256].

Peroxisome proliferator-activated receptors (PPAR)

The GR that mediates glucocorticoid effects in the treatment of IBD is a member of the so-called steroid or nuclear receptor superfamily. Other members of this family have gained increasing attention in the recent years. Particularly PPARγ and PPARα have been shown to have NF-κB-inhibiting activities, and could be possible tools for the treatment of IBD in the future. They are further examples for a multisite treatment approach.

PPARs – like GR – are ligand-activated receptors. They have been discovered to be regulators of lipid and lipoprotein metabolism [257]. However, in recent years it was shown that they also regulate cellular proliferation, differentiation and apoptosis [257], features that may be very important during repair processes after or during intestinal inflammation. Three family members are known. Besides PPARα and PPARγ, PPARδ is encoded by a separate gene and expressed in most tissues. PPARs form heterodimers with the retinoid X receptor (RXR) and bind to PPAR response elements (PPRE) in the promoters of target genes.

PPARγ

As mentioned, PPARγ is a member of the nuclear hormone receptor family and a ligand-activated transcription factor. High expression is found in adipose tissue, the adrenal gland, the spleen and, interestingly, in the colon [257–262]. PPARγ is involved in the induction of adipocyte differentiation and glucose-homeostasis [262]. PPARγ is also expressed in differentiated macrophages, whereas there is no expression in monocytes [263].

Thiazolidinediones were identified as synthetic ligands of PPARγ [262, 264–273]. Besides pharmacologically developed ligands natural ligands such as free fatty acids and the prostaglandin D2 metabolite 15-deoxy-Δ12,14 prostaglandin J2 bind to the PPARγ protein and stimulate the transcription of target genes [274–279]. Prostaglandin D2 metabolites cannot be detected in adipose tissue; however, they are important intermediate products of arachidonic acid metabolism in macrophages and antigen-presenting cells [280].

In activated macrophages a significant-upregulation of PPARγ was found [281–283]. An activation of PPARγ by its ligands 15Δ-PGJ2 or thiazolidinediones inhibited *iNOS*, *gelatinase B* and *scavenger receptor A* genes. This inhibition is partially mediated by an antagonism to the transcription factors AP-1, STAT-1 and NF-κB [283]. Furthermore it could be demonstrated that PPARγ inhibits the expression of a number of proinflammatory cytokines in monocytes [283, 284].

Besides macrophages and adipocytes, colonic epithelial cells express high levels of PPARγ mRNA and protein [258, 285–290]. The physiological function of PPARγ in intestinal epithelial cells is not well understood. A recent study by Su and co-workers showed that the expression of proinflammatory cytokines was reduced by incubation with PPARγ ligands, which was mediated by inhibition of NF-κB activation [291]. The administration of thiazolidinediones during the recovery phase in an acute model of DSS (dextran sulphate sodium)-induced colitis in mice was followed by a dramatic improvement in histological signs of inflammation [291]. Clinical trials to test the efficacy of thiazolidinediones in IBD are under way.

When activated, PPARγ molecules form heterodimers with another transcription factor of the nuclear receptor superfamily, the retinoid-X-receptor (RXR). Heterozygous PPARγ and RXRα knockout mice display a significantly enhanced susceptibility to 2,4,6-trinitrobenzene sulfonic acid (TNBS)-induced colitis compared with their wild-type littermates, indicating a role for the RXR/PPARγ heterodimer in protection against colon inflammation [292]. The administration of both PPARγ and RXR agonists also reduced TNBS-induced colitis, reflected by a decrease in TNF and IL-1β mRNA levels and a reduction of NF-κB DNA-binding activity [292]. A synergistic effect of PPARγ and RXR ligands was observed.

In addition to their NF-κB antagonistic properties ligands for PPARγ, similar to GR have been proven to induce apoptosis in a number of different cell types and cell lines [257, 293–303]. However, it is not clear whether the induction of apoptosis is simply mediated by the inhibition of the antiapoptotic NF-κB or by a yet-incompletely elucidated specific mechanism. In addition it is necessary to clarify whether the induction of apoptosis by PPARγ ligands plays a role in the regulation of the human immune system. It is important to note that PPARγ activators have also been discussed as inductors of colon polyp formation [289], which could be a major problem in the therapy of IBD patients, increasing their risk of developing colon cancer. Future studies are necessary to clarify this problem.

PPARα

PPARα is another member of the PPAR family. Recently it has been shown that dehydroepiandrosterone (DHEA) could be a natural ligand for PPARα. DHEA and its sulphated metabolite (DHEAS) are the most abundant steroid hormones in the body. They are predominantly synthesized in the adrenal glands in response to adrenocorticotrophin (ACTH) from its precursors cholesterol and pregnenolone, and can be further metabolized via androstenedione into androsterone and via testosterone into 17β-estradiol [304]. DHEA inhibits activation of NF-κB and secretion of IL-6 and IL-12 via the activation of PPARα [305–307]. Furthermore DHEA stimulates the production of IL-10 in murine spleen cells [308].

Treatment with 50–200 mg/day DHEA was shown to be effective in patients with lupus erythematosus [309–312]. On the other hand DHEAS concentrations are decreased in patients with IBD [313, 314].

In a pilot trial treatment with DHEA was safe and effective in patients with refractory active CD or UC [315]. In this study a dose of 200 mg/day DHEA in all patients was used.

Ligands for PPARα are at present being developed by several major pharmaceutical companies. Future studies are necessary to clarify whether these ligands are favorable compared to the endogenous ligand DHEA, and whether PPARα ligation is followed by antiapoptotic or proapoptotic stimuli [316].

The data for both members of the PPAR family are so far incomplete and controlled randomized clinical trials are needed. However, they show clearly that possibilities for multi-site anti-inflammatory therapies are not limited to GR. PPAR ligands could prove to have great potential for the treatment of IBD.

Inhibition of NF-κB-mediated *trans*-activation as a central target of IBD therapy

The discussion of GR functions showed that one of the most important anti-inflammatory mechanisms mediated by glucocorticoid therapy is the inhibition of the proinflammatory transcription factor NF-κB. Furthermore, the first genetic mutations associated with susceptibility to CD were found in NOD2 [317, 318], which is a NF-κB-activating protein [319–321]. Therefore the NF-κB system needs more detailed consideration.

Molecular mechanisms of NF-κB activation

Transcription factors of the NF-κB/Rel family form dimeric complexes which control the expression of a variety of inducible genes involved in inflammation and proliferation [322, 323]. The prototypic heterodimeric complex NF-κB consists of the subunits p50 and p65 (RelA) [324, 325]. The inactive NF-κB dimer is present in the cytosol bound to inhibitory proteins, termed IκB [326, 327] (Fig. 6). IκBα, IκBβ and IκBε have similar functions in inhibiting the translocation of the NF-κB dimer [328]. The activation of NF-κB by inflammatory cytokines and microorganisms requires the release of IκB from the complex [324–327, 329]. The release of IκB is induced by

phosphorylation of IκB at two conserved amino-terminal serine residues by a multiprotein IκB-kinase complex containing IκB-kinase alpha (IKKα), beta (IKKβ) and gamma (IKKγ) (Fig. 6) [330–332]. This is followed by a poly-ubiquination of the IκB proteins by a specialized E3 ubiquitin ligase complex (E3IκB) [333] which makes them accessible to proteolytic degradation by the 26S proteasome (Fig. 6) [328]. The removal of IκB proteins exposes nuclear localization signals (NLS) followed by translocation of the activated NF-κB into the nucleus [330]. There, the activated NF-κB dimer interacts with regulatory NF-κB elements in promoters and enhancers [324, 325, 329, 330] (Fig. 6). Among the genes *trans*-activated by the NF-κB dimer, interestingly, is IκBα [328]. This usually limits NF-κB action. If IκB does not find a binding partner in the cytosol it translocates to the nucleus, binds activated NF-κB and mediates re-shuttling of the complex to the cytosol.

NF-κB activation in IBD

There is evidence that NF-κB transcription factors might play an important role in the inflammatory process of IBD. It was shown that the administration of antisense phosphothioate oligonucleotides to the p65 subunit of NF-κB abrogates colitis in IL-10-deficient mice and in the TNBS-colitis model [334]. Inhibition of the proteasome complex which is responsible for the rapid degradation of IκB prevented NF-κB activation and attenuated the colonic and splenic injury and inflammation in the PG/PS model [335]. In the DSS model of chronic colitis the DSS-induced intestinal inflammation was characterized by an increase of NF-κB activity [336]. Blocking NF-κB activation by administering gliotoxin, a fungal product, was accompanied by a significant suppression of intestinal inflammation and mRNA expression of TNF-α and IL-1α *in vivo* [336].

NF-κB activation was demonstrated in cultured rat intestinal epithelial cells (IEC-6) by IL-1β and TNF-α [207, 337]. Dexamethasone prevented epithelial cells from being activated by these mediators [207, 337]. In mucosal biopsies from patients suffering from IBD, activation of NF-κB was demonstrated to be mainly localized in two cell types in the intestinal mucosa by double-labeling techniques: (1) in lamina propria macrophages and (2) in epithelial cells [208].

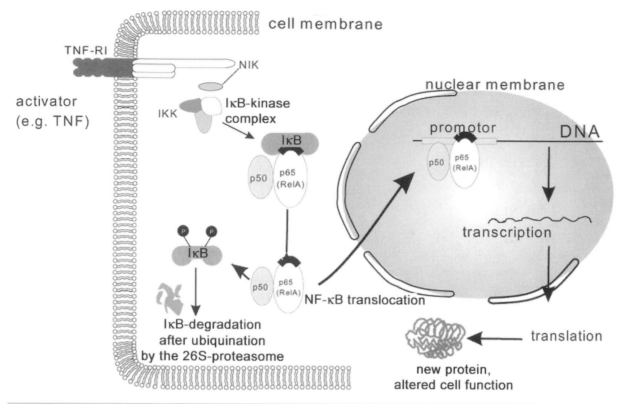

Figure 6. Principles of NF-κB activation: In the cytoplasm the NF-κB complex is associated with the inhibitory protein IκB. Activation of NF-κB is induced by a number of different signals, as for example IL-1 and TNF-α. These signals activate an IκB-kinase complex that contains the IκB-kinases IKK-α (IKK1) and IKK-β (IKK2). IKK-α and IKK-β are phosphorylated, leading to a recruitment of IκB and phosphorylation of IκB at serine32 and serine36. This is followed by release of IκB from the complex. Consecutively a rapid proteolytic degradation of IκB and a translocation of the activated NF-κB into the nucleus takes place. In the nucleus the activated NF-κB dimer interacts with regulatory NF-κB elements in promoters and enhancers, leading to alteration in transcription rates and altered cell function. When the degradation of IκB is blocked by inhibitors of the proteasome complex IκB reassociates with the NF-κB dimer and NF-κB activation is inhibited.

Furthermore, mutations in *NOD2*, a gene which is mainly expressed in monocytes/macrophages and activates NF-κB, has been shown to be associated with susceptibility to CD [317, 318].

A variety of genes are induced in the inflamed mucosa which have been shown to be regulated by NF-κB, including the genes encoding *TNF-α* [171, 329, 338–341], *IL-1β* [171, 184, 339, 341–345], *IL-6* [346, 347], *IL-8* [348, 349], *macrophage colony-stimulating factor (M-CSF)* [329], *macrophage granulocyte colony-stimulating factor (GM-CSF)* [329], *monocyte chemotactic protein-1 (MCP-1)* [325, 350], *vascular cell adhesion molecule-1 (VCAM1)* [351, 352] and *intercellular adhesion molecule-1 (ICAM1)* [325]. Some of these gene products such as TNF-α and IL-1, are also able to activate NF-κB [324, 325], leading to a positive autoregulatory loop [184].

NF-κB and co-factors

As mentioned above, one of the most important effects of glucocorticoids (and ligands for other nuclear receptors) in the treatment of inflammatory diseases is the suppression of the *trans*-activating ability of NF-κB. Nuclear receptors (GR and PPAR), as well as NF-κB depend on the co-activators CREP-binding protein (CBP) and steroid receptor coactivator-1 (SRC-1) for their transcriptional activity [99, 100]. It has been suggested that some of the inhibitory affect of GR action is mediated by a nuclear competition for limited amounts of the co-activators CBP and SRC-1 [100]. This means that the presence of activated GR would induce binding of CBP and/or SRC-1 and that as a consequence activated NF-κB (p65) does not find a sufficient number of co-activator molecules to be transcriptionally active. A heterozygous mutation in CBP is sufficient to induce Rubinstein–Taybi syndrome, illustrating the critical importance of a certain amount of CBP protein in the nucleus [353].

It is not clear whether direct protein–protein interactions between NF-κB and the GR occur or whether both proteins could be bound to a common interacting protein such as CBP.

Glucocorticoids are also known to directly induce IκBa gene transcription [97]. However, it has been reported that in many cases this is not sufficient to reduce or abolish NF-κB DNA-binding activity. In addition, glucocorticoids are able to inhibit the expression of NF-κB target genes in the absence of protein synthesis, indicating that IκB induction may contribute to the inhibition of NF-κB activation but the interaction described above is more important [97].

Pathways leading to NF-κB activation

A number of different pathways have been described that are able to activate NF-κB and induce its *trans*-activating activity. In many of these pathways the IKK complex and subsequent degradation of IκB is involved. Extracellular signals can induce IKK activation by specific cell surface receptors. However, alternative pathways have been recently described, in which the signal transduction cascade is initiated by intracellular receptors or detection systems [319–321].

TNF signaling as a prototype of cell-surface receptor-initiated NF-κB activation

TNF is an important mediator of mucosal inflammation and is thought to play a key role in the pathophysiology of IBD [354–356]. The TNF system is complex and has a number of regulatory mechanisms. Besides the induction of other proinflammatory cytokines TNF has pleiotropic functions mediating induction of apoptosis, cell proliferation, modulating viral replication, allergy, and inducing insulin resistance [357, 358]. The TNF homotrimer consisting of three 17 kDa units transduces these cellular responses through two distinct receptors: type I (p60 or p55), which are expressed on all cell types, and type II (p80 or p75), which are expressed only on cells of the immune system and endothelial cells. Both receptors can induce NF-κB and AP-1 as well as mitogen-activated protein (MAP) kinase

activation [357–362]. The activation of NF-κB by ligated TNF receptors is mediated first by recruitment of an adaptor protein (TRADD), activation of a seronine–threonine kinase (RIP) followed by activation of TNF receptor associated factor (TRAF) 2 (Fig. 7). TRAF-2 recruits the IκBα-kinase complex (IKK) to the TNF receptor [357]. It also associates with NF-κB inducing kinase (NIK), which can be a component of the IKK complex, at least when it is overexpressed (Fig. 7). NIK then activates IKKα by phosphorylation of Ser 176 [357]. However, IKKα phosphorylation after TNF receptor ligation can also occur without the presence of NIK. Besides IKKα the IKK complex contains IKKβ, which has a very similar structure to IKKα and the unrelated IKKγ. Binding of TNF to its receptors induces phosphorylation of all three kinases. The presence of IKKβ and IKKγ seems to bee essential for TNF-mediated NF-κB activation [357]. The activated IKK complex then phosphorylates IκB, leading to its ubiquination and degradation.

The TNF-receptor–IKK–NF-κB cascade is prototypic for a cell-surface-receptor-initiated NF-κB activation. It has been speculated the inhibition of the interaction of the TNF homotrimer with its receptors may prevent NF-κB activation, and may be beneficial in inflammatory diseases. As this point of intervention is different to glucocorticoids, which take action in the nucleus, it was assumed early that anti-TNF treatment could prevent NF-κB-mediated effects in steroid-resistant refractory patients. Several methods of intervention are possible and have found their way into clinical trials. The synthesis of TNF itself can be reduced, neutralizing antibodies to TNF can be administered and recombinant soluble TNF receptor can also block TNF signaling cascades.

In 1993, for the first time, a mouse/human chimeric antibody was described, which was generated in mice and had a high affinity to human TNF. This chimeric antibody (cA2) was initially used in clinical studies with patients suffering from rheumatoid arthritis, and showed very positive effects [363–369]. A pilot study in patients with severe, steroid-dependent CD showed a similar rapid improvement of the patients' symptoms [370]. A number of studies have since proved the efficacy of the anti-TNF treatment, and it can be regarded as an established therapy for patients with a glucocorticoid-dependent or -resistant disease course [371–388].

One of the most likely mechanisms by which the administration of anti-TNF antibodies reduces joint

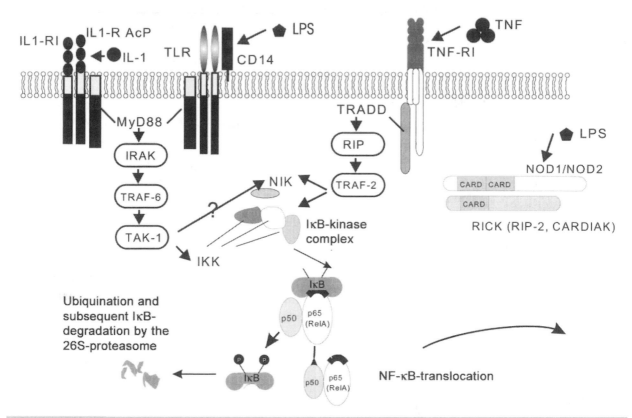

Figure 7. Pathways of NF-κB activation. TNF-RI (binding TNF) and the IL-1 receptor family (binding IL-1α or IL-1β to IL-1RI and extracellular LPS to TLRs) utilize distinct but analogous signaling cascades resulting in IKK activation, IκB degradation and finally in NF-κB translocation and activation. Both bind adaptor proteins (TRADD associates to TNF-RI, MyD88 associates with IL-1RI and TLRs). This is followed by a recruitment of a seronine–threonine kinase (RIP and IRAK respectively) that are phosphorylated. Both pathways then utilize TRAF factors (TRAF-2 and TRAF-6) leading to IKK activation. A new pathway leading to NF-κB activation has gained attention by the demonstration of an association of polymorphisms in the NOD2 gene with the susceptibility for Crohn's disease. NOD1 and NOD2 are potential intracellular receptors for LPS, binding LPS in a leucin-rich domain. After binding their CARD domain interacts with the CARD domain of RICK, followed by IKK-complex activation. Potential targets for therapeutic intervention may be defined in the future by further elucidation of the pathways shown.

and mucosal inflammation is reduced activation of NF-κB. The antibody prevents circulating TNF from binding to its receptor, subsequent IKK activation, IκB phosphorylation and NF-κB activation. However, this may not be the whole story, as a positive effect of the anti-TNF antibody administration is still observed up to 1 year after the antibody has been cleared from the circulation [355]. It has been suggested that anti-TNF therapy may also induce apoptosis in activated lymphocytes and macrophages. On the other hand, in glucocorticoid responders, long-lasting remissions can be achieved when no therapeutic glucocorticoids are administered, indicating that the effector needs not be present for a long-lasting change of immune mechanisms.

NF-κB activation induced by the IL-1 receptor family

Like TNF, IL-1 is a central regulator of immune functions. It plays a major role in both systemic and local immune responses to bacteria and bacterial wall products such as LPS [359, 389–391]. For IL-1 two receptors (IL-1RI and IL-1RII) are known that mediate cellular responses. These receptors belong to a family of receptors based on homologous molecule structures within the intracellular signaling domain. Other family members include the IL-18 receptor and, perhaps more importantly, the recently discovered Toll-like receptors (TLR), which recognize different bacterial products (TLR4: lipopolysaccharides (LPS), TLR2: Gram-positive bacteria, bacterial proteins, TLR9: bacterial DNA) [392–400].

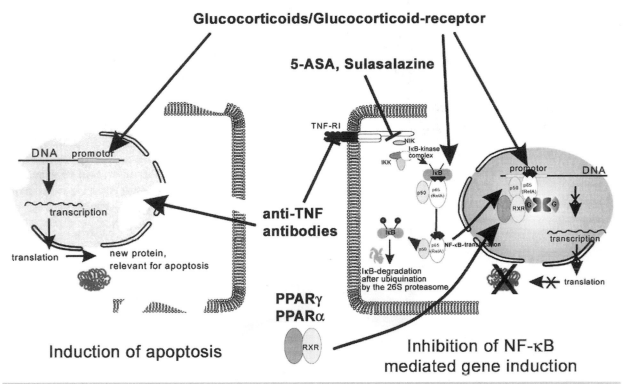

Figure 8. Summary: Multi target therapies for inflammatory bowel disease act on two major pathways they induce apoptosis and/or inhibit the activation of NF-κB.

The type I IL-1 receptor (IL-1RI) is an 80 kDa high-affinity receptor present on most cells of the immune system, including monocytes/macrophages and lymphocytes. The receptor consists of a 319 AA aminoterminal extracellular domain, a 219 AA carboxyl-terminal intracellular domain, and a transmembrane domain containing a short region of uncharged AA [390]. The cytoplasmic domain of IL-1RI shows homology to the IL-18 receptor and the TLR family. The region between AA 513 and 529 of the IL-1RI molecule appears to be crucial for NF-κB activation. Both biologically active isoforms of IL-1, α and β, can bind to IL-1RI. A so-called IL-1 receptor associated protein (IL-1RAcP) is necessary for IL-1 receptor function. IL-1RAcP does not bind either IL-1α or IL-1β, but it increases their binding affinity to the IL-1RI and, more importantly, it activates additional signal transduction pathways that are not activated in cells expressing IL-1RI alone [390]. The type II IL-1 receptor (IL-1RII) is a 60 kDa receptor with a very short cytoplasmic domain lacking signal transduction capabilities even though it can bind IL-1 with high affinity. Mammalian TLR are homologs of *Drosophila* Toll receptor and are also members of the IL-1 receptor family with the ability to activate NF-κB. To date, 10 TLRs (TLR 1-10) have been described.

The first event in IL-1 signal transduction following IL-1 binding to IL-1RI is the formation of the IL-1R and IL-1R-AcP complex [390] (Fig. 7). This induces a rapid and stable association of an adapter protein called MyD88 with the receptor complex. MyD88 allows the interaction of IL-1 receptor associated kinase (IRAK) with the complex (Fig. 7). The association of MyD88 with IRAK is rapid and transient, followed by a phosphorylation of IRAK resulting in reduced affinity for MyD88 and its release from the IL-1RI complex [390]. To date three IRAK molecules (IRAK, IRAK-2 and IRAK-M) are known. Phosphorylated IRAK and IRAK-2 subsequently associate with the downstream signaling protein TNF receptor-associated factor 6 (TRAF6), a member of the TNF receptor-associated factor family. Activation of TRAF6 is followed by activation of NIK (Fig. 7). As mentioned (see above) NIK may form a complex with IKKα, IKKβ, and IKKγ. Ligands that bind to TLR proteins activate NF-κB by using similar signal transduction pathways.

Because of the importance of IL-1 receptor family members for NF-κB activation, future therapy strategies may well target this system. Interesting targets for a therapeutic intervention are not only the IL-1/IL-1R system but also the LPS recognizing TLR4 and the bacterial DNA-binding TLR9. Targeting IRAK or MyD88 may also turn out to be an interesting strategy.

NF-κB activation by NOD1 and NOD2

Recent data indicate an association of the susceptibility for CD with polymorphisms or mutations in the NOD2 gene [317, 318]. For the first time a genetic mutation involved in the pathogenesis of IBD could be demonstrated. It is intriguing that that mutated protein is expressed mainly in monocytes, binds LPS and is capable of NF-κB activation.

NOD1 and NOD2 as well as Apaf1 are members of a family of intracellular proteins that contain an N-terminal caspase recruitment domain (CARD) [319–321]. NOD1 and NOD2 (now termed CARD 15) both respond to LPS with NF-κB activation independent of TLR4 and MyD88 function [320] (Fig. 7). However, their preferences for different LPS forms and different bacteria seem to differ [320]. After binding of LPS to a leucin-rich domain in the NOD1 or NOD2 (CARD 15) protein the CARD domain of NOD interacts with the corresponding CARD domain of a protein called RICK (also called RIP2 and CARDIAK). RICK is a protein kinase that is able to activate NF-κB in a IKK-dependent pathway (Fig. 7). IκBα, IKKα, IKKβ as well as IKKγ seem to be necessary for NOD-RICK mediated NF-κB activation [319]. Based upon these results NOD1 and NOD2 (CARD 15) are likely to be members of an intracellular recognition system for LPS regulating NF-κB activation.

Side-effects of NF-κB blockade

We all are aware of the immunosuppressive side-effects of a systemic glucocorticoid therapy that can lead to fatal consequences in the case of infections. One of the reasons for the observed immunosuppression is the induction of apoptosis in activated lymphocyte and monocyte populations. As the inhibition of NF-κB is one of the most important mechanisms of glucocorticoid (and PPAR-ligand) mediated effects, it is clear also that NF-κB inhibition may contribute to the side-effects.

The disruption of the p65 gene in mice is followed by embryonic lethality at 15–16 days of gestation and a massive degeneration of the liver by programmed cell death or apoptosis at this early time point [401]. TNF-mediated gene induction is absent in those mice, whereas a basic NF-κB-dependent transcription of genes is conserved [401]. This indicates the p65 subunit is essential for inducible, but not basal, transcription in NF-κB-regulated pathways. Mice lacking the p50 subunit, in contrast, show no developmental abnormalities [402]. However, they exhibit multifocal defects in various forms of immune responses, e.g. a lack of proliferation of B cells in response to bacterial lipopolysaccharide and a defect in basal and specific antibody production [402].

From these observations it can be concluded that a systemic complete blockade of NF-κB activation could be a dangerous treatment approach. In a DSS model of colitis, treatment with 2×20 μg/day of the NF-κB inhibitor gliotoxin was followed by reduced survival of the mice despite improved histology in the colon [336].

It may therefore be better to achieve a local (mucosal) NF-κB inhibition. Curcumin, a substance derived from the plant *Curcuma longa*, which is used as a spice in India, inhibits IκB degradation and thereby NF-κB activation [403–409]. As the absorption rate of *Curcumin* from the gut is low, a local NF-κB inhibition could be potentially achieved with this drug. Like 'topical' steroids such as budesonide this 'local' NF-κB inhibition would avoid systemic side-effects.

Another possibility that has been discussed would be the development of tissue-specific IKK inhibitors; however, so far there is no clear evidence for a clear tissue-specificity of IKK activation pathways. Until a local or tissue specific direct NF-κB inhibition becomes possible indirect and systemic approaches such as therapy with anti-TNF antibodies must be evaluated. Taken together, NF-κB seems to play a key role for the treatment of chronic and acute inflammatory diseases and is the final target of a number of successful multi-site therapeutic approaches. Inhibition of NF-κB at different cellular levels has provided therapeutic alternatives in the past and will provide new alternatives to glucocorticoid therapy in the future. This may finally lead to an optimized therapy for individual patients with their specific course of IBD. The understanding of the mechanisms involved in NF-κB activation on the one hand, and GR and PPAR-mediated suppression of NF-κB activation on the other, is essential for this future development.

References

1. Schleimer RP. An overview of glucocorticoid anti-inflammatory actions. Eur J Clin Pharmacol 1993; 45: S3–7; discussion S43—4.
2. Barnes PJ, Adcock I. Anti-inflammatory actions of steroids: molecular mechanisms. Trends Pharmacol Sci 1993; 14: 436–41.
3. Barnes PJ. Anti-inflammatory actions of glucocorticoids: molecular mechanisms. Clin Sci (Colch) 1998; 94: 557–72.
4. Kirwan JR. Effects of long-term glucocorticoid therapy in rheumatoid arthritis. Z Rheumatol 2000; 59: II: 85–9.
5. van der Velden VH. Glucocorticoids: mechanisms of action and anti-inflammatory potential in asthma. Mediators Inflamm 1998; 7: 229–37.
6. Spahn JD, Leung DY. The role of glucocorticoids in the management of asthma. Allergy Asthma Proc 1996; 17: 341–50.
7. Lombardino JG. Mechanism of action of drugs for treating inflammation and arthritis. Eur J Rheumatol Inflamm 1983; 6: 24–35.
8. Friend DR. Review article: Issues in oral administration of locally acting glucocorticosteroids for treatment of inflammatory bowel disease. Aliment Pharmacol Ther 1998; 12: 591–603.
9. Adcock IM, Ito K. Molecular mechanisms of corticosteroid actions. Monaldi Arch Chest Dis 2000; 55: 256–66.
10. Kumar R, Thompson EB. The structure of the nuclear hormone receptors. Steroids 1999; 64: 310–19.
11. Webster JC, Cidlowski JA. Mechanisms of glucocorticoid-receptor-mediated repression of gene expression. Trends Endocrinol Metab 1999; 10: 396–402.
12. Glass CK, Rosenfeld MG. The coregulator exchange in transcriptional functions of nuclear receptors. Genes Dev 2000; 14: 121–41.
13. Newton R. Molecular mechanisms of glucocorticoid action: what is important? Thorax 2000; 55: 603–13.
14. McKay LI, Cidlowski JA. Molecular control of immune/inflammatory responses: interactions between nuclear factor-kappa B and steroid receptor-signaling pathways. Endocrinol Rev 1999; 20: 435–59.
15. Truelove S, Witts L. Cortisone in ulcerative colitis: preliminary report on a therapeutic trial. Br Med J 1954; 2: 375–8.
16. Truelove S, Witts L. Cortisone and corticotrophin in ulcerative colitis. Br Med J 1959; 10: 387–94.
17. Jones J, Lennard-Jones J. Corticosteroids and corticotrophin in the treatment of Crohn's disease. Gut 1966; 7: 181–7.
18. Roberts G, Naish J. Corticosteroids in Crohn's disease. Gut 1968; 9: 736.
19. Lennard-Jones J. Toward optimal use of corticosteroids in ulcerative colitis and Crohn's disease. Gut 1983; 24: 177–81.
20. Jewell D. Corticosteroids for the management of ulcerative colitis and Crohn's disease. Gastroenterol Clin N Am 1989; 18: 21–34.
21. Routes J, Claman H. Corticosteroids in inflammatory bowel disease. A review. J Clin Gastroenterol 1987; 9: 529–35.
22. Hanauer S, Baert F. Medical therapy of inflammatory bowel disease. Med Clin N Am 1994; 78: 1413–26.
23. Malchow H, Ewe K, Brandes J et al. European Cooperative Crohn's Disease Study (ECCDS): results of drug treatment. Gastroenterology 1984; 86: 249–66.
24. Brattsand R, Linden M. Cytokine modulation by glucocorticoids: mechanisms and actions in cellular studies. Aliment Pharmacol Ther 1996; 10: 81–92.
25. Arzt E, Paez Pereda M, Costas M et al. Cytokine expression and molecular mechanisms of their auto/paracrine regulation of anterior pituitary function and growth. Ann NY Acad Sci 1998; 840: 525–31.
26. Arzt E, Kovalovsky D, Igaz LM et al. Functional cross-talk among cytokines, T-cell receptor, and GR transcriptional activity and action. Ann NY Acad Sci 2000; 917: 672–7.
27. Barnes PJ. Novel approaches and targets for treatment of chronic obstructive pulmonary disease. Am J Respir Crit Care Med 1999; 160: S72–9.
28. Venkatesh VC, Ballard PL. Glucocorticoids and gene expression. Am J Respir Cell Mol Biol 1991; 4: 301–3.
29. Weinberger C, Hollenberg SM, Rosenfeld MG, Evans RM. Domain structure of human glucocorticoid receptor and its relationship to the v-erb-A oncogene product. Nature 1985; 318: 670–2.
30. Hollenberg SM, Weinberger C, Ong ES et al. Primary structure and expression of a functional human glucocorticoid receptor cDNA. Nature 1985; 318: 635–41.
31. Weinberger C, Hollenberg SM, Ong ES et al. Identification of human glucocorticoid receptor complementary DNA clones by epitope selection. Science 1985; 228: 740–2.
32. Evans R. The steroid and thyroid hormone receptor superfamily. Science 1988; 240: 889–95.
33. Arriza JL, Weinberger C, Cerelli G et al. Cloning of human mineralocorticoid receptor complementary DNA: structural and functional kinship with the glucocorticoid receptor. Science 1987; 237: 268–75.
34. Evans R. Molecular characterization of the glucocorticoid receptor. Recent Prog Horm Res 1989; 45: 1–22.
35. Lamberts S, Koper J, Biemond P, den-Holder F, de-Jong F. Cortisol receptor resistance: the variability of its clinical presentation and response to treatment. J Clin Endocrinol Metab 1992; 74: 313–21.
36. Lamberts SW, Huizenga AT, de Lange P, de Jong FH, Koper JW. Clinical aspects of glucocorticoid sensitivity. Steroids 1996; 61: 157–60.
37. Okret S, Dong Y, Tanaka H, Cairns B, Gustafsson J. The mechanism for glucocorticoid-resistance in a rat hepatoma cell variant that contains functional glucocorticoid receptor. J Steroid Biochem Mol Biol 1991; 40: 353–61.
38. Schlaghecke R, Beuscher D, Kornely E, Specker C. Effects of glucocorticoids in rheumatoid arthritis. Diminished glucocorticoid receptors do not result in glucocorticoid resistance. Arthritis Rheum 1994; 37: 1127–31.
39. Muller M, Renkawitz R. The glucocorticoid receptor. Biochim Biophys Acta 1991; 1088: 171–82.
40. Muller M, Baniahmad C, Kaltschmidt C, Renkawitz R. Multiple domains of the glucocorticoid receptor involved in synergism with the CACCC box factor(s). Mol Endocrinol 1991; 5: 1498–503.
41. Baniahmad C, Muller M, Altschmied J, Renkawitz R. Cooperative binding of the glucocorticoid receptor DNA binding domain is one of at least two mechanisms for synergism. J Mol Biol 1991; 222: 155–65.
42. Baumann H, Paulsen K, Kovacs H et al. Refined solution structure of the glucocorticoid receptor DNA-binding domain. Biochemistry 1993; 32: 13463–71.
43. Luisi BF, Xu WX, Otwinowski Z, Freedman LP, Yamamoto KR, Sigler PB. Crystallographic analysis of the interaction of the glucocorticoid receptor with DNA. Nature 1991; 352: 497–505.
44. Pan T, Freedman LP, Coleman JE. Cadmium-113 NMR studies of the DNA binding domain of the mammalian glucocorticoid receptor. Biochemistry 1990; 29: 9218–25.
45. Freedman LP, Luisi BF, Korszun ZR, Basavappa R, Sigler PB, Yamamoto KR. The function and structure of the metal coordination sites within the glucocorticoid receptor DNA binding domain. Nature 1988; 334: 543–6.
46. Freedman LP, Yamamoto KR, Luisi BF, Sigler PB. More fingers in hand. Cell 1988; 54: 444.

47. Luisi BF, Schwabe JW, Freedman LP. The steroid/nuclear receptors: from three-dimensional structure to complex function. Vitam Horm 1994; 49: 1–47.

48. Giguere V, Hollenberg SM, Rosenfeld MG, Evans RM. Functional domains of the human glucocorticoid receptor. Cell 1986; 46: 645–52.

49. Hollenberg SM, Giguere V, Evans RM. Identification of two regions of the human glucocorticoid receptor hormone binding domain that block activation. Cancer Res 1989; 49: 2292–4.

50. Hollenberg SM, Giguere V, Segui P, Evans RM. Colocalization of DNA-binding and transcriptional activation functions in the human glucocorticoid receptor. Cell 1987; 49: 39–46.

51. Dahlman-Wright K, Baumann H, McEwan IJ et al. Structural characterization of a minimal functional transactivation domain from the human glucocorticoid receptor. Proc Natl Acad Sci USA 1995; 92: 1699–703.

52. Dahlman-Wright K, McEwan IJ. Structural studies of mutant glucocorticoid receptor transactivation domains establish a link between transactivation activity *in vivo* and alpha-helix-forming potential *in vitro*. Biochemistry 1996; 35: 1323–7.

53. McEwan IJ, Wright AP, Dahlman-Wright K, Carlstedt-Duke J, Gustafson JA. Direct interaction of the tau 1 transactivation domain of the human glucocorticoid receptor with the basal transcriptional machinery. Mol Cell Biol 1993; 13: 399–407.

54. McEwan IJ, Dahlman-Wright K, Amlof T, Ford J, Wright AP, Gustafsson JA. Mechanisms of transcription activation by nuclear receptors: studies on the human glucocorticoid receptor tau 1 transactivation domain. Mutat Res 1995; 333: 15–22.

55. Henriksson A, Almlof T, Ford J, McEwan IJ, Gustafson JA, Wright AP. Role of the Ada adaptor complex in gene activation by the glucocorticoid receptor. Mol Cell Biol 1997; 17: 3065–73.

56. Ford J, McEwan IJ, Wright AP, Gustafsson JA. Involvement of the transcription factor IID protein complex in gene activation by the N-terminal transactivation domain of the glucocorticoid receptor *in vitro*. Mol Endocrinol 1997; 11: 1467–75.

57. Guarente L. Transcriptional coactivators in yeast and beyond. Trends Biochem Sci 1995; 20: 517–21.

58. Zeiner M, Gehring U. A protein that interacts with members of the nuclear hormone receptor family: identification and cDNA cloning. Proc Natl Acad Sci USA 1995; 92: 11465–9.

59. Onate SA, Tsai SY, Tsai MJ, O'Malley BW. Sequence and characterization of a coactivator for the steroid hormone receptor superfamily. Science 1995; 270: 1354–7.

60. Chakravarti D, LaMorte VJ, Nelson MC et al. Role of CBP/P300 in nuclear receptor signalling. Nature 1996; 383: 99–103.

61. Jantzen HM, Strahle U, Gloss B et al. Cooperativity of glucocorticoid response elements located far upstream of the tyrosine aminotransferase gene. Cell 1987; 49: 29–38.

62. Beato M, Truss M, Chavez S. Control of transcription by steroid hormones. Ann NY Acad Sci 1996; 784: 93–123.

63. Beato M. Gene regulation by steroid hormones. Cell 1989; 56: 335–44.

64. Abbinante N, Simpson L, Leikauf G. Corticosteroids increase secretory leukocyte protease inhibitor transcript levels in airway epithelial cells. Am J Physiol 1995; 268: L601–6.

65. Colotta F, Dower SK, Sims JE, Mantovani A. The type II 'decoy' receptor: a novel regulatory pathway for interleukin 1. Immunol Today 1994; 15: 562–6.

66. Colotta F, Mantovani A. Induction of the interleukin-1 decoy receptor by glucocorticoids. Trends Pharmacol Sci 1994; 15: 138–9.

67. Colotta F, Re F, Muzio M et al. Interleukin-1 type II receptor: a decoy target for IL-1 that is regulated by IL-4. Science 1993; 261: 472–5.

68. Purton JF, Boyd RL, Cole TJ, Godfrey DI. Intrathymic T cell development and selection proceeds normally in the absence of glucocorticoid receptor signaling. Immunity 2000; 13: 179–86.

69. Kofler R. The molecular basis of glucocorticoid-induced apoptosis of lymphoblastic leukemia cells. Histochem Cell Biol 2000; 114: 1–7.

70. Hulkko SM, Wakui H, Zilliacus J. The pro-apoptotic protein death-associated protein 3 (DAP3) interacts with the glucocorticoid receptor and affects the receptor function. Biochem J 2000; 349: 885–93.

71. Jamieson CA, Yamamoto KR. Crosstalk pathway for inhibition of glucocorticoid-induced apoptosis by T cell receptor signaling. Proc Natl Acad Sci USA 2000; 97: 7319–24.

72. Tolosa E, King LB, Ashwell JD. Thymocyte glucocorticoid resistance alters positive selection and inhibits autoimmunity and lymphoproliferative disease in MRL-lpr/lpr mice. Immunity 1998; 8: 67–76.

73. Cidlowski JA, King KL, Evans-Storms RB, Montague JW, Bortner CD, Hughes FM, Jr. The biochemistry and molecular biology of glucocorticoid-induced apoptosis in the immune system. Recent Prog Horm Res 1996; 51: 457–90.

74. Nieto MA, Gonzalez A, Gambon F, Diaz-Espada F, Lopez-Rivas A. Apoptosis in human thymocytes after treatment with glucocorticoids. Clin Exp Immunol 1992; 88: 341–4.

75. Wyllie AH, Morris RG. Hormone-induced cell death. Purification and properties of thymocytes undergoing apoptosis after glucocorticoid treatment. Am J Pathol 1982; 109: 78–87.

76. Wyllie AH, Morris RG, Smith AL, Dunlop D. Chromatin cleavage in apoptosis: association with condensed chromatin morphology and dependence on macromolecular synthesis. J Pathol 1984; 142: 67–77.

77. Ramdas J, Liu W, Harmon JM. Glucocorticoid-induced cell death requires autoinduction of glucocorticoid receptor expression in human leukemic T cells. Cancer Res 1999; 59: 1378–85.

78. Ramdas J, Harmon JM. Glucocorticoid-induced apoptosis and regulation of NF-kappaB activity in human leukemic T cells. Endocrinology 1998; 139: 3813–21.

79. Drouin J, Sun YL, Chamberland M et al. Novel glucocorticoid receptor complex with DNA element of the hormone-repressed POMC gene. EMBO J 1993; 12: 145–56.

80. Charron J, Drouin J. Glucocorticoid inhibition of transcription from episomal proopiomelanocortin gene promotor. Proc Natl Acad Sci USA 1986; 83: 8903–7.

81. Malkoski SP, Handanos CM, Dorin RI. Localization of a negative glucocorticoid response element of the human corticotropin releasing hormone gene. Mol Cell Endocrinol 1997; 127: 189–99.

82. Malkoski SP, Dorin RI. Composite glucocorticoid regulation at a functionally defined negative glucocorticoid response element of the human corticotropin-releasing hormone gene. Mol Endocrinol 1999; 13: 1629–44.

83. Murphy EP, Conneely OM. Neuroendocrine regulation of the hypothalamic pituitary adrenal axis by the nurr1/nur77 subfamily of nuclear receptors. Mol Endocrinol 1997; 11: 39–47.

84. Newton R, Barnes P, Adcock I. Transcription factors. In: Barnes PJ, Rodger IW, Thomson NC, eds. Asthma: Basic mechanisms and clinical management. London: Academic Press, 1998: 459–74.

85. Schule R, Rangarajan P, Kliewer S, Ransone LJ, Bolado J, Yang N, Verma IM, Evans RM. Functional antagonism between oncoprotein c-Jun and the glucocorticoid receptor. Cell 1990; 62: 1217–26.

86. Jonat C, Rahmsdorf HJ, Park KK *et al.* Antitumor promotion and antiinflammation: down-modulation of AP-1 (Fos/Jun) activity by glucocorticoid hormone. Cell 1990; 62: 1189–204.

87. Yang-Yen HF, Chambard JC, Sun YL *et al.* Transcriptional interference between c-Jun and the glucocorticoid receptor: mutual inhibition of DNA binding due to direct protein–protein interaction. Cell 1990; 62: 1205–15.

88. Konig H, Ponta H, Rahmsdorf HJ, Herrlich P. Interference between pathway-specific transcription factors: glucocorticoids antagonize phorbol ester-induced AP-1 activity without altering AP-1 site occupation *in vivo*. EMBO J 1992; 11: 2241–6.

89. Caldenhoven E, Liden J, Wissink S *et al.* Negative cross-talk between RelA and the glucocorticoid receptor: a possible mechanism for the antiinflammatory action of glucocorticoids. Mol Endocrinol 1995; 9: 401–12.

90. Ray A, Prefontaine KE. Physical association and functional antagonism between the p65 subunit of transcription factor NF-kappa B and the glucocorticoid receptor. Proc Natl Acad Sci USA 1994; 91: 752–6.

91. Ray A, Siegel MD, Prefontaine KE, Ray P. Anti-inflammation: direct physical association and functional antagonism between transcription factor NF-KB and the glucocorticoid receptor. Chest. 1995; 107: 139S.

92. Scheinman RI, Gualberto A, Jewell CM, Cidlowski JA, Baldwin AS, Jr. Characterization of mechanisms involved in transrepression of NF-kappa B by activated glucocorticoid receptors. Mol Cell Biol 1995; 15: 943–53.

93. McKay LI, Cidlowski JA. CBP (CREB binding protein) integrates NF-kappaB (nuclear factor-kappaB) and glucocorticoid receptor physical interactions and antagonism. Mol Endocrinol 2000; 14: 1222–34.

94. McKay LI, Cidlowski JA. Cross-talk between nuclear factor-kappa B and the steroid hormone receptors: mechanisms of mutual antagonism. Mol Endocrinol 1998; 12: 45–56.

95. Brostjan C, Anrather J, Csizmadia V *et al.* Glucocorticoid-mediated repression of NFkappaB activity in endothelial cells does not involve induction of IkappaBalpha synthesis. J Biol Chem 1996; 271: 19612–16.

96. Wissink S, van Heerde EC, Schmitz ML *et al.* Distinct domains of the RelA NF-kappaB subunit are required for negative cross-talk and direct interaction with the glucocorticoid receptor. J Biol Chem 1997; 272: 22278–84.

97. Wissink S, van Heerde EC, van der Burg B, van der Saag PT. A dual mechanism mediates repression of NF-kappaB activity by glucocorticoids. Mol Endocrinol 1998; 12: 355–63.

98. Kamei Y, Xu L, Heinzel T *et al.* A CBP integrator complex mediates transcriptional activation and AP-1 inhibition by nuclear receptors. Cell 1996; 85: 403–14.

99. Sheppard KA, Rose DW, Haque ZK *et al.* Transcriptional activation by NF-kappaB requires multiple coactivators. Mol Cell Biol 1999; 19: 6367–78.

100. Sheppard KA, Phelps KM, Williams AJ *et al.* Nuclear integration of glucocorticoid receptor and nuclear factor-kappaB signaling by CREB-binding protein and steroid receptor coactivator-1. J Biol Chem 1998; 273: 29291–4.

101. Kurokawa R, Kalafus D, Ogliastro MH *et al.* Differential use of CREB binding protein-coactivator complexes. Science 1998; 279: 700–3.

102. Horvai AE, Xu L, Korzus E *et al.* Nuclear integration of JAK/STAT and Ras/AP-1 signaling by CBP and p300. Proc Natl Acad Sci USA 1997; 94: 1074–9.

103. Glass CK, Rose DW, Rosenfeld MG. Nuclear receptor coactivators. Curr Opin Cell Biol 1997; 9: 222–32.

104. Ray DW, Suen CS, Brass A, Soden J, White A. Structure/function of the human glucocorticoid receptor: tyrosine 735 is important for transactivation. Mol Endocrinol 1999; 13: 1855–63.

105. Radoja N, Komine M, Jho SH, Blumenberg M, Tomic-Canic M. Novel mechanism of steroid action in skin through glucocorticoid receptor monomers. Mol Cell Biol 2000; 20: 4328–39.

106. Oshima H, Simons SS, Jr. Modulation of transcription factor activity by a distant steroid modulatory element. Mol Endocrinol 1992; 6: 416–28.

107. Zeng H, Plisov SY, Simons SS, Jr. Ability of the glucocorticoid modulatory element to modify glucocorticoid receptor transactivation indicates parallel pathways for the expression of glucocorticoid modulatory element and glucocorticoid response element activities. Mol Cell Endocrinol 2000; 162: 221–34.

108. Kaul S, Blackford JA, Jr., Chen J, Ogryzko VV, Simons SS, Jr. Properties of the glucocorticoid modulatory element binding proteins GMEB-1 and -2: potential new modifiers of glucocorticoid receptor transactivation and members of the family of KDWK proteins. Mol Endocrinol 2000; 14: 1010–27.

109. Jimenez-Lara AM, Heine MJ, Gronemeyer H. Cloning of a mouse glucocorticoid modulatory element binding protein, a new member of the KDWK family. FEBS Lett 2000; 468: 203–10.

110. Theriault JR, Charette SJ, Lambert H, Landry J. Cloning and characterization of hGMEB1, a novel glucocorticoid modulatory element binding protein. FEBS Lett 1999; 452: 170–6.

111. Zeng H, Jackson DA, Oshima H, Simons SS, Jr. Cloning and characterization of a novel binding factor (GMEB-2) of the glucocorticoid modulatory element. J Biol Chem 1998; 273: 17756–62.

112. Zeng H, Kaul S, Simons SS, Jr. Genomic organization of human GMEB-1 and rat GMEB-2: structural conservation of two multifunctional proteins. Nucleic Acids Res 2000; 28: 1819–29.

113. Oakley RH, Cidlowski JA. Homologous down regulation of the glucocorticoid receptor: the molecular machinery. Crit Rev Eukaryot Gene Expr. 1993; 3: 63–88.

114. Burnstein KL, Cidlowski JA. Regulation of gene expression by glucocorticoids. Annu Rev Physiol 1989; 51: 683–99.

115. Burnstein KL, Jewell CM, Cidlowski JA. Human glucocorticoid receptor cDNA contains sequences sufficient for receptor down-regulation. J Biol Chem 1990; 265: 7284–91.

116. Burnstein KL, Bellingham DL, Jewell CM, Powell-Oliver FE, Cidlowski JA. Autoregulation of glucocorticoid receptor gene expression. Steroids 1991; 56: 52–8.

117. Burnstein KL, Cidlowski JA. The down side of glucocorticoid receptor regulation. Mol Cell Endocrinol 1992; 83: C1–8.

118. Burnstein KL, Cidlowski JA. Multiple mechanisms for regulation of steroid hormone action. J Cell Biochem 1993; 51: 130–4.

119. Webster JC, Cidlowski JA. Downregulation of the glucocorticoid receptor. A mechanism for physiological adaptation to hormones. Ann NY Acad Sci 1994; 746: 216–20.

120. Webster JC, Jewell JE, Bodwell JE, Munck A, Sar M, Cidlowski JA. Mouse glucocorticoid receptor phosphorylation status influences multiple functions of the receptor protein. J Biol Chem 1997; 272: 9287–93.

121. Bamberger CM, Bamberger AM, de Castro M, Chrousos GP. Glucocorticoid receptor beta, a potential endogenous inhibitor of glucocorticoid action in humans. J Clin Invest 1995; 95: 2435–41.

122. Bamberger CM, Else T, Bamberger AM, Beil FU, Schulte HM. Regulation of the human interleukin-2 gene by the alpha and beta isoforms of the glucocorticoid receptor. Mol Cell Endocrinol 1997; 136: 23–8.

123. Bamberger CM, Bamberger AM, Wald M, Chrousos GP, Schulte HM. Inhibition of mineralocorticoid activity by the beta-isoform of the human glucocorticoid receptor. J Steroid Biochem Mol Biol 1997; 60: 43–50.

124. Bamberger CM, Schulte HM, Chrousos GP. Molecular determinants of glucocorticoid receptor function and tissue sensitivity to glucocorticoids. Endocrinol Rev 1996; 17: 245–61.

125. Oakley RH, Sar M, Cidlowski JA. The human glucocorticoid receptor beta isoform. Expression, biochemical properties, and putative function. J Biol Chem 1996; 271: 9550–9.

126. Oakley RH, Webster JC, Sar M, Parker CR, Jr, Cidlowski JA. Expression and subcellular distribution of the beta-isoform of the human glucocorticoid receptor. Endocrinology 1997; 138: 5028–38.

127. Oakley RH, Jewell CM, Yudt MR, Bofetiado DM, Cidlowski JA. The dominant negative activity of the human glucocorticoid receptor beta isoform. Specificity and mechanisms of action. J Biol Chem 1999; 274: 27857–66.

128. Sousa AR, Lane SJ, Cidlowski JA, Staynov DZ, Lee TH. Glucocorticoid resistance in asthma is associated with elevated *in vivo* expression of the glucocorticoid receptor beta-isoform. J Allergy Clin Immunol 2000; 105: 943–50.

129. Christodoulopoulos P, Leung DY, Elliott MW *et al*. Increased number of glucocorticoid receptor-beta-expressing cells in the airways in fatal asthma. J Allergy Clin Immunol 2000; 106: 479–84.

130. Hamid QA, Wenzel SE, Hauk PJ *et al*. Increased glucocorticoid receptor beta in airway cells of glucocorticoid-insensitive asthma. Am J Respir Crit Care Med 1999; 159: 1600–4.

131. Gagliardo R, Chanez P, Vignola AM *et al*. Glucocorticoid receptor alpha and beta in glucocorticoid dependent asthma. Am J Respir Crit Care Med 2000; 162: 7–13.

132. Carlstedt-Duke J. Glucocorticoid receptor beta: View II. Trends Endocrinol Metab 1999; 10: 339–42.

133. Vottero A, Chrousos GP. Glucocorticoid Receptor beta: View I. Trends Endocrinol Metab 1999; 10: 333–8.

134. Stahl M, Ludwig D, Fellermann K, Stange EF. Intestinal expression of human heat shock protein 90 in patients with Crohn's disease and ulcerative colitis. Dig Dis Sci 1998; 43: 1079–87.

135. Shimada T, Hiwatashi N, Yamazaki H, Kinouchi Y, Toyota T. Relationship between glucocorticoid receptor and response to glucocorticoid therapy in ulcerative colitis. Dis Colon Rectum 1997; 40: S54–8.

136. Rogler G, Meinel A, Lingauer A *et al*. Glucocorticoid receptors are down-regulated in inflamed colonic mucosa but not in peripheral blood mononuclear cells from patients with inflammatory bowel disease. Eur J Clin Invest 1999; 29: 330–6.

137. Rosewicz S, McDonald AR, Maddux BA, Goldfine ID, Miesfeld RL, Logsdon CD. Mechanism of glucocorticoid receptor down-regulation by glucocorticoids. J Biol Chem 1988; 263: 2581–4.

138. Okret S, Poellinger L, Dong Y, Gustafsson JA. Down-regulation of glucocorticoid receptor mRNA by glucocorticoid hormones and recognition by the receptor of a specific binding sequence within a receptor cDNA clone. Proc Natl Acad Sci USA 1986; 83: 5899–903.

139. Cidlowski JA, Cidlowski NB. Regulation of glucocorticoid receptors by glucocorticoids in cultured HeLa S3 cells. Endocrinology. 1981; 109: 1975–82.

140. Honda M, Orii F, Ayabe T *et al*. Expression of glucocorticoid receptor beta in lymphocytes of patients with gluco-

corticoid-resistant ulcerative colitis. Gastroenterology 2000; 118: 859–66.

141. Stange EF. Glucocorticoid receptor activity in inflammatory bowel disease: hindsight or foresight? Eur J Clin Invest 1999; 29: 278–9.

142. Boumpas DT, Paliogianni F, Anastassiou ED, Balow JE. Glucocorticosteroid action on the immune system: molecular and cellular aspects. Clin Exp Rheumatol 1991; 9: 413–23.

143. Almawi WY, Melemedjian OK, Rieder MJ. An alternate mechanism of glucocorticoid anti-proliferative effect: promotion of a Th2 cytokine-secreting profile. Clin Transplant 1999; 13: 365–74.

144. Kirsch AH, Mahmood AA, Endres J *et al*. Apoptosis of human T-cells: induction by glucocorticoids or surface receptor ligation *in vitro* and *ex vivo*. J Biol Regul Homeost Agents 1999; 13: 80–9.

145. Lanza L, Scudeletti M, Puppo F *et al*. Prednisone increases apoptosis in *in vitro* activated human peripheral blood T lymphocytes. Clin Exp Immunol 1996; 103: 482–90.

146. King LB, Ashwell JD. Signaling for death of lymphoid cells. Curr Opin Immunol 1993; 5: 368–73.

147. Chapman MS, Askew DJ, Kuscuoglu U, Miesfeld RL. Transcriptional control of steroid-regulated apoptosis in murine thymoma cells. Mol Endocrinol 1996; 10: 967–78.

148. Van Houten N, Blake SF, Li EJ *et al*. Elevated expression of Bcl-2 and Bcl-x by intestinal intraepithelial lymphocytes: resistance to apoptosis by glucocorticoids and irradiation. Int Immunol 1997; 9: 945–53.

149. Franchimont D, Galon J, Gadina M *et al*. Inhibition of Th1 immune response by glucocorticoids: dexamethasone selectively inhibits IL-12-induced Stat4 phosphorylation in T lymphocytes. J Immunol 2000; 164: 1768–74.

150. Girndt M, Sester U, Kaul H, Hunger F, Kohler H. Glucocorticoids inhibit activation-dependent expression of costimulatory molecule B7-1 in human monocytes. Transplantation 1998; 66: 370–5.

151. Wagner DH, Jr, Hagman J, Linsley PS, Hodsdon W, Freed JH, Newell MK. Rescue of thymocytes from glucocorticoid-induced cell death mediated by CD28/CTLA-4 costimulatory interactions with B7-1/B7-2. J Exp Med 1996; 184: 1631–8.

152. Rogler G, Hausmann M, Vogl D *et al*. Isolation and phenotypic characterization of colonic macrophages. Clin Exp Immunol 1998; 112: 205–15.

153. Rogler G, Hausmann M, Spottl T *et al*. T-cell co-stimulatory molecules are upregulated on intestinal macrophages from inflammatory bowel disease mucosa. Eur J Gastroenterol Hepatol 1999; 11: 1105-1111.

154. Andus T, Rogler G, Daig R, Falk W, Schölmerich J, Gross V. The role of macrophages. In: Tygat GNJ, Bartelsman JFWM, van Deventer SJH, eds. Inflammatory Bowel Disease. Dordrecht: Kluwer, 1995: 281–97

155. Lee SH, Starkey PM, Gordon S. Quantitative analysis of total macrophage content in adult mouse tissues. Immunochemical studies with monoclonal antibody F4/80. J Exp Med 1985; 161: 475-489.

156. Donnellan WL. The structure of the colonic mucosa. The epithelium and subepithelial reticulohistiocytic complex. Gastroenterology 1965; 49: 496-514.

157. Rogler G, Andus T, Aschenbrenner E *et al*. Alterations of the phenotype of colonic macrophages in inflammatory bowel disease. Eur J Gastroenterol Hepatol 1997; 9: 893–9.

158. Mahida YR, Patel S, Gionchetti P, Vaux D, Jewell DP. Macrophage subpopulations in lamina propria of normal and inflamed colon and terminal ileum. Gut 1989; 30: 826–34.

159. Malizia G, Calabrese A, Cottone M *et al*. Expression of leukocyte adhesion molecules by mucosal mononuclear

phagocytes in inflammatory bowel disease. Gastroenterology 1991; 100: 150–9.

160. Tanner AR, Arthur MJ, Wright R. Macrophage activation, chronic inflammation and gastrointestinal disease. Gut 1984; 25: 760–83.

161. Thyberg J, Graf W, Klingenstrom P. Intestinal fine structure in Crohn's disease. Lysosomal inclusions in epithelial cells and macrophages. Virchows Arch A Pathol Anat Histol 1981; 391: 141–52.

162. Meuret G, Bitzi A, Hammer B. Macrophage turnover in Crohn's disease and ulcerative colitis. Gastroenterology 1978; 74: 501–3.

163. Hirata I, Murano M, Nitta M et al. Estimation of mucosal inflammatory mediators in rat DSS-induced colitis. Possible role of PGE(2) in protection against mucosal damage. Digestion 2001; 63: 73–80.

164. Nieto N, Torres MI, Fernandez MI et al. Experimental ulcerative colitis impairs antioxidant defense system in rat intestine. Dig Dis Sci 2000; 45: 1820–7.

165. Raab Y, Sundberg C, Hallgren R, Knutson L, Gerdin B. Mucosal synthesis and release of prostaglandin E2 from activated eosinophils and macrophages in ulcerative colitis. Am J Gastroenterol 1995; 90: 614–20.

166. van Heeckeren AM, Rikihisa Y, Park J, Fertel R. Tumor necrosis factor alpha, interleukin-1 alpha, interleukin-6, and prostaglandin E2 production in murine peritoneal macrophages infected with *Ehrlichia risticii*. Infect Immun 1993; 61: 4333–7.

167. Yamashita S. Studies on changes of colonic mucosal PGE2 levels and tissue localization in experimental colitis. Gastroenterol Jpn 1993; 28: 224–35.

168. Schreiber S, Raedler A, Stenson WF, MacDermott RP. The role of the mucosal immune system in inflammatory bowel disease. Gastroenterol Clin N Am 1992; 21: 451–502.

169. Donowitz M. Arachidonic acid metabolites and their role in inflammatory bowel disease. An update requiring addition of a pathway. Gastroenterology 1985; 88: 580–7.

170. Eliakim R, Karmeli F, Razin E, Rachmilewitz D. Role of platelet-activating factor in ulcerative colitis. Enhanced production during active disease and inhibition by sulfasalazine and prednisolone. Gastroenterology 1988; 95: 1167–72.

171. Reinecker HC, Steffen M, Witthoeft T et al. Enhanced secretion of tumour necrosis factor-alpha, IL-6, and IL-1 beta by isolated lamina propria mononuclear cells from patients with ulcerative colitis and Crohn's disease. Clin Exp Immunol 1993; 94: 174–81.

172. Grimm MC, Elsbury SK, Pavli P, Doe WF. Interleukin 8: cells of origin in inflammatory bowel disease. Gut 1996; 38: 90–8.

173. Mahida YR, Wu K, Jewell DP. Enhanced production of interleukin 1-beta by mononuclear cells isolated from mucosa with active ulcerative colitis of Crohn's disease. Gut 1989; 30: 835–8.

174. Rogler G, Andus T. Cytokines in inflammatory bowel disease. World J Surg. 1998; 22: 382–9.

175. Gross V, Andus T, Leser HG, Roth M, Scholmerich J. Inflammatory mediators in chronic inflammatory bowel diseases.. Klin Wochenschr. 1991; 69: 981–7.

176. Andus T, Gross V, Casar I et al. Activation of monocytes during inflammatory bowel disease. Pathobiology 1991; 59: 166–70.

177. Stylianou E, Nie M, Ueda A, Zhao L. c-Rel and p65 transactivate the monocyte chemoattractant protein-1 gene in interleukin-1 stimulated mesangial cells. Kidney Int 1999; 56: 873–82.

178. Vincenti MP, Coon CI, Brinckerhoff CE. Nuclear factor kappaB/p50 activates an element in the distal matrix metalloproteinase 1 promoter in interleukin-1beta-stimu-lated synovial fibroblasts. Arthritis Rheum 1998; 41: 1987–94.

179. Martin T, Cardarelli PM, Parry GC, Felts KA, Cobb RR. Cytokine induction of monocyte chemoattractant protein-1 gene expression in human endothelial cells depends on the cooperative action of NF-kappa B and AP-1. Eur J Immunol 1997; 27: 1091–7.

180. Mori N, Prager D. Transactivation of the interleukin-1alpha promoter by human T-cell leukemia virus type I and type II Tax proteins. Blood 1996; 87: 3410–17.

181. Parry GC, Mackman N. Transcriptional regulation of tissue factor expression in human endothelial cells. Arterioscler Thromb Vasc Biol 1995; 15: 612–21.

182. Kunsch C, Lang RK, Rosen CA, Shannon MF. Synergistic transcriptional activation of the IL-8 gene by NF-kappa B p65 (RelA) and NF-IL-6. J Immunol 1994; 153: 153–64.

183. Dunn SM, Coles LS, Lang RK, Gerondakis S, Vadas MA, Shannon MF. Requirement for nuclear factor (NF)-kappa B p65 and NF-interleukin-6 binding elements in the tumor necrosis factor response region of the granulocyte colony-stimulating factor promoter. Blood 1994; 83: 2469–79.

184. Hiscott J, Marois J, Garoufalis J et al. Characterization of a functional NF-kappa B site in the human interleukin 1 beta promoter: evidence for a positive autoregulatory loop. Mol Cell Biol 1993; 13: 6231–40.

185. Kunsch C, Rosen CA. NF-kappa B subunit-specific regulation of the interleukin-8 promoter. Mol Cell Biol 1993; 13: 6137–46.

186. Roebuck KA, Carpenter LR, Lakshminarayanan V, Page SM, Moy JN, Thomas LL. Stimulus-specific regulation of chemokine expression involves differential activation of the redox-responsive transcription factors AP-1 and NF-kappaB. J Leukoc Biol 1999; 65: 291–8.

187. Baeuerle PA, Baltimore D. NF-kappa B: ten years after. Cell 1996; 87: 13–20.

188. McKay DM, Perdue MH. Intestinal epithelial function: the case for immunophysiological regulation. Cells and mediators (1). Dig Dis Sci 1993; 38: 1377–87.

189. McKay DM, Perdue MH. Intestinal epithelial function: the case for immunophysiological regulation. Implications for disease (2). Dig Dis Sci 1993; 38: 1735–45.

190. Perdue MH, McKay DM. Integrative immunophysiology in the intestinal mucosa. Am J Physiol 1994; 267: G151–65.

191. Selby WS, Janossy G, Mason DY, Jewell DP. Expression of HLA-DR antigens by colonic epithelium in inflammatory bowel disease. Clin Exp Immunol 1983; 53: 614–18.

192. Bland PW, Whiting CV. Induction of MHC class II gene products in rat intestinal epithelium during graft-versus-host disease and effects on the immune function of the epithelium. Immunology 1992; 75: 366–71.

193. Bland PW, Warren LG. Antigen presentation by epithelial cells of the rat small intestine. II. Selective induction of suppressor T cells. Immunology 1986; 58: 9–14.

194. Bland PW, Warren LG. Antigen presentation by epithelial cells of the rat small intestine. I. Kinetics, antigen specificity and blocking by anti-Ia antisera. Immunology 1986; 58: 1–7.

195. Mayer L, Shlien R. Evidence for function of Ia molecules on gut epithelial cells in man. J Exp Med 1987; 166: 1471–83.

196. Panja A, Barone A, Mayer L. Stimulation of lamina propria lymphocytes by intestinal epithelial cells: evidence for recognition of nonclassical restriction elements. J Exp Med 1994; 179: 943–50.

197. Jung HC, Eckmann L, Yang SK et al. A distinct array of proinflammatory cytokines is expressed in human colon epithelial cells in response to bacterial invasion. J Clin Invest 1995; 95: 55–65.

198. Eckmann L, Reed SL, Smith JR, Kagnoff MF. *Entamoeba histolytica* trophozoites induce an inflammatory cytokine response by cultured human cells through the paracrine

action of cytolytically released interleukin-1 alpha. J Clin Invest 1995; 96: 1269–79.

199. Gibson P, Rosella O. Interleukin 8 secretion by colonic crypt cells *in vitro*: response to injury suppressed by butyrate and enhanced in inflammatory bowel disease. Gut 1995; 37: 536–43.

200. Daig R, Rogler G, Aschenbrenner E *et al*. Human intestinal epithelial cells secrete interleukin-1 receptor antagonist and interleukin-8 but not interleukin-1 or interleukin-6. Gut 2000; 46: 350–8.

201. Shirota K, LeDuy L, Yuan SY, Jothy S. Interleukin-6 and its receptor are expressed in human intestinal epithelial cells. Virchows Arch B Cell Pathol Incl Mol Pathol 1990; 58: 303–8.

202. Bocker U, Damiao A, Holt L *et al*. Differential expression of interleukin 1 receptor antagonist isoforms in human intestinal epithelial cells. Gastroenterology 1998; 115: 1426–38.

203. Warhurst AC, Hopkins SJ, Warhurst G. Interferon gamma induces differential upregulation of alpha and beta chemokine secretion in colonic epithelial cell lines. Gut 1998; 42: 208–13.

204. Yang SK, Eckmann L, Panja A, Kagnoff MF. Differential and regulated expression of C-X-C, C-C, and C-chemokines by human colon epithelial cells. Gastroenterology 1997; 113: 1214–23.

205. Eckmann L, Jung HC, Schurer-Maly C, Panja A, Morzycka-Wroblewska E, Kagnoff MF. Differential cytokine expression by human intestinal epithelial cell lines: regulated expression of interleukin 8. Gastroenterology 1993; 105: 1689–97.

206. Parikh AA, Salzman AL, Kane CD, Fischer JE, Hasselgren PO. IL-6 production in human intestinal epithelial cells following stimulation with IL-1 beta is associated with activation of the transcription factor NF-kappa B. J Surg Res 1997; 69: 139–44.

207. Jobin C, Panja A, Hellerbrand C *et al*.Inhibition of proinflammatory molecule production by adenovirus- mediated expression of a nuclear factor kappaB super-repressor in human intestinal epithelial cells. J Immunol 1998; 160: 410–18.

208. Rogler G, Brand K, Vogl D *et al*. Nuclear factor kappaB is activated in macrophages and epithelial cells of inflamed intestinal mucosa. Gastroenterology 1998; 115: 357–69.

209. Schreiber S, Nikolaus S, Hampe J. Activation of nuclear factor kappa B inflammatory bowel disease. Gut 1998; 42: 477–84.

210. Cavicchi M, Whittle BJ. Regulation of induction of nitric oxide synthase and the inhibitory actions of dexamethasone in the human intestinal epithelial cell line, Caco-2: influence of cell differentiation. Br J Pharmacol 1999; 128: 705–15.

211. Zareie M, Brattsand R, Sherman PM, McKay DM, Perdue MH. Improved effects of novel glucocorticosteroids on immune-induced epithelial pathophysiology. J Pharmacol Exp Ther 1999; 289: 1245–9.

212. Willoughby CP, Piris J, Truelove SC. Tissue eosinophils in ulcerative colitis. Scand J Gastroenterol 1979; 14: 395–9.

213. Dvorak AM, Monahan RA, Osage JE, Dickersin GR. Crohn's disease: transmission electron microscopic studies. II. Immunologic inflammatory response. Alterations of mast cells, basophils, eosinophils, and the microvasculature. Hum Pathol 1980; 11: 606–19.

214. Bischoff SC, Wedemeyer J, Herrmann A *et al*. Quantitative assessment of intestinal eosinophils and mast cells in inflammatory bowel disease. Histopathology 1996; 28: 1–13.

215. Geboes K. From inflammation to lesion. Acta Gastroenterol Belg 1994; 57: 273–84.

216. Sarin SK, Malhotra V, Sen Gupta S, Karol A, Gaur SK, Anand BS. Significance of eosinophil and mast cell counts in rectal mucosa in ulcerative colitis. A prospective controlled study. Dig Dis Sci 1987; 32: 363–7.

217. Choy MY, Walker-Smith JA, Williams CB, MacDonald TT. Activated eosinophils in chronic inflammatory bowel disease. Lancet 1990; 336: 126–7.

218. Seegert D, Rosenstiel P, Pfahler H, Pfefferkorn P, Nikolaus S, Schreiber S. Increased expression of IL-16 in inflammatory bowel disease. Gut 2001; 48: 326–32.

219. Louahed J, Zhou Y, Maloy WL *et al*. Interleukin 9 promotes influx and local maturation of eosinophils. Blood 2001; 97: 1035–42.

220. Jinquan T, Jing C, Jacobi HH *et al*. CXCR3 expression and activation of eosinophils: role of IFN-gamma-inducible protein-10 and monokine induced by IFN-gamma. J Immunol 2000; 165: 1548–56.

221. Schwingshackl A, Duszyk M, Brown N, Moqbel R. Human eosinophils release matrix metalloproteinase-9 on stimulation with TNF-alpha. J Allergy Clin Immunol 1999; 104: 983–9.

222. Velazquez JR, Lacy P, Mahmudi-Azer S, Moqbel R. Effects of interferon-gamma on mobilization and release of eosinophil- derived RANTES. Int Arch Allergy Immunol 1999; 118: 447–9.

223. Miyamasu M, Hirai K, Takahashi Y *et al*. Chemotactic agonists induce cytokine generation in eosinophils. J Immunol 1995; 154: 1339–49.

224. Hansel TT, Braun RK, De Vries IJ *et al*. Eosinophils and cytokines. Agents Actions Suppl. 1993; 43: 197–208

225. Yamashita N, Koizumi H, Murata M, Mano K, Ohta K. Nuclear factor kappa B mediates interleukin-8 production in eosinophils. Int Arch Allergy Immunol 1999; 120: 230–6.

226. Jang AS, Choi IS, Koh YI *et al*. Effects of prednisolone on eosinophils, IL-5, eosinophil cationic protein, EG2+ eosinophils, and nitric oxide metabolites in the sputum of patients with exacerbated asthma. J Korean Med Sci 2000; 15: 521–8.

227. Miyamasu M, Misaki Y, Izumi S *et al*. Glucocorticoids inhibit chemokine generation by human eosinophils. J Allergy Clin Immunol 1998; 101: 75–83.

228. Shidham VB, Swami VK. Evaluation of apoptotic leukocytes in peripheral blood smears. Arch Pathol Lab Med 2000; 124: 1291–4.

229. Arai Y, Nakamura Y, Inoue F, Yamamoto K, Saito K, Furusawa S. Glucocorticoid-induced apoptotic pathways in eosinophils: comparison with glucocorticoid-sensitive leukemia cells. Int J Hematol 2000; 71: 340–9.

230. Nittoh T, Fujimori H, Kozumi Y, Ishihara K, Mue S, Ohuchi K. Effects of glucocorticoids on apoptosis of infiltrated eosinophils and neutrophils in rats. Eur J Pharmacol 1998; 354: 73–81.

231. Walsh GM. Mechanisms of human eosinophil survival and apoptosis. Clin Exp Allergy 1997; 27: 482–7.

232. Adachi T, Motojima S, Hirata A *et al*. Eosinophil apoptosis caused by theophylline, glucocorticoids, and macrolides after stimulation with IL-5. J Allergy Clin Immunol 1996; 98: S207–15.

233. Schleimer RP, Bochner BS. The effects of glucocorticoids on human eosinophils. J Allergy Clin Immunol 1994; 94: 1202–13.

234. Jaye DL, Parkos CA. Neutrophil migration across intestinal epithelium. Ann NY Acad Sci 2000; 915: 151–61.

235. Kim B, Barnett JL, Kleer CG, Appelman HD. Endoscopic and histological patchiness in treated ulcerative colitis. Am J Gastroenterol 1999; 94: 3258–62.

236. Bartram CI, Talbot IC. Coloncoscopic biopsies in colitis. Abdom Imaging 1995; 20: 384–6.

237. Mitsuyama K, Toyonaga A, Sasaki E *et al*. IL-8 as an important chemoattractant for neutrophils in ulcerative

colitis and Crohn's disease. Clin Exp Immunol 1994; 96: 432–6.

238. Grisham MB, Granger DN. Neutrophil-mediated mucosal injury. Role of reactive oxygen metabolites. Dig Dis Sci 1988; 33: 6S–15S.

239. Lewis DC, Walker-Smith JA, Phillips AD. Polymorphonuclear neutrophil leucocytes in childhood Crohn's disease: a morphological study. J Pediatr Gastroenterol Nutr 1987; 6: 430–8.

240. Kane SP, Vincenti AC. Mucosal enzymes in human inflammatory bowel disease with reference to neutrophil granulocytes as mediators of tissue injury. Clin Sci (Colch) 1979; 57: 295–303.

241. Fauci AS, Dale DC, Balow JE. Glucocorticosteroid therapy: mechanisms of action and clinical considerations. Ann Intern Med 1976; 84: 304–15.

242. van der Saag PT, Caldenhoven E, van de Stolpe A. Molecular mechanisms of steroid action: a novel type of cross-talk between glucocorticoids and NF-kappa B transcription factors. Eur Respir J Suppl. 1996; 22: 146–53s.

243. Wheller SK, Perretti M. Dexamethasone inhibits cytokine-induced intercellular adhesion molecule-1 up-regulation on endothelial cell lines. Eur J Pharmacol 1997; 331: 65–71.

244. Wissink S, van de Stolpe A, Caldenhoven E, Koenderman L, van der Saag PT. NF-kappa B/Rel family members regulating the ICAM-1 promoter in monocytic THP-1 cells. Immunobiology 1997; 198: 50–64.

245. Tessier P, Audette M, Cattaruzzi P, McColl SR. Up-regulation by tumor necrosis factor alpha of intercellular adhesion molecule 1 expression and function in synovial fibroblasts and its inhibition by glucocorticoids. Arthritis Rheum 1993; 36: 1528–39.

246. Fattal-German M, Ladurie FL, Cerrina J, Lecerf F, Berrih-Aknin S. Modulation of ICAM-1 expression in human alveolar macrophages *in vitro*. Eur Respir J 1996; 9: 463–71.

247. Atsuta J, Plitt J, Bochner BS, Schleimer RP. Inhibition of VCAM-1 expression in human bronchial epithelial cells by glucocorticoids. Am J Respir Cell Mol Biol 1999; 20: 643–50.

248. Summers RW, Switz DM, Sessions JT, Jr et al. National Cooperative Crohn's Disease Study: results of drug treatment. Gastroenterology 1979; 77: 847–69.

249. Jue DM, Jeon KI, Jeong JY. Nuclear factor kappaB (NF-kappaB) pathway as a therapeutic target in rheumatoid arthritis. J Korean Med Sci 1999; 14: 231–8.

250. MacDermott RP. Progress in understanding the mechanisms of action of 5-aminosalicylic acid. Am J Gastroenterol 2000; 95: 3343–5.

251. Nikolaus S, Folsch U, Schreiber S. Immunopharmacology of 5-aminosalicylic acid and of glucocorticoids in the therapy of inflammatory bowel disease. Hepatogastroenterology 2000; 47: 71–82.

252. Wahl C, Liptay S, Adler G, Schmid RM. Sulfasalazine: a potent and specific inhibitor of nuclear factor kappa B. J Clin Invest 1998; 101: 1163–74.

253. Liptay S, Bachem M, Hacker G, Adler G, Debatin KM, Schmid RM. Inhibition of nuclear factor kappa B and induction of apoptosis in T- lymphocytes by sulfasalazine. Br J Pharmacol 1999; 128: 1361–9.

254. Weber CK, Liptay S, Wirth T, Adler G, Schmid RM. Suppression of NF-kappaB activity by sulfasalazine is mediated by direct inhibition of IkappaB kinases alpha and beta. Gastroenterology 2000; 119: 1209–18.

255. Munkholm P, Langholz E, Davidsen M, Binder V. Frequency of glucocorticoid resistance and dependency in Crohn's disease. Gut 1994; 35: 360–2.

256. Munkholm P, Langholz E, Davidsen M, Binder V. Disease activity courses in a regional cohort of Crohn's disease patients. Scand J Gastroenterol 1995; 30: 699–706.

257. Chinetti G, Fruchart JC, Staels B. Peroxisome proliferator-activated receptors (PPARs): nuclear receptors at the crossroads between lipid metabolism and inflammation. Inflamm Res 2000; 49: 497–505.

258. Fajas L, Auboeuf D, Raspe E et al. The organization, promoter analysis, and expression of the human PPARgamma gene. J Biol Chem 1997; 272: 18779–89.

259. Kliewer SA, Willson TM. The nuclear receptor PPARgamma – bigger than fat. Curr Opin Genet Dev 1998; 8: 576–81.

260. Kliewer SA, Forman BM, Blumberg B et al. Differential expression and activation of a family of murine peroxisome proliferator-activated receptors. Proc Natl Acad Sci USA 1994; 91: 7355–9.

261. Lemberger T, Braissant O, Juge-Aubry C et al. PPAR tissue distribution and interactions with other hormone-signaling pathways. Ann NY Acad Sci 1996; 804: 231–51.

262. Tontonoz P, Hu E, Graves RA, Budavari AI, Spiegelman BM. mPPAR gamma 2: tissue-specific regulator of an adipocyte enhancer. Genes Dev 1994; 8: 1224–34.

263. Chinetti G, Griglio S, Antonucci M et al. Activation of proliferator-activated receptors alpha and gamma induces apoptosis of human monocyte-derived macrophages. J Biol Chem 1998; 273: 25573–80.

264. Wiesenberg I, Chiesi M, Missbach M, Spanka C, Pignat W, Carlberg C. Specific activation of the nuclear receptors PPARgamma and RORA by the antidiabetic thiazolidinedione BRL 49653 and the antiarthritic thiazolidinedione derivative CGP 52608. Mol Pharmacol 1998; 53: 1131–8.

265. Murphy GJ, Holder JC. PPAR-gamma agonists: therapeutic role in diabetes, inflammation and cancer. Trends Pharmacol Sci 2000; 21: 469–74.

266. Fujiwara T, Horikoshi H. Troglitazone and related compounds: therapeutic potential beyond diabetes. Life Sci 2000; 67: 2405–16.

267. Spiegelman BM. PPAR-gamma: adipogenic regulator and thiazolidinedione receptor. Diabetes 1998; 47: 507–14.

268. Berger J, Bailey P, Biswas C et al. Thiazolidinediones produce a conformational change in peroxisomal proliferator-activated receptor-gamma: binding and activation correlate with antidiabetic actions in db/db mice. Endocrinology 1996; 137: 4189–95.

269. Pershadsingh HA. Pharmacological peroxisome proliferator-activated receptorgamma ligands: emerging clinical indications beyond diabetes. Expert Opin Investig Drugs 1999; 8: 1859–72.

270. Willson TM, Lehmann JM, Kliewer SA. Discovery of ligands for the nuclear peroxisome proliferator-activated receptors. Ann NY Acad Sci 1996; 804: 276–83.

271. Lehmann JM, Moore LB, Smith-Oliver TA, Wilkison WO, Willson TM, Kliewer SA. An antidiabetic thiazolidinedione is a high affinity ligand for peroxisome proliferator-activated receptor gamma (PPAR gamma). J Biol Chem 1995; 270: 12953–6.

272. Willson TM, Wahli W. Peroxisome proliferator-activated receptor agonists. Curr Opin Chem Biol 1997; 1: 235–41.

273. De Vos P, Lefebvre AM, Miller SG et al. Thiazolidinediones repress ob gene expression in rodents via activation of peroxisome proliferator-activated receptor gamma. J Clin Invest 1996; 98: 1004–9.

274. Kliewer SA, Lenhard JM, Willson TM, Patel I, Morris DC, Lehmann JM. A prostaglandin J2 metabolite binds peroxisome proliferator-activated receptor gamma and promotes adipocyte differentiation. Cell 1995; 83: 813–19.

275. Kliewer SA, Sundseth SS, Jones SA et al. Fatty acids and eicosanoids regulate gene expression through direct interactions with peroxisome proliferator-activated receptors alpha and gamma. Proc Natl Acad Sci USA 1997; 94: 4318–23.

276. Forman BM, Tontonoz P, Chen J, Brun RP, Spiegelman BM, Evans RM. 15-Deoxy-delta 12, 14-prostaglandin J2 is

a ligand for the adipocyte determination factor PPAR gamma. Cell 1995; 83: 803–12.

277. Forman BM, Chen J, Evans RM. The peroxisome proliferator-activated receptors: ligands and activators. Ann NY Acad Sci 1996; 804: 266–75.

278. Forman BM, Chen J, Evans RM. Hypolipidemic drugs, polyunsaturated fatty acids, and eicosanoids are ligands for peroxisome proliferator-activated receptors alpha and delta. Proc Natl Acad Sci USA 1997; 94: 4312–17.

279. Krey G, Braissant O, L'Horset F et al. Fatty acids, eicosanoids, and hypolipidemic agents identified as ligands of peroxisome proliferator-activated receptors by coactivator-dependent receptor ligand assay. Mol Endocrinol 1997; 11: 779–91.

280. Urade Y, Ujihara M, Horiguchi Y, Ikai K, Hayaishi O. The major source of endogenous prostaglandin D2 production is likely antigen-presenting cells. Localization of glutathione-requiring prostaglandin D synthetase in histiocytes, dendritic, and Kupffer cells in various rat tissues. J Immunol 1989; 143: 2982–9.

281. Ricote M, Huang JT, Welch JS, Glass CK. The peroxisome proliferator-activated receptor (PPARgamma) as a regulator of monocyte/macrophage function. J Leukoc Biol 1999; 66: 733–9.

282. Ricote M, Huang J, Fajas L et al. Expression of the peroxisome proliferator-activated receptor gamma (PPARgamma) in human atherosclerosis and regulation in macrophages by colony stimulating factors and oxidized low density lipoprotein. Proc Natl Acad Sci USA 1998; 95: 7614–19.

283. Ricote M, Li AC, Willson TM, Kelly CJ, Glass CK. The peroxisome proliferator-activated receptor-gamma is a negative regulator of macrophage activation. Nature 1998; 391: 79–82.

284. Jiang C, Ting AT, Seed B. PPAR-gamma agonists inhibit production of monocyte inflammatory cytokines. Nature 1998; 391: 82–6.

285. Fajas L, Fruchart JC, Auwerx J. PPARgamma3 mRNA: a distinct PPARgamma mRNA subtype transcribed from an independent promoter. FEBS Lett 1998; 438: 55–60.

286. DuBois RN, Gupta R, Brockman J, Reddy BS, Krakow SL, Lazar MA. The nuclear eicosanoid receptor, PPARgamma, is aberrantly expressed in colonic cancers. Carcinogenesis 1998; 19: 49–53.

287. Sarraf P, Mueller E, Jones D et al. Differentiation and reversal of malignant changes in colon cancer through PPARgamma. Nat Med 1998; 4: 1046–52.

288. Sarraf P, Mueller E, Smith WM et al. Loss-of-function mutations in PPAR gamma associated with human colon cancer. Mol Cell 1999; 3: 799–804.

289. Saez E, Tontonoz P, Nelson MC et al. Activators of the nuclear receptor PPARgamma enhance colon polyp formation. Nat Med 1998; 4: 1058–61.

290. Lefebvre M, Paulweber B, Fajas L et al. Peroxisome proliferator-activated receptor gamma is induced during differentiation of colon epithelium cells. J Endocrinol 1999; 162: 331–40.

291. Su CG, Wen X, Bailey ST et al. A novel therapy for colitis utilizing PPAR-gamma ligands to inhibit the epithelial inflammatory response. J Clin Invest 1999; 104: 383–9.

292. Desreumaux P, Dubuquoy L, Nutten S et al. Attenuation of colon inflammation through activators of the retinoid X receptor (RXR)/peroxisome proliferator-activated receptor gamma (PPARgamma) heterodimer. A basis for new therapeutic strategies. J Exp Med 2001; 193: 827–38.

293. Rohn TT, Wong SM, Cotman CW, Cribbs DH. 15-Deoxy-delta12,14-prostaglandin J2, a specific ligand for peroxisome proliferator-activated receptor-gamma, induces neuronal apoptosis. Neuroreport 2001; 12: 839–43.

294. Marx J. Cancer research. Anti-inflammatories inhibit cancer growth – but how? Science 2001; 291: 581–2.

295. Tsubouchi Y, Sano H, Kawahito Y et al. Inhibition of human lung cancer cell growth by the peroxisome proliferator-activated receptor-gamma agonists through induction of apoptosis. Biochem Biophys Res Commun 2000; 270: 400–5.

296. Okura T, Nakamura M, Takata Y, Watanabe S, Kitami Y, Hiwada K. Troglitazone induces apoptosis via the p53 and Gadd45 pathway in vascular smooth muscle cells. Eur J Pharmacol 2000; 407: 227–35.

297. McCarty MF. Activation of PPARgamma may mediate a portion of the anticancer activity of conjugated linoleic acid. Med Hypotheses 2000; 55: 187–8.

298. Kawahito Y, Kondo M, Tsubouchi Y et al. 15-Deoxy-delta(12,14)-PGJ(2) induces synoviocyte apoptosis and suppresses adjuvant-induced arthritis in rats. J Clin Invest 2000; 106: 189–97.

299. Padilla J, Kaur K, Harris SG, Phipps RP. PPAR-gamma-mediated regulation of normal and malignant B lineage cells. Ann NY Acad Sci 2000; 905: 97–109.

300. Miller RT, Anderson SP, Corton JC, Cattley RC. Apoptosis, mitosis and cyclophilin-40 expression in regressing peroxisome proliferator-induced adenomas. Carcinogenesis 2000; 21: 647–52.

301. Chang TH, Szabo E. Induction of differentiation and apoptosis by ligands of peroxisome proliferator-activated receptor gamma in non-small cell lung cancer. Cancer Res 2000; 60: 1129–38.

302. Wu GD. A nuclear receptor to prevent colon cancer. N Engl J Med 2000; 342: 651–3.

303. Takahashi N, Okumura T, Motomura W, Fujimoto Y, Kawabata I, Kohgo Y. Activation of PPARgamma inhibits cell growth and induces apoptosis in human gastric cancer cells. FEBS Lett 1999; 455: 135–9.

304. Kroboth PD, Salek FS, Pittenger AL, Fabian TJ, Frye RF. DHEA and DHEA-S: a review. J Clin Pharmacol 1999; 39: 327–48.

305. Straub RH, Scholmerich J, Zietz B. Replacement therapy with DHEA plus corticosteroids in patients with chronic inflammatory diseases – substitutes of adrenal and sex hormones. Z Rheumatol 2000; 59: 108–18.

306. Poynter ME, Daynes RA. Peroxisome proliferator-activated receptor alpha activation modulates cellular redox status, represses nuclear factor-kappaB signaling, and reduces inflammatory cytokine production in aging. J Biol Chem 1998; 273: 32833–41.

307. Poynter ME, Daynes RA. Age-associated alterations in splenic iNOS regulation: influence of constitutively expressed IFN-gamma and correction following supplementation with PPARα lpha activators or vitamin E. Cell Immunol 1999; 195: 127–36.

308. Cheng GF, Tseng J. Regulation of murine interleukin-10 production by dehydroepiandrosterone. J Interferon Cytokine Res 2000; 20: 471–8.

309. van Vollenhoven RF, Morabito LM, Engleman EG, McGuire JL. Treatment of systemic lupus erythematosus with dehydroepiandrosterone: 50 patients treated up to 12 months. J Rheumatol 1998; 25: 285–9.

310. van Vollenhoven RF, Engleman EG, McGuire JL. Dehydroepiandrosterone in systemic lupus erythematosus. Results of a double-blind, placebo-controlled, randomized clinical trial. Arthritis Rheum 1995; 38: 1826–31.

311. van Vollenhoven RF, Engleman EG, McGuire JL. An open study of dehydroepiandrosterone in systemic lupus erythematosus. Arthritis Rheum 1994; 37: 1305–10.

312. van Vollenhoven RF, Park JL, Genovese MC, West JP, McGuire JL. A double-blind, placebo-controlled, clinical

trial of dehydroepiandrosterone in severe systemic lupus erythematosus. Lupus 1999; 8: 181–7

313. Straub RH, Vogl D, Gross V, Lang B, Scholmerich J, Andus T. Association of humoral markers of inflammation and dehydroepiandrosterone sulfate or cortisol serum levels in patients with chronic inflammatory bowel disease. Am J Gastroenterol 1998; 93: 2197–202.

314. de la Torre B, Hedman M, Befrits R. Blood and tissue dehydroepiandrosterone sulphate levels and their relationship to chronic inflammatory bowel disease. Clin Exp Rheumatol 1998; 16: 579–82.

315. Andus T, Klebl F, Rogler G, Bregenzer N, Scholmerich J, Straub RH. Successful treatment of active Crohn's disease with oral dehydroepiandrosterone (DHEA): An open controlled pilot trial. Gastroenterology 2001; 120: A1440

316. Diep QN, Touyz RM, Schiffrin EL. Docosahexaenoic acid, a peroxisome proliferator-activated receptor- alpha ligand, induces apoptosis in vascular smooth muscle cells by stimulation of p38 mitogen-activated protein kinase. Hypertension 2000; 36: 851–5.

317. Hugot JP, Chamaillard M, Zouali H et al. Association of NOD2 leucine-rich repeat variants with susceptibility to Crohn's disease. Nature 2001; 411: 599–603.

318. Ogura Y, Bonen DK, Inohara N et al. A frameshift mutation in NOD2 associated with susceptibility to Crohn's disease. Nature 2001; 411: 603–6.

319. Ogura Y, Inohara N, Benito A, Chen FF, Yamaoka S, Nunez G. Nod2, a Nod1/Apaf-1 family member yhat is restricted to monocytes and activates NF-kappa B. J Biol Chem 2001; 276: 4812–18.

320. Inohara N, Ogura Y, Chen FF, Muto A, Nunez G. Human nod1 confers responsiveness to bacterial lipopolysaccharides. J Biol Chem 2001; 276: 2551–4.

321. Inohara N, Koseki T, del Peso L et al. Nod1, an Apaf-1-like activator of caspase-9 and nuclear factor-kappaB. J Biol Chem 1999; 274: 14560–1.

322. Lenardo MJ, Baltimore D. NF-kappa B: a pleiotropic mediator of inducible and tissue-specific gene control. Cell 1989; 58: 227–9.

323. Baeuerle PA. The inducible transcription activator NF-kappa B: regulation by distinct protein subunits. Biochim Biophys Acta 1991; 1072: 63–80.

324. Grilli M, Chiu JJ, Lenardo MJ. NF-kappa B and Rel: participants in a multiform transcriptional regulatory system. Int Rev Cytol 1993; 143: 1–62.

325. Baeuerle PA, Henkel T. Function and activation of NF-kappa B in the immune system. Annu Rev Immunol 1994; 12: 141–79.

326. Baeuerle PA, Baltimore D. I kappa B: a specific inhibitor of the NF-kappa B transcription factor. Science 1988; 242: 540–6.

327. Cheng Q, Cant CA, Moll T et al. NK-kappa B subunit-specific regulation of the I kappa B alpha promoter. J Biol Chem 1994; 269: 13551–7.

328. Huxford T, Malek S, Ghosh G. Structure and mechanism in NF-kappa B/I kappa B signaling. Cold Spring Harb Symp Quant Biol 1999; 64: 533–40.

329. Muller JM, Ziegler-Heitbrock HW, Baeuerle PA. Nuclear factor kappa B, a mediator of lipopolysaccharide effects. Immunobiology 1993; 187: 233–56.

330. Maniatis T. Catalysis by a multiprotein IkappaB kinase complex. Science 1997; 278: 818–19.

331. Mercurio F, Zhu H, Murray BW et al. IKK-1 and IKK-2: cytokine-activated IkappaB kinases essential for NF-kappaB activation. Science 1997; 278: 860–6.

332. Woronicz JD, Gao X, Cao Z, Rothe M, Goeddel DV. IkappaB kinase-beta: NF-kappaB activation and complex formation with IkappaB kinase-alpha and NIK. Science 1997; 278: 866–9.

333. Karin M, Delhase M. The I kappa B kinase (IKK) and NF-kappa B: key elements of proinflammatory signalling. Semin Immunol 2000; 12: 85–98.

334. Neurath MF, Pettersson S, Meyer zum Buschenfelde KH, Strober W. Local administration of antisense phosphorothioate oligonucleotides to the p65 subunit of NF-kappa B abrogates established experimental colitis in mice. Nat Med 1996; 2: 998–1004.

335. Conner EM, Brand S, Davis JM et al. Proteasome inhibition attenuates nitric oxide synthase expression, VCAM- 1 transcription and the development of chronic colitis. J Pharmacol Exp Ther 1997; 282: 1615–22.

336. Herfarth H, Brand K, Rath HC, Rogler G, Scholmerich J, Falk W. Nuclear factor-kappa B activity and intestinal inflammation in dextran sulphate sodium (DSS)-induced colitis in mice is suppressed by gliotoxin. Clin Exp Immunol 2000; 120: 59–65.

337. Jobin C, Hellerbrand C, Licato LL, Brenner DA, Sartor RB. Mediation by NF-kappa B of cytokine induced expression of intercellular adhesion molecule 1 (ICAM-1) in an intestinal epithelial cell line, a process blocked by proteasome inhibitors. Gut 1998; 42: 779–81.

338. Beutler B, Van Huffel C. An evolutionary and functional approach to the TNF receptor/ligand family. Ann NY Acad Sci 1994; 730: 118–33.

339. Stevens C, Walz G, Singaram C, et al. Tumor necrosis factor-alpha, interleukin-1 beta, and interleukin-6 expression in inflammatory bowel disease. Dig Dis Sci 1992; 37: 818–26.

340. MacDonald TT, Hutchings P, Choy MY, Murch S, Cooke A. Tumour necrosis factor-alpha and interferon-gamma production measured at the single cell level in normal and inflamed human intestine. Clin Exp Immunol 1990; 81: 301–5.

341. Pullman WE, Elsbury S, Kobayashi M, Hapel AJ, Doe WF. Enhanced mucosal cytokine production in inflammatory bowel disease. Gastroenterology 1992; 102: 529–37.

342. Dinarello CA. The biological properties of interleukin-1. Eur Cytokine Netw 1994; 5: 517–31.

343. Dinarello CA. Role of pro- and anti-inflammatory cytokines during inflammation: experimental and clinical findings. J Biol Regul Homeost Agents 1997; 11: 91–103.

344. Youngman KR, Simon PL, West GA et al. Localization of intestinal interleukin 1 activity and protein and gene expression to lamina propria cells. Gastroenterology 1993; 104: 749–58.

345. Andus T, Daig R, Vogl D et al. Imbalance of the interleukin 1 system in colonic mucosa – association with intestinal inflammation and interleukin 1 receptor antagonist genotype 2. Gut 1997; 41: 651–7.

346. Kishimoto T, Akira S, Narazaki M, Taga T. Interleukin-6 family of cytokines and gp130. Blood 1995; 86: 1243–54.

347. Kusugami K, Fukatsu A, Tanimoto M et al. Elevation of interleukin-6 in inflammatory bowel disease is macrophage- and epithelial cell-dependent. Dig Dis Sci 1995; 40: 949–59.

348. Daig R, Andus T, Aschenbrenner E, Falk W, Scholmerich J, Gross V. Increased interleukin 8 expression in the colon mucosa of patients with inflammatory bowel disease. Gut 1996; 38: 216–22.

349. Baggiolini M, Dewald B, Moser B. Interleukin-8 and related chemotactic cytokines – CXC and CC chemokines. Adv Immunol 1994; 55: 97–179.

350. Reinecker HC, Loh EY, Ringler DJ, Mehta A, Rombeau JL, MacDermott RP. Monocyte-chemoattractant protein 1 gene expression in intestinal epithelial cells and inflammatory bowel disease mucosa. Gastroenterology 1995; 108: 40–50.

351. Iademarco MF, McQuillan JJ, Rosen GD, Dean DC. Characterization of the promoter for vascular cell adhesion molecule-1 (VCAM-1). J Biol Chem 1992; 267: 16323–9.

352. Neish AS, Williams AJ, Palmer HJ, Whitley MZ, Collins T. Functional analysis of the human vascular cell adhesion molecule 1 promoter. J Exp Med 1992; 176: 1583–93.

353. Murata T, Kurokawa R, Krones A et al. Defect of histone acetyltransferase activity of the nuclear transcriptional coactivator CBP in Rubinstein–Taybi syndrome. Hum Mol Genet 2001; 10: 1071–6.

354. Papadakis KA, Targan SR. Role of cytokines in the pathogenesis of inflammatory bowel disease. Annu Rev Med 2000; 51: 289–98.

355. Targan SR. Biology of inflammation in Crohn's disease: mechanisms of action of anti-TNF-a therapy. Can J Gastroenterol 2000; 14(Suppl. C): 13–16C.

356. Plevy SE, Landers CJ, Prehn J et al. A role for TNF-alpha and mucosal T helper-1 cytokines in the pathogenesis of Crohn's disease. J Immunol 1997; 159: 6276–82.

357. Aggarwal BB. Tumour necrosis factors receptor associated signalling molecules and their role in activation of apoptosis, JNK and NF-kappaB. Ann Rheum Dis 2000; 59(Suppl. 1): I6–16.

358. Darnay BG, Aggarwal BB. Signal transduction by tumour necrosis factor and tumour necrosis factor related ligands and their receptors. Ann Rheum Dis 1999; 58(Suppl. 1): I2–13.

359. Cao Z, Tanaka M, Regnier C et al. NF-kappa B activation by tumor necrosis factor and interleukin-1. Cold Spring Harb Symp Quant Biol 1999; 64: 473–83.

360. Chan KF, Siegel MR, Lenardo JM. Signaling by the TNF receptor superfamily and T cell homeostasis. Immunity 2000; 13: 419–22.

361. Gravestein LA, Borst J. Tumor necrosis factor receptor family members in the immune system. Semin Immunol 1998; 10: 423–34.

362. Malek NP, Pluempe J, Kubicka S, Manns MP, Trautwein C. Molecular mechanisms of TNF receptor-mediated signaling. Recent Results Cancer Res 1998; 147: 97–106.

363. Lorenz HM, Antoni C, Valerius T et al. In vivo blockade of TNF-alpha by intravenous infusion of a chimeric monoclonal TNF-alpha antibody in patients with rheumatoid arthritis. Short term cellular and molecular effects. J Immunol 1996; 156: 1646–53.

364. Lorenz HM. TNF inhibitors in the treatment of arthritis. Curr Opin Investig Drugs 2000; 1: 188–93.

365. Maini RN, Elliott M, Brennan FM, Williams RO, Feldmann M. Targeting TNF alpha for the therapy of rheumatoid arthritis. Clin Exp Rheumatol 1994; 12(Suppl. 11): S63–6.

366. Maini RN, Elliott MJ, Brennan FM et al. Monoclonal anti-TNF alpha antibody as a probe of pathogenesis and therapy of rheumatoid disease. Immunol Rev 1995; 144: 195–223.

367. Maini RN, Elliott MJ, Brennan FM, Feldmann M. Beneficial effects of tumour necrosis factor-alpha (TNF-alpha) blockade in rheumatoid arthritis (RA). Clin Exp Immunol 1995; 101: 207–12.

368. Maini RN, Elliott M, Brennan FM, Williams RO, Feldmann M. TNF blockade in rheumatoid arthritis: implications for therapy and pathogenesis. Apmis 1997; 105: 257–63.

369. Maini RN, Taylor PC, Paleolog E et al. Insights into the pathogenesis of rheumatoid arthritis from application of anti-TNF therapy. Nihon Rinsho Meneki Gakkai Kaishi 2000; 23: 487–9.

370. van Dullemen HM, van Deventer SJ, Hommes DW et al. Treatment of Crohn's disease with anti-tumor necrosis factor chimeric monoclonal antibody (cA2). Gastroenterology 1995; 109: 129–35.

371. Lang KA, Peppercorn MA. Promising new agents for the treatment of inflammatory bowel disorders. Drugs R D 1999; 1: 237–44.

372. Rutgeerts P, Baert F. New strategies in the management of inflammatory bowel disease. Acta Clin Belg 1999; 54: 274–80.

373. Ricart E, Panaccione R, Loftus EV, Tremaine WJ, Sandborn WJ. Successful management of Crohn's disease of the ileoanal pouch with infliximab. Gastroenterology 1999; 117: 429–32.

374. Sandborn WJ, Hanauer SB. Antitumor necrosis factor therapy for inflammatory bowel disease: a review of agents, pharmacology, clinical results, and safety. Inflamm Bowel Dis 1999; 5: 119–33.

375. Heresbach D, Semana G, Gosselin M, Bretagne MG. An immunomodulation strategy targeted towards immunocompetent cells or cytokines in inflammatory bowel diseases (IBD). Eur Cytokine Netw 1999; 10: 7–15.

376. Evans RC, Clarke L, Heath P, Stephens S, Morris AI, Rhodes JM. Treatment of ulcerative colitis with an engineered human anti-TNFalpha antibody CDP571. Aliment Pharmacol Ther 1997; 11: 1031–5.

377. van Deventer SJ, Camoglio L. Monoclonal antibody therapy of inflammatory bowel disease. Pharm World Sci 1997; 19: 55–9.

378. Schreiber S, Campieri M, Colombel JF et al. Use of anti-tumour necrosis factor agents in inflammatory bowel disease. European guidelines for 2001–2003. Int J Colorectal Dis 2001; 16: 1–11; discussion 12–13.

379. Kam LY, Targan SR. TNF-alpha antagonists for the treatment of Crohn's disease. Expert Opin Pharmacother 2000; 1: 615–22.

380. Mikula CA. Anti-TNF alpha: new therapy for Crohn's disease. Gastroenterol Nurs 1999; 22: 245–8.

381. Shanahan F. Anti-TNF therapy for Crohn's disease: a perspective (infliximab is not the drug we have been waiting for). Inflamm Bowel Dis 2000; 6: 137–39.

382. Rutgeerts PJ, Targan SR. Introduction: anti-TNF strategies in the treatment of Crohn's disease. Aliment Pharmacol Ther 1999; 13(Suppl. 4): 1.

383. van Deventer SJ. Anti-TNF antibody treatment of Crohn's disease. Ann Rheum Dis 1999; 58(Suppl. 1): I114–20.

384. D'Haens G, Van Deventer S, Van Hogezand R et al. Endoscopic and histological healing with infliximab anti-tumor necrosis factor antibodies in Crohn's disease: A European multicenter trial. Gastroenterology 1999; 116: 1029–34.

385. Baert FJ, Rutgeerts PR. Anti-TNF strategies in Crohn's disease: mechanisms, clinical effects, indications. Int J Colorectal Dis 1999; 14: 47–51.

386. Hommes DW, van Dullemen HM, Levi M et al. Beneficial effect of treatment with a monoclonal anti-tumor necrosis factor-alpha antibody on markers of coagulation and fibrinolysis in patients with active Crohn's disease. Haemostasis 1997; 27: 269–77.

387. van Hogezand RA, Verspaget HW. The future role of anti-tumour necrosis factor-alpha products in the treatment of Crohn's disease. Drugs 1998; 56: 299–305.

388. van Hogezand RA, Verspaget HW. New therapies for inflammatory bowel disease: an update on chimeric anti-TNF alpha antibodies and IL-10 therapy. Scand J Gastroenterol Suppl. 1997; 223: 105–7.

389. Kimbrell DA, Beutler B. The evolution and genetics of innate immunity. Nat Rev Genet 2001; 2: 256–67.

390. Daun JM, Fenton MJ. Interleukin-1/Toll receptor family members: receptor structure and signal transduction pathways. J Interferon Cytokine Res 2000; 20: 843–55.

391. O'Neill L. The Toll/interleukin-1 receptor domain: a molecular switch for inflammation and host defence. Biochem Soc Trans 2000; 28: 557–63.

392. Imler JL, Hoffmann JA. Toll and Toll-like proteins: an ancient family of receptors signaling infection. Rev Immunogenet 2000; 2: 294–304

393. Kaisho T, Akira S. Critical roles of Toll-like receptors in host defense. Crit Rev Immunol 2000; 20: 393–405.

394. Beutler B, Poltorak A. Positional cloning of Lps, and the general role of toll-like receptors in the innate immune response. Eur Cytokine Netw 2000; 11: 143–52.

395. Means TK, Golenbock DT, Fenton MJ. The biology of Toll-like receptors. Cytokine Growth Factor Rev 2000; 11: 219–32.

396. Beutler B. Endotoxin, toll-like receptor 4, and the afferent limb of innate immunity. Curr Opin Microbiol. 2000; 3: 23–8.

397. Beutler B. Tlr4: central component of the sole mammalian LPS sensor. Curr Opin Immunol 2000; 12: 20–6.

398. Qureshi ST, Gros P, Malo D. The Lps locus: genetic regulation of host responses to bacterial lipopolysaccharide. Inflamm Res 1999; 48: 613–20.

399. Hemmi H, Takeuchi O, Kawai T *et al.* A Toll-like receptor recognizes bacterial DNA. Nature 2000; 408: 740–5.

400. Du X, Poltorak A, Wei Y, Beutler B. Three novel mammalian toll-like receptors: gene structure, expression, and evolution. Eur Cytokine Netw 2000; 11: 362–71.

401. Beg AA, Sha WC, Bronson RT, Ghosh S, Baltimore D. Embryonic lethality and liver degeneration in mice lacking the RelA component of NF-kappa B. Nature 1995; 376: 167–70.

402. Sha WC, Liou HC, Tuomanen EI, Baltimore D. Targeted disruption of the p50 subunit of NF-kappa B leads to multifocal defects in immune responses. Cell 1995; 80: 321–30.

403. Xu YX, Pindolia KR, Janakiraman N, Chapman RA, Gautam SC. Curcumin inhibits IL1 alpha and TNF-alpha induction of AP-1 and NF-κB DNA-binding activity in bone marrow stromal cells. Hematopathol Mol Hematol 1997; 11: 49–62.

404. Plummer SM, Holloway KA, Manson MM *et al.* Inhibition of cyclo-oxygenase 2 expression in colon cells by the chemopreventive agent curcumin involves inhibition of NF-kappaB activation via the NIK/IKK signalling complex. Oncogene 1999; 18: 6013–20.

405. Pan MH, Lin-Shiau SY, Lin JK. Comparative studies on the suppression of nitric oxide synthase by curcumin and its hydrogenated metabolites through down-regulation of IkappaB kinase and NFkappaB activation in macrophages. Biochem Pharmacol 2000; 60: 1665–76.

406. Kumar A, Dhawan S, Hardegen NJ, Aggarwal BB. Curcumin (Diferuloylmethane) inhibition of tumor necrosis factor (TNF)-mediated adhesion of monocytes to endothelial cells by suppression of cell surface expression of adhesion molecules and of nuclear factor-kappaB activation. Biochem Pharmacol 1998; 55: 775–83.

407. Jobin C, Bradham CA, Russo MP *et al.* Curcumin blocks cytokine-mediated NF-kappa B activation and proinflammatory gene expression by inhibiting inhibitory factor I-kappa B kinase activity. J Immunol 1999; 163: 3474-83.

408. Han SS, Chung ST, Robertson DA, Ranjan D, Bondada S. Curcumin causes the growth arrest and apoptosis of B cell lymphoma by downregulation of egr-1, c-myc, bcl-XL, NF-kappa B, and p53. Clin Immunol 1999; 93: 152–61.

409. Brennan P, O'Neill LA. Inhibition of nuclear factor kappaB by direct modification in whole cells–mechanism of action of nordihydroguaiaritic acid, curcumin and thiol modifiers. Biochem Pharmacol 1998; 55: 965–73.

27 | Targeted therapies for inflammatory bowel disease

SANDER J.H. VAN DEVENTER

Introduction

Medical treatment of inflammatory bowel disease (IBD) has traditionally consisted of administration of anti-inflammatory drugs such as sulfasalazine, mesalazine, glucocorticosteroids, and more recently immunomodulating drugs including azathioprine, methotrexate, and cyclosporine. None of these drugs has been primarily designed for use in IBD, and for most the precise mechanisms of action are unknown. The development of drugs for IBD has long been hindered by the lack of suitable animal models and lack of knowledge of the regulation of (immune-mediated) mucosal inflammation. In the past decade the cells involved in mucosal inflammation, and many of the proteins that lymphocytes, monocytes and antigen-presenting cells use to communicate, have been characterized. Mice that either lack or over-express these proteins often develop IBD, and this has not only greatly improved basic knowledge, but also provided elegant models for testing of therapeutic interventions. Concurrently, the rapid development of biotechnology has resulted in new classes of drugs that are now commonly known as 'biologicals'. The term 'biologicals' originally referred to a group of therapeutically administered endogenous proteins such as antibodies, cytokines, and naturally occurring cytokine-neutralizing proteins. However, most biologicals have been extensively modified to increase the therapeutic effects or to increase half-life, and compounds such as antisense oligonucleotides, that do not occur naturally, are usually also categorized as biologicals. Hence, a better operational definition for biological therapies is that these approaches all use peptides, proteins or nucleic acids in order to specifically target cell activation, or the consequences thereof. Biological therapies differ from traditional small molecules in several aspects. Because biological therapies specifically interfere with a single target, the clinical efficacy of such interventions directly reflects the pathogenic importance of such targets. As a result this class of therapeutic agents has greatly contributed to current understanding of the pathogenesis of IBD. Current biotechnology allows rapid development of biologicals (antibodies, peptides, cytokines, antisense oligonucleotides) for clinical intervention studies, thereby greatly decreasing drug development time. Most of these compounds are highly species-specific and because extensive animal testing is usually not feasible, the path from bench to bedside becomes even shorter.

A second line of targeted therapies has been a result of rapidly increased understanding of the pathways through which receptors on the cell membrane transmit signals to the nucleus, resulting in the transcriptional activation of specific genes (the signal transduction pathways). Specific inhibitors of components of these pathways have been generated, and some have anti-inflammatory properties in preclinical models. Finally, gene therapy allows very specific manipulation of cell function, and although no gene therapy trials have been initiated in IBD, preclinical development has been initiated.

In this chapter the fundamentals and therapeutic efficacy of targeted therapies are discussed. Although IBD has become a test bed for development of targeted therapies for chronic inflammatory diseases, and the number of approaches and clinical trials is overwhelming, it should be noted that only one of these approaches (treatment with TNF-α-neutralizing antibodies) has at present been approved for use in Crohn's disease (CD).

Therapeutic targets in IBD

The development of biological therapies has been facilitated by remarkable progress in the understanding of the pathogenesis of mucosal inflammatory mechanisms (Fig. 1). This has largely been a consequence of the availability of mouse models of IBD, most of which resulted from genetic targeting [1]. Many of the observations originally made in mice

Stephan R. Targan, Fergus Shanahan and Loren C. Karp (eds.), Inflammatory Bowel Disease: From Bench to Bedside, 2nd Edition, 553–571.
© 2003 *Kluwer Academic Publishers. Printed in Great Britain*

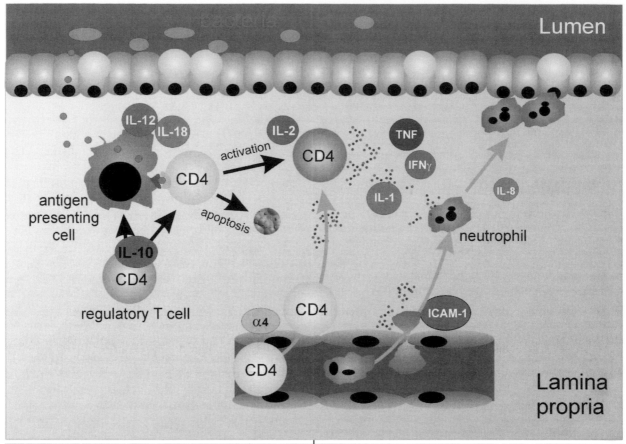

Figure 1. Crohn's disease is thought to result from uncontrolled immune activation following presentation of intestinal antigens by antigen-presenting cells. This requires the recognition of the antigen/HLA complex by the lymphocyte T cell receptor, the expression of membrane-bound expressed co-stimulatory molecules, and cytokines such as IL-12 and IL-18. Activated T lymphocytes produce proinflammatory cytokines that recruit and activate other immune cells. Normally, this reaction is controlled by induction of apoptosis of activated lymphocytes, and by regulatory T lymphocytes. Therapeutically, this inflammation can be controlled by blocking of cytokines (IL-12, IL-18, TNF-α), by induction of apoptosis or by interfering with neutrophil of lymphocyte recruitment.

have subsequently been confirmed in patients with IBD. Based on these data it is now possible to construct models of the inflammatory mechanisms that define specific targets (Fig. 1). Important differences exist between the disease mechanisms in CD and ulcerative colitis (UC), and the development of biological therapies for these diseases may diverge considerably. Certain disease mechanisms in IBD are also found in other chronic inflammatory diseases, such as rheumatoid arthritis, multiple sclerosis, and psoriasis, and biologicals that are developed in parallel for these indications may prove to be effective in CD or UC. Finally, the fields of immune suppression and transplantation have identified molecular targets that are involved in cell activation or trafficking, enabling the development of therapeutic interventions that can be applied in IBD. In

general, three groups of therapeutic targets for biological therapies can be defined: neutralization of proinflammatory cytokines, application of anti-inflammatory cytokines, and interference with cell activation or cell trafficking.

Neutralization of proinflammatory cytokines

In the final decades of the last century the pivotal insight emerged that inflammatory reactions are mediated by families of proteins with multiple, often redundant, autocrine, paracrine and endocrine activities, and these are now named cytokines. The two prototype pro-inflammatory cytokines are tumor necrosis factor α (TNF-α) and interleukin-1β (IL-

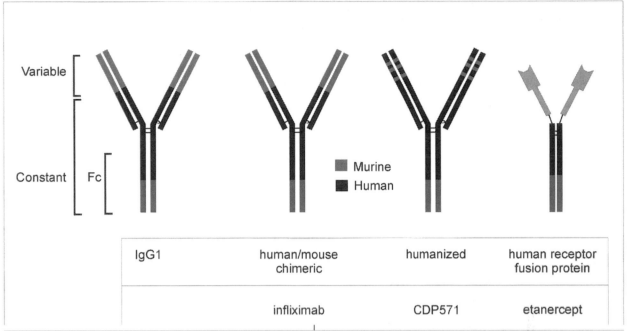

Figure 2. Three different TNF-α-neutralizing molecules. CDP571 contains less mouse protein than infliximab and presumably is less immunogenic. Etanercept is not an antibody, but a fusion protein of two TNF-α p75 receptors and an IgG1 tail.

1β) (for extensive reviews of their biological activities see refs 2 and 3). In addition, a system of T lymphocyte- and natural killer cell-activation cytokines has been discovered, which links innate and adaptive immunity, and includes the cytokines IL-12, IL-18 and interferon-γ (Fig. 3) [4]. Virtually all current experimental anticytokine approaches in IBD have targeted one of these cytokines.

Interleukin-1β

IL-1β, the first endogenous pyrogen to be identified, is produced by professional inflammatory cells, but also by many parenchymal cells. Generation of the mature form of IL-1β is dependent on cleavage of the IL-1β propeptide by IL-1 converting enzyme (ICE), a caspase that is also necessary for activation of IL-18 [5]. IL-1β is recognized by a specific receptor, the IL-1β type I receptor, which is widely expressed, and signal transduction is dependent on the presence of a second membrane protein, the IL-1 receptor associated protein [6]. Signal transduction proceeds through activation of TRAF6 and several other components that are shared with the endotoxin and the IL-18 signal transduction pathways [7]. IL-1β induces a wide range of secondary cytokines and

chemokines, increases eicosanoid production, and up-regulates cell adhesion molecules and tissue factor (thereby activating the coagulation cascade). The potent inflammatory effects of IL-1β potentially can damage the host, but are tightly controlled *in vivo* by a naturally occurring antagonist, IL-1 receptor antagonist (IL-1RA), by a membrane-bound decoy receptor (IL-1RII) and by soluble receptors (Fig. 2).

Increased concentrations of IL-1β are detected in the mucosa of patients with active CD and UC, and it has been suggested that the latter disease is characterized by an imbalance of IL-1β/IL-1RA production [8–10]. This imbalance may be a result of a combination of genetic polymorphisms that are associated with a high IL-1β and a low IL-1RA production [11]. However, the specificity of the increased mucosal IL-1β/IL-1RA production ratio for UC has been questioned [12]. In a neutrophil-dependent model of IBD (immune complex colitis in rabbits), IL-1RA showed remarkable therapeutic efficacy, but no clinical trials in IBD have been reported [13]. IL-1RA can be produced in sufficient amounts for large-scale clinical use, and was tested for efficacy in three clinical trials in patients with sepsis syndrome. Although the drug was found to be safe, no effect on the primary outcome, 28-day all-

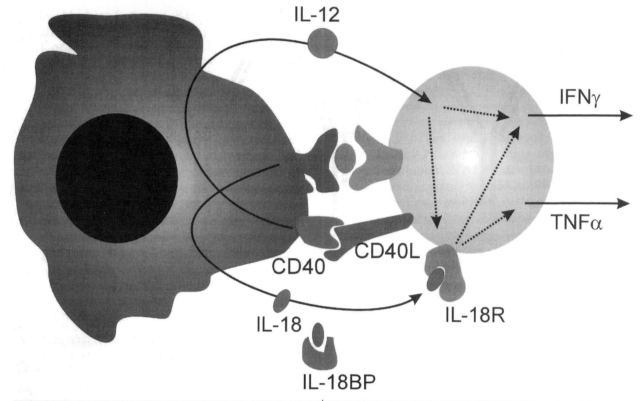

Figure 3. IL-12 and IL-18 both cause Th1 differentiation of CF4$^+$ T lymphocytes, eventually leading to increased production of IFN-γ and TNF-α. IL-12 can be blocked using specific antibodies, whereas IL-18 is blocked both by antibodies and by a naturally occurring protein named IL-18 binding protein.

cause mortality, was observed. A clinical study in rheumatoid arthritis showed long-term efficacy, with a significant effect on the progression of joint erosions. Hence, despite its short half-life, systemically administered IL-1RA can modulate compartmentalized inflammatory disease in the long term. In view of these data, IL-1RA remains an attractive candidate drug for the treatment of IBD.

Tumor necrosis factor-α

The tumor necrosis factor family of cytokines and receptors is involved in development of the immune system, inflammation, and apoptosis. Members of this family that have been implicated in the pathogenesis of IBD include lymphotoxin-β, fas and TNF-α [14]. TNF-α is a 17 kDa cytokine that is mainly produced by monocytes and lymphocytes upon a variety of stimuli. The two most important signal transduction pathways that lead to transcription of the TNF-α gene involve activation of NF-κB and MAP kinases (see below). Several small molecules

influence transcription and translation of TNF-α by interfering with intracellular targets. An increase of the intracellular cAMP concentration by inhibition of phosphodiesterase reduces TNF-α transcription, and this mechanism causes the reduction of TNF-α production by pentoxifyllin and by thalidomide (analogs) [15–18]. TNF-α is translated as an immature protein with an unusually long signal peptide, which retains the protein within the extracellular membrane, where it forms homotrimers. Membrane-bound homotrimeric TNF-α is biologically active (mainly through interaction with the type II TNF receptor – see below) but can only exert paracrine effects. A specific metalloproteinase, TNF-α converting enzyme (TACE), cleaves the TNF molecule extracellularly, thereby liberating homotrimeric soluble TNF-α [19–22]. TNF-α is recognized by two receptors, TNFRI, which is expressed by a wide variety of cells, and is considered responsible for signaling inflammation and apoptosis, and TNFRII, which is mainly expressed by white blood cells [23, 24]. Signaling through TNFRI activates two distinct pathways, leading to inflammatory responses and apoptosis respectively (see Fig. 5). It is of importance to realize that induction of apoptosis is both activated (through activation of the death domain) and inhibited (by NF-κB) by TNF-α, and the net result depends on the inflammatory context and the type of cell studied [25].

The importance of TNF-α for chronic mucosal inflammation has been clearly established and is discussed in chapters 4, 5, and 7. For this reason TNF-α has become a major therapeutic target (using small molecules, antibodies and designed proteins) in IBD.

Small molecular TNF-α inhibitors

Phosphodiesterase inhibitors

Methylxanthine compounds are vasodilators, inhibit platelet aggregation and thromboxane A_2 synthesis, and were initially designed to treat intermittent claudication resulting from large vessel atherosclerosis. The best-known drug in this class is pentoxifylline, a non-specific phosphodiesterase inhibitor, that was subsequently found to diminish the production of proinflammatory cytokines *in vitro* as well as *in vivo* [18, 26]. This finding led to a series of clinical trials in patients with sepsis and chronic inflammatory diseases. In patients with active CD, oxpentifylline (a pentoxifylline derivative) reduced the production of TNF-α by peripheral blood mononuclear cells, but had no effect on disease activity [27]. Rolipram is a specific inhibitor of the type 4 phosphodiesterase and inhibits cAMP-dependent signaling through cAMP-response element-binding factor (CREB) [15, 28]. This not only causes a reduction of the production of proinflammatory cytokines, but also reduces T lymphocyte chemotaxis. Rolipram is effective in various animal models of chronic T lymphocyte-dependent inflammatory disease, such as adjuvant arthritis and multiple sclerosis, and was shown to reduce mucosal TNF-α production in dextran sulfate-induced colitis, thereby preventing tissue damage [29, 30]. The clinical efficacy of rolipram in IBD has not been investigated.

Thalidomide

Thalidomide was introduced in Europe as a sedative, but its use was soon abandoned because of teratogenicity. It has long been known that thalidomide has immunomodulatory effects, and thalidomide is used in erythema nodosum leprosum, a T lymphocyte-mediated complication of lepra that is characterized by high circulating concentrations of TNF-α and IFN-γ. More recently, thalidomide has been clinically used in rheumatoid arthritis, Behçet's disease, systemic lupus erythematosus, multiple myeloma, and therapy-refractory tuberculosis [31–35]. Oral ulcerations secondary to CD and those occurring in AIDS do respond favorably to thalidomide administration [36]. Two open-label trials have explored the potential efficacy of thalidomide in CD [37, 38]. Both included patients with chronic active, steroid-unresponsive disease, and patients received daily thalidomide doses ranging from 100 to 300 mg. Both studies reported a substantial reduction of the CD activity index, and one study suggested that thalidomide could have steroid-sparing effects [37]. The results of these two uncontrolled studies suggest that thalidomide may have beneficial effects in patients with chronic active CD. It remains to be seen whether this clinical effect is related to a reduction of TNF-α production. In previous studies in HIV-infected patients and patients with tuberculosis no inhibition of TNF-α production by thalidomide treatment has been observed [33]. In addition to inhibiting TNF-α, thalidomide also affects the production of IL-10 and IL-12, and activates T lymphocytes and down-regulates the expression of T lymphocyte chemokine receptors [16, 39–41]. Thalidomide analogs with more specific phosphodiesterase-inhibiting and T lymphocyte-stimulating properties have been synthesized, allowing a more specific targeting [42].

TACE inhibitors

TNF-α converting enzyme (TACE) is a metalloproteinase that cleaves membrane-bound TNF between alanine at position 76 and valine at position 77, thereby releasing soluble trimeric TNF-α [19, 21, 22]. Several metalloproteinase inhibitors more or less specifically inhibit TACE, which results in a reduction of the release of soluble TNF-α, while the number of membrane-bound TNF-α molecules is unaffected. TACE inhibitors indeed inhibit the release of TNF-α in various mouse models of inflammatory disease, and one of these compounds reduced inflammatory tissue damage in TNBS-induced colitis in rats [43]. However, although in the latter model the severity of colitis was attenuated, this was not associated with a reduction of TNF-α production. Therefore, it is likely that the TACE inhibitor used in this experiment reduced inflammation by a non-specific inhibition of metalloproteinases other than TACE. Most TACE inhibitors available not only interfere with cleavage of TNF-α, but also reduce the shedding of TNF receptors that occurs in activated mononuclear cells. Shedding of TNF receptors dampens the biological effects of TNF-α, because of the reduced number of potential TNF-α binding sites, and because soluble receptors retain the ability to bind and neutralize TNF-α. It has been suggested that the reduced shedding of TNF receptors caused a paradoxical increase of disease activity in collagen-induced arthritis in mice that were treated with a TACE inhibitor [44]. In endotoxin-challenged human volunteers, pretreatment with an oral TACE inhibitor significantly reduced the release of TNF-α, but also interfered with the shedding of TNF receptors [45, 46]. Results from clinical trials with TACE inhibitors have not been published.

TNF-α-binding molecules

The development of TNF-binding molecules mainly resulted from the hypothesis that the mortality of sepsis was caused by the proinflammatory effects of TNF-α. Indeed, administration of TNF-α neutralizing antibodies reduced mortality in certain (primate) sepsis models, particularly those induced by injection of large numbers of Gram-negative bacteria or endotoxin [47]. However, the clinical efficacy of TNF-α neutralizing antibodies in sepsis has been disappointing, and with a few exceptions drug development for this indication has been discontinued [48]. Nonetheless, this line of research has led to the development of two classes of TNF neutralizing proteins that are currently used in chronic inflammatory diseases. The first class includes TNF neutralizing antibodies. The first generation of these antibodies was induced in mice that were immunized with human TNF-α, resulting in the generation of hybridomas that produced murine high-affinity anti-human TNF-α antibodies. Because (repeated) administration of mouse antibodies in humans causes immunogenic responses, all currently available antibodies have been modified in order to reduce mouse-specific protein sequences. By 'grafting' the variable (antibody-binding) regions on a human IgG tail, human–mouse chimeric antibodies were generated, in which the percentage of mouse protein was reduced to 25–30% (Fig. 2) [49]. Human–mouse chimeric antibodies may induce antibody responses (human antichimeric antibodies: HACA), and because these antibodies are directed against the murine antigen-binding domains of the antibody, they frequently interfere with ligand-binding, and hence reduce the biological activity. A further refinement was the 'humanization' of antibodies, in which only the hypervariable (mouse-derived) complemen-

tary-determining regions (CDRs) of the antibody are inserted in a human antibody backbone. Such antibodies contain about 5% of mouse protein, and although experience is still limited, the available data suggest that humanization indeed reduces the incidence of immunogenic responses [50]. Finally, by several techniques, cytokine-neutralizing antibodies can be generated that consist entirely of human protein sequences. One of the major obstacles in this development is the difficulty of generating high-affinity antibodies. In addition, for reasons that are incompletely understood, some completely human antibodies are still immunogenic when administered to humans. Nonetheless, high-affinity human anti-TNF-α antibodies are now available and being tested in clinical trials [51]. Apart from complete antibodies, F(ab)2 fragments have been used, which have a significantly shorter half-life, which may be enhanced by coupling to polyethylene glycol (PEG) [52, 53]. All TNF-α neutralizing antibodies that are currently developed for clinical use are of the IgG class. Human IgG_1, but not IgG_4, antibodies are able to bind and activate complement, and it has been reported that TNF-α/antibody immune complex formation and subsequent complement activation may cause febrile responses. However, no such reactions have been observed in the large number of patients treated with TNF-α neutralizing antibodies of the IgG_1 class.

A second class of TNF-α neutralizing proteins consists of recombinant soluble (PEG-linked) receptors, or dimeric TNF type I or II receptors which are fused on an IgG_1 antibody tail [54]. Clinical studies have been performed with the latter two constructs. In sepsis patients the dimeric TNFR1/IgG_1 construct did not significantly reduce mortality, and the TNFRII/IgG_1 construct (etanercept) caused a dose-dependent *increase* in mortality. No definitive explanation for this finding has been provided, but it should be noted that TNF-α-binding proteins and antibodies have the ability to retain TNF-α within the circulation, and may even shuttle compartmentalized TNF-α form tissue sites into the blood. As long as the bound TNF-α is effectively neutralized, this does not cause adverse effects. Although the TNFRII/IgG_1 construct has a high TNF-α binding affinity, compared to TNRI/IgG_1 constructs or TNF-α-neutralizing antibodies, it has a high 'off' rate, which implies that bound ligand (TNF-α) is relatively easily released. By such a mechanism TNFRII/IgG_1 constructs may act as a TNF 'sponge', and this may explain the deleterious effect of the use of such constructs in sepsis patients. Etanercept has been administered to a large number of rheumatoid arthritis patients without causing adverse effects, but a small number of treated patients developed severe sepsis. Because all currently reported clinical trials in IBD have used anti-TNF-α antibodies, the further discussion is restricted to this class of TNF-α binding proteins.

CDP571

CDP571 is a humanized high-affinity IgG$_4$ antibody that has been used in clinical trials in rheumatoid arthritis patients, in UC and in CD. Most reported data concern short-term studies, and the antibody has been demonstrated to be safe and well tolerated. In a small trial in patients with active CD a single CDP571 dose (5 mg/kg) reduced the median Crohn Disease Activity Index (CDAI) from 263 to 167 and 29% of patients were in remission 2 weeks after the start of treatment [55]. At a larger dose (10 or 20 mg/ kg every 8–12 weeks) CDP517 induced a response in about 45% of patients with active CD (27% in placebo-treated patients) that seemed to be maintained by repeated infusions [56]. Interestingly, patients treated with the lower 10 mg/kg dose with the longer interval (12 weeks) showed the best responses. A third trial investigated the potential steroid-sparing effects of CDP571. Patients with CD in remission (CDAI < 150), who were using corticosteroids and had previously failed an attempt to taper the steroid dose, were treated with CDP571 (an induction dose of 20 mg/kg, followed by 10 mg/kg at week 8) or placebo. After 40 weeks, in 44% of CDP571-treated patients, but in only 22% of placebo-treated patients, corticosteroids could be successfully discontinued [57]. Hence, CDP571 is effective in chronic steroid-dependent CD.

Infliximab

Infliximab is a first-generation human–mouse chimeric antibody, with a high affinity for human TNF-α. The antibody binds soluble as well as membrane-bound TNF-α and potently interfered with the biological activity of TNF-α *in vitro*. The rationale for the use of anti-TNF-α antibodies in chronic inflammatory disease came from pivotal studies in collagen-induced arthritis in mice and by using human synovial explants obtained from patients with rheumatoid arthritis. Subsequent clinical studies demonstrated that intravenous administration of infliximab (10 or 20 mg/kg) to patients with severe therapy-refractory rheumatoid arthritis

resulted in dramatic and rather prolonged (weeks) clinical responses. These responses were associated with a rapid reduction of C-reactive protein serum concentrations and of the erythrocyte sedimentation rate, and with a marked functional improvement. It has been subsequently reported that these clinical responses can be maintained by repeated infliximab infusions (every 4 or 8 weeks), which were generally well tolerated. Importantly, long-term treatment with infliximab and etanercept reduces radiological progression of joint destruction. Hence, in rheumatoid arthritis, TNF-α neutralizing proteins are not merely anti-inflammatory, but also modify the natural course of the disease. The (pre)clinical development of infliximab for sepsis, as well as the initial results in rheumatoid arthritis patients, revealed that the drug was well tolerated and no serious side-effects were observed. The first clinical experience with infliximab in CD was obtained in a child with therapy-refractory Crohn's colitis associated with severe perianal disease and a remarkable clinical and endoscopic response to infliximab infusion was reported (two 10 mg/kg doses were infused within a 2-week period) [58]. Similar findings were reported in an open-label study including 10 patients who received a single dose of 10 or 20 mg/kg [59]. In this study rapid endoscopic improvement was observed in several patients, C-reactive protein concentrations decreased, as well as mucosal concentrations of secretory phospholipase A$_2$. In addition, it was demonstrated that the increased intravascular generation of thrombin, which occurs in active CD, was rapidly normalized by infliximab treatment. Because the proinflammatory effects of thrombin are well known, this latter effect is considered to add to the anti-inflammatory effects of TNF-α neutralization. Two controlled clinical trials have reported the efficacy of infliximab in chronic active CD and in patients with fistulas. The first study included 108 patients with active CD who were randomised to receive a single infusion of infliximab (either 5, 10, or 20 mg/kg) or placebo [60]. All included patients had failed prior medical treatment, and most were treated with corticosteroids or immunomodulatory drugs at enrolment. Four weeks after the infusion a clinical response, defined as a reduction of the CDAI by more than 70 points, was observed in 65% of all infliximab-treated patients combined, as opposed to 17% of placebo-treated patients. Moreover, in about one-third of infliximab-treated patients a complete clinical remission was induced. Non-responding patients received an open-label infusion (10 mg/kg) and all responding patients were re-randomized to receive 8-weekly infusions of infliximab (10 mg/kg) or placebo, for a total of four infusions. Analysis of the second part of this study revealed that the therapeutic response was gradually lost in placebo-treated patients, but therapeutic responses and remissions were well maintained by repeated infliximab infusions [61].

Remarkably, clinical responses following administration of infliximab correlate well to endoscopic responses, and in some patients all mucosal lesions disappear [62].

Because healing of perianal fistulas was observed in infliximab-treated patients, a second controlled trial in patients with enterocutaneous or perianal fistulas was undertaken. Although previous uncontrolled trials had suggested that antibiotics, 6-mercaptopurine (6-MP) and cyclosporine were useful in the treatment of perianal fistulas, this trial represented the first controlled clinical trial in CD patients with fistulas. Administration of infliximab at three time points (0, 2, and 6 weeks) resulted in the closure of all fistulas in 46% of treated patients, as compared to 13% of patients who received placebo infusions in addition to standard medical therapy [63]. The median time to closure was 14 days in infliximab-treated patients (more than 40 days in the placebo group) and the duration of the response was about 3 months. These two controlled trials clearly demonstrated the efficacy of infliximab in chronic active (therapy-refractory) CD and in fistulas secondary to CD, and were the basis of the approval of the drug for these indications both in North America and Europe. Subsequently, a dose-escalating clinical trial in pediatric patients suggested that the efficacy of treatment of children was similar to that in adults. Systemic complications of CD, such as spondyloarthritis and erythema nodosum, as well as 'metastatic' CD, have been reported to respond favorably to infliximab treatment, and CD in ileoanal reservoirs has also been successfully treated [64–66]. The experience in UC is very limited, but some patients may show therapeutic responses [67]. A large controlled clinical trial has been initiated.

Side-effects of anti-TNF-α antibodies

Infliximab treatment is associated with several side-effects. As expected, some patients (about 13%) develop HACA, which usually are low titer and do not necessarily preclude future treatment. Concurrent treatment with corticosteroids or immunosuppressive drugs reduces the incidence of HACA

induction (unpublished data). About 25% of patients who received infliximab infusions after having being treated in the initial clinical trials developed a clinical reaction characterized by fever and severe muscle and joint tenderness, which is now referred to as 'delayed hypersensitivity reaction'. These reactions are caused by a rapid induction of very high titers of HACA, even in patients who had not shown any HACA response either during the initial treatment or shortly before the repeat infusion. Delayed hypersensitivity reactions occur only after a long 'drug holiday', and have not been observed in patients who were repeatedly infused at 4–12-week intervals. Patients with delayed hypersensitivity reactions do not develop end-organ damage and respond well to treatment with corticosteroids or NSAID. Nonetheless, such patients should not receive subsequent infliximab infusions, because the high-titer HACA interfere with the TNF-α-binding capacity of infliximab. Non-HACA-related infusion reactions include headache, (localized) urticaria, and wheezing, all occurring during or rapidly after the infusion. These reactions can be managed by reducing the infusion rate (the 5 mg/kg dose is usually administered within 2 h), and by administration of corticosteroids or antihistamines. Occasionally skin rashes occur in infliximab-treated patients and about 9% of all infused patients (transiently) develop anti-dsDNA antibodies, which is only rarely associated with lupus-like clinical features such as the typical butterfly rash, pleuritis, or arthritis. A comparable incidence of anti-dsDNA antibody formation has been reported following CDP571 treatment, and this may represent a class-specific side-effect. Although lymphomas have occurred in infliximab-treated patients, most cases concerned patients who had an increased lymphoma risk because of the underlying disease (AIDS, rheumatoid arthritis). The background incidence of lymphomas in patients with CD is low, but two patients have been reported who were diagnosed with lymphomas after infliximab treatment. It should be noted that the incidence of lymphomas associated with immunosuppressive drugs is affected by the underlying disease (the incidence is high in rheumatoid arthritis and transplant patients) and by the duration of follow-up. Because of the wide confidence limits and the short follow-up period it is at present not possible to reliably estimate the lymphoma risk in anti-TNF-α antibody-treated patients.

TNF-α is known to have a pivotal role in the immune response to infections, in particular those from intracellular pathogens, and many investigators predicted that TNF-α neutralizing therapies would result in a greatly increased infection rate. This prediction has not been substantiated, and it is now known that the infection rate in infliximab-treated patients with CD is only slightly increased. However, neutralization of TNF-α can have serious consequences in patients with current intracellular infections, in particular tuberculosis, or in immuno-compromised patients, and such conditions should be excluded before initiation of treatment (by chest X-ray and PPD skin test). After more than 140 000 patients had been infused with infliximab, 70 cases of tuberculosis have been reported [68]. Many of these were extrapulmonary, and in most cases the cause was reactivation of latent disease. The effect of treatment using TNF-α neutralizing proteins on the safety and efficacy of vaccinations, in particular those with life-attenuated microorganisms, is not known, and the experience in pregnant women is very limited.

Clinical use of TNF neutralizing proteins

Although TNF-α neutralizing therapies are an important step forward in the medical treatment of CD, many questions remain to be answered. What is the long-term effect of repeated infusions and what are the side-effects of such strategies? Does infliximab treatment modify the natural course of CD and can surgery be prevented? Why are about one-third of CD patients refractory to infliximab therapy? Do standard immunosuppressive therapies, such as 6-MP/azathioprine and methotrexate synergize with TNF-α neutralizing treatments in CD? Obviously, it is important to know the answers, and several clinical trials addressing these questions have been initiated.

At present, because of the high costs and the uncertainty about long-term side-effects, anti-TNF-α antibodies are second- or third-line therapies of IBD. Before considering such therapies it is mandatory to ensure that patients are appropriately managed, and in steroid-refractory or -dependent patients treatment with azathioprine or methotrexate should be considered first. It is important to exclude underlying fibrotic stenoses, inflammatory infiltrates, short bowel syndrome, and gastrointestinal infections. The approved infliximab dose in active CD is 5 mg/kg administered as a 2 h infusion. Data reported by large IBD centers indicate that the response rate in clinical practice is similar to the results of controlled clinical trials (about two-thirds

of patients showing a response, one-third a clinical remission). Patients who do not respond may be offered a second dose, but the majority of these patients are genuinely refractory to anti-TNF-α therapy or have complications such as bowel stenosis. Only relatively small clinical studies have reported the effects of repeated anti-TNF-α administrations, and at present the best strategy for repeated treatment of responding patients is uncertain. Because most patients will relapse 8–12 weeks after a single infliximab dose, I usually prescribe three doses (5 mg/kg) with an 8-week interval, and in order to reduce side-effects and prolong the duration of remission I treat all patients with either azathioprine (2.5 mg/kg per day orally) or methotrexate (25 mg/week subcutaneously). If relapse occurs after the third infliximab infusion, patients can be retreated at an interval that is somewhat shorter than the observed relapse-free interval after the last dose. Infliximab is very useful in treating patients with perianal fistulas, but only in the context of appropriate (multidisciplinary) management. Before institution of treatment abscesses should be appropriately drained, setons should be inserted whenever appropriate, and removed after one or two infliximab doses.

In conclusion, anti-TNF-α strategies are an important addition to the therapeutic armamentarium in CD and may induce important therapeutic responses in difficult-to-treat patients. Successful application of these therapies requires optimal baseline treatment including appropriately dosed immunomodulatory drugs in most patients. Short-term side-effects occur in a minority of patients, are usually not severe, and do not preclude further treatment in most patients. All patients considered for infliximab therapy should be screened for (latent) tuberculosis. The incidence and nature of long-term side-effects of this class of drugs remains uncertain, because of the relatively short follow-up of anti-TNF-α antibody-treated patients.

Interference with the IL-12/IL-18/IFN-γ axis

IL-12 and IL-18 are cytokines that cause Th1 differentiation of T lymphocytes following antigen-dependent stimulation (Fig. 3). Th1-differentiated T lymphocytes are characterized by the production of IL-2 and IFN-γ. Increased mucosal concentrations of IFN-γ occur in CD, and more recently increased production of both IL-12 and IL-18 has been demonstrated to be a specific feature of CD (as opposed to UC). Although IFN-γ has long been considered to be a proinflammatory cytokine, and in some animal models of IBD anti-IFN-γ antibodies decrease disease activity, recent data from animal models have led to a more differentiated view. Mice that are IFN-γ or IFN-γ receptor-deficient are not protected against the induction of colitis by intracolonic administration of TNBS, and IFN-γ may have anti-inflammatory effects by stimulating apoptosis of activated T lymphocytes. In a small series of patients with CD, administration of low doses of IFN-γ did not exacerbate disease activity. Nonetheless, anti-human IFN-γ antibodies have been generated for clinical use, and studies in CD patients are planned.

IL-12 is a heterodimeric cytokine that is composed of a p35 and a p40 chain. The heterodimeric p75 molecule is recognized by a specific receptor expressed by T lymphocytes and NK cells. In mice, homodimeric p40 is able to antagonize p75, and recently it has been demonstrated that p40 may form heterodimers with proteins other than p35. Hence, several cytokines that share the IL-12 p40 chain have now been identified, and these seem to have different biological activities. For example, experiments performed in p35- and p40-deficient mice demonstrated that the presence of p40 (in the absence of IL-12 p75) is protective in TNBS colitis. This is of importance, because most anti-IL-12 antibodies developed for clinical use bind p40. On the other hand, in wild-type mice anti-p40 antibodies were protective in TNBS-induced colitis, and the mechanism of action was related to the induction of apoptosis. Anti-human IL-12 antibodies have been generated, but no clinical results have been reported.

More recently, IL-18 has been identified as a major IFN-γ inducer. Within the intestinal mucosal of patients with CD, epithelial as well as lamina propria cells produce increased amounts of IL-18. Like IL-1, IL-18 is translated as a propeptide that needs to be cleaved by ICE in order to generate the mature bioactive protein. The IL-18 receptor with its associated proteins, as well as the associated signaling pathways, are very similar to the IL-1 receptor. IL-18 is antagonized by a naturally occurring soluble protein, IL-18 binding protein, that has a very high affinity. IL-18 antibodies, as well as recombinant IL-18 binding protein, are currently being tested for efficacy in various animal models of chronic inflammation.

Anti-inflammatory cytokines

IL-10

IL-10 is a small homodimeric cytokine that antagonizes production of proinflammatory cytokines by T lymphocytes as well as monocytes, decreases expression of HLA class II molecules, and strongly reduces T lymphocyte proliferation. The importance of IL-10 for regulation of mucosal immune responses became apparent when mice made IL-10 deficient by homologous recombination developed cachexia and anemia as a consequence of chronic inflammatory disease of the small and large intestines. The mucosal inflammation in these mice responds to treatment with anti-TNF or anti-IFN-γ antibodies, but remarkably, IL-10 administration is protective only when administered early in the course of the disease. Recombinant human IL-10 was found to be safe in human volunteers when administered intravenously or subcutaneously, and down-regulated the production of TNF-α and other proinflammatory cytokines in *ex-vivo* stimulation experiments. In endotoxin-challenged volunteers, IL-10 pretreatment resulted in a decrease of the production of TNF-α, IL-6 and IL-8, and activation of the coagulation system was prevented. A short-term phase II study in patients with active CD demonstrated that intravenously administered IL-10 was well tolerated, and suggested a beneficial clinical effect. Two large long-term clinical studies were performed in CD patients [69, 70]. One study enrolled mild to moderately active CD patients, who were not using corticosteroids or azathioprine, and daily subcutaneous doses of IL-10 or placebo were administered. The second study enrolled chronic active patients who had failed treatment with corticosteroids or immunosuppressive drugs. In both studies a moderate reduction of disease activity was observed at rhIL-10 doses between 5 and 10 μg/kg. At higher doses patients started to experience side-effects and therapeutic effects were lost. In a search for a possible mechanism, blood from patients being treated with IL-10 was stimulated *ex vivo* with endotoxin or phytohemagglutin (PHA). A dose-dependent reduction of endotoxin-induced TNF-α production was found, but after PHA stimulations in patients treated with IL-10 doses above 10 μg/kg resulted in an increased production of TNF-α and IFN-γ. These data indicate that IL-10 dose-dependently decreased the production of TNF-α by monocytes, but at higher doses increased the production of TNF-α and IFN-γ by lymphocytes (most likely CD8[+] T lymphocytes and NK cells). In retrospect, a similar increase in IFN-γ production by IL-10 was also found in endotoxin-challenged volunteers (who received a single rhIL-10 dose of 25 µg/kg) [71]. Hence, when systemically administered, rhIL-10 at higher doses caused side effects that interfered with therapeutic efficacy. This has led to the development of methods that would more efficiently deliver IL-10 into the intestinal mucosa, for example by genetically modifying gut-homing T lymphocytes to express IL-10.

IL-11

Interleukin 11 (IL-11) is a member of the IL-6 family of cytokines. These cytokines activate cells through activation of heterodimeric membrane receptors, which consist of the transmembrane protein gp130, and cytokine-specific α-unit (the IL-11 receptor α-chain in case of IL-11). IL-11 is produced by mesenchymal cells and has a wide spectrum of biological activities, including the stimulation of thrombopoiesis, and the protection of the gut epithelium from injury induced by irradiation and chemotherapeutic drugs. IL-11 also suppresses TNF-α production, probably through interference with NF-κB signaling. In the HLA-B27 transgenic rat model, rhIL-11 reduced the severity of colitis, and reduced the mucosal production of TNF-α, IL-1β and IFN-γ. In a multicenter controlled clinical trial, enrolling 76 patients with active CD, the safety and activity of several doses (5, 15, 40 µg/kg, administered two or five times weekly) of rhIL-11 were investigated. Treatment was well tolerated, and an increase in thrombocyte count was observed in patients who received the higher doses or were most frequently treated. The highest clinical responses were observed in the patient group that received 16 µg/kg per week, in whom a therapeutic response (a decrease of the CDAI ⩾ 100 points) was observed in 5/12 patients (42%). Based on these preliminary results, further controlled clinical trials were started.

Interference with activation or recruitment of inflammatory leukocytes

Inflammatory bowel disease is characterized by an influx of inflammatory cells into the intestinal mucosa. The mechanisms responsible for recruitment of neutrophils and monocytes, and the more specific 'homing' of lymphocytes, have been characterized and provided well-defined therapeutic targets.

Anti-CD4 antibodies

In view of the large body of evidence for a dominant role of CD4+ T lymphocytes in the initiation and control of mucosal immune responses, it is somewhat surprising that so few studies have aimed to alter T lymphocyte function using monoclonal antibodies. This may be a result of the unfavorable safety profiles of some of these interventions (i.e. OKT3 treatment). In an open-label dose-escalating study 12 patients with active CD were infused with seven daily doses of a depleting anti-CD4 antibody (cMT412). In patients who received daily doses of 10 and 30 mg (for a total dose of 100 and 210 mg, respectively), transient reductions of the circulating CD4 counts were induced, and a moderate therapeutic effect was observed. In the 4 patients who received a 100 mg daily dose (a total dose of 700 mg) a long-lasting reduction (months) of the CD4+ lymphocyte count was induced, and all patients had a clinical response. Although the antibody infusion was associated with mild acute toxicity, the long duration of depletion of circulating CD4+ count is a severe drawback of this therapy. It should be noted that non-depleting anti-CD4+ antibodies with a good safety profile have been clinically tested for other indications. Interest in anti-CD4+ antibodies may revive in view of the finding of therapeutic synergism of antibodies that target CD4 and TNF-α in collagen-induced arthritis in mice. In addition, other surface molecules expressed by T lymphocytes (CD2, CD40) are attractive therapeutic targets and are developed for use in inflammatory diseases.

ICAM1 antisense oligonucleotides

Antisense oligonucleotides are short stretches of single-stranded DNA (18–25 bases) designed to target specific mRNA. Binding of the antisense oligonucleotide to the target mRNA results in the formation of a RNA/DNA hybrid that is rapidly degraded by RNAse H. Single-strand oligonucleotides are rapidly degraded within plasma, and either large amounts need to be infused, or the (phosphorothioate) backbone needs to be modified in order to resist breakdown. Alternatively, the oligonucleotides can be administered locally. A general side-effect of oligonucleotides with a phosphorothioate backbone is prolongation of the activated partial thromboplastin time (PTT) through inhibition of the intrinsic tenase activity, and very high doses may also activate complement. ISIS 2302 is an antisense oligonucleotide that specifically hybridizes to human mRNA encoding the adhesion molecule ICAM1, which is important for the binding of neutrophils to cytokine-stimulated endothelium. Because this neutrophil–endothelial cell interaction is necessary for transmigration of neutrophils into the tissue, this intervention is expected to specifically inhibit neutrophil influx into the mucosal in IBD. Indeed, preclinical studies in mice have demonstrated that administration of a murine analog of ISIS 2302 (ISIS 3082) ameliorated dextran sulfate-induced colitis in mice. A small controlled clinical study included 20 patients with active steroid-refractory CD who were treated with 13 infusions of ISIS 2302 (0.5, 1, or 2 mg/kg) or placebo in a period of 26 days. At the end of the study 47% of all ISIS 2302-treated patients, and 20% of placebo-treated patients, were in remission (CDAI < 150). Unfortunately, a subsequent larger controlled study failed to confirm these promising data [72].

Anti-α_4 antibodies

The homing of intestinal T- and B lymphocytes is in large part a consequence of interaction of the $\alpha_4\beta_7$ integrin and the mucosal addressin MadCAM1 [73–75]. Antibodies that block this interaction interfere with recruitment of potential proinflammatory mononuclear cells into the mucosa, and in animal models of intestinal inflammation this principle has been demonstrated to have anti-inflammatory effects [76]. Clinical studies using anti–α_4-antibodies in CD have been initiated.

Inhibitors of signal transduction pathways

Inflammation is a result of altered expression of many genes, as a consequence of cell activation by various stimuli such as bacterial products, osmotic stress, oxygen radicals, radiation, or cytokines. These stimuli activated two major families of transcription activators, i.e. activator protein-1 (AP-1) and the NF-κB family, that regulate the fate of the cell (proliferation or apoptotic cell death) and the transcription of inflammatory cytokines (Fig. 4). In their turn the transcription activators are activated by

interacting networks of mitogen-activated protein kinases (MAPK). At least 12 mammalian MAPK members have been recognized, and it has become apparent that these kinases are activated in a three-step process that involves a MAP-kinase-kinase-kinase (MKKK), a MAP kinase-kinase (MKK) and a MAP kinase (Fig. 4). Although the MKKK–MKK–MAPK pathways extensively interact, specificity is conferred by the limited MAPK specificity of MKK and the presence of 'scaffold' proteins that anchor specific MKKK/MKK/MAPK proteins. Scaffolding results in the formation of multi-protein activation complexes that control signal transduction pathways. Development of specific protein kinase inhibitors is hindered by their redundancy and the presence of isoforms with different expression patterns and biological effects, but recently great progress has been made. Clinical development has been most rapid for MAPK p38 inhibitors, many of which are based on anti-inflammatory pyridinyl imidazole compounds. Several other small molecular inhibitors of the p38 MAP kinase have been developed, which act either by preventing phosphorylation of the kinase, or by blocking activation of kinases downstream of p38 through steric hindrance. The prototype MAPK p38 inhibitor is SB 203580, which inhibits LPS-induced TNF-α production, and is effective in several animal models of acute and chronic inflammation. SB 203580 is not very specific for MAPK p38, but second- and third-generation specific p38 inhibitors are currently in clinical development. This class of small molecular compound is expected to have anti-inflammatory effects resulting from inhibition of several proinflammatory cytokines, including TNF-α. Specific inhibitors of C-jun aminoterminal kinases (JNK), the major route for AP-1 activation, have not been reported, but are likely to be developed. These molecules are expected to have an anti-inflammatory profile that differs from MAPK inhibitors. Of the three JNK isomers, JNK2 is specifically involved in Th1 differentiation, and JNK2 inhibitors will be attractive candidate drugs for treatment of CD, multiple sclerosis and rheumatoid arthritis.

In conclusion, inhibition of specific protein kinases may be a potent anti-inflammatory strategy, and several (orally effective) lead compounds have been developed. However, the (long-term) safety of these compounds is unknown.

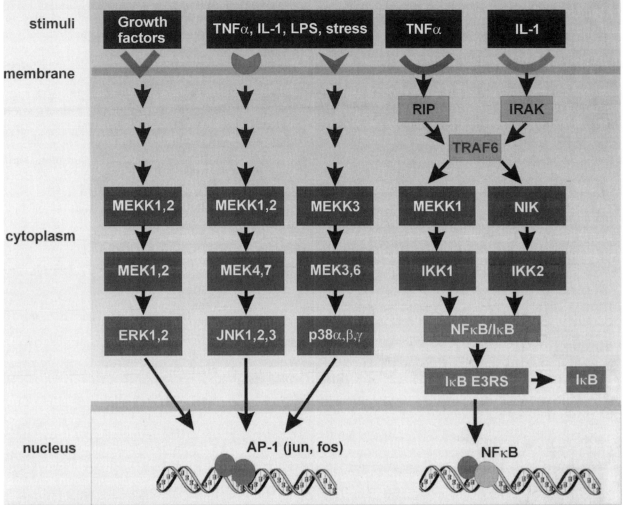

Figure 4. MAP kinases transmit signals from activated membrane receptors to the nucleus, causing increased transcription of multiple genes involved in inflammation. Three major pathways have been identified, leading to activation of ERK1,2, JNK1,2,3, and p38α,β,γ, respectively.

NF-κB

In resting cells dimeric NF-κB is bound to IκB, which prevents translocation to the nucleus. A multi-unit protein kinase, the IκB kinase (two isoforms, IKK1 and IKK2 have been identified) that is activated by proinflammatory stimuli is able to phosphorylate IκB, thereby rendering IκB a target for a ubiquitin ligase complex. The subsequent ubiquination of IκB results in degradation within the 26S proteasome. The free NF-κB migrates into the nucleus and binds to a specific motif within the promoter of several genes involved in inflammation, including the TNF-α gene (Fig. 5). By regulating the degradation of IκB the IKK complex critically controls activation of the

TNF-α gene, and this has recently received substantial attention as a therapeutic target. In addition, low molecular weight NF-κB inhibitors have been developed, and these are able to reduce production of proinflammatory cytokines in animal models. Another interesting approach is interference with NF-κB activation by interfering with the degradation of IκB, either by preventing IKK activity or by reducing the production of NF-κB components such as the p65 protein. Curcumin, a food derivative, has been demonstrated to down-regulate NF-κB translocation through an effect that is located upstream of IKK activation, whereas interference with the production of NF-κB p65 protein by local adminis-

Activation of Rel/NFkB

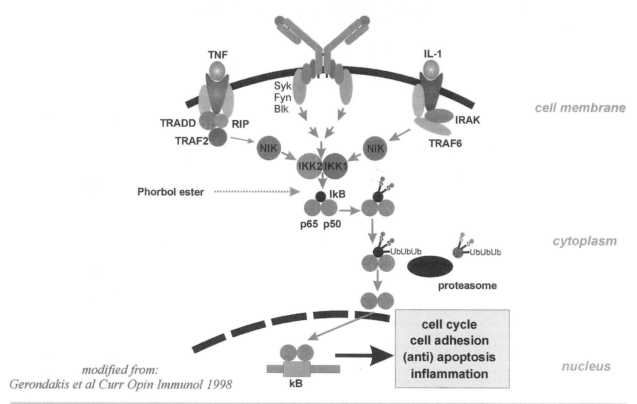

modified from:
Gerondakis et al Curr Opin Immunol 1998

Figure 5. Activation of several cytokine receptors, including the TNF-α p55 receptor and the IL-1 receptor causes activation of the NF-κB receptor, IκB is phosphorylated and degraded in the proteasome, thereby freeing the NF-κB, that is now able to translocate into the nucleus, where it activates many genes involved in cell adhesion, apoptosis and inflammation.

tration of antisense oligonucleotides reduced the severity of TNBS-induced colitis in mice. The efficacy of this latter approach in IBD is currently being investigated in clinical trials. Finally, the anti-inflammatory effects of IL-10 may in part be related to interference with NF-κB signaling.

Gene therapy

The principle of gene therapy is simple: introduction of a functionally active gene into somatic cells in order to express a therapeutic protein. Early gene therapy projects were designed to correct 'inborn errors of metabolism' or to counteract abnormal proliferation of cancer cells. More recently, gene therapy techniques are also being applied to alter the course of chronic inflammatory diseases. Because IBD are under complex polygenic control, and the pivotal genes have not been characterized, there is at present no reason to believe that these disease can be cured by gene therapy. However, as will be discussed, gene therapy can be used to alter the function of cells that are critically involved in the regulation of mucosal inflammation. One of the critical factors for success of gene therapy in chronic inflammatory diseases is the long-lasting and sufficient expression of the therapeutic gene in the target tissue, and many early gene therapy protocols failed simply because no therapeutic protein was expressed. When applied in chronic inflammatory diseases the intervention itself should not elicit inflammatory responses and long-term expression is necessary. Because the *in-vivo* efficiency of transfection using naked DNA is low, most gene therapy projects have been performed using viral vectors. These differ greatly in their efficacy and immunogenicity, and the duration of expression of the therapeutic gene.

Adenovirus [77, 78]

Most gene therapy trials have used adenovirus-derived vectors for gene delivery. Adenovirus is a double-stranded virus that causes common cold and gastroenteritis in humans. Of the more than 50 known serotypes, type 2 (Ad2) and type 5 (Ad5) have been used to construct vectors. The double-stranded 30–40 kbp adenovirus genome is flanked by two inverted terminal repeat sequences that contain the origins for DNA replication. The genome encodes for 'early' (E1–4) and 'late' genes. Because viral gene therapy vectors should be replication-incompetent, and because the products of early genes are immunogenic, in most currently used vectors one or more of these genes has been deleted. Production of such defective viruses is achieved using 'packaging' cell lines that encode for the deleted genes. The adenovirus particle is an icosahedral virion and has no envelope. From each penton base a trimeric fiber protein protrudes that ends in a 'knob' structure, which binds to the receptors on target cells (a 'ball with spikes'). The most important cellular receptor for adenovirus is the Coxsackie/adenovirus receptor (CAR). Viral entry requires a second interaction of the capsid with cell surface αV integrins, leading to endocytosis of the particle. Once in the cell nucleus, adenovirus DNA remains extrachromosomal and is transiently (days to weeks) transcribed.

The advantage of adenoviral vectors is the ability to accommodate large DNA cassettes, and large amounts of vector can be produced and purified. A major disadvantage is the relatively short duration of expression (days to weeks) of the transgene, and the immunogenicity of virtually all currently available vectors. Of particular importance for application in the gut is that epithelial cells express only low amounts of the CAR, and hence transfection efficiency is low even when locally applied. It is possible to increase the transfection efficiency by re-targeting adenoviral vectors through alterations of the knob structure, or by application of bispecific antibodies that bind both to the knob structure and to a cellular receptor. Despite these alterations it is doubtful whether adenoviral vectors will be useful in chronic inflammatory diseases, in particular because these vectors themselves are immunogenic and cause inflammatory responses.

Adeno-associated virus

Adeno-associated viruses (AAV) [79] are parvoviruses, and five human serotypes have been identified. These viruses are widely prevalent and, despite the fact that most adult humans have been infected with AAV, the virus is not known to cause a disease. AAV is a DNA virus that is packaged in a non-enveloped icosahedral capsid. The viral genome is a small (4.7 kb) linear DNA flanked by two terminal repeats. It is transcribed in three regions that produce seven transcripts. Because the primary cellular receptor for AAV is heparan sulfate, AAV is able to infect a wide range of (non-dividing) cells. Within the cell the single-stranded DNA needs to be converted into a duplex, and subsequently is integrated at a specific locus on chromosome 19. The second strand formation is the rate-limiting step in AAV infection, and is greatly enhanced by the presence of adeno (helper) virus. This ability of adenovirus has been traced back to a product of the E4 gene, and based on this knowledge adenovirus-free systems for AAV production have been developed. Site-specific integration in chromosome 19 is a potential advantage of AAV-based viral vectors, but in most vectors the *rep* gene, that is necessary for site-specific integration, is deleted; consequently AAV-based vectors integrate non-specifically. The great advantage of AAV vectors is the efficient and long-term transduction of a wide range of cells, including the intestinal epithelium, and the absence of immunogenic responses. Long-term therapeutic expression (up to a year) of coagulation factor IX has been reported in factor IX-deficient mice and hemophilic dogs, and clinical trials in patients suffering from hemophilia B are ongoing [80]. Long-lasting expression of β-galactosidase within the small bowel of rats has been achieved using orally administered AAV vectors [81]. The gene was expressed by the epithelium, as well as by lamina propria cells, and treated rats became lactose-tolerant (normal adult rats do not express lactase). Because the turnover of the small bowel epithelium is rapid, the longevity of the β-galactosidase expression presumably indicates that epithelial stem cells were infected. As compared to adenovirus vectors, the maximal size of the therapeutic gene in AAV vectors is limited, and large-scale production and purification are more difficult. Despite these technical difficulties, AAV vectors are promising tools for (mucosa) targeted gene therapy in the intestinal tract.

Retroviruses

Retroviruses [82] are a large family of viruses that include lentiviruses and oncoviruses. They consist of a core nucleocapsid that is enclosed in a phospholipid envelope containing the specific glycoproteins that interact with cell surface receptors. The viral genome is present as two single-stranded RNA strands, that end in long terminal repeats (LTR) containing the promoter and enhancer elements for viral transcription. The wild-type genome of the murine leukemia viruses that are frequently used for vector construction contains three genes, *gag*, *pol*, and *env*. These encode reverse transcriptase, the nucleocapsid and envelope proteins as well as a packaging signal (ψ) that is necessary for viral assembly at the cellular membrane. The most frequently used retroviral vector is based on the murine Moloney leukemia virus (MMLV), which is non-pathogenic in humans. In this vector almost the entire viral genome can be replaced by a gene of interest. Non-infectious vectors are produced in 'packaging' cell lines that encode *gag, pol*, and *env*. MMLV-based vectors are sensitive to inactivation by complement, infect only dividing cells, and when genes are expressed under the control of viral promoters, these may be silenced by methylation of deletion of proviral DNA. Despite these disadvantages, using MMLV-based vectors, *ex-vivo*-transduced hematopoietic stem cells have been demonstrated to express therapeutic genes for many months. At present MMLV-based vectors are the most attractive tools for targeting T lymphocytes, and it has recently been demonstrated that human peripheral blood CD4[+] T lymphocytes acquire a T regulatory phenotype after transfection with an MMLV vector containing IL-10 [83]. Such approaches may be effective in a range of T lymphocyte-dependent chronic inflammatory diseases, including CD. Recent improvements in retroviral vector technology include cellular retargeting by replacing the retroviral envelope gene with the vesicular stomatitis virus G envelope protein ('pseudotyping') that is recognized by a ubiquitously expressed membrane phospholipid [84]. In addition, lentiviral vectors are now available that are able to integrate into the genome of non-dividing cells and can enter intestinal epithelial cells through the apical membrane. These characteristics render these vectors extremely interesting tools for intestinal gene therapy.

Conclusion

New therapies for IBD have resulted from specific interference with mucosal proinflammatory cascades. Biotechnology, in particular the ability to rapidly generate monoclonal antibodies, has dramatically shortened the time to develop new interventions. In 1992 the first patient with CD was infused with infliximab, and today this therapy is approved and widely used in North America and Europe. Several other interventions, including the administration of 'regulatory' cytokines (IL-10) and antisense oligonucleotides (blocking ICAM1 and NF-κB p65) have also been tested in clinical trials. More recently, small molecules that block signal transduction pathways, and gene therapy approaches, have become available for clinical testing in IBD. Clearly, many of these new interventions will eventually fail on the route to clinical application. However, some of the drugs that make their way into clinical practice will become new standards of treatment, infliximab being a prominent example. These new therapies come with new and sometimes unexpected toxicities, and are expensive. It is conceivable that within the near future small molecules with therapeutic profiles similar to anti-TNF-α antibodies will become available at lower costs. Using these new therapies, remission induction can now be achieved in most patients with active IBD. The new biological therapies have been less successful in maintaining remissions, and this remains an unmet therapeutic need.

References

1. Elson CO, Cong Y, Brandwein S *et al*. Experimental models to study molecular mechanisms underlying intestinal inflammation. Ann NY Acad Sci 1998; 859: 85–95.
2. Dinarello CA. Biologic basis for interleukin-1 in disease. Blood 1996; 87: 2095–147.
3. Beutler BA. The role of tumor necrosis factor in health and disease. J Rheumatol 1999; 26: 16–21.
4. Dinarello CA. Interleukin-1 beta, interleukin-18, and the interleukin-1 beta converting enzyme. Ann NY Acad Sci 1998; 856: 1–11.
5. Fantuzzi G, Dinarello CA. Interleukin-18 and interleukin-1 beta: two cytokine substrates for ICE (caspase-1). J Clin Immunol 1999; 19: 1–11.
6. Dinarello CA. Interleukin-1, interleukin-1 receptors and interleukin-1 receptor antagonist. Int Rev Immunol 1998; 16: 457–99.
7. Thomassen E, Bird TA, Renshaw BR, Kennedy MK, Sims JE. Binding of interleukin-18 to the interleukin-1 receptor homologous receptor IL-1Rrp1 leads to activation of signaling pathways similar to those used by interleukin-1. J Interferon Cytokine Res 1998; 18: 1077–88.

8. Brynskov J, Tvede N, Andersen CB, Vilien M. Increased concentrations of interleukin 1beta, interleukin-2, and soluble interleukin-2 receptors in endoscopical mucosal biopsy specimens with active inflammatory bowel disease. Gut 1992; 33: 55–8.

9. Mahida YR, Wu K, Jewell DP. Enhanced production of interleukin 1-beta by mononuclear cells isolated from mucosa with active ulcerative colitis or Crohn's disease. Gut 1989; 30: 835–8.

10. Casini-Raggi V, Kam L, Chong YJ, Fiocchi C, Pizarro TT, Cominelli F. Mucosal imbalance of IL-1 and IL-1 receptor antagonist in inflammatory bowel disease. A novel mechanism of chronic intestinal inflammation. J Immunol 1995; 154: 2434–40.

11. Stokkers PC, van Aken BE, Basoski N, Reitsma PH, Tytgat GN, van Deventer SJ. Five genetic markers in the interleukin 1 family in relation to inflammatory bowel disease. Gut 1998; 43: 33–9.

12. Andus T, Daig R, Vogl D et al. Imbalance of the interleukin 1 system in colonic mucosa – association with intestinal inflammation and interleukin 1 receptor agonist genotype 2. Gut 1997; 41: 651–7.

13. Cominelli F, Nast CC, Duchini A, Lee M. Recombinant interleukin-1 receptor antagonist blocks the proinflammatory activity of endogenous interleukin-1 in rabbit immune colitis. Gastroenterology 1992; 103: 65–71.

14. Wallach D, Varfolomeev EE, Malinin NL, Goltsev YV, Kovalenko AV, Boldin MP. Tumor necrosis factor receptor and Fas signaling mechanisms. Annu Rev Immunol 1999; 17: 331–67.

15. Bielekova B, Lincoln A, McFarland H, Martin R. Therapeutic potential of phosphodiesterase-4 and -3 inhibitors in Th1-mediated autoimmune diseases. J Immunol 2000; 164: 1117–24.

16. Corral LG, Kaplan G. Immunomodulation by thalidomide and thalidomide analogues. Ann Rheum Dis 1999; 58: I107–13.

17. Muller GW, Shire MG, Wong LM et al. Thalidomide analogs and PDE4 inhibition. Bioorg Med Chem Lett 1998; 8: 2669–74.

18. Reimund JM, Dumont S, Muller CD et al. In vitro effects of oxpentifylline on inflammatory cytokine release in patients with inflammatory bowel disease. Gut 1997; 40: 475–80.

19. Black RA, Rauch CT, Kozlosky CJ et al. A metalloproteinase disintegrin that releases tumour-necrosis factor-alpha from cells. Nature 1997; 385: 729–33.

20. Killar L, White J, Black R, Peschon J. Adamalysins. A family of metzincins including TNF-alpha converting enzyme (TACE). Ann NY Acad Sci 1999; 878: 442–52.

21. Moss ML, Jin SL, Milla ME et al. Cloning of a disintegrin metalloproteinase that processes precursor tumour-necrosis factor-alpha [Published erratum appears in Nature 1997; 386: 738]. Nature 1997; 385: 733–6.

22. Moss ML, Jin SL, Becherer JD et al. Structural features and biochemical properties of TNF-alpha converting enzyme (TACE). J Neuroimmunol 1997; 72: 127–9.

23. Tartaglia LA, Rothe M, Hu YF, Goeddel DV. Tumor necrosis factor's cytotoxic activity is signaled by the p55 TNF receptor. Cell 1993; 73: 213–16.

24. Tartaglia LA, Goeddel DV, Reynolds C et al. Stimulation of human T-cell proliferation by specific activation of the 75-kDa tumor necrosis factor receptor. J Immunol 1993; 151: 4637–41.

25. Beg AA, Baltimore D. An essential role for NF-kappaB in preventing TNF-alpha-induced cell death [See comments]. Science 1996; 274: 782–4.

26. Levi M, Ten Cate H, Bauer KA et al. Inhibition of endotoxin-induced activation of coagulation and fibrinolysis by

27. pentoxifylline or by a monoclonal anti-tissue factor antibody in chimpanzees. J Clin Invest 1994; 93: 114–20.

27. Bauditz J, Haemling J, Ortner M, Lochs H, Raedler A, Schreiber S. Treatment with tumour necrosis factor inhibitor oxpentifylline does not improve corticosteroid dependent chronic active Crohn's disease [See comments]. Gut 1997; 40: 470–4.

28. MacKenzie SJ, Houslay MD. Action of rolipram on specific PDE4 cAMP phosphodiesterase isoforms and on the phosphorylation of cAMP-response-element-binding protein (CREB) and p38 mitogen-activated protein (MAP) kinase in U937 monocytic cells. Biochem J 2000; 347: 571–8.

29. Zou LP, Deretzi G, Pelidou SH et al. Rolipram suppresses experimental autoimmune neuritis and prevents relapses in Lewis rats. Neuropharmacology 2000; 39: 324–33.

30. Hartmann G, Bidlingmaier C, Siegmund B et al. Specific type IV phosphodiesterase inhibitor rolipram mitigates experimental colitis in mice. J Pharmacol Exp Ther 2000; 292: 22–30.

31. Singhal S, Mehta J, Desikan R et al. Antitumor activity of thalidomide in refractory multiple myeloma [See comments] [Published erratum appears in N Engl J Med 2000; 342: 364]. N Engl J Med 1999; 341: 1565–71.

32. Postema PT, den Haan P, van Hagen PM, van Blankenstein M. Treatment of colitis in Behcet's disease with thalidomide. Eur J Gastroenterol Hepatol 1996; 8: 929–31.

33. Bekker LG, Haslett P, Maartens G, Steyn L, Kaplan G. Thalidomide-induced antigen-specific immune stimulation in patients with human immunodeficiency virus type 1 and tuberculosis. J Infect Dis 2000; 181: 954–65.

34. Tramontana JM, Utaipat U, Molloy A et al. Thalidomide treatment reduces tumor necrosis factor alpha production and enhances weight gain in patients with pulmonary tuberculosis. Mol Med 1995; 1: 384–97.

35. Sato EI, Assis LS, Lourenzi VP, Andrade LE. Long-term thalidomide use in refractory cutaneous lesions of systemic lupus erythematosus. Rev Assoc Med Brasil 1998; 44: 289–93.

36. Jacobson JM, Spritzler J, Fox L et al. Thalidomide for the treatment of esophageal aphthous ulcers in patients with human immunodeficiency virus infection. National Institute of Allergy and Infectious Disease AIDS Clinical Trials Group. Immunol Today 1999; 20: 538–40.

37. Vasiliauskas EA, Kam LY, Abreu-Martin MT et al. An open-label pilot study of low-dose thalidomide in chronically active, steroid-dependent Crohn's disease. Gastroenterology 1999; 117: 1278–87.

38. Ehrenpreis ED, Kane SV, Cohen LB, Cohen RD, Hanauer SB. Thalidomide therapy for patients with refractory Crohn's disease: an open-label trial. Gastroenterology 1999; 117: 1271–7.

39. Haslett PA, Klausner JD, Makonkawkeyoon S et al. Thalidomide stimulates T cell responses and interleukin 12 production in HIV-infected patients. AIDS Res Hum Retroviruses 1999; 15: 1169–79.

40. Verbon A, Juffermans NP, Speelman P et al. A single oral dose of thalidomide enhances the capacity of lymphocytes to secrete gamma interferon in healthy humans. Surg Endosc 2000; 14: 721–5.

41. Juffermans NP, Verbon A, Olszyna DP, van Deventer SJ, Speelman P, van Der Poll T. Thalidomide suppresses upregulation of human immunodeficiency virus coreceptors CXCR4 and CCR5 on $CD4^+$ T cells in humans. J Infect Dis 2000; 181: 2067–70.

42. Corral LG, Haslett PA, Muller GW et al. Differential cytokine modulation and T cell activation by two distinct classes of thalidomide analogues that are potent inhibitors of TNF-alpha. J Immunol 1999; 163: 380–6.

43. Sykes AP, Bhogal R, Brampton C *et al*. The effect of an inhibitor of matrix metalloproteinases on colonic inflammation in a trinitrobenzenesulphonic acid rat model of inflammatory bowel disease. Aliment Pharmacol Ther 1999; 13: 1535–42.

44. Williams LM, Gibbons DL, Gearing A, Maini RN, Feldmann M, Brennan FM. Paradoxical effects of a synthetic metalloproteinase inhibitor that blocks both p55 and p75 TNF receptor shedding and TNF alpha processing in RA synovial membrane cell cultures. J Clin Invest 1996; 97: 2833–41.

45. Dekkers PE, Lauw FN, ten Hove T *et al*. The effect of a metalloproteinase inhibitor (GI5402) on tumor necrosis factor-alpha (TNF-alpha) and TNF-alpha receptors during human endotoxemia. Blood 1999; 94: 2252–8.

46. Dekkers PE, ten Hove T, Lauw FN *et al*. The metalloproteinase inhibitor GI5402 inhibits endotoxin-induced soluble CD27 and CD16 release in healthy humans. Infect Immun 2000; 68: 3036–9.

47. Tracey KJ, Abraham E. From mouse to man: or what have we learned about cytokine-based anti-inflammatory therapies? Shock 1999; 11: 224–5.

48. Abraham E. Why immunomodulatory therapies have not worked in sepsis. Nursing 1999; 29: 59–63; quiz 64.

49. Knight DM, Trinh H, Le J *et al*. Construction and initial characterization of a mouse–human chimeric anti-TNF antibody. Cytokine 1995; 7: 15–25.

50. Holliger P, Bohlen H. Engineering antibodies for the clinic. Mol Immunol 1993; 30: 1443–53.

51. Kempeni J. Preliminary results of early clinical trials with the fully human anti-TNFalpha monoclonal antibody D2E7. Cancer Metastasis Rev 1999; 18: 411–19.

52. Bendele AM, McComb J, Gould T *et al*. Combination benefit of PEGylated soluble tumor necrosis factor receptor type I (PEG sTNF-RI) and dexamethasone or indomethacin in adjuvant arthritic rats. Clin Exp Rheumatol 1999; 17: 553–60.

53. Edwards CK, 3rd. PEGylated recombinant human soluble tumour necrosis factor receptor type I (r-Hu-sTNF-RI): novel high affinity TNF receptor designed for chronic inflammatory diseases. J Rheumatol 2000; 27: 601–9.

54. Epstein WV. Treatment of rheumatoid arthritis with a tumor necrosis factor receptor-Fc fusion protein [Letter; comment]. J Immunol 1998; 160: 4098–103.

55. Stack WA, Mann SD, Roy AJ *et al*. Randomised controlled trial of CDP571 antibody to tumour necrosis factor-alpha in Crohn's disease [See comments]. Lancet 1997; 349: 521–4.

56. Sandborn WJ, Feagan BG, Hanauer SB *et al*. An engineered human antibody to TNF (CDP571) for active Crohn's disease: a randomized double-blind placebo-controlled trial. Gastroenterology 2001; 120: 1330–8.

57. Feagan BG, Sandborn WJ, Baker JP *et al*. A randomized, double-blind, placebo-controlled, multi-center trial of the engineered human antibody to TNF (CDP571) for steroid sparing and maintenance of remission in patients with steroid-dependent Crohn's disease. Gastroenterology 2000; 118: A655.

58. Derkx B, Taminiau J, Radema S *et al*. Tumour-necrosis-factor antibody treatment in Crohn's disease [Letter] [See comments]. Lancet 1993; 342: 173–4.

59. Van Dullemen HM, Van Deventer SJH, Hommes DW *et al*. Treatment of Crohn's disease with anti-tumor necrosis factor chimeric monoclonal antibody (cA2). Gastroenterology 1995; 109: 129–35.

60. Targan SR, Hanauer SB, Vandeventer SJH *et al*. A short-term study of chimeric monoclonal antibody Ca2 to tumor necrosis factor alpha for Crohns-disease. N Engl J Med 1997; 337: 1029–35.

61. Rutgeerts P, D'Haens G, Targan S *et al*. Efficacy and safety of retreatment with anti-tumor necrosis factor antibody (infliximab) to maintain remission in Crohn's disease. Gastroenterology 1999; 117: 761–9.

62. D'Haens G, Van Deventer S, Van Hogezand R *et al*. Endoscopic and histological healing with infliximab anti-tumor necrosis factor antibodies in Crohn's disease: a European multicenter trial. Gastroenterology 1999; 116: 1029–34.

63. Present DH, Rutgeerts P, Targan S *et al*. Infliximab for the treatment of fistulas in patients with Crohn's disease. N Engl J Med 1999; 340: 1398–405.

64. Ricart E, Panaccione R, Loftus EV, Tremaine WJ, Sandborn WJ. Successful management of Crohn's disease of the ileoanal pouch with infliximab. Gastroenterology 1999; 117: 429–32.

65. Brandt J, Haibel H, Cornely D *et al*. Successful treatment of active ankylosing spondylitis with the anti-tumor necrosis factor alpha monoclonal antibody infliximab (In process citation). Arthritis Rheum 2000; 43: 1346–52.

66. Van der Linde K, Meijssen MA, Van Bodegraven AA *et al*. Infliximab for treatment of perineal metastatic crohn's disease. Gastroenterology 2000; 118: A588.

67. Sands BE, Tremaine WJ, Sandborn WJ *et al*. Infliximab in the treatment of severe, steroid-refractory ulcerative colitis: a pilot study. Inflamm Bowel Dis 2001; 7: 83–8.

68. Keane J, Gershon S, Wise RP *et al*. Tuberculosis associated with infliximab, a tumor necrosis factor alpha-neutralizing agent. N Engl J Med 2001; 345: 1098–104.

69. Schreiber S, Fedorak RN, Nielsen OH *et al*. Safety and efficacy of recombinant human interleukin 10 in chronic active Crohn's disease. Crohn's Disease IL-10 Cooperative Study Group. Gastroenterology 2000; 119: 1461–72.

70. Fedorak RN, Gangl A, Elson CO *et al*. Recombinant human interleukin 10 in the treatment of patients with mild to moderately active Crohn's disease. Interleukin 10 Inflammatory Bowel Disease Cooperative Study Group. Gastroenterology 2000; 119: 1473–82.

71. Lauw FN, Pajkrt D, Hack CE, Kurimoto M, van Deventer SJ, van Der Poll T. Proinflammatory effects of IL-10 during human endotoxemia. J Infect Dis 2000; 182: 888–94.

72. Schreiber S, Nikolaus S, Malchow H *et al*. Absence of efficacy of subcutaneous antisense ICAM-1 treatment of chronic active Crohn's disease. Gastroenterology 2001; 120: 1339–46.

73. Mebius RE, Streeter PR, Michie S, Butcher EC, Weissman IL. A developmental switch in lymphocyte homing receptor and endothelial vascular addressin expression regulates lymphocyte homing and permits CD4$^+$ CD3$^-$ cells to colonize lymph nodes. Proc Natl Acad Sci USA 1996; 93: 11019–24.

74. Berg EL, McEvoy LM, Berlin C, Bargatze RF, Butcher EC. L-selectin-mediated lymphocyte rolling on MAdCAM-1 [See comments]. Nature 1993; 366: 695–8.

75. Berlin C, Berg EL, Briskin MJ *et al*. Alpha 4 beta 7 integrin mediates lymphocyte binding to the mucosal vascular addressin MAdCAM-1. Cell 1993; 74: 185.

76. Podolsky DK, Lobb R, King N *et al*. Attenuation of colitis in the cotton-top tamarin by anti-alpha 4 integrin monoclonal antibody. J Clin Invest 1993; 92: 372–80.

77. Richards CD, Braciak T, Xing Z, Graham F, Gauldie J. Adenovirus vectors for cytokine gene expression. Ann NY Acad Sci 1995; 762: 282–92; discussion 292–3.

78. Wilson JM. Adenoviruses as gene-delivery vehicles. N Engl J Med 1996; 334: 1185–7.

79. Flotte TR, Carter BJ. Adeno-associated virus vectors for gene therapy. Gene Ther 1995; 2: 357–62.

80. Chao H, Samulski R, Bellinger D, Monahan P, Nichols T, Walsh C. Persistent expression of canine factor IX in hemophilia B canines. Gene Ther 1999; 6: 1695–704.

81. During MJ, Xu R, Young D, Kaplitt MG, Sherwin RS, Leone P. Peroral gene therapy of lactose intolerance using an adeno-associated virus vector [See comments]. Nat Med 1998; 4: 1131–5.

82. Laine F, Blouin V, Ferry N. Evaluation of recombinant retrovirus and adenovirus for gene transfer to normal and pathologic intestine. Gastroenterol Clin Biol 1999; 23: 221–8.

83. Te Velde AA, Van Montfrans C, Spits H, Hooijberg E, Van Deventer SJH. Therapeutic potential of genetically modified T-lymphocytes in Crohn's disease. Gastroenterology 2000; 118: A873.

84. Abe A, Chen ST, Miyanohara A, Friedmann T. *In vitro* cell-free conversion of noninfectious Moloney retrovirus particles to an infectious form by the addition of the vesicular stomatitis virus surrogate envelope G protein. J Virol 1998; 72: 6356–61.

28 | Role of antibiotics and probiotics in the management of inflammatory bowel disease

PHILIPPE MARTEAU AND FERGUS SHANAHAN

Introduction

An infectious cause or contribution to the primary pathogenesis of inflammatory bowel disease (IBD) has not been demonstrated, although many studies have followed that track [1]. However, the deleterious role of some microorganisms from the endogenous flora is also now well established in the majority of models of colitis or enteritis [1–4]. Antibiotics have a well-established role in the management of complications of IBD such as abscess and pouchitis. Whether antibiotics are of use as a primary therapy for either Crohn's disease (CD) or ulcerative colitis (UC) is less clear. An alternative way of influencing intestinal ecology is the use of probiotics or prebiotics. Probiotics are defined as living non-pathogenic microorganisms which, when ingested, exert a positive influence on host health or physiology [5, 6]. Prebiotics have been defined as non-digestible food ingredient that beneficially affects the host by selectively stimulating the growth and/or activity of one or a limited number of bacteria in the colon, that have the potential to improve host health [7]. As some animal studies have shown that probiotics or prebiotics may help in preventing or curing experimental colitis, clinical trials have begun in IBD.

This chapter focuses on the use of metronidazole and ciprofloxacin in CD and pouchitis. In addition, existing data on the use of other antimicrobial agents and on the potential for probiotics in IBD is reviewed.

Background – rationale for therapeutic manipulation of enteric flora in IBD

Although the etiology is unclear, considerable advances have been made in understanding the pathogenesis of CD and UC. This involves an interaction between three contributory cofactors: host susceptibility, mucosal immunity and the resident enteric bacterial flora. Experimental models suggest that the inflammatory response in IBD is the result of abnormal immunologic reactivity to normal flora in a genetically susceptibile host, rather than an appropriate immune response to an abnormal or pathogenic flora [2–4]. Although a specific pathogenic infection has not been implicated that could account for most cases of IBD, heterogeneity may exist and enteric infections might also act as cofactors influencing mucosal immune development and/or have an impact on the timing or clinical onset and phenotype of IBD.

The mucosal immune system senses and interprets the local microenvironment; under normal circumstances it exhibits a restrained response to commensal flora (tolerance) which is coupled with the capacity to react effectively to episodic challenge from pathogenic bacteria (immunity). This requires exquisitely precise regulation. In susceptible individuals, IBD may arise due to a breakdown in immunologic tolerance to the normal enteric bacteria [1, 2]. The pattern of the pathologic immunoinflammatory response is determined by the profile of mucosal cytokines generated which is, in part, genetically regulated and probably influenced by previous immunologic experience including types and timing of exposure to childhood mucosal infections. CD is associated with type 1 helper T cell (Th1) cytokines, such as interferon-γ, tumor necrosis factor (TNF)-α, and interleukin-(IL)-12, although there is some evidence that the profile of mucosal cytokines in early lesions may differ from that of chronic lesions [1, 8, 9]. Ulcerative colitis, in contrast, does not fit easily into the Th1/Th2 paradigm; it does not represent a Th1 response and appears, at least in established disease, to be a modified Th2 response associated with cytokines such as IL-5 and IL-10 [8–10].

Stephan R. Targan, Fergus Shanahan and Loren C. Karp (eds.), Inflammatory Bowel Disease: From Bench to Bedside, 2nd Edition, 573–585.

Most currently available drug therapies for either CD or UC suppress or modulate the host immune and inflammatory response at both systemic and mucosal levels [11]. Until recently, little attention has been directed toward modifying the enteric microenvironment. A striking example of the importance of controlling environmental influences on IBD is the adverse effect of smoking on the clinical course of CD [12]. In addition, the impact of environmental infections on the mucosal immuno-inflammatory response is dramatically illustrated by the apparent capacity of helminthic infections to switch mucosal cytokine production in patients with CD from a Th1 profile toward a Th2 [13]. Indeed, one of the suggested reasons for the increase in prevalence of CD within developed countries within recent decades is reduced exposure to helminthic and other parasitic infections [14].

For patients with established disease, therapeutic modification of the resident bacterial flora with antibiotics or probiotics has recently attracted considerable scientific and clinical research interest and offers another opportunity to influence the mucosal cytokine milieu. However, modification of the enteric flora is not a simple exercise – the flora within the human intestine are complex and dynamic with 400–500 bacterial species accounting for 1–2 kg of intestinal content and a collective metabolism tantamount to that of a virtual organ the neglected organ [15, 16]. While antibiotics may appear an obvious method for modifying the flora, they are too non-specific, pose a risk of overgrowth with pathogens such as *Clostridium difficile*, and the potential for development of antibiotic resistance. Probiotics offer the advantage of more measured and controlled

manipulation of the flora in IBD and they have properties beyond a simple antimicrobial effect [4–6, 17–18]. In addition, probiotics offer the prospect of genetically modified organisms designed for delivery of important biological molecules including IL-10, vaccines and other biologically important molecules [18–20].

The rationale for therapeutic modification of the enteric flora in patients with established IBD is based on two main lines of evidence. First, is the beneficial conditioning influence of the commensal bacterial flora on intestinal structure and function under normal circumstances. Second is a body of evidence implicating the enteric flora in driving the mucosal inflammatory response in susceptible individuals (Table 1) [21–38].

Epithelial cells have been described as sensors of pathogenic infection, and cytokine signaling by the epithelium has been well described in the context of enteric pathogenic infections [39]. However, bidirectional dialog between the host and the normal flora is also evident [22, 40]. Indeed, evidence for influence of the enteric flora on mucosal integrity is well illustrated in germfree animals, where there is reduced epithelial turnover, vascularity, luminal enzyme activity, mucosal-associated lymphoid tissue and thickness of bowel wall. In addition, there are alterations in peristalsis and immune function [23]. Thus, the flora exchange regulatory signals not only with the epithelium but with the subepithelial cells within the intestine [4, 41, 42]. Evidence implicating the resident bacterial flora as an essential cofactor driving the inflammatory process in IBD is based on observational yet persuasive data from human studies and direct experimental results using animal

Table 1. Rationale for therapeutic manipulation of enteric flora in IBD

Observational and experimental lines of evidence	References
Conditioning effects of resident flora on mucosal structure and function including epithelial turnover, blood flow, peristalsis, immune development and function	4, 16, 21–23
Lesions in IBD occur in areas of highest bacterial exposure	
Clinical response to diversion of fecal stream, relapse on restoration	24, 25
Experimental induction of inflammation by exposure to fecal material	26, 27
Immunologic reactivity to flora in patients with IBD (loss of tolerance)	28–33
Attenuation of inflammation in animal models of IBD when germfree	34, 35
Experimental transfer of colitis with T cells reactive to bacterial antigens	36
Influence of antibiotics and probiotics in experimental animals and in pouchitis	37, 38

*References are representative, not comprehensive.

models (Table 1). Perhaps the most persuasive argument is the transfer of enterocolitis using T cells that are reactive to enteric bacteria in an animal model of IBD [36].

In summary, although the lessons of *Helicobacter pylori* and peptic ulcer disease are sobering, and a search for a specific infectious etiology for IBD will continue [4, 8, 43], the bulk of evidence suggests that IBD is not a simple struggle between microbe and humans but rather a more complex interplay amongst genes, commensals and immune cells. There is a sound rationale for therapeutic alteration of the enteric flora and, as discussed below, the evidence for its efficacy as an adjunct to existing therapies is promising.

Metronidazole

Metronidazole is a nitroimidazole compound that has a clinically useful antimicrobial spectrum against anaerobes, particularly gut anaerobes, as well as certain intestinal protozoan infections. Metronidazole is a prodrug which has no antimicrobial properties until it is activated by bacterial enzymes [44]. The size of the bacterial flora in the colon and the proportion of anaerobes in comparison with the small bowel may account for differences in efficacy of metronidazole in colonic and small bowel CD.

The actual mode of action of metronidazole in CD is uncertain and may not be limited to its antimicrobial activity [4, 44] as metronidazole also has immunomodulatory effects and tissue-healing properties [46].

A role for metronidazole in CD was first suggested by Ursing and Kamme in 1975 [47]. Since then, its clinical usefulness in CD has been the subject of few well-designed studies but much debate. Metronidazole has some beneficial effect in ileocolonic CD. As discussed later, this has been shown in randomized controlled trials. Metronidazole has also been shown to be effective in perineal CD, although a randomized controlled study proving the efficacy in this setting has not been performed. Metronidazole is not effective in isolated small bowel CD but decreases the risk of recurrence of ileal lesions after ileocolonic resection for CD. Open studies and two randomized controlled trials have shown that it is not effective in UC when used alone or as an adjunct to corticosteroids [48–50]. The results of the randomized trials are summarized in Table 2.

Ileocolonic Crohn's disease

Blichfeldt *et al.* [51] evaluated metronidazole as adjunctive therapy (patients were allowed to use prednisone or salazosulfapyridine) compared to placebo in a double-blind, crossover study. They found no overall benefit of metronidazole except in the subset of six patients with colitis only, in which there was considerable improvement. The Cooperative Crohn's Disease Study in Sweden [52] compared metronidazole, 800 mg/day, as primary therapy to sulfasalazine, 3 g/day. Although this was a double-blind, crossover study, there was no placebo control. The authors found metronidazole and sulfasalazine to be equally effective therapy. Small bowel disease alone did not benefit, as only two subjects of 12 in this subset on metronidazole improved. Of note, in this trial, just over half the patients responded to either therapy and only 25% of metronidazole patients achieved quiescent disease. Ambrose *et al.* [53] compared metronidazole alone, metronidazole plus cotrimoxazole, cotrimoxazole alone and placebo in a randomized trial of 1 month involving 72 patients. No difference of response was observed between the four groups. In a 16-week randomized, placebo-controlled trial by Sutherland *et al.* [54], two different doses of metronidazole were compared with placebo in patients with active CD. By the end of the trial there was no difference in attaining remission in either of the metronidazole groups compared to placebo (27% for both metronidazole groups versus 25% for placebo). However, more individual patients on metronidazole showed some improvement in their Crohn's Disease Activity Index (CDAI) compared with patients using placebo. Prantera *et al.* [55] compared, in a 12-week randomized trial, the efficacy of a combination of metronidazole (250 mg four times daily) plus ciprofloxacin (500 mg twice daily) vs methylprednisolone (0.7–1 mg/kg followed by tapering) in 41 patients with active CD. Clinical remission was observed in 45.5% of the patients receiving the antibiotics vs 63% in the steroid group (n.s.). There were more side-effects in the antibiotic group (27.3% vs 10.6%). The authors concluded that, despite the high incidence of adverse events, this combination of antibiotics could be an alternative to steroids in the treatment of acute CD for the patients who tolerate the drugs.

Rutgeerts *et al.* performed two randomized controlled trails demonstrating that metronidazole and ornidazole are significantly effective in the prevention of postoperative recurrence of CD after ileal resection [56, 57]. In the first trial, 60 patients

were treated with prednisone (with decreasing dose) plus mesalazine plus either ciprofloxacin (500–750 mg twice a day) or placebo for 6 months. Both treatments were equally effective during the first 3 months; however, after 6 months treatment failure was less frequent in the ciprofloxacin group (21% vs 44%, $p = 0.02$), although endoscopic and histologic findings were not different. It is at present difficult to draw firm conclusions on the efficacy of ciprofloxacin in UC from this single study, and the study design has been criticized, especially because of the associated treatments [79]. Confirmatory studies are needed.

Hurst *et al.* [64] reported that eight out of 11 patients with pouchitis who had not tolerated or responded to metronidazole responded to ciprofloxacin. In an open trial, Gionchetti *et al.* [80] treated 18 patients suffering from refractory pouchitis with rifaximin (a broad-spectrum non-absorbable antibiotic) plus ciprofloxacin for 15 days; 16/18 either improved ($n = 10$) or went into remission ($n = 6$).

Side-effects

Ciprofloxacin appears to be safe for short-term or long-term use in IBD patients [81]. The most common side-effects include nausea, vomiting and skin reactions. Tendinitis and rupture, usually of the Achilles tendon, are very rare, but clinicians should be aware that steroids are predisposing factors [81]. All new quinolones including ciprofloxacin are contraindicated for use in pregnant women, based on the arthropathogenicity of these medications observed in immature animals [82].

Antimycobacterial therapy

Based on the sporadic finding of mycobacteria, especially *Mycobacterium paratuberculosis*, in tissue from patients with CD, several authors have tried various antituberculous drugs to treat patients. There have been anecdotal reports of remissions of CD after antimycobacterial therapy [83–85]; however, the randomized controlled trials and open studies have yielded less convincing results (Table 3).

Elliott *et al.* [86] performed a double-blind placebo-controlled study evaluating sulfadoxine, 1.5 g, plus pyrimethamine, 75 mg, once weekly in patients with steroid-resistant active CD. Sulfadoxine was chosen because this group of investigators had isolated a sulfadoxine-sensitive *Mycobacterium kansaii* species from tissue from a patient with CD. There was no difference in outcome between therapy with this antibiotic regimen versus placebo. Shaffer *et al.* [87] evaluated rifampin, 10 mg/kg per day, plus ethambutol, 15 mg/kg per day, as primary therapy for CD in a double-blind, placebo-controlled crossover study. They found no significant difference between rifampin plus ethambutol therapy compared to placebo in terms of clinical status and CDAI levels. Twenty-seven patients were enrolled but only 14 completed the study. Ten of the 14 patients completing the trial had relapses, five of whom were on active drug. Three of the four patients who withdrew from the trial because they required surgery

Table 3. Randomized placebo-controlled trials with antimycobacterial therapy in Crohn's disease

Drugs	No. of patients	Duration of treatment	Remission (antibiotic vs placebo)	Ref.
Sulfadoxine + pyrimethamine	51	12 months	No effect	86
Rifampicin + ethambuthol (crossover)	27	12 months	No effect	87
Rifabutin	24	6 months	No effect	94
Clofazimin	49	12 months	No effect	88
Rifampicin + ethambuthol + isoniazid	130	24 months	No effect	89, 90
Rifampicin + ethambuthol + clofazimin + dapsone	40	9 months	72 % vs 33 %*	91
Clarithromycin (crossover)	15	3 months	71.4 % vs 12.5 %*	96
Clarithromycin + ethambuthol	31	3 months	No effect	97

*$p < 0.05$

were using active drug. Afdhal et al. [88] reported that clofazimin (which is bactericidal against Mycobacterium leprae, Mycobacterium avium and Mycobacterium ulcerans) in a dose of 100 mg/day for 8 months was not more effective than the placebo. In the largest trial [89, 90], 130 subjects were randomized double-blind to receive for up to 2 years either rifampicin, isoniazid, and ethambutol or identical placebos. The effect of the treatment on the course of the disease was assessed in a number of ways including the Harvey–Bradshaw index, the number of episodes of surgery required, radiological change, the total steroid dosage during the study, and the number of days of which prednisone was above 10 mg. Efficacy was evaluated after 2 years, and more recently after 5 years in 81% of the patients. No benefit was observed in the treated group. During the study period, 17 patients in the antituberculous group had experienced adverse events (vs three in the placebo group), and the treatment had to be stopped because of adverse events in nine. Two subsequent randomized controlled trials have been more optimistic but remain preliminary. Prantera et al. [91] treated, for 9 months, 40 corticodependent patients with active CD with rifampicin, ethambutol, clofazimin and dapsone or placebos. After 9 months of treatment, 4/19 patients treated with the antibiotics vs 11/17 in the placebo group still needed corticosteroids ($p = 0.03$); eight patients had anemia related to dapsone therapy, and two of them had to stop the treatment because of this adverse event. Borgaonkar et al. performed a meta-analysis of the trials using antituberculous agents to treat CD [92], and calculated that the pooled odds ratio for maintenance of remission in treatment vs control for all studies was 1.1 (n.s.). However, they considered that the studies could be divided into two subgroups based upon the method by which corticosteroids were used to induce remission. The studies by Afdhal et al. [88] and by Prantera et al. [91] used corticosteroids with subsequent tapering while the other did not. Pooling of these two trials yielded an odds ratio for maintenance of remission in treatment vs control of 3.37 (95% confidence interval 1.38–8.24). The authors concluded that this regimen might be effective.

Mycobacterium paratuberculosis is generally resistant to standard antituberculous drugs, and infections are difficult to eradicate. This may explain the absence of efficacy of usual antituberculous agents in CD and stimulated pursuit of drugs active against this microorganism, especially rifabutin, clarithromycin, and azithromycin [93]. Rifabutin alone was compared to placebo by Basilisco et al. [94] in 24 subjects treated for 6 months; the study was interrupted because of the occurrence of allergies, but no difference in efficacy was observed between the two groups. Gui et al. [95] performed an open study in 52 patients with severe CD who received clarithromycin or azithromycin together with rifabutin for a mean of 18 months. A reduction of CDAI at 6 and 24 months and of C-reactive protein was observed, and only two out of 19 patients who were steroid-dependent at the beginning of the study continued to require steroids. Graham et al. [96] treated in a crossover study 15 patients with CD with 1 g/day clarithromycin or placebo for 3 months. They reported that remission could be achieved by about 40% of the patients with severe disease [96]. However, more recently, the same group reported that a combination of clarithromycin and ethambutol for 3 months was not more effective than placebo in 31 patients followed 1 year [97].

Other antibiotics

Moss et al. [98] evaluated in an open fashion the effects of five antibiotics (ampicillin, tetracyclin, clindamycin, cephalotin, and erythromycin) in 44 patients with CD. Criteria used for patient selection or for antibiotic selection were unclear. The authors reported that, by 6 months, 41 of 44 patients significantly improved. Of 35 patients evaluated radiographically, 15 patients showed either no improvement or deteriorated. Savidge [99] reported on the use of trimethoprim-sulfamethoxazole in treating eight patients with active UC in an open fashion. Two patients failed therapy, five patients achieved complete clinical remission (all within 1 week), and one patient had some improvement. The treatment duration was from 2 to 26 weeks. Ambrose et al. [53] reported on four groups of patients with acutely active CD randomized to either placebo therapy, trimethoprim-sulfamethoxazole plus placebo, metronidazole plus placebo, or trimethoprim-sulfamethoxazole plus metronidazole. This study suggested no benefit of any antibiotic combination compared to placebo. Saverymuttu et al. [100] reported a randomized trial comparing prednisolone, 0.5 mg/kg per day, plus a normal diet to an elemental diet plus framycetin, colistin, and nystatin (three non-absorbable antibiotics) in 32 patients with apparently active CD. The premise of the study was that intestinal decontamination lowers the antigenic load and improves disease activity. There was a similar rate of improvement in both groups based on radiolabeled fecal leukocyte excretion and changes in CDAI. However, statistical analysis was not included in this report. To provide intestinal decontamination, Burke *et al.* [101] treated patients with active UC with 7 days of oral tobramycin adjunctively to corticosteroids and sulfasalazine. Compared with placebo, the group receiving tobramycin had a greater remission rate. The concurrent use of the standard therapies, however, precludes a clear conclusion as to what effect the tobramycin had.

Dickinson *et al.* [102] reported a double-blind, placebo-controlled study of 7 days with oral vancomycin in acute exacerbation of idiopathic colitis. The rationale for using vancomycin was to eradicate *Clostridium difficile*, which had been implicated as an exacerbating factor in some patients with idiopathic colitis, and to treat the overgrowth of Grampositive flora in the bowels of UC patients. Forty patients (33 with UC and seven with CD) requiring hospitalization were randomized to vancomycin, 500 mg every 6 hours, or placebo. There was no significant difference in the outcome between vancomycin- and placebo-treated patients. Interestingly, no patients had *C. difficile* cultured from their stool. This report showed that vancomycin was of no benefit and that *C. difficile* is not an important factor in most patients with exacerbation of idiopathic colitis. Other studies have also found that only four of 44 patients with UC [103] and two of 169 patients with IBD (neither of whom had active disease [104]) were found to have *C. difficile* toxin in their stool.

Dapsone, which is used to treat leprosy, was used in six patients with active CD. Within 3 months, four of six patients achieved complete remission [105]. Prantera *et al.* [106] treated a patient with a 12-year history of Crohn's ileocolitis, during a flare of Crohn's proctitis, with dapsone, 75 mg/day. The proctitis was dramatically improved within 2 weeks, and complete remission was achieved, including healing of all known intestinal disease, during 12 months of therapy. The same author later performed a case study of five patients treated with dapsone; two improved and one went into remission [107]. He later performed a randomized controlled study with four antimycobacterial drugs including dapsone [91], and reported that it was effective (see above).

Rifaximin

Gionchetti *et al.* [108] performed a 10-day double-blind controlled trial comparing the efficacy of rifaximin and placebo in 28 patients with severe refractory UC; 64% of the patients receiving rifaximin improved vs 42% in the control group (n.s.). Rifaximin resulted in a significant reduction in stool frequency, rectal bleeding, and endoscopic score compared to placebo. This therapeutic response was surprisingly high, even in the control group, if one considers that the patients had severe colitis. Further studies are thus needed to confirm this report. In another study the same authors reported that a combination of rifaximin plus ciprofloxacin was helpful in subjects with refractory pouchitis [80].

In a 5-day randomized controlled study, Casellas *et al.* compared the efficacy of amoxicillin–clavulanic acid, methylprednisolone or a combination of both in 30 patients with active UC [109]. The release of IL-8 by the inflamed intestinal mucosa was decreased by the antibiotic.

Probiotics

Rationale

Probiotics are live microbial food ingredients that alter the enteric microflora and have a beneficial effect on health [5, 6]. They include bacteria such as lactobacilli, bifidobacteria, *Escherichia coli*, etc., or yeast such as *Saccharomyces* [110]. The effects can be either direct effects due to the expression *in vivo* of intrinsic metabolic properties of the microorganism or to some part of its architecture, or indirect effects due to modifications of the endogenous flora or of the immune system [110]. The tolerance is usually excellent, although several cases of infection have been published [110–113]. Although the mechanisms involved in many effects are often not understood, the survival of the strains in the gastrointestinal tract, and in some cases its adhesion to the mucosa, seem important pharmacokinetic factors [114, 115]. Several studies have shown interesting effects of probiotics in animals models of IBD [4, 19, 37, 116–118]. Intracolonic administration of *Lactobacillus reuteri* R2LC to rats with acetic acid-induced colitis significantly decreased the disease while *Lactobacillus* HLC was ineffective [116]. Administration of *L. reuteri* R2LC and *L. plantarum* DSM 9843 to rats with methotrexate-induced enterocolitis reduced intestinal permeability, bacterial translocation and plasma endotoxin levels compared with rats with enterocolitis and no treatment [117]. A strain of *L. salivarius* (ssp *salivarius* UCC118) diminished the rate of progression from inflammation through dysplasia to colon cancer in the IL-10-deficient model, when compared to non-probiotic-fed animals [118].

Clinical trials

Many of the clinical trials using probiotics in IBD have been published only in preliminary abstract form, but information is rapidly increasing.

Ulcerative colitis

McCann *et al.* [119] were the first to suggest, from their experience in open treatment of 10 subjects, that long-term administration of *Escherichia coli* strain Nissle 1917, and other bacterial strains including *Lactobacillus acidophilus*, and *Bifidobacterium bifidum* may help maintaining remission in UC. Two randomized controlled trials were then performed comparing the efficacy of this strain to mesalazine for the maintenance of remission in UC [120, 121]. Kruis *et al.* [120] included, in a 12-week double-blind double dummy study, 120 patients with inactive UC. Half of them received 1.5 g/day of mesalazine, and the other half received 200 mg/day of mutaflor (Ardeypharm GmbH, Herdecke, Germany) which contains 25×10^9 viable *E. coli* bacteria per 100 mg. After 12 weeks, 11.3% of the subjects receiving mesalazine and 16% of those receiving *E. coli* had relapsed, and this difference was not significant. Rembacken *et al.* published a second trial in which *E. coli* strain Nissle 1917 was also compared to mesalazine in 116 patients with active UC [121]. Patients with active colitis were randomized to receive 2.4 g/day of mesalazine or 200 mg/day of mutaflor in enteric capsules, which release the *E. coli* in the terminal ileum. All patients were also given a 1-week course of oral gentamicin 240 mg/day to suppress their native *E. coli* flora, and either rectal or oral steroids according to the extent of their disease. Remission was attained in 75% of the patients in the mesalazine group vs 68% in the *E. coli* group (difference n.s.). When remission was reached, the steroids were tapered and stopped over 4 months, and the dose of mesalazine was reduced to 1.2 g/day. Relapse occurred in 73% of the patients in the mesalazine group vs 67% in the *E. coli* group (difference n.s.). These two trials demonstrate that the tolerance was good, but can only suggest that *E. coli*

strain Nissle 1917 may be helpful in UC. Indeed, none of the trials compared this strain to placebo, the statistical power of the first study was low, as the follow-up was short, and as the efficacy of the mesalazine second study was rather low. Ishikawa *et al.* [122] gave to 21 subjects suffering from UC 100 ml/day of fermented milk for 1 year. Eleven received *B. bifidum* YIT 4007, *B. breve* YIT 4065, and *L. acidophilus* YIT 0168 in the milk and the other 10 did not. They reported that the probiotic mixture was well tolerated and that there were less relapses in the group receiving (27%) than in the control group (90%). The bifidobacteria were recovered from the feces of the subjects.

Pouchitis

Pouchitis has been shown to be associated with reduced counts of bifidobacteria and lactobacilli, suggesting that it may result from an imbalance of the endogenous flora [123]. Gionchetti *et al.* performed a randomized double-blind study comparing the effect of a probiotic mixture: VSL#3 and placebo to prevent recurrence of chronic relapsing pouchitis [38]. Eligible patients had chronic relapsing pouchitis defined as at least three relapses per year. When they entered the study they were in remission, and no other treatment was allowed. Remission had been induced by 1 month of antibiotic treatment with ciprofloxacin and rifabutin. VSL#3 (CSL, Milan, Italy) contains 300 billion viable lyophilized bacteria per gram of four strains of lactobacilli (*L. casei, L. plantarum, L. acidophilus, L. delbrueckii* subsp. *bulgaricus*), three strains of bifidobacteria (*B. longum, B. breve, B. infantis*), and one strain *of Streptococcus salivarius* subsp. *thermophilus*. The treatment (6 g/day) was given for 9 months. Forty patients entered the study. A relapse occurred in 15% of the subjects in the VSL#3 group vs 100% in the placebo group ($p < 0.001$). No side-effects were observed. The mechanism of this therapeutic effect is not yet established; however, the authors showed that the fecal concentration of lactobacilli, bifidobacteria and streptococci increased in the VSL#3 group and, in another study, that continuous treatment with VSL#3 increases the tissue levels of IL-10 in patients with chronic pouchitis [124]. The same authors studied the effect of VSL#3 to prevent pouchitis. Forty patients who had colectomy and ileo-pouch–anal anastomosis for UC were randomized to receive either VSL#3 (3 g/day) or placebo immediately after ileostomy closure and for 1 year. Pouchitis occurred in 10% of the patients in the VSL#3 group vs 40% of those in the placebo group ($p < 0.01$). Friedman *et al.* treated 10 patients with pouchitis with a mixture of *Lactobacillus rhamnosus* strain GG and fructro-oligosaccharides for 1 month and reported that this short term treatment was effective in all cases [125].

Crohn's disease

Several trials suggested that *Saccharomyces boulardii*, a probiotic yeast [6, 126] has some efficacy in the treatment of CD [127, 128]. Plein and Hotz [127] performed a pilot double-blind controlled study testing the efficacy of *S. boulardii* on symptoms of CD. Twenty patients with active moderate CD were randomized to receive for 7 weeks, together with the standard treatment, either *S. boulardii* or a placebo. A significant reduction in the frequency of bowel movements and in disease activity was observed in the group receiving *S. boulardii* but not in the placebo group. Guslandi *et al.* [128] treated 32 patients with CD in clinical remission either with 1 g/day of *S. boulardii* plus mesalazine 2 g/day or mesalazine 3 g/day in a double-blind randomized study. A clinical relapse was observed less frequently in the group who received the probiotic (1/16 at 1 year) than in the mesalazine group (6/16, $p < 0.05$). In an open study a 10-day administration of *Lactobacillus* GG to 14 children with active or inactive CD resulted in an increase in IgA-secreting cells to β-lactoglobulin and casein, which indicates an interaction between the probiotic and the local immune system [129]. The lactobacillus did not influence the disease activity; however, the study group was too small and the study duration was too short to assess accurately a clinical effect [129].

Campieri *et al.* compared the efficacy of a combination of rifaximin 1.8 g/day for 3 months followed by VSL#3 probiotic therapy vs mesalazine 4 g/day in the prevention of postoperative recurrence of CD [130]. Forty patients were randomized; after 1 year 20% of the patients treated with the probiotic had a severe endoscopic relapse vs 40% of the patients treated with mesalazine.

Malchow treated in a double-blind controlled pilot study 28 subjects suffering from CD of the colon with *E. coli* strain Nissle 1917 or placebo [131]. The probiotic was well tolerated, and the rate of relapse was lower in the probiotic group (33%) than in the placebo group (63%).

Conclusion

The notion that IBD might have an infectious etiology has recurred over the years. Part of the appeal in finding an infectious agent is that simple and possibly curative therapy could be offered to patients. However, convincing evidence for a role for viruses, bacteria, or mycobacteria in the etiopathogenesis of these diseases is lacking. There are no convincing data supporting the use of antimicrobial agents as primary therapy in IBD. An exception may be metronidazole in CD. Despite the lack of randomized, controlled trials of metronidazole for perineal CD, the open data available and general clinical experience are convincing. The role of metronidazole in other clinical forms of CD is less clear. Well-designed studies have been sparse, and many trials have been inadequately powered or methodologically flawed. The first trials with probiotics are encouraging but much work is required before they can be recommended for routine use. The properties of the constituents of probiotic preparations need clarification and mechanistic studies are needed. Most importantly, for both probiotic and antibiotic strategies, the most urgent requirement is an improved understanding of the normal flora and its interaction with the host in health and disease.

References

1. Fiocchi C. Inflammatory bowel disease: etiology and pathogenesis. Gastroenterology 1998; 115: 182–205.
2. Shanahan F. Mechanisms of immunologic sensation of intestinal contents. Am J Physiol (Gastrointest Liver Physiol) 2000; 278: G191–6.
3. French N, Pettersson S. Microbe-host interactions in the alimentary tract: the gateway to understanding inflammatory bowel disease. Gut 2000; 47: 162–3.
4. Shanahan F. Probiotics and inflammatory bowel disease: is there a scientific rationale? Inflam Bowel Dis 2000; 6: 107–15.
5. Fuller R. Probiotics in man and animal. J Appl Bacteriol 1989; 66: 365–78.
6. Marteau P, De Vrese M, Cellier C, Schhrezenmeir J. Protection from gastrointestinal diseases using probiotics. Am J Clin Nutr 2001; 73: 430S–6S.
7. Salminen S, Bouley C, Boutron-Ruault MC *et al.* Functional food science and gastrointestinal physiology and function. Br J Nutr 1998; 80(Suppl. 1): 147–71.
8. Elson CO. Commensal bacteria as targets in Crohn's disease. Gastroenterology 2000; 119: 254–7.
9. Desreumaux P, Brandt E, Bambiez L *et al.* Distinct cytokine patterns in early and chronic ileal lesions of Crohn's disease. Gastroenterology 1997; 113: 118–26.
10. Stallmach A, Strober W, MacDonald TT *et al.* Induction and modulation of gastrointestinal inflammation. Immunol Today 1998; 19: 438–41.
11. Sands BE. Therapy of inflammatory bowel disease. Gastroenterology 2000; 118: S68–82.

12. Timmer A, Sutherland LR, Martin F. Oral contraceptive use and smoking are risk factors for relapse in Crohn's disease. Gastroenterology 1998; 114: 1143–50.

13. Summers RW, Urban J, Elliott D, Qadir K et al. Th2 conditioning by *Trichuris suis* appears safe and effective in modifying the mucosal immune response in inflammatory bowel disease. Gastroenterology 1999; 116: A828 (Abstract).

14. Elliott DE, Urban JF Jr, Argo CK, Weinstock JV. Does the failure to acquire helminthic parasites predispose to Crohn's disease? FASEB J 2000; 14: 1848–55.

15. Bocci V. The neglected organ: bacterial flora has a crucial immunostimulatory role. Perspect Biol Med 1992; 35: 251–60.

16. Berg RD. The indigenous gastrointestinal microflora. Trends Microbiol. 1996; 4: 430–5.

17. Bengmark S. Ecological control of the gastrointestinal tract. The role of probiotic flora. Gut 1998; 42: 2–7.

18. Dugas B, Mercenier A, Lenoir-Wijnkoop I et al. Immunity and probiotics. Immunol Today 1999; 20: 387–90.

19. Steidler L, Hans W, Schotte L et al. Treatment of murine colitis by *Lactococcus lactis* secreting interleukin-10. Science 2000; 289: 1352–5.

20. Shanahan F. Therapeutic manipulation of gut flora. Science 2000; 289: 1311–12.

21. MacDonald TT, Pattersson S. Bacterial regulation of intestinal immune responses. Inflam Bowel Dis 2000; 6: 116–22.

22. Gordon JI, Hooper LV, McNevin SM et al. Epithelial cell growth and differentiation III. Promoting diversity in the intestine: conversations between the microflora, epithelium, and diffuse GALT. Am J Physiol 273 (Gastrointest Liver Physiol 1997; 36): G565–70.

23. Midtvedt T. Microbial functional activities. In: Hanson LA, Yolken RH (eds). Intestinal Microflora, Nestle Nutrition Workshop Series. Philadelphia: Lippincott-Raven, 1999; 42: 79–96.

24. Janowitz HD, Croen EC, Sacher DB. The role of the fecal stream in Crohn's disease: an historical and analytical review. Inflam Bowel Dis 1998; 4: 29–39.

25. Rutgeerts P, Geboes K, Peeters M et al. Effect of faecal stream diversion on recurrence of Crohn's disease in the neoterminal ileum. Lancet 1991; 338: 771–4.

26. Harper PH, Lee ECG, Kettlewell MGW et al. Role of the faecal stream in the maintenance of Crohn's colitis. Gut 1985; 26: 279–84.

27. D'Haens GR, Geboes K, Peeters M et al. Early lesions of recurrent Crohn's disease caused by infusion of intestinal contents in excluded ileum. Gastroenterology 1998; 114: 262–7.

28. Shanahan F. Antibody 'markers' in Crohn's disease: opportunity or overstatement? Gut 1997; 40: 557–8.

29. Shanahan F. Immunologic and genetic links in Crohn's disease. Gut 2000; 46: 6–7.

30. Duchmann R, Kaiser I, Hermann E et al. Tolerance exists towards resident intestinal flora but is broken in active inflammatory bowel disease (IBD). Clin Exp Immunol 1995; 102: 448–55.

31. Duchmann R, Schmitt E, Knolle P et al. Tolerance towards resident intestinal flora in mice is abrogated in experimental colitis and restored by treatment with interleukin-10 or antibodies to interleukin-12. Eur J Immunol 1996; 26: 934–8.

32. MacPherson A, Khoo UY, Forgacs I et al. Mucosal antibodies in inflammatory bowel disease are directed against intestinal bacteria. Gut 1996; 38: 365–75.

33. Duchmann R, May E, Heike M et al. T cell specificity and cross reactivity toward enterobacteria, *Bacteroides*, *Bifido-*

34. *bacterium*, and antigens from resident intestinal flora in humans. Gut 1999; 44: 812–18.

34. Blumberg RS, Saubermann LJ, Strober W. Animal models of mucosal inflammation and their relation to human inflammatory bowel disease. Curr Opin Immunol 1999; 11: 648–56.

35. Arseneau KO, Pizarro TT, Cominelli F. Discovering the cause of inflammatory bowel disease: lessons from animal models. Curr Opin Gastroenterology 2000; 16: 310–17.

36. Cong Y, Brandwein SL, McCabe RP et al. CD4+ T cells reactive to enteric bacterial antigens in spontaneously colitic C3H/HeJBir mice: increased T helper cell type 1 response and ability to transfer disease. J Exp Med 1998; 187: 855–64.

37. Madsen KL, Doyle JS, Jewell LD et al. *Lactobacillus* species prevents colitis in interleukin 10 gene-deficient mice. Gastroenterology 1999; 116: 1107–14.

38. Gionchetti P, Rizzello F, Venturi A et al. Oral bacteriotherapy as maintenance treatment in patients with chronic pouchitis: a double-blind, placebo-controlled trial. Gastroenterology 2000; 119: 305–9.

39. Kagnoff MF, Eckmann L. Epithelial cells as sensors for microbial infection. J Clin Invest 1997; 100: 6–10.

40. Bry L, Falk PG, Midtvedt T, Gordon JI. A model system of host–microbial interactions in an open mammalian ecosystem. Science 1996; 273: 1380–3.

41. Mourelle M, Salas A, Guarnier F et al. Stimulation of transforming growth factor-β1 by enteric bacteria in the pathogenesis of rat intestinal fibrosis. Gastroenterology 1988; 114: 519–26.

42. Haller D, Bode C, Hammes WP et al. Non-pathogenic bacteria elicit a differential cytokine response by intestinal epithelial cell/leucocyte co-cultures. Gut 2000; 47: 79–87.

43. Sutton CL, Kim J, Yamane A et al. Identification of a novel bacterial sequence associated with Crohn's disease. Gastroenterology 2000; 119: 23–31.

44. Freeman CD, Klutman NE, Lamp KC. Metronidazole. A therapeutic review and update. Drugs 1997; 54: 679–708.

45. Krook A, Jarnerot G, Danielsson D. Clinical effect of metronidazole and sulfasalazine on Crohn's disease in relation to changes in the fecal flora. Scand J Gastroenterol 1981; 16: 569–75.

46. Borden EB, Sammartano RJ, Dembe C, Boley SJ. The effect of metronidazole on wound healing in rats. Surgery 1985; 97: 331–6.

47. Ursing B, Kamme C. Metronidazole therapy for Crohn's disease. Lancet 1975; 1: 775–7.

48. Davies PS, Rhodes J, Heatley RV, Owen E. Metronidazole in the treatment of chronic proctitis. A controlled study. Gut 1987; 18: 680–1.

49. Gilat T, Suissa A, Leichtman G et al. A comparative study of metronidazole and sulfasalazine in active, not severe ulcerative colitis. An Israeli multicenter study. J Clin Gastroenterol 1987; 9: 415–17.

50. Chapman RW, Selby WS, Jewel DP. Controlled trial of intravenous metronidazole as an adjunct to corticosteroids in severe ulcerative colitis. Gut 1986; 27: 1210–2.

51. Blichfeldt P, Blomhoff JP, Myhre E, Gjone E. Metronidazole in Crohn's disease. Scand J Gastroenterol 1978; 13: 123–7.

52. Rosen A, Ursing B, Alm T et al. A comparative study of metronidazole and sulfasalazine for active Crohn's disease: the Cooperative Crohn's Disease Study in Sweden. II. Result. Gastroenterology 1982; 83: 550–62.

53. Ambrose NS, Allan RN, Keighley MR et al. Antibiotic therapy for treatment in relapse of intestinal Crohn's disease. A prospective randomized study. Dis Colon Rectum 1985; 28: 81–5.

54. Sutherland L, Singleton J, Sessions J *et al.* Double blind, placebo controlled trial of metronidazole in Crohn's disease. Gut 1991; 32: 1071–5.

55. Prantera C, Zannoni F, Scribano ML *et al.* An antibiotic regimen for the treatment of active Crohn's disease: a randomized,controlled clinical trial of metronidazole plus ciprofloxacin. Am J Gastroenterol 1996; 91: 328–32.

56. Rutgeerts P, Hiele M, Geboes K *et al.* Controlled trial of metronidazole treatment for prevention of Crohn's recurrence after ileal resection. Gastroenterology 1995; 108: 1617–21.

57. Rutgeerts P, D'Haens G, Baert F *et al.* Nitroimidazol antibiotics are efficacious for prophylaxis of postoperative recurrence of Crohn's disease: a placebo controlled trial. Gastroenterology 1999; 116: G3506.

58. Bernstein LH, Frank SM, Brandt LJ, Boley SJ. Healing of perineal Crohn's disease with metronidazole. Gastroenterology 1980; 79: 357–65.

59. Brandt LJ, Bernstein LH, Boley SJ, Frank MS. Metronidazole therapy for the perineal Crohn's disease: a follow-up study. Gastroenterology 1982; 83: 33–7.

60. Jakobovits J, Schuster MM. Metronidazole therapy for Crohn's disease and associated fistulae. Am J Gastroenterol 1984; 79: 533–40.

61. McKee RF, Keenan RA. Perianal Crohn's disease: is it all bad news? Dis Colon Rectum 1996; 39: 136–42.

62. Sandborn W, McLeod R, Jewell D. Pharmacotherapy for inducing and maintaining remission in pouchitis. Cochrane Database Syst Rev 2000; 2: CD001176.

63. Madden MV, McIntyre AS, Nicholls RJ. Double-blind crossover trial of metronidazole versus placebo in chronic unremitting pouchitis. Dig Dis Sci 1994; 39: 1193–6.

64. Hurst RD, Molinari M, Chung TP, Rubin M, Michelassi F. Prospective study of the incidence, timing and treatment of pouchitis in 104 consecutive patients after restorative proctocolectomy. Arch Surg 1996; 131: 497–500.

65. Simchuk EJ, Thirlby RC. Risk factors and true incidence of pouchitis in patients after ileal pouch–anal anastomoses. World J Surg 2000; 24: 851–6.

66. Nygaard K, Bergan T, Bjorneklett A, Hoverstad T, Lassen J, Aase S. Topical metronidazole treatment in pouchitis. Scand J Gastroenterol 1994; 29: 462–7.

67. Duffy LF, Daum F, Fisher SE *et al.* Peripheral neuropathy in Crohn's disease patients treated with metronidazole. Gastroenterology 1985; 88: 681–4.

68. Burtin P, Taddio A, Ariburnu O, Einarson TR, Koren G. Safety of metronidazole in pregnancy: a metaanalysis. Am J Obstet Gynecol 1995; 172: 525–9.

69. Krause JR, Ayuyang HQ, Ellis LD. Occurrence of three cases of carcinoma in individuals with Crohn's disease treated with metronidazole. Am J Gastroenterol 1985; 80: 978–82.

70. Falagas ME, Walker AM, Jick H, Ruthazer R, Griffith J, Snydman DR. Late incidence of cancer after metronidazole use: a matched metronidazole user/nonuser study. Clin Infect Dis 1998; 26: 384–8.

71. Caro-Paton T, Carvajal A, Martin de Diego I, Martin-Arias LH, Alvarez Requejo A, Rodriguez Pinilla E. Is metronidazole teratogenic? A meta-analysis. Br J Clin Pharmacol 1997; 44: 179–82.

72. Yoshimura T, Kurita C, Usami E *et al.* Immunomodulatory action of levofloxacin on cytokine production by human peripheral blood mononuclear cells. Chemotherapy 1996; 42: 459–64.

73. Turunen U, Färkkilä M, Seppäl PA. Long-term treatment of perianal or fistulous Crohn's disease with ciprofloxacin. Scand J Gastroenterol 1989; 24(Suppl. 158): 144.

74. Colombel JF, Lemann M, Cassagnou M *et al.* A controlled trial comparing ciprofloxacin with mesalazine for the treatment of active Crohn's disease. Groupe d'Etudes Therapeutiques des Affections Inflammatoires Digestives (GETAID). Am J Gastroenterol 1999; 94: 674–8.

75. Solomon MJ, McLeod RS, O'Connor BI, Steinhart AH, Greenberg GR, Cohen Z. Combination ciprofloxacin and metronidazole in severe perianal Crohn's disease. Can J Gastroenterol 1993; 7: 571–2.

76. Greenbloom SL, Steinhart AH, Greenberg GR. Combination ciprofloxacin and metronidazole for active Crohn's disease. Can J Gastroenterol 1998; 12: 53–6.

77. Prantera C, Berto E, Scribano ML, Falasco G. Use of antibiotics in the treatment of active Crohn's disease: experience with metronidazole and ciprofloxacin. Ital J Gastroenterol Hepatol 1998; 30: 602–6.

78. Turunen UM, Farkkila MA, Hakala K *et al.* Long-term treatment of ulcerative colitis with ciprofloxacin: a prospective, double-blind, placebo-controlled study. Gastroenterology 1998; 115: 1072–8.

79. Present DH. Ciprofloxacin as a treatment for ulcerative colitis – not yet. Gastroenterology 1998; 115: 1289–91.

80. Gionchetti P, Rizzello F, Venturi A *et al.* Antibiotic combination therapy in patients with chronic, treatment-resistant pouchitis. Aliment Pharmacol Ther 1999; 13: 713-1-8.

81. Segev S, Yaniv I, Haverstock D, Reinhart H. Safety of long-term therapy with ciprofloxacin: data analysis of controlled clinical trials and review. Clin Infect Dis 1999; 28: 299–308.

82. Bomford JAL, Ledger JC, O'Keefe BJ, Reiter Ch. Ciprofloxacin use during pregnancy. Drugs 1993; 45(Suppl. 3): 461–2.

83. Picciotto A, Gesu GP, Schito GC, Testa R, Varagona G, Celle G. Antimycobacterial chemotherapy in inflammatory bowel disease. Biomed Pharmacother 1989; 43: 141–3.

84. Warren JB, Rees HC, Cox TM. Remission of Crohn's disease with tuberculosis chemotherapy. N Engl J Med 1986; 314: 182.

85. Schultz MG, Rieder HL, Hersh T, Riepe S. Remission of Crohn's disease with antimycobacterial chemotherapy. Lancet 1987; 2: 1391–2.

86. Elliott PR, Burnham WR, Berghouse LM, Lennard-Jones JE, Langman MJ. Sulphadoxine–pyrimethamine therapy in Crohn's disease. Digestion 1982; 23: 132–4.

87. Shaffer JL, Hughes S, Linaker BD, Baker RD, Turnberg LA. Controlled trial of rifampicin and ethambutol in Crohn's disease. Gut 1984; 25: 203–5.

88. Afdhal NH, Long A, Lennon J, Crowe J, O'Donoghue DP. Controlled trial of antimycobacterial therapy in Crohn's disease. Clofazimine versus placebo. Dig Dis Sci 1991; 36: 449–53.

89. Swift GL, Srivastava ED, Stone R *et al.* Controlled trial of anti-tuberculous chemotherapy for two years in Crohn's disease. Gut 1994; 35: 363–8.

90. Thomas GA, Swift GL, Green JT *et al.* Controlled trial of antituberculous chemotherapy in Crohn's disease: a five year follow up study. Gut 1998; 42: 497–500.

91. Prantera C, Kohn A, Mangiarotti R, Andreoli A, Luzi C. Antimycobacterial therapy in Crohn's disease: results of a controlled, double-blind trial with a multiple antibiotic regimen. Am J Gastroenterol 1994; 89: 513–18.

92. Borgaonkar MR, MacIntosh DG, Fardy JM. A meta-analysis of antimycobacterial therapy for Crohn's disease. Am J Gastroenterol 2000; 95: 725–9.

93. Hulten K, Almashhrawi A, El-Zaatari FA, Graham DY. Antibacterial therapy for Crohn's disease: a review emphasizing therapy directed against mycobacteria. Dig Dis Sci 2000; 45: 445–56.

94. Basilisco G, Ranzi T, Campanini C *et al.* Controlled trial of rifabutin in Crohn's disease. Curr Ther Res 1989; 46: 242–50.

95. Gui GP, Thomas PR, Tizard ML, Lake J, Sanderson JD, Hermon-Taylor J. Two-year-outcomes analysis of Crohn's disease treated with rifabutin and macrolide antibiotics. J Antimicrob Chemother 1997; 39: 393–400.

96. Graham DY, Al-Assi MT, Robinson M. Prolonged remission in Crohn's disease following therapy for *Mycobacterium paratuberculosis* infection. Gastroenterology 1995; 108: A826.

97. Goodgame RW, Kimball K, Akram S, Graham DY, Ou Ching-Nan. Randomized controlled trial of clarithromycin and ethambutol in the treatment of Crohn's disease. Gastroenterology 1999; 116: G3150.

98. Moss AA, Carbone JV, Kressel HY. Radiologic and clinical assessment of broad-spectrum antibiotic therapy in Crohn's disease. Am J Roentgenol 1978; 131: 787–90.

99. Savidge RS. Trimethoprim and sulphamethoxazole in ulcerative colitis. Postgrad Med J 1969; 45(Suppl.): 101–4.

100. Saverymuttu S, Hodgson HJ, Chadwick VS. Controlled trial comparing prednisolone with an elemental diet plus nonabsorbable antibiotics in active Crohn's disease. Gut 1985; 26: 994–8.

101. Burke DA, Axon ATR, Clayden SA, Dixon MF, Johnston D, Lacey RW. The efficacy of tobramycin in the treatment of ulcerative colitis. Aliment Pharmacol Ther 1990; 4: 123–9.

102. Dickinson RJ, O'Connor HJ, Pinder I, Hamilton I, Johnston D, Axon ATR. Double blind controlled trial of oral vancomycin as adjunctive treatment in acute exacerbations of idiopathic colitis. Gut 1985; 26: 1380–4.

103. Meyers S, Mayer L, Bottone E, Desmond E, Janowitz HD. Occurrence of *Clostridium difficile* toxin during the course of inflammatory bowel disease. Gastroenterology 1981; 80: 697–700.

104. Bartlett JG, Laughon BE, Bayless TM. Role of microbial agents in relapses of idiopathic inflammatory bowel disease. In: Bayless TM, ed. Current Management of Inflammatory Bowel Disease. Toronto: BC Decker, 1987: 86–93.

105. Ward M, McManus JPA. Dapsone in Crohn's disease. Lancet 1975; 1: 1236: 7.

106. Prantera C, Argentieri R, Mangiarotti R, Levenstein S. Dapsone and remission of Crohn's disease. Lancet 1988; 1: 536.

107. Prantera C, Bothamley G, Levenstein S, Mangiarotti R, Argentieri R. Crohn's disease and mycobacteria: two cases of Crohn's disease with high anti-mycobacterial antibody levels cured by dapsone therapy. Biomed Pharmacother 1989; 43: 295–9.

108. Gionchetti P, Rizzello F, Ferrieri A *et al.* Rifaximin in patients with moderate or severe ulcerative colitis refractory to steroid-treatment: a double-blind, placebo-controlled trial. Dig Dis Sci 1999; 44: 1220–1.

109. Casellas F, Borruel N, Papo M *et al.* Antiinflammatory effects of enterically coated amoxicillin–clavulanic acid in active ulcerative colitis. Inflam Bowel Dis 1998; 4: 1–5.

110. Marteau P, Pochart P, Bouhnik Y, Rambaud JC. Fate and effects of some transiting microorganisms in the human gastrointestinal tract. World Rev Nutr Diet 1993; 74: 1–21.

111. Donohue DC, Salminen S, Marteau P. Safety of probiotic bacteria. In: Salminen S, von Wright A, eds, Lactic Acid Bacteria – Microbiology and Functional Aspects, 2nd edn. New York: Marcel Dekker, 1998, 369–84.

112. Rautio M, Jousimies-Somer H, Kauma H *et al.* Liver abscess due to a *Lactobacillus rhamnosus* strain indistinguishable from *L. rhamnosus* strain GG. Clin Infect Dis 1999; 28: 1159–60.

113. Hennequin C, Kauffmann-Lacroix C, Jobert A *et al.* Possible role of catheters in *Saccharomyces boulardii* fungemia. Eur J Clin Microbiol Infect Dis 2000; 19: 16–20.

114. Marteau P, Vesa T. Pharmacokinetics of probiotics and biotherapeutic agents in humans. Biosci Microflora 1998; 17: 1–6.

115. Vesa T, Pochart P, Marteau P. Pharmacokinetics of *Lactobacillus plantarum* NCIMB 8826, *Lactobacillus fermentum* KLD, and *Lactococcus lactis* MG 1363 in the human gastrointestinal tract. Aliment Pharmacol Ther 2000; 14: 823–8.

116. Fabia R, Ar'Rajab A, Johansson ML, Willen R, Andersson R. The effect of exogenous administration of *Lactobacillus reuteri* R2LC and oat fiber on acetic acid-induced colitis in the rat. Scand J Gastroenterol 1993; 28: 155–62.

117. Mao Y, Nobaeck S, Kasravi B *et al.* The effects of *Lactobacillus* strains and oat fiber on methotrexate-induced enterocolitis in rats. Gastroenterology 1996; 111: 334–44.

118. Collins JK, Murphy L, O'Mahony L, Dunne C, O'Sullivan GC, Shanahan F. A controlled trial of probiotic treatment of IL-10 knockout mice. Gastroenterology 1999; 116: G2981.

119. McCann ML, Abrams RS, Nelson RP Jr. Recolonization therapy with nonadhesive *Escherichia coli* for treatment of inflammatory bowel disease. Ann NY Acad Sci 1994; 730: 243–5.

120. Kruis W, Schütz E, Fric P, Fixa B, Judmaier G, Stolte M. Double-blind comparison of an oral *Escherichia coli* preparation and mesalazine in maintaining remission of ulcerative colitis. Aliment Pharmacol Ther 1997; 11: 853–8.

121. Rembacken BJ, Snelling AM, Hawkey PM, Chalmers DM, Axon AT. Non-pathogenic *Escherichia coli* versus mesalazine for the treatment of ulcerative colitis: a randomised trial. Lancet 1999; 354: 635–9.

122. Ishikawa H, Imaoka A, Umesaki Y, Tanaka R, Ohtani T. Randomized controlled trial of the effect of *Bifidobacterium*-fermented milk on ulcerative colitis. Gastroenterology 2000; 118: A4171.

123. Ruseler van Embden JGH, Schouten WR, van Lieshout LMC. Pouchitis: result of microbial imbalance? Gut 1994; 35: 658–64.

124. Gionchetti P, Orsla O, Rizzello F *et al. In vivo* effect of a highly concentrated probiotic on IL-10 pelvic ileal–pouch tissue levels. Gastroenterology 1999; 116: A723

125. Friedman G, George J. Treatment of refractory 'pouchitis' with prebiotic and probiotic therapy. Gastroenterology 2000; 118: G4167.

126. Elmer GW, Surawicz CM, McFarland LV. Biotherapeutic agents. A neglected modality for the treatment and prevention of selected intestinal and vaginal infections. J Am Med Assoc 1996; 275: 870–6.

127. Plein K, Hotz J. Therapeutic effects of *Saccharomyces boulardii* on mild residual symptoms in a stable phase of Crohn's disease with special respect to chronic diarrhea – a pilot study. Z Gastroenterol 1993; 31: 129–34.

128. Guslandi M, Mezzi G, Sorghi M, Testoni PA. *Saccharomyces boulardii* in maintenance treatment of Crohn's disease. Dig Dis Sci 2000; 45: 1462–4.

129. Malin M, Suomalainen H, Saxelin M, Isolauri E. Promotion of IgA immune response in patients with Crohn's disease by oral bacteriotherapy with *Lactobacillus* GG. Ann Nutr Metab 1996; 40: 137–45.

130. Campieri M, Rizzello F, Venturi A *et al.* Combination of antibiotic and probiotic treatment is efficacious in prophylaxis of post-operative recurrence of Crohn's disease: a randomized controlled study vs mesalamine. Gastroenterology 2000; 118: G4179.

131. Malchow HA. Crohn's disease and *Escherichia coli* . A new approach in therapy to maintain remission of colonic Crohn's disease? J Clin Gastroenterol 1997; 25: 653–8.

29 | Nutrition in inflammatory bowel disease

GREGG W. VAN CITTERS AND HENRY C. LIN

Nutrition in the pathogenesis of inflammatory bowel disease (IBD)

The properly nourished body is central to establishing and maintaining a state of 'wellness'. Nutrients are required in varying amounts to fuel the complex interplay of physiological responses responsible for growth, development, maintenance, immunity, and repair. When quantity or quality of food is lacking, or when ingested food is not properly processed, the consequences may include malnutrition, stunted growth, impaired immune response, or gastrointestinal symptoms. With the intestinal mucosa serving as the first point of contact with ingested food, the intestinal response to a meal includes an immune reaction to food antigens. The outcome of such an immune response may determine whether a heightened state of immune response is present for a short or long duration of time.

Nutrients as pathogenetic factors

Since the primary function of the intestines is to digest and absorb food and food itself is a source of foreign antigens, it is intuitive to first consider dietary agents as potential causative factors for disturbances in the immune response of the digestive system. A large number of studies have sought correlation between diet and onset or activity of IBD [1–10]. Because animal models for these diseases generally express an IBD-like mucosal abnormality within a short period of time, interventional studies involving chronic exposure to potentially antigenic foods have not been possible. Although there is strong evidence to support a role for genetic predisposition in the etiology of IBD, genetic markers for subgroups of patients with IBD have only recently been identified [11–25], making controlled, prospective, longitudinal studies of the effect of diet in genetically at-risk patient population thus far only a dream. Thus, studies performed to date have been cross-sectional and have the inherent weakness that the recall necessary to describe the diet is accomplished years after the onset of symptoms, while the disease may have been silently developing for years prior to symptom manifestation.

Most of the evidence for a relationship between diet and ulcerative colitis (UC) is with the use of a 'Western' diet, particularly ω-6 fats [1, 2, 4, 6, 8, 9], and the strongest relationship between diet and Crohn's disease (CD) is with the use of refined carbohydrates, particularly sucrose [4, 5, 10]. Improvement of inflammation and inflammatory mediators with ω-3 oils in some [3, 9, 26–29] but not all [30] studies suggests a potential relationship between altered fatty acid balance in the diet and disease activity, although it is premature to project these findings to the pathogenesis of disease. It is difficult to conclude causation from diet in these studies since physicians and patients often treat gastrointestinal distress by dietary restriction. These restrictions often dictate a shift to more refined, easily digested and absorbed foods such as simple starches and sugars. Thus, it is always difficult to discern whether the increased consumption of refined carbohydrates among Crohn's patients preceded or followed the onset of disease.

Food allergies and intolerances

Because IBD are autoimmune disorders, it is also attractive to consider the possibility that the disease or symptoms may be precipitated by food allergies or intolerances. Again, little evidence is available to support this conclusion. True food allergies as a cause of food intolerance are relatively rare [31, 32] and studies have failed to show significant associations between food allergens and IBD much beyond what would be expected in normal populations [32, 33]. Food intolerances may be more difficult to assess. Blinding subjects to food is challenging, elimination diet and food challenge tests are difficult

Stephan R. Targan, Fergus Shanahan and Loren C. Karp (eds.), Inflammatory Bowel Disease: From Bench to Bedside, 2nd Edition, 587–604.
© 2003 *Kluwer Academic Publishers. Printed in Great Britain*

and dietary adherence even more so [34, 35]. In addition, self-reporting without objective follow-up testing invariably leads to an unnecessarily long list of suspected offending foods [36].

Malnutrition in IBD

Malnutrition is prevalent in the setting of both active [37–39] and quiescent [40] IBD. Protein–energy malnutrition, trace nutrient deficiencies, and dehydration are common in active disease. Deficiencies of micronutrients such as essential fatty acids [41] and vitamins and trace minerals [40], are likely to linger following an acute episode or develop over a period of time in quiescent disease because of maldigestion or malabsorption.

Epidemiology of malnutrition in IBD

Childhood and adolescence

Information on the incidence and prevalence of IBD among the young is scarce. One study describes six apparent cases of IBD in infants at a single hospital between 1990 and 1993 [42]. Although it is difficult to quantify the number of cases of IBD among this population, it is generally accepted that nutritional deficiencies are common, if not universal, at least among children with CD [43]. The most obvious consequence of malnutrition in this population is growth retardation. Many studies have been conducted examining the efficacy of enteral nutrition versus conventional medical therapy such as steroids [44–46], or the use of enteral supplementation as adjunctive therapy [47–50]. In general, enteral supplementation of an oral diet increases calories and deposition of lean tissue, and may increase linear growth velocity [50]. Elemental diets do not appear to have any advantage over polymeric (peptide) diets [48], and both appear to be superior to parenteral nutrition in terms of bowel health [51, 52].

Short bowel syndrome

Nutritional deficiency is *sine qua non* of short bowel syndrome. The severity of deficiency is related to the extent of small bowel resection, and patients with < 100 cm remaining without colon in continuity typically require parenteral nutrition to sustain life [53–55]. Fluid and electrolyte balance is critical in this population, particularly in the setting of jejunostomy where there is no colonic salvage of nutrients, fluid, and electrolytes, and may require intravenous supplementation to oral intake [54, 55]. General protein–calorie malnutrition and micronutrient deficiencies may also be present [56–60].

Eating disorders

Disordered eating patterns may be present in the setting of IBD [61], most commonly to avoid symptoms but a concurrent true eating disorder should also be considered. While it is possible that disordered eating may mask underlying IBD [62], IBD patients who present with persistent weight loss in the absence of grossly active disease, and who fit the profile to be at risk of an eating disorder, should be carefully screened for the possibility of an overlapping disease. Developing adolescents may be at particularly high risk for concurrent IBD and an eating disorder [63].

Causes of malnutrition

Numerous factors can contribute to malnutrition in the patient with IBD. Symptoms of IBD may reduce appetite and prevent adequate food intake. Chronic diarrhea may be the most persistent and debilitating symptom of IBD, affecting more than 90% of IBD patients [64]. Inadequate intake may be quite common (up to half of patients with CD) [65]. Alterations of energy metabolism have been observed in CD [66]. Stress of chronic or acute inflammation is associated with a variety of pathophysiological changes that reduce food intake and alter nutrient metabolism. Concurrent mucosal dysfunction, such as protein-losing enteropathy or relative disaccharidase deficiency, may contribute to diarrhea and loss of nutrients, electrolytes, and fluids. Medications may induce nausea, vomiting, or anorexia. Small intestinal bacterial overgrowth may prevent digestion and absorption of nutrients in addition to generating considerable flatus and osmotically active metabolites that contribute to discomfort and diarrhea. Fistulas and bypass tracts interfere with normal absorption and motility, and may harbor bacteria. Finally, motility dysfunction in the form of rapid gastrointestinal transit may cause severe maldigestion and malabsorption by limiting contact time of the luminal contents with the mucosal surface. Rapid transit may result from intrinsic motility defects, secondary impairment from chronic inflammation or intestinal surgery.

Resting energy expenditure (REE)

Abnormal REE is not typically an important factor since patients with active CD do not have higher REE compared to predicted energy expenditure [67] or compared to healthy controls [68]. Similarly, total energy expenditure in CD patients is not different from expected values, and any potential alterations in REE are compensated for by changes in activity [69].

IBD symptoms that affect nutrition

Gastrointestinal symptoms associated with IBD that may limit food intake include pain, nausea, vomiting, abdominal distension, gas, and diarrhea. The menstrual cycle may exacerbate gastrointestinal symptoms [70] leading to monthly periods of reduced food intake. Accelerated intestinal transit [71, 72] or inflammation [73] may exaggerate nutrient-triggered release of gut peptides that can slow gastric emptying and trigger excessive satiety [74–78].

Iatrogenic food aversion and food–drug interactions

Nutrient–medication interactions are more challenging to overcome since the use of drugs may not be elective. Commonly encountered interactions include the inhibition of folate absorption by sulfasalazine [79]; the inhibition of calcium absorption and the promotion of urinary calcium excretion by steroids [80]; and the loss of essential fatty acids [81], fat-soluble vitamins [82], and minerals [83] with the use of bile acid-binding resins that are commonly prescribed in short bowel patients. In addition, nausea, vomiting, or anorexia may be common side-effects of some IBD drugs [84, 85]. Until medications can be tapered or replaced with alternatives, nutrient supplements can be given to make up for losses (see ref. 86) and anti-emetic or orexigenic agents can be offered to ameliorate drug-induced appetite suppression.

Inflammatory stress

Cytokines such as interleukin-1 (IL-1), IL-6, and tumor necrosis factor (TNF) are produced in response to inflammation and serve as triggers for the synthesis of acute-phase proteins. Malnutrition *per se* increases expression of IL-6 [87, 88], α_2-macroglobulin [87] and IL-1β [88]. A vicious cycle of wasting may therefore occur in IBD, with cytokine-induced malnutrition and malnutrition-induced increases in cytokine expression working in concert against nutritional repletion. Metabolic responses to cytokines and acute-phase proteins include catabolism of muscle protein and amino acids, sequestration of iron and zinc, elevated gluconeogenesis and acute-phase protein synthesis secondary to increased amino acid flux into the liver, impaired fatty acid uptake by adipose tissue, net loss of nitrogen and electrolytes combined with fluid and sodium retention, loss of vitamins by increased degradation or inactivation, and general activation of the immune system (reviewed in ref. 89).

Mucosal dysfunction

Mucosal diseases such as protein-losing enteropathy [90–92] and relative disaccharidase deficiency [93] may coexist with inflamed bowel. Depending on disease activity, physicians and dietitians may advise patients to refrain from foods that exacerbate symptoms. Many physicians dogmatically place patients on dairy restriction, but genetic deficiency of brush-border lactase may be the only reason to limit intake of milk [94–96]. Recent evidence indicates that cytokines regulate expression of brush-border disaccharidases other than lactase [97], which may explain intolerance to carbohydrates other than lactose in active IBD.

Small intestinal bacterial overgrowth

Bacteria are essential to optimal intestinal function. While the colon may contain up to 10^{11} colony-forming units (CFU), the small intestine is relatively devoid of bacterial flora. When the normal gut flora moves proximally to colonize the small intestine and is allowed to proliferate unchecked, diarrhea and excessive flatus may result when bacteria gain access to the still-unassimilated food. Bacterial overgrowth of the proximal small intestine may directly impair absorption of nutrients [98], generate metabolites such as short-chain fatty acids that contribute to the luminal osmotic load [99], and produce large volumes of metabolic gases (e.g. hydrogen, methane, carbon dioxide) by fermentation of unabsorbed nutrient substrates. Colonization of the small bowel is facilitated by disease or surgical removal of ileocecal valve [100–102] that normally provide a natural sphincter preventing excessive bacterial movement into the small intestine. Small intestinal dysmotility associated with aging may contribute to bacterial overgrowth in the elderly patient [103]. Chronic intestinal inflammation may impair the natural defenses against bacterial build-up in the small intestine including loss of 'intestinal housekeeper waves' and epithelial secretory antibodies. Alcohol abuse has also been associated with gastric overgrowth of bacteria [104].

Small intestinal bacterial overgrowth may contribute to increased intestinal permeability [105–109]. Increased permeability could contribute to the exaggerated immune response characteristic of CD by permitting bacterial translocation across the normally tight epithelial barrier. Additionally, increased epithelial permeability may contribute to malabsorption by permitting entry of macromolecules normally digested to constituent substrates at the epithelium.

Diversion of the luminal content

Intestinal diversions such as intestino-intestinal fistulas reroute the luminal contents and may diminish digestive and absorptive capacity. In addition, an intestino-cutaneous fistula may result in loss of large amounts of fluid, electrolytes and nutrients. Medical and nutritional therapy leading to closure of fistulas improves nutritional status [110]. Fistulas may cause malnutrition severe enough to be fatal to the patient [111, 112].

Surgical perturbations

Surgical perturbations interfere with fat absorption, speed transit, and facilitate bacterial overgrowth into the small intestine. Patients with surgically altered intestinal anatomy often complain of persistent diarrhea [113]. Ileal resection may lead to loss of intestinal uptake of bile acids, contributing to solute- and bile acid-stimulated diarrhea [114–117] and change motility and transit [118]. Resection of less than 100 cm of ileum causes watery diarrhea [119] resulting from the entry of incompletely absorbed bile salts into the colon to stimulate secretory diarrhea. Disease or resection may interrupt bile acid recirculation to account for the chronic diarrhea in some IBD patients [120]. Failure of bile salt replacement [121] or bile acid sequestrant therapy in patients with disease or resection of the distal small intestine requires an alternative explanation for their diarrhea.

Resection of more than 100 cm of ileum leads to a loss of bile acids in excess of the rate of hepatic synthesis [122]. With such severe depletion of the bile acid pool, the micellar phase in fat digestion and absorption is impaired [122] and digestion of fat in the small intestine becomes incomplete, to result in steatorrhea [119, 123]. When the fatty stool reaches the colon the resident bacteria break down the fats

into long-chain fatty acids that stimulate secretion in the colonic mucosa, contributing to a fatty acid-induced secretory diarrhea [64, 122, 124].

Rapid transit

Chronic diarrhea is associated with malnutrition [125]. Digestion and absorption of a meal depends on adequate residence time in the small intestine [125], which permits optimal nutrient availability and uptake. Accelerated intestinal transit diminishes time available for digestion of nutrient macromolecules and absorption of the end-products of nutrient digestion by the small intestine, resulting in greater stool volume and diarrhea [126]. Improper digestion and absorption of luminal contents displace nutrient substrates to the colon for metabolism by colonic bacteria. The resulting production of osmotically active substances may draw water into the lumen [127]. Each of these factors may contribute to abnormal speeding of transit of the luminal contents to further exacerbate the diarrhea by diminishing the time available for absorption of water and electrolytes. Standard anti-diarrheal treatments, including opiates and α_2-adrenergic agonists, may slow intestinal transit to increase contact time between the luminal contents and the absorptive mucosal surface [124, 128].

Intestinal transit of a meal is normally regulated by the system of nutrient-triggered inhibitory feedback or 'brakes' distributed along the small bowel (Fig. 1A). Proximal and/or distal gut braking systems may be impaired by inflammation or tissue destruction during active disease, or may be missing entirely in IBD patients with small bowel resection. Resection of 50–70% of the proximal small intestine preserves weight with slightly lowered capacity to absorb fat and protein [129], but removal of the distal small intestine causes severe steatorrhea [129, 130]. Ileocecal bypass markedly accelerates transit compared to distal resection with intact ileocecal junction [101], leading to significant steatorrhea.

Read *et al.* [131] and Spiller *et al.* [132, 133] described slowing of gastric emptying and intestinal transit in response to direct infusion of fat emulsion into the distal jejunum as the 'ileal brake'. Fat is the most potent trigger of the ileal brake [134]. The braking response depends specifically on the availability of fatty acids as the end-product of fat digestion [131, 132] and is proportional to the length of intestine (i.e. the number of nutrient receptors) exposed to a given load of fat [135]. Thus, the inhibitory feedback response triggered by fat (the

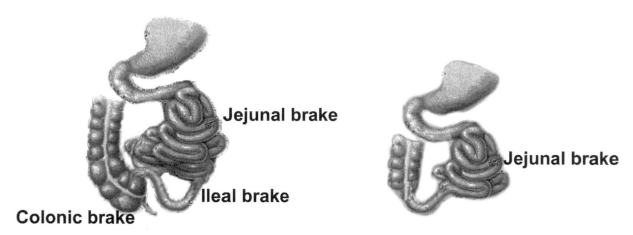

Figure 1. A: Normal transit control. Ileal brake is the most potent controller of gastrointestinal transit, with complementary assistance from companion braking systems. **B:** Abnormal transit control after colectomy with ileal resection. Loss of ileal and colonic brakes leads to uncontrolled transit. Jejunal brake may not be able to compensate if end products of digestion are unavailable (transit may be too fast to permit adequate digestion). The result is diarrhea worsened by steatorrhea. These effects explain malnutrition even when the length of the small intestine is still adequate. The effect would be worse if the patient had extensive intestinal resections.

ileal brake) allows adequate time for digestion of nutrients in the proximal gut. In the setting of ileal disease [136] or resection, accelerated transit through the proximal gut [134] speeds up, leaving little time for adequate digestion of fat or other nutrient macromolecules.

Although distal small intestine inhibitory feedback has been considered the sole nutrient-triggered control mechanism governing intestinal transit, companion braking systems have been recently described in the proximal small intestine (jejunal brake) [137] and the colon (colonic brake) [138] (Fig. 1B). The ileal brake inhibits transit more potently than the jejunal brake [139] to explain the greater steatorrhea seen in the loss of the distal rather than proximal one-half of the small intestine [129]. The colonic brake, most potently triggered by protein, slows distal small intestine motility by peptide YY release [140]. Thus, interaction between the ileal and the jejunal and colonic brakes is required for normal control of gastrointestinal transit. Impairment or loss of the ileal brake may be ameliorated as long as there is healthy jejunum and colon present in continuity. Greater frequency and weight of stools in patients with ileoanal pouches [141] or ileoanal anastomoses [142, 143] may be secondary to loss of the colonic brake.

In the absence of the ileum and colon, transit control is entirely dependent on the jejunal brake.

Since residence time of the luminal contents in this setting may be inadequate for complete digestion of fat, the jejunal brake may be silent because of a lack of availability of the necessary trigger. The consequence of such total brake failure is maldigestion and malabsorption of the luminal contents secondary to uncontrolled speed of transit. Thus, rapid transit is an under-appreciated but critically important explanation for chronic diarrhea and malnutrition in IBD.

Importance of nutritional management in IBD

Except in severe cases of malnutrition where protein–energy malnutrition is strikingly evident, many nutritional deficiencies may be latent in IBD. Disturbances in energy, lipid, cholesterol, and bone metabolism may all be present but screening for them is not typically done. Protein–energy malnutrition and disturbances in energy metabolism may prolong or exacerbate a disease flare by failing to provide substrates for tissue repair. Intestinal barrier function is compromised in the malnourished patient, increasing the magnitude of the acute-phase response [144]. Essential fatty acid deficiency, typically obvious only in the form of a dermatitis, may alter membrane fluidity, affecting numerous cellular transport and signaling processes, and altering synthesis of lipid signaling molecules such as prostaglandins and leukotrienes. Interrupted also, in time, be a complication of malnutrition since both digestive and absorptive capacity are reduced by protein–calorie malnutrition. Such a complication would result in a vicious cycle of impairment whereby the patient's symptoms and physical signs of malnutrition would progressively worsen. In addition, diarrhea may reflect deficiency or electrolyte imbalance that require specific intervention. A number of excellent reviews are available on the physical findings associated with nutritional deficiencies [168–172].

Laboratory studies

Laboratory studies should be used to confirm suspicions of nutritional deficiencies and to identify subclinical deficiencies. Protein–energy malnutrition should be assessed with anthropometric measurements and serum albumin and prealbumin. Fat malabsorption can be quantified with 24-hour stool collection for fecal fat. Non-specific indicators of fat malabsorption include low serum concentrations of fat-soluble vitamins and β-carotene and low serum concentrations of essential fatty acids. Mean corpuscular hemoglobin and volume may be associated with low folate and vitamin B_{12} concentrations. In this case, low concentrations of the water-soluble vitamins should also be suspected. Screening should include iron, zinc, magnesium, and copper concentrations [173] in addition to electrolytes.

Calcium homeostasis may be upset, particularly in the setting of fat malabsorption [173] and colonic resection [174]. Altered bone metabolism should be suspected for all IBD patients [175, 176], particularly those with a history of glucocorticoid therapy [177]. At the minimum, for the patient-at-risk, serum calcium, phosphate, alkaline phosphatase measurements, and bone densitometry should be obtained. Signs of metabolic bone disease should lead to a referral to an endocrinologist for aggressive management. The risk for abnormal bone metabolism and nephrolithiasis is elevated in IBD patients with hyperoxaluria and hypercalciuria [178].

Diarrhea should be given a specific diagnosis as well as quantified in volume. Factors contributing to diarrhea in the IBD patient include concurrent mucosal disease, small intestinal bacterial overgrowth, and rapid gastrointestinal transit. Protein-losing enteropathy can be evaluated by direct measurement of protein content in whole-gut lavage [90] or more practically, by elevated α_1-antitrypsin clearance [92]. Disaccharidase deficiencies can be detected with carbohydrate challenge testing, measuring breath excretion of gaseous byproducts of carbohydrate fermentation [94, 95].

The lactulose breath hydrogen test [179–181] can be used to distinguish between small intestinal bacterial overgrowth and rapid gastrointestinal transit by carefully examining the timing and magnitude of the rise in breath hydrogen in response to oral lactulose and by comparing breath hydrogen profiles before and after antibiotic treatment. In an unoperated patient, rapid transit will show a premature rise of modest magnitude with a hydrogen profile demonstrating usually only a single peak, whereas small intestinal bacterial overgrowth typically manifests as a premature rise of great magnitude with a hydrogen profile demonstrating double peaks (small and large intestine). The picture is complicated in the IBD patient with ileocolonic resection, as rapid transit may coexist with bacterial overgrowth. In this setting it is advisable to treat the patient with a short course of poorly absorbed antibiotic [182] and re-evaluate after a time period suitable for recolonization by normal flora. If bacterial overgrowth was the primary cause of diarrhea there should be resolution of symptoms and a normalized breath hydrogen test. If rapid transit were to be an important contributor to diarrhea, then rapid transit will still show in the breath hydrogen test as an early and moderate rise in breath hydrogen. Although a potential drawback of the lactulose breath hydrogen test for quantifying rapid transit is that oral lactulose may contribute to a shorter absolute value for the transit time [181] by increasing the osmotic load, this effect does not usually limit the usefulness of the test. Within each diagnostic unit it is the relative rather than the absolute value of the transit time that distinguishes a normal from an abnormal result. Glucose may be used instead of lactulose for the breath hydrogen test [183, 184]. However, since even a large load of glucose can be normally absorbed by the proximal small intestine, complete absorption of the test substance may reduce the sensitivity of the glucose breath hydrogen test for diagnosing small intestinal bacterial overgrowth involving only the distal one-half of the small bowel.

Treating malnutrition in IBD

Regardless of the nutritional approach, treatment should include a psychosocial component. The therapeutic strategy should be developed in cooperation with the patient. Patients should be educated about their disease and encouraged to build their support systems, including family involvement and self-help groups [157]. A psychiatric referral should be considered if there is suspicion of confounding eating disorder.

Nutritional management in IBD

Nutrition has at least two applications in the clinical management of IBD. As a primary therapy, nutrition can be used to induce remission as well as to sustain the patient. As an adjunct therapy, nutrition can correct deficiencies and modulate the immune response to maintain long-term remission.

Nutrition as primary therapy

Bowel rest has often been suggested as a therapeutic approach to calming the inflammatory response during a flare of CD, particularly when clinical manifestations include complications such as obstructive or fistulating disease. Specifically, the role of bowel rest in inducing or maintaining a remission has been pursued but remains controversial [50, 147, 185–187]. Greenberg et al. [185] randomized 51 CD patients in acute flare who were unresponsive to medical management to receive total parenteral nutrition (TPN) only, enteral nutrition (EN) only, or a mixture of oral and parenteral nutrition. They found no difference between groups in remission induction or maintenance of remission at 1 year. Similarly, Wright and Adler [147] found no effect of nutrient delivery route on the short-term outcome of CD patients hospitalized for disease exacerbations. Pediatric CD patients showed similar rates of remission and relapse but had improved relapse and linear growth rates when nocturnal EN feedings were continued in conjunction with the resumption of normal oral intake [50]. When TPN plus bowel rest was coupled with aggressive medical management [186], remission was induced and maintained in most CD patients (UC patients overwhelmingly required surgical intervention). Within 1 week following major upper gastrointestinal surgery there was no clinical difference detected in patients receiving TPN plus bowel rest compared with patients receiving only EN [187].

TPN is typically the preferred nutritional support method for CD patients with active disease or complications. TPN may result in a more favorable outcome where bowel obstruction is a prominent

finding [145]. TPN may also improve recovery from bowel resections when used perioperatively [188]. Caution should be used in interpreting clinical signs when TPN is given in the context of a CD flare, as primary acute-phase indicators may be falsely improved with TPN [189]. Additionally, TPN plus bowel rest may contribute to mucosal atrophy [190], allowing bacterial overgrowth [191] and translocation [192] and increased release of macrophage tumor necrosis factor (TNF-α) [193], a putative mediator of the autoimmune response in both UC [23] and CD [16]. Therefore, because TPN therapy is not necessarily associated with less costly outcomes [194], may not avoid surgical interventions, and is associated with significant morbidity and mortality [191, 195, 196], the anticipated benefits of TPN therapy must be carefully weighed against these risks.

Enteral nutrition alone, whether elemental [197], polymeric [196, 198], or whole protein [45], may be as effective as bowel rest plus TPN for inducing or maintaining remission in CD [147, 199, 200]. However, it remains controversial whether EN may be as effective as steroid therapy in inducing [201–206] or maintaining [46, 197, 202, 207, 208] remission. Meta-analyses of studies involving EN and/or steroid therapy [201, 204, 207] found that EN was no better than, and often inferior to, steroid therapy. Peptide-based diets may be as effective as prednisolone in improving CD activity scores after brief periods of treatment [202, 205], although steroid therapy is clearly superior in the long term. Larger and longer studies controlled for disease activity, location, and bowel resection location and extent are needed to better determine whether EN is effective in inducing or maintaining remission of IBD.

Nutrition as adjunct therapy

The above studies suggest that nutritional support, regardless of route of delivery, can be effective primary therapy for IBD for brief periods. Because malnutrition and its detrimental effects are so prevalent in IBD, supplemental nutrition may improve patient outcomes over extended periods. Although nutritional interventions are not conclusively superior to medical management of IBD, they may enhance the capability of drugs such as steroids or immunomodulators to induce or maintain remission [186, 195, 209–211]. TPN is most effective as an adjunct therapy when absorptive capacity is compromised, as with active jejunoileal disease or short

The future of nutrition in IBD

Many, if not most, patients with IBD suffer from some degree of malnutrition. As such, greater awareness of the problem of malnutrition and the application of more effective treatments are both critically important to achieving the clinician's goal of improved overall health of patients with IBD. A common cause of malnutrition in both active and quiescent IBD may be chronic diarrhea, as chronic diarrhea may be associated with accelerated intestinal transit, a mechanism for poor assimilation of both food and oral drugs. Accordingly, the future of the management of malnutrition is to deal with both the issues of what the patient needs as well as how to get it in.

References

1. Anonymous. Dietary and other risk factors of ulcerative colitis. A case–control study in Japan. Epidemiology Group of the Research Committee of Inflammatory Bowel Disease in Japan. J Clin Gastroenterol 1994; 19:166–71.
2. Anonymous. A case–control study of ulcerative colitis in relation to dietary and other factors in Japan. Epidemiology Group of the Research Committee of Inflammatory Bowel Disease in Japan. J Gastroenterol 1995; 30(Suppl. 8):9–12.
3. O'Morain C, Tobin A, Suzuki Y, O'Riordan T. Risk factors in inflammatory bowel disease. Scand J Gastroenterol (Suppl.) 1989; 170: 58–60.
4. Persson PG, Ahlbom A, Hellers G. Diet and inflammatory bowel disease: a case–control study. Epidemiology 1992; 3: 47–52.
5. Probert CS, Bhakta P, Bhamra B, Jayanthi V, Mayberry JF. Diet of South Asians with inflammatory bowel disease. Arq Gastroenterol 1996; 33: 132–5.
6. Reif S, Klein I, Lubin F, Farbstein M, Hallak A, Gilat T. Pre-illness dietary factors in inflammatory bowel disease. Gut 1997; 40: 754–60.
7. Russel MG, Stockbrugger RW. Epidemiology of inflammatory bowel disease: an update. Scand J Gastroenterol 1996; 31: 417–27.
8. Russel MG, Engels LG, Muris JW et al. Modern life in the epidemiology of inflammatory bowel disease: a case-control study with special emphasis on nutritional factors. Eur J Gastroenterol Hepatol 1998; 10: 243–9.
9. Shoda R, Matsueda K, Yamato S, Umeda N. Epidemiologic analysis of Crohn disease in Japan: increased dietary intake of n-6 polyunsaturated fatty acids and animal protein relates to the increased incidence of Crohn disease in Japan. Am J Clin Nutr 1996; 63: 741–5.
10. Tragnone A, Valpiani D, Miglio F et al. Dietary habits as risk factors for inflammatory bowel disease. Eur J Gastroenterol Hepatol 1995; 7: 47–51.
11. Achord JL, Gunn CHJ, Jackson JF. Regional enteritis and HLA concordance in multiple siblings. Dig Dis Sci 1982; 27: 330–2.
12. Roth MP, Petersen GM, McElree C, Feldman E, Rotter JI. Geographic origins of Jewish patients with inflammatory bowel disease. Gastroenterology 1989; 97: 900–4.
13. Orholm M, Iselius L, Sorensen TI, Munkholm P, Langholz E, Binder V. Investigation of inheritance of chronic inflam-

matory bowel diseases by complex segregation analysis. Br Med J 1993; 306: 20–4.
14. Yang H, McElree C, Roth MP, Shanahan F, Targan SR, Rotter JI. Familial empirical risks for inflammatory bowel disease: differences between Jews and non-Jews. Gut 1993; 34: 517–24.
15. Gilberts EC, Greenstein AJ, Katsel P, Harpaz N, Greenstein RJ. Molecular evidence for two forms of Crohn disease. Proc Natl Acad Sci USA 1994; 91: 12721–4.
16. Plevy SE, Targan SR, Yang H, Fernandez D, Rotter JI, Toyoda H. Tumor necrosis factor microsatellites define a Crohn's disease-associated haplotype on chromosome 6. Gastroenterology 1996; 110: 1053–60.
17. Ohmen JD, Yang HY, Yamamoto KK et al. Susceptibility locus for inflammatory bowel disease on chromosome 16 has a role in Crohn's disease, but not in ulcerative colitis. Hum Mol Genet 1996; 5: 1679–83.
18. Reinshagen M, Loeliger C, Kuehnl P et al. HLA class II gene frequencies in Crohn's disease: a population based analysis in Germany. Gut 1996; 38: 538–42.
19. De La Concha EG, Fernandez-Arquero M, Santa-Cruz S et al. Positive and negative associations of distinct HLA-DR2 subtypes with ulcerative colitis (UC). Clin Exp Immunol 1997; 108: 392–5.
20. McLeod RS, Steinhart AH, Siminovitch KA et al. Preliminary report on the Mount Sinai Hospital Inflammatory Bowel Disease Genetics Project. Dis Colon Rectum 1997; 40: 553–7.
21. Mirza MM, Lee J, Teare D et al. Evidence of linkage of the inflammatory bowel disease susceptibility locus on chromosome 16 (IBD1) to ulcerative colitis. J Med Genet 1998; 35: 218–21.
22. Bouma G, Oudkerk PM, Crusius JB et al. Evidence for genetic heterogeneity in inflammatory bowel disease (IBD); HLA genes in the predisposition to suffer from ulcerative colitis (UC) and Crohn's disease (CD). Clin Exp Immunol 1997; 109: 175–9.
23. Bouma G, Crusius JB, Garcia-Gonzalez MA et al. Genetic markers in clinically well defined patients with ulcerative colitis (UC). Clin Exp Immunol 1999; 115: 294–300.
24. Cavanaugh JA, Callen DF, Wilson SR et al. Analysis of Australian Crohn's disease pedigrees refines the localization for susceptibility to inflammatory bowel disease on chromosome 16. Ann Hum Genet 1998; 62: 291–8.
25. Papo M, Quer JC, Gutierrez C et al. Genetic heterogeneity within ulcerative colitis determined by an interleukin-1 receptor antagonist gene polymorphism and antineutrophil cytoplasmic antibodies. Eur J Gastroenterol Hepatol 1999; 11: 413–20.
26. Endres S, Ghorbani R, Kelley VE et al. The effect of dietary supplementation with n-3 polyunsaturated fatty acids on the synthesis of interleukin-1 and tumor necrosis factor by mononuclear cells. N Engl J Med 1989; 320: 265–71.
27. Kim YI. Can fish oil maintain Crohn's disease in remission? Nutr Rev 1996; 54: 248–52.
28. Salomon P, Kornbluth AA, Janowitz HD. Treatment of ulcerative colitis with fish oil n–3-omega-fatty acid: an open trial. J Clin Gastroenterol 1990; 12: 157–61.
29. Stenson WF, Cort D, Rodgers J et al. Dietary supplementation with fish oil in ulcerative colitis. Ann Intern Med 1992; 116: 609-614.
30. Lorenz-Meyer H, Bauer P, Nicolay C et al. Omega-3 fatty acids and low carbohydrate diet for maintenance of remission in Crohn's disease. A randomized controlled multicenter trial. Study Group Members (German Crohn's Disease Study Group). Scand J Gastroenterol 1996; 31: 778–85.
31. Burr ML, Merrett TG. Food intolerance: a community survey. Br J Nutr 1983; 49: 217–19.

32. Young E, Stoneham MD, Petruckevitch A, Barton J, Rona R. A population study of food intolerance. Lancet 1994; 343: 1127–30.

33. Bischoff SC, Herrmann A, Manns MP. Prevalence of adverse reactions to food in patients with gastrointestinal disease. Allergy 1996; 51: 811–18.

34. Giaffer MH, Cann P, Holdsworth CD. Long-term effects of elemental and exclusion diets for Crohn's disease. Aliment Pharmacol Ther 1991; 5: 115–25.

35. Pearson M, Teahon K, Levi AJ, Bjarnason I. Food intolerance and Crohn's disease. Gut 1993; 34: 783–7.

36. Ballegaard M, Bjergstrom A, Brondum S, Hylander E, Jensen L, Ladefoged K. Self-reported food intolerance in chronic inflammatory bowel disease. Scand J Gastroenterol 1997; 32: 569–71.

37. Dieleman LA, Heizer WD. Nutritional issues in inflammatory bowel disease. Gastroenterol Clin N Am 1998; 27: 435–51.

38. Han PD, Burke A, Baldassano RN, Rombeau JL, Lichtenstein GR. Nutrition and inflammatory bowel disease. Gastroenterol Clin N Am 2000; 28: 423–43.

39. Sturniolo GC, Mestriner C, Lecis PE et al. Altered plasma and mucosal concentrations of trace elements and antioxidants in active ulcerative colitis. Scand J Gastroenterol 1998; 33: 644–9.

40. Geerling BJ, Badart-Smook A, Stockbrugger RW, Brummer RJ. Comprehensive nutritional status in patients with long-standing Crohn disease currently in remission. Am J Clin Nutr 1998; 67: 919–26.

41. Esteve-Comas M, Nunez MC, Fernandez-Banares F et al. Abnormal plasma polyunsaturated fatty acid pattern in non-active inflammatory bowel disease. Gut 1993; 34: 1370–3.

42. Dady IM, Thomas AG, Miller V, Kelsey AJ. Inflammatory bowel disease in infancy: an increasing problem? J Pediatr Gastroenterol Nutr 1996; 23: 569–76.

43. Seidman E, LeLeiko N, Ament M et al. Nutral issues in pediatric inflammatory bowel disease. J Pediatr Gastroenterol Nutr 1991; 12: 424–38.

44. Thomas AG, Taylor F, Miller V. Dietary intake and nutritional treatment in childhood Crohn's disease. J Pediatr Gastroenterol Nutr 1993; 17: 75–81.

45. Ruuska T, Savilahti E, Maki M, Ormala T, Visakorpi JK. Exclusive whole protein enteral diet versus prednisolone in the treatment of acute Crohn's disease in children. J Pediatr Gastroenterol Nutr 1994; 19: 175–80.

46. Papadopoulou A, Rawashdeh MO, Brown GA, McNeish AS, Booth IW. Remission following an elemental diet or prednisolone in Crohn's disease. Acta Paediatr 1995; 84: 79–83.

47. Polk DB, Hattner JA, Kerner JA, Jr. Improved growth and disease activity after intermittent administration of a defined formula diet in children with Crohn's disease. J Parent Ent Nutr 1992; 16: 499–504.

48. Beattie RM, Schiffrin EJ, Donnet-Hughes A et al. Polymeric nutrition as the primary therapy in children with small bowel Crohn's disease. Alimen Pharmacol Ther 1994; 8: 609–15.

49. Khoshoo V, Reifen R, Neuman MG, Griffiths A, Pencharz PB. Effect of low- and high-fat, peptide-based diets on body composition and disease activity in adolescents with active Crohn's disease. J Parent Ent Nutr 1996; 20: 401–5.

50. Wilschanski M, Sherman P, Pencharz P, Davis L, Corey M, Griffiths A. Supplementary enteral nutrition maintains remission in paediatric Crohn's disease. Gut 1996; 38: 543–8.

51. Rossi TM, Lee PC, Young C, Tjota A. Small intestinal mucosa changes, including epithelial cell proliferative activity, of children receiving total parenteral nutrition (TPN). Dig Dis Sci 1993; 38: 1608–13.

52. Hirose S, Hirata M, Azuma N, Shirai Z, Mitudome A, Oda T. Carnitine depletion during total parenteral nutrition despite oral L-carnitine supplementation. Acta Paediatr Jpn 1997; 39: 194–200.

53. Gagliardi E, Brathwaite CE. Nutral implications of significant small bowel resection. N Jersey Med 1995; 92: 155–7.

54. Nightingale JM. The short-bowel syndrome. Eur J Gastroenterol Hepatol 1995; 7: 514–20.

55. Nightingale JM, Lennard-Jones JE, Gertner DJ, Wood SR, Bartram CI. Colonic preservation reduces need for parenteral therapy, increases incidence of renal stones, but does not change high prevalence of gall stones in patients with a short bowel. Gut 1992; 33: 1493–7.

56. Woolf GM, Miller C, Kurian R, Jeejeebhoy KN. Nutral absorption in short bowel syndrome. Evaluation of fluid, calorie, and divalent cation requirements. Dig Dis Sci 1987; 32: 8–15.

57. Engels LG, van den Hamer CJ, van Tongeren JH. Iron, zinc, and copper balance in short bowel patients on oral nutrition. Am J Clin Nutr 1984; 40: 1038–41.

58. Edes TE, Walk BE, Thornton WHJ, Fritsche KL. Essential fatty acid sufficiency does not preclude fat-soluble-vitamin deficiency in short-bowel syndrome. Am J Clin Nutr 1991; 53: 499–502.

59. Someya N, Yoshida T, Haraguchi Y, Tanaka K. A case of short bowel syndrome in which remarkable amelioration of mental deterioration was achieved by administration of trace elements. Gastroenterol Jpn 1985; 20: 465–9.

60. Hiroi K, Goto Y, Ishikawa J, Kida K, Matsuda H. A case of beriberi accompanying short bowel. Acta Paediatr Jpn 1995; 37: 84–7.

61. Gryboski JD. Eating disorders in inflammatory bowel disease. Am J Gastroenterol 1993; 88: 293–6.

62. Holaday M, Smith KE, Robertson S, Dallas J. An atypical eating disorder with Crohn's disease in a fifteen-year-old male: a case study. Adolescence 1994; 29: 865–73.

63. Mallett P, Murch S. Anorexia nervosa complicating inflammatory bowel disease. Arch Dis Childh 1990; 65: 298–300.

64. Musch MW, Chang EB. Diarrhea in inflammatory bowel diseases. In: Targan SR, Shanahan F, eds. Inflammatory Bowel Disease: From Bench to Bedside. Baltimore, MD: Williams Wilkins, 1994: 239–54.

65. Rigaud D, Angel LA, Cerf M et al. Mechanisms of decreased food intake during weight loss in adult Crohn's disease patients without obvious malabsorption. Am J Clin Nutr 1994; 60: 775–81.

66. Muller MJ, Schmidt LU, Korber J et al. Reduced metabolic efficiency in patients with Crohn's disease. Dig Dis Sci 1993; 38: 2001–9.

67. Chan AT, Fleming CR, O'Fallon WM, Huizenga KA. Estimated versus measured basal energy requirements in patients with Crohn's disease. Gastroenterology 1986; 91: 75–8.

68. Mingrone G, Greco AV, Benedetti G et al. Increased resting lipid oxidation in Crohn's disease. Dig Dis Sci 1996; 41: 72–6.

69. Stokes MA, Hill GL. Total energy expenditure in patients with Crohn's disease: measurement by the combined body scan technique. J Parent Ent Nutr 1993; 17: 3–7.

70. Kane SV, Sable K, Hanauer SB. The menstrual cycle and its effect on inflammatory bowel disease and irritable bowel syndrome: a prevalence study. Am J Gastroenterol 1998; 93: 1867–72.

71. Annese V, Bassotti G, Napolitano G, Usai P, Andriulli A, Vantrappen G. Gastrointestinal motility disorders in patients with inactive Crohn's disease. Scand J Gastroenterol 1997; 32: 1107–17.

psychosocial function. Am J Gastroenterol 1995; 90: 1450–4.

156. Berin MC, Perdue MH. Effect of psychoneural factors on intestinal epithelial function. Can J Gastroenterol 1997; 11: 353–7.

157. Talal AH, Drossman DA. Psychosocial factors in inflammatory bowel disease. Gastroenterol Clin N Am 1995; 24: 699–716.

158. Guyatt G, Mitchell A, Irvine EJ et al. A new measure of health status for clinical trials in inflammatory bowel disease. Gastroenterology 1989; 96: 804–10.

159. Drossman DA, Leserman J, Li ZM, Mitchell CM, Zagami EA, Patrick DL. The rating form of IBD patient concerns: a new measure of health status. Psychosom Med 1991; 53: 701–12.

160. Drossman DA, Li Z, Leserman J, Patrick DL. Ulcerative colitis and Crohn's disease health status scales for research and clinical practice. J Clin Gastroenterol 1992; 15: 104–12.

161. Johnston KR, Govel LA, Andritz MH. Gastrointestinal effects of sorbitol as an additive in liquid medications. Am J Med 1994; 97: 185–91.

162. Breitenbach RA, Simon J. Cases from the aerospace medicine resident teaching file. Case 59. A case of 'unbearable' gremlinenteritis [Clinical Conference]. Aviat Space Environ Med 1994; 65: 432–3.

163. Goldberg LD, Ditchek NT. Chewing gum diarrhea. Am J Dig Dis 1978; 23: 568.

164. Lin HC, Sanders SL, Gu YG, Doty JE. Erythromycin accelerates solid emptying at the expense of gastric sieving. Dig Dis Sci 1994; 39: 124–8.

165. Eisenberg DM, Kessler RC, Foster C, Norlock FE, Calkins DR, Delbanco TL. Unconventional medicine in the United States. Prevalence, costs, and patterns of use. N Engl J Med 1993; 328: 246–52.

166. Borins M. The dangers of using herbs. What your patients need to know. Postgrad Med 1999; 104: 91–5.

167. Foster S, Tyler VE. Tyler's Honest Herbal: A Sensible Guide to the Use of Herbs and Related Remedies. 4th edn. Binghamton, NY: Haworth Press, Inc., 1999.

168. Wright RA, Heymsfield S. Nutral Assessment. Boston: Blackwell Scientific Publications, 1984.

169. Bates CJ. Diagnosis and detection of vitamin deficiencies. Br Med Bull 1999; 55: 643–57.

170. Balint JP. Physical findings in nutritional deficiencies. Pediatr Clin N Am 1998; 45: 245–60.

171. Touger-Decker R. Oral manifestations of nutrient deficiencies. Mount Sinai J Med 1998; 65: 355–61.

172. Ehrenpreis ED, Popovich TL, Cravero R. A practical guide to the recognition of nutritional deficiencies. Compr Ther 1997; 23: 218–22.

173. Ovesen L, Chu R, Howard L. The influence of dietary fat on jejunostomy output in patients with severe short bowel syndrome. Am J Clin Nutr 1983; 38: 270–7.

174. Hylander E, Ladefoged K, Jarnum S. Calcium absorption after intestinal resection. The importance of a preserved colon. Scand J Gastroenterol 1990; 25: 705–10.

175. Pigot F, Roux C, Chaussade S et al. Low bone mineral density in patients with inflammatory bowel disease. Dig Dis Sci 1992; 37: 1396–403.

176. Silvennoinen J, Lamberg-Allardt C, Karkkainen M, Niemela S, Lehtola J. Dietary calcium intake and its relation to bone mineral density in patients with inflammatory bowel disease. J Intern Med 1996; 240: 285–92.

177. Robinson RJ, al-Azzawi F, Iqbal SJ, Kryswcki T, Almond L, Abrams K et al. Osteoporosis and determinants of bone density in patients with Crohn's disease. Dig Dis Sci 1998; 43: 2500–6.

178. Kuczera M, Wiecek A, Kokot F. Markers of bone turnover in patients with nephrolithiasis. Int Urol Nephrol 1997; 29: 523–8.

179. Staniforth DH, Rose D. Statistical analysis of the lactulose/breath hydrogen test in the measurement of orocaecal transit: its variability and predictive value in assessing drug action. Gut 1989; 30: 171–5.

180. Riordan SM, McIver CJ, Walker BM, Duncombe VM, Bolin TD, Thomas MC. The lactulose breath hydrogen test and small intestinal bacterial overgrowth. Am J Gastroenterol 1996; 91: 1795–803.

181. Miller MA, Parkman HP, Urbain JL et al. Comparison of scintigraphy and lactulose breath hydrogen test for assessment of orocecal transit: lactulose accelerates small bowel transit. Dig Dis Sci 1997; 42: 10–18.

182. Attar A, Flourie B, Rambaud JC et al. Antibiotic efficacy in small intestinal bacterial overgrowth-related chronic diarrhea: a crossover, randomized trial. Gastroenterology 1999; 117: 794–7.

183. Sellin JH, Hart R. Glucose malabsorption associated with rapid intestinal transit. Am J Gastroenterol 1992; 87: 584–9.

184. de BD, Chaussain M, Badoual J, Raymond J, Dupont C. Small-bowel bacterial overgrowth in children with chronic diarrhea, abdominal pain, or both. J Pediatr 1996; 128: 203–7.

185. Greenberg GR, Fleming CR, Jeejeebhoy KN, Rosenberg IH, Sales D, Tremaine WJ. Controlled trial of bowel rest and nutritional support in the management of Crohn's disease. Gut 1988; 29: 1309–15.

186. Sitzmann JV, Converse RLJ, Bayless TM. Favorable response to parenteral nutrition and medical therapy in Crohn's colitis. A report of 38 patients comparing severe Crohn's and ulcerative colitis. Gastroenterology 1990; 99: 1647–52.

187. Reynolds JV, Kanwar S, Welsh FK et al. 1997 Harry M. Vars Research Award. Does the route of feeding modify gut barrier function and clinical outcome in patients after major upper gastrointestinal surgery? J Parent Ent Nutr 1997; 21: 196–201.

188. Steffes C, Fromm D. Is preoperative parenteral nutrition necessary for patients with predominantly ileal Crohn's disease? Arch Surg 1992; 127: 1210–12.

189. Carlson GL, Gray P, Barber D, Shaffer JL, Mughal M, Irving MH. Total parenteral nutrition modifies the acute phase response to Crohn's disease. J Roy Coll Surg Edinb 1994; 39: 360–4.

190. Mukau L, Talamini MA, Sitzmann JV. Elemental diets may accelerate recovery from total parenteral nutrition-induced gut atrophy. J Parent Ent Nutr 1994; 18: 75–8.

191. Kaufman SS, Loseke CA, Lupo JV et al. Influence of bacterial overgrowth and intestinal inflammation on duration of parenteral nutrition in children with short bowel syndrome. J Pediatr 1997; 131: 356–61.

192. Weber TR. Enteral feeding increases sepsis in infants with short bowel syndrome. J Pediatr Surg 1995; 30: 1086–8.

193. Pappo I, Bercovier H, Berry E, Gallilly R, Feigin E, Freund HR. Antitumor necrosis factor antibodies reduce hepatic steatosis during total parenteral nutrition and bowel rest in the rat. J Parent Ent Nutr 1995; 19: 80–2.

194. Eisenberg JM, Glick HA, Buzby GP, Kinosian B, Williford WO. Does perioperative total parenteral nutrition reduce medical care costs?. J Parent Ent Nutr 1993; 17: 201–9.

195. Galandiuk S, O'Neill M, McDonald P, Fazio VW, Steiger E. A century of home parenteral nutrition for Crohn's disease. Am J Surg 1990; 159: 540–4.

196. Gonzalez-Huix F, de Leon R, Fernandez-Banares F et al. Polymeric enteral diets as primary treatment of active Crohn's disease: a prospective steroid controlled trial. Gut 1993; 34: 778–82.

197. Teahon K, Bjarnason I, Pearson M, Levi AJ. Ten years' experience with an elemental diet in the management of Crohn's disease. Gut 1990; 31: 1133–7.

198. Giaffer MH, North G, Holdsworth CD. Controlled trial of polymeric versus elemental diet in treatment of active Crohn's disease. Lancet 1990; 335: 816–19.

199. Gonzalez-Huix F, Fernandez-Banares F, Esteve-Comas M *et al.* Enteral versus parenteral nutrition as adjunct therapy in acute ulcerative colitis. Am J Gastroenterol 1993; 88: 227–32.

200. Jones VA. Comparison of total parenteral nutrition and elemental diet in induction of remission of Crohn's disease. Long-term maintenance of remission by personalized food exclusion diets. Dig Dis Sci 1987; 32: 100S–7S.

201. Fernandez-Banares F, Cabre E, Esteve-Comas M, Gassull MA. How effective is enteral nutrition in inducing clinical remission in active Crohn's disease? A meta-analysis of the randomized clinical trials. J Parent Ent Nutr 1995; 19: 356–64.

202. Gorard DA, Hunt JB, Payne-James JJ *et al.* Initial response and subsequent course of Crohn's disease treated with elemental diet or prednisolone. Gut 1993; 34: 1198–202.

203. Lindor KD, Fleming CR, Burnes JU, Nelson JK, Ilstrup DM. A randomized prospective trial comparing a defined formula diet, corticosteroids, and a defined formula diet plus corticosteroids in active Crohn's disease. Mayo Clin Proc 1992; 67: 328–33.

204. Messori A, Trallori G, D'Albasio G, Milla M, Vannozzi G, Pacini F. Defined-formula diets versus steroids in the treatment of active Crohn's disease: a meta-analysis. Scand J Gastroenterol 1996; 31: 267–72.

205. Okada M, Yao T, Yamamoto T, Takenaka K, Imamura K, Maeda K *et al.* Controlled trial comparing an elemental diet with prednisolone in the treatment of active Crohn's disease. Hepato-Gastroenterology 1990; 37: 72–80.

206. Zoli G, Care M, Parazza M *et al.* A randomized controlled study comparing elemental diet and steroid treatment in Crohn's disease. Alimen Pharmacol Ther 1997; 11: 735–40.

207. Griffiths AM, Ohlsson A, Sherman PM, Sutherland LR. Meta-analysis of enteral nutrition as a primary treatment of active Crohn's disease. Gastroenterology 1995; 108: 1056–67.

208. O'Brien CJ, Giaffer MH, Cann PA, Holdsworth CD. Elemental diet in steroid-dependent and steroid-refractory Crohn's disease. Am J Gastroenterol 1991; 86: 1614–18.

209. Abad-Lacruz A, Gonzalez-Huix F, Esteve M *et al.* Liver function tests abnormalities in patients with inflammatory bowel disease receiving artificial nutrition: a prospective randomized study of total enteral nutrition vs total parenteral nutrition. J Parent Ent Nutr 1990; 14: 618–21.

210. Cosgrove M, Jenkins HR. Experience of percutaneous endoscopic gastrostomy in children with Crohn's disease. Arch Dis Childh 1997; 76: 141–3.

211. di Costanzo J, Cano N, Martin J *et al.* Treatment of external gastrointestinal fistulas by a combination of total parenteral nutrition and somatostatin. J Parent Ent Nutr 1987; 11: 465–70.

212. Fernandez-Banares F, Mingorance MD, Esteve M, *et al.* Serum zinc, copper, and selenium levels in inflammatory bowel disease: effect of total enteral nutrition on trace element status. Am J Gastroenterol 1990; 85: 1584–9.

213. Goode HF, Robertson DA, Kelleher J, Walker BE. Effect of fasting, self-selected and isocaloric glucose and fat meals and intravenous feeding on plasma zinc concentrations. Ann Clin Biochem 1991; 28(Pt 5): 442–5.

214. Myung SJ, Yang SK, Jung HY *et al.* Zinc deficiency manifested by dermatitis and visual dysfunction in a patient with Crohn's disease. J Gastroenterol 1998; 33: 876–9.

215. Rannem T, Ladefoged K, Hylander E, Hegnhoj J, Staun M. Selenium depletion in patients with gastrointestinal diseases: are there any predictive factors? Scand J Gastroenterol 1998; 33: 1057–61.

216. Tominaga M, Iida M, Aoyagi K, Kohrogi N, Matsui T, Fujishima M. Red cell folate concentrations in patients with Crohn's disease on parenteral nutrition. Postgrad Med J 1989; 65: 818–20.

217. Touloukian RJ, Gertner JM. Vitamin D deficiency rickets as a late complication of the short gut syndrome during infancy. J Pediatr Surg 1981; 16: 230–5.

218. Zak J, Burns D, Lingenfelser T, Steyn E, Marks IN. Dry beriberi: unusual complication of prolonged parenteral nutrition. J Parent Ent Nutr 1991; 15: 200–1.

219. Riordan AM, Hunter JO, Cowan RE *et al.* Treatment of active Crohn's disease by exclusion diet: East Anglian multicentre controlled trial. Lancet 1993; 342: 1131–4.

220. Lykins TC, Stockwell J. Comprehensive modified diet simplifies nutrition management of adults with short-bowel syndrome. J Am Diet Assoc 1998; 98: 309–15.

221. Holman RT. Control of polyunsaturated acids in tissue lipids. J Am Coll Nutr 1986; 5: 183–211.

222. Gerster H. Can adults adequately convert alpha-linolenic acid (18: 3n-3) to eicosapentaenoic acid (20: 5n-3) and docosahexaenoic acid (22: 6n-3)?. Int J Vit Nutr Res 1998; 68: 159–73.

223. Spector AA. Essentiality of fatty acids. Lipids 1999; 34(Suppl): S1–3.

224. Fisher M, Upchurch KS, Levine PH *et al.* Effects of dietary fish oil supplementation on polymorphonuclear leukocyte inflammatory potential. Inflammation 1986; 10: 387–92.

225. McCall TB, O'Leary D, Bloomfield J, O'Morain CA. Therapeutic potential of fish oil in the treatment of ulcerative colitis. Aliment Pharmacol Ther 1989; 3: 415–24.

226. Kuroki F, Iida M, Matsumoto T, Aoyagi K, Kanamoto K, Fujishima M. Serum n3 polyunsaturated fatty acids are depleted in Crohn's disease. Dig Dis Sci 1997; 42: 1137–41.

227. Geerling BJ, Houwelingen AC, Badart-Smook A, Stockbrugger RW, Brummer, RJ. Fat intake and fatty acid profile in plasma phospholipids and adipose tissue in patients with Crohn's disease, compared with controls. Am J Gastroenterol 1999; 94: 410–17.

228. Belluzzi A, Brignola C, Campieri M, Pera A, Boschi S, Miglioli M. Effect of an enteric-coated fish-oil preparation on relapses in Crohn's disease. N Engl J Med 1996; 334: 1557–60.

229. Belluzzi A, Campieri M, Brignola C, Gionchetti P, Miglioli M, Barbara L. Polyunsaturated fatty acid pattern and fish oil treatment in inflammatory bowel disease [Letter]. Gut 1993; 34: 1289–90.

230. Hawthorne AB, Daneshmend TK, Hawkey CJ *et al.* Treatment of ulcerative colitis with fish oil supplementation: a prospective 12 month randomised controlled trial. Gut 1992; 33: 922–8.

231. Almallah YZ, Richardson S, O'Hanrahan T *et al.* Distal procto-colitis, natural cytotoxicity, and essential fatty acids. Am J Gastroenterol 1998; 93: 804–9.

232. Greenfield SM, Green AT, Teare JP *et al.* A randomized controlled study of evening primrose oil and fish oil in ulcerative colitis. Aliment Pharmacol Ther 1993; 7: 159–66.

233. Lee TH, Hoover RL, Williams JD *et al.* Effect of dietary enrichment with eicosapentaenoic and docosahexaenoic acids on *in vitro* neutrophil and monocyte leukotriene generation and neutrophil function. N Engl J Med 1985; 312: 1217–24.

234. Matthews DE, Marano MA, Campbell RG. Splanchnic bed utilization of glutamine and glutamic acid in humans. Am J Physiol 1993; 264: E848–54.

235. Reeds PJ, Burrin DG, Jahoor F *et al.* Enteral glutamate is almost completely metabolized in first pass by the gastrointestinal tract of infant pigs [Published errata appear in Am J Physiol 1996; 271: section E following table of contents]. Am J Physiol 1996; 270: E413–18.

236. Den Hond E, Hiele M, Peeters M, Ghoos Y, Rutgeerts P. Effect of long-term oral glutamine supplements on small intestinal permeability in patients with Crohn's disease. J Parent Ent Nutr 1999; 23: 7–11.

237. Byrne TA, Morrissey TB, Gatzen C *et al.* Anabolic therapy with growth hormone accelerates protein gain in surgical patients requiring nutritional rehabilitation. Ann Surg 1993; 218: 400–16.

238. Byrne TA, Morrissey TB, Nattakom TV, Ziegler TR, Wilmore DW. Growth hormone, glutamine, and a modified diet enhance nutrient absorption in patients with severe short bowel syndrome. J Parent Ent Nutr 1995; 19: 296–302.

239. Byrne TA, Persinger RL, Young LS, Ziegler TR, Wilmore, DW. A new treatment for patients with short-bowel syndrome. Growth hormone, glutamine, and a modified diet. Ann Surg 1995; 222: 243–54.

240. Scolapio JS, Camilleri M, Fleming CR *et al.* Effect of growth hormone, glutamine, and diet on adaptation in short-bowel syndrome: a randomized, controlled study. Gastroenterology 1997; 113: 1074–81.

241. Wilmore DW, Lacey JM, Soultanakis RP, Bosch RL, Byrne, TA. Factors predicting a successful outcome after pharmacologic bowel compensation. Ann Surg 1997; 226: 288–92.

242. Lin HC, Van Citters GW, Heimer F, Bonorris G. Slowing of gastrointestinal transit by oleic acid: a preliminary report of a novel, nutrient-based treatment in humans. Dig Dis Sci 2001; 46: 223–9.

243. Van Citters GW, Lin HC. Oleic acid improves drug absorption in patients with inflammatory bowel disease. Gastroenterology 1998; 114: A1105 (Abstract).

30 | Medical management of ulcerative colitis

WILLIAM J. SANDBORN

Introduction

The optimal medical treatment of patients with ulcerative colitis (UC) requires that the treating physician obtain a history and perform any necessary diagnostic procedures, and then prescribe an appropriate medication regimen based on a knowledge of clinical pharmacology and the evidence from controlled clinical trials. This chapter will review the results from clinical trials that assessed the efficacy of medications used to treat UC and then provide an integrated therapeutic approach to the medical treatment of specific disease settings for patients with UC.

Pretreatment evaluation of the patient

Prior to initiating or altering the medical treatment regimen of patients with UC, the physician should evaluate the patient [1]. This evaluation begins with a medical history to determine the age of onset, the duration of disease, the extent of disease, the disease course over time, prior and current medication use (including duration and dose), and the symptoms currently being experienced by the patient. At the time of diagnosis the patients should undergo colonoscopy with mucosal biopsy and small bowel X-ray to provide a baseline characterization of the UC and to exclude Crohn's disease (CD). Infectious and medication-associated causes of colitis should be excluded. In patients with an established diagnosis of UC it is useful to repeat these tests when patients relapse and fail to respond to empiric therapy with 5-aminosalicylates and/or corticosteroids, prior to instituting immune modifier therapy or referring the patient for surgery. Adherence to this methodical approach allows the treating physician to make observations that would lead to a change in therapy such as: a change in the proximal extent of colitis; endoscopic findings of severe colitis; features that are more compatible with a diagnosis of CD; infectious

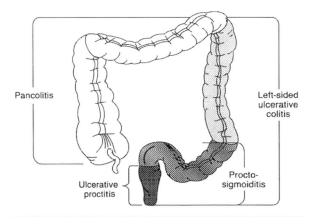

Figure 1. Distinguishing the various states of ulcerative colitis – proctitis, proctosigmoiditis, left-sided colitis, and pancolitis – depends on both the degree of mucosal inflammation and the extent of colonic mucosal involvement. (Reprinted with permission from: Miner PB, Peppercorn MA, Targan SR. A rational approach to 5-aminosalicylic acid therapy in ulcerative colitis. Hosp Pract 1993; 28(Suppl 3): 3–24.)

colitis or medication-associated colitis; and patients with UC in endoscopic remission who may be experiencing symptoms of concomitant irritable bowel syndrome.

Classification of the patient according to the anatomic extent of involvement is shown in Fig. 1 [2]. Determining the extent of involvement is important because many 5-aminosalicylate-based medications and corticosteroid preparations are delivered topically, and do not distribute uniformly throughout the colon at a high concentration. The expected sites of drug delivery for various topically delivered 5-aminosalicylate formulations are shown in Table 1 [3]. Suppositories can be expected to release medication only in the rectum (approximately the last 10 cm of the colon) [4, 5]. Enemas will reach the ascending colon/splenic flexure in approximately 80–90% of patients (Fig. 2) [6–13].

Stephan R. Targan, Fergus Shanahan and Loren C. Karp (eds.), Inflammatory Bowel Disease: From Bench to Bedside, 2nd Edition, 605–629.
© 2003 *Kluwer Academic Publishers. Printed in Great Britain*

Table 1. 5-Aminosalicylate preparations

Generic name	Proprietary name	Formulation	Sites of delivery	Daily dose Active	Daily dose Maintenance	Indication
Mesalamine	Rowasa Salofalk	Enema suspension	Distal to splenic flexure	4 g	1–4 g	Active distal UC, remission maintenance distal UC
Mesalamine	Rowasa Canasa	Suppository	Rectum	1–1.5 g	0.5–1 g	Active proctitis, remission maintenance distal UC
Mesalamine	Asacol	Eudragit-s-coated tablets (release at pH $\geqslant 7.0$)	Terminal ileum, colon	1.6–4.8 g	0.8–4.8 g	Active UC, remission maintenance UC
Mesalamine	Salofalk Mesasal Claversal	Mesalamine in a sodium /glycerine buffer coated with Eudragit-l (release at pH $\geqslant 6.0$)	Distal jejunum, proximal ileum	1.5–4 g	0.75–4 g	Active UC, remission maintenance UC
Mesalamine	Pentasa	Ethylcellulose-coated microgranules (time and pH-dependent release)	Duodenum, jejenum, ileum, colon	2–4 g	1.5–4	Active UC, remission maintenance UC
Olsalazine	Dipentum	5-ASA dimer linked by azo-bond	Colon	2–3 g	1 g	Active UC, remission maintenance UC
Sulfasalazine	Azulfadine	5-ASA linked to sulfa-pyridine by azo-bond	Colon	2–4 g	2–4 g	Active UC, remission maintenance UC
Balsalazide	Colazide Colazal	5-ASA linked to inert carrier by azo-bond	Colon	2–6.75 g	2–6.75 g	Active UC, maintenance UC

Reprinted after modification with permission from: Loftus EV, Sandborn WJ. Drug therapy for inflammatory bowel disease. Contemp Intern Med 1995; 7: 21–34.

The Truelove and Witts classification can be used to determine whether patients have mild to moderately active or severely active UC (Table 2) [14]. This assessment of disease severity is important in determining whether or not to hospitalize the patient and whether steroid therapy is mandatory. Other disease activity indexes such as the Sutherland Index or the Mayo Index are more useful for distinguishing patients with remission, mildly active disease, and moderately active disease for the purposes of assessing efficacy of sulfasalazine and other 5-aminosalicylate-based medications (Table 3) [15, 16].

Goals of treatment

The primary goals of medical therapy are to induce and then maintain significant clinical improvement or remission, resulting in a reduction or resolution of the signs and symptoms of active UC. Secondary goals, which often occur in parallel with clinical changes, are induction of endoscopic improvement and remission. The efficacy of various medical therapies in achieving these endpoints in patients with UC is reviewed in the following sections.

5-Aminosalicylate-based medications

Sulfasalazine, oral mesalamine (Pentasa, Asacol, Salofalk, Mesasal, Claversal) rectal mesalamine (Rowasa, Canasa, Salofalk, Pentasa), olsalazine, and balsalazide are all drugs that deliver 5-aminosalicylate to the colon (Table 1) [3]. The clinical pharmacology of these medications is reviewed in detail elsewhere in this book.

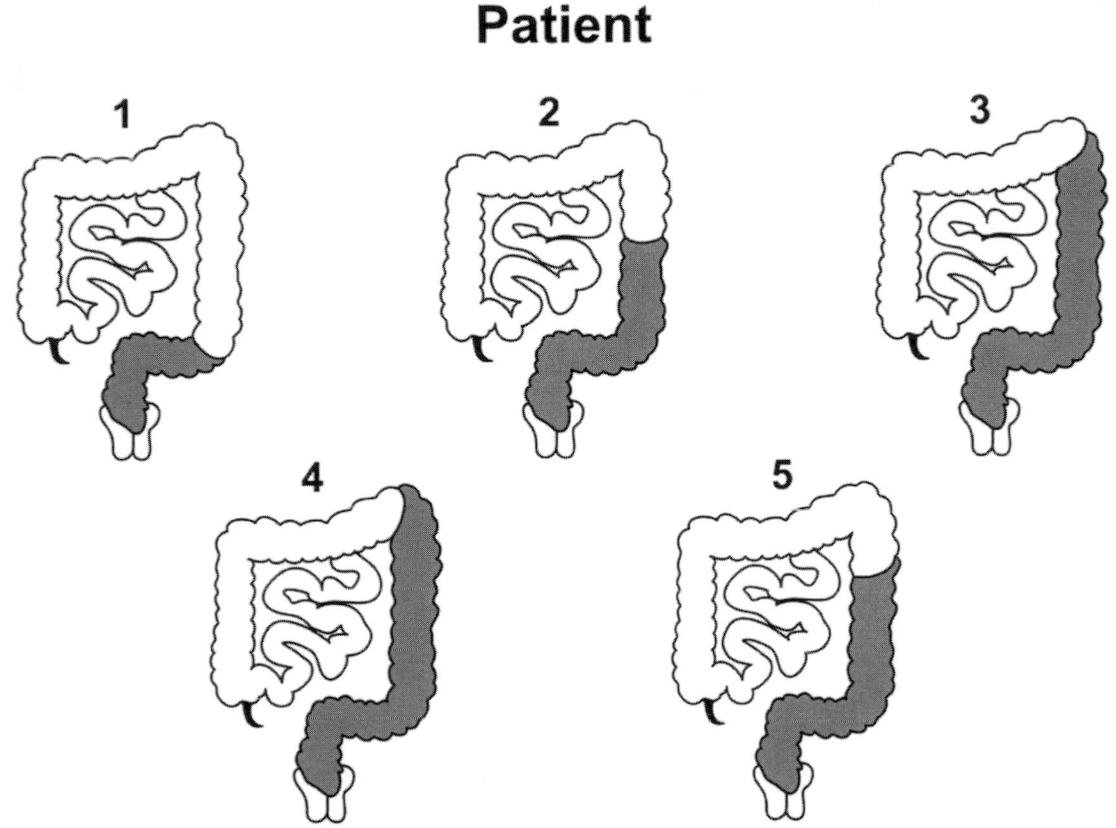

Patient

Figure 2. The individual colonic spread of radiolabeled low-viscosity 100 ml budesonide enemas in five patients with distal ulcerative colitis 15 min after administration. The filled areas of the colon represent areas where radioactivity was found. Modified with permission from: Nyman-Pantelidis M, Nillson A, Wagner GW, Borga O. Pharmacokinetics and retrograde colonic spread of budesonide enemas in patients with distal ulcerative colitis. Aliment Pharmacol Ther 1994; 8: 617–22.

Table 2. Truelove and Witts criteria for evaluating the severity of ulcerative colitis*

Variable	Mild disease	Severe disease	Fulminant disease
Stools (number/day)	< 4	> 6	> 10
Blood in stool	Intermittent	Frequent	Continuous
Temperature (°C)	Normal	> 37.5	> 37.5
Pulse (beats/min)	Normal	> 90	> 90
Hemoglobin	Normal	< 75% of normal value	Transfusion required
Erythrocyte sedimentation rate (mm/h)	≤ 30	> 30	> 30
Colonic features on X-ray		Air, edematous wall, thumbprinting	Dilatation
Clinical signs		Abdominal tenderness	Abdominal distention and tenderness

*Moderate disease includes features of both mild and severe disease.
Reprinted with permission from: Truelove SC, Witts LT. Cortisone in ulcerative colitis: final report on a therapeutic trial. Br Med J 1955; 2: 1041–8.

Table 3. Mayo scoring system for assessment of ulcerative colitis activity

Stool frequency*
0 = Normal no. stools for this for this patient
1 = 1–2 stools more than normal
2 = 3–4 stools more than normal
3 = 5 or more stools more than normal
* Each patient served as his or her own control to establish the degree of abnormality of the stool frequency

Rectal bleeding**
0 = No blood seen
1 = Streaks of blood with stool less than half the time
2 = Obvious blood with stool most of the time
3 = Blood alone passed
** The daily bleeding score represented the most severe day of bleeding

Findings of flexible proctosigmoidoscopy
0 = Normal or inactive disease
1 = Mild disease (erythema, decreased vascular pattern, mild friability)
2 = Moderate disease (marked erythema, absent vascular pattern, friability, erosions)
3 = Severe disease (spontaneous bleeding, ulceration

Physician's global assessment***
0 = Normal
1 = Mild disease
2 = Moderate disease
3 = Severe disease
*** The physician's global assessment acknowledged the three other criteria, the patient's daily record of abdominal discomfort and general sense of well-being, and other observations, such as physical findings and the patient's performance status

A total Mayo ulcerative colitis activity score of 0–2 points indicates remission/minimally active disease; a score of 3–5 points indicates mildly active disease; a score of 6–10 points indicates moderately active disease; and a score of 11–12 may indicate moderate or severe disease, depending on the patient's Truelove and Witt's score. Reprinted with permission from: Schroeder KW, Tremaine WJ, Ilstrup DM. Coated oral 5-aminosalicylic acid therapy for mildly to moderately active ulcerative colitis. N Engl J Med 1987; 317: 1625–9.

Sulfasalazine

In 1942 Svartz reported on both the therapeutic results and the toxic effects of a novel sulfanilamide preparation, sulfasalazine, in patients with UC [17]. Sulfasalazine is composed of 5-aminosalicylate linked to sulfapyridine by a diazo bond. Placebo-controlled trials demonstrated that sulfasalazine administered orally at doses of 2–6 g/day or as a 3 g enema was effective in inducing remission in patients with mildly to moderately active UC and ulcerative proctitis [18–21]. Studies comparing sulfasalazine with a combination of low-dose oral and rectal steroids for active UC concluded that steroid therapy acted more rapidly, and perhaps was more effective, than sulfasalazine [22, 23]. Additional placebo-controlled trials demonstrated that sulfasalazine at doses of 2–4 g/day was effective in maintaining remission in patients with UC, and that the 4 g dose was more effective whereas the 2 g dose was better tolerated [24–26]. One placebo-controlled trial failed to demonstrate a maintenance benefit [27]. Com-

parative studies of sulfasalazine versus a high-fiber diet or mast cell stabilizers such as cromoglycate also showed maintenance benefits for sulfasalazine [28–31]. Approximately 10–20% of orally administered sulfasalazine is absorbed systemically with the remainder passing unaltered to the colon [32]. Sulfasalazine undergoes metabolism in the colon by bacterial azoreductase enzymes to 5-aminosalicylate and sulfapyridine [33, 34]. The active moiety of sulfasalazine was determined to be the poorly absorbed molecule 5-aminosalicylate and not the well-absorbed molecule sulfapyridine [32, 35–38].

Adverse events occurring in patients with inflammatory bowel disease (IBD) treated with sulfasalazine include: headache, epigastric pain, nausea and vomiting, cyanosis, skin rash, fever, hepatitis, autoimmune hemolysis, transient reticulosis, aplastic anemia, leukopenia, agranulocytosis, folate deficiency, pancreatitis, systemic lupus erythematosus, sulfonamide-induced toxic epidermal necrolysis, Stevens-Johnson syndrome, pulmonary dysfunction, and male infertility [39, 40]. For the most part the side-effects from sulfasalazine can be attributed to the systemic absorption of sulfa-pyridine, and they occur more commonly in patients who are genetically predisposed to 'slow' acetylation of sulfapyridine to *N*-acetylsulfapyridine in the liver [39]. Headache, nausea and vomiting, and epigastric pain often appear to be related to the sulfasalazine dose, and it is frequently possible to desensitize patients by discontinuing sulfasalazine for 1–2 weeks, and then restarting at 0.125–0.25 g/day and increasing by 0.125 g/week up to a maintenance dose of 2 g/day [40]. Sulfasalazine therapy may also lead to a paradoxical worsening of diarrhea in patients with UC [41].

Rectal mesalamine (5-aminosalicylate)

After it was demonstrated that mesalamine (5-ami-nosalicylate; 5-ASA) was the active moiety of sulfa-salazine (discussed above), oral and rectal drug delivery systems were devised to avoid absorption of mesalamine in the proximal small intestine, instead targeting the colon as the site of drug release. Placebo-controlled trials demonstrated that mesala-mine administered rectally as a suspension enema at doses of 1–4 g/day or as a suppository at doses of 0.5–1.5 g/day was effective in inducing remission in patients with mildly to moderately active left-sided UC, ulcerative proctosigmoiditis, and ulcerative proctitis [4, 15, 42–44]. There does not appear to be a dose response across this range of mesalamine doses [42, 45]. Studies comparing novel foam or suppository formulations of mesalamine to standard mesalamine enemas or suppositories have shown equivalent results [46–48]. Relatively small studies comparing rectally administered 5-ASA with rectal steroids demonstrated similar efficacy rates [49–59]. However, a meta-analysis suggested that rectally administered mesalamine is superior to rectal ster-oids for inducing remission [45]. Other small comparative studies have suggested that rectally administered mesalamine is equivalent to oral sulfasalazine, 4-aminosalicylate, and bismuth but not sucralfate [22, 23, 60–63]. A comparison of oral mesalamine 2.4 g/day, rectal mesalamine 4 g/day, and a combination of the two therapies demonstrated a benefit for rectal mesalamine and combination therapy [64]. Whether this result represents a mesalamine dose response or an advantage for rectal delivery of mesalamine is unclear. Additional placebo-controlled trials demonstrated that mesalamine administered rectally as 1 or 4 g enemas or 0.5 or 1 g suppositories was effective in maintaining remission in patients with left-sided UC, distal UC, and ulcerative proctitis [65–69]. There is little evidence of a mesalamine dose response in maintenance therapy, but more frequent dosing intervals (twice-daily suppositories or daily enemas) are associated with lower relapse rates than less frequent dosing intervals of once-daily suppositories or enemas every second or third night [66, 68, 70]. Comparative studies suggest that rectal mesalamine 4 g is superior to oral mesalamine 1.5 or 2 g and that rectal mesalamine 4 g in combination with oral mesalamine 1.6 g is super-ior to monotherapy with oral mesalamine 1.6 g for maintaining remission [71–73]. It is unclear whether this represents a dose response or an advantage for rectal delivery of mesalamine.

Oral mesalamine (5-ASA)

Placebo-controlled trials demonstrated that oral mesalamine administered at doses of 1.6–4.8 g/day (Asacol 1.6–4.8 g/day, Pentasa 2–4 g/day) was effec-tive in inducing remission in patients with mildly to moderately active UC [16, 74–76]. Meta-analyses indicate that a dose response for oral mesalamine probably exists [77, 78]. Comparative studies have demonstrated that oral mesalamine at doses of 0.8–4.0 g/day has comparable efficacy to sulfasalazine 2.0–4.0 g/day, but that side-effects occur more frequently in sulfasalazine-treated patients [79–81]. Additional placebo-controlled trials demonstrated that oral mesalamine at doses of 0.8–4.0 g/day was effective in maintaining remission in patients with UC [82, 83]. Comparative studies of oral mesalamine versus sulfasalazine demonstrated comparable efficacy for maintaining remission in UC, again with fewer side-effects for oral mesalamine [84–88]. More recent comparative studies for maintaining remis-sion in patients with UC have suggested that oral mesalamine may be equivalent to dietary fiber and probiotic bacteria [88–91].

Olsalazine

Olsalazine is a dimer, composed of two 5-ASA molecules linked by a diazo bond. Placebo-controlled trials demonstrated that olsalazine adminis-tered orally at doses of 0.75–3 g/day or rectally as a 1 g enema was not consistently effective in inducing remission in patients with mildly to moderately active UC, due to a higher than expected dropout rate in olsalazine-treated patients for worsened diarrhea [92–97]. The worsened diarrhea is a result of ileal secretion [98]. In contrast to the placebo-controlled trials, studies that compared olsalazine with sulfasalazine for active UC for the most part concluded that the two agents had comparable efficacy [99–102]. Additional placebo controlled trials demonstrated that olsalazine at doses of 1–2 g/day was effective in maintaining remission in patients with UC [103, 104]. Comparative studies of olsalazine against oral mesalamine and sulfasalazine demonstrated similar efficacy for maintenance of remission in patients with UC [105–110].

Balsalazide

Balsalazide is composed of 5-ASA linked to an inert carrier molecule by a diazo bond. A comparative study of balsalazide 6.75 g/day with oral mesalamine (Asacol) 2.4 g/day in patients with active UC demonstrated similar efficacy [112]. Maintenance studies in patients with UC demonstrated that balsalazide 4 g/day was more effective than 2 g/day, balsalazide 3 g/day had similar efficacy to balsalazide 6 g/day and to oral mesalamine (Asacol) 1.2 g/day, and balsalazide 2 g/day had similar efficacy to sulfasalazine 2 g/day in maintaining remission [111, 113–115].

Toxicity of mesalamine, olsalazine, and balsalazide

Adverse events attributable to 5-ASA occur infrequently in patients with IBD treated with mesalamine, olsalazine, and balsalazide. Rare but serious events include pulmonary toxicity, pericarditis, hepatitis, and pancreatitis [116–119]. Interstitial nephritis has been reported in patients treated with mesalamine but whether the mesalamine causes the renal lesion is unclear [120–123]. Several studies have demonstrated that renal tubular proteinuria may be related to the disease activity of the IBD [124, 125]. Hanauer *et al.* reported on the safety of Asacol in 2940 patients with UC at doses up to 7.2 g/day for up to 5.2 years and concluded that there were no clinically significant dose or duration effects on renal function [126]. A minority of patients will experience worsening diarrhea and abdominal pain due to a hypersensitivity reaction to 5-ASA, and treatment with olsalazine will lead to an ileal secretory diarrhea in some patients, as discussed above [127].

Corticosteroid-based medications

Cortisone is produced by the adrenal cortex, and prednisone must be activated in the liver to hydrocortisone and prednisolone, respectively. Prednisolone and methylprednisolone have the same glucocorticoid and anti-inflammatory activity as hydrocortisone but less mineralocorticoid activity. Rectal administration of hydrocortisone, prednisolone, methylprednisolone, and betamethasone; oral administration of cortisone, prednisone, and prednisolone; and intravenous administration of prednisolone, methylprednisolone, and corticotropin are all methods of delivering corticosteroids for a systemic effect (Table 4). In contrast to systemically administered corticosteroids, rectal administration of beclomethasone, tixicortol, budesonide, and prednisolone metasulfobenzoate; and oral administration of fluticasone and controlled colonic release budesonide are all methods of delivering corticosteroids directly to the colon for a non-systemic effect (Table 4). Topical administration of beclomethasone, fluticasone, tixocortol, or budesonide to the colon results in a predominantly non-systemic effect because these newer corticosteroids have high affinities for the glucocorticoid receptors and undergo extensive first-pass hepatic metabolism. Topical administration of prednisolone metasulfobenzoate and tixocortol to the colon results in a predominantly non-systemic effect because they are poorly absorbed.

Oral corticosteroids (systemic effect)

In 1954 and 1955 Truelove and colleagues reported the preliminary and final results of a placebo-controlled trial which demonstrated that a tapering dose of cortisone beginning at 100 mg/day was effective in inducing remission in patients with mildly to severely active UC [14, 128]. Studies comparing sulfasalazine with a combination of low-dose oral and rectal steroids for active UC concluded that steroid therapy acted more rapidly, and perhaps was more effective, than sulfasalazine [22, 23]. A dose-ranging study demonstrated that prednisone 40–60 mg/day was more effective than 20 mg/day, and that 60 mg/day was no more effective than 40 mg/day but resulted in a greater frequency of side-effects [129]. A subsequent study demonstrated that a single daily dose of prednisone 40 mg was equally effective as prednisone 10 mg four times daily [130]. Placebo-controlled trials of cortisone 25 mg twice daily and prednisone

Table 4. Rectal corticosteroid preparations

Generic name	Proprietary name	Formulation	Sites of delivery	Site and mechanism of action	Daily dose (mg)	Indication
Hydrocortisone acetate	Anusol-HC 25 mg	Suppository 25 mg	Rectum	Systemic	50–100	Active proctitis
Hydrocortisone	Cortenema	Enema 100 mg/60ml	Distal to splenic flexure	Systemic	100	Active distal UC
Hydrocortisone acetate	Cortifoam	Foam 80 mg/ 900 mg foam	Distal rectum	Systemic	80–160	Active proctitis in the distal rectum
Hydrocortisone acetate	Colifoam*	Foam 125 ml/5 ml foam	Distal to splenic flexure	Systemic	125–250	Active distal UC
Hydrocortisone acetate	Proctocort	Suppository 30 mg	Rectum	Systemic	60–120	Active proctitis
Hydrocortisone acetate + pramoxine hydrochloride (local anesthetic)	Proctofoam HC	Topical aerosol 1% hydrocortisone (approx. 7 mg) 1% pramoxine (approx. 7 mg)	Anus, distal rectum	Systemic	7–28	Active procitis
Prednisolone phosphate	Predsol enema*	Enema 20 mg/100 ml	Distal to splenic flexure	Systemic	20	Active distal UC
Betamethasone valerate	Betnesol*	Enema 5 mg/100 ml	Distal to splenic flexure	Systemic	5	Active distal UC
Prednisolone metasulpho-benzoate	Predenema*	Enema 20 mg/100 ml	Distal to splenic flexure	Non-systemic: poorly absorbed	20	Active distal UC
Prednisolone metasulpho-benzoate	Predfoam*	Foam 20 mg/20 ml foam	Distal to splenic flexure	Non-systemic: poorly absorbed	20	Active distal UC
Tixocortol pivalate	Rectovalone*	Enema 250 mg/100 ml	Distal to splenic flexure	Non-systemic: poorly absorbed and first pass metabolism	250	Active distal UC
Budesonide	Entocort enema*	Enema 2 mg/100 ml	Distal to splenic flexure	Non-systemic: first pass metabolism	2	Active distal UC

*Indicates not available in the United States.

at doses of 15 mg/day or 40 mg every other day failed to demonstrate a maintenance benefit for oral corticosteroids [131–133].

Intravenous corticosteroids and corticotropin (ACTH)

Patients with severe UC and those refractory to oral coticosteroids are hospitalized and treated with intravenous corticosteroids. The rationale for this practice is altered corticosteroid absorption and metabolism in patients with UC. Oral administration of a 40 mg dose of prednisolone resulted in a lower peak and a slower rate of decrease in the plasma concentration of prednisolone in patients with severe UC compared with the time versus concentration curve observed in healthy volunteers; although total prednisolone absorption was similar [134]. In contrast, intravenous administration of prednisolone to patients with UC resulted in serum concentrations similar to volunteers [135]. Continuous infusion of prednisolone resulted in greater mean serum concentrations over time compared to bolus intravenous dosing; and both intravenous dosing strategies resulted in greater mean serum concentrations than oral dosing [135]. Uncontrolled studies have reported that approximately 60% of patients hospitalized for severe UC will respond to intravenous corticosteroid therapy [136–138]. Dosing strategies have included prednisolone 60 mg/day in four divided doses [136], betamethasone 3 mg twice daily [138], and hydrocortisone 300–400 mg/day [139–141]. Methylprednisolone 40–60 mg/day is preferred by many clinicians because it has minimal mineralocorticoid effect. There was no apparent advantage in increasing the dose of methylprednisolone to 1000 mg/day [142]. No placebo-controlled trials of intravenous corticosteroid therapy for severe UC have been performed.

A comparative study of intramuscular corticotropin (adrenal corticotropin hormone, ACTH) 80 U/day and cortisone 200 mg/day demonstrated a similar overall benefit in patients with active UC and in the subgroup of patients with a first attack, with a possible advantage for corticotropin in patients in patients with a relapse of established colitis [131]. Subsequent studies in patients with severe UC showed that overall the response to corticotropin 80–120 U/day is similar to hydrocortisone 300–400 mg/day, with trends toward better response to hydrocortisone in patients recently treated with cortico-

steroids and better response to corticotropin in patients not recently treated with corticosteroids [139–141].

Rectal corticosteroids (systemic effect)

Hydrocortisone, prednisolone, methylprednisolone, and betamethasone administered directly to the rectum as enemas or suppositories are well absorbed (similar to oral dose) [143, 144] and can result in suppression of the adrenal axis [49, 145–148]. Placebo-controlled trials have demonstrated efficacy for rectal administration of hydrocortisone 100 mg and prednisolone 5 mg in patients with active ulcerative proctitis or proctosigmoiditis [149–151]. Relatively small studies comparing rectally administered 5-ASA with rectal hydrocortisone 100–178 mg/day or prednisolone 20–30 mg/day, demonstrated similar efficacy rates in patients with active ulcerative proctitis or proctosigmoiditis [49–57, 59, 152, 153]. However, a meta-analysis suggested that rectally administered mesalamine is superior to rectal steroids for inducing remission [45]. Other small comparative studies have suggested that rectally administered hydrocortisone 100 mg, prednisolone 20–30 mg, or betamethasone 5 mg is equivalent to oral prednisone, oral sulfasalazine, and rectal 4-aminosalicylate, sodium cromoglycate, hydrocortisone foam 100 mg, and Ridogrel in patients with active ulcerative proctitis or proctosigmoiditis [23, 154–160]. Rectal hydrocortisone 100 mg every 2 nights each week for 6 months did not demonstrate a maintenance benefit compared with placebo [149].

Rectal corticosteroids (non-systemic effect)

Placebo-controlled trials demonstrated that budesonide administered rectally in a suspension enema at doses of 2–8 mg/day was effective in inducing remission in patients with mildly to moderately active left-sided UC, ulcerative proctosigmoiditis, and ulcerative proctitis; a 0.5 mg/day dose was not effective [48, 161–164]. Relatively small studies comparing rectally administered budesonide 2.0-2.5 mg/day with other rectal steroids (methylprednisolone 20 mg, prednisolone 25–31 mg, hydrocortisone 100–125 mg) demonstrated similar efficacy rates [147, 148, 163, 165–167]. Similarly, relatively small studies comparing rectally administered budesonide 2 mg/day with rectal 5-ASA 1–4 g/day demonstrated similar efficacy rates [58, 168]. Other small comparative studies have demonstrated that rectally administered non-systemic corticosteroids (prednisolone metasulfobenzoate 20 mg, beclomethasone 0.5–3 mg, tixocortol 250 mg) are equivalent to oral prednisolone, oral 5-ASA, rectal betamethasone 5 mg, rectal hydrocortisone 100 mg, rectal prednisolone 30 mg, rectal 5-ASA, and Ridogrel but not sucralfate [59, 157, 169–174]. Rectal budesonide 2 mg 2 nights each week for 6 months did not demonstrate a maintenance benefit compared with placebo [164].

Oral corticosteroids (non-systemic effect)

A placebo-controlled trial demonstrated that oral fluticasone 20 mg/day was not effective in inducing remission in patients with mildly to moderately active distal UC [175]. A study comparing oral fluticasone 20 mg/day with prednisolone 40 mg/day tapered to 10–20 mg/day in patients with active UC showed a greater benefit and more rapid response in the prednisolone group [176]. A comparative study of controlled colonic release budesonide 10 mg and prednisolone 40 mg/day and tapered to 0 mg demonstrated similar response rates in the two groups, with fewer side-effects in the budesonide group [177].

Toxicity of corticosteroids

Corticosteroid toxicity occurred frequently in patients with active CD treated with prednisone at an initial dose of 60 mg/day tapered over 17 weeks. Toxicities observed included a moon face in 47%, acne in 30%, infection in 27%, ecchymoses in 17%, hypertension in 15%, hirsutism in 7%, petechial bleeding in 6%, and striae in 6% [178]. A similar short-term toxicity profile can be expected in patients with UC.

Prolonged corticosteroid therapy at low to intermediate doses (doses frequently utilized in patients with steroid-dependent UC) is associated with the potential for multiple serious side-effects [179]. Hypertension occurs in up to 20% of patients [180]. New-onset diabetes mellitus requiring initiation of hypoglycemic therapy occurs at a frequency 2.23 times greater than in the general population [181]. Infection occurs at a frequency of 13–20% [182]. Osteonecrosis occurs at a frequency of approximately 5% [183]. The frequency of steroid-associated osteoporosis may be as high as 50% [184]. Neurologic side-effects occur often and can include myopathy at a frequency of 7% and psychosis at a frequency of 3–5% [185]. Ophthalmologic side-effects also occur often and can include cataracts at a frequency of 22% (dose-dependent) and glaucoma (frequency unclear, response genetically determined) [186, 187]. These frequencies of side-effects from prolonged exposure to corticosteroids were generally confirmed in a study of patients with UC who had undergone colectomy for medically refractory disease [188].

Immune modifer medications

The antimetabolites 6-mercaptopurine (Purinethol), its pro-drug azathioprine (Imuran), and methotrexate; the calcineurin inhibitors cyclosporine (Sandimmune, Neoral) and tacrolimus (FK506, Prograf); and the T-cell inhibitor mycophenolate mofetil (Cellcept) are all medications with immune modifier activity. The clinical pharmacology of these medications is reviewed in detail elsewhere in this book.

Azathioprine and 6-mercaptopurine

The first uncontrolled reports of the treatment of UC with 6-mercaptopurine (6-MP) and azathioprine (AZA) date back to the early 1960s [189–191]. A placebo-controlled trial of AZA 2.5 mg/kg per day in combination with a tapering dose of corticosteroids in 80 patients with active UC showed no benefit at 1 month and a trend toward a benefit at 1 year that was not significant [192, 193]. A comparative study of AZA 2.5 mg/kg per day versus sulfasalazine 65 mg/kg per day in patients with active UC showed similar efficacy for the two agents [194]. Two small placebo-controlled trials suggested that AZA at 1.5 mg/kg per day and 2.0–2.5 mg/kg per day was steroid-sparing in patients with steroid-dependent UC [195, 196]. Finally, a placebo-controlled withdrawal trial in patients maintained with AZA 100 mg/day demonstrated a maintenance of remission benefit [197]. These studies have been supplemented by five recently published open series of AZA and 6-MP therapy for UC [198–202]. Overall, these controlled and uncontrolled studies demonstrate that 6-MP and AZA are effective for steroid-sparing and maintenance of remission, and probably for inducing remission in patients with chronically active and treatment-refractory UC.

Adverse events occurring in patients with IBD treated with 6-MP and AZA include: pancreatitis

(3%); fever, rash, arthralgias, malaise, nausea, diarrhea, leukopenia (2–5%); thrombocytopenia, infection, and hepatitis [203–205]. It appears that there is not an increased risk of malignancy when AZA/6-MP is used as a monotherapy in IBD, and in three large series only one lymphoma occurred in 1308 patients [203, 206, 207].

Methotrexate

Two uncontrolled reports of the treatment of UC with methotrexate date occurred in the late 1980s and early 1990s [208, 209]. These studies suggested that intramuscular methotrexate 25 mg/week might be beneficial whereas oral methotrexate 15 mg/week appeared less promising. In patients with CD these uncontrolled observations regarding dose response and route of administration have been substantiated, with placebo-controlled trials demonstrating efficacy for intramuscular methotrexate 15–25 mg/week but not for oral methotrexate 12.5–15 mg/week [210–213]. In patients with UC a single placebo-controlled trial of oral methotrexate 12.5 mg/week did not demonstrate efficacy for either inducing or maintaining remission [214]. Whether intramuscular or subcutaneous methotrexate at doses of 15–25 mg/week would be effective for patients with UC is unknown, although the uncontrolled study discussed above is encouraging [208]. Based on the currently available evidence, patients with UC should not be treated with methotrexate.

Cyclosporine

The use of oral cyclosporine for UC was first reported in 1984 [215]. Subsequently multiple uncontrolled studies have reported a beneficial effect of cyclosporine administered at relatively high doses (5–15 mg/kg per day orally or 2–7 mg/kg per day intravenously) in patients with severe UC unresponsive to intravenous corticosteroids [216–221]. A placebo-controlled trial demonstrated that the addition of intravenous cyclosporine administered at a dose of 4 mg/kg per day as a continuous infusion to intravenous corticosteroids was effective for inducing remission in patients with severe steroid-refractory UC (82% versus 0% response) [222]. However, only 45% of the patients treated with cyclosporine had avoided colectomy after 6 months of follow-up [223], an observation confirmed by other uncontrolled studies [217–219, 224]. Maintenance therapy

with AZA or 6-MP in patients with UC who require treatment with cyclosporine appears to reduce the rate of relapse and colectomy [217, 225, 226]. Two more recent controlled trials have demonstrated that monotherapy with intravenous cyclosporine 4 mg/kg per day has efficacy comparable to intravenous corticosteroids or intravenous corticosteroids combined with intravenous cyclosporine in patients with active refractory UC [227, 228]. Overall, these studies demonstrate that intravenous cyclosporine is effective in inducing remission in patients with severe, steroid-refractory UC, but that the benefit is of limited duration unless AZA or 6-MP is initiated for maintenance of remission. Uncontrolled pilot studies of low-dose cyclosporine enemas suggested a potential beneficial effect in patients with active left-sided UC [229–232], but a placebo-controlled trial was negative [233].

Adverse events occurring in patients with IBD treated with cyclosporine include: hypertension, headaches, paresthesias, seizures, gingival hyperplasia, hypertrichosis, anaphylaxis, opportunistic infection, and renal insufficiency [217, 221, 234, 235]. There is an increased risk of opportunistic infection in patients with IBD treated with intravenous cyclosporine combined with corticosteroids and AZA or 6-MP; *Pneumocystis carinii* pneumonia, invasive apergillosis, lung abscess, mycotic aneurysm, and overwhelming sepsis have all been reported, with death rates ranging from 1% to 2% in larger series [217, 234–237]. There does not appear to be an increase in perioperative morbidity or mortality in patients with UC who receive intravenous cyclosporine and then require colectomy within a short period of time [238]. Another study reported that 20% of 99 patients with IBD treated with intravenous cyclosporine had a decrease in estimated renal function greater than 30% [239]. Results from a previous study suggest that patients with autoimmune diseases treated with intravenous cyclosporine have a significant likelihood of having histologic evidence of irreversible nephrotoxicity on renal biopsy (which to date has not been performed in patients with IBD) [240].

Tacrolimus

Small uncontrolled case series have suggested that tacrolimus may be beneficial in patients with refractory UC [241–243]. To date no controlled trials of tacrolimus have been performed in patients with UC. Given the similarities in mechanism of action to cyclosporine, it is reasonable to believe that tacrolimus would have similar efficacy and toxicity as cyclosporine in this patient group.

Mycophenolate mofetil

A small controlled trial reported that mycophenolate mofetil 15 mg/kg per day had similar efficacy as azathioprine 2.5 mg/kg per day in patients with chronically active CD [244]. In contrast, a small controlled trial of mycophenolate mofetil 20 mg/kg per day versus AZA 2.0 mg/kg per day in patients with chronically active UC demonstrated a superior outcome with azathioprine [245]. Similarly, an uncontrolled study did not report a benefit with mycophenolate in patients with UC [246]. Based on the currently available evidence, patients with UC should not be treated with mycophenolate mofetil.

Miscellaneous agents

4-Aminosalicylate (4-ASA)

4-Aminosalicylate (para-aminosalicylate, PAS) is an isomer of 5-ASA, the active component of sulfasalazine. Controlled trials with oral or rectal enema formulations of 4-ASA have shown superiority to placebo and equivalence to corticosteroids and 5-ASA [61, 154, 247–252].

Nicotine

Epidemiologic studies have demonstrated that non-smokers are at increased risk to develop UC. There are multiple potential mechanistic explanations for this beneficial effect [253]. Two placebo-controlled trials of transdermal nicotine patches reported that the highest tolerated dose of nicotine (up to 25 mg/24 h and 22 mg/24 h, respectively) was effective in patients with active UC [254, 255]. Similarly, a controlled trial of transdermal nicotine at the highest tolerated dose (up to 25 mg/16 h) showed equivalence to prednisolone for active UC [256]. A controlled trial using a lower dose of transdermal nicotine (15 mg/16 h) for maintenance of remission was negative [257]. Two uncontrolled studies of nicotine enemas for active distal UC reported a beneficial clinical effect and a reduction in both blood concentrations of nicotine (by first-pass hepatic metabolism of nicotine) and side-effects [258, 259]. Side-effects from transdermal nicotine occur frequently and include contact dermatitis, nausea, vomiting, headaches, sleep disturbance, diaphoresis, tremor, and lightheadedness [253–255].

Heparin

The inflammatory bowel diseases have been associated with a hypercoagulable state, and heparin has been proposed as a potential therapy in UC both for its anticoagulant and anti-inflammatory effects [260]. Four uncontrolled trials have suggested that both intravenous and subcutaneous heparin may be of benefit in patients with active UC [261–264]. A placebo-controlled trial of subcutaneous porcine heparin 10 000 units two or three times daily in patients with active UC reported a response rate of 42% for the heparin group and 19% for the placebo group [265]. Paradoxically, heparin appears to improve active UC rather than to exacerbate bleeding from the friable and ulcerated colonic mucosa.

Anti-tumor necrosis factor α antibody

Placebo-controlled trials have demonstrated that the mouse/human chimeric monoclonal antibody to tumor necrosis factor (TNF)-α, infliximab, and the humanized antibody to TNF, CDP571, are effective for the treatment of CD [266–269]. Two small studies conducted in patients with active UC have suggested a potential beneficial effect [270, 271]. Use of anti-TNF-α antibodies for the treatment of UC in clinical practice is premature at the present time.

Short-chain fatty acids

Luminal n-butyrate and other short-chain fatty acids (SCFA) produced by bacterial carbohydrate fermentation are the major luminal source of energy for colonocytes, and colonocytes from patients with UC may have reduced capacity to oxidize SCFA [272]. Two small and poorly designed controlled trials suggested that SCFA enemas may be beneficial in active distal UC [273, 274]. Subsequently, four placebo-controlled trials with larger sample sizes have been conducted [275–278]. Two of two studies comparing butyrate enemas to placebo [275, 276], and two of three studies comparing SCFA enemas to placebo [276–278] failed to demonstrate efficacy in patients with active left-sided UC.

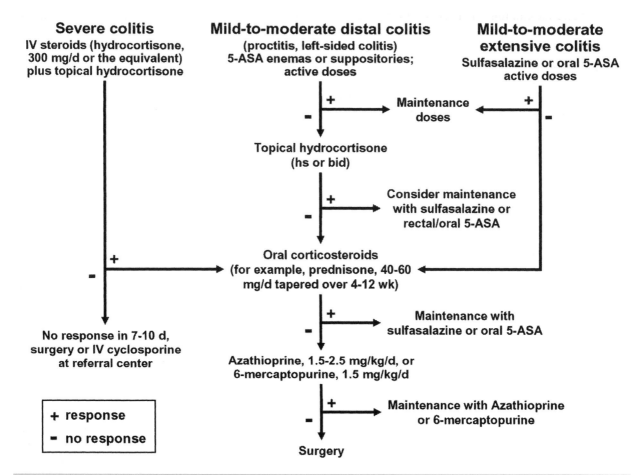

Figure 3. Suggested treatment guidelines for ulcerative colitis are offered in this algorithm. Reprinted after modification with permission from: Loftus EV, Sandborn WJ. Drug therapy for inflammatory bowel disease. Contemp Intern Med 1995; 7: 21–34.

avoided due to a high frequency of diarrhea in patients with active UC.

Sulfasalazine therapy is associated with more side effects but is less expensive than oral mesalamine or balsalazide. In one study the combination of mesalamine enemas 4 g/day and oral mesalamine 2.4 g/day was more effective than either agent alone [64] and another study demonstrated that combination therapy results in greater colonic tissue concentrations of 5-ASA [306]. Based on these data, many clinicians use rectal and oral mesalamine in combination to induce remission and then continue the oral mesalamine for maintenance of remission. In patients who fail to respond to oral or rectal mesalamine, sulfasalazine, or balsalazide, rectal corticosteroids can be tried. When all of these treatment approaches are ineffective, then oral prednisone is added to the other

oral and rectal therapies. The preferred initial prednisone dosing regimen is 40 mg/day administered as a single dose. The optimal tapering strategy has not been determined, but experienced clinicians will typically treat the patient with prednisone 40 mg/day for 2–4 weeks, then taper by 5 mg/week to a daily dose of 20 mg/day, then slow the taper to 2.5 mg/week until prednisone is discontinued.

Once the patients have achieved clinical remission, a long-term maintenance of remission strategy must be undertaken to avoid relapse. Again, patient preferences with regard to rectal therapy must be considered. Rectal mesalamine may be more efficacious than orally administered sulfasalazine or mesalamine for maintaining remission [71, 72]. Again, for patients who will accept rectal therapy, mesalamine suppositories (500 mg once or twice daily) for proctitis and mesalamine enemas (4 g nightly, every other night or every third night) for distal colitis are the treatment of choice. For patients who prefer oral therapy, oral mesalamine 1.6–4.8 g/day, sulfasalazine 2–4 g/day, olsalazine 1.0 g/day, and balsalazide 3.0–6.75 g/day are all equivalent first-line maintenance treatments [77, 78, 113]. Sulfasalazine therapy is associated with more side-effects but is less expensive than oral mesalamine, olsalazine, or balsalazide. In one study the combination of mesalamine enemas 4 g/day and oral mesalamine 1.2 g/day was more effective than oral mesalamine alone [73]; however, most patients find maintenance with both oral and rectal mesalamine unacceptable. There is not agreement among expert clinicians as to whether patients should taper rectal mesalamine to the least frequent effective dose interval, or oral mesalamine, sulfasalazine, olsalazine, or balsalazide to the lowest effective dose; or instead continue maintenance therapy with the same dose interval or dose required to induce remission. The former strategy is less expensive and may improve patient compliance by reducing the amount and frequency of medication administered, whereas the latter strategy may result in effective maintenance of remission in a larger proportion of patients. Rectal corticosteroids are not effective for maintaining remission and should not be used for that indication. Clinical trials have not demonstrated that oral corticosteroids at low to moderate doses are effective for maintaining remission. Nevertheless, some patients who respond to higher doses of prednisone will relapse with steroid tapering and can be maintained nearly asymptomatic by increasing the prednisone dose back to 15–25 mg/day. These patients are classified as 'steroid-dependent'. Because of the toxicity associated with long-term corticosteroid therapy, this is not an acceptable form of maintenance therapy and such patients should be treated for refractory disease as described below.

Extensive ulcerative colitis

Oral administration of medications that deliver 5-ASA to the colon is the treatment of choice in patients with mildly to moderately active extensive UC. Oral mesalamine 2.0-4.8 g/day, sulfasalazine 2–4 g/day, and balsalazide 6.75 g/day are all equivalent first-line treatments [77, 78, 112]. Sulfasalazine therapy is associated with more side effects but is less expensive than oral mesalamine or balsalazide. Olsalazine should be avoided due to a high frequency

of diarrhea in patients with active UC. There appears to be a dose response for oral medications that deliver 5-ASA [77]. There is not agreement among expert clinicians as to whether the preferred strategy is to begin with the lowest dose proven to be effective for active disease, increasing the dose in those patients who fail to respond; or rather to begin with the maximally tolerated dose and then titrate the dose downward when the patient comes into clinical remission. When treatment with one of these agents at an optimal dose has failed, then oral prednisone is added to the oral mesalamine, sulfasalazine, or balsalazide. The preferred initial prednisone dosing regimen is 40 mg/day administered as a single dose, with tapering as described above for proctitis/distal UC.

Once the patients have achieved clinical remission, a long-term maintenance of remission strategy must be undertaken to avoid relapse. Oral therapy with a drug that delivers 5-ASA to the colon is the treatment of choice. Oral mesalamine 1.6–4.8 g/day, sulfasalazine 2–4 g/day, olsalazine 1.0 g/day, and balsalazide 3.0–6.75 g/day are all equivalent first-line maintenance treatments [77, 78, 113]. Sulfasalazine therapy is associated with more side-effects but is less expensive than oral mesalamine, olsalazine, or balsalazide. As described above for patients with proctitis/distal UC, there is not agreement among expert clinicians as to whether patients with extensive UC should taper oral mesalamine, sulfasalazine, olsalazine, or balsalazide to the lowest effective dose; or instead continue maintenance therapy with the same dose required to induce remission. Clinical trials have demonstrated that oral corticosteroids at low to moderate doses are not effective for maintaining remission. As discussed above for proctitis/distal UC, treatment with prednisone 15–25 mg/day in patients with extensive UC who are 'steroid-dependent' is not acceptable because of the toxicity associated with long-term corticosteroid therapy. Such patients should be treated for refractory disease as described below.

Refractory ulcerative colitis

Patients with mildly to moderately active UC who fail to respond to oral prednisone at a dose of 40–60 mg/day in combination with mesalamine, sulfasalazine, or balsalazide can be considered to have refractory UC. One potential approach to treatment is hospitalization for intravenous administration of corticosteroids. The rationale for this treatment approach is a clinical trial that demonstrated greater mean serum prednisolone concentrations with intravenous compared to oral dosing [135].

The mainstay of treatment in patients who have failed combination therapy with maximal doses of oral and rectal mesalamine and oral corticosteroids is AZA or 6-MP. The prodrug AZA is approximately 50% 6-MP by molecular weight, requiring a conversion factor of 2 to convert a dose of AZA to a therapeutically equivalent dose of 6-MP. The doses of AZA and 6-MP shown to be effective for UC and CD in controlled trials range from 100 mg/day to 3.0 mg/kg per day. For patients with normal AZA and 6-MP metabolism (based on normal thiopurine methyltransferase (TPMT) activity), a starting AZA dose of 2.0–2.5 mg/kg per day or 6-MP dose of 1.0–1.5 mg/kg per day is recommended (see Chapter 25 on Clinical pharmacology for further details). Patients with decreased TPMT activity should have their starting AZA or 6-MP dose reduced by 50% to 1.0–1.25 mg/kg per day and 0.5–0.75 mg/kg per day, respectively. Patients with absent TPMT activity should not be treated with AZA or 6-MP. AZA and 6-MP are slow-acting antimetabolite drugs, requiring at least 1–2 months and perhaps 3–4 months to reach the full clinical effect. Thus, concomitant therapy with corticosteroids should not be tapered below a dose of 15–20 mg/day for 2–3 months in patients who are beginning AZA or 6-MP. Concomitant therapy with mesalamine, sulfasalazine, olsalazine, or balsalazide is continued in most cases. Measurement of a total leukocyte count every 1–2 months as long as patients are receiving AZA or 6-MP is mandatory to monitor for leukopenia. Indications for treatment with AZA or 6-MP in patients with UC include: induction of remission in steroid-refractory disease; steroid sparing in steroid-dependent disease; and maintenance of remission in patients who have failed maintenance therapy with high-dose mesalamine, sulfasalazine, olsalazine, or balsalazide.

Transdermal nicotine may be of benefit as an alternative to AZA or 6-MP in patients with active UC refractory to mesalamine, sulfasalazine, olsalazine, balsalazide, and corticosteroids. Because nonsmokers frequently experience side-effects from nicotine when initally beginning therapy, a dose escalation strategy in which patients are treated with 7 mg/day of transdermal nicotine for 1 week, then 14 mg/day for 1 week, then 21 mg/day is recommended. Clinical trials have demonstrated efficacy for transdermal nicotine over 4–6 weeks of treatment. The role of maintenance therapy with transdermal nicotine beyond 6 weeks is unknown.

Severe ulcerative colitis

Severe UC is defined using the 'Truelove and Witts criteria' (Table 1) [14]. Toxic (fulminant) colitis is defined as the sudden extension of mucosal inflammation through all layers of the colonic wall to the serosa and presents clinically as focal visceral tenderness to deep palpation. Megacolon is defined as dilation of the colon (5–6 cm or more) demonstrated by X-ray and presents clinically as abdominal distension, decreased or absent bowel sounds, and in some cases decreased stool frequency. Approximately 10% of all patients with UC will develop a severe flare at some point in their disease course, whereas only 1–2% progress to toxic (fulminant) colitis and/or megacolon. The mortality for severe UC is 2%, but remains approximately 30% for toxic (fulminant) colitis.

In patients with severe or toxic colitis, hospitalization is mandatory. The treatment regimen outlined by Truelove and Jewell, consisting of intravenous fluids, electrolyte supplements, bowel rest, transfusion if indicated, intravenous antibiotics, intravenous corticosteroids, and rectal corticosteroids, remains in use today [136], although controlled trials have demonstrated that intravenous antibiotics are not of benefit. Sixty percent of patients treated with this regimen will be symptom-free by the end of 5 days, 15% will have significant improvement, and 25% will not improve and should be treated with cyclosporine or surgery.

Most patients hospitalized with severe UC should continue to receive a normal diet. Two randomized controlled trials have demonstrated that bowel rest does not affect the outcome of severe UC in patients treated with intravenous prednisone [307, 308]. Patients with toxic colitis or megacolon should be made nil per os because of the potential for eminent surgical intervention. Peripheral or central intravenous nutrition should be instituted if there is evidence of malnutrition. The goal of intravenous nutrition is to replace nutritional deficits rather than for any primary therapeutic benefit.

Factors which have been implicated in the development of toxic megacolon should be avoided including barium enema, narcotic antidiarrheals (codeine, tincture of opium, loperamide, and diphenoxylate), anticholinergic agents, antidepressants, and electrolyte imbalance. Patients should be monitored frequently. Abdominal X-ray may be indicated daily in patients with severe colitis and twice daily in patients with megacolon. Frequent physical examination by both an experienced gastroenterologist and surgeon is also of great importance, as is frequent monitoring of the complete blood count, electrolytes, and nutritional parameters.

Mesalamine, sulfasalazine, olsalazine, and balsalazide should in general be temporarily discontinued in patients hospitalized with severe or toxic UC because of the possibility of a drug-induced exacerbation of colitis which can be indistinguishable from a flare of colitis. Controlled clinical trials have demonstrated that antibiotics have no role in the treatment of severe UC unless a specific infection is suspected. Nevertheless, many authorities continue to advocate broad-spectrum antibiotic therapy with either a combination of metronidazole, an aminoglycoside, and a broad-spectrum penicillin or with a third-generation cephalosporine. Intravenous corticosteroid therapy should be initiated with hydrocortisone 300–400 mg/day or methylprednisolone 40–60 mg/day. There are no controlled data to determine the frequency of administration but a pharmacokinetic study showed that corticosteroid blood levels are better maintained within the presumptive therapeutic range when administered as a continuous infusion rather than as intermittent bolus therapy. For patients who have not been recently treated with steroids there is some evidence to suggest that they may respond better to intravenous ACTH administered at a dose of 40 units every 8 h than to conventional corticosteroids.

Patients with severe UC who fail to respond to 7–10 days of intravenous corticosteroid therapy may be considered for 'rescue' therapy with intravenous cyclosporine at a dose of 4 mg/kg per day administered as a continuous infusion over 24 h. This dose should be adjusted to maintain a whole blood cyclosporine A concentration (high-performance liquid chromatography or monoclonal radioimmunoassay) of approximately 300–350 ng/ml. Patients with known infection, hypocholesterolemia (risk of seizure), or significant renal insufficiency should not be treated with cyclosporine. Significant abdominal pain is probably a relative indication since this may represent transmural inflammation and potentially early perforation. Patients who fail to respond within 7–10 days should undergo colectomy. Patients who respond to intravenous cyclosporine should be discharged on oral cyclosporine at a dose approximately twice the total daily dose that they received

intravenously. This may be administered as standard oral cyclosporine (Sandimmune) or as the microemulsion oral formulation of cyclosporine (Neoral). Again, the oral cyclosporine dose should be adjusted to maintain a whole blood concentration of cyclosporine A in the range of approximately 300–350 ng/ml. Oral cyclosporine should be overlapped for 3–4 months with the slow-acting immune modifier agents AZA or 6-MP, which are then continued long-term for maintenance of remission. Corticosteroids can be tapered over 2–3 months. Prophylaxis for *Pneumocystis carrini* pneumonia with trimethoprim/sulfomethoxazole is recommended while patients are receiving triple-drug immunosuppression.

Conclusions

Initial treatment of mild to moderately active UC may be sulfasalazine, oral or rectal mesalamine, balsalazide, corticosteroid enemas, or oral corticosteroids. Patients with persistent mild to moderate symptoms of active UC in spite of these therapies (treatment-refractory) may require AZA/6-MP, and in some cases intravenous corticosteroid or transdermal nicotine. Patients with severely active UC should be treated with intravenous conventional corticosteroids, and intravenous cyclosporine may be considered in those who do not respond. Remission should be maintained with sulfasalazine, oral or rectal mesalamine, olsalazine, or balsalazide, and in some cases with AZA/6-MP.

References

1. Tremaine WJ, Sandborn WJ. Practice guidelines for inflammatory bowel disease: an instrument for assessment. Mayo Clin Proc 1999; 74: 495–501.
2. Miner PB Jr, Peppercorn MA, Targan SR. A rational approach to 5-aminosalicylic acid therapy in ulcerative colitis. Hosp Pract (Off Ed) 1993; 28(Suppl.)3: 1–24.
3. Loftus EV Jr, Sandborn WJ. Drug therapy for inflammatory bowel disease. Contemp Intern Med 1995; 7: 21–34.
4. Williams CN, Haber G, Aquino JA. Double-blind, placebo-controlled evaluation of 5-ASA suppositories in active distal proctitis and measurement of extent of spread using 99mTc-labeled 5-ASA suppositories. Dig Dis Sci 1987; 32: 71–5S.
5. Jay M, Beihn RM, Digenis GA, Deland FH, Caldwell L, Mlodozeniec AR. Disposition of radiolabelled suppositories in humans. J Pharm Pharmacol 1985; 37: 266–8.
6. Chapman NJ, Brown ML, Phillips SF *et al*. Distribution of mesalamine enemas in patients with active distal ulcerative colitis. Mayo Clin Proc 1992; 67: 245–8.
7. Tiel-van Buul MM, Mulder CJ, van Royen EA, Wiltink EH, Tytgat GN. Retrograde spread of mesalazine (5-aminosalicylic acid)-containing enema in patients with ulcerative colitis. Clin Pharmacokinet 1991; 20: 247–51.

8. Jay M, Digenis GA, Foster TS, Antonow DR. Retrograde spreading of hydrocortisone enema in inflammatory bowel disease. Dig Dis Sci 1986; 31: 139–44.

9. Campieri M, Lanfranchi GA, Brignola C *et al.* Retrograde spread of 5-aminosalicylic acid enemas in patients with active ulcerative colitis. Dis Colon Rectum 1986; 29: 108–10.

10. Kruis W, Bull U, Eisenburg J, Paumgartner G. Retrograde colonic spread of sulphasalazine enemas. Scand J Gastroenterol 1982; 17: 933–8.

11. Nyman-Pantelidis M, Nilsson A, Wagner ZG, Borga O. Pharmacokinetics and retrograde colonic spread of budesonide enemas in patients with distal ulcerative colitis. Aliment Pharmacol Ther 1994; 8: 617–22.

12. Swarbrick ET, Loose H, Lennard-Jones JE. Enema volume as an important factor in successful topical corticosteroid treatment of colitis. Proc R Soc Med 1974; 67: 753–4.

13. van Bodegraven AA, Boer RO, Lourens J, Tuynman HA, Sindram JW. Distribution of mesalazine enemas in active and quiescent ulcerative colitis. Aliment Pharmacol Ther 1996; 10: 327–32.

14. Truelove SC, Witts LJ. Cortisone in ulcerative colitis. Final report on a therapeutic trial. Br Med J 1955; 2: 1041–8.

15. Sutherland LR, Martin F, Greer S *et al.* 5-Aminosalicylic acid enema in the treatment of distal ulcerative colitis, proctosigmoiditis, and proctitis. Gastroenterology 1987; 92: 1894–8.

16. Schroeder KW, Tremaine WJ, Ilstrup DM. Coated oral 5-aminosalicylic acid therapy for mildly to moderately active ulcerative colitis. A randomized study. N Engl J Med 1987; 317: 1625–9.

17. Svartz N. Salazopyrin, a new sulfanilamide preparation: A. Therapeutic results in rheumatic polyarthritis. B. Therapeutic results in ulcerative colitis. C. Toxic manifestations in treatment with sulfanilamide preparation. Acta Med Scand 1942; 110: 557–90.

18. Baron JH, Connell AM, Lennard-Jones JE, Jones FA. Sulphasalazine and salicylazosulphadimidine in ulcerative colitis. Lancet 1962; 1: 1094–6.

19. Dick AP, Grayson MJ, Carpenter RG, Petrie A. Controlled trial of sulphasalazine in the treatment of ulcerative colitis. Gut 1964; 5: 437–42.

20. Palmer KR, Goepel JR, Holdsworth CD. Sulphasalazine retention enemas in ulcerative colitis: a double-blind trial. Br Med J (Clin Res Ed) 1981; 282: 1571–3.

21. Fruhmorgen P, Demling L. On the efficacy of ready-made-up commercially available salicylazosulphapyridine enemas in the treatment of proctitis, proctosigmoiditis and ulcerative colitis involving rectum, sigmoid and descending colon. Hepatogastroenterology 1980; 27: 473–6.

22. Truelove SC, Watkinson G, Draper G. Comparison of corticosteroid and sulphasalazine in the treatment of ulcerative colitis. Br Med J 1962; 2: 1708–11.

23. Lennard-Jones JE, Longmore AJ, Newell AC *et al.* An assessment of prednisone, salazopyrine and topical hydrocortisone hemisuccinate used as outpatient treatment for ulcerative colitis. Gut 1960; 1: 217–22.

24. Misiewicz JJ, Lennard-Jones JE, Connell AM, Parson JH, Avery Jones F. Controlled trial of sulphasalazine in maintenance therapy for ulcerative colitis. Lancet 1965; 1: 185–8.

25. Dissanayake AS, Truelove SC. A controlled therapeutic trial of long-term maintenance treatment of ulcerative colitis with sulphazalazine (Salazopyrin). Gut 1973; 14: 923–6.

26. Azad Khan AK, Howes DT, Piris J, Truelove SC. Optimum dose of sulphasalazine for maintenance treatment in ulcerative colitis. Gut 1980; 21: 232–40.

27. Riis P, Anthonisen P, Wulff HR, Folkenborg O, Bonnevie O, Binder V. The prophylactic effect of salazosulphapyridine in ulcerative colitis during long-term treatment. A double-

blind trial on patients asymptomatic for one year. Scand J Gastroenterol 1973; 8: 71–4.

28. Davies PS, Rhodes J. Maintenance of remission in ulcerative colitis with sulphasalazine or a high-fibre diet: a clinical trial. Br Med J 1978; 1: 1524–5.

29. Dronfield MW, Langman MJ. Comparative trial of sulphasalazine and oral sodium cromoglycate in the maintenance of remission in ulcerative colitis. Gut 1978; 19: 1136–9.

30. Willoughby CP, Heyworth MF, Piris J, Truelove SC. Comparison of disodium cromoglycate and sulphasalazine as maintenance therapy for ulcerative colitis. Lancet 1979; 1: 119–22.

31. Davies PS, Rhodes J, Counsell B, Evans BK. Maintenance of remission in ulcerative colitis. Effect of an orally absorbed mast cell stabilizer. Am J Gastroenterol 1980; 74: 150–3.

32. Das KM, Eastwood MA, McMAnus JPA, Sircus W. The metabolism of salicylazosulphapyridine in ulcerative colitis II. The relationship between metabolites and the progress of the disease studied in out-patients. Gut 1973; 14: 637–41.

33. Peppercorn MA, Goldman P. The role of intestinal bacteria in the metabolism of salicylazosulfapyridine. J Pharmacol Exp Ther 1972; 181: 555–62.

34. Azad Khan AK, Guthrie G, Johnston HH, Truelove SC, Williamson DH. Tissue and bacterial splitting of sulphasalazine. Clin Sci 1983; 64: 349–54.

35. Das KM, Eastwood MA, McManus JP, Sircus W. The metabolism of salicylazosulphapyridine in ulcerative colitis. I. The relationship between metabolites and the response to treatment in inpatients. Gut 1973; 14: 631–41.

36. Azad Khan AK, Piris J, Truelove SC. An experiment to determine the active therapeutic moiety of sulphasalazine. Lancet 1977; 2: 892–5.

37. van Hees PA, Bakker JH, van Tongeren JH. Effect of sulphapyridine, 5-aminosalicylic acid, and placebo in patients with idiopathic proctitis: a study to determine the active therapeutic moiety of sulphasalazine. Gut 1980; 21: 632–5.

38. Klotz U, Maier K, Fischer C, Heinkel K. Therapeutic efficacy of sulfasalazine and its metabolites in patients with ulcerative colitis and Crohn's disease. N Engl J Med 1980; 303: 1499–502.

39. Das KM, Eastwood MA, McManus JP, Sircus W. Adverse reactions during salicylazosulfapyridine therapy and the relation with drug metabolism and acetylator phenotype. N Engl J Med 1973; 289: 491–5.

40. Taffet SL, Das KM. Sulfasalazine. Adverse effects and desensitization. Dig Dis Sci 1983; 28: 833–42.

41. Shanahan F, Targan S. Sulfasalazine and salicylate-induced exacerbation of ulcerative colitis [Letter]. N Engl J Med 1987; 317: 455.

42. Campieri M, Gionchetti P, Belluzzi A *et al.* Optimum dosage of 5-aminosalicylic acid as rectal enemas in patients with active ulcerative colitis. Gut 1991; 32: 929–31.

43. Hanauer SB. Dose-ranging study of mesalamine (PENTASA) enemas in the treatment of acute ulcerative proctosigmoiditis: results of a multicentered placebo- controlled trial. The U.S. PENTASA Enema Study Group. Inflam Bowel Dis 1998; 4: 79–83.

44. Sutherland LR, Martin F. 5-Aminosalicylic acid enemas in treatment of distal ulcerative colitis and proctitis in Canada. Dig Dis Sci 1987; 32: 64–6S.

45. Marshall JK, Irvine EJ. Rectal corticosteroids versus alternative treatments in ulcerative colitis: a meta-analysis. Gut 1997; 40: 775–81.

46. Marteau P, Florent C. Comparative, open, randomized trial of the efficacy and tolerance of slow-release 5-ASA suppositories once daily versus conventional 5-ASA suppositories twice daily in the treatment of active cryptogenic proctitis:

French Pentasa Study Group. Am J Gastroenterol 2000; 95: 166–70.

47. Campieri M, Paoluzi P, D'Albasio G, Brunetti G, Pera A, Barbara L. Better quality of therapy with 5-ASA colonic foam in active ulcerative colitis. A multicenter comparative trial with 5-ASA enema. Dig Dis Sci 1993; 38: 1843–50.

48. Gionchetti P, Rizzello F, Venturi A *et al.* Comparison of mesalazine suppositories in proctitis and distal proctosigmoiditis. Aliment Pharmacol Ther 1997; 11: 1053–7.

49. Danish 5-ASA Group. Topical 5-aminosalicylic acid versus prednisolone in ulcerative proctosigmoiditis. A randomized, double-blind multicenter trial. Dig Dis Sci 1987; 32: 598–602.

50. Campieri M, Lanfranchi GA, Bazzocchi G G *et al.* Treatment of ulcerative colitis with high-dose 5-aminosalicylic acid enemas. Lancet 1981; 2: 270–1.

51. Porro GB, Ardizzone S, Petrillo M, Fasoli A, Molteni P, Imbesi V. Low Pentasa dosage versus hydrocortisone in the topical treatment of active ulcerative colitis: a randomized, double-blind study. Am J Gastroenterol 1995; 90: 736–9.

52. Mulder CJ, Tytgat GN, Wiltink EH, Houthoff HJ. Comparison of 5-aminosalicylic acid (3 g) and prednisolone phosphate sodium enemas (30 mg) in the treatment of distal ulcerative colitis. A prospective, randomized, double-blind trial. Scand J Gastroenterol 1988; 23: 1005–8.

53. Farup PG, Hovde O, Halvorsen FA, Raknerud N, Brodin U. Mesalazine suppositories versus hydrocortisone foam in patients with distal ulcerative colitis. A comparison of the efficacy and practicality of two topical treatment regimens. Scand J Gastroenterol 1995; 30: 164–70.

54. Friedman LS, Richter JM, Kirkham SE, DeMonaco HJ, May RJ. 5-Aminosalicylic acid enemas in refractory distal ulcerative colitis: a randomized, controlled trial. Am J Gastroenterol 1986; 81: 412–18.

55. Lee FI, Jewell DP, Mani V *et al.* A randomised trial comparing mesalazine and prednisolone foam enemas in patients with acute distal ulcerative colitis. Gut 1996; 38: 229–33.

56. Campieri M, Gionchetti P, Belluzzi A *et al.* Efficacy of 5-aminosalicylic acid enemas versus hydrocortisone enemas in ulcerative colitis. Dig Dis Sci 1987; 32: 67–70S.

57. Lucidarme D, Marteau P, Foucault M, Vautrin B, Filoche B. Efficacy and tolerance of mesalazine suppositories vs. hydrocortisone foam in proctitis. Aliment Pharmacol Ther 1997; 11: 335–40.

58. Lemann M, Galian A, Rutgeerts P *et al.* Comparison of budesonide and 5-aminosalicylic acid enemas in active distal ulcerative colitis. Aliment Pharmacol Ther 1995; 9: 557–62.

59. Cobden I, al Mardini H, Zaitoun A, Record CO. Is topical therapy necessary in acute distal colitis? Double-blind comparison of high-dose oral mesalazine versus steroid enemas in the treatment of active distal ulcerative colitis. Aliment Pharmacol Ther 1991; 5: 513–22.

60. Kam L, Cohen H, Dooley C, Rubin P, Orchard J. A comparison of mesalazine suspension enema and oral sulfasalazine for treatment of active distal ulcerative colitis in adults. Am J Gastroenterol 1996; 91: 1338–42.

61. Campieri M, Lanfranchi GA, Bertoni F *et al.* A double-blind clinical trial to compare the effects of 4-aminosalicylic acid to 5-aminosalicylic acid in topical treatment of ulcerative colitis. Digestion 1984; 29: 204–8.

62. Pullan RD, Ganesh S, Mani V *et al.* Comparison of bismuth citrate and 5-aminosalicylic acid enemas in distal ulcerative colitis: a controlled trial. Gut 1993; 34: 676–9.

63. Campieri M, Gionchetti P, Belluzzi A *et al.* Sucralfate, 5-aminosalicylic acid and placebo enemas in the treatment of distal ulcerative colitis. Eur J Gastroenterol Hepatol 1991; 3: 41–4.

64. Safdi M, DeMicco M, Sninsky C *et al.* A double-blind comparison of oral versus rectal mesalamine versus combination therapy in the treatment of distal ulcerative colitis. Am J Gastroenterol 1997; 92: 1867–71.

65. Biddle WL, Greenberger NJ, Swan JT, McPhee MS, Miner PB Jr. 5-Aminosalicylic acid enemas: effective agent in maintaining remission in left-sided ulcerative colitis [Published erratum appears in Gastroenterology 1989; 96: 1630]. Gastroenterology 1988; 94: 1075–9.

66. Miner P, Daly R, Nester T and the Rowasa Study Group. The effect of varying the dose intervals of mesalamine enemas for the prevention of relapse in distal ulcerative colitis. Gastroenterology 1994; 106: A736.

67. D'Arienzo A, Panarese A, D'Armiento FP *et al.* 5-Aminosalicylic acid suppositories in the maintenance of remission in idiopathic proctitis or proctosigmoiditis: a double-blind placebo-controlled clinical trial. Am J Gastroenterol 1990; 85: 1079–82.

68. D'Albasio G, Paoluzi P, Campieri M *et al.* Maintenance treatment of ulcerative proctitis with mesalazine suppositories: a double-blind placebo-controlled trial. Italian IBD Study Group. Am J Gastroenterol 1998; 93: 799–803.

69. Marteau P, Crand J, Foucault M, Rambaud JC. Use of mesalazine slow release suppositories 1 g three times per week to maintain remission of ulcerative proctitis: a randomised double blind placebo controlled multicentre study. Gut 1998; 42: 195–9.

70. Sutherland L, Martin F. 5-Aminosalicylic acid enemas in the maintenance of distal ulcerative colitis and proctitis. Can J Gastroenterol 1987; 1: 3–6.

71. D'Albasio G, Trallori G, Ghetti A *et al.* Intermittent therapy with high-dose 5-aminosalicylic acid enemas for maintaining remission in ulcerative proctosigmoiditis. Dis Colon Rectum 1990; 33: 394–7.

72. Mantzaris GJ, Hatzis A, Petraki K, Spiliadi C, Triantaphyllou G. Intermittent therapy with high-dose 5-aminosalicylic acid enemas maintains remission in ulcerative proctitis and proctosigmoiditis. Dis Colon Rectum 1994; 37: 58–62.

73. D'Albasio G, Pacini F, Camarri E *et al.* Combined therapy with 5-aminosalicylic acid tablets and enemas for maintaining remission in ulcerative colitis: a randomized double-blind study. Am J Gastroenterol 1997; 92: 1143–7.

74. Sninsky CA, Cort DH, Shanahan F *et al.* Oral mesalamine (Asacol) for mildly to moderately active ulcerative colitis. A multicenter study. Ann Intern Med 1991; 115: 350–5.

75. Sutherland LR, Robinson M, Onstad G *et al.* A double-blind, placebo controlled, multicenter study of the efficacy and safety of 5-aminosalicylic acid tablets in the treatment of ulcerative colitis. Can J Gastroenterol 1990; 4: 463–7.

76. Hanauer S, Schwartz J, Robinson M *et al.* Mesalamine capsules for treatment of active ulcerative colitis: results of a controlled trial. Pentasa Study Group. Am J Gastroenterol 1993; 88: 1188–97.

77. Sutherland LR, May GR, Shaffer EA. Sulfasalazine revisited: a meta-analysis of 5-aminosalicylic acid in the treatment of ulcerative colitis. Ann Intern Med 1993; 118: 540–9.

78. Sutherland LR, Roth DE, Beck PL. Alternatives to sulfasalazine: a meta-analysis of 5-ASA in the treatment of ulcerative colitis. Inflam Bowel Dis 1997; 3: 65–78.

79. Munakata A, Yoshida Y, Muto T *et al.* Double-blind comparative study of sulfasalazine and controlled-release mesalazine tablets in the treatment of active ulcerative colitis. J Gastroenterol 1995; 30(Suppl. 8): 108–11.

80. Rachmilewitz D. Coated mesalazine (5-aminosalicylic acid) versus sulphasalazine in the treatment of active ulcerative colitis: a randomised trial. Br Med J 1989; 298: 82–6.

81. Riley SA, Mani V, Goodman MJ, Herd ME, Dutt S, Turnberg LA. Comparison of delayed release 5 aminosalicylic acid (mesalazine) and sulphasalazine in the treatment of

156. Grace RH, Gent AE, Hellier MD. Comparative trial of sodium cromoglycate enemas with prednisolone enemas in the treatment of ulcerative colitis. Gut 1987; 28: 88–92.
157. Halpern Z, Sold O, Baratz M, Konikoff F, Halak A, Gilat T. A controlled trial of beclomethasone versus betamethasone enemas in distal ulcerative colitis. J Clin Gastroenterol 1991; 13: 38–41.
158. Lennard-Jones JE. Betamethasone 17-valerate and prednisolone 21-phosphate retention enemas in proctocolitis. Br Med J 1971; 3: 84–6.
159. Ruddell WS, Dickinson RJ, Dixon MF, Axon AT. Treatment of distal ulcerative colitis (proctosigmoiditis) in relapse: comparison of hydrocortisone enemas and rectal hydrocortisone foam. Gut 1980; 21: 885–9.
160. Van Outryve M, Huble F, Van Eeghem P, De Vos M. Comaprison of ridogrel versus prednisolone, both administered rectally, for the treatment of active ulcerative colitis. Gastroenterology 1996; 110: A1035.
161. Danielsson A, Lofberg R, Persson T et al. A steroid enema, budesonide, lacking systemic effects for the treatment of distal ulcerative colitis or proctitis. Scand J Gastroenterol 1992; 27: 9–12.
162. Hanauer SB, Robinson M, Pruitt R et al. Budesonide enema for the treatment of active, distal ulcerative colitis and proctitis: a dose-ranging study. U.S. Budesonide Enema Study Group. Gastroenterology 1998; 115: 525–32.
163. Bayless T, Sninsky C, US Budesonide Enema Study Group. Budesonide enema is an effective alternative to hydrocortisone enema in active distal ulcerative colitis. Gastroenterology 1995; 108: A778.
164. Lindgren S, Suhr O, Persson T, Pantzar N. Treatment of active distal ulcerative colitis (UC) and maintenance of remission with Entocort enema: a randomised controlled dosage study. Gut 1997; 41: A223.
165. Danish Budesonide Study Group. Budesonide enema in distal ulcerative colitis. A randomized dose–response trial with prednisolone enema as positive control. Scand J Gastroenterol 1991; 26: 1225–30.
166. Lofberg R, Ostergaard TO, Langholz E et al. Budesonide versus prednisolone retention enemas in active distal ulcerative colitis [Published erratum appears in Aliment Pharmacol Ther 1995; 9: 213]. Aliment Pharmacol Ther 1994; 8: 623–9.
167. Tarpila S, Turunen U, Seppala K et al. Budesonide enema in active haemorrhagic proctitis – a controlled trial against hydrocortisone foam enema. Aliment Pharmacol Ther 1994; 8: 591–5.
168. Lamers C, Meijer J, Engels L et al. Comparative study of the topically acting glucocorticoid budesonide and 5-aminosalicylic acid enema therapy of proctitis and proctosigmoiditis. Gastroenterology 1991; 100: A223.
169. Hamilton I, Pinder IF, Dickinson RJ, Ruddell WS, Dixon MF, Axon AT. A comparison of prednisolone enemas with low-dose oral prednisolone in the treatment of acute distal ulcerative colitis. Dis Colon Rectum 1984; 27: 701–2.
170. Hanauer SB, Kirsner JB, Barrett WE. The treatment of left-sided ulcerative colitis with tixicortol pivalate. Gastroenterology 1986; A1449.
171. Mulder CJ, Endert E, van der HH et al. Comparison of beclomethasone dipropionate (2 and 3 mg) and prednisolone sodium phosphate enemas (30 mg) in the treatment of ulcerative proctitis. An adrenocortical approach. Neth J Med 1989; 35: 18–24.
172. Mulder CJ, Fockens P, Van der Heide H, Tytgat GNJ. A controlled randomized trial of beclomethasone dipropionate (3 mg) versus 5-ASA (1 g) versus the combination of both (3 mg/1 g) as retention enemas in active distal ulcerative colitis. Gastroenterology 1994; 106: A739.
173. Riley SA, Gupta I, Mani V. A comparison of sucralfate and prednisolone enemas in the treatment of active distal ulcerative colitis. Scand J Gastroenterol 1989; 24: 1014–18.
174. van der Heide H, van den Brandt-Gradel V, Tytgat GN et al. Comparison of beclomethasone dipropionate and prednisolone 21-phosphate enemas in the treatment of ulcerative proctitis. J Clin Gastroenterol 1988; 10: 169–72.
175. Angus P, Snook JA, Reid M, Jewell DP. Oral fluticasone propionate in active distal ulcerative colitis. Gut 1992; 33: 711–14.
176. Hawthorne AB, Record CO, Holdsworth CD et al. Double blind trial of oral fluticasone propionate v prednisolone in the treatment of active ulcerative colitis. Gut 1993; 34: 125–8.
177. Lofberg R, Danielsson A, Suhr O et al. Oral budesonide versus prednisolone in patients with active extensive and left-sided ulcerative colitis. Gastroenterology 1996; 110: 1713–18.
178. Singleton JW, Law DH, Kelley ML Jr, Mekhjian HS, Sturdevant RA. National Cooperative Crohn's Disease Study: adverse reactions to study drugs. Gastroenterology 1979; 77: 870–82.
179. Talar-Williams C, Sneller MC. Complications of corticosteroid therapy. Eur Arch Dotorhinolaryngol 1994; 251: 131–6.
180. Whitworth JA. Mechanisms of glucocorticoid-induced hypertension [Clinical conference]. Kidney Int 1987; 31: 1213–24.
181. Gurwitz JH, Bohn RL, Glynn RJ, Monane M, Mogun H, Avorn J. Glucocorticoids and the risk for initiation of hypoglycemic therapy. Arch Intern Med 1994; 154: 97–101.
182. Stuck AE, Minder CE, Frey FJ. Risk of infectious complications in patients taking glucocorticosteroids. Rev Infect Dis 1989; 11: 954–63.
183. Mankin HJ. Nontraumatic necrosis of bone (osteonecrosis). N Engl J Med 1992; 326: 1473–9.
184. Lukert BP, Raisz LG. Glucocorticoid-induced osteoporosis. Rheum Dis Clin N Am 1994; 20: 629–50.
185. Lacomis D, Samuels MA. Adverse neurologic effects of glucocorticosteroids. J Gen Intern Med 1991; 6: 367–77.
186. Urban RC Jr, Dreyer EB. Corticosteroid-induced glaucoma. Int Ophthalmol Clin 1993; 33: 135–9.
187. Urban RC Jr, Cotlier E. Corticosteroid-induced cataracts. Surv Ophthalmol 1986; 31: 102–10.
188. Kusunoki M, Moeslein G, Shoji Y et al. Steroid complications in patients with ulcerative colitis. Dis Colon Rectum 1992; 35: 1003–9.
189. Bean RHD. The treatment of chronic ulcerative colitis with 6-mercaptopurine. Med J Austral 1962; 2: 592–3.
190. McKay IR, Wall AJ, Goldstein G. Response to azathioprine in ulcerative colitis. Report of 7 cases. Am J Dig Dis 1966; 11: 536–45.
191. Bowen GE, Irons GV, Rhodes JB, Kirsner JB. Early experiences with azathioprine in ulcerative colitis. A note of caution. J Am Med Assoc 1966; 195: 166–70.
192. Jewell DP, Truelove SC. Azathioprine in ulcerative colitis: an interim report on a controlled therapeutic trial. Br Med J 1972; 1: 709–12.
193. Jewell DP, Truelove SC. Azathioprine in ulcerative colitis: final report on controlled therapeutic trial. Br Med J 1974; 4: 627–30.
194. Caprilli R, Carratu R, Babbini M. Double-blind comparison of the effectiveness of azathioprine and sulfasalazine in idiopathic proctocolitis. Preliminary report. Am J Dig Dis 1975; 20: 115–20.
195. Kirk AP, Lennard-Jones JE. Controlled trial of azathioprine in chronic ulcerative colitis. Br Med J (Clin Res Ed) 1982; 284: 1291–2.

196. Rosenberg JL, Wall AJ, Levin B, Binder HJ, Kirsner JB. A controlled trial of azathioprine in the management of chronic ulcerative colitis. Gastroenterology 1975; 69: 96–9.

197. Hawthorne AB, Logan RF, Hawkey CJ et al. Randomised controlled trial of azathioprine withdrawal in ulcerative colitis. Br Med J 1992; 305: 20–2.

198. Adler DJ, Korelitz BI. The therapeutic efficacy of 6-mercaptopurine in refractory ulcerative colitis. Am J Gastroenterol 1990; 85: 717–22.

199. Steinhart AH, Baker JP, Brzezinski A, Prokipchuk EJ. Azathioprine therapy in chronic ulcerative colitis. J Clin Gastroenterol 1990; 12: 271–5.

200. Lobo AJ, Foster PN, Burke DA, Johnston D, Axon AT. The role of azathioprine in the management of ulcerative colitis. Dis Colon Rectum 1990; 33: 374–7.

201. George J, Present DH, Pou R, Bodian C, Rubin PH. The long-term outcome of ulcerative colitis treated with 6-mercaptopurine. Am J Gastroenterol 1996; 91: 1711–14.

202. Ardizzone S, Molteni P, Imbesi V, Bollani S, Bianchi PG, Molteni F. Azathioprine in steroid-resistant and steroid-dependent ulcerative colitis [Published erratum appears in J Clin Gastroenterol 1998; 26: 231]. J Clin Gastroenterol 1997; 25: 330–3.

203. Present DH, Meltzer SJ, Krumholz MP, Wolke A, Korelitz BI. 6-Mercaptopurine in the management of inflammatory bowel disease: short- and long-term toxicity. Ann Intern Med 1989; 111: 641–9.

204. Connell WR, Kamm MA, Ritchie JK, Lennard-Jones JE. Bone marrow toxicity caused by azathioprine in inflammatory bowel disease: 27 years of experience. Gut 1993; 34: 1081–5.

205. Kirschner BS. Safety of azathioprine and 6-mercaptopurine in pediatric patients with inflammatory bowel disease. Gastroenterology 1998; 115: 813–21.

206. Connell WR, Kamm MA, Dickson M, Balkwill AM, Ritchie JK, Lennard-Jones JE. Long-term neoplasia risk after azathioprine treatment in inflammatory bowel disease. Lancet 1994; 343: 1249–52.

207. Bouhnik Y, Lemann M, Mary JY et al. Long-term follow-up of patients with Crohn's disease treated with azathioprine or 6-mercaptopurine. Lancet 1996; 347: 215–19.

208. Kozarek RA, Patterson DJ, Gelfand MD, Botoman VA, Ball TJ, Wilske KR. Methotrexate induces clinical and histologic remission in patients with refractory inflammatory bowel disease. Ann Intern Med 1989; 110: 353–6.

209. Baron TH, Truss CD, Elson CO. Low-dose oral methotrexate in refractory inflammatory bowel disease. Dig Dis Sci 1993; 38: 1851–6.

210. Feagan BG, Rochon J, Fedorak RN et al. Methotrexate for the treatment of Crohn's disease. North American Crohn's Study Group Investigators. N Engl J Med 1995; 332: 292–7.

211. Feagan BG, Fedorak RN, Irvine EJ et al. A comparison of methotrexate with placebo for the maintenance of remission in Crohn's disease. North American Crohn's Study Group Investigators. N Engl J Med 2000; 342: 1627–32.

212. Oren R, Moshkowitz M, Odes S et al. Methotrexate in chronic active Crohn's disease: a double-blind, randomized, Israeli multicenter trial. Am J Gastroenterol 1997; 92: 2203–9.

213. Arora S, Katkov W, Cooley J et al. Methotrexate in Crohn's disease: results of a randomized, double-blind, placebo-controlled trial. Hepatogastroenterology 1999; 46: 1724–9.

214. Oren R, Arber N, Odes S et al. Methotrexate in chronic active ulcerative colitis: a double-blind, randomized, Israeli multicenter trial. Gastroenterology 1996; 110: 1416–21.

215. Gupta S, Keshavarzian A, Hodgson HJ. Cyclosporin in ulcerative colitis [Letter]. Lancet 1984; 2: 1277–8.

216. Lichtiger S, Present DH. Preliminary report: cyclosporin in treatment of severe active ulcerative colitis. Lancet 1990; 336: 16–19.

217. Cohen RD, Stein R, Hanauer SB. Intravenous cyclosporin in ulcerative colitis: a five-year experience. Am J Gastroenterol 1999; 94: 1587–92.

218. Hermida-Rodriguez C, Cantero PJ, Garcia-Valriberas R, Pajares Garcia JM, Mate-Jimenez J. High-dose intravenous cyclosporine in steroid refractory attacks of inflammatory bowel disease. Hepatogastroenterology 1999; 46: 2265–8.

219. Hyde GM, Thillainayagam AV, Jewell DP. Intravenous cyclosporin as rescue therapy in severe ulcerative colitis: time for a reappraisal? Eur J Gastroenterol Hepatol 1998; 10: 411–13.

220. Santos J, Baudet S, Casellas F, Guarner L, Vilaseca J, Malagelada JR. Efficacy of intravenous cyclosporine for steroid refractory attacks of ulcerative colitis. J Clin Gastroenterol 1995; 20: 285–9.

221. Sandborn WJ. A critical review of cyclosporine therapy in inflammatory bowel disease. Inflam Bowel Dis 1995; 1: 48–63.

222. Lichtiger S, Present DH, Kornbluth A et al. Cyclosporine in severe ulcerative colitis refractory to steroid therapy. N Engl J Med 1994; 330: 1841–5.

223. Kornbluth A, Lichtiger S, Present D, Hanauer S. Long-term results of oral cyclosporin in patients with severe ulcerative colitis: a double-blind, randomized, multi-center trial. Gastroenterology 1994; 106: A714.

224. Stack WA, Long RG, Hawkey CJ. Short- and long-term outcome of patients treated with cyclosporin for severe acute ulcerative colitis. Aliment Pharmacol Ther 1998; 12: 973–8.

225. Ramakrishna J, Langhans N, Calenda K, Grand RJ, Verhave M. Combined use of cyclosporine and azathioprine or 6-mercaptopurine in pediatric inflammatory bowel disease. J Pediatr Gastroenterol Nutr 1996; 22: 296–302.

226. Fernandez-Banares F, Bertran X, Esteve-Comas M et al. Azathioprine is useful in maintaining long-term remission induced by intravenous cyclosporine in steroid-refractory severe ulcerative colitis. Am J Gastroenterol 1996; 91: 2498–9.

227. Svanoni F, Bonassi U, Bagnolo F, Caporuscio S. Effectiveness of cyclosporine A (CsA) in the treatment of active refractory ulcerative colitis (UC). Gastroenterology 1998; 114: A1096.

228. D'Haens G, Lemmens L, Hiele M et al. Intravenous cyclosporine (CyA) monotherapy versus intravenous methylprednisolone (MP) in severe ulcerative colitis: a randomized, double blind controlled trial. Gastroenterology 1998; 114: A963.

229. Sandborn WJ, Tremaine WJ, Schroeder KW, Steiner BL, Batts KP, Lawson GM. Cyclosporine enemas for treatment-resistant, mildly to moderately active, left-sided ulcerative colitis. Am J Gastroenterol 1993; 88: 640–5.

230. Ranzi T, Campanini MC, Velio P, Quarto dP, Bianchi P. Treatment of chronic proctosigmoiditis with cyclosporin enemas [Letter; comment]. Lancet 1989; 2: 97.

231. Brynskov J, Freund L, Thomsen OO, Andersen CB, Rasmussen SN, Binder V. Treatment of refractory ulcerative colitis with cyclosporin enemas [Letter; see comments]. Lancet 1989; 1: 721–2.

232. Winter TA, Dalton HR, Merrett MN, Campbell A, Jewell DP. Cyclosporin A retention enemas in refractory distal ulcerative colitis and 'pouchitis'. Scand J Gastroenterol 1993; 28: 701–4.

233. Sandborn WJ, Tremaine WJ, Schroeder KW et al. A placebo-controlled trial of cyclosporine enemas for mildly to moderately active left-sided ulcerative colitis. Gastroenterology 1994; 106: 1429–35.

31 | Surgical management of ulcerative colitis

IAN LINDSEY AND NEIL J. McC MORTENSEN

Introduction

The past 25 years have seen great changes in the management of ulcerative colitis (UC) with the introduction of a new procedure, ileal pouch–anal anastomosis (IPAA), and a gradual development in terms of refinement of its technique. These include older refinements such as methods of anastomosis, pouch design, and the plane of rectal dissection, as well as more recent ones, including laparoscopic-assisted IPAA, omission or otherwise of a loop ileostomy and IPAA for selected patients with Crohn's disease (CD).

This chapter reviews the history of surgery for UC, and examines indications and goals of surgery, the various surgical options, and focuses detailed attention on aspects of IPAA, now considered the gold standard for surgery.

History and evolution of surgery for ulcerative colitis

In the early 1900s major surgery was hazardous, and severe UC was treated by irrigating the colon with fluids introduced via appendicostomy [1], then subsequently by cecostomy [2]. As abdominal surgery became safer, more invasive excisional procedures evolved to allow surgeons to gain better long-term control of the disease in severe cases. In 1944 Strauss and Strauss established proctocolectomy and end-ileostomy, although there was major morbidity related to the ileostomy [3].

These difficulties were largely alleviated by the development of the everted ileostomy in 1952 by Brooke [4]. The field of stomal therapy was pioneered in the late 1950s at the Cleveland Clinic, leading to progress in the development of better stomal appliances and improved patient education [5].

However, the ileostomy remained 'incontinent', and this led to the development by Kock in the late 1960s of the 'continent' ileostomy with an intra-abdominal reservoir [6]. Although addition of a nipple valve further improved its continence [7], the high complication and reoperation rate and the emergence of IPAA led to its decline except in a few dedicated units.

Ileorectal anastomosis (IRA) was described by Devine [8] and championed by Aylett [9] in the UK in the 1960s as a means of avoiding an ileostomy. However, a high incidence of inflammation in the rectal stump, with need for subsequent rectal excision, added to the development of dysplasia and cancer in the rectum, has largely led to its abandonment in UC [10].

IPAA has naturally evolved as a procedure to eliminate mucosal disease in UC while maintaining intestinal continuity and preserving anal continence [11]. It was born of a combination of two major surgical concepts, each of which had a long history of development. Ileoanal anastomosis was attempted as early as 1900 but functional outcome was very poor [12]. Nissen [13] revisited the procedure in 1933, as did Ravitch and Sabiston [14] in 1947 with similar results. Soave [15] in 1964 popularized colonic pull-through after distal rectal mucosectomy for Hirschd-prung's disease in children. In 1973 Safaie-Shirafi and Soper [16] performed distal rectal mucosal stripping with straight ileoanal anastomosis for familial adenomatous polyposis, and in 1977 Martin et al. [17] performed similar procedures in patients with UC. However, straight ileoanal anastomosis was plagued by high stool frequency, urgency and incontinence.

The concept of improving the stool frequency of an ileoanal anastomosis by construction of an ileal reservoir originated well prior to the latest of these developments. Valiente and Bacon (1955) [18] described a triple-limbed ileal pouch in dogs combined with an ileoanal anastomosis. Karlan et al. [19] (1959) constructed a double-barrel pouch in dogs with good effect. Parks and Nicholls (1978) [11] performed the first ileal reservoir in combination

Stephan R. Targan, Fergus Shanahan and Loren C. Karp (eds.), Inflammatory Bowel Disease: From Bench to Bedside, 2nd Edition, 631–641.
© 2003 Kluwer Academic Publishers. Printed in Great Britain

colon. No terminal ileum is resected in division of the ileum and colon and construction of the end ileostomy. The inferior mesenteric artery is preserved and individual sigmoid vessels are taken. The distal sigmoid is divided to allow easy reach to the anterior abdominal wall, the staple line is inverted with sutures, and the end of the stump brought out just into the subcutaneous tissue extra-fascially in the lowest part of the abdominal wound, securing the serosa to the fascia. A blow-out of the stump, a risk especially if the rectum is diseased, results in wound infection rather than pelvic sepsis. If the stump is badly diseased and will not hold sutures it can be brought out 5–7 cm beyond the abdominal wall and covered with moist gauze, and at 7–10 days amputated flush to mature a mucous fistula, with sufficient adherence to the abdominal wall. No breach is made in the pelvic planes, allowing dissection in virgin territory at the second stage.

Diverting loop ileostomy and 'blowhole' colostomy

Turnbull *et al.* [32] described this operation in the setting of multiple sealed perforations and distended, friable bowel, the setting of severe acute colitis, on the basis that colectomy was hazardous because of the risk of gross fecal spillage. These days, better medical management and earlier surgical referral have made this option almost redundant, but on rare occasions it may be useful, and is included for historical reasons.

Technical points

The lie of the transverse colon is gaged with supine abdominal X-ray and a radiopaque marker at the umbilicus, the abdomen is entered via a small lower midline incision and a loop ileostomy is fashioned. A new vertical left paramedian incision is made over the dilated transverse colon and, before the colon is opened, the omentum and seromuscular layer of the colon is sutured carefully to the parietal peritoneum. The bowel is opened and a skin-level colostomy is matured. The colon is removed electively 6 months later.

Other emergency procedures

Emergency proctocolectomy and end-ileostomy

This was once advocated as the operation of choice in the setting of acute colitis [33] but subtotal colectomy is now preferred. Although controlled data are unlikely to become available, the risks of bleeding, damage to autonomic nerves and pelvic sepsis are likely to be higher than elective rectal dissection [30], and the option of future pouch surgery is eliminated. It may occasionally be required for massive bleeding or for limited severe acute proctosigmoiditis, where subtotal colectomy alone is unlikely to deal with the acute surgical problem.

Emergency colectomy and ileorectal anastomosis (IRA)

This option is rarely advised.

Emergency IPAA and loop ileostomy

Since this is major challenging reconstructive surgery with significant risk of complications even in the elective setting, this operation should not be undertaken in the acute setting.

Surgical goals and options: elective setting

There are several surgical options for UC, and each has its particular advantages and disadvantages. Generally these relate to avoidance or otherwise of the following: a permanent ileostomy; a rectal excision with its risks of nerve damage and bleeding; surveillance of the rectal stump and risk of rectal cancer; anorectal function; a perineal dissection with its risks of non-healed perineal wound; staged multiple operations and their impact on work and life; complex surgery with its risks of complications.

Total abdominal colectomy and IRA

IRA has gone out of fashion since the emergence of IPAA, having been popularized by Aylett in the 1960s and 1970s as the only surgical alternative to permanent ileostomy [9]. The main reason for declining interest in IRA is the cumulative requirement for rectal excision (primarily for poor function but also because of dysplasia and cancer in the rectum). This requirement ranges from 11% to 57% [34] (mean about 25%), and is proportional to length of follow-up. Poor function may result from persistent proctitis or rectal stricture, although the overall functional results are similar to IPAA, and most patients' function is slightly superior to those published for IPAA. The risk of cancer in the retained rectum is the greatest fear of the surgeon undertaking IRA, this risk increasing with time and estimated to be about 5% at 15–20 years [34]. Patients require diligent follow-up for sigmoidoscopic surveillance of the rectum, yet may develop rectal cancer despite this.

IRA does have its attractions, because it is simple, has low mortality and morbidity, both ileostomy and the complications of a rectal dissection are avoided, its functional results are similar to IPAA and the option of future restorative surgery is available [34].

If IRA is to be performed, several preconditions must be met. The rectum must be relatively spared and be distensible, the anal sphincters must be adequate to deal with liquid stool and IRA should not be contemplated when there is dysplasia or cancer in the colon or rectum.

Perhaps IRA finds its niche in two circumstances assuming the above preconditions are met. First, in the adolescent [35] or young adult, who wishes to avoid a stoma or a pelvic dissection while growing up or having a family. Psychological as well as sexual function and fertility difficulties may be avoided, the procedure acting as a 'bridge' to later IPAA.

Secondly, a diagnosis of indeterminate colitis may influence the surgeon to perform IRA on the basis that, if the patient has UC, IPAA is still feasible, yet if CD develops, IRA is an excellent restorative option if rectum is supple and (relatively) spared [36]. The advantages are avoidance of a stoma, biopsy of the rectum without confounding effects of diversion on rectal histology, and keeping future options open. The disadvantages are the risk of anastomotic leak, and lack of information on the natural history of the diverted rectal disease.

Subtotal colectomy and permanent end-ileostomy

Most patients after urgent subtotal colectomy and ileostomy are keen to undergo IPAA in order to have their ileostomy closed. However, it should be recognized that, occasionally, the now-healthy asymptomatic patient does not wish to submit to further major surgery. Because of the long-term risks of cancer in the retained rectum [34] and difficulty in surveillance, the patient should be actively discouraged from this course of action. The notion of future proctectomy (with or without reconstruction) should be raised with the patient at the first outpatient review.

Proctocolectomy and permanent end-ileostomy (PC)

Prior to the advent of IPAA this proctocolectomy and ileostomy (PC) was considered the gold standard in UC and its attractions are several. Unless the patient is very ill PC can be performed as a single operation. It eliminates all colonic and rectal mucosal disease and therefore UC symptoms and cancer risk. In the hands of a well-trained colorectal surgeon this is a relatively straightforward operation. For these reasons it is the alternative of choice to IPAA, and even in specialized centers a substantial proportion of patients will undergo this operation. In Oxford just under a quarter of our patients elect to undergo PC.

The overriding disadvantage, of course, is the presence of a permanent ileostomy, which most patients, especially younger ones, want to avoid at all costs. However, a subset of patients will decline IPAA because of its complexities and risks, and this may relate to their age, social or work circumstances. In some patients IPAA is contraindicated because of age, poor sphincter function or advanced colon or rectal cancer.

It is difficult to compare the benefits and drawbacks of PC and IPAA. The procedures are offered to different population groups with different expectations, which introduces selection bias. Additionally, the yardsticks by which we measure outcomes are different and thus difficult to directly compare, although some have tried to do so using quality-of-life instruments. Satisfaction with an ileostomy can be high, particularly for patients over 60. However, we also know that IPAA patients experience less difficulty performing daily activities, less restriction in sport and sexual activity than those with permanent ileostomy [37] and therefore overall may have a greater quality of life.

Technical points

Colonic mobilization is conducted preserving the omentum. Low ligation of the inferior mesenteric vessels is performed. Rectal dissection is carried out carefully to avoid damaging the nerves governing sexual and bladder function. Either close rectal or mesorectal dissection may be employed, since close rectal dissection has not shown an advantage over mesorectal dissection in protecting the pelvic nerves. An intersphincteric perineal dissection is performed.

Care is taken in fashioning the permanent end-ileostomy to minimize stoma-related complications.

PSC it is important to properly manage the UC because PSC patients are candidates for liver transplantation. Brooke ileostomy should be avoided in those not suitable for transplantation since 50% of these patients will bleed from peristomal varices [60]. In those candidates for transplantation, IPAA is controversial due to the high risk of chronic pouchitis despite immuno-suppressive therapy [61].

Technical issues and controversies

Staging of surgery: one, two or three stages?

IPAA is a complex reconstructive operation with a low pelvic anastomosis. The risk of leak is significant and pelvic sepsis is a major cause of poor function and pouch failure. Surgeons have been reluctant to perform this operation without the protection of a covering loop ileostomy to mitigate the consequences of pelvic sepsis. However, closure of ileostomy has its complications and increases overall hospital stay. Omission of ileostomy has been shown to be reasonable in selected low-risk cases when compared against use of a loop ileostomy in higher-risk patients [62].

Of high-risk factors considered by surgeons including high-dose steroids (> 20 mg), hypoalbuminemia and anemia, only steroids have consistently shown to be a reliable factor. However, since it is not legitimate to compare high- and low-risk groups, because of the inherent biases, it remains open as to whether the low-risk patient is best served by protective loop ileostomy or not. A randomized trial after exclusion of these high-risk patients would answer this question, but not surprisingly the one small trial addressing this issue was inconclusive [63].

Single-stage surgery is seen most often in large North American tertiary colorectal units and has obvious advantages for the patient when it is safe to perform. The major drawback is the inability to clearly distinguish UC from CD, particularly when preoperative information is equivocal or when proctocolectomy is performed for severe disease, and there is a small risk of inadvertent pouch construction for CD [31].

Laparoscopic-assisted or open surgery for IPAA?

The role of laparoscopic-assisted IPAA is being debated. There are doubts about the true advantages of minimal access in terms of speed of recovery. However, being a benign disease, minimal access surgery for inflammatory bowel disease (IBD) in principle has a lot to recommend it.

Laparoscopically assisted IPAA is certainly feasible, and some impressive results have been published [64]. Laparoscopic-assisted subtotal colectomy has been reported for acute severe colitis with results comparable to matched open controls [65]. The issues are those of surgical morbidity and mortality, potentially less surgical stress, with faster recovery and less immune suppression, as well as fewer adhesions and better cosmesis.

The data comparing open to laparoscopically assisted IPAA are inadequate. Reported series in the literature are either retrospective reviews detailing general experience, morbidity and mortality results, as well as duration of ileus and length of stay, or non-randomized comparisons with matched open controls. Results are similar to those reported in the open literature. Data from randomized controlled trials are awaited.

It would be useful to know if immune suppression is less in minimal-access surgery. IBD patients are often immune-suppressed because of their underlying illness, poor nutrition and medical therapies. Difficulties exist in knowing which parameter best directly reflects the surgical stress response. Differences in serum interleukin-6 (IL-6) after open and laparoscopically assisted colonic surgery for IBD have consistently shown trends to increased IL-6 levels after open surgery but none with statistical significance [66–69]. This may be because of the heterogeneity of the data as there is a high variability of IL-6 response, particularly in open cases [68, 69]. Recently, granulocyte elastase (GE) has been studied as an alternative marker, in comparison to IL-6 and C-reactive protein (CRP), after open and laparoscopically assisted surgery for IBD [69]. It was found to be significantly elevated ($p < 0.05$) on days 1, 2 and 3 in open surgery compared to laparoscopically assisted patients. This marker shows promise, but clearly further research is required. Other studies have demonstrated a poor correlation between serum CRP and the extent of tissue damage [66–68].

Fewer adhesions appear to form after laparoscopic surgery when compared to open surgery. There is both anecdotal and scientific evidence to support this from observations at laparoscopy and from animal studies [70–75]. There are no data on the incidence of adhesions after laparoscopic surgery for IBD, but any reduction would clearly be an advantage, particularly during IPAA, when adhesions formed at subtotal colectomy and ileostomy can be problematic.

Preservation of body image in this often-young group of patients is an advantage of the laparoscopic approach. A comparative non-randomized study of 22 patients undergoing laparoscopic or open resection for IBD showed that cosmetic score was significantly higher in the laparoscopic group ($p < 0.01$), and that body image correlated strongly with cosmesis and quality of life [76].

Close rectal or mesorectal dissection?

A particular concern to male patients contemplating IPAA is the risk of impotence secondary to pelvic nerve damage. If surgery is to be acceptable to patients then the risk of nerve damage and impotence must be kept to a minimum. Close rectal or perimuscular dissection is a surgical technique first described by Dowling and Lee at Oxford in 1972 [77]. By convention the mesorectal plane is used for rectal cancer surgery, and by some surgeons for IBD. Close rectal dissection is conducted in the non-anatomical perimuscular plane in an effort to avoid damage to the pelvic autonomic nerves, which lie immediately outside the mesorectal plane. It is, however, a more challenging dissection.

According to recent data there appears to be no statistically significant difference in the rates of complete or partial impotence between those undergoing mesorectal and close rectal dissection [51]. This is useful information since many surgeons operate in the mesorectal plane out of convenience and familiarity, and it is important for such surgeons to be clear that they are not disadvantaging their patients by using this plane.

Mucosectomy and handsewn anastomosis or double-stapling?

The intense debate that this issue generated during the 1980s has largely subsided. The debate was centered on the question of whether it is safe to leave a 'columnar cuff' of mucosa in the upper half of the anal canal, as is done after double-stapling, or whether complete extirpation of all columnar epithelium down to the dentate line is necessary by mucosectomy.

On one side of the argument the 'musosectomists' argue that, to eliminate or reduce the risk of columnar cuff dysplasia and cancer in the longer term, as well as that of recurrent colitis in the cuff ('cuffitis'), mucosectomy is necessary [78]. Double-stapling leaves potential disease-bearing columnar mucosa in the anal canal and sometimes inadvertently leaves a short rectal stump.

Antagonists to this view, however, favor the technical ease and speed of double-stapling with the elimination of the perineal phase of surgery. They cite the superior nocturnal continence subsequent to avoidance of the manual disturbance of the anal sphincters [79] and preservation of the important anal transition zone with its sensory discriminatory function [80]. They also point to the hitherto-unrecognized variability in transitional zone anatomy [81] as well as data showing that mucosectomy is often incomplete and can leave residual islands of columnar mucosa behind [82].

A paucity of good randomized data has hindered clarification of this issue [83]. However, it is fair to say that, after 15 years of follow-up of the double-stapled operation, the incidence of columnar cuff dysplasia and cancer is small [84], and most of the few cases of cancer [85] have been in patients undergoing mucosectomy. We routinely practice double-stapling but recognize the technical requirement to be able to undertake mucosectomy in certain circumstances, as well as the need to closely follow up double-stapled patients in the longer term.

Pouch design: J, S or W configuration?

There are several options in pouch design for IPAA, including the J, S and W pouches, and in essence these are double, treble and quadruple 15–20 cm single limbs of ileum turned back on themselves a multiple of times to create a reservoir of variable volume. Although, early on, pouches were composed of many different configurations, the J pouch is now the most widely used, because its ease of construction is a major advantage. W pouches probably carry a small advantage over J pouches in terms of pouch frequency, but this was during the phase of routine mucosectomy, when tension on J pouches using mucosectomy was greater than currently [86]. This advantage has been largely offset by the more common use of double-stapling, and the difference in stool frequency between different pouch configurations is regarded as negligible.

References

1. Brown JY. Value of complete physiological rest of large bowel in treatment of certain ulcerations and obstetrical lesions of this organ. Surg Gynecol Obstet 1913; 16: 610–16.
2. Brooke BN. Ulcerative Colitis and its Surgical Treatment. Edinburgh: E&S Livingstone, 1954.
3. Strauss AA, Strauss SF. Surgical treatment of ulcerative colitis. Surg Clin N Am 1944; 24: 211–24.

Introduction

The term 'pouchitis' was coined by Kock et al. [1] in 1977 to describe an inflammatory condition of the continent ileal reservoir in patients who have undergone a proctocolectomy. This procedure was first described in 1969 [2]. In 1980 Parks et al. and Utsunomiya et al. [3, 4] independently described a procedure consisting of a proctocolectomy with ileal reservoir and anal anastomosis. With minor modifications the ileal pouch–anal anastomosis (IPAA) is currently the surgical option of choice in patients with familial adenomatous polyposis (FAP) and ulcerative colitis (UC) with either dysplasia or disease refractory to medical therapy.

The functional outcome after IPAA is acceptable. The median number of bowel movements in 24 h is six. Soiling at night occurs in approximately one-third of patients and 24% need to wear a pad occasionally [5]. Despite these numbers, the health-related quality of life after IPAA has consistently been comparable to normal populations and better than in those with active UC or inflammatory bowel disease (IBD) in general [5–7]. However, Tiainen et al. found that the health-related quality of life decreased with poor functional status, increased number of bowel movements and chronic pouchitis [5].

Pouchitis is the most common long-term complication of IPAA in UC [8]. Its definition and diagnostic criteria have evolved over time and its etiology is unknown. This chapter will review the current knowledge base for this frequent and sometimes debilitating form of IBD.

Diagnosis

The diagnosis of pouchitis should be made on a combination of clinical, endoscopic and histologic grounds. Patients will usually present with diarrhea, watery stools, fecal urgency, abdominal cramps and occasional rectal bleeding. An endoscopy with biopsies of the pouch is done to confirm the diagnosis. The neoterminal ileum above the pouch should be normal; inflammation and ulceration here raises the suspicion of possible Crohn's disease (CD). Inflammation of the pouch mucosa with granularity, edema, mucosal hemorrhages, contact bleeding and superficial ulcers is present in pouchitis with varying degrees of severity [9]. Inflammation is either uniform throughout the pouch or more severe in the distal pouch [10].

In 1987 the Mayo Clinic defined pouchitis as a clinical syndrome of watery, frequent, at times bloody stool accompanied by urgency, incontinence, abdominal cramps, malaise and fever. The symptoms must be present for at least 2 days and should be relieved within 48 h with metronidazole therapy [8]. While this definition is sensitive for pouchitis, it is not specific and may include other clinical entities such as CD, pouch ischemia and anastomotic stricture.

The St Marks Hospital developed a diagnostic criteria for pouchitis based on a triad of diarrhea (6 or more stools/day), endoscopic findings (four or more of edema, granularity, friability, loss of vascular pattern, mucosal hemorrhage or ulceration), and a minimum grade of 4 on a 6-point histopathologic index (polymorphonuclear leukocyte infiltration and percent ulceration per low-power field) [11]. This definition was very specific, but would exclude less severe cases of pouchitis.

In 1994 Sandborn et al. developed the Pouchitis Disease Activity Index (PDAI) incorporating the Mayo Clinic definition and the pouchitis triad and histopathologic index defined by the St Marks group [12]. The PDAI attempts to provide a standardized definition of pouchitis based on clinical, endoscopic and histologic markers (Table 1), with pouchitis defined as a score of seven or more points. Diarrhea was defined based on an increase from the baseline number of bowel movements. Other clinical manifes-

Stephan R. Targan, Fergus Shanahan and Loren C. Karp (eds.), Inflammatory Bowel Disease: From Bench to Bedside, 2nd Edition, 643–658.
© 2003 *Kluwer Academic Publishers. Printed in Great Britain*

Genetics: pANCA and extraintestinal manifestations

The association of the serologic marker antineutrophil cytoplasmic antibody-perinuclear staining pattern (pANCA) with pouchitis is controversial. The prevalence of pANCA in UC patients is 60% [34]. Whether this number is decreased after proctocolectomy [35, 36] or unchanged [37–40] is a matter of debate. The literature is also divided as to whether there is a correlation between pANCA and the development of pouchitis. Four studies have found that the prevalence of pANCA is higher than expected in IPAA patients with pouchitis (89–100%) and lower than expected in patients without pouchitis (18–74%) [34, 38, 39, 41]. However, six more recent studies have shown that there is no correlation between pANCA and the occurrence of pouchitis [36, 40, 42–45]. Whether the failure of these later studies to demonstrate an association is based on the definitions of pouchitis used, the ANCA assay methodology, disease heterogenicity or a true absence of association remains to be determined.

However, pANCA levels are increased in patients with primary sclerosing cholangitis (PSC) [46]. PSC, in turn, is a risk factor for pouchitis [35, 47, 48]. Patients with PSC who undergo IPAA have a 63% chance of developing pouchitis versus only 32% for those without PSC. The cumulative risk of developing pouchitis in PSC patients is also higher at 1, 2, 5 and 10 years than in UC patients without pouchitis (22%, 43%, 61% and 79% respectively versus 15.5%, 22.5%, 36% and 45.5%) [48].

Extraintestinal manifestations (EIM) are also increased in patients with pouchitis [42, 49–51]. The increased incidence of pouchitis in patients with PSC and other EIM suggests that there may be a particular genotype of UC that has a stronger predisposition to develop pouchitis. pANCA may or may not be a serological marker for that genotype. These correlations also support the theory that pouchitis may be either a recurrence of UC in the pouch or a third, new form of IBD.

Missed diagnosis of Crohn's disease

Patients with pouchitis may have findings that overlap with CD. Often, ulcerations and fistulas occur at the site of anastomotic suture lines and have features consistent with CD [9, 52]. However, histologic and endoscopic studies of refractory pouchitis have shown no evidence of CD [9, 53]. Multiple investiga-

tors have suggested that a diagnosis of CD should never be made based on findings in the pouch. This diagnosis requires disease in the neoterminal ileum above the pouch, the presence of fistulas, reexamination of the original proctocolectomy specimen or disease in the remaining gut consistent with CD.

Fecal stasis and bacterial overgrowth

After colectomy the ileal reservoir develops a microbial flora count that is between what is expected in the normal terminal ileum and the colon [54]. This finding, as well as the response of the inflamed pouch mucosa to antibiotics (see below) has led to the theory that pouchitis is the result of inflammation caused by fecal stasis and bacterial overgrowth in the new ileal reservoir. Studies of the ileal pouch have varied. Some authors found that patients with pouchitis did indeed have greater counts of anaerobic and/or aerobic bacteria, when compared to controls without pouchitis [55–59]. Others have found an increase in the bacterial count in all ileal pouches when compared to ileostomy controls and the normal colon, but without a significant difference between those with and without pouchitis [60–64]. This suggests that, if a relationship exists between bacterial overgrowth and pouchitis, it is not a direct one.

Fecal bile acids

Alterations in bile acid metabolism occur after IPAA. Natori *et al.* found increased levels of cholic acid and chenodeoxycholic acid and decreased levels of the secondary bile acids deoxycholic acid and lithocholic acid in ileal pouches versus healthy controls. However, these secondary bile acids were greater in the ileal pouch compared to ileostomy patients, suggesting that a degree of normalization occurs in pouch patients secondary to fecal stasis and bacterial overgrowth in the pouch [65].

Bile acids were found to be cytotoxic to epithelial cells [66], suggesting they have a role in pouchitis and colonic metaplasia. However, later studies by the same author showed that the ileal dialysate was not cytotoxic to the epithelial monolayers. Epithelial resistance and histologic structure was actually preserved, suggesting the presence of a protective factor in the dialysate [67]. Further studies also disputed the role of bile acids in pouchitis by demonstrating no difference in the total bile acid concentration or daily fecal bile acid output in pouchitis patients versus those with a healthy ileal reservoir [52, 64, 68].

Short-chain fatty acids (SCFA)

Short-chain fatty acids (acetate, propionate, butyrate), are products of anaerobic bacterial fermentation of carbohydrates. They are the major source of energy for the colonic mucosa [69] and are involved in crypt cell production and the absorption of water and electrolytes [70]. While patients with IPAA have been found to have the same mean total concentrations of SCFA as normal controls [71] some authors have found decreased levels of SCFA in both active ulcerative colitis [72, 73] and active pouchitis [74–77]. However, Sandborn *et al.* found no difference in the total fecal SCFA concentrations between patients with and without pouchitis, no correlation between fecal bacterial concentrations and total fecal SCFA, and no correlation between fecal concentrations of bacteria or SCFA and chronic inflammation or villous atrophy [64].

Ischemia

Construction of the ileal pouch may require division of mesenteric vessels to avoid tension on the anastomosis, resulting in some degree of ischemia in the pouch [78]. This ischemia may not be a single postoperative injury, but chronic transient damage aggravated by distension of the pouch. Mild endoscopic and histologic changes consistent with ischemia have been found in the ileal reservoirs of IPAA patients [52, 79]. Patients with pouchitis were also found to have lower rates of mucosal blood flow on endoscopic Doppler readings in the pouch than healthy controls [80].

The villi of the small intestine are reported to contain the highest concentration of xanthine dehydrogenase of any tissue [81]. It has been hypothesized that transient ischemia in the pouch leads to conversion of xanthine dehydrogenase to xanthine oxidase. During subsequent reperfusion, xanthine oxidase catalyzes the formation of oxygen free radicals, possibly leading to cellular injury and pouchitis [82–84]. However, the same surgical techniques are used in both UC and FAP patients, the latter of whom have far fewer episodes of pouchitis. It is unlikely that ischemia is itself a direct cause of pouchitis, but it may play a role in the susceptible host.

Epidemiology

Incidence

The cumulative risk of having one or more episode of pouchitis varies from 15% to 53% in patients with UC. This variation in range likely results from the different diagnostic criteria used for pouchitis over the years [48, 85–91]. The rate is much lower in patients with FAP, ranging from 3% to 14% [85, 87, 92]. The rates of refractory pouchitis range from 4.5% to 5.5%, with severe intractable pouchitis leading to excision of the pouch in 0.3% to 1.3% of patients. Fig. 1 shows the clinical outcome of 100 UC patients at the Mayo Clinic who underwent IPAA [13].

Predictive factors

Penna *et al.* found a cumulative risk of pouchitis in UC patients to be 15.5%, 22.5%, 36% and 45.5% at 1, 2, 5 and 10 years after IPAA, respectively. This risk was much higher in patients who had PSC, whose risk at 1, 2, 5 and 10 years was 22%, 43%, 61% and 79% respectively [48]. Stahlberg *et al.* found similar results with a cumulative risk of 51% at 4 years. All six patients (100%) with PSC developed pouchitis, and extracolonic manifestations as a whole were a predictive factor for pouchitis [89].

Multiple other studies lend support to the belief that there is an increased incidence of pouchitis in patients with EIMs [42, 49–51]. Lohmuller *et al.* studied 734 patients who underwent IPAA. Patients who had preoperative EIM had a 39% incidence of pouchitis versus an incidence of 26% for those who did not. Those who developed EIM postoperatively had a 53% incidence of pouchitis versus 25% in those who did not.

As in UC smoking has been found to be protective against the development of pouchitis. Merrett *et al.* found an incidence of pouchitis of 33% in ex-smokers, 25% in non-smokers and 6% in current smokers [93]. These findings have been supported by others [49, 89].

The role of the extent of preoperative UC on the development of pouchitis is more controversial. Samarasekera *et al.* found no correlation between distal colitis or more extensive disease and the incidence of pouchitis in 177 patients studied [94]. However, Schmidt *et al.* found that colonic extension had a statistically significant association with the development of pouchitis after IPAA with a linear

Treatment

The treatment of pouchitis is predominantly empiric given the few controlled trials available. In a review of medical therapy in pouchitis, Sandborn *et al.* identified only four randomized controlled trials for the treatment of pouchitis [116]. Antibiotics are the mainstay of treatment, lending credence to theories of bacterial overgrowth and fecal stasis having a primary role in the pathogenesis of pouchitis. Other treatments are based on therapy used in UC as well as pathophysiologic changes noted in the pouch. Table 2 lists the treatment options available [117].

Antibiotics

Metronidazole is the first-line therapy for pouchitis. Support for metronidazole comes from a '*N*-of-1'

randomized trial [118] and a randomized controlled crossover trial which demonstrated a 73% response (defined as a decrease in stool frequency) in 13 patients with chronic pouchitis. The placebo response was 9% [119]. Hurst *et al.* found that 41 of 52 patients (79%) with acute pouchitis responded to a 7-day course of metronidazole at 250 mg orally three times a day with complete relief [92]. Two small series found metronidazole to have a response rate of 100% when given as a topical solution instilled at 75–150 mg daily [120] or 40–160 mg daily [121]. The 20% of patients who fail to respond to oral metronidazole, or who suffer from side-effects such as dysgeusia, dyspepsia, nausea and peripheral neuropathy, can be tried on alternate antibiotics.

Hurst *et al.* found that 11 of 52 patients did not respond to metronidazole. These patients were then given ciprofloxacin at 500 mg twice a day, with eight

Table 2. Treatment options for pouchitis

Class		Example
1. Antibiotics	A.	Metronidazole
	B.	Ciprofloxacin
	C.	Amoxicillin/clavulanic acid
	D.	Erythromycin
	E.	Tetracycline
	F.	Rifaximin
2. Probiotics	A.	Lactobacilli, Bifidobacteria, *Streptococcus salivarius* subsp. *thermophilus*
3. 5-Aminosalicylates	A.	Mesalamine enemas
	B.	Sulfasalazine
	C.	Oral mesalamine
4. Corticosteroids	A.	Conventional corticosteroid enemas
	B.	Budesonide enemas
	C.	Oral corticosteroids
5. Nutritional agents	A.	Short-chain fatty acid enemas or suppositories
	B.	Glutamine suppositories
6. Immune modifier agents	A.	Cyclosporine enemas
	B.	Azathioprine
7. Oxygen free radical inhibitor	A.	Allopurinol
8. Smoking/nicotine	A.	Smoking
	B.	?Transdermal nicotine
9. Antidiarrheal/antimicrobial	A.	Bismuth subsalicylate
	B.	Bismuth carbomer enemas
10. Surgical options	A.	Ileal pouch exclusion
	B.	Ileal pouch excision

Modified with permission from: Sandborn WJ. Pouchitis following ileal pouch–anal anastomosis: definition, pathogenesis, and treatment. Gastroenterology 1994; 107: 1856–60.

(73%) responding. This gave an overall antibiotic response rate of 96% [86]. Gionchetti *et al.* used rifaximin 1 g twice a day in combination with ciprofloxacin 500 mg twice a day for 15 days in 18 patients with chronic treatment-resistant pouchitis [122]. Six of 18 (33%) had complete remission defined as a PDAI of 0. Ten of 18 (55.6%) had clinical improvement with a decrease of three points on their PDAI, for a total response rate of 88.8%. Other antibiotics used with some success include amoxicillin/clavulanic acid, erythromycin and tetracycline [123].

An initial episode of pouchitis should be treated with metronidazole 250 mg three times a day for 7–10 days. Response should be seen within 2–3 days. Responders who have repeat episodes and are able to tolerate the medication should be re-treated with the same regimen. Some patients with chronic pouchitis will require anywhere from 250 mg every third day to 250 mg three times daily to maintain their response. Others may develop resistance and require a rotating schedule of three or more antibiotics. If antibiotics fail, other therapeutic options should be considered (Fig. 2) [117].

5-Aminosalicylates (5-ASA)

Anecdotal reports suggest a benefit from oral and topical mesalamine [9, 52, 124]. Miglioli *et al.* describe three patients with pouchitis after IPAA for UC. They were given 5-ASA as a suppository or enema at 1.2–4 g daily. After 20–30 days a clinical and endoscopic improvement was noted with partial histological recovery [125].

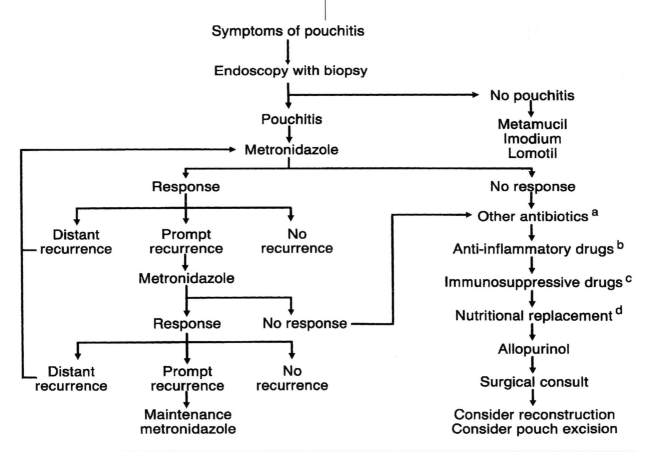

Figure 2. Treatment algorithm for pouchitis. Other antibiotics[a] indicates: ciprofloxacin, rifaximin, amoxicillin/clavulanate, erythromycin, tetracycline, and cycling of multiple antibiotics. Anti-inflammatory drugs[b] indicates: mesalamine enemas, sulfasalazine, and oral mesalamine. Immunosuppressive drugs[c] indicates: steroid enemas, oral steroids, budesonide suppositories, azathioprine, and cyclosporine enemas. Nutritional replacement[d] indicates: SCFA enemas and glutamine suppositories. Probiotics are not available in the United States. Reproduced with permission from: Sandborn WJ. Pouchitis following ileal pouch–anal anastomosis: definition, pathogenesis, and treatment. Gastroenterology 1994; 107: 1856–60.

The bacteria required to split the azo bond in sulfasalazine and release the 5-ASA moiety are present in the reservoir of patients after IPAA [126], suggesting sulfasalazine will be a viable treatment modality. Pentasa may also achieve some release of mesalamine into the ileal pouch. However, no trials were found in the literature for oral 5-ASA agents in the treatment of pouchitis.

Corticosteroids

When antibiotics fail, oral and topical corticosteroids have been tried with limited anecdotal success [52, 124]. A small trial of budesonide suppositories was conducted in 10 patients with active pouchitis. After 1.5 mg/day for 4 weeks all patients had clinical and endoscopic improvement or remission, but six (60%) relapsed within 8 weeks [127].

Immunosuppressive therapy

Immunosuppressives have been anecdotally surprisingly ineffective, as well as poorly studied. MacMillan *et al.* did report a small retrospective series of four patients with chronic pouchitis [128]. Patients were treated with varying doses of azathioprine or 6-mercaptopurine. Within 6 months of starting therapy, steroids were discontinued and a sustained response was maintained for up to 3 years. Cyclosporine (CSA) enemas were used in 12 patients with distal UC and one patient with pouchitis while continuing prior therapy. This 250 mg CSA retention enema resulted in symptomatic and endoscopic but not histologic improvement within 8 weeks in the patient with pouchitis [129].

Transplant data demonstrate that immunosuppression is not protective against pouchitis. Zins *et al.* report seven patients with IPAA who underwent orthotopic liver transplantation for PSC [130]. Five of the seven had chronic or recurrent pouchitis prior to transplant, of whom four continued to have chronic pouchitis after transplant despite a triple immunosuppressive regimen of prednisone, azathioprine and either cyclosporine or FK506. One patient who had been free of pouchitis prior to transplant developed a single acute episode post-transplant. Rowley *et al.* report a series of four patients with IPAA and orthotopic liver transplant for PSC. One of the four developed chronic pouchitis despite cyclosporine use [131].

Bismuth

Bismuth carbomer foam enemas showed promising results in an open-label trial [132]. Twelve patients with treatment-refractory chronic pouchitis were treated with 230 mg elemental bismuth containing carbomer foam enemas. The enemas were given nightly for 45 days. Ten of 12 (83%) patients had a clinical response with a decrease in their PDAI by 2 or more points. Of these 10, six (60%) maintained their remission over 12 months while receiving an enema every third night. No side-effects were reported.

However, a randomized double-blind placebo-controlled trial in 40 patients demonstrated no difference between placebo and bismuth carbomer foam enema in the treatment of chronic pouchitis [133]. Twenty patients received a placebo enema containing gum resin, and 20 received 270 mg of elemental bismuth complexed with carbomer delivered as foam enemas for 3 weeks. No patients achieved remission (PDAI of 0) but nine patients (45%) in each group achieved a clinical response with a three-point decrease in their PDAI. The authors site low concentrations of bismuth in the enemas, short duration of treatment, therapeutic efficacy of gum resin (given the high placebo rate of 45%) or a true treatment failure to explain the lack of efficacy of bismuth. As in UC and CD, promising pilot studies do not always translate into positive randomized controlled trials.

A retrospective series of 13 patients with chronic pouchitis studied the effect of oral bismuth subsalicylate tablets (Pepto-Bismol) on disease course. All patients were receiving antibiotics (metronidazole or ciprofloxacin) but remained symptomatic. All patients had an initial dose of eight chewable bismuth subsalicylate tablets (each 262 mg) per day for 4 weeks. Eleven of the 13 had a clinical response with a decrease in stool frequency, fecal incontinence and/or abdominal cramping. One patient reduced the dose secondary to bloating while the seven others reduced their dose because of equal efficacy at the lower dose. Five of the 11 responders were able to discontinue antibiotic use after 4 weeks [134]. Thus, bismuth appears safe and efficacious and warrants further trials.

Allopurinol

Allopurinol is a xanthine oxidase inhibitor. The theoretical basis for its use in pouchitis is to inhibit the production of free radicals and thus inhibit mucosal injury. A small trial by Levin *et al.* demonstrated a 50% response rate in acute and chronic pouchitis [83]. Eight patients with acute pouchitis received 300 mg twice daily of allopurinol. Four had resolution of symptoms. Fourteen patients with chronic pouchitis were treated with the same dose for 28 days; seven of the 14 had a clinical response. These findings lend credence to the theory of ischemic damage and free radical injury contributing to the pathogenesis of pouchitis. A randomized controlled trial of allopurinol for the treatment of pouchitis is currently ongoing in Scandinavia.

Nutritional agents

Fiber

Thrilby *et al.* demonstrated that oral fiber supplementation has no benefit on stool frequency, pouch function, bloating or stool consistency in patients after IPAA [135]. Fiber is equally unlikely to be of benefit in the treatment of pouchitis.

SCFA/glutamine

SCFA (acetate, propionate, butyrate) are products of anaerobic bacterial fermentation. They are the major source of energy for the colonic mucosa [69] while glutamine is the major energy source for enterocytes. Data for their use in the treatment of pouchitis are limited and mostly negative. Two small series used the same SCFA enema formulation of 60 mM sodium acetate, 30 mM sodium propionate and 40 mM sodium *n*-butyrate in a combined total of 10 patients with chronic pouchitis [136, 137]. Only three patients had a clinical response while two patients actually showed worsening of their clinical symptoms. In contrast, den Hoed *et al.* described a patient with treatment-refractory pouchitis who was given a similar SCFA enema combination twice daily for 4 weeks. After this treatment she had complete resolution of her symptoms and remained symptom-free during 2 years of follow-up [138]. Another series used either butyrate or glutamine suppositories for 10 days in patients with chronic pouchitis. Six of the nine (67%) patients treated with butyrate, and four of the 10 (40%) patients treated with glutamine, failed, remaining symptomatic without measurable clinical response [77]. Given the lack of a placebo control it is unclear whether these two therapies are equally effective or equally ineffective.

Smoking/nicotine

Smoking has been found to be protective against pouchitis [49, 89, 93]. However, to date there have been no trials of nicotine enemas or transdermal nicotine patch for the treatment of pouchitis.

Probiotics

Probiotics are live organisms, usually bacteria, found as commensals in the human gastrointestinal tract. Based on the hypothesis that an imbalance in these organisms may result in inflammatory conditions such as pouchitis, Gionchetti *et al.* conducted a randomized double-blind placebo-controlled trial of the probiotic VSL-3 (Sitia-Yomo, Milano, Italy) [139]. Forty patients with chronic pouchitis in remission (PDAI of 0) received either placebo or a 6 g daily oral dose of VSL-3 for 9 months. VSL-3 contains 5×10^{11}/g of viable lyophilized bacteria consisting of four strains of lactobacilli (*L. acidophilus*, *L. delbrueckii* subsp. *bulgaricus*, *L. plantarum*, *L. casei*), three strains of bifidobacteria (*B. infantis*, *B. longum*, *B. breve*) and one strain of *Streptococcus salivarius* subsp. *thermophilus*. Seventeen (85%) of the patients who received VSL-3 were free of recurrence (defined as an increase in the PDAI by 2 or more points) as opposed to none of the 20 patients who received placebo. No side-effects were reported. The VSL-3-treated group was found to have an increase in fecal concentrations of lactobacilli, bifidobacteria and *S. thermophilus* by day 15. The safety and efficacy of this therapy for chronic pouchitis appears promising; however, currently the formulation has limited availability.

Crohn's disease

When CD is diagnosed in the pouch, treatment is along the lines of Crohn's elsewhere in the gastrointestinal tract. Berrebi *et al.* report a series of two patients with IPAA diagnosed with CD in the reservoir. Both responded to corticosteroid and azathioprine therapy, with eventual maintenance on azathioprine alone [140]. Recently, Ricart *et al.* reported a series of seven patients with IPAA for UC who were subsequently diagnosed with CD. These patients had active inflammatory or fistulizing CD in the pouch and were refractory to conventional therapy. They were treated with varying doses of the murine chimeric anti-tumor necrosis factor (TNF)-α antibody, infliximab. Six patients had a complete response with closure of all fistulous tracts, and one had a partial response [141].

Pouch excision

Pouch excision is rare, and occurs more commonly for pouch dysfunction than for true chronic pouchitis. However, Penna *et al.* estimate that approximately 1.3% of patients who undergo IPAA for UC will need a pouch excision for chronic treatment-refractory pouchitis [48]. Sachar noted that resorting to pouch removal for confirmed refractory pouchitis is largely a quality-of-life decision for the patients themselves, and should be made in conjunction with a supportive gastroenterologist and surgeon [142].

Summary

Pouchitis is an idiopathic inflammatory disease of the ileal reservoir in patients who have undergone IPAA. Approximately half of all UC patients who undergo this procedure will have at least one episode of pouchitis, with approximately 15% experiencing a chronic course. PSC and other EIM increase the likelihood of developing pouchitis while smoking is protective. Similar genetic and autoimmune mechanisms to UC appear to occur in an ileal reservoir that demonstrates increasingly colon-like adaptations with respect to bacterial content and mucosal characteristics. While most patients have a good response to antibiotic therapy, those with chronic disease become a therapeutic challenge with the specter of dysplasia looming in the foreground.

References

1. Kock NG, Darle N, Hulten L, Kewenter J, Myrvold H, Philipson B. Ileostomy. Curr Prob Surg 1977; 14: 1–52.
2. Kock NG. Intra-abdominal 'reservoir' in patients with permanent ileostomy. Preliminary observations on a procedure resulting in fecal 'continence' in five ileostomy patients. Arch Surg 1969; 99: 223–31.
3. Parks AG, Nicholls RJ, Belliveau P. Proctocolectomy with ileal reservoir and anal anastomosis. Br J Surg 1980; 67: 533–8.
4. Utsunomiya J, Iwama T, Imajo M et al. Total colectomy, mucosal proctectomy, and ileoanal anastomosis. Dis Colon Rectum 1980; 23: 459–66.
5. Tiainen J, Matikainen M. Health-related quality of life after ileal J-pouch–anal anastomosis for ulcerative colitis: long-term results. Scand J Gastroenterol 1999; 34: 601–5.
6. Martin A, Dinca M, Leone L et al. Quality of life after proctocolectomy and ileo-anal anastomosis for severe ulcerative colitis. Am J Gastroenterol 1998; 93: 166–9.
7. Provenzale D, Shearin M, Phillips-Bute BG et al. Health-related quality of life after ileoanal pull-through evaluation and assessment of new health status measures. Gastroenterology 1997; 113: 7–14.
8. Pemberton JH, Kelly KA, Beart RW, Jr, Dozois RR, Wolff BG, Ilstrup DM. Ileal pouch–anal anastomosis for chronic ulcerative colitis. Long-term results. Ann Surg 1987; 206(4): 504–13.
9. Di Febo G, Miglioli M, Lauri A et al. Endoscopic assessment of acute inflammation of the ileal reservoir after restorative ileo-anal anastomosis. Gastrointest Endosc 1990; 36: 6–9.
10. Setti Carraro PG, Talbot IC, Nicholls JR. Patterns of distribution of endoscopic and histological changes in the ileal reservoir after restorative proctocolectomy for ulcerative colitis. A long-term follow-up study. Int J Colorect Dis 1998; 13: 103–7.
11. Moskowitz RL, Shepherd NA, Nicholls RJ. An assessment of inflammation in the reservoir after restorative proctocolectomy with ileoanal ileal reservoir. Int J Colorect Dis 1986; 1: 167–74.
12. Sandborn WJ, Tremaine WJ, Batts KP, Pemberton JH, Phillips SF. Pouchitis after ileal pouch–anal anastomosis: a Pouchitis Disease Activity Index. Mayo Clin Proc 1994; 69: 409–15.
13. Sandborn W. Pouchitis: Definition, Risk Factors, Frequency, Natural History, Classification, and Public Health Perspective. Lancaster, England: Kluwer Academic Publishers; 1997.
14. Moonka D, Furth EE, MacDermott RP, Lichtenstein GR. Pouchitis associated with primary cytomegalovirus infection. Am J Gastroenterol 1998; 93: 264–6.
15. Munoz-Juarez M, Pemberton JH, Sandborn WJ, Tremaine WJ, Dozois RR. Misdiagnosis of specific cytomegalovirus infection of the ileoanal pouch as refractory idiopathic chronic pouchitis: report of two cases. Dis Colon Rectum 1999; 42: 117–20.
16. Solomon MJ, McLeod RS, O'Connor BI, Cohen Z. Assessment of peripouch inflammation after ileoanal anastomosis using endoluminal ultrasonography. Dis Colon Rectum 1995; 38: 182–7.
17. Woolfson K, McLeod RS, Walfisch S, Yip K, Cohen Z. Pelvic pouch emptying scan: an evaluation of scintigraphic assessment of the neorectum. Int J Colorect Dis 1991; 6: 29–32.
18. de Silva HJ, Millard PR, Soper N, Kettlewell M, Mortensen N, Jewell DP. Effects of the faecal stream and stasis on the ileal pouch mucosa. Gut 1991; 32: 1166–9.
19. Merrett MN, Soper N, Mortensen N, Jewell DP. Intestinal permeability in the ileal pouch. Gut 1996; 39: 226–30.
20. Apel R, Cohen Z, Andrews CW, Jr, McLeod R, Steinhart H, Odze RD. Prospective evaluation of early morphological changes in pelvic ileal pouches. Gastroenterology 1994; 107: 435–43.
21. Stallmach A, Moser C, Hero-Gross R et al. Pattern of mucosal adaptation in acute and chronic pouchitis. Dis Colon Rectum 1999; 42: 1311–7.
22. Campbell AP, Merrett MN, Kettlewell M, Mortensen NJ, Jewell DP. Expression of colonic antigens by goblet and columnar epithelial cells in ileal pouch mucosa: their association with inflammatory change and faecal stasis. J Clin Pathol 1994; 47: 834–8.
23. de Silva HJ, Millard PR, Kettlewell M, Mortensen NJ, Prince C, Jewell DP. Mucosal characteristics of pelvic ileal pouches. Gut 1991; 32: 61–5.
24. Shepherd NA, Healey CJ, Warren BF, Richman PI, Thomson WH, Wilkinson SP. Distribution of mucosal pathology and an assessment of colonic phenotypic change in the pelvic ileal reservoir. Gut 1993; 34: 101–5.

25. Lichtman SN, Wang J, Hummel B, Lacey S, Sartor RB. A rat model of ileal pouch–rectal anastomosis. Inflam Bowel Dis 1998; 4: 187–95.

26. de Silva HJ, Jones M, Prince C, Kettlewell M, Mortensen NJ, Jewell DP. Lymphocyte and macrophage subpopulations in pelvic ileal pouches. Gut 1991; 32: 1160–5.

27. Gionchetti P, Campieri M, Belluzzi A et al. Mucosal concentrations of interleukin-1 beta, interleukin-6, interleukin-8, and tumor necrosis factor-alpha in pelvic ileal pouches. Dig Dis Sci 1994; 39: 1525–31.

28. Patel RT, Bain I, Youngs D, Keighley MR. Cytokine production in pouchitis is similar to that in ulcerative colitis. Dis Colon Rectum 1995; 38: 831–7.

29. Schreiber S, Gionchetti P, Hampe J et al. Pouchitis shares similarities with ulcerative colitis in the pattern of cytokine transcription factor activation. Gastroenterology 1997; 112: A10086.

30. Kuhbacher T, Gionchetti P, Hampe J. Pouchitis shares similarities with ulcerative colitis in the pattern of cytokine transcription factor activation. Gut 1997 1997; 41(Suppl. 3): A–P148.

31. Stallmach A, Schafer F, Hoffmann S et al. Increased state of activation of CD4 positive T cells and elevated interferon gamma production in pouchitis. Gut 1998; 43: 499–505.

32. Gertner DJ, Rampton DS, Madden MV, Talbot IC, Nicholls RJ, Lennard-Jones JE. Increased leukotriene B4 release from ileal pouch mucosa in ulcerative colitis compared with familial adenomatous polyposis. Gut 1994; 35: 1429–32.

33. Boerr LA, Sambuelli AM, Filinger E et al. Increased mucosal levels of leukotriene B4 in pouchitis: evidence for a persistent inflammatory state. Eur J Gastroenterol Hepatol 1996; 8: 57–61.

34. Sandborn WJ, Landers CJ, Tremaine WJ, Targan SR. Antineutrophil cytoplasmic antibody correlates with chronic pouchitis after ileal pouch–anal anastomosis. Am J Gastroenterol 1995; 90: 740–7.

35. Aitola P, Matikainen M, Mattila J, Tomminen T, Hiltunen KM. Chronic inflammatory changes in the pouch mucosa are associated with cholangitis found on peroperative liver biopsy specimens at restorative proctocolectomy for ulcerative colitis. Scand J Gastroenterol 1998; 33: 289–93.

36. Esteve M, Mallolas J, Klaassen J et al. Antineutrophil cytoplasmic antibodies in sera from colectomised ulcerative colitis patients and its relation to the presence of pouchitis. Gut 1996; 38: 894–8.

37. Reumaux D, Colombel JF, Duclos B et al. Antineutrophil cytoplasmic auto-antibodies in sera from patients with ulcerative colitis after proctocolectomy with ileo-anal anastomosis. Adv Exp Med Biol 1993; 336: 523–5.

38. Patel RT, Stokes R, Birch D, Ibbotson J, Keighley MR. Influence of total colectomy on serum antineutrophil cytoplasmic antibodies in inflammatory bowel disease. Br J Surg 1994; 81: 724–6.

39. Yang P, Oresland T, Jarnerot G, Hulten L, Danielsson D. Perinuclear antineutrophil cytoplasmic antibody in pouchitis after proctocolectomy with ileal pouch–anal anastomosis for ulcerative colitis. Scand J Gastroenterol 1996; 31: 594–8.

40. Freeman HJ, Roeck B, Devine DV, Carter CJ. Atypical perinuclear antineutrophil cytoplasmic antibodies after colectomy in inflammatory bowel disease. Can J Gastroenterol 1997; 11: 305–10.

41. Vecchi M, Gionchetti P, Bianchi MB et al. p-ANCA and development of pouchitis in ulcerative colitis patients after proctocolectomy and ileoanal pouch anastomosis [Letter; published erratum appears in Lancet 1994; 344: 1168]. Lancet 1994; 344: 886–7.

42. Aisenberg J, Wagreich J, Shim J et al. Perinuclear antineutrophil cytoplasmic antibody and refractory pouchitis. A case–control study. Dig Dis Sci 1995; 40: 1866–72.

43. Brett PM, Yasuda N, Yiannakou JY et al. Genetic and immunological markers in pouchitis. Eur J Gastroenterol Hepatol 1996; 8: 951–5.

44. Kaditis AG, Perrault J, Sandborn WJ, Landers CJ, Zinsmeister AR, Targan SR. Antineutrophil cytoplasmic antibody subtypes in children and adolescents after ileal pouch–anal anastomosis for ulcerative colitis. J Pediatr Gastroenterol Nutr 1998; 26: 386–92.

45. Yasuda N, Thomas P, Ellis H, Herbst F, Nicholls J, Ciclitira P. Perinuclear anti-neutrophil cytoplasmic antibodies in ulcerative colitis after restorative protocolectomy do not correlate with the presence of pouchitis. Scand J Gastroenterol 1998; 33: 509–13.

46. Duerr RH, Targan SR, Landers CJ et al. Neutrophil cytoplasmic antibodies: a link between primary sclerosing cholangitis and ulcerative colitis. Gastroenterology 1991; 100: 1385–91.

47. Kartheuser AH, Dozois RR, Wiesner RH, LaRusso NF, Ilstrup DM, Schleck CD. Complications and risk factors after ileal pouch–anal anastomosis for ulcerative colitis associated with primary sclerosing cholangitis. Ann Surg 1993; 217: 314–20.

48. Penna C, Dozois R, Tremaine W et al. Pouchitis after ileal pouch–anal anastomosis for ulcerative colitis occurs with increased frequency in patients with associated primary sclerosing cholangitis. Gut 1996; 38: 234–9.

49. Klenzak J, Isaacs K, Koruda M. Predicting pouchitis: race, extraintestinal manifestations of disease and tobacco use. Am J Gastroenterol 1997; 92: A1679 #385.

50. Lohmuller JL, Pemberton JH, Dozois RR, Ilstrup D, van Heerden J. Pouchitis and extraintestinal manifestations of inflammatory bowel disease after ileal pouch–anal anastomosis. Ann Surg 1990; 211: 622–7; discussion 627–9.

51. ter Borg EJ, Nadorp JH, Elbers JR. Ileal pouch arthritis: a case report. Eur J Gastroenterol Hepatol 1996; 8: 957–9.

52. Shepherd NA, Hulten L, Tytgat GN, Nicholls RJ, Nasmyth DG, Hill MJ et al. Pouchitis. Int J Colorect Dis 1989; 4: 205–29.

53. Subramani K, Harpaz N, Bilotta J et al. Refractory pouchitis: does it reflect underlying Crohn's disease? Gut 1993; 34: 1539–42.

54. Gorbach SL, Nahas L, Weinstein L, Levitan R, Patterson JF. Studies of intestinal microflora. IV. The microflora of ileostomy effluent: a unique microbial ecology. Gastroenterology 1967; 53: 874–80.

55. Santavirta J, Mattila J, Kokki M, Matikainen M. Mucosal morphology and faecal bacteriology after ileoanal anastomosis. Int J Colorect Dis 1991; 6: 38–41.

56. Onderdonk AB, Dvorak AM, Cisneros RL et al. Microbiologic assessment of tissue biopsy samples from ileal pouch patients. J Clin Microbiol 1992; 30: 312–7.

57. McLeod RS, Antonioli D, Cullen J et al. Histologic and microbiologic features of biopsy samples from patients with normal and inflamed pouches. Dis Colon Rectum 1994; 37: 26–31.

58. Ruseler-van Embden JG, Schouten WR, van Lieshout LM. Pouchitis: result of microbial imbalance? Gut 1994; 35: 658–64.

59. Becker J, Onderdonk A. Bacterial dysbiosis in the pathogenesis of ileal pouchitis. Gastroenterology 1994; 106(Suppl. 4): A650.

60. Kelly DG, Phillips SF, Kelly KA, Weinstein WM, Gilchrist MJ. Dysfunction of the continent ileostomy: clinical features and bacteriology. Gut 1983; 24: 193–201.

61. O'Connell PR, Rankin DR, Weiland LH, Kelly KA. Enteric bacteriology, absorption, morphology and emptying after ileal pouch–anal anastomosis. Br J Surg 1986; 73: 909–14.

62. Luukkonen P, Valtonen V, Sivonen A, Sipponen P, Jarvinen H. Fecal bacteriology and reservoir ileitis in patients oper-

action utilizing an intravenous loading protocol for AZA was not successful in a controlled clinical trial [49].

Another unresolved issue is the duration of therapy following induction of remission. In one study, patients who had been in remission on AZA or 6-MP for at least 4 years had the same rate of relapse whether treatment was continued or stopped [50]. The series compared patients who had voluntarily discontinued immunomodulation compared to patients who continued on therapy. However, no randomized or prospective data have been generated to assess the ultimate duration of treatment benefits. Many experienced clinicians continue therapy on an indefinite basis.

Despite the clinical efficacy of AZA and 6-MP in CD, a substantial proportion of patients fail to respond to therapy. A meta-analysis of eight randomized, placebo-controlled trials of these agents in the induction of remission in active CD found the overall response rate to be 54% for 6-MP or AZA treatment, compared with 33% for placebo [45]. Inducing leukopenia has been suggested as a means of improving clinical efficacy [51]. The role of therapeutic drug monitoring for 6-thioguanine (6-TGN) nucleotides and 6-methylmercaptopurine has not yet been established in prospective controlled trials, although several series suggest that levels of 6-TGN metabolites and 6-methlylmercaptopurine will predict therapeutic efficacy and toxicity, respectively [52–55]. 6-TGN concentrations greater than 230–250 pmol/8×10^8 red blood cells (RBC) appear to correlate with efficacy, whereas concentrations greater than 500 pmol/8×10^8 RBC correlate with myelosuppression [52, 54, 55]. Differing assays of metabolites may provide different therapeutic ranges and, as yet, comparisons between assays have not been described. A prospective, randomized, controlled trial is needed to test the hypothesis that, compared to standard dosing, 6-MP/AZA dosing adjusted to achieve target therapeutic 6-TGN concentrations will enhance treatment efficacy (and decrease toxicity).

Methotrexate

Methotrexate (MTX), an inhibitor of dihydrofolate reductase and other folate-dependent enzymes, has anti-inflammatory properties that are possibly related to decreased interleukin-1 (IL-1) production, decreased neutrophil chemotaxis, decreased eicosanoid production and other actions including

increased lymphocyte apoptosis [56]. In the first reported uncontrolled study, patients with refractory CD were treated with 25 mg intramuscularly, weekly for 12 weeks, followed by 7.5–15 mg per os weekly. Disease activity (measured by clinical indices) improved, as did endoscopic healing. The dose of MTX was selected arbitrarily, based on studies in asthma, and is higher than doses used to treat rheumatoid arthritis [57]. A dose response has not been defined for MTX in CD, but despite excellent absorption there continues to be more evidence in favor of parenteral administration than for the oral route [58].

Subsequent to the original reports of efficacy for MTX in CD a placebo-controlled trial was performed in steroid-refractory patients that confirmed benefits of the 25 mg dose when administered intramuscularly or subcutaneously, weekly, for 16 weeks. Twice as many MTX-treated patients entered remission (39.4% vs 19.1%; $p = 0.06$) despite cessation of steroids [59]. Patients who achieved remission in this trial and others recruited after open-label MTX were then enrolled in a trial of maintenance therapy. Patients were randomized to MTX 15 mg intramuscularly, weekly, or placebo for 40 weeks. After 40 weeks, 26/40 (65%) of the MTX-treated patients remained in remission, compared with 14/36 (39%) of the placebo-treated patients ($p = 0.01$) [60]. These well-designed studies establish the role of MTX in the treatment of active CD and in the maintenance of remission of quiescent CD.

Mycophenolate mofetil

Mycophenolic acid, the active moiety of mycophenolate mofetil, inhibits inosine monophosphate dehydrogenase and depletes guanine nucleotides in lymphocytes [61]. Mycophenolate mofetil has been employed as part of immunosuppression regimens in cardiac and renal transplantation and other diseases [61]. Uncontrolled studies reported efficacy in the treatment of steroid-dependent, luminal CD and perianal CD [62, 63]. In a randomized, open-label trial, 70 patients with chronically active CD (CDAI > 150) were treated with prednisolone and either mycophenolate (15 mg/kg per day) or azathioprine (2.5 mg/kg per day), and were followed for 6 months [64]. Corticosteroids were tapered according to a standard protocol to a dose of 5 mg/day, which was maintained throughout the study. The two treatment groups had comparable decreases in the CDAI score at 6 months (125 and 152 points in the AZA and mycophenolate groups respectively). Mycophenolate therapy was well tolerated. In the subgroup of patients with more severe disease (CDAI >300), mycophenolate appeared to decrease clinical activity faster than AZA. The short follow-up period, and the concurrent use of low-dose steroids, do not allow any conclusions regarding any maintenance benefit from mycophenolate. A study of 6-MP or AZA non-responders who were treated with mycophenolate reported low efficacy and high rates of discontinuation due to adverse effects [65]. Preliminary data also suggest that initial responders eventually relapse [66]. The are no long-term data on mycophenolate with regard to CD maintenance, steroid-sparing, or safety.

Cyclosporine

Cyclosporine, an important immunosuppressive agent in transplantation, selectively inhibits helper T lymphocytes. Cyclosporine inhibits calcineurin-stimulated events, such as transcription of IL-2, IL-3, IL-4, interferon gamma (IFN-γ) and tumor necrosis factor α (TNF-α) [67–69]. Cyclosporine has low and variable bioavailability, although the newer, micro-emulsion formulation (Neoral) has improved bioavailability compared with the gelatin capsule formulation (Sandimmune) [70]. The relatively narrow therapeutic margin and unpredictable absorption have made the study of cyclosporine difficult for the treatment of CD.

Although initial trials demonstrated optimism for the potential of oral cyclosporine at doses of 5–7.5 mg/kg in active, steroid-refractory CD [71], subsequent maintenance trials failed to demonstrate any prolonged benefits at non-toxic doses [72, 73]. These poor results may have been related to the poor and variable absorption of the Sandimmune formulation. However, when employed intravenously at doses similar to those used for UC (mg/kg continuous intravenous infusion), cyclosporine has been used effectively for steroid-refractory and fistulizing CD with response rates between 60% and 80% in uncontrolled series [74–77]. Nevertheless, cyclosporine therapy has, for the most part, been supplanted by the use of infliximab for refractory and fistulizing CD.

Tacrolimus

Tacrolimus (FK506) is an immunosuppressive agent used in transplantation and in the treatment of various autoimmune disorders [78]. Similar to cyclosporine, tacrolimus inhibits calcineurin-mediated synthesis of IL-2 and other cytokines by T helper lymphocytes [67]. A potential advantage for tacrolimus compared with cyclosporine is better small intestinal absorption, even by diseased small bowel [79]. Uncontrolled studies have reported success of tacrolimus in combination with AZA or 6-MP therapy in some patients with refractory ulcerative colitis (UC) and CD [80]. Tacrolimus combined with AZA or 6-MP and perianal surgery as needed was effective therapy for refractory perianal CD [81]. Similar to the role of cyclosporine in UC, tacrolimus may have a role as 'bridging' therapy to long-term maintenance therapy with AZA or 6-MP [81]. However, no controlled trials have yet been reported that assess tacrolimus for any CD indication.

Anti-TNF therapies

The pleiotropic cytokine, TNF-α, has been implicated as a central mediator in the pathogenesis of rheumatoid arthritis, CD, and other inflammatory disorders [82, 83]. TNF-α induces up-regulation of proinflammatory mediators (IL-1, nitric oxide, and prostaglandins), metalloproteinases and adhesion molecules [82]. In several animal models of IBD neutralization of TNF-α by monoclonal antibodies ameliorates mucosal inflammation [84, 85] and a transgenic mouse that over expresses TNF develops a Crohn's-like bowel disease [86]. In CD a high number of mucosal and lamina propria cells express TNF-α [87–90]. Nevertheless, the most convincing evidence for the central role of TNF-α in human CD came from the dramatic results of therapy with anti-TNF-α monoclonal antibodies.

Infliximab

Infliximab is a high-affinity, chimeric (75% human, 25% murine), anti-TNF-α monoclonal IgG$_1$ antibody consisting of a murine antigen-binding region and a human constant region. Infliximab binds and neutralizes soluble TNF-α [91] by blocking its binding to the p55 and p75 cellular receptors [92]. Infliximab also binds transmembrane TNF-α and causes lysis of TNF-α-expressing murine myeloma cells by both antibody-dependent cellular cytotoxicity and complement-dependent cytotoxicity effector mechanisms [93]. Infliximab has also been shown to induce apoptosis (programmed cell death) of cells bearing surface TNF [94].

Following an initial promising case report [95], a pilot study was conducted in 10 patients with active, steroid-refractory Crohn's ileocolitis who received a single infusion of open-label infliximab (10 mg/kg in eight patients, 20 mg/kg in two patients). The mean CDAI score fell from 257 before treatment to 69 at week 8, and clinical response was accompanied by mucosal healing in all but one patient [96]. In an open-label, dose-escalating study of 20 patients with active, steroid-refractory CD, infliximab was administered sequentially to groups of five patients at doses of 1, 5, 10 and 20 mg/kg. At 4 and 8 weeks the rates of clinical response (defined as a CDAI decline > 70 points) were 90% and 45% respectively. At 4 and 8 weeks clinical remission (defined as a CDAI < 150) was seen in 40% and 25% of patients. The 1 mg/kg dose appeared less effective, but no dose–response effect was seen with the 5, 10 or 20 mg/kg doses [97].

Subsequently, in a 12-week, randomized, double-blind, placebo-controlled trial in moderate–severe CD (CDAI 220–400), 108 patients received a single intravenous infusion of placebo or infliximab (5, 10 or 20 mg/kg) [98]. The primary endpoint was clinical response, defined as a CDAI reduction of ≥ 70 points at 4 weeks. Clinical response was 81%, 50%, 64% and 17% for the 5 mg/kg, 10 mg/kg, 20 mg/kg and placebo groups respectively. Overall clinical response was 65% for the infliximab groups combined ($p < 0.001$ versus placebo). At 12 weeks 41% of the infliximab-treated patients versus 12% of the patients in the placebo group maintained a clinical response ($p = 0.008$). At 4 weeks clinical remission, defined by CDAI score below 150, occurred in 33% of the infliximab-treated patients versus 4% of the placebo-treated patients ($p = 0.005$). By 12 weeks the difference in the rates of clinical remission was not significant (24% in the infliximab group versus 8% in the placebo group, $p = 0.31$). Symptomatic improvement was accompanied by reductions in C-reactive protein (CRP) that began to rise again at 12 weeks.

In a secondary stage of the trial, patients not achieving a clinical response at 4 weeks received open-label infliximab at a dose of 10 mg/kg. Among the placebo-treated non-responders, response and remission rates were 58% and 47% respectively at 4 weeks after the second infusion, i.e. similar to the rates seen in the initial, blinded study. Among the infliximab-treated non-responders, response and remission rates were 34% and 17% respectively, indicating that this group was less likely to respond to infliximab. The fall in clinical response/remission rates, and the CRP increase at 12 weeks, suggest that by that point the effect of infliximab has waned and disease relapses. This trial confirmed the efficacy of infliximab for treatment of moderate–severe CD, with the 5 mg/kg dose showing the best results [98].

In contrast to the lack of correlation between clinical improvement and mucosal healing with steroid treatment of CD [99], infliximab induced both endoscopic healing [100] and decreased histologic disease activity [101] coinciding with reductions in clinical indices and CRP. These findings, coupled with the sustained response observed in some patients, suggest a potential disease-modifying effect of infliximab. This effect may be mediated by lysis of TNF-α-expressing cells, rather than by simple neutralization of soluble or transmembrane TNF-α by circulating antibody [94].

The duration of clinical benefits after a single infusion of infliximab averages 8 weeks with a larger inter-individual range [102]. To evaluate the role of re-treatment, 73 patients who had demonstrated a clinical response to an initial infusion of infliximab or placebo in the induction of remission trial [98], were randomized to re-treatment with infliximab ($n = 37$) or placebo ($n = 36$) [103]. Beginning at 12 weeks after the first infusion, patients received repeat infusions of placebo or infliximab (10 mg/kg) at 8-week intervals (weeks 12, 20, 28 and 36). At 44 weeks the rates of clinical remission were 53% for the infliximab-treated patients and 20% for the placebo-treated patients ($p = 0.013$) [103]. The corresponding rates of clinical response were 62% for the infliximab-treated patients and 37% for the placebo-treated patients, although this difference did not reach statistical significance. Discontinuation of the study medication due to loss of efficacy occurred in 12/36 (33.3%) of patients in the placebo group, compared with 4/37 (10.8%) of the infliximab-treated patients. There was a trend for improved rates of clinical response in patients receiving concurrent treatment with 6-MP or AZA [103]. Our experience at the University of Chicago demonstrates that infliximab allows steroid tapering [102]. Although infliximab appears to be effective in maintaining disease remission, long-term safety data are lacking. However, we are reassured by the 2-year safety experience from combination treatment with infliximab in rheumatoid arthritis at doses up to 10 mg/kg administered monthly concomitant with MTX [104].

Infliximab has also been evaluated in a large study to assess treatment of fistulizing CD [105]. Ninety-four patients with draining abdominal or perianal fistulas were enrolled in an 18-week-long, randomized, double-blind, placebo-controlled trial comparing placebo, infliximab 5 mg/kg or infliximab 10 mg/kg, in a schedule of three intravenous infusions at weeks 0, 2 and 6. Forty percent of the patients were former or current users of AZA or 6-MP, and 30% of patients were using antibiotics. The primary endpoint, a reduction of $\geqslant 50\%$ from baseline in the number of draining fistulas for at least 4 weeks, was achieved by 68% of patients who received infliximab 5 mg/kg and by 56% of patients who received infliximab 10 mg/kg, versus 26% of placebo-treated patients ($p = 0.002$ and $p = 0.02$ respectively). Closure of all fistulas was observed in 55% of patients on the 5 mg/kg dose and 38% of patients on the 10 mg/kg dose, and 13% of placebo-treated patients ($p = 0.001$ and $p = 0.04$ respectively). Infliximab was more beneficial in non-users of AZA or 6-MP (odds ratio of response: 1.8 and 8.3 for users and non-users respectively). This finding is not surprising since immunomodulators have shown efficacy in the treatment of perianal disease. Compared with the placebo-treated patients the infliximab-treated patients had significant decreases in the score on the Perianal Disease Activity Index at weeks 2 and 8. In the responders the median time to response with infliximab was 14 days, compared with 42 days for patients responding to placebo. The median duration of response was 12 weeks. Five patients (all on infliximab) suffered serious adverse reactions; four of these patients were assigned to the 10 mg/kg dose and, of these, three had infectious complications (pneumonia, furunculosis and anal abscess). The study again confirmed that 5 mg/kg was also an optimal dose for treatment of fistulizing CD, although the optimal number and timing of infusions will need to be addressed in future studies [105].

The most frequently reported events in infliximab-treated patients have been headache, nausea and upper respiratory infections [106]. Acute infusion reactions consisting of fever, chills, pruritus, urticaria and shortness of breath or dyspnea occurred in 16% of infliximab-treated patients. Most infusion reactions were mild, and all patients recovered with treatment (e.g. diphenhydramine) and/or discontinuation of the infusion. Human antichimeric antibodies (HACA) developed in 13% of patients and correlated with the occurrence of infusion reactions. Concurrent immunomodulatory therapy with AZA, 6-MP or MTX protected against both infusion reactions and the development of HACA. It is uncertain what role HACA have regarding efficacy, duration of response or risk of infusion reactions. Many patients in clinical trials were re-treated despite the presence of HACA. Other immunologic responses include antibodies to double-stranded DNA that developed in 9% of patients, but only a few patients have developed lupus-like syndromes that appear to behave similar to other reports of drug-induced lupus [106]. The formation of anti-DNA antibodies may be a class effect of related preparations of monoclonal antibodies as they have also been seen with etanercept [107].

A second type of delayed reactions occurred in patients who had received an initial infliximab infusion, followed by a second infusion 6–24 months later. In contrast to the acute infusion reactions these patients had features of a serum sickness-like illness that occurred 3–12 days after the second infusion. These 'delayed hypersensitivity reactions' presented with severe arthralgias, myalgias, fever, rash, and leukocytosis. All patients recovered, although several required hospitalization and treatment with high-dose corticosteroids. Of note, these patients had no evidence of HACA prior to the inciting infusion but rapidly developed high HACA titers coinciding with the delayed hypersensitivity reaction. Thus far there are no reports of these patients receiving subsequent infliximab infusions.

Of 771 patients who have received infliximab in clinical trials (including trials in rheumatoid arthritis), six patients have developed lymphoproliferative disorders, including a 60-year-old patient with CD for 30 years who had also been receiving AZA and who developed a B-cell non-Hodgkin's lymphoma. A 29-year-old patient with CD for 4 years developed Hodgkin's disease 2 weeks after receiving an infliximab infusion at a dose of 5 mg/kg. In this case the rapid emergence of lymphoma makes a causative role for infliximab unlikely. Such reports linking infliximab to lymphoma must be examined carefully, as patients with CD are at increased risk for lymphoma as a result of their underlying disease and immunosuppressive therapies [108]. Overall, the available data provide no firm evidence linking infliximab treatment to infections, malignancy or autoimmune disorders [106].

The ultimate role for infliximab in CD has yet to be defined. The drug has been marketed in the US for only 2 years, and FDA approval has been limited to single infusions of 5 mg/kg for active disease not responding to 'conventional' therapy or as a series of three infusions for fistulizing disease. Nevertheless, most patients who respond to infliximab lose their clinical response by 8–12 weeks and do benefit from repeated infusions. In contrast, infliximab is approved for three initial doses at 0, 2 and 6 weeks followed by maintenance therapy every 8 weeks. The rheumatoid arthritis patients are treated concurrently with MTX and have a lower incidence of HACA formation and infusion reactions. Thus, it is likely that repeated early infusions (and possibly concurrent immune modulation) allow the development of tolerance whereas, as has been noted in the patients with delayed hypersensitivity reactions, single infusions may be tolerizing and increase the risk of delayed hypersensitivity when subsequent infusions are delayed beyond 8–12 weeks.

We currently reserve infliximab therapy for patients who have failed or cannot tolerate therapy with AZA, 6-MP or MTX, and administer repeat infusions of infliximab at approximately 8-week intervals, or as needed according to the duration of the clinical response. Additional indications include patients who are intolerant of steroid therapy, or who have significant symptoms despite steroids, who cannot wait for the long-term response to conventional immune modulators. We have observed that most patients who respond require ongoing therapy with infliximab despite concurrent AZA, 6-MP or MTX. The response to infliximab is probably decreased in patients with intestinal strictures, especially in the presence of proximal bowel dilation [109]. For patients with fistulizing CD we utilize infliximab after a stepwise approach, starting with antibiotics and surgical drainage of purulence and possible placement of setons to prevent re-accumulation of fluctuance. We use infliximab along with AZA or 6-MP maintenance therapy, but also recognize that some patients may achieve long-term results after a single infliximab infusion. Patients are re-treated with infliximab on an as-needed basis to control recurrent fistula drainage.

CDP571

CDP571 is a humanized, high-affinity, anti-TNF-α monoclonal IgG$_4$ antibody that contains the complementarity-determining region of a murine anti-TNF-α antibody linked to a human γ4 heavy chain and κ light chain [110]. CDP571 contains 95% human and 5% murine sequences, and thus has the theoretical advantage of less immunogenicity than infliximab. CDP571 has anti-TNF-α neutralizing

activity but does not fix complement or mediate antibody-dependent cytotoxicity [107].

In a double-blind, placebo-controlled study, 31 patients with mild–moderately active CD (CDAI 150–400) were randomly assigned to receive a single infusion of CDP571 ($n = 21$; 5 mg/kg) or placebo ($n = 10$) and were followed for 8 weeks. The primary endpoint was the change in CDAI after 2 weeks. In the CDP571-treated group, median CDAI fell from 263 to 167 ($p = 0.0003$), whereas in placebo-treated patients the change was not significant (253 and 247, before and after treatment respectively). Six patients in the CDP571-treated group, but no patients in the placebo group, achieved remission (DCAI < 150) at 2 weeks (n.s.) [111]. In the CDP571-treated patients there were significant improvements in the Harvey–Bradshaw score, erythrocyte sedimentation rate and α_1-glycoprotein at 2 weeks, but these improvements were not sustained at follow-up at 4, 6 and 8 weeks. The decline in clinical and laboratory parameters starting at 4 weeks paralleled the progressive fall in CDP571 plasma concentrations.

In a larger, dose-ranging trial, 169 patients with moderate–severely active CD were randomized to placebo or four different regimens of CDP571 (10 or 20 mg/kg at week 0; and 10 mg/kg at weeks 8 and 16, or 10 mg/kg at week 12), and were followed for 24 weeks. At week 2 clinical improvement (defined as a CDAI decrease of > 70 points from baseline) occurred in 15/56 (27%) of the placebo group, 29/54 (54%) of the 10 mg/kg group ($p = 0.005$), and 21/57 (37%) of the 20 mg/kg group. Of interest, the group that received CDP571 at 12-week intervals experienced a significantly longer time before withdrawal from the trial, whereas there were no differences between CDP571 from placebo for patients receiving drug at shorter intervals. Two of 13 (15%) placebo-treated patients with draining fistulas had closure of $\geq 50\%$ of fistulas, compared with 12/24 (50%) of CDP571-treated patients ($p = 0.074$). Among CDP571-treated patients, anti-CDP571 and anti-double-stranded DNA antibodies developed in 9% and 7% of patients respectively [112]. No patients developed HACA.

A second randomized, double-blind, placebo-controlled trial examined the steroid-sparing properties of CDP571 [113]. Seventy-one patients with steroid-dependent CD received CDP571 (20 mg/kg at week 0, and 10 mg/kg at week 8) or placebo. At week 40, 17/39 (43.6%) of CDP571-treated patients were in remission and off steroids, compared with 7/32 (21.9%) of placebo-treated patients ($p = 0.049$). In the CDP571-treated group, anti-CDP571 and anti-double-stranded DNA antibodies developed in 2.6% and 6.7% of patients respectively.

Etanercept

Etanercept is a genetically engineered fusion protein that contains two identical chains of the recombinant extracellular human p75 TNFR monomer fused to the Fc domain of human IgG_1 [114]. Etanercept binds soluble TNF-α and blocks its binding to TNF-α receptors [114, 115]. *In vitro*, etanercept binds to transmembrane TNF-α, but does not result in antibody-dependent or complement-dependent cytotoxicity [107]. In a pilot study, 10 patients with active CD (CDAI 220–450) were treated with etanercept 25 mg subcutaneously twice a week for 12 weeks [116]. Clinical results demonstrated about 50% improvement that was not accompanied by mucosal healing. A larger study, yet to be reported, did not substantiate differences between etanercept and placebo in patients with chronic active CD (Sandborn, W, personal communication).

The success of anti-TNF-α therapy clearly points to TNF-α as a pivotal mediator in the pathogenesis of CD, yet many questions remain as to the precise mechanisms of anti-TNF-α strategies in CD. An understanding of the relative roles of soluble and transmembrane TNF-α, and the identification of the cellular source(s) of TNF-α in CD, may allow the design of better-targeted anti-TNF-α approaches. Comparative studies of non-responders, responders, and long-term responders to infliximab will illuminate the role of TNF and other mediators in the entire disease spectrum of CD. The suggestion of lower efficacy with higher doses of infliximab suggests that 'too much' anti-TNF-α therapy may be detrimental to therapeutic efficacy. Of equal importance, excessive amounts of anti-TNF-α therapies may interfere with the homeostatic role of TNF-α at the systemic level, and may predispose to infection and abnormal immune surveillance of neoplasia. Recently, the FDA has required warnings for both infliximab and etanercept regarding risks of demyelinating neurologic sequelae, as well as risks of miliary tuberculosis in high-risk populations. As with other targeted therapies in CD (topical mesalamine and corticosteroids), targeting anti-TNF therapy to the mucosal level could potentially improve efficacy and minimize toxicity.

Thalidomide

Thalidomide, a drug originally released as a sedative and antiemetic, has multiple immunomodulatory and anti-inflammatory properties, has been re-approved by the FDA for treatment of lepromatous leprosy and has been used to treat aphthous stomatitis [117, 118]. Thalidomide suppresses production of TNF-α [119, 120] and IL-12 [121], but also has other pharmacologic actions, including anti-angiogenesis, that are potentially relevant to IBD [122]. In an open-label trial [123], 16 male and six female patients with steroid-refractory luminal ($n = 9$) and refractory fistulizing ($n = 13$) CD received thalidomide 200 mg/day ($n = 18$) or 300 mg/day ($n = 4$) for 12 weeks. The dose was reduced if patients developed excessive sedation. For lumenal disease, clinical response was defined as a reduction in the CDAI score of > 150 points, and remission was defined by a CDAI score < 150. For fistulizing disease, response was defined as a clinical improvement of $\geqslant 1+$ in three parameters of the goal interval score (GIS) [47], and remission as a score of $\geqslant 2+$ in all three parameters of the GIS. All 14 patients completing 12 weeks of treatment had a clinical response, and nine were in remission (three luminal and six fistula patients). Two patients with fistulizing disease resistant to infliximab responded to thalidomide. Median daily prednisone dose decreased from 26 mg initially, to 7.5 mg at week 12 ($p < 0.05$). Electromyography (EMG) was performed in all patients who completed the trial, and showed evidence of a mild sensorimotor axonal and demyelinating polyneuropathy in two patients. Although the most frequent adverse effect was sedation, peripheral neuropathy was the major limiting factor to long-term use [123]. In another open-label study 12 male patients with steroid-refractory, treatment-resistant CD received a different thalidomide formulation at 50 mg/day ($n = 6$) or 100 mg/day ($n = 6$) for 12 weeks [124]. At the end of the trial 70% of patients had had a clinical response (defined as a reduction in the CDAI score of $\geqslant 100$ points and a reduction of steroid usage by $\geqslant 50\%$), and 20% of patients had achieved remission (defined as a reduction in CDAI score of $\geqslant 100$ points and a CDAI score of < 150 and complete withdrawal of steroids). The median decrease in the CDAI score was 142 points ($p = 0.002$), and there was also a trend for improvement in the IBDQ index. Improvement in the CDAI and IBDQ was seen quickly, within 1–2 weeks of therapy. Drowsiness and peripheral neuropathy, again, were the most common adverse effects, seen in 58% and 42% of binds ICAM1 mRNA and inhibits ICAM1 expression [163]. In a pilot, dose-escalating trial, 20 patients with active, steroid-treated CD were randomized to ISIS 2302 (13 intravenous infusions of 0.5, 1, or 2 mg/kg over 26 days) or placebo, and were followed for 5 months [164]. Steroids were tapered according to the discretion of a blinded investigator, and not according to a standard protocol. ISIS 2302 was well tolerated. The only apparent drug-related adverse effects were transient, dose-related elevations in activated partial thromboplastin time. A dose-related reduction in qualitative intestinal mucosal ICAM1 expression was seen during the treatment period. Corticosteroid usage was significantly lower in the ISIS 2302-treated group, although changes in the scores of the CDAI, endoscopic index of severity and IBDQ did not differ significantly between the two groups. More recently a multicenter trial comparing subcutaneously administered ISIS 2302 (0.5 mg/kg per day for 2 days, 1 week, 2 weeks or 4 weeks) to placebo in patients with steroid-refractory CD, was terminated after interim analysis failed to detect any differences in the rates of remission, CDAI change, or steroid usage at week 14 [165]. A multi-center, double-blind, placebo-controlled trial in 299 patients with active, steroid-dependent CD, randomized patients to ISIS 2302 at 2 mg/kg intravenously three times weekly for 4 weeks, ISIS for 2 weeks, or placebo did not demonstrate significant benefits, although this was possibly related to underdosing of the drug [166].

The α_4 integrins are important mediators of leukocyte migration across vascular endothelium. The integrin $\alpha_4\beta_7$ is a key mucosal homing molecule expressed by a specific subset of gut-homing, memory T cells. $\alpha_4\beta_7$ is involved in both lymphocyte rolling and adhesion to the endothelium, where it binds to mucosal addressin cell adhesion molecule-1 (MAdCAM1) [167]. Antegren is a recombinant, humanized antibody to α_4 with activity against the integrins $\alpha_4\beta_1$ and $\alpha_4\beta_7$. A double-blind, placebo-controlled trial randomized 30 patients with moderately active CD (CDAI 150–400), to a single infusion of Antegren ($n = 18$) or placebo ($n = 12$) [168]. At 2 weeks, seven patients in the Antegren group were in remission (CDAI < 150), compared with one patient in the placebo group ($p = 0.1$). The mean CDAI scores at 0 and 2 weeks in the Antegren group were 258 and 213 ($p = 0.02$), whereas there was no significant change in the placebo group. In this small study, Antegren therapy was safe and well tolerated, with a trend for efficacy.

Probiotics

A body of evidence from experimental and clinical studies indicates a critical role for intestinal microflora in the pathogenesis of CD. In several animal models, germfree animals are protected from intestinal inflammation [169–172], whereas colitis is rapidly induced upon exposure to specific pathogen-free enteric bacteria [169, 171, 173]. In CD patients who have undergone bowel resection with ileo-colonic anastomoses, ileal inflammation is absent when the fecal stream is diverted by a proximal ileostomy [174]. Ileal inflammation occurs after reversal of the ileostomy, or after infusion of ileostomy contents into the bypassed ileum [174, 175]. Antibiotics and bowel rest (see Chapter 29 on Nutritional Therapies) have a role in the management of CD. Probiotics are living microbial feed supplements that benefit the host by changing the microbial balance. In IL-10$^{-/-}$ mice, repopulation of the colon with *Lactobacillus* species restored concentrations to normal and attenuated the colitis [176]. IL-10$^{-/-}$ mice that were exposed to the small intestinal parasitic worm *Heligmosomoides polygyrus* had attenuated colitis [177]. The mechanisms behind the beneficial effects of probiotics could include secretion of antimicrobial products, inhibition of bacterial adherence to the epithelium, alteration of luminal pH, induction of host growth factors, and immunomodulatory effects, such as altered cytokine patterns [178–181]. Collectively, these data point to the importance of bacteria in the initiation and progression of intestinal inflammation. and suggest that modifying the microbial milieu may suppress intestinal inflammation.

Recently, a randomized trial assessed *Saccharomyces boulardii*, a non-pathogenic yeast, in the maintenance treatment of CD. Thirty-two patients with inactive CD of the ileum or colon received a 6-month maintenance therapy with *S. boulardii* 1 g q.d. and mesalamine 1 g b.i.d., or mesalamine alone at a dose of 1 g t.i.d. Treatment with *S. boulardii* was associated with a decrease in the rate of relapse at 6 months from 37.5% (6/16) to 6% (1/16) ($p = 0.04$) [182].

Nutritional approaches

A novel enteric-coated fish oil preparation has been evaluated for clinically quiescent CD patients who had evidence of subclinical disease activity manifest by increased acute phase reactants [183]. Seventy-eight patients were randomized in a 1-year double-blind and placebo-controlled trial investigating enteric-coated fish oil containing 2.7 g of n-3 fatty acids or placebo. After 1 year 59% of patients randomized to fish oil remained in remission compared to 26% of patients in the placebo group ($p = 0.001$). The only side-effect of the fish oil was diarrhea leading four patients to withdraw from the trial. This novel approach to CD requires confirmation. The study group was unique in that patients were in clinical remission, but appeared to have an increased risk of relapse according to the Italian laboratory index. It remains to be determined whether fish oil will have relapse-preventing properties in other clinical settings of CD or if other formulations of n-3 fatty acids will have similar benefits.

Clinical applications

The variety of potential approaches to the medical management of CD must be placed into the context of the clinical disease severity, location and complications. Recent guidelines have been determined based upon evidence from clinical trials as well as clinical experience. Unfortunately, while data from clinical trials can assist in the framework of therapeutic options, large gaps in our evidence base make it impossible to treat all CD patients according to evidence alone [1]. In addition, there are no discrete means of defining clinical disease activity. While, in clinical trials, the CDAI is often employed, this is a cumbersome instrument that is rarely used in clinical practice. Furthermore, there are no validated instruments to separate mild/mild–moderate/moderate/ moderate–severe/severe/or refractory disease states. Clinical experience and good clinical judgement are necessary to manage individual cases. In general, most clinicians invoke a therapeutic pyramid for 'step-up' therapies similar to treatment of rheumatoid arthritis; however, such an algorithm has not been prospectively evaluated. In addition, many patients are treated with combination therapies that have not been tested together in clinical trials.

Supportive and symptomatic therapy

Many gastrointestinal symptoms are non-specific such as frequent bowel movements, abdominal pain, dyspepsia, etc., and the frequency of non-specific abdominal symptoms and irritable bowel syndrome (IBS) is high in the general population. Therefore, an important premise for the treatment of CD is to discriminate between symptoms or signs related to *inflammation* versus symptoms that are related to IBS, a chronic pain syndrome (e.g. fibromyalgia) or anatomic changes (intestinal resection, post-cholecystectomy, etc.). Inflammatory symptoms include bleeding, fevers, night sweats or extraintestinal complaints such as swollen joints or skin lesions (erythema nodosum, pyoderma gangrenosum). Signs include abdominal tenderness or mass, the presence of fecal leukocytes, elevated WBC, ESR or CRP and the mucosal features are confirmed by ulceration demonstrated by radiographic or endoscopic studies. Penetrating complications (i.e. fistula or abscess) are confirmed by CT scan, MRI or ultrasound.

Diarrhea should be evaluated from a pathophysiologic basis to define the optimal management. The presence of fecal leukocytes defines inflammatory diarrhea. Quantification of stool volume, fecal fat, electrolytes and osmolarity assists in determining both causation and treatment approaches. After intestinal resection, fecal fat determinations are helpful to determine the appropriateness of either a low-fat diet or supplementation with bile salt sequestrants. Antidiarrheals such as loperamide or diphenoxylate are useful for many patients with mild symptoms or after short resections, but should be avoided in patients with obstructive symptoms or severe disease (due to the potential of inducing toxic megacolon). Antispasmodics are helpful for patients with mild cramping.

Chronic pain is a common problem for patients with CD. Likewise, iatrogenic narcotic tolerance is an unfortunate consequence of prolonged use of addictive agents. We limit narcotic use to the perioperative period and treat chronic pain with low doses of tricyclic antidepressants or with consultation from a pain-management service.

Dietary advice is dependent upon the individual's symptoms. We are particularly cognizant that fat malabsorption may cause diarrhea and is a contributor to nephrolithiasis. Low-fat diets may be indicated for patients with extensive ileal disease or ileal resection. We recommend low-residue diets for patients with evidence of luminal narrowing or abdominal cramping. In contrast, patients with colon resections or constipation benefit from the addition of soluble fiber or stool bulking agents.

hospitalized patients, response occurs rapidly for patients who have been refractory to oral steroids.

Maintenance of remission

Clinical remission refers to asymptomatic patients or those without inflammatory sequelae. Symptoms due to surgical resection, malabsorption, or irritable bowel syndrome may persist in the absence of active inflammation. Clinical remissions may be induced by medical therapy or surgical resection (in the absence of residual disease).

It is becoming clear that sequential therapy for CD is effective and depends upon the inductive approach utilized to induce a clinical remission. Patients who have responded to an aminosalicylate can continue on the same therapy as long as they continue to respond [15]. Similarly, disease activity that responds to antibiotics typically recurs after cessation of treatment [34]. Therefore, we usually continue antibiotics at the lowest dose that controls symptoms but are observant for side-effects such as paresthesias with metronidazole.

It is equally apparent that corticosteroids do not maintain remissions in CD [22]. Furthermore, aminosalicylates have not been efficacious at maintaining remissions after steroid-induced remissions [5, 14]. Therefore, the majority of patients requiring steroid therapy will benefit from long-term management with either a purine analog [184, 185, 190] or MTX [60]. The duration of treatment with AZA or 6-MP has not been evaluated in prospective trials; nor has the safety of MTX been evaluated for more than 2 years [191]. Long-term (at least 4–5 years) therapy with a purine analog does appear to be efficacious in uncontrolled series, although optimal dosing has not been established for maintenance therapy [50, 192].

The issue of maintenance therapy after infliximab remains speculative. Repeat dosing is necessary for the majority of patients, yet it is unclear whether the addition of immunomodulation improves long-term outcomes [102, 103].

Another category of maintenance therapy for CD includes potential prophylaxis against postoperative recurrence. Without therapy there is a predictable recurrence of endoscopically visible inflammation at, and proximal to, an ileocolonic anastomosis [193]. Definitions of postoperative recurrence have included the presence of endoscopic lesions, clinical recurrence or radiographic recurrence. Clinical trials have evaluated various end-points and have enrolled different types of patients. Nevertheless, there con-

tinues to be an expanding body of evidence in favor of postoperative therapy to delay endoscopic and clinical recurrence of CD [194]. In several trials sulfasalazine at doses above 3 g daily [7] and mesalamine, 3 g daily [195], reduced the risk of postoperative recurrence for up to 3 years in subgroups of patients. However, a recent large multicenter trial did not find any benefits to postoperative 4 g mesalamine daily except for patients with isolated ileal disease [17]. We also performed a trial comparing placebo, a mesalamine (3 g/day) and 6-MP (50 mg/day) and found that both mesalamine and 6-MP were beneficial at delaying endoscopic and clinical postoperative recurrence for at least 2 years [16]. Additional trials of antibiotics are necessary as short-term administration of high-dose metronidazole, 20 mg/kg, was able to reduce recurrence for up to 1 year, but longer duration trials at lower, more tolerable doses, are necessary to evaluate antibiotic therapy [39].

It is clear that environmental factors can influence the risk of postoperative recurrence, with cigarette smoking having a detrimental impact on postoperative maintenance [196]. At present, aside from advising cigarette smokers to discontinue smoking, there is not sufficient evidence to recommend any specific postoperative regimen for individual patients. We therefore attempt to assess an individual's pattern of disease and will recommend postoperative therapy for patients with short-duration, rapidly recurring, or penetrating CD, although we recognize that, at present, it is not possible to treat based upon our current evidence base.

Management of perianal disease

Perianal complications are sufficiently common in CD that discussion of their management deserves mention. The only controlled trial, to date, for treatment of perianal CD examined fistula healing with infliximab and, as mentioned above, a series of three infusions was efficacious in ceasing drainage from fistula for an average of 12 weeks [105]. However, most clinicians still do not consider infliximab a first-line approach to perianal CD, due to the cost and uncertainties regarding long-term use.

Most experienced clinicians approach perianal CD in collaboration with surgeons to ascertain that abscesses have been adequately drained. Persistent drainage from perianal fistulas improves with the use of antibiotics such as metronidazole or ciprofloxacin, either alone or in combination [33, 37, 38]. Once therapy has terminated, however, the majority of patients relapse [34], necessitating long-term treatment. There is also evidence that long-term use of a purine analog can maintain improvement in perianal disease [47]. Prior to the use of infliximab we, and others, had found that intravenous cyclosporine [75, 76] or oral tacrolimus [197, 198] could also reduce fistula output, although relapse was common after ceasing therapy.

Conclusions

At the present time one cannot treat CD on the basis of evidence, alone. There are far too many questions that have not been addressed in clinical trials and unique individual clinical scenarios. A primary need is to understand the etiopathogenesis of CD and to identify subtypes (patterns of disease) with predictable responses to individual or combination therapies. Even with our most common approaches there is controversy regarding the ultimate clinical benefits of aminosalicylate therapy in CD. Optimal dosing and formulations have yet to be established. Recognition that corticosteroid therapy inevitably leads to relapse or steroid-dependence will, eventually, require a more aggressive use of immunomodulators or steroid-sparing alternative treatments. Unfortunately, we have yet to identify optimal dosing regimens or duration of treatment with conventional (AZA, 6-MP, MTX) or novel (infliximab) immunomodulators. Additional data with all of these are needed to assess safety and efficacy with these agents during pregnancy and lactation. Antibiotics remain a great 'underground' therapy for CD, and there is emerging potential for nutritional and probiotic therapies that will need to be assessed in controlled, comparative trials. The postoperative 'model' of anastomotic recurrence offers a more homogeneous group of patients that still require subgrouping to define optimal postoperative treatment strategies. Therapies need to be evaluated both sequentially and in combination, according to disease location, subtype and genetic pattern. Furthermore, as novel approaches become available, new markers for disease activity or genetic markers to predict response may ultimately help to individualize and optimize medical treatment.

References

1. Hanauer SB, Meyers S. Management of Crohn's disease in adults. Am J Gastroenterol 1997; 92: 559–66.

2. Camma C *et al.* Mesalamine in the maintenance treatment of Crohn's disease: a meta-analysis adjusted for confounding variables. Gastroenterology 1997; 113: 1465–73.

3. Greenfield SM *et al.* Review article. The mode of action of the aminosalicylates in inflammatory bowel disease. Aliment Pharmacol Ther 1993; 7: 369–83.

4. Wikberg M, Ulmius J, Ragnarsson G. Review article. Targeted drug delivery in treatment of intestinal diseases. Aliment Pharmacol Ther 1997; 11(Suppl 3.): 109–15.

5. Summers RW *et al.* National Cooperative Crohn's Disease Study: results of drug treatment. Gastroenterology 1979; 77: 847–69.

6. Malchow H *et al.* European Cooperative Crohn's Disease Study (ECCDS): results of drug treatment. Gastroenterology 1984; 86: 249–66.

7. Ewe K *et al.* Postoperative recurrence of Crohn's disease in relation to radicality of operation and sulfasalazine prophylaxis: a multicenter trial. Digestion 1989; 42: 224–32.

8. Singleton JW *et al.* Mesalamine capsules for the treatment of active Crohn's disease: results of a 16-week trial. Pentasa Crohn's Disease Study Group. Gastroenterology 1993; 104: 1293–301.

9. Hanauer S, Stromberg U. A meta-analysis of 4 g Pentasa trials in active Crohn's disease. Aliment Pharmacol Ther 2002 (In press).

10. Colombel JF *et al.* A controlled trial comparing ciprofloxacin with mesalazine for the treatment of active Crohn's disease. Groupe d'Etudes Therapeutiques des Affections Inflammatoires Digestives (GETAID). Am J Gastroenterol 1999; 94: 674–8.

11. Thomsen OO *et al.* A comparison of budesonide and mesalamine for active Crohn's disease. International Budesonide-Mesalamine Study Group. N Engl J Med 1998; 339: 370–4.

12. Tremaine WJ *et al.* A randomized, double-blind, placebo-controlled trial of the oral mesalamine (5-ASA) preparation, Asacol, in the treatment of symptomatic Crohn's colitis and ileocolitis. J Clin Gastroenterol 1994; 19: 278–82.

13. Prantera C *et al.* Mesalamine in the treatment of mild to moderate active Crohn's ileitis: results of a randomized, multicenter trial. Gastroenterology 1999; 116: 521–6.

14. Modigliani R *et al.* Mesalamine in Crohn's disease with steroid-induced remission: effect on steroid withdrawal and remission maintenance. Groupe d'Etudes des Affections Inflammatoires Digestives. Gastroenterology 1996; 110: 688 93.

15. Hanauer SB *et al.* Long-term management of Crohn's disease with mesalamine capsules (Pentasa). Pentasa Crohn's Disease Compassionate Use Study Group. Am J Gastroenterol 1993; 88: 1343–51.

16. Korelitz B *et al.* Postoperative prophylaxis with 6MP, 5-ASA or placebo in Crohn's disease: a 2 year multicenter trial. Gastroenterology 1998; 114: A688 (Abstract).

17. Lochs H *et al.* Prophylaxis of postoperative relapse in Crohn's disease with mesalamine. European Cooperative Crohn's Disease Study VI. Gastroenterology, 2000; 118: 264–73.

18. Hanauer SB. Review articles: drug therapy: inflammatory bowel disease. N Engl J Med 1996; 334: 841–8.

19. Barnes PJ. Anti-inflammatory actions of glucocorticoids: molecular mechanisms. Clin Sci 1998; 94: 557–72.

20. Kornbluth A *et al.* How effective is current medical therapy for severe ulcerative and Crohn's colitis? An analytic review of selected trials. J Clin Gastroenterol 1995. 20: 280–4.

21. Munkholm P *et al.* Frequency of glucocorticoid resistance and dependency in Crohn's disease. Gut 1994; 35: 360–2.

22. Steinhart, AH *et al.* Corticosteroids for maintaining remission of Crohn's disease. Cochrane Database Syst Rev 2000; 2.

108. Bickston SJ *et al.* The relationship between infliximab treatment and lymphoma in Crohn's disease. Gastroenterology 1999; 117: 1433–7.

109. Lichtenstein GR *et al.* Response to infliximab is decreased in the presence of intestinal strictures in patients with Crohn's disease. Am J Gastroenterol 1999; 94: 2676 (Abstract).

110. Stephens S *et al.* Comprehensive pharmacokinetics of a humanized antibody and analysis of residual anti-idiotypic responses. Immunology 1995; 85: 668–74.

111. Stack WA *et al.* Randomised controlled trial of CDP571 antibody to tumour necrosis factor-alpha in Crohn's disease. Lancet 1997; 349: 521–4.

112. Sandborn WJ *et al.* A randomized controlled trial of CDP571, a humanized antibody to TNFa in moderately to severely active Crohn's disease. Gastroenterology 2000; 118: A655 (Abstract).

113. Feagan BG *et al.* A randomized, double-blind, placebo-controlled, multi-center trial of engineered human antibody to TNF (CDP571) for steroid sparing and maintenance of remission in patients with steroid-dependent Crohn's disease. Gastroenterology 2000; 118: A655 (Abstract).

114. Mohler KM *et al.* Soluble tumor necrosis factor (TNF) receptors are effective therapeutic agents in lethal endotoxemia and function simultaneously as both TNF carriers and TNF antagonists. J Immunol 1993; 151: 1548–61.

115. Mohler KM *et al.* Protection against a lethal dose of endotoxin by an inhibitor of tumour necrosis factor processing. Nature 1994; 370: 218–20.

116. D'Haens G *et al.* Etanercept (TNF receptor fusion protein, Enbrel) is effective and well tolerated in active refractory Crohn's disease: results of a single center pilot trial. Gastroenterology 2000; 118: A656 (Abstract).

117. Corral LG, Kaplan G. Immunomodulation by thalidomide and thalidomide analogues. Ann Rheum Dis 1999; 58(Suppl. 1): I107–13.

118. Calabrese L, Fleischer AB. Thalidomide: current and potential clinical applications. Am J Med 2000; 108: 487–95.

119. Sampaio EP *et al.* Thalidomide selectively inhibits tumor necrosis factor alpha production by stimulated human monocytes. J Exp Med 1991; 173: 699–703.

120. Moreira AL *et al.* Thalidomide exerts its inhibitory action on tumor necrosis factor alpha by enhancing mRNA degradation. J Exp Med 1993; 177: 1675–80.

121. Moller DR *et al.* Inhibition of IL-12 production by thalidomide. J Immunol 1997; 159: 5157–61.

122. Sands BE, Podolsky DK. New life in a sleeper: thalidomide and Crohn's disease. Gastroenterology 1999; 117: 1485–8.

123. Ehrenpreis ED *et al.* Thalidomide therapy for patients with refractory Crohn's disease: an open-label trial. Gastroenterology 1999; 117: 1271–7.

124. Vasiliauskas EA *et al.* An open-label pilot study of low-dose thalidomide in chronically active, steroid-dependent Crohn's disease. Gastroenterology 1999; 117: 1278–87.

125. De Waal Malefyt R *et al.* Interleukin-10. Curr Opin Immunol 1992; 4: 314–20.

126. De Vries JE. Immunosuppressive and anti-inflammatory properties of interleukin 10. Ann Med 1995; 27: 537–41.

127. Kuhn R *et al.* Interleukin-10-deficient mice develop chronic enterocolitis. Cell 1993; 75: 263–74.

128. Davidson NJ *et al.* T helper cell 1-type CD4+ T cells, but not B cells, mediate colitis in interleukin 10-deficient mice. J Exp Med 1996; 184: 241–51.

129. Van Deventer SJ, Elson CO, Fedorak RN. Multiple doses of intravenous interleukin 10 in steroid-refractory Crohn's disease. Crohn's Disease Study Group. Gastroenterology 1997; 113: 383–9.

130. Fedorak RN *et al.* Safety, tolerance and efficacy of multiple doses of subcutaneous interleukin-10 in mild to moderate active Crohn's disease (STAMM-CD). Gastroenterology 1998; 114: A974 (Abstract).

131. Schreiber S *et al.* A safety and efficacy study of recombinant human interleukin-10 (rHuIL-10) treatment in 329 patients with chronic active Crohn's disease (CACD). Gastroenterology 1998; 114: A1080 (Abstract).

132. Colombel J *et al.* Safety and tolerance of subcutaneous recombinant human interleukin-10 (IL-10) in subjects with Crohn's disase after first ileal or ileocecal resection. Gastroenterology 1998; 116: A689 (Abstract).

133. Rogy MA *et al.* Transfer of interleukin-4 and interleukin-10 in patients with severe inflammatory bowel disease of the rectum. Hum Gene Ther 2000; 11: 1731–41.

134. Steidler L *et al.* Treatment of murine colitis by *Lactococcus lactis* secreting interleukin-10. Science 2000; 289: 1352–5.

135. Keith JC Jr *et al.* IL-11, a pleiotropic cytokine: exciting new effects of IL-11 on gastrointestinal mucosal biology. Stem Cells 1994; 12(Suppl. 1): 79–89.

136. Qiu BS, Pfeiffer CJ, Keith JC Jr. Protection by recombinant human interleukin-11 against experimental TNB-induced colitis in rats. Dig Dis Sci 1996; 41: 1625–30.

137. Keith JC *et al.* Oral delivery of recombinant human interleukin-11 decreases clinical signs and histologic lesions in animal models of inflammatory bowel disease. Gastroenterology 2000; 118: A701 (Abstract).

138. Sands BE *et al.* Preliminary evaluation of safety and activity of recombinant human interleukin 11 in patients with active Crohn's disease. Gastroenterology 1999; 117: 58–64.

139. Trinchieri G. Interleukin-12: a cytokine produced by antigen-presenting cells with immunoregulatory functions in the generation of T-helper cells type 1 and cytotoxic lymphocytes. Blood 1994; 84: 4008–27.

140. Monteleone G *et al.* Interleukin 12 is expressed and actively released by Crohn's disease intestinal lamina propria mononuclear cells. Gastroenterology 1997; 112: 1169–78.

141. Parronchi P *et al.* Type 1 T-helper cell predominance and interleukin-12 expression in the gut of patients with Crohn's disease. Am J Pathol 1997; 150: 823–32.

142. Fuss IJ *et al.* Disparate CD4+ lamina propria (LP) lymphokine secretion profiles in inflammatory bowel disease. Crohn's disease LP cells manifest increased secretion of IFN-gamma, whereas ulcerative colitis LP cells manifest increased secretion of IL-5. J Immunol 1996; 157: 1261–70.

143. Neurath MF *et al.* Antibodies to interleukin 12 abrogate established experimental colitis in mice. J Exp Med 1995; 182: 1281–90.

144. Ehrhardt RO *et al.* Induction and prevention of colonic inflammation in IL-2-deficient mice. J Immunol 1997; 158: 566–73.

145. Davidson NJ *et al.* IL-12, but not IFN-gamma, plays a major role in sustaining the chronic phase of colitis in IL-10-deficient mice. J Immunol 1998; 161: 3143–9.

146. Simpson SJ *et al.* T cell-mediated pathology in two models of experimental colitis depends predominantly on the interleukin 12/Signal transducer and activator of transcription (Stat)-4 pathway, but is not conditional on interferon gamma expression by T cells. J Exp Med 1998; 187: 1225–34.

147. Liu Z *et al.* Anti-interleukin 12 antibody prevents experimental colitis in SCID mice reconstituted with CD45RBHIGH CD4+ T cells. Gastroenterology 2000; 118: A576 (Abstract).

148. Barnes PJ, Karin M. Nuclear factor-kappaB: a pivotal transcription factor in chronic inflammatory diseases. N Engl J Med 1997; 336: 1066–71.

149. Schottelius AJ, Baldwin AS Jr. A role for transcription factor NF-kappa B in intestinal inflammation. Int J Colorectal Dis 1999; 14: 18–28.

150. Neurath MF *et al.* Local administration of antisense phosphorothioate oligonucleotides to the p65 subunit of NF-kappa B abrogates established experimental colitis in mice. Nat Med 1996; 2: 998–1004.

151. Rogler G *et al.* Nuclear factor kappaB is activated in macrophages and epithelial cells of inflamed intestinal mucosa. Gastroenterology 1998; 115: 357–69.

152. Schreiber S, Nikolaus S, Hampe J. Activation of nuclear factor kappa B inflammatory bowel disease. Gut 1998; 42: 477–84.

153. Podolsky DK *et al.* Attenuation of colitis in the cotton-top tamarin by anti-alpha 4 integrin monoclonal antibody. J Clin Invest 1993; 92: 372–80.

154. Wong PY *et al.* Antibodies to intercellular adhesion molecule-1 ameliorate the inflammatory response in acetic acid-induced inflammatory bowel disease. J Pharmacol Exp Ther 1995; 274: 475–80.

155. Palmen MJ *et al.* Anti-CD11b/CD18 antibodies reduce inflammation in acute colitis in rats. Clin Exp Immunol 1995; 101: 351–6.

156. Hesterberg PE *et al.* Rapid resolution of chronic colitis in the cotton-top tamarin with an antibody to a gut-homing integrin alpha 4 beta 7. Gastroenterology 1996; 111: 1373–80.

157. Picarella, D *et al.* Monoclonal antibodies specific for beta 7 integrin and mucosal addressin cell adhesion molecule-1 (MAdCAM-1) reduce inflammation in the colon of scid mice reconstituted with CD45RBhigh CD4+ T cells. J Immunol 1997; 158: 2099–106.

158. Bennett CF *et al.* An ICAM-1 antisense oligonucleotide prevents and reverses dextran sulfate sodium-induced colitis in mice. J Pharmacol Exp Ther 1997; 280: 988–1000.

159. Cronstein BN, Weissmann G. The adhesion molecules of inflammation. Arthritis Rheum 1993; 36: 147–57.

160. Gonzalez-Amaro R *et al.* Pentoxifylline inhibits adhesion and activation of human T lymphocytes. J Immunol 1998; 161: 65–72.

161. Malizia G *et al.* Expression of leukocyte adhesion molecules by mucosal mononuclear phagocytes in inflammatory bowel disease. Gastroenterology 1991; 100: 150–9.

162. Nakamura S *et al.* In situ expression of the cell adhesion molecules in inflammatory bowel disease. Evidence of immunologic activation of vascular endothelial cells. Lab Invest 1993; 69: 77–85.

163. Bennett CF *et al.* Inhibition of endothelial cell adhesion molecule expression with antisense oligonucleotides. J Immunol 1994; 152: 3530–40.

164. Yacyshyn BR *et al.* A placebo-controlled trial of ICAM-1 antisense oligonucleotide in the treatment of Crohn's disease. Gastroenterology 1998; 114: 1133–42.

165. Schreiber S *et al.* Anti-sense ICAM-1 (ISIS-2032) for subcutaneous treatment of chronic active Crohn's disease (CACD): Lack of efficacy in a prospective, double-blind, multicenter randomized trial. Gastroenterology 2000; 118: A568 (Abstract).

166. Yacyshyn BR *et al.* Double-blinded, randomized, placebo-controlled trial of the remission inducing and steroid sparing properties of two schedules of ISIS 2032 (ICAM-1 antisense) in active, steroid-dependent Crohn's disease. Gastroenterology, 2000; 118: A570 (Abstract).

167. Salmi M, Jalkanen S. Molecules controlling lymphocyte migration to the gut. Gut 1999; 45: 148–53.

168. Gordon FH *et al.* Randomised double-blind placebo-controlled trial of recombinant humanised antibody to α_4 integrin (AntegrenTM) in active Crohn's disease. Gastroenterology 1999; 116: A726 (Abstract).

169. Rath HC *et al.* Normal luminal bacteria, especially Bacteroides species, mediate chronic colitis, gastritis, and arthritis in HLA-B27/human beta2 microglobulin transgenic rats. J Clin Invest 1996; 98: 945–53.

170. Dianda L *et al.* T cell receptor-alpha beta-deficient mice fail to develop colitis in the absence of a microbial environment. Am J Pathol 1997; 150: 91–7.

171. Sellon RK *et al.* Resident enteric bacteria are necessary for development of spontaneous colitis and immune system activation in interleukin-10-deficient mice. Infect Immun 1998; 66: 5224–31.

172. Contractor NV *et al.* Lymphoid hyperplasia, autoimmunity, and compromised intestinal intraepithelial lymphocyte development in colitis-free gnotobiotic IL-2-deficient mice. J Immunol 1998; 160: 385–94.

173. Sartor RB. Postoperative recurrence of Crohn's disease: the enemy is within the fecal stream. Gastroenterology 1998; 114: 398–400.

174. Rutgeerts P *et al.* Effect of faecal stream diversion on recurrence of Crohn's disease in the neoterminal ileum. Lancet 1991; 338: 771–4.

175. D'Haens GR *et al.* Early lesions of recurrent Crohn's disease caused by infusion of intestinal contents in excluded ileum. Gastroenterology 1998; 114: 262–7.

176. Madsen KL *et al.* Lactobacillus species prevents colitis in interleukin 10 gene-deficient mice. Gastroenterology 1999; 116: 1107–14.

177. Elliott DE *et al.* Helminthic parasites inhibit spontaneous colitis in IL-10 deficient mice. Gastroenterology 2000; 118: A863 (Abstract).

178. Campieri M, Gionchetti P. Probiotics in inflammatory bowel disease: new insight to pathogenesis or a possible therapeutic alternative? Gastroenterology 1999; 116: 1246–9.

179. Gionchetti P *et al.* In vivo effect of a highly concentrated probiotic on IL-10 pelvic ileal-pouch tissue levels. Gastroenterology 1999; 116: A723 (Abstract).

180. O'Mahony L *et al.* Probiotics, mononuclear cells, and epithelial cells: an anti-inflammatory network. Gastroenterology 2000; 118: A102 (Abstract).

181. Schultz M *et al.* Oral administration of *Lactobacillus* GG (L.GG) induces an antiinflammatory, TH-2 mediated systemic immune response towards intestinal organisms. Gastroenterology 2000; 118: A781 (Abstract).

182. Guslandi M. Flare-up of Crohn's disease is prevented by Saccharomyces boulardii. Gastroenterology 2000; 118: A779 (Abstract).

183. Belluzzi A *et al.* Effect of an enteric-coated fish-oil preparation on relapses in Crohn's disease. N Engl J Med 1996; 334: 1557–60.

184. Candy S *et al.* A controlled double blind study of azathioprine in the management of Crohn's disease. Gut 1995; 37: 674–8.

185. Markowitz J *et al.* A multicenter trial of 6-mercaptopurine and prednisone in children with newly diagnosed Crohn's disease. Gastroenterology 2000; 119: 895–902.

186. Valentine JF, Sninsky CA. Prevention and treatment of osteoporosis in patients with inflammatory bowel disease. Am J Gastroenterol 1999; 94: 878–83.

187. Han PD *et al.* Nutrition and inflammatory bowel disease. Gastroenterol Clin North Am 1999; 28: 423–43, ix.

188. Felder JB, Adler DJ, Korelitz BI. The safety of corticosteroid therapy in Crohn's disease with an abdominal mass. Am J Gastroenterol 1991; 86: 1450–5.

189. Chun A *et al.* Intravenous corticotrophin vs. hydrocortisone in the treatment of hospitalized patients with Crohn's disease: a randomized double-blind study and follow-up. Inflam Bowel Dis 1998; 4: 177–81.

190. Ewe K *et al.* Azathioprine combined with prednisolone or monotherapy with prednisolone in active Crohn's disease. Gastroenterology 1993; 105: 367–72.

may be delayed while the nutritional status of the severely malnourished patient is improved, or abscesses and inflammatory masses are treated. Percutaneous drainage of intra-abdominal abscesses is an important component of the management of CD patients. Doing this may avoid a multiple-staged operation and a temporary stoma [3]. If there are associated medical conditions they should be treated. Finally, patient education is an important aspect of surgical management. The patient should be prepared both physically and psychologically for surgery.

An ileostomy is frequently required in patients with CD; it may be permanent or temporary. Pre-operative marking of the stoma is essential since how well the stoma functions may have a profound effect on outcome and the patient's acceptance of it [4]. When siting a stoma it should be placed away from scars and creases and in a location where the patient can visualize it adequately when he/she is sitting or lying. If not, the patient may have difficulty changing the appliance. Both stoma placement and siting of incisions are extremely important in patients with CD. These patients will often have multiple operations, possibly require stoma revisions in the future and may have significant weight gain or loss in the future. Thus, not only must the stoma be placed well initially, but other sites, say in the left lower quadrant, should be preserved. For this reason midline incisions are preferred.

Temporary ileostomies may be constructed in a number of situations. If surgery is performed as an emergency, because of a free perforation, abscess or obstruction, it may be unwise to perform an anastomosis because of the risk of it not healing. In this situation the proximal end can be brought out as an ileostomy or colostomy or the anastomosis can be performed with a proximal defunctioning ileostomy. Loop ileostomies are often indicated in patients who have severe perianal disease unresponsive to more conservative surgical procedures or medical therapy. While it is unusual that it will be possible to close the stoma in the future, this will allow the perianal sepsis to settle before performing a proctectomy. Psychologically patients may not be willing to have a permanent stoma initially and may be more accepting of a stoma knowing that there is a possibility, albeit remote, of it being temporary. In the past Harper and colleagues advocated performing a split ileostomy so that medication could be delivered to the defunctioned colon through the distal limb of the ileostomy [5]. However, that approach has failed to gain acceptance at other centers and there is little evidence to support its use.

Laparoscopic surgery for Crohn's disease

With the recent introduction of laparoscopic techniques it is possible to perform gastrointestinal resections laparoscopically. CD is an ideal indication for the laparoscopic approach since it is a benign disease and the concerns related to cancer recurrence do not apply [6–11]. In addition it may produce an improved cosmetic result, which is an important consideration in this, often young and single, patient population. There tends to be less pain and higher patient satisfaction with laparoscopic procedures. On the other hand the patient may have multiple adhesions from previous operations, or a large inflammatory mass, abscess or fistula or obstructed bowel which may preclude a laparoscopic approach. The other issues related to a laparoscopic approach are that it may be more difficult to assess the extent of the disease, particularly small bowel skip lesions, and operative time tends to be longer. However, these issues are of less concern now as more surgeons attain greater experience generally with laparoscopic techniques. There is, however, no consistent evidence that hospital stays are shortened significantly or that return to work occurs earlier following laparoscopy.

As laparoscopic techniques have become more widely adopted the indications have widened. It is well accepted that the laparoscopic approach for performing defunctioning stomas offers real advantages over an open approach. The former can be performed easily with the stoma being brought out through one of the port sites. Currently, terminal ileal and right colon resections, segmental resections of the small and large bowel, proctectomy and reconstruction of the gastrointestinal tract following a Hartmann procedure are being performed. Although it is possible to perform subtotal colectomy and pouch procedures, the benefit of this approach is less obvious with these procedures because of the increased time taken to perform them.

Most proponents advocate performing laparoscopic-assisted resections so that the bowel is exteriorized through a small incision at one of the port sites and the mesentery, which is often thickened, is divided extracorporeally. The early experience suggests that laparoscopic resections are safe, although patient selection is important [6–10]. Reissman *et al.* [6] reported on a series of 72 patients who had laparoscopic surgery for inflammatory bowel dis-

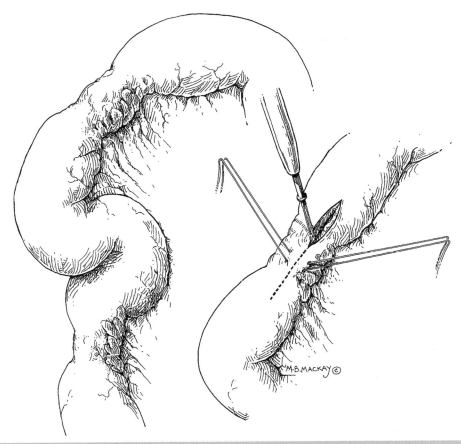

Figure 1. A short stricture due to small bowel Crohn's disease which is amenable to strictureplasty. After insertion of stay sutures, a longitudinal incision on the antimesenteric side of the small bowel is made over the length of the stricture.

ease. The conversion rate was 10% with a complication rate of 18%. The latter was not higher than that observed in a cohort of patients having open surgery. Bauer and colleagues reported the results of 18 patients who had ileal or ileocolic resections for CD. The conversion rate was 22% with no significant complications reported [7]. Ludwig *et al.* reported a conversion rate of 19% and complication rate of 3% in a cohort of 31 patients having various procedures for CD [8]. In a series from the University of Toronto, MacRae and colleagues reported no deaths in 42 patients who had ileocolic resections, and complications in six patients: anastomotic bleeding in three patients, and an enterotomy, intra-abdominal seroma, port-site hematoma and phlegmon in one patient each [9]. Included in this group were seven patients with phlegmons and abscesses, 10 with enteroenteral fistula, one with an enterovesical fistula, four with extensive adhesions, four with small bowel disease elsewhere and four who had had an ileocolic resection previously [9].

Postoperative maintenance therapy

Various medical therapies have been studied in the postoperative setting. While medical therapy is usually prescribed by gastroenterologistis, postoperative maintenance therapies may be prescribed by surgeons. Mesalamine or 5-acetylsalicylic acid (5-ASA) is theoretically an ideal agent for use as maintenance therapy because it has few side-effects and no long-term toxicity. Since most recurrences occur in the pre-anastomotic bowel, formulations where 5-ASA is released and active in the distal small bowel appear to be most effective. There are three trials which have shown that 5-ASA is beneficial in decreasing the symptomatic and/or endoscopic recurrence rates, while a fourth failed to show benefit [12–15]. A meta-analysis by Camma and colleagues, which included the first three trials, revealed an absolute risk reduction of 13% in the postoperative recurrence rate [16]. However, the follow-up time varied in the combined trials, as did the baseline recurrence rate, so it is difficult to interpret this absolute risk reduction. However, it seems that 5-ASA in the postoperative setting is safe but results in a modest reduction in the risk of recurrence. It is also difficult to determine which patients may benefit from it. In a trial performed at our center, 5-ASA appeared to be most effective in those patients with disease limited to the colon, but these patients were also the ones with the lowest risk of recurrence. Korelitz and colleagues performed a three-arm trial in 131 patients comparing 5-ASA (Pentasa 3 g/day) to 6-mercaptopurine (6-MP) 50 mg/day to placebo. Both the symptomatic and endoscopic rates of recurrence were reduced in both treatment groups, although more so in the group receiving 6-MP. Thus, at 24 months, the symptomatic recurrence rates in the 5-ASA and 6-MP groups were 61% and 53% respectively compared to 70% in the placebo group [17].

Two other trials have investigated the use of metronidazole or budesonide in the postoperative setting, but both drugs were ineffective in decreasing recurrence of disease [18, 19]. Because of the side-effects of metronidazole it is poorly tolerated by patients. Although, overall budesonide was of no benefit, it was effective in the subgroup of patients in whom the indication for surgery was inflammatory disease [19]. Fish oil has also shown some benefit in the postoperative setting in one small trial [20].

Surgery for small bowel Crohn's disease

Although CD may affect any part of the small bowel, the terminal ileum is most frequently involved. At the other end of the spectrum there may be multiple skip lesions throughout the small bowel. The pattern of disease may also vary, with some patients having primarily fibrostenotic, inflammatory or fistulizing disease. In a review of 500 patients operated on at the Cleveland Clinic between 1966 and 1973, Farmer and colleagues observed that obstruction was the indication for surgery in 55% and intestinal fistula and abscess in 32% of patients with small bowel disease [21]. The indications in patients with ileocolic disease were similar. Others have reported that patients will continue to manifest with the same patterns of disease after resection [22].

Depending on the site of the disease, and indication for surgery, the surgical approach may vary. However, resection is performed in most patients with small bowel or ileocolic disease. Although strictureplasty is used in only select patients, it has been a valuable addition to the surgical armamentarium in CD. Bypass procedures (the so-called Eisenhower procedure) were popular in the 1960s but they are rarely performed now because of the high rate of recrudescence of the disease in the short term and the increased risk of small bowel cancer in the long term. At present the only indication for a bypass procedure would be a gastrojejunostomy for duodenal CD. In the unusual situation where the surgeon feels it is unsafe to resect small intestinal disease, a defunctioning ileostomy would be preferable to a bypass procedure. However, this situation is rarely encountered today because of improved imaging techniques and the ability to percutaneously drain abscesses preoperatively.

Bowel resection

For disease involving the terminal ileum the resection usually encompasses the terminal ileum and cecum since the disease usually extends to or into the cecum. The decision whether a primary anastomosis will be performed will depend on whether the procedure is performed electively or as an emergency; this includes the status of the patient, including his/her nutritional status; whether he/she is on high doses of steroids or immunosuppressive agents; and the local conditions of the bowel including whether the bowel is obstructed or whether there is an abscess present. In suboptimal conditions it may be prudent to bring out the proximal end of the bowel as an ileostomy or to perform an anastomosis and a proximal defunctioning ileostomy with the plan to reanastomose the bowel at a later date.

While surgery is often successful in treating the complications of the disease, and improving patients' quality of life, recurrence of the disease is a frequent occurrence and therefore a major concern. Recurrence rates vary depending on the criteria used to define recurrence [23]. Thus, endoscopic recurrence rates varying from 29% to 93% at 1 year have been reported [12, 24, 25]. The reported clinical or symptomatic recurrence rates, which are probably most relevant, range from 6% to 16% per year [26]. In our own study of 76 patients who were followed prospectively, the symptomatic recurrence rate was approximately 12% at 1 year and 47% at 3 years [12]. Thereafter there was a decrease in the yearly recurrence rate, which has also been reported by others. It appears that there are various patient factors which

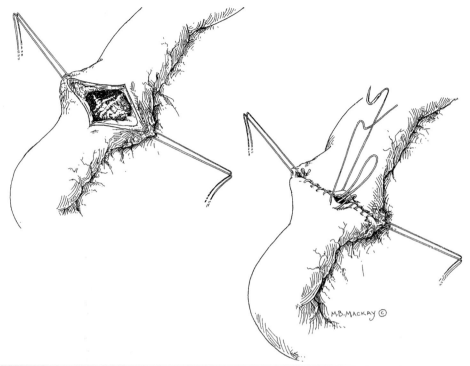

Figure 2. To perform a Heinecke–Mikulicz strictureplasty, the longitudinal incision is closed transversely. This can be done using a running inverting suture.

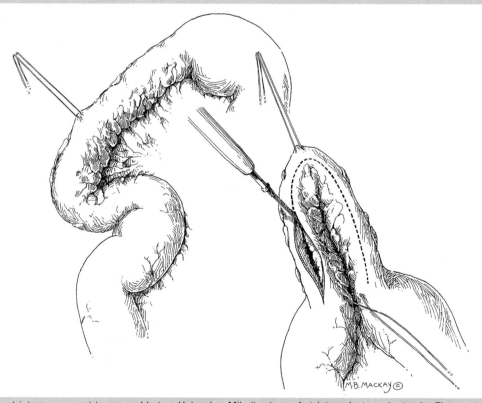

Figure 3. Long strictures may not be amenable to a Heinecke–Mikulicz type of strictureplasty so instead a Finney strictureplasty is preferred. A longitudinal incision is made over the whole length of the stricture along the antimesenteric border of the bowel.

may affect the recurrence rate, including the number of previous operations and the indication for surgery [27]. Smokers also appear to have a higher risk of recurrence [28].

Recognizing that recurrence following surgery is a significant problem, surgeons have looked at various maneuvers which might decrease the risk. There are conflicting data regarding the effect of microscopic disease at the resection margin [23]. However, given that CD is an intestinal disease, that it is focal in distribution, and that histologic abnormalities have been demonstrated in segments of bowel which appear to be grossly normal, the significance of microscopic disease at the resection margin is questionable.

The length of the resection margin has also generated conflicting and controversial results. In the 1970s, Krause and co-workers [29] advocated a radical approach of excising 10–30 cm of normal bowel proximal and distal to the affected area. This was based on a retrospective study with follow-up ranging from 7 to 19 years where recurrence rates of 29% and 84% respectively were reported in patients having radical or limited surgery. However, the two approaches were performed at different hospitals so the possibility of selection biases is real. Fazio and colleagues recently published the results of a randomized controlled trial in which 152 patients were randomized to one of two groups: proximal resection margins of 2 cm in length or 12 cm in length [30]. After a mean follow-up of 56 months the recurrence rate (as defined by the need for a further resection) was 25% in the limited resection group compared to 18% in the extended-resection group, a difference which was not statistically significant. Thus, the approach accepted by most surgeons is to resect the bowel which is grossly involved plus a margin of several centimeters of normal bowel. Frozen sections are usually unnecessary.

While there is theoretical concern that obstruction to the fecal stream may be important in the recurrence of CD preanastomotically, at present there is little evidence to suggest that the type of anastomosis alters the risk. Only one trial of 86 patients has addressed this. Cameron and colleagues randomized patients who had an ileocolic resection to an end-to-end anastomosis or end-to-side anastomosis [31]. After a mean follow-up of 47 months the recurrence rates in the two groups were similar at 23% and 31% respectively. It is hypothesized that a side-to-side anastomosis may be wider, and therefore lead to less fecal stasis than an end-to-end anastomosis. There

are no published randomized controlled trials comparing the two techniques. Munoz-Juarez and colleagues reviewed the experience of 138 patients who had ileocolic resections at the Mayo Clinic and Birmingham General Hospital [32]. There were 69 patients who had stapled side-to-side anastomoses and they were age- and gender-matched to 69 patients who had end-to-end sutured anastomoses. The groups were similar with the exception of mean follow-up (20 vs. 35 months) which may account for the difference in symptomatic recurrence rates of 18% in the stapled and 48% in the sutured group. Two studies have reported similar findings [33, 34]. On the other hand, two other studies have found no difference in recurrence rates when the data were analyzed actuarially [35, 36]. The discrepancies in the reports may be due to the studies being retrospective, with variable criteria for diagnosing recurrence and anastomotic techniques and, finally, follow-up may differ between the groups.

There may be special concerns related to the surgical management of fistulas and abscesses. Hopefully, as discussed previously, abscesses will have been recognized and drained percutaneously preoperatively. If not, anastomosis of the bowel is not advised unless there is a small contained abscess within the mesentery of the resected bowel. The most common fistulas are enterocolonic or enteroenteric, often occurring in segments of bowel which are otherwise normal. Other sites of fistulization are those to the bladder, skin, vagina and less commonly ones involving the stomach and duodenum [37, 38] (also Waly A, McLeod RS, O'Connor BI, Cohen Z, unpublished). In our experience about one-third of patients have multiple fistulas (Waly *et al.*, unpublished). Resection of the involved segment of CD is always required and, in many instances, the fistula can be removed in continuity with the CD. However, if it is into a segment of bowel remote from the CD, the bowel may be repaired or a short segment may have to be resected depending on the amount of surrounding reaction. The bowel may be primarily anastomosed unless there is associated sepsis. In our series only 22% of our patients required an ileostomy, with those having multiple fistulas being more likely to require a defunctioning ileostomy (Waly *et al.*, unpublished).

Strictureplasty

Strictureplasty was first advocated in the 1980s for the treatment of fibrotic strictures in CD [39].

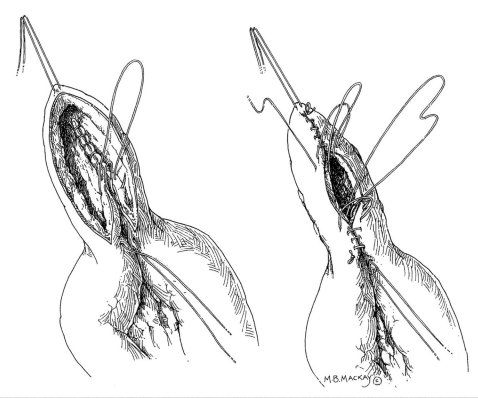

Figure 4. To complete the Finney strictureplasty the bowel is folded on itself and again closed with a running suture beginning with the posterior aspect of the anastomosis and completing it anteriorly.

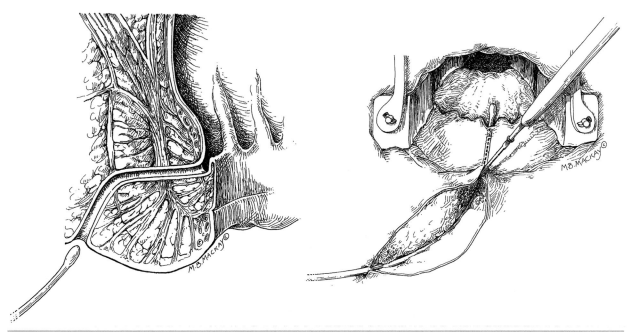

Figure 5. A typical transphincteric fistula arising from a gland at the dentate line and traversing across both the internal and external sphincters and ischiorectal fossa. A fistulotomy is performed by passing a probe through the external opening along the tract to the internal opening, which in this case is in the posterior midline. A fistulotomy is performed by cutting down on to the fistula tract in its entirety. The bed of the fistula tract may be curetted but it is not excised. In performing fistulotomy in this patient a part of the internal and external sphincters will be divided as well as the overlying skin and subcutaneous tissue.

Although resection of the diseased segment is still the preferred surgical option for most patients, strictureplasties have been used with increasing frequency, especially in patients who have multiple skip lesions or have had multiple resections in the past. As a consequence the largest experience has been with strictureplasties performed in the small bowel. However, they may also be performed for strictures involving a previous ileocolic anastomosis, as well as those in the duodenum and colon. Strictureplasty is less applicable to strictures in the colon, since there is usually involvement of the rest of the colon which requires resection. One must also always be cautious that a stricture in the colon is not cancerous.

Two types of strictureplasties have been described: the so-called Heinicke–Mickulitz which is performed for short strictures and the Finney for longer strictures. In performing a strictureplasty a longitudinal incision is made the length of the stricture. The base of the strictureplasty should be biopsied to ensure it is not a malignant stricture. Our preference is to suture the bowel using a one-layer continuous absorbable suture. Because the bowel is usually thickened and fibrotic there is a risk of fracture if a stapler is used (Figs. 1–4).

Recently Michelassi *et al.* described a side-to-side isoperistaltic strictureplasty for management of a long segment of disease or multiple strictures in the midsmall bowel [40]. The bowel is divided and a side-to-side anastomosis is performed, thus avoiding a resection, a blind loop or a bypassed segment. Although they reported no complications with this technique it has been used in only a small number patients so one must be cautious in its application. Another recent report, from Poggioli *et al.* described a strictureplasty in which a side-to-side anastomosis is performed between the diseased terminal ileum and the right colon [41]. This technique again has been used in only five patients; therefore the utility of this technique is also yet to be determined.

Despite the concerns of anastomosing diseased bowel, the short-term complication rate following this procedure is low with reported complication rates ranging from 1% to 14% [42–47]. In our own series of 43 patients in whom 154 strictureplasties were performed between 1985 and 1994, there was only one confirmed leak and one other suspected leak [43]. The other important variable is the long-term outcome in these patients. The largest series reported in the literature is from the Cleveland Clinic [44]. They reported on 116 patients in whom 452

strictureplasties had been performed. In 99% obstructive symptoms were relieved. With a median follow-up of 3 years 24% of their patients had developed symptomatic recurrences and 15% required reoperation. In our series 14 of 43 patients (33%) required reoperation after a mean follow-up of 55 months. However, in most of these patients there was progression of disease and the original strictureplasties were still patent. Stebbing *et al.*, reporting on experience at Oxford, also noted that only 3.7% of strictureplasty sites restenosed and required reoperation [45]. In our own series none of the following variables, including type of strictureplasty, number of previous operations, site of the stricture and whether a resection was performed in conjunction with the strictureplasty, had an effect on long-term outcome. Yamamoto *et al.* found that young age at surgery (<37 years) was a poor prognostic variable [46]. Tichansky *et al.* reviewed 15 series containing 506 patients in whom 1825 strictureplasties were performed. They found a lower reoperative rate in those patients who had Finney rather than Heineke–Mikulicz strictureplasties, and in whom the disease was not active and there was no preoperative weight loss [47].

Given that the procedure can be performed safely, and that a conservative approach to CD is advocated, strictureplasty has an important role in the surgical management of patients with CD. However, at the present time its use is generally limited to those patients who have multiple skip lesions or who have had multiple resections previously. It is contraindicated in patients with long strictures, abscesses or fistulizing disease. In the future, however, further evaluation of this procedure compared with resection is warranted, especially with respect to long-term outcome. Another question which remains unanswered is whether these patients should receive maintenance therapy. There are no data from randomized controlled trials, and opinion seems to be divided on this question. However, since most of these patients do have extensive disease, it has been our practice recently to advise prophylaxis with an immunosuppressive such as Imuran.

Surgery for gastroduodenal disease

Gastroduodenal disease is rarely seen in isolation. Yamamoto *et al.* reported that gastroduodenal disease occurred in association with disease else-

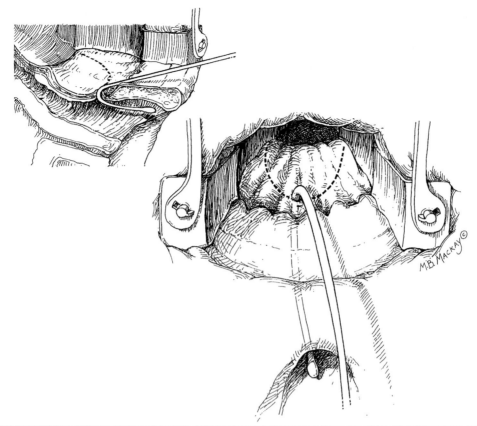

Figure 6. A rectovaginal fistula arising from the dentate line and passing through the rectovaginal septum. Note how thin the rectovaginal septum is and hence most rectovaginal fistula tracts are usually completely epithelialized.

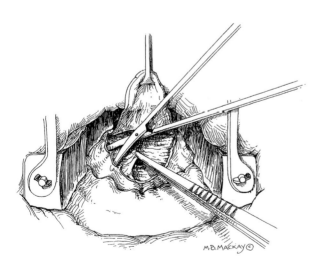

Figure 7. Low rectovaginal fistulas may be closed using a flap advancement procedure. A flap advancement procedure is performed by elevating a flap of mucosa, submucosa and internal sphincter beginning just below the fistula opening.

where in 96% of patients [48]. The most common and significant complication of gastroduodenal CD is stricture formation. Most patients with a stricture will not respond to medical therapy and will require surgery. Whereas in the past the preferred option for gastroduodenal disease was a bypass procedure (usually gastrojejunostomy), strictureplasty is the preferred option now where it is technically possible. The advantage of strictureplasty is that the pylorus is preserved, and hopefully there is slower transit time and less diarrhea. This is an important consideration in this patient population who frequently have had resection of other parts of their small bowel or colon. Because surgery for gastroduodenal Crohn's is performed infrequently, the reported series are small. Yamamoto and colleagues reported the results of 10 patients who had a strictureplasty for duodenal obstruction [48]. In four patients the strictureplasty included a pyloroplasty. Eight patients had a good result: one patient required a Roux Y duodeno-jejunostomy because of anastomotic breakdown and one required a gastrojejunostomy due to persistent symptoms of obstruction.

When strictureplasty is not possible, gastrojejunostomy is the procedure of choice [49, 50]. Because of the risk of marginal ulceration with long-term follow-up, vagotomy has been advocated. With the availability of proton-pump inhibitors and H_2 blockers, vagotomy may not be necessary, but there are no data to make recommendations for or against the addition of vagotomy.

Fistula to the duodenum most commonly occur secondary to CD elsewhere [51]. Fistulas arising from the colon or from a previous ileocolonic anastomosis comprise the commonest sites due to the proximity of these structures to the duodenum. Because the duodenum is usually not involved with disease, the duodenum and colon/ileum may be separated and the fistula closed primarily. There is often associated induration so it is important to mobilize the duodenum widely and excise the tissue surrounding the fistula opening before attempting closure. Results are excellent in most patients.

Surgery for large bowel disease

Both the manifestations and the indications for surgery in large bowel disease differ from those in small bowel disease. Farmer *et al.* reported that the indication for surgery in patients with colonic CD was poor response to medical therapy in 26%, presence of internal fistula and abscesses in 23%, toxic megacolon in 20% and perianal disease in 19% [21]. Just as the indications for surgery are quite diverse, the pattern of involvement in colonic disease may be quite variable with some patients having predominantly right-sided involvement, others having colonic involvement with sparing of the rectum and others having pancolitis. Furthermore, the disease may be complicated by the presence of perianal disease.

Most patients requiring surgery for colonic disease will require a resection. If there is sparing of the rectum, and no or minimal perianal disease, then a colectomy and ileorectal or ileosigmoid anastomosis can be performed. Proctocolectomy and ileostomy will be required for patients with pancolitis or those with severe perianal disease. The obvious advantage of performing an anastomosis is that a stoma is avoided. However, the reported recurrence rates are significantly higher in those patients in whom a colectomy and anastomosis is performed. Andrews *et al.* reported recurrence rates of 46% and 60% at 5 and 10 years respectively in patients who had ileorectal anastomoses compared with rates of 10% and 21% in those who had a proctocolectomy and ileostomy [52].

Despite the higher recurrence rates, colectomy and ileorectal anastomosis has an important role in the management of patients with CD, since many patients are young and would prefer to avoid having an ileostomy. However, patients must be carefully selected. Patients who have significant perianal disease or severe rectal disease are not candidates. Longo *et al.* reviewed 131 patients who underwent colectomy and ileorectal anastomosis (IRA) at the Cleveland Clinic, and found that the presence of small bowel disease preoperatively was the only predictive factor of need for further surgery [53]. The age at surgery, duration of disease, steroid use, presence of proctitis and perianal disease did not affect outcome. However, it is quite likely that this was a highly selected group of patients, and those with significant rectal or perianal disease would not have been included. From the results of reported series it can be anticipated that approximately 50–65% of patients will develop recurrence of their disease. In some patients the recurrence may be confined to the small bowel so a further resection and anastomosis is possible. Thus, the Cleveland Clinic reported that 86% of their patients had a functioning IRA at 5 years and 48% at 10 years. Similarly Buchmann and colleagues reported that 70% of their 105 patients had a functioning IRA at 7 years, while Ambrose *et al.* reported that 66% of their patients had a functioning IRA at 9.5 years [54, 55].

Proctocolectomy is the procedure of choice for those patients with pancolitis or extensive perianal disease. In those patients with perianal disease with associated sepsis it may be prudent to perform a subtotal colectomy and ileostomy, and subsequently perform the proctectomy when the sepsis has settled. This may minimize the risk of an unhealed perineal wound. The major complication of this operation is the risk of an unhealed perineal wound which has been reported to occur in up to 20% of patients. Pelvic nerve injury is a rare but important complication. As stated previously, the recurrence rates following proctocolectomy and ileostomy are lower than with colectomy and ileorectal anastomosis.

At the time of surgery, measures to decrease the potential for sepsis should be employed, including an adequate mechanical bowel preparation and prophylactic antibiotics. Tapering of steroids and improving

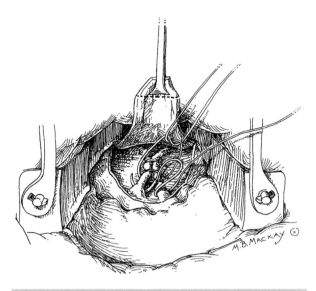

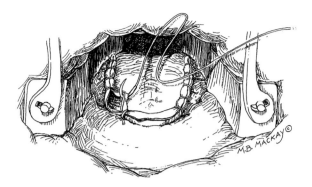

Figure 9. The flap is then brought down beyond the fistula opening and sutured.

Figure 8. Once the flap of the tissue has been elevated the fistula tract is curetted and the fistula is closed.

the general status of the patient with parenteral nutrition may be helpful. An intersphincteric dissection of the anorectum along anatomical planes, and meticulous hemostasis, are also important in preventing the perineal wound problems that are frequent complications after proctectomy in patients with CD.

Another controversy that exists is whether there is a role for segmental resection in Crohn's colitis. Segmental colonic disease occurs uncommonly, so most reported series are small, it is difficult to draw conclusions, and treatment may have to be individualized.

Ileal pouch procedure

The ileal pouch–anal anastomosis (IPAA) has become the surgical procedure of choice for most patients with UC. When it was first introduced there was a high complication rate but today it can be performed safely with relatively few complications, low failure rate and good functional results. However, it has generally been performed only in patients with UC and familial adenomatous polyposis. CD has been considered a contraindication because of the risk of small bowel and perianal involvement. Failure rates of 30–50% have also been reported in small series of patients with CD [56–59]. Only one recent report has suggested that the procedure can be performed safely in patients with CD with a complication rate similar to that in patients with UC. Panis and colleagues performed ileal pouches in 31 patients with CD who had no evidence of associated anoperineal or small bowel disease [60]. The results were compared to those of 71 patients with UC who underwent IPAA in a similar time period. Among the 31 CD patients, 19% developed septic complications including three pouch–perineal fistulas, one pouch–vaginal fistula and one extrasphincteric abscess. Two patients developed CD of the reservoir. Two of the five patients required pouch excision. At follow-up at 5 years the functional results were similar in the two groups of patients [60].

Although this report suggests that selected CD patients may have a satisfactory outcome with a pouch procedure, one must be somewhat cautious in the interpretation of these results. Since perianal disease frequently complicates Crohn's colitis these patients are a highly selected group, or alternatively may have indeterminant colitis. Others have reported satisfactory results in patients with indeterminant colitis [61]. Thus, generally CD remains a contraindication to performing a pouch procedure. However, in patients in whom there is uncertainty regarding the diagnosis, this procedure may be considered. Patients must be carefully selected and fully informed that their risk of complications and failure may be higher. Maintenance medical therapy should also be considered if the diagnosis of CD is suspected. However, while there is theoretical appeal to this strategy, at present there is little evidence to support this approach [62]. Another option would be to perform a subtotal colectomy and ileostomy, and delay construction of the pouch for several years,

sion is necessary. However, in very selected patients local repair of the fistula may be undertaken. Medical treatment alone is usually unsuccessful in the treatment of these fistulas because it is a short tract which epithelializes. Similarly, spontaneous closure virtually never occurs. Medical treatment may have a role in inducing a remission of the rectal disease so that a local repair can be undertaken, or improving the consistency of stool so there is less discharge through the fistula opening.

The choice of treatment depends on two factors: patient symptoms and the disease status of the rectum. If the fistula is small and low-lying the patient may experience relatively minor symptoms and no treatment other than medical management of any rectal disease is indicated, although spontaneous closure of the fistula for long periods would be unusual. However, if the patient has persistent fecal or purulent discharge from the vagina, or has gross incontinence, treatment is indicated.

A local repair of the fistula should be undertaken only when the disease is in remission and the rectal tissue is healthy. In the Cleveland Clinic experience 40% of patients were amenable to local repair of the rectovaginal fistula [85]. In these patients repair was successful after one attempt in 54% and 68% overall. The type of repair performed largely depends on the preference of the individual surgeon. Our preference, where possible, is to perform a mucosal flap advancement via the rectum (Figs. 6–9). Meticulous surgical technique is mandatory. We also recommend temporary fecal diversion with a loop ileostomy in most patients, although in the Cleveland Clinic series protection with a stoma did not affect outcome. If patients are carefully selected, excellent results may be achieved.

Summary

Surgery plays an important role in the management of CD, and likely will continue to do so until the etiology of CD is elucidated and more specific medical therapies are available. In most instances surgery leads to an improvement in quality of life and allows patients to regain normal physical well-being without experiencing the side-effects and dysutility of taking medication. Thus, the need for surgery should not be considered a failure of management. Instead, there is a role for both medical therapy and surgical therapy. Because of the variable patterns of disease seen in CD, as well as the individual concerns

of patients, treatment may have to be individualized. Optimally, care should be given, using a team approach including gastroenterologists, surgeons and paramedical personnel such as nurses, enterostomal therapists, and psychiatrists. Care should also be provided as a continuum. In order, however, to achieve excellent results, patients require careful preoperative evaluation and management, and surgeons must be familiar with the various patterns of disease and the complications that they may encounter.

References

1. Binder V, Both H, Hansen PK, Hendriksen C, Kreiner S, Torp-Pedersen K. Incidence and prevalence of ulcerative colitis and Crohn's disease in the county of Copenhagen 1962 to 1978. Gastroenterology 1982; 83: 563–8.
2. Freeney PC. Crohn's disease and ulcerative colitis. Evaluation with double contrast barium enema examination and endoscopy. Postgrad Med 1986; 80: 139–56.
3. Doemeny JM, Burke DR, Meranze SG. Percutaneous drainage of abscesses in patients with Crohn's disease. Gastrointest Radiol 1988; 13: 237–41.
4. McLeod RS, Lavery IC, Leatherman JR et al. Factors affecting quality of life with a conventional ileostomy. World J Surg 1986; 10: 474–80.
5. Harper PH, Truelove SC, Lee ECG, Kettlewell MGW, Jewell DP. Split ileostomy and ileocolostomy for Crohn's disease of the colon and ulcerative colitis: a 20 year survey. Gut 1983; 24: 106–13.
6. Reissman P, Salky BA, Pfeifer J, Edye M, Jagelman DG, Wexner SD. Laparoscopic surgery in the management of inflammatory bowel disease. Am J Surg 1996; 171: 47–51.
7. Bauer JJ, Harris MT, Grumbach NM, Gorfine SR. Laparoscopic-assisted intestinal resection for Crohn's disease. J Clin Gastroenterol 1996; 23: 44–6.
8. Ludwig KA, Milsom JW, Church JM, Fazio VW. Preliminary experience with laparoscopic intestinal surgery for Crohn's disease. Am J Surg 1996; 171: 52–6.
9. Poritz LS, Friedlich M, MacRae HM. Is it safe to begin doing laparoscopic colon surgery with ileocolic resections for Crohn's disease? Can J Surg 2000; 43(Suppl.): 6.
10. Poulin EC, Schlachta CM, Mamazza J, Seshadri PA. Should enteric fistulas from Crohn's disease or diverticulitis be treated laparoscopically or by open surgery. A matched cohort study. Dis Colon Rectum 2000; 43: 621–6.
11. Wexner SD, Moscovitz ID. Laparoscopic colectomy in diverticular and Crohn's disease. Surg Clin N Am 2000; 80: 1299–319.
12. McLeod RS, Wolff BG, Steinhart AH et al. Prophylactic mesalamine treatment decreases postoperative recurrence of Crohn's disease. Gastroenterology 1995; 109: 404–13.
13. Caprilli R, Andreoli A, Capurso L et al. Oral mesalamine (5-ASA: Asacol) for the prevention of post-operative recurrence of Crohn's disease. Aliment Pharmacol Ther 1994; 8: 35–45.
14. Brignola C, Cottone M, Pera A et al. The Italian Cooperative Study Group. Mesalamine in the prevention of endoscopic recurrence after intestinal resection for Crohn's disease. Gastroenterology 1995; 108: 345–9.
15. Lochs H, Mayer M, Fleig WE et al. Prophylaxis of postoperative relapse in Crohn's disease with mesamaline:

European Cooperative Crohn's Disease Study VI. Gastroenterology 2000; 118: 264–73.

16. Camma C, Guinta M, Rosselli M, Rosselli M, Cottone M. Mesalamine in the maintenance treatment of Crohn's disease: a meta-analysis adjusted for confounding variables. Gastroenterology 1997; 113: 1465–73.

17. Korelitz B, Hanauer S, Rutgeerts P *et al.* Post-operative prophylaxis with 6-MP, 5-ASA or placebo in Crohn's disease: a 2-year multicenter trial. Gastroenterology 1998; 114: A1011 (Abstract)

18. Rutgeerts P, Hiele M, Geboes K *et al.* Controlled trial of metronidazole treatment in the prevention of Crohn's recurrence after ileal resection. Gastroenterology 1996; 108: 1617–21.

19. Hellers G, Lofberg R, Rutgeerts P *et al.* Oral budesonide for prevention of recurrence following ileocecal resection of Crohn's disease: a one year placebo controlled trial. Gastroenterology 1996; 110: A923.

20. Belluzzi A, Campieri M, Belloli C *et al.* New enteric coated preparation Ω-3 fatty acids for preventing post surgical recurrence in Crohn's disease. Gastroenterology 1998; 112: A930.

21. Farmer RG, Hawk WA, Turnbull RB Jr. Indications for surgery in Crohn's disease. Gastroenterology 1976; 71: 245–50.

22. Greenstein AJ, Lachman P, Sachar DB *et al.* Perforating and non-perforating indications for repeated operations in Crohn's disease: evidence for two clinical forms. Gut 1988; 29: 588–92.

23. McLeod RS. Resection margins and recurrent Crohn's disease. Hepatogastroenterology 1990; 37: 63–5.

24. Rutgeerts P, Geobes K, Vantrappen G, Kerremans R, Coengrachts JL, Coremans G. Natural history of recurrent Crohn's disease at the ileocolonic anastomosis after curative surgery. Gut 1984; 25: 665–72.

25. Olaison G, Smedh K, Sjodahl R. Natural course of Crohn's disease after ileocolic resection: endoscopically visualized ileal ulcers preceding symptoms. Gut 1992; 33: 331–5.

26. Williams JG, Wong WD, Rothenberger DA, Goldberg SM. Recurrence of Crohn's disease after resection. Br J Surg 1991; 78: 10–19.

27. Sachar DB, Wolfson DM, Greenstein AJ, Stczynski R, Janowitz HD. Risk factors of postoperative recurrence of Crohn's disease. Gastroenterology 1983; 85: 917–21.

28. Benoni C, Nilsson A. Smoking and inflammatory bowel disease: comparison with systemic lupus erythematosus. A case control study. Scand J Gastroent 1990; 25: 751–5.

29. Krause U, Ejerblad S, Bergman L. Crohn's disease: a long-term study of the clinical course in 186 patients. Scand J Gastroent 1985; 20: 516–24.

30. Fazio VW, Marchetti F, Church JM *et al.* Effect of resection margins on the recurrence of Crohn's disease in the small bowel. Ann Surg 1996; 224: 563–73.

31. Cameron JL, Hamilton SR, Coleman J, Sitzman JV, Bayless TM. Patterns of ileal recurrence in Crohn's disease. Ann Surg 1992; 215: 546–52.

32. Munoz-Juarez M, Yamamoto T, Wolff BG, Keighley MRB. Wide lumen stapled anastomosis versus conventional end-to-end anastomosis in the treatment of Crohn's disease. Dis Colon Rectum 2001; 44: 20–5.

33. Hashemi M, Novell JR, Lewis AA. Side-to-side anastomosis may delay recurrence in Crohn's disease. Dis Colon Rectum 1998; 41: 1293–6.

34. Kusunoki M, Ikeuchi H, Yanagi H, Shoji Y, Yamamura T. A comparison of stapled and hand-sewn anastomosis in Crohn's disease. Dig Surg 1998; 15: 679–82.

35. Scott NA, Sue-Ling HM, Hughes LM. Anastomotic configuration does not affect recurrence of Crohn's disease after ileocolonic resection. Int J Colorectal Dis 1995; 10: 67–9.

36. Moskovicz D, McLeod RS, Greenberg GR, Cohen Z. Operative and environmental risk factors for recurrence of Crohn's disease. Int J Colorectal Dis 1999; 14: 224–6.

37. Saint-Marc O, Tiret E, Vaillant JC, Frileux P, Parc R. Surgical management of internal fistulas in Crohn's disease. J Am Coll Surg 1996; 183: 97–100.

38. Michelassi F, Stella M, Balestracci T, Giuliant F, Marogna P, Block GE. Incidence, diagnosis and treatment of enteric and colorectal fistulae in patients with Crohn's disease. Ann Surg 1993; 218: 660–6.

39. Lee ECG, Papaioannou N. Minimal surgery for chronic obstruction in patients with extensive or universal Crohn's disease. Ann R Coll Surg 1982; 64: 519–21.

40. Michelassi F, Hurst RD, Melis M *et al.* Side-to-side isoperistaltic strictureplasty in extensive Crohn's strictures: a prospective longitudinal study. Ann Surg 2000; 232: 401–8.

41. Poggioli G, Stocchi L, Laureti S *et al.* Conservative surgical management of terminal ileitis. Dis Colon Rectum 1997; 40: 234–9.

42. Spencer MP, Nelson H, Wolff BG, Dozois RR. Strictureplasty for obstructive Crohn's disease: the Mayo experience. Mayo Clin Proc 1994; 69: 33–6.

43. Serra J, Cohen Z, McLeod RS. Natural history of strictureplasty in Crohn's disease: 9-year experience. Can J Surg 1995; 38: 481–5.

44. Fazio VW, Tjandra JJ, Lavery IC, Church JM, Milsom JW, Oakley JR. Long-term follow-up of strictureplasty in Crohn's disease. Dis Colon Rectum 1993; 36: 355–61.

45. Stebbing JF, Jewell DP, Kettlewell GW, Mortensen NJ. Long-term results of recurrence and reoperation after strictureplasty for obstructive Crohn's disease. Br J Surg 1995; 82: 1471–4.

46. Yamamoto T, Keighley MRB. Factors Affecting the incidence of postoperative septic complications and recurrence after strictureplasty for jejunoileal Crohn's disease. Am J Surg 1999; 178: 240–5.

47. Tichansky D, Cagir B, Yoo E, Marcus SM, Fry RD. Strictureplasty for Crohn's disease. Meta-analysis. Dis Colon Rectum 2000; 43: 911–19.

48. Yamamoto T, Allan RN, Keighley MRB. An audit of gastroduodenal Crohn disease: clinicopathologic features and management. Scand J Gastroenterol 1999; 34: 1019–24.

49. Ross TM, Fazio VW, Farmer RG. Long-term results of surgical treatment for Crohn's disease of the duodenum. Ann Surg 1983; 197: 399–406.

50. Murray JM, Schoetz DJ, Nugent FW, Coller JA, Veidenheimer MC. Surgical management of Crohn's disease involving the duodenum. Am J Surg 1984; 147: 58–65.

51. Jacobson IM, Schapiro RH, Warshaw AL. Gastric and duodenal fistulas in Crohn's disease. Gastoenterology 1985; 89: 1347–52.

52. Andrews HA, Lewis P, Allan RN. Prognosis after surgery for colonic Crohn's disease. Br J Surg 1989; 76: 1184–90.

53. Longo WE, Oakley JR, Lavery IC, Church JM, Fazio VW. Outcome of ileorectal anastomosis for Crohn's colitis. Dis Colon Rectum 1992; 35: 1066–71.

54. Buchmann P, Weterman IT, Keighley MR *et al.* The Prognosis of ileorectal anastomosis in Crohn's disease. Br J Surg 1981; 68: 7–10.

55. Ambrose NS, Keighley MR, Alexander-Williams J, Allan RN. Clinical impact of colectomy and ileorectal anastomosis in the managment of Crohn's disease. Gut 1984; 25: 223–7.

56. Deutsch AA, McLeod RS, Cullen J, Cohen Z. Results of the pelvic pouch procedure in patients with Crohn's disease. Dis Colon Recum 1991; 34: 475–7.

57. Hyman NH, Fazio VW, Tukson WB, Lavery IC. Consequences of ileal pouch–anal anastomosis for Crohn's colitis. Dis Colon Rectum 1991; 34: 653–7.

58. Grobler SP, Hosie KB, Affie E, Thompson H, Keighley MRB. Outcome of restorative proctocolectomy when the diagnosis is suggestive of Crohn's disease. Gut 1993; 34: 1384–8.

59. Peyregne V, Francois Y, Gilly F-N, Descos J-L, Flourie B, Vignal J. Outcome of ileal pouch after secondary diagnosis of Crohn's disease. Int J Colorectal Dis 2000; 15: 49–53.

60. Panis Y, Poupard B, Nemeth J, Lavergne A, Hautefeuille P, Valleur P. Ileal pouch/anal anastomosis for Crohn's disease. Lancet 1996; 347: 854–7.

61. Pezim ME, Pemberton JH, Beart RW *et al.* Outcome of 'indeterminant' colitis following ileal pouch anal anastomosis. Dis Colon Rectum 1989; 32: 653–8.

62. Ricart E, Panaccione R, Loftus EV, Tremaine WJ, Sandborn WJ. Successful management of Crohn's disease of the ileoanal pouch with infliximab. Gastroenterology 1999; 117: 429–32.

63. Hobbiss JH, Schofield PF. Management of perianal Crohn's disease. J R Soc Med 1982; 75: 414–17

64. Fielding JF. Perianal lesions in Crohn's disease. J R Coll Surg Edinb 1972; 17: 27–32

65. Rankin GB, Watts HD, Melnyk CS, Kelley ML Jr. National Cooperative Crohn's Disease Study. Extraintestinal manifestations and perianal complications. Gastroenterology 1979; 77: 914–20.

66. Marks CG, Ritchie JK, Lockhart-Mummery HE. Anal fistulas in Crohn's disease. Br J Surg 1981; 68: 525–7.

67. Buchmann P, Alexander-Williams J. Classification of perianal Crohn's disease. Clin Gastroenterol 1980; 9: 323–30.

68. Solomon MJ, McLeod RS, O'Connor BI, Steinhart AH, Greenberg GR, Cohen Z. Combination ciprofloxacin and metronidazole in severe perianal Crohn's disease. Can J Gastroenterol 1993; 7: 571–3.

69. Van Outryve MJ, Pelckmans PA, Michielsen PP, Van Maercke YM. Value of transrectal ultrasonography in Crohn's disease. Gastroenterology 1991; 101: 1171–7.

70. Solomon MJ, McLeod RS, Cohen EK, Cohen Z. Anal wall thickness under normal and inflammatory conditions of the anorectum as determined by endoluminal ultrasonography. Am J Gastroenterol 1995; 90: 574–8.

71. Haggett PJ, Moore NR, Shearman JD, Travis SP, Jewell DP, Mortensen NJ. Pelvic and perineal complications of Crohn's disease: assessment using magnetic resonance imaging. Gut 1995; 36: 407–10.

72. Jenss H, Starlinger M, Skaleij M. Magnetic resonance imaging in perianal Crohn's disease. Lancet 1992; 340: 1286.

73. Lunniss PJ, Barker PG, Sultan AH *et al.* Magnetic resonance imaging of fistula-in-ano. Dis Colon Rectum 1994; 37: 708–18.

74. Bergstrand O, Ewerth S, Hellers G, Holmstrom B, Ullman J, Wallberg P. Outcome following treatment of anal fistulae in Crohn's disease. Acta Chir Scand Suppl 1980; 500: 43–4.

75. Bernard D, Morgan S, Tasse D. Selective surgical management of Crohn's disease of the anus. Can J Surg 1986; 29: 318–21.

76. Sohn N, Korelitz BI. Local operative treatment of anorectal Crohn's disease. J Clin Gastroenterol 1982; 4: 395–9.

77. Sohn N, Korelitz BI, Weinstein MA. Anorectal Crohn's disease: definitive surgery for fistulas and recurrent abscesses. Am J Surg 1980; 139: 394–7.

78. Nordgren S, Fasth S, Hulten L. Anal fistulas in Crohn's disease: incidence and outcome of surgical treatment. Int J Colorectal Dis 1992; 7: 214–18.

79. Present DH, Rutgeerts P, Tergan S *et al.* Infliximab for the treatment of fistulas in patients with Crohn's disease. N Engl J Med 1999; 340: 1398–405.

80. Williams JG, MacLeod CA, Rothenberger DA, Goldberg SM. Seton treatment of high anal fistulae. Br J Surg 1991; 78: 1159–61.

81. Matos D, Lunniss PJ, Phillips RK. Total sphincter conservation in high fistula in ano: results of a new approach. Br J Surg 1993; 80: 802–4.

82. Winter AM, Banks PA, Petros JG. Healing of transsphincteric perianal fistulas in Crohn's disease using a new technique. Am J Gastroenterol 1993; 88: 2022–5.

83. Grant DR, Cohen Z, McLeod RS. Loop ileostomy for anorectal Crohn's disease. Can J Surg 1986; 29: 32–5.

84. Zelas P, Jagelman DG. Loop ileostomy in the management of Crohn's colitis in the debilitated patient. Ann Surg 1980; 191: 164–8.

85. Hull TL, Fazio VW. Surgical approaches to low anovaginal fistula in Crohn's disease. Am J Surg 1997; 173: 95–8.

35 | Postoperative prevention of recurrence of Crohn's disease

FILIP BAERT, GEERT D'HAENS AND PAUL RUTGEERTS

Introduction

Important progress is being made in unraveling the inflammatory cascade involved in the pathophysiology of the chronic inflammation seen in Crohn's disease (CD). However, the exact pathogenesis and potential causes remain unknown. Due to its chronic nature, and tendency to re-occur after a so-called 'curative' resection, the management of this condition is largely medical. Surgery remains, however, a very important and sometimes inevitable tool in management. The disease almost invariably recurs at the anastomosis, in a case of classic ileocecal resection on the ileal side. This disease process occurs during the first days after surgery and contact of the mucosa with the fecal stream. Risk factors for recurrence have been studied and several agents have been tested in an attempt to prevent recurrence. The advent of a wide array of new biological agents, possibly interacting with the key steps in the early pathophysiological events, may bring CD recurrence prevention even more into focus.

Definitions and diagnosis

It is important to distinguish CD recurrence from relapse of CD (Table 1).

Crohns's disease recurrence

This can be defined as the appearance of objective signs – defined radiologically, endoscopically or by histology – of CD in the gut of a patient who has had a resection of all macroscopic diseased bowel segments.

The recurrence documented by ileocolonoscopy or radiology can be either symptomatic or asymptomatic. If clinical symptoms reappear after a so-called 'curative' surgery (see below), reappearance of macroscopic recurrent CD should be documented before clinical recurrence of CD is proven. Clinical

Table 1. Definitions

Recurrence
Endoscopic recurrence
Clinical recurrence
Surgical recurrence

Relapse

Types of surgery
Radical ('curative') resection
Local or segmental resection
Bypass surgery

recurrence can in some instances lead to a new resection, sometimes called surgical recurrence.

Crohn's disease relapse

This is the appearance of the clinical features (signs or symptoms) of CD after a symptom-free interval (period of remission), in patients with known disease; provided that other non-related causes of these symptoms have been excluded.

Types of surgery

The term recurrence can be used only after a radical or curative resection. A radical resection involves the excision of a sufficient length of normal bowel from either side of the diseased gut together with lymph nodes draining the region to remove all the disease. Nowadays the segment of normal bowel removed is rather limited (5–15 cm) in order to avoid short bowel syndrome upon repeated surgery. This type of resection is called 'curative resection'. Local or segmental resections are designed to remove segments of CD which are causing the symptoms such as fistulas and strictures. No attempt is made to carry out a curative resection, and areas of inflammation may be left behind. Bypass operations divert the fecal stream

Stephan R. Targan, Fergus Shanahan and Loren C. Karp (eds.), Inflammatory Bowel Disease: From Bench to Bedside, 2nd Edition, 697–709.

from the diseased segment to improve the inflammation in the dysfunctioning gut.

The diagnosis of recurrent CD on pure clinical grounds is not often evident, especially early after surgery. The symptoms of recurrent disease are not always easily distinguishable from symptoms due the postoperative state and to cholerrheic diarrhea. The baseline is the state at 3 months after resection. Most patients have recovered completely by that time. The CD activity index (CDAI) is an instrument which is not really valid in the postoperative setting.

As outlined above, endoscopic examinations have been the most sensitive routine tool to document macroscopic recurrence. Given the correlation between clinical course and endoscopic appearance, this test has become the gold standard to document lesions, and offers the additional benefit of the potential to take biopsies. The majority of pharmaceutical recurrence prevention trials have indeed used endoscopic parameters as an endpoint. The severity of endoscopic recurrence can be classified as 'mild' or 'severe', but a more detailed score has been developed by Rutgeerts *et al.* (see Table 2) and has been adopted in most clinical trials [1]. Recently, several efforts have been made to develop more sensitive methods to detect recurrence and likelihood of recurrence at an even earlier phase. An adjunct to routine endoscopic investigation may be offered by endoscopic fluorescence imaging. With this technique (injection of sodium fluoresceine and mucosal illumination with blue light), bright fluorescent spots looking macroscopically normal were found to correspond with superficial erosive inflammatory lesions on histological examination [2].

Alternatively radiolabeled granulocyte scintigraphy was found to be reliable to detect early postoperative asymptomatic recurrence in a small group of patients [3].

Table 2. Endosopic recurrence severity index

i0: No macroscopic recurrence in the neoterminal ileum
i1: Less than five aphthous ulcers (< 5 mm)
i2: More than five aphthae with normal mucosa in between, or ulceration confined to the anastomosis
i3: Diffuse aphthous ileitis with a diffuse inflamed ileum
i4: Diffuse ileitis with larger ulcers, irregularity and narrowing

Pathogenesis

All systematic endoscopic and histologic studies are concordant and describe early recurrent lesions in the ileum in 70–80% of patients in the first year following a 'curative' ileocecal resection.

It is not at all clear what makes the ileal mucosa so vulnerable to recurrent lesions. CD has been shown to be a disease affecting the entire intestine. Even in the macroscopically normal-appearing ileum in CD mucosal architectural changes: epithelial bridge formation and goblet cell hyperplasia can be present. Inflammatory lesions in the section margins are not predictive of recurrence but perineural inflammatory changes might be of importance. The combined presence of bacteria and bile acids, a break in the mucosa of the suture, reflux of colonic contents and the organization of the mucosal immune cells may be contributing factors.

Diversion of intestinal contents through a proximal ileostomy protects the neoterminal ileum and ileocolonic anastomosis from recurrence [4], suggesting that luminal contents, probably the bacterial flora, trigger flares of CD. This is also strongly suggested by the finding that, in the same model, infusion of ileal contents through a normal diverted ileocolonic anastomosis induces inflammation characterized by mixed inflammatory infiltrate and cytokine up-regulation as early as 1 week after surgery [5].

The role of the fecal stream

We recently demonstrated that the mucosa in the neoterminal ileum remains unaffected as long as the fecal stream is diverted (via loop ileostomy). After 8 days of perfusion of ileal effluent into the efferent loop of the loop ileostomy through the ileocolonic anastomosis into the colon, a massive influx of inflammatory cells into the mucosal compartment of the neoterminal ileum took place. The microscopic lesions showed a focal distribution and included villous architectural changes, limited patchy surface epithelial cell damage, and necrosis and accumulation of eosinophils and mononuclear cells in the lamina propria in the top of the villi. Further characterization of mononuclear cells showed increased macrophage activation (CD68), antigen presentation, epithelioid transformation and active transendothelial leukocyte recruitment into the mucosal compartment. This study provided further evidence for the involvement of fecal contents in the induction of early lesions in recurrent CD [5].

In an earlier study we demonstrated that recurrent Crohn's lesions in the neoterminal ileum did not appear as long as the fecal stream was diverted, whereas the majority of patients (71%) developed mucosal lesions 6 months after intestinal continuity had been restored [4]. The same phenomenon was observed in a study in Oxford, in which ileal fluid was infused into defunctioned colon previously affected by CD [6].

In spite of the evidence that luminal contents provides a continuous stimulus responsible for persistent inflammation, it remains unclear which component of the fecal stream could be the principal culprit. A few elegant studies provide interesting clues. When ileal effluent was ultrafiltrated prior to infusion into defunctioned colon, no signs of recurrent inflammation developed, suggesting that intact bacteria or large dietary particles (>0.22 μm) must be responsible for the inflammatory response [6, 7]. Experimental models of inflammatory bowel disorders in immunologically altered rodents (transgenic, knockout, spontaneous) require the presence of normal luminal bacteria, especially *Bacteroides* spp. In HLA-B27 transgenic rats *Bacteroides* spp. preferentially induce colitis [8], and in humans *B. fragilis* is increased in CD ileal resections [9]. Besides *Bacteroides* spp. the human neoterminal ileum is also heavily colonized by *Escherichia coli* and *Clostridium* spp. (i.e. a colonic-like flora) after ileocolonic resection [10]. Two clinical studies indicate that the reduction of the load of anaerobic bacteria during intake of nitroimidazole antibiotics (metronidazole and ornidazole) led to less severe endoscopic recurrence [11, 12]. All these studies suggest a potential role of bacteria in inducing CD recurrence.

In addition, other experiments focused on dietary components as a factor in luminal-content-induced recurrence. For instance ubiquitous titanium dioxide and aluminosilicate particles used as food and pharmaceutical additives induce persistent intestinal injury [13]. Further studies, possibly using the infusion model, may elucidate the main responsible components in the fecal stream.

It has also been suggested that increased intestinal permeability, leading to enhanced penetration of antigens, may be a basic feature of CD [14]. This hypothesis was not, however, confirmed by investigators in France. They were unable to find a correlation between enhanced permeability 6 weeks postoperatively and endoscopic recurrence again 6 weeks later [15].

Early immunologic changes

A major factor in the development of intestinal inflammation is the delicate balance of cytokines. In the inflamed mucosa of full-blown CD, a typical Th1-pattern of cytokines has been observed, with abundant presence of tumor necrosis factor alpha (TNF-α), interleukin-1 (IL-1) and interferon gamma (IFN-γ). This pattern is different from the one observed in early ileal Crohn's lesions, where low levels of IFN and high levels of IL-4, a typical immunoregulatory T-helper 2 cytokine, were demonstrated [16]. IL-4 attenuates the barrier function of the intestinal epithelium and may induce an enhanced penetration of noxious agents. In addition, incubation of monocytes/macrophages with IL-4 stimulates IL-12 and TNF production by these cells and may explain a switch from a Th2 toward a more typical Th1 response [17]. The same group of investigators also demonstrated that ileal CD recurrence was associated with an enhanced IL-5 and immunoglobulin E (IgE) production accompanied by eosinophilic infiltration, a finding which suggested the involvement of an allergic mechanism [18].

Predilection for the neoterminal ileum

It remains unclear why postoperative recurrence of CD preferably develops in the ileum immediately proximal to the ileocolonic anastomosis. Scanning electron-microscopic studies have shown that a triad consisting of mucosal architectural alterations, epithelial bridge formation and goblet cell hyperplasia can be found in the majority of biopsies taken from resection specimens, both in the affected area and in the unaffected proximal ileal section margin. Macroscopic recurrence of CD would merely represent a transition from (electron-)microscopic towards endoscopically visible disease [19].

Reflux of colonic content after removal of the ileocecal valve may play a key role in this phenomenon. In addition, stasis and bacterial overgrowth may be involved. In the absence of a classic ileocolonic anastomosis, e.g. with primary ileostomies, the risk of severe recurrence is indeed much lower [20]. An alternative explanation has been sought in the inflammatory changes often encountered in the enteric nervous system. Even in the absence of microscopic inflammation in the ileal resection margins, subtle inflammation surrounding neural structures is common and may 'guide' the inflammation to the more proximal ileal segments [21]. Our group showed that the presence and severity of neuritis in the ileal section margin were predictive of recurrent CD 3 months postoperatively [22].

Postoperative recurrence is not exclusively located in the neoterminal ileum. Recurrent inflammation in the colon after an ileal or ileocecal resection is rare, but may occur. We reported on a series of 18 patients in whom the rectum was the major site of symptomatic CD recurrence, often without accompanying ileal recurrence [23].

Incidence, natural history and characteristics of recurrence

For the assessment of recurrence rates an actuarial analysis has to be used. This implies the calculation of the number of patients with recurrent disease over the number of patients at risk in each year of follow-up allowing recurrence in previous years.

Systematic endoscopic study data are available only for the neoterminal ileum and ileocolonic anastomosis after ileal or ileocolonic resections. Recurrent lesions can be visualized as early as a few weeks to months after resection in the neoterminal ileum proximal to the anastomosis with a post-anastomotic colon mostly free of macroscopic disease, although microscopic colonic lesions can also be identified [1]. Severe endoscopic recurrence is seen in about 30% of patients 3 months after surgery and 50–94% of patients at 12 months, as shown in the placebo arms of the postoperative recurrence prevention trials [24].

Symptoms recur later after curative resection averaging about 10% of the patients per follow-up year if one looks at figures of older follow-up series. In the same postoperative prevention drug studies the symptomatic recurrence rates in the placebo groups are higher and amount to 23–26% at 1 year and about 40% at 2 years [24]. Recurrence of tissue lesions precedes the appearance of recurrent symptoms. The severity and extent of tissue recurrence predicts the time to clinical relapse. Patients without lesions or presenting only a few aphthous ulcers at ileocolonoscopy at 1 year are not at risk for early symptomatic relapse, but more than half of the patients presenting with diffuse aphthous or ulcerative ileitis will have symptomatic relapse within 1–3 years after operation. Patients with ulcers confined to the immediate preanastomotic region are probably prone to develop fibrostenosis of the anastomosis [25].

There is convincing evidence that in patients with postoperative recurrence the evolution of CD mimics the natural evolution of CD at its onset. The evolution goes from preulcerative inflammation over aphthoid ulcers to more extensive ulceration and nodularity, to result in complications including stenosis and fissures which can be complicated by abscesses and fistulas.

The clinical presentation of recurrent Crohn's ileitis is often strikingly similar to the preoperative presentation. As early as 1971 de Dombal *et al.* suggested that there might be several subtypes of CD: an 'indolent' one, which tends to recur slowly, and an 'aggressive' one, recurring soon after surgical resection [26]. This hypothesis was further elaborated in a retrospective analysis at the Mount Sinai Hospitals in New York, in which patients were classified into a subgroup with 'perforating' CD (including fistulas and abscesses), and a non-perforating or stenosing subgroup. Second operations for perforating indications were performed more often among cases whose surgical indication had been perforation initially. Reoperation for perforating disease was required earlier for non-perforating CD [27]. We have not been able to reproduce this finding in a group of North American patients in whom recurrence was defined radiologically and not based on reoperation. In this same study the *length* of ileal recurrence measured on small bowel X-rays before resection and at the time of symptomatic recurrence was comparable before surgery and at the time of clinical recurrence. In seven patients who had sequential small bowel studies without intervening surgery, the length of measured inflammation remained unchanged, a finding which demonstrates that the extent of disease rarely changes once it is established [28].

Risk factors for symptomatic recurrence after resection for Crohn's disease (Table 3)

Several studies have looked for the potential risk factors for CD recurrence. We will discuss the main risk factors found and reproduced in several studies. The only independent factors generally reproduced in multivariate analyses are location of the disease prior to surgery, pattern of the disease and smoking status.

Many other factors such as gender, duration of disease, first or subsequent resection, type of anastomosis and extent of the resection (see below), contraceptive pill use, age at onset of disease, presence of granulomas, blood tranfusions, or a

Table 3. Risk factors for Crohn's disease recurrence

Risk factors for recurrence
Active smoking (especially in women)
Location of disease ileocolitis > ileitis > colitis
Ileostomy ≪ Ileocolonic anastomosis

No risk factors for recurrence
Type of anastomosis (hand-sewn versus stapled;
    end-to-end versus end-to-side or side-to-side)
Resection free margins
First versus second or third resection

family history have not been found to be risk factors in multivariate analyses in several studies [29, 30].

Location of diseased segment

The anatomic site of bowel resection is without doubt an important determinant of recurrence. The highest rates are found after resection for ileocolitis or ileitis involving an ileocolonic anastomosis. Lower rates are found after colonic resection with colo-colic anastomosis. Surprisingly CD also recurs in the ileum after right colonic resection with ileocolonic anastomosis even when the ileum was not diseased prior to surgery. The rate of symptomatic recurrence proximal to an ileostomy is the lowest. It is uncertain whether the rate is really lower or whether the evolution of recurrent lesions is slower.

Reoperation rates after resection with ileocolonic anastomosis range from 25% to 60% at 5 years and 42% to 91% at 15 years. After colo-colic anastomosis the rates range between 8.5% and 42% at 5 years and 22% to 40% at 15 years. Reoperation for end-ileostomies still amounts to 25% at 5 years and 45% at 10 years.

The rate of recurrence of CD in the neoterminal ileum after ileorectal anastomosis seems comparable to that after more proximal ileocolonic anastomosis but the disease more often spreads distally with anorectal complications as the main manifestation [20, 31].

The behavior of Crohn's disease

CD has been divided into three categories according to its behavior: an inflammatory type, a fibrostenotic type (forming strictures) and a perforating type (forming fistulas and abscesses). Perforating disease

was found to be a good predictor of recurrence as described by studies from de Dombal and coauthors [26] in Leeds and Greenstein *et al.* [27] in New York. De Dombal *et al.* as early as 1971 described a biphasic symptomatic recurrence graph, but offered no clear explanation. The Mount Sinai investigators distinguished perforating indications for resection and non-perforating indications. Perforating indications included acute free perforation, subacute perforation with abscess formation, and chronic perforation with intestinal fistula formation. Non-perforating indications comprised intestinal obstruction, medical intractability, hemorrhage, and toxic dilation without perforation.

Operations for perforating indications in their retrospective analyses were followed by repeated resection much earlier than operations for non-perforating indications. Time to first reoperation was 4.7 years in the perforating group and 8.8 years in the non-perforating group. Time to second reoperation averaged 2.3 years for perforating versus 5.2 years for non-perforating indications. Second operations in the perforating indication group were undertaken for perforating indications again in 64% of the patients with ileitis and 77% of the patients with ileocolitis. A third resection in patients with perforating indications for second resection was carried out for perforating complications in 81% overall. Another study confirms perforating disease as a significant predictor for clinical and surgical recurrence.

Not all investigators have confirmed this dichotomy of CD behavior.

It should be stated that many of these studies are based on retrospective series dating back to the 1970s or earlier. Today, with the broader use of immunosuppressive and the new biological agents, it is probably fair to look at clinical recurrence rather than surgical recurrence. We studied the correlation between preoperative disease and recurrent ileitis in terms of length and all three types of disease behavior. We found that the majority of patients with initial fibrostenotic disease, and all patients with inflammatory disease, had recurrence with the same disease pattern. Perforating disease presented again with symptoms with any of the three features. There was a striking correlation between the pre- and postsurgical extent of ileal disease ($r = 0.70$; $p < 0.0001$). We could not confirm perforating disease as being a more aggressive type in terms of onset of clinical recurrence [28].

Smoking status

Generally speaking smoking has a deleterious effect on CD. The most important risk factor for clinical recurrence and reoperation generally reproduced in all studies is smoking. In an Italian series by M. Cottone in 1994 the 6-year clinical recurrence-free rate after surgery was 60% (95 CI 43–72%) for non-smokers, 41% (95% CI 11–70%) for ex-smokers and 27% (95% CI 17–37%) for smokers [32].

The need for repeated surgery 5 years after surgery averages 20% in non-smokers versus 36% in smokers, as shown by Sutherland *et al.* in 1990. At 10 years these rates amount to 41% and 70% respectively [33]. The risk is particularly high in female smokers with small bowel disease (odd ratio 9.2). Another study confirms the high risk with a higher cumulative recurrence risk in heavy smokers (> 15 cigarettes/day).

The risk of excisional surgery associated with smoking seems to be increased only in patients not given immunosuppressive drugs, as shown by the French Getaid Group [34]. It seems that the effects of smoking can be antagonized by long-term immunosuppression.

Prevention

General measures and surgical factors

Only one strategy has resulted in a long-term disease-free perianastomotic region thus far. Diversion of intestinal contents through a proximal ileostomy protects the neoterminal ileum and ileocolonic anastomosis from recurrence [4]. All other strategies can help to reduce the incidence of CD recurrence but will never prevent it completely.

As mentioned above, active smokers have a substantially higher risk of having recurrence after a radical resection. There is approximately a twofold increased risk of recurrence, and the risk is dependent on the number of cigarettes smoked. Ex-smokers have a similar risk to that of non-smokers, and giving up smoking soon after surgery is associated with a lower probability of recurrence [35, 36].

There is no role for the continuation of steroid use in general postoperatively. Steroid therapy should be completely tapered and stopped prior to or immediately after surgery.

Several surgical factors have been studied. Surgeons have looked at various strategies to decrease the risk of postsurgical recurrence. Contrary to what was originally believed, the pathological features of the section margins and of the resected bowel loops do not affect the incidence of recurrence. Neither the presence of granulomas in the resection specimen, nor the presence or absence of 'disease-free' resection margins (i.e. with or without inflammatory activity) have been shown to influence recurrence rates or severity, although the presence of neural inflammation may be a predictor of early recurrence [22, 37, 38].

A recent clinical trial in which patients were randomized to 2 or 10 cm margins, performed at the Cleveland Clinic, detected no difference in recurrence rates [39]. The type of anastomosis (end-to-end versus end-to-side ileocolonic anastomosis) also has also no effect on the rate of recurrence [31]. In some centers an end-to-end ileocolonic anastomosis is preferred, because anastomotic strictures can more easily be treated endoscopically with this construction. Given these findings, resections should be as limited as possible and surgically safe. The recurrence rates of CD are much lower after surgical resection with ileostomy than after resection with ileocolonic anastomosis [40–42], unless the fecal stream is diverted from the anastomosis [21]. In a group of 182 patients with an end-ileostomy for CD 64% of those with ileocolitis as initial presentation had recurrence in the neoterminal ileum after 20 years, versus 15% of those with initial colitis ($p < 0.001$) [43]. The number of interventions seems to be of little importance with regard to recurrence. In a Swedish study the cumulative recurrence rates at 10 years were 65% after the second intervention versus 60% after the third one. This supports the hypothesis that disease behavior remains unchanged throughout the patient's history. The same study reported that an ileorectal anastomosis may carry an increased risk for postoperative recurrence, up to 70% at 10 years [44].

Medical intervention

It seems obvious that if one can prevent the recurrence of new lesions in the remaining bowel symptomatic relapse will also be prevented. Eventually this would lead to cure of the disease. Prophylactic therapy after resection for CD should therefore aim primarily at keeping the remaining bowel completely free of the disease. A secondary endpoint could be the prevention of symptomatic recurrence only. We are at present far from reaching the primary goal.

Standard anti-inflammatory approaches with glucocorticosteroids or 5-acetylsalicylic (5-ASA) formulations are unable to prevent tissue recurrence. Studies with 5-ASA formulations show that in the short term the most severe endoscopic lesions can be prevented, but the evolution seems only to be somewhat delayed. The problem with 5-ASA treatment may be the delivery of the highest concentrations to the site of the ileocolonic anastomosis.

A major drawback of prophylactic studies available at present is the lack of good patient selection at inclusion. We present a summary of the current available evidence (see also Table 4)

Sulfasalazine and 5-ASA

Prophylactic therapy with sulfasalazine has been shown not to be beneficial in all but one study.

By far the largest number of recurrence prevention trials has been performed with mesalamine (5-ASA). This medication is considered safe and well tolerated, but is rather expensive when used chronically in appropriate doses. Postoperative prevention studies with 5-ASA have produced varying results, possibly because of different pharmacological preparations, different doses and time point at the start of the postoperative treatment (from less than 10 days to 8 weeks following surgery). In addition, endpoints of the studies differed in that they used endoscopic, clinical and/or radiologic endpoints as primary criteria. Finally patient selection in the diferent studies may be an important bias.

An Italian study by Caprilli and colleagues demonstrated a preventive effect of 2.4 g/day of Asacol, with a significant reduction in the 2-year endoscopic and clinical recurrence rate. The authors observed a 39% prevention of all recurrences and 55% prevention of severe recurrences. This study, however, was not blinded, and therefore may have been subject to bias. Moreover recurrence rates in the group without treatment were rather low [45]. In another Italian study, by Brignola *et al.*, using 3 g of Pentasa per day, severe endoscopic recurrence was seen in 56% of patients compared to 24% in the treatment group ($p < 0.008$) [46]. A large Canadian multicenter trial with an appropriate placebo group confirmed these results to a certain extent: the overall 3-year symptomatic recurrence was 27% on 1.5 g mesalamine twice daily (Salofalk) started within 8 weeks after curative resection as compared to 47% on placebo. The most important limitation of this study was the time point at which therapy was initiated. Eight weeks after surgery some patients undoubtedly already had microscopic (and endoscopic) signs of Crohn's recurrence. Based on the placebo results in this study one could argue that 53% of the patients received unnecessary treatment for 3 years [47].

Mesalamine in a slow-release formulation (Pentasa) was also compared with placebo more recently in the German-Austrian double-blind ECCDS IV study. Using 4 g Pentasa/day and examining at clinical parameters (Crohn's Disease Activity Index, CDAI) to determine recurrence and all types of resections for CD were included. In this study, after

Table 4. Summary of postoperative recurrence trials: active compound, endpoints and key results

Study	Product	Start	Endpoints	Result
Caprilli *et al* [45] ($n = 110$)	Asacol 2.4 g/day × 2 years	< 15 days	Endo 6, 12, 24 months Clin 6, 12, 24 months	24 months: 52% vs 85% ($p < 0.002$) 24 months: 18% vs 41% ($p = 0.006$)
Brignola *et al.* [46] ($n = 77$)	Pentasa 3 g/day × 1 year	< 30 days	Endo 12 months	Severe 24% vs 56% ($p < 0.008$)
McLeod *et al.* [47] ($n = 163$)	Salofalk 3 g/day × 1 year	< 8 weeks	Endo + clin + RX	Clin at 3 years 27% vs 47%
Lochs *et al.* [48] ($n = 318$)	Pentasa 4 g/day × 18 months	< 10 days	Clin 18 months	No effect, except for small bowel alone
Rutgeerts *et al.* [11] ($n = 60$)	Metron 20 mg/kg × 3 months	< 7 days	Endo 3, 12 months Clin 12, 24, 36 months	12 months 52% vs 75% 12 months 4% vs 25%
Rutgeerts *et al.* [12] ($n = 71$)	Ornidazole 1 g/day × 1 year	< 7 days	Endo 3, 12 months	12 months 64% vs 94% ($p = 0.059$)
Korelitz *et al.* [51] ($n = 118$)	Placebo vs Pentasa 3 g vs. 6-MP 50 mg	< 7 days	Endo 6, 12, 24 months Clin 12, 24 months	24 months 90% vs 80% vs 68% ($p = 0.04$) Only for 6-MP significant

Endo = endoscopic; Clin = clinical.

18 months, clinical relapse rates were not significantly lower in Pentasa- than in placebo-treated patients. Subgroup analysis, however, did show a significant effect on patients operated on for small bowel disease alone [48].

In a meta-analysis adjusted for confounding variables, not including Lochs' data, the advantage of taking mesalamine in the postoperative setting of CD was estimated to offer a reduction in recurrence rates of approximately 13% [24]. This implies that eight patients would have to be treated with doses up to 3–4 g/day for a period of 2–3 years at a considerable cost in order to prevent one clinical postoperative recurrence.

Nitroimidazole antibiotics

Metronidazole is effective to control active CD. It has also been shown that high concentrations of anaerobic bacteria are present in the terminal ileum in CD after ileal resection, and bacterial antigens possibly play a role in the induction of Crohn's inflammation. For these reasons Rutgeerts and colleagues performed a controlled trial with metronidazole 20 mg/kg per day or placebo started within a week after resection, and continued for 3 months. At 12 weeks 75% of patients had recurrent lesions in the neoterminal ileum in the placebo group versus 52% in the metronidazole group. Interestingly, metronidazole reduced the clinical recurrence rates at 1 year (4% versus 25%), but not at 2 and 3 years. Unfortunately, the rate of adverse events in the metronidazole-treated patients was considerable [11]. Therefore we conducted a follow-up study using ornidazole 500 mg b.i.d. given for a full year after surgery. At 3 months 74% of placebo-treated patients had severe endoscopic recurrence (i2–i4) versus 41% of ornidazole-treated patients ($p = 0.02$). At 1 year 94% of the placebo patients had i2–i4 versus 62% of the ornidazole patients [12]. However, given the toxicity of nitroimidazole antibiotics when given for a long time and/or in high doses, they can probably only be used as initial short-term prevention therapy.

6-Mercaptopurine

Immunomodulators such as azathioprine and 6-mercaptopurine (6-MP) are the most potent agents in the maintenance treatment of CD [49, 50]. It was therefore logical that the benefit of these agents to prevent postsurgical recurrence was tested. One hundred eighteen patients were enrolled in a North American–European multicenter trial with randomization to 50 mg 6-mercaptopurine/day, 3 g Pentasa (12 tablets each 250 mg)/day or placebo in a double-blind, double-dummy fashion. Follow-up lasted 2 years with clinical check-ups and ileocolonoscopies 6, 12 and 24 months after surgery. During the trial a considerable number of patients dropped out of the study because of adverse events or lack of compliance (16 in the Pentasa group, 16 in the 6-MP group and 11 in the placebo group). Intent-to-treat analysis showed absence of endoscopic relapse in 32% of the patients on 6-MP ($p = 0.04$), in 20% on Pentasa (n.s.) and in 10% on placebo at 2 years. Severe endoscopic relapse at 2 years (score $>$i2) was more frequently observed with placebo and Pentasa than with 6-MP ($p = 0.01$ vs placebo and 0.07 vs Pentasa). The clinical relapse rate was reduced by both Pentasa and 6-MP, but statistical significance was achieved only with 6-MP ($p = 0.04$). The authors concluded that 6-MP is the strongest recurrence prevention therapy to date, and that higher doses may lead to even lower recurrence rates [51].

A small non-randomized study in the pediatric age group also showed statistical benefit (using the Kaplan–Meyer recurrence free curve) when treating patients with 6-MP started postoperatively [52].

Interleukin 10

IL-10 was a promising candidate to prevent CD recurrence as it is considered an anti-inflammatory cytokine potentially able to reset the imbalance between the T helper 1 lymphocytes (producing the proinflammatory cytokines) and the T helper 2 lymphocytes (producing the anti-inflammatory cytokines). However, a placebo-controlled trial with IL-10 given subcutaneously for the first 3 months after surgery showed no benefit for the active treatment. This study, however, had a very limited follow-up of 3 months and also included a large subgroup of patients with inactive disease who are known to have a low risk of recurrence anyway [53]. Further studies in higher-risk groups, and using other ways to reduce IL-10 or other cytokine and anticytokine strategies, are certainly warranted.

Steroids

Classic glucocorticosteroids have never been shown to prevent postoperative CD recurrence. The new topically acting glucocorticosteroid budesonide did not prevent the development of new lesions at 1 year after resection [54, 55]. Standard glucocorticosteroids or budesonide should therefore be tapered and discontinued within 4 weeks after resection.

Algorithm to prevent Crohn's disease recurrence

Postoperative Crohn's recurrence prevention should start in practice when the indication for surgery is considered (Fig. 1). Elective surgery should be performed only after informing patients of the risks and benefits of surgery, including the risk for postoperative Crohn's recurrence. When the risk for clinical recurrence is considered high the threshold to decide for surgery should be higher and postoperative management should be discussed earlier. In all cases active smokers should be advised to quit smoking.

Risk factors for recurrence are discussed above. In addition to the known risk factors patients undergoing a second or third resection and patients with longer enteric segments involved should also be considered patients at higher risk since recurrence in these patients will have more important consequences.

Outside clinical trials our practical management will differ according to the estimated risk of recurrence:

1. Patients considered low risk (non-smokers, fibrostenotic disease, first resections, short segments of disease) will not be treated medically after surgery. However, we will suggest patients undergo a routine ileocolonoscopy (and or small bowel X-ray) 6–12 months after surgery. Treatment will then be tailored according to the objective recurrence signs. Patients with no or mild ileal lesions will have an annual clinical follow-up. Thereafter endoscopy will be performed only when symptoms suggestive for recurrence appear. Patients with more severe lesions, but with a limited extent of the ileum involved (e.g. < 10 cm), will be treated with 5-ASA at 3–4 g daily and followed up clinically each year. Patients with severe lesions (ulcerations, narrowing) and a longer ileal segment involved will be put on azathioprine or 6 MP with 2-monthly control of white blood count and followed up clinically every 6 months. When already symptomatic at the initial postoperative endoscopy budesonide in an ileal release form will be added in a dosage of 9 mg/day, and tapered as soon as the symptoms resolve.

2. Patients considered at high risk for postoperative Crohn's recurrence will be offered routine treatment. When steroids are taken before surgery they will be tapered and stopped. Immunomodulator treatment (azathioprine or 6-MP) will be continued postoperatively. Patients not on immunomodulators will be started on 6-MP (1 mg/kg daily) or azathioprine (2 mg/kg daily) as soon as oral intake starts after surgery. As always blood counts should be monitored at regular intervals. High-risk patients will be followed clinically every 6 months. Endoscopy or X-ray will be performed only when clinically indicated. Asymptomatic patients will be continued on immunomodulator treatments for at least a few years before the treatment is stopped. In patients becoming symptomatic despite immunomodulator treatment dosages can be optimized according to metabolite levels. Alternatively methotrexate and/or an anti-TNF agent can be considered.

Management of clinical recurrence

It is imperative to treat patients with relapse due to disease recurrence in an aggressive manner. There is no place for 5-ASA therapy at that time. Progression of the disease must be prevented by all means, since reoperation will lead to more functional loss and diarrhea, which becomes more difficult to treat. Many symptoms which then develop are not related to CD itself. We always start with a combination of budesonide 9 mg/day o.m. and azathioprine 2.5 mg/kg per day o.m. for 3 months and then discontinue the steroids and keep the patient on immunosuppression indefinitely. When an anastomotic stenosis develops amenable to dilation, this should be considered. Patients who undergo balloon dilation of an anastomotic stenosis have longer remissions if they are treated with a short course of budesonide controlled ileal release and further azathioprine maintenance than if they remain untreated [56].

In as many as 60% of patients the disease will remain controlled using azathioprine monotherapy. In these patients thorough tissue healing may also be achieved [57]. If the disease flares despite azathioprine one should check on compliance, optimize the dose and should not discontinue azathioprine too early because of failure. In that situation reinduction with glucocorticosteroids is an option, but here anti-TNF antibodies (Remicade) will play a key role.

Future approaches

Future studies should be designed in such way that only high-risk patients are included, so that the best

Consider risk factors for recurrence, inform patient. If active smoker, advice to quit smoking !

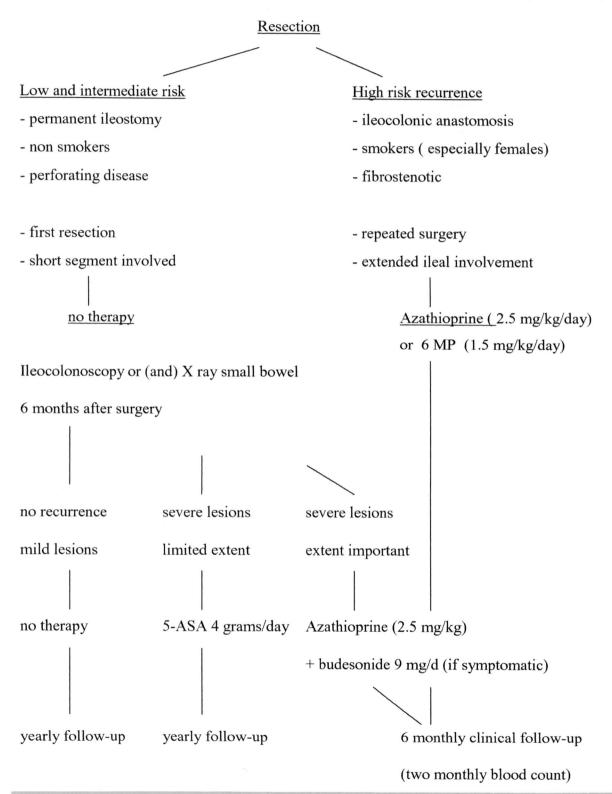

Figure 1. Algorithm for the medical prophylaxis of Crohn's recurrence after resection.

prophylactic therapy can emerge. Among the classic drugs, optimizing 5-ASA by delivering a higher dosage to the anastomotic region may be more efficient [58]. Immunosuppression and immuno-modulation are still the most attractive approaches to the prevention of recurrent CD, and they have been tested suboptimally so far.

Several potential new candidate drugs are being explored. IL-10 is still a good candidate for prevention of recurrence because of its immunoregulatory effects, but one small study showed no efficacy for this cytokine in prevention. Monoclonal antibodies to TNF should be effective for recurrence prevention but data are lacking. Whether this therapy will be able to change the natural history of CD remains uncertain.

Some authors advocate that the current subcutaneous route of delivery is insufficient to counteract inflammation in the bowel wall. Completely novel ways to deliver larger amounts of compounds including IL-10 are being developed. Among others genetically modified T cells delivering high levels of IL-10 to the gut are just one of the exciting possibilities emerging [59].

Combination therapies also are appealing; those we are currently studying include a combination of metronidazole and azathioprine for prevention of recurrent lesions in the tissue.

Given the importance of the fecal stream and the intestinal flora in the pathogenesis of recurrence the administration of probiotics early after surgery is a safe and potentially active treatment option [60].

Summary

Although the therapy of CD is primarily medical, surgery still plays an important role in its management. The high incidence of postoperative CD recurrence is, however, a major drawback. We provide a clear and practical algorithm which will help the clinician to decide when and what kind of prophylactic treatment is indicated. Strategies to prevent recurrence start with a careful selection of patients to send for surgery, based on the known risk factors of recurrence. Current evidence suggests only a moderate effect of the known active agents in the prevention of postoperative CD recurrence. Only patients at higher risk for recurrence should continue on, or be treated with, immunosuppressives (6-MP or azathioprine) after surgery. All others can be followed clinically, or alternatively should undergo an ileocolonoscopy 3–12 months after surgery. If severe endoscopic recurrence is seen, therapy is indicated to prevent the imminent clinical symptoms, or eventually a new resection. Much is anticipated from newer biological agents potentially interacting with earlier steps in the pathogenesis of recurrent CD.

References

1. Rutgeerts P, Geboes K, Vantrappen G, Beyls J, Kerremans R, Hiele M. Predictability of the postoperative course of Crohn's disease. Gastroenterology 1990; 99: 956–63.
2. Maunoury V, Mordon S, Geboes K *et al.* Endoscopic fluorescence imaging for the study of anastomotic recurrences in Crohn's disease: correlation with histological findings. Gastroenterology 1999; 116; A689.
3. Biacone L, Scopinaro F, Ierardi M *et al.* 99m Tc-HMPOA granulocyte scintigraphy in the early detection of postoperative asymptomatic recurrence of Crohn's disease. Dig Dis Sci 1997; 42: 1549–56.
4. Rutgeerts P, Geboes K, Peeters M *et al.* Effect of fecal stream diversion on recurrence of Crohn's disease in the neoterminal ileum. Lancet 1991; 338: 771–4.
5. D'Haens G, Geboes K, Peeters M, Baert F, Penninckx F. Early lesions of recurrent Crohn's disease caused by infusion of intestinal contents in excluded ileum. Gastroenterology 1998; 114: 262–7.
6. Fasoli R, Kettlewell MGW, Mortensen N, Jewell DP. Response to fecal challenge in defunctioned colonic Crohn's disease: prediction of long-term response. Br J Surg 1990; 77: 616–17.
7. Harper PH, Lee ECG, Kettlewell MGW, Bennett MK, Jewell DP. Role of fecal stream in the maintenance of Crohn's colitis. Gut 1985; 26: 279–84.
8. Rath HC, Herfarth HH, Ikeda JS *et al.* Normal luminal bacteria, especially *Bacteroides* species, mediate chronic colitis, gastritis and arthritis in HLA-B27/β$_2$-microglobulin transgenic rats. J Clin Invest 1996; 98: 945–53.
9. Keighly MR, Arabi Y, Dimock F, Burdon DW, Allan RN, Alexander-Williams J Influence of inflammatory bowel disease on intestinal microflora. Gut 1978; 19: 1099–104.
10. Lederman E, Neut C, Desreumaux P *et al.* Bacterial overgrowth in the neoterminal ileum after ileocolonic resection for Crohn's disease. Gastroenterology 1997; 112: A2865.
11. Rutgeerts P, Peeters M, Hiele M *et al.* A placebo controlled trial of metronidazole for recurrence prevention of Crohn's disease after resection of the terminal ileum. Gastroenterology 1995; 108: 1617–21.
12. Rutgeerts P, D'Haens G, Baert F *et al.* Nitroimidazol antibiotics are efficacious for prophylaxis of postoperative recurrence of Crohn's disease: a placebo controlled trial. Gastroenterology 1999; 116: A808.
13. Powell JJ, Ainley CC, Mason IM *et al.* Characterization of inorganic microparticles in pigment cells of human gut associated lymphoid tissue. Gut 1996; 38: 390–5.
14. Wyatt J, Vogelsang H, Hubl W, Waldhoer T, Lochs H. Intestinal permeability and the prediction of relapse in Crohn's disease. Lancet. 1993; 341: 1437–9.
15. Klein O, Houdret N, Desreumaux P *et al.* Intestinal permeability is not predicitive of endoscopic recurrence in patients operated on for Crohn's disease. Gastroenterology 1996; 112: A1096.
16. Desreumaux P, Brandt E, Gambiez L *et al.* Distinct cytokine patterns in early and chronic ileal lesions of Crohn's disease. Gastroenterology 1997; 113: 118–26.

36 | The molecular pathology of inflammatory bowel disease-associated neoplasia and preneoplasia

STEPHEN MELTZER

Introduction

Molecular alterations underlying inflammatory bowel disease-associated neoplasia and preneoplasia (IBDN) have been studied extensively over the past 10 years. Perhaps the most interesting facet of these studies has been the emergence of IBDN as a distinct form of colorectal neoplasia, with both similarities to and differences from sporadic colorectal neoplasia and preneoplasia (SCN). This finding of differences between IBDN and SCN should not surprise IBD clinicians, who are quite familiar with the known biologic differences between these two forms of neoplasia. For example, it is widely held that the interval between dysplasia and frank carcinoma is only a few years in IBDN, contrasted with 10–15 years or longer for SCN. Furthermore, frank carcinoma in IBDN often evolves from flat dysplastic lesions, whereas SCN is commonly believed to evolve from polypoid dysplasias (adenomas). Finally, IBDN develops in a setting of intense mucosal inflammation, often after 20 or more years of non-dysplastic IBD; SCN typically develops on a substratum of non-inflamed colonic mucosa.

Investigations of IBDN, however, have closely paralleled the investigative paradigm established in SCN by Bert Vogelstein and his colleagues [1]. Early in the history of these analyses, proto-oncogenes of the *ras* family were studied [2–5]. Later, loss of heterozygosity (LOH) was evaluated, and evaluations of tumor-suppressor genes (TSG) evolved directly from these LOH studies [1, 6–10]. Subsequently, the unique form of mutation known as microsatellite instability (MSI) was evaluated in IBDN, and the ramifications of this form of mutation were investigated [11–16]. This form of mutation comprises length mutations in oligonucleotide repeat sequences, typically in non-coding regions of genomic DNA. The ability of MSI to target specific coding regions was also evaluated in IBDN [17–19]. MSI is caused by inactivation or defective function of DNA mismatch repair (MMR) genes [20–24]. Finally, gene inactivation by promoter hypermethylation was studied in IBDN [25]. Hypermethylation appears to be of pivotal importance in IBDN, since it inactivates TSG such as the cyclin-dependent kinase inhibitor p16 [26] along with MMR genes [25]. In the future comprehensive new molecularly based taxonomies may augment traditional approaches to classifying IBDN. In particular, gene expression 'signatures', or profiles of the expression levels of thousands of genes generated by cDNA microarrays, promise to shed light not only on new taxonomies, but also on novel molecular genetic pathways involved in IBDN [27–35]. Genes involved in these pathways offer the potential to serve as biomarkers of cancer risk and disease progression; moreover, they present promising targets of future molecular and pharmacologic cancer prevention and treatment strategies.

Abnormal DNA content (aneuploidy)

Much of the groundwork for future investigations of neoplastic progression in ulcerative colitis was laid with studies of DNA content, or ploidy, which can be determined using flow cytometric measurement of disaggregated nuclei [9, 36–43]. This is a very valuable tool in detecting clonality of tissues or cells. The earliest reports of flow cytometric DNA analysis in ulcerative colitis were published from Stockholm in 1984 [44] and in a later survey by the same group [45]. The prevalence of aneuploidy in this series of 51 patients correlated well with disease duration and the presence of histologic dysplasia or carcinoma. Similar findings were reported by other investigators [38, 46, 47]. A higher prevalence of DNA aneuploidy was found in dysplastic than in nondysplastic tissues,

Stephan R. Targan, Fergus Shanahan and Loren C. Karp (eds.), Inflammatory Bowel Disease: From Bench to Bedside, 2nd Edition, 711–718.
© 2003 *Kluwer Academic Publishers. Printed in Great Britain*

but this difference did not achieve statistical significance [45]. A prospective study on aneuploidy in ulcerative colitis was published in 1987 [48]. In this study 53 patients with long-standing universal ulcerative colitis were followed for a mean of 3.5 years. Four of five patients with aneuploidy developed dysplasia; aneuploidy preceded dysplasia by 1 year in one patient and antedated a Dukes A carcinoma by 1 year in another patient.

The precise predictive value of aneuploidy has yet not been consistently substantiated [49, 50]. Other publications on aneuploidy in ulcerative colitis have included elegant mapping studies, some of which combine ploidy studies with molecular analyses [38, 40, 51, 52]. These systematic investigations demonstrated large areas of colonic mucosa containing identical aneuploid DNA content. This evidence strongly suggests that these large areas of epithelium arose from a single abnormal progenitor cell, in agreement with the clonal theory of cancer proffered above.

In summary, measurement of DNA content is a well-established technique that has been shown to correlate often, if imperfectly, with the clinical progression of premalignant lesions in ulcerative colitis. In this respect it shows potential as a clinical prognostic tool to be used in conjunction with conventional histologic analysis.

Proto-oncogenes in IBD neoplasia

Proto-oncogenes are the normal forms of genes, expressed in normal cells under physiologic circumstances, which become activated to their oncogenic forms (i.e. into oncogenes) by various molecular mechanisms in tumors [53]. Even though there are two alleles of each proto-oncogene in each cell, only one allele need be activated in order for a carcinogenic effect to be exerted. In this respect proto-oncogene mutations function as dominant mutations, and oncogenes are often referred to as 'dominant oncogenes'. One group of proto-oncogenes is known as the *ras* family, comprising three genes: Kirsten *ras* (Ki-*ras* or K-*ras*), Harvey *ras* (Ha-*ras* or H-*ras*), and neuroblastoma *ras* (N-*ras*). These genes are activated in tumors by point mutations of codons 12, 13, and 61. Mutations in *ras* family genes have been reported in SCN, particularly in K-*ras* and less frequently in H-*ras* [54–59]. Mutations in SCN are most frequent in codons 12 and 13 of K-*ras* and H-*ras* [54–60]. Studies of IBDN lesions identified the

first major contrast between these lesions and SCN: namely, a paucity of K-*ras* and H-*ras* mutations [2–5, 43, 61–63]. Reasons for this apparent contrast are unclear, but this finding was the first of many to suggest that molecular pathways underlying the two forms of colonic neoplasia might differ.

Gene amplification in IBD neoplasia

Gene amplification is the process of duplication and reduplication of genomic DNA regions, sometimes encompassing large regions of chromosomes and multiple genes [64]. Certain cellular proto-oncogenes (such as c-myc, N-myc, c-myb, EGF-R, and c-erbB-2) are activated by DNA amplification in human tumors [59, 61, 65–72]. These extra genomic copies of genes often result in increased levels of mRNA or protein expression of the genes encoded. However, relatively few studies of gene amplification in IBDN have been published. One study found no amplification of common proto-oncogenes in IBDN [61].

Tumor suppressor genes and loss of heterozygosity in IBD neoplasia

TSG can be considered the opposites of proto-oncogenes. TSG suppress tumor formation by various mechanisms, either by preventing entry into the cell division cycle, promoting programmed cell death (apoptosis), leading to cellular growth arrest, or interrupting proliferative signals to the cellular interior [73]. TSG are present in normal form in all cells of the body, but in contrast to proto-oncogenes, which are activated, they become inactivated in tumors [73]. However, because inactivation of only one copy (allele) still leaves a remaining active copy, both alleles must be inactivated in order for tumorigenesis to proceed. For this reason, TSGs are sometimes referred to as *recessive* oncogenes or *anti*-oncogenes.

LOH, also known as allelic deletion, is the process of deletion of one allele of genomic DNA, often encompassing large chromosomal regions [7, 59, 74]. Because LOH may remove one functional copy of a TSG, it is a hallmark of TSG inactivation. However, LOH may also occur non-specifically, in random fashion, and affect any portion of the genome [6, 7]. When LOH occurs frequently at a particular chromosomal locus it is widely believed to represent a non-random event and to imply the presence of a potential TSG at that locus [74, 75].

Generally speaking, LOH frequency must exceed a 'background' frequency in order for non-randomness to be assumed, but this frequency varies from study to study and among different tumor types [7, 76–87]. For SCN this background LOH rate approximates 20% [7]. Thus, LOH rates in SCN significantly higher than 20% imply the existence of a TSG at a given locus.

In IBDN, LOH has been observed frequently at chromosomal arms 5q, 8p, 9p, 13q, 17p, and 18q [8, 15, 16, 88–93]. These loci house the TSGs adenomatous polyposis coli (APC) (5q), p16/p15/p14 (9p), retinoblastoma (Rb or RB1) (13q), p53 or TP53 (17p), and DPC4 or SMAD4 (18q). 18q also contains the gene deleted in colon cancer (DCC) [94]. LOH in IBDN has been shown to affect large areas of colonic mucosa [9, 88]. This finding suggests that the LOH originated in a single progenitor cell, conferring a growth advantage on it and leading to its clonal expansion .

Point mutational inactivation of tumor suppressor genes in IBD neoplasia

p53

The classic paradigm for TSG inactivation was discovered in sporadic colon neoplasia (SCN) by the Vogelstein group [1]. According to this model, one allele of a TSG is removed by LOH, while the remaining allele is inactivated by point mutation. The prototypical TSG fitting this paradigm is p53. p53 is a TSG which encodes a nuclear DNA-binding transcriptional activator with multiple growth-suppressive functions, including induction of apoptosis, exit from the cell cycle, and growth arrest [95]. Approximately 50% of all human tumors show inactivation of p53 [96]. In SCN, p53 inactivation constitutes a relatively late event, occurring only in large, severely dysplastic, often villous adenomas [75]. In contrast to SCN, IBDN is characterized by the relatively early occurrence of p53 inactivation [8–10, 12, 97–99]. p53 mutations have even been described in non-dysplastic IBD mucosa [98]. As with LOH, p53 mutations can populate large regions of colonic mucosa, again suggesting a single event in a parent cell leading to clonal expansion of that cell due to a growth advantage over surrounding non-mutant cells [98]. An analogous finding has been reported for LOH affecting the p53 gene locus on

chromosome 17p, which can occur in non-dysplastic mucosa and occupy large portions of colonic mucosa in IBDN [9].

Adenomatous polyposis coli

APC, which stands for adenomatous polyposis coli, is the TSG responsible for the familial colorectal cancer syndrome known as familial adenomatous polyposis, or FAP [100–102]. When mutant in the germline, APC causes this syndrome. However, APC is also widely regarded as the 'gatekeeper' gene for sporadic colon cancer [103]. 'Gatekeeper' signifies a somatic event that occurs extremely early and frequently in a given tumor type: a gatekeeper event is the *sine qua non* of a tumor, without which the neoplastic process cannot initiate in that particular organ or cell type [104]. APC mutation, usually accompanied by LOH of its locus on chromosome 5q, occurs in 80% of sporadic colon cancers and adenomatous polyps [103, 105–108]. Mutations in APC tend to cluster in a region comprising the proximal two-thirds of exon 15, known as the mutation cluster region or MCR [109]. APC mutations in the MCR occur even in the smallest benign colonic adenomas, less than 0.5 cm in diameter [103]. Herein lies one of the most striking contrasts between SCN and IBDN: in IBDN, APC mutations in the MCR occur in less than 5% of colorectal dysplasias and cancers [63, 110]. 5q-LOH occurs in IBDN, but also at a much lower frequency than in SCN [15, 92]. Moreover, when 5q-LOH or APC mutations do occur in IBDN, they are found late in neoplastic progression [15, 90, 92, 110]. These findings contrast with p53 mutation or 17p-LOH, which represent early events in IBDN and late events in SCN [8–10, 12, 97–99].

One interesting aspect of APC is a particular germline sequence variant, I1307K [111]. This alteration, occurring in codon 1307, leads to the replacement of isoleucine by lysine [111]. However, this amino acid substitution itself does not alter protein function appreciably. Rather, the underlying nucleic acid substitution (replacement of a thymidine by an adenine) creates a microsatellite tract (see below). This microsatellite tract itself, along with surrounding regions within the gene, becomes prone to secondary mutations, which occur somatically [111]. Patients with this germline sequence variant have an increased likelihood of developing colon cancer within their lifetimes, presumably because APC is the gatekeeper gene in this organ, and somatic APC mutations occurring in colon epithelium are more likely than in other organ epithelia to lead to cancer development [111]. This germline mutation is more frequent in Ashkenazi Jews than in other populations [112–114]. However, it is extremely rare in Ashkenazi Jews with IBD, occurring in only 1.5% of this group, and it is found in only 0.8% of all IBD patients [115]. Thus, this germline mutation does not likely account for a significant proportion of neoplasia arising in the setting of chronic IBD.

Microsatellite instability in IBD neoplasia

Microsatellite instability (MSI) comprises length mutations in oligonucleotide repeat portions of the genome [116–118]. This phenomenon is a manifestation of defective DNA mismatch repair, or MMR [119–121]. When DNA MMR genes are mutated in the germline they result in the genetic disorder known as hereditary non-polyposis colorectal cancer (HNPCC) [119]. HNPCC is characterized by a greatly increased risk of developing carcinomas of the endometrium, stomach, right side of the colon, and other anatomic sites [122, 123]. However, DNA MMR gene inactivation and MSI also occur in sporadic tumors affecting the colorectum, endometrium, stomach, and other organs [124–129]. MSI has been classified into three types: (a) MSI-high or MSI-H, i.e. MSI affecting 40% or more of oligonucleotide repeat sites in a particular analysis; (b) MSI-low or MSI-L, connoting MSI affecting less than 40% of these loci; and (c) MSI-negative or microsatellite-stable (MSS), meaning MSI affecting none of the loci analyzed.

MSI-H is widely regarded as 'true' MSI, i.e. reflecting an underlying defect in MMR [130, 131]. MSI-L may occur even in the absence of an underlying MMR defect and may represent a random, non-specific event, analogous to the occurrence of LOH at or below its background frequency for a given tumor type [132]. The vast majority of tumors with documented DNA MMR gene defects are MSI-H, rather than MSI-L [132].

IBDN have been studied for MSI. In one study MSI was found in 19% of IBD-associated dysplastic and cancerous lesions, and in 21% of patients with IBDNs [11]. In other published studies the prevalence of MSI in IBDNs was somewhat higher [13, 14, 16].

The most prevalent molecular mechanism underlying MSI in sporadic human tumors is inactivation of DNA MMR genes. Germline mutations in at least six MMR genes have been described in patients with HNPCC, who have tumors characterized by a high frequency of MSI (MSI-H) [20, 119, 120, 133–141]. However, mutations in MMR genes are rare in sporadic tumors with MSI [24, 142, 143]. Recently, an alternative mode of MMR gene inactivation has been described in these tumors: hypermethylation of the hMLH1 mismatch repair gene promoter region [144–148]. Hypermethylation of hMLH1 occurs in 80% of SCN with MSI [144, 146, 149]. It has also been described in endometrial and gastric tumors with MSI, where it may occur early in tumorigenesis [145, 147, 148, 150]. Approximately 50% of IBDN with high-frequency MSI (MSI-H neoplasms) show hypermethylation of hMLH1 [25]. Thus, this epigenetic alteration constitutes an important example of the contrast in molecular pathways between IBDN and SCN.

References

1. Fearon ER, Vogelstein B. A genetic model for colorectal tumorigenesis. Cell 1990; 61: 759–67.
2. Meltzer SJ, Mane SM, Wood PK *et al.* Activation of c-Ki-ras in human gastrointestinal dysplasias determined by direct sequencing of polymerase chain reaction products. Cancer Res 1990; 50: 3627–30.
3. Burmer GC, Levine DS, Kulander BG, Haggitt RC, Rubin CE, Rabinovitch PS. c-Ki-ras mutations in chronic ulcerative colitis and sporadic colon carcinoma. Gastroenterology 1990; 99: 416–20.
4. Bell SM, Kelly SA, Hoyle JA *et al.* c-Ki-ras gene mutations in dysplasia and carcinomas complicating ulcerative colitis. Br J Cancer 1991; 64: 174–8.
5. Burmer GC, Rabinovitch PS, Loeb LA. Frequency and spectrum of c-Ki-ras mutations in human sporadic colon carcinoma, carcinomas arising in ulcerative colitis, and pancreatic adenocarcinoma. Environ Health Perspect 1991; 93: 27–31.
6. Kern SE, Fearon ER, Tersmette KW *et al.* Clinical and pathological associations with allelic loss in colorectal carcinoma [Corrected; published erratum appears in J Am Med Assoc 1989; 262: 1952]. J Am Med Assoc 1989; 261: 3099–103.
7. Vogelstein B, Fearon ER, Kern SE *et al.* Allelotype of colorectal carcinomas. Science 1989; 244: 207–11.
8. Greenwald BD, Harpaz N, Yin J *et al.* Loss of heterozygosity affecting the p53, Rb, and mcc/apc tumor suppressor gene loci in dysplastic and cancerous ulcerative colitis. Cancer Res 1992; 52: 741–5.
9. Burmer GC, Rabinovitch PS, Haggitt RC *et al.* Neoplastic progression in ulcerative colitis: histology, DNA content, and loss of a p53 allele. Gastroenterology 1992; 103: 1602–10.
10. Burmer GC, Crispin DA, Kolli VR *et al.* Frequent loss of a p53 allele in carcinomas and their precursors in ulcerative colitis. Cancer Commun 1991; 3: 167–72.

11. Suzuki H, Harpaz N, Tarmin L *et al.* Microsatellite instability in ulcerative colitis-associated colorectal dysplasias and cancers. Cancer Res 1994; 54: 4841–4.

12. Kern SE, Redston M, Seymour AB *et al.* Molecular genetic profiles of colitis-associated neoplasms. Gastroenterology 1994; 107: 420–8.

13. Brentnall TA, Crispin DA, Bronner MP *et al.* Microsatellite instability in nonneoplastic mucosa from patients with chronic ulcerative colitis. Cancer Res 1996; 56: 1237–40.

14. Cravo ML, Albuquerque CM, Salazar de Sousa L *et al.* Microsatellite instability in non-neoplastic mucosa of patients with ulcerative colitis: effect of folate supplementation. Am J Gastroenterol 1998; 93: 2060–4.

15. Fogt F, Vortmeyer AO, Goldman H, Giordano TJ, Merino MJ, Zhuang Z. Comparison of genetic alterations in colonic adenoma and ulcerative colitis-associated dysplasia and carcinoma. Hum Pathol 1008; 29: 131–6.

16. Fogt F, Urbanski SJ, Sanders ME *et al.* Distinction between dysplasia-associated lesion or mass (DALM) and adenoma in patients with ulcerative colitis. Hum Pathol 2000; 31: 288–91.

17. Souza RF, Garrigue-Antar L, Lei J *et al.* Alterations of transforming growth factor-beta 1 receptor type II occur in ulcerative colitis-associated carcinomas, sporadic colorectal neoplasms, and esophageal carcinomas, but not in gastric neoplasms. Hum Cell 1996; 9: 229–36.

18. Souza RF, Lei J, Yin J *et al.* A transforming growth factor beta 1 receptor type II mutation in ulcerative colitis-associated neoplasms. Gastroenterology 1997; 112: 40 5.

19. Grady W, Rajput A, Myerof L, Markowitz S. What's new with RII? Gastroenterology 1997; 112: 297–302.

20. Leach FS, Nicolaides NC, Papadopoulos N *et al.* Mutations of a mutS homolog in hereditary nonpolyposis colorectal cancer. Cell 1993; 75: 1215–25.

21. Fishel R, Kolodner RD. Identification of mismatch repair genes and their role in the development of cancer. Curr Opin Genet Dev 1995; 5: 382–95.

22. Jiricny J. Colon cancer and DNA repair: have mismatches met their match? Trends Genet 1994; 10: 164–8.

23. Parsons R, Li GM, Longley MJ *et al.* Hypermutability and mismatch repair deficiency in RER+ tumor cells. Cell 1993; 75: 1227–36.

24. Liu B, Nicolaides NC, Markowitz S *et al.* Mismatch repair gene defects in sporadic colorectal cancers with microsatellite instability. Nat Genet 1995; 9: 48–55.

25. Fleisher AS, Esteller M, Harpaz N *et al.* Microsatellite instability in inflammatory bowel disease-associated neoplastic lesions is associated with hypermethylation and diminished expression of the DNA mismatch repair gene, hMLH1. Cancer Res 2000; 60: 4864–8.

26. Hsieh CJ, Klump B, Holzmann K, Borchard F, Gregor M, Porschen R. Hypermethylation of the p16INK4a promoter in colectomy specimens of patients with long-standing and extensive ulcerative colitis Cancer Res 1998; 58: 3942–5.

27. Schena M, Shalon D, Davis RW, Brown PO. Quantitative monitoring of gene expression patterns with a complementary DNA microarray. Science 1995; 270: 467–70.

28. DeRisi J, Penland L, Brown PO *et al.* Use of cDNA microarray to analyse gene expression patterns in human cancer. Nature Genetics 1996; 14: 457–60.

29. Heller RA, Schena M, Chai A *et al.* Discovery and analysis of inflammatory disease-related genes using cDNA microarrays. Proc Natl Acad Sci USA 1997; 94: 2150–5.

30. Chuaqui RF, Cole KA, Emmert-Buck MR, Merino MJ. Histopathology and molecular biology of ovarian epithelial tumors Ann Diagn Pathol 1998; 2: 195–207.

31. Duggan DJ, Bittner M, Chen Y, Meltzer P, Trent J. M. Expression profiling using cDNA microarrays. Nat Genet 1999; 21: 10–4.

32. Friend SH. How DNA microarrays and expression profiling will affect clinical practice Br Med J 1999; 319: 1306–7.

33. Golub TR, Slonim DK, Tamayo P *et al.* Molecular classification of cancer: class discovery and class prediction by gene expression monitoring. Science 1999; 286: 531–7.

34. Khan J, Saal LH, Bittner ML, Chen Y, Trent JM, Meltzer PS. Expression profiling in cancer using cDNA microarrays. Electrophoresis 1999; 20: 223–9.

35. Khan J, Bittner ML, Chen Y, Meltzer PS, Trent JM. DNA microarray technology: the anticipated impact on the study of human disease. Biochim Biophys Acta 1999; 1423: M17–28.

36. Fozard JB, Quirke P, Dixon MF, Giles GR, Bird C. C. DNA aneuploidy in ulcerative colitis Gut 1986; 27: 1414–8.

37. Fozard JB, Quirke P, Dixon MF. DNA aneuploidy in ulcerative colitis. Gut 1987; 28: 642–4.

38. Levine DS, Rabinovitch PS, Haggitt RC *et al.* Distribution of aneuploid cell populations in ulcerative colitis with dysplasia or cancer. Gastroenterology 1991; 101: 1198–210.

39. Porschen R, Robin U, Schumacher A *et al.* DNA aneuploidy in Crohn's disease and ulcerative colitis: results of a comparative flow cytometric study. Gut 1992; 33: 663–7.

40. Rubin CE, Haggitt RC, Burmer GC *et al.* DNA aneuploidy in colonic biopsies predicts future development of dysplasia in ulcerative colitis. Gastroenterology 1992; 103: 1611–20.

41. Navratil E, Stettler C, Paul G *et al.* Assessment of dysplasia, mucosal mucins, p53 protein expression, and DNA content in ulcerative colitis patients with colectomy and ileorectal anastomosis. Scand J Gastroenterol 1995; 30: 361–6.

42. Klump B, Holzmann K, Kuhn A *et al.* Distribution of cell populations with DNA aneuploidy and p53 protein expression in ulcerative colitis Eur J Gastroenterol Hepatol 1997; 9: 789–94.

43. Holzmann K, Klump B, Borchard F *et al.* Comparative analysis of histology, DNA content, p53 and Ki-ras mutations in colectomy specimens with long-standing ulcerative colitis. Int J Cancer 1998; 76: 1–6.

44. Hammarberg C, Slezak P, Tribukait B. Early detection of malignancy in ulcerative colitis. A flow-cytometric DNA study. Cancer 1984; 53: 291–5.

45. Hammarberg C, Rubio C, Slezak P, Tribukait B, Ohman U. Flow-cytometric DNA analysis as a means for early detection of malignancy in patients with chronic ulcerative colitis. Gut 1984; 25: 905–8.

46. Melville DM, Jass JR, Shepherd NA *et al.* Dysplasia and deoxyribonucleic acid aneuploidy in the assessment of precancerous changes in chronic ulcerative colitis. Observer variation and correlations. Gastroenterology 1988; 95: 668–75.

47. Melville DM, Jass JR, Morson BC *et al.* Observer study of the grading of dysplasia in ulcerative colitis: comparison with clinical outcome. Hum Pathol 1989; 20: 1008–14.

48. Lofberg R, Tribukait B, Ost A, Brostrom O, Reichard H. Flow cytometric DNA analysis in longstanding ulcerative colitis: a method of prediction of dysplasia and carcinoma development? Gut 1987; 28: 1100–6.

49. Rutegard J, Ahsgren L, Stenling R, Roos G. DNA content and mucosal dysplasia in ulcerative colitis. Flow cytometric analysis in patients with dysplastic or indeterminate morphologic changes in the colorectal mucosa. Dis Colon Rectum 1989; 32: 1055–19.

50. Rutegard J, Ahsgren L, Stenling R, Roos G. DNA content in ulcerative colitis. Flow cytometric analysis in a patient series from a defined area. Dis Colon Rectum 1988; 31: 710–5.

51. Levine DS, Reid BJ, Haggitt RC, Rubin CE, Rabinovitch PS. Correlation of ultrastructural aberrations with dysplasia and flow cytometric abnormalities in Barrett's epithelium. Gastroenterology 1989; 96: 355–67.

52. Reid BJ, Blount PL, Rubin CE *et al*. Flow-cytometric and histological progression to malignancy in Barrett's esophagus: prospective endoscopic surveillance of a cohort. Gastroenterology 1992; 102: 1212–9.

53. Kahn S, Yamamoto F, Almoguera C *et al*. The c-K-ras gene and human cancer (Review). Anticancer Res 1987; 7: 639–52.

54. Bos JL, Fearon ER, Hamilton SR *et al*. Prevalence of ras gene mutations in human colorectal cancers. Nature 1987; 327: 293–7.

55. Forrester K, Almoguera C, Han K, Grizzle WE, Perucho M. Detection of high incidence of K-ras oncogenes during human colon tumorigenesis. Nature 1987; 327: 298–303.

56. Burmer GC, Rabinovitch PS, Loeb LA. Analysis of c-Ki-ras mutations in human colon carcinoma by cell sorting, polymerase chain reaction, and DNA sequencing. Cancer Res 1989; 49: 2141–6.

57. Delattre O, Olschwang S, Law DJ *et al*. Multiple genetic alterations in distal and proximal colorectal cancer. Lancet 1989; 2: 353–6.

58. Bodmer WF, Cottrell S, Frischauf AM *et al*. Genetic analysis of colorectal cancer. Princess Takamatsu Symp 1989; 20: 49–59.

59. Meltzer SJ, Ahnen DJ, Battifora H, Yokota J, Cline MJ. Protooncogene abnormalities in colon cancers and adenomatous polyps [Published erratum appears in Gastroenterology 1987; 93: 223]. Gastroenterology 1987; 92: 1174–80.

60. Almoguera C, Shibata D, Forrester K, Martin J, Arnheim N, Perucho M. Most human carcinomas of the exocrine pancreas contain mutant c-K-ras genes. Cell 1988; 53: 549–54.

61. Meltzer SJ, Zhou D, Weinstein WM. Tissue-specific expression of c-Ha-ras in premalignant gastrointestinal mucosae. Exp Mol Pathol 1989; 51: 264–74.

62. Redston MS, Papadopoulos N, Caldas C, Kinzler KW, Kern SE. Common occurrence of APC and K-ras gene mutations in the spectrum of colitis-associated neoplasias. Gastroenterology 1995; 108: 383–92.

63. Suzui M, Ushijima T, Yoshimi N *et al*. No involvement of APC gene mutations in ulcerative colitis-associated rat colon carcinogenesis induced by 1-hydroxyanthraquinone and methylazoxymethanol acetate. Mol Carcinogenet 1997; 20: 389–93.

64. Feinberg AP. The molecular biology of human cancer. Prog Clin Biol Res 1985; 198: 279–92.

65. Slamon DJ, Clark GM, Wong SG, Levin WJ, Ullrich A, McGuire WL. Human breast cancer: correlation of relapse and survival with amplification of the HER-2/neu oncogene. Science 1987; 235: 177–82.

66. Lu SH, Hsieh LL, Luo FC, Weinstein IB. Amplification of the EGF receptor and c-myc genes in human esophageal cancers. Int J Cancer 1988; 42: 502–5.

67. Mallet MK, Mane SM, Meltzer SJ, Needleman SW. c-myc amplification coexistent with activating N-ras point mutation in the biphenotypic leukemic cell line Red-3. Leukemia 1989; 3: 511-1-5.

68. Bigner SH, Friedman HS, Vogelstein B, Oakes WJ, Bigner DD. Amplification of the c-myc gene in human medulloblastoma cell lines and xenografts [Published erratum appears in Cancer Res 1990; 50: 3809]. Cancer Res 1990; 50: 2347–50.

69. Jiang W, Kahn SM, Tomita N, Zhang YJ, Lu SH, Weinstein IB. Amplification and expression of the human cyclin D gene in esophageal cancer. Cancer Res 1992; 52: 2980–3.

70. Zhang YJ, Jiang W, Chen CJ *et al*. Amplification and overexpression of cyclin D1 in human hepatocellular carcinoma. Biochem Biophys Res Commun 1993; 196: 1010–6.

71. Oliner JD, Pietenpol JA, Thiagalingam S, Gyuris J, Kinzler KW, Vogelstein B. Oncoprotein MDM2 conceals the activa-tion domain of tumour suppressor p53. Nature 1993; 362: 857–60.

72. Kauraniemi P, Hedenfalk I, Persson K *et al*. MYB oncogene amplification in hereditary BRCA1 breast cancer. Cancer Res 2000; 60: 5323–8.

73. Weinberg R. Tumor suppressor genes. Science 1991; 254: 1138–461.

74. Vogelstein B, Fearon ER, Hamilton SR *et al*. Genetic alterations during colorectal-tumor development. N Engl J Med 1988; 319: 525–32.

75. Baker SJ, Preisinger AC, Jessup JM *et al*. p53 gene mutations occur in combination with 17p allelic deletions as late events in colorectal tumorigenesis. Cancer Res 1990; 50: 7717–22.

76. Devilee P, van Vliet M, van Sloun P *et al*. Allelotype of human breast carcinoma: a second major site for loss of heterozygosity is on chromosome 6q. Oncogene 1991; 6: 1705–11.

77. Sato T, Saito H, Morita R, Koi S, Lee J, Nakamura Y. Allelotype of human ovarian cancer. Cancer Res 1991; 51: 5118 – 22.

78. Aoki T, Mori T, Du X, Nisihira T, Matsubara T, Nakamura Y. Allelotype study of esophageal carcinoma. Genes Chromosomes Cancer 1994; 10: 177–82.

79. Nawroz H, van der Riet P, Hruban RH, Koch W, Ruppert JM, Sidransky D. Allelotype of head and neck squamous cell carcinoma. Cancer Res 1994; 54: 1152–5.

80. Seymour AB, Hruban RH, Redston M *et al*. Allelotype of pancreatic adenocarcinoma. Cancer Res 1994; 54: 2761–4.

81. Field JK, Kiaris H, Risk JM *et al*. Allelotype of squamous cell carcinoma of the head and neck: fractional allele loss correlates with survival [Published erratum appears in Br J Cancer 1996; 74: 1153]. Br J Cancer 1995; 72: 1180–8.

82. Rosin MP, Cairns P, Epstein JI, Schoenberg MP, Sidransky D. Partial allelotype of carcinoma in situ of the human bladder. Cancer Res 1995; 55: 5213–16.

83. Califano JA, Johns MMr, Westra WH *et al*. An allelotype of papillary thyroid cancer. Int J Cancer 1996; 69: 442–4.

84. Johns MMr, Westra WH, Califano JA, Eisele D, Koch WM, Sidransky D. Allelotype of salivary gland tumors. Cancer Res 1996; 56: 1151–4.

85. Hammoud ZT, Kaleem Z, Cooper JD, Sundaresan R, Patterson GA, Goodfellow PJ. Allelotype analysis of esophageal adenocarcinomas: evidence for the involvement of sequences on the long arm of chromosome 4. Cancer Res 1996; 65: 4499–502.

86. Dolan K, Garde J, Gosney J *et al*. Allelotype analysis of oesophageal adenocarcinoma: loss of heterozygosity occurs at multiple sites. Br J Cancer 1998; 78: 950–7.

87. Yustein AS, Harper JC, Petroni GR, Cummings OW, Moskaluk CA, Powell SM. Allelotype of gastric adenocarcinoma. Cancer Res 1999; 59: 1437–41.

88. Chang M, Tsuchiya K, Batchelor RH *et al*. Deletion mapping of chromosome 8p in colorectal carcinoma and dysplasia arising in ulcerative colitis, prostatic carcinoma, and malignant fibrous histiocytomas. Am J Pathol 1994; 144: 1–6.

89. Hoque AT, Hahn SA, Schutte M, Kern SE. DPC4 gene mutation in colitis associated neoplasia. Gut 1997; 40: 120–2.

90. Fogt F, Vortmeyer AO, Stolte M *et al*. Loss of heterozygosity of the von Hippel Lindau gene locus in polypoid dysplasia but not flat dysplasia in ulcerative colitis or sporadic adenomas. Hum Pathol 1998; 29: 961–4.

91. Zou TT, Lei J, Shi YQ *et al*. FHIT gene alterations in esophageal cancer and ulcerative colitis (UC). Oncogene 1997; 15: 101–5.

92. Tomlinson I, Ilyas M, Johnson V *et al.* comparison of the genetic pathways involved in the pathogenesis of three types of colorectal cancer. J Pathol 1998; 184: 148–52.

93. Odze RD, Brown CA, Hartmann CJ, Noffsinger AE Fogt F. Genetic alterations in chronic ulcerative colitis-associated adenoma-like DALMs are similar to non-colitic sporadic adenomas. Am J Surg Pathol 2000; 24: 1209–16.

94. Fearon EKC, Nigro J, Kern S *et al.* Identification of a chromosome 18q gene that is altered in colorectal cancers. Science 1989; 247: 49–56.

95. Wang XW, Harris CC. p53 tumor-suppressor gene: clues to molecular carcinogenesis. J Cell Physiol 1997; 173: 247–55.

96. Harris CC. p53: at the crossroads of molecular carcinogenesis and molecular epidemiology. J Invest Dermatol Symp Proc 1996; 1: 115–18.

97. Yin J, Harpaz N, Tong Y *et al.* J. p53 point mutations in dysplastic and cancerous ulcerative colitis lesions. Gastroenterology 1993; 104: 1633–9.

98. Brentnall TA, Crispin DA, Rabinovitch PS *et al.* Mutations in the p53 gene: an early marker of neoplastic progression in ulcerative colitis. Gastroenterology 1994; 107: 369–78.

99. Harpaz N, Peck AL, Yin J *et al.* p53 protein expression in ulcerative colitis-associated colorectal dysplasia and carcinoma. Hum Pathol 1994; 25: 1069–74.

100. Groden J, Thliveris A, Samowitz W *et al.* Identification and characterization of the familial adenomatous polyposis coli gene. Cell 1991; 66: 589–600.

101. Joslyn G, Carlson M, Thliveris A *et al.* Identification of deletion mutations and three new genes at the familial polyposis locus. Cell 1991; 66: 601–13.

102. Kinzler KW, Nilbert MC, Su LK *et al.* Identification of FAP locus genes from chromosome 5q21. Science 1991; 253: 661–5.

103. Powell SM, Zilz N, Beazer-Barclay Y *et al.* APC mutations occur early during colorectal tumorigenesis. Nature 1992; 359: 235–7.

104. Sidransky D. Is human patched the gatekeeper of common skin cancers? Nat Genet 1996; 14: 7–8.

105. Nakamura Y, Nishisho I, Kinzler KW *et al.* Mutations of the adenomatous polyposis coli gene in familial polyposis coli patients and sporadic colorectal tumors. Princess Takamatsu Symp 1991; 22: 285–92.

106. Cho KR, Vogelstein B. Suppressor gene alterations in the colorectal adenoma–carcinoma sequence. J Cell Biochem Suppl 1992; 16G: 137–41.

107. Baba S. Recent advances in molecular genetics of colorectal cancer. World J Surg 1997; 21: 678–87.

108. Ilyas M, Tomlinson IP. Genetic pathways in colorectal cancer. Histopathology 1996; 28: 389–99.

109. Miyoshi Y, Nagase H, Ando H *et al.* Somatic mutations of the APC gene in colorectal tumors: mutation cluster region in the APC gene. Hum Mol Genet 1992; 1: 229–33.

110. Tarmin L, Yin J, Harpaz N *et al.* Adenomatous polyposis coli gene mutations in ulcerative colitis-associated dysplasias and cancers versus sporadic colon neoplasms. Cancer Res 1995; 55: 2035–8.

111. Laken SJ, Petersen GM, Gruber SB *et al.* Familial colorectal cancer in Ashkenazim due to a hypermutable tract in APC. Nat Genet 1997; 17: 79–83.

112. Frayling IM, Beck NE, Ilyas M *et al.* The APC variants I1307K and E1317Q are associated with colorectal tumors, but not always with a family history. Proc Natl Acad Sci USA 1998; 95: 10722–7.

113. Gryfe R, Di Nicola N, Gallinger S, Redston M. Somatic instability of the APC I1307K allele in colorectal neoplasia. Cancer Res 1998; 58: 4040–3.

114. Woodage T, King SM, Wacholder S *et al.* The APCI1307K allele and cancer risk in a community-based study of Ashkenazi Jews. Nat Genet. 20: 62–5, 1998.

115. Yin J, Harpaz N, Souza RF *et al.* Low prevalence of the APC I1307K sequence in Jewish and non-Jewish patients with inflammatory bowel disease. Oncogene 1999; 18: 3902–4.

116. Ionov Y, Peinado MA, Malkhosyan S, Shibata D, and Perucho M. Ubiquitous somatic mutations in simple repeated sequences reveal a new mechanism for colonic carcinogenesis. Nature 1993; 363: 558–61.

117. Aaltonen LA, Peltomaki P, Leach FS *et al.* Clues to the pathogenesis of familial colorectal cancer. Science 1993; 260: 812–16.

118. Thibodeau SN, Bren G, Schaid D. Microsatellite instability in cancer of the proximal colon. Science 1993; 260: 816–19.

119. Aaltonen LA, Peltomaki P. Genes involved in hereditary nonpolyposis colorectal carcinoma Anticancer Res 1994; 14: 1657–60.

120. Bronner CE, Baker SM, Morrison PT *et al.* Mutation in the DNA mismatch repair gene homologue hMLH1 is associated with hereditary non-polyposis colon cancer. Nature 1994; 368: 258–61.

121. Koi M, Umar A, Chauhan DP *et al.* Human chromosome 3 corrects mismatch repair deficiency and microsatellite instability and reduces *N*-methyl-*N'*-nitro-*N*-nitrosoguanidine tolerance in colon tumor cells with homozygous hMLH1 mutation [Published erratum appears in Cancer Res 1995; 55: 201]. Cancer Res 1994; 54: 4308–12.

122. Vasen HFA, Mecklin J-P, Kahn PM, Lynch HT. Hereditary non-polyposis colorectal cancer. Lancet 1991; 338: 887.

123. Benatti P, Sassatelli R, Roncucci L *et al.* Tumour spectrum in hereditary non-polyposis colorectal cancer (HNPCC) and in families with 'suspected HNPCC'. A population-based study in northern Italy. Colorectal Cancer Study Group. Int J Cancer 1993; 54: 371–7.

124. Peltomaki P, Lothe RA, Aaltonen LA *et al.* Microsatellite instability is associated with tumors that characterize the hereditary non-polyposis colorectal carcinoma syndrome. Cancer Res 1993; 53: 5853–5.

125. Meltzer SJ, Yin J, Manin B *et al.* Microsatellite instability occurs frequently and in both diploid and aneuploid cell populations of Barrett's-associated esophageal adenocarcinomas. Cancer Res 1994; 54: 3379–82.

126. Rhyu MG, Park WS, Meltzer SJ. Microsatellite instability occurs frequently in human gastric carcinoma. Oncogene 1994; 9: 29–32.

127. Berg PE, Liu J, Yin J, Rhyu MG, Frantz CN, Meltzer, SJ. Microsatellite instability is infrequent in neuroblastoma. Cancer Epidemiol Biomarkers Prev 1995; 4: 907–9.

128. Brentnall TA, Chen R, Lee JG *et al.* Microsatellite instability and K-ras mutations associated with pancreatic adenocarcinoma and pancreatitis. Cancer Res 1995; 55: 4264–7.

129. Eshleman JR, Markowitz SD. Microsatellite instability in inherited and sporadic neoplasms. Curr Opin Oncol 1995; 7: 83–9.

130. Boland CR, Thibodeau SN, Hamilton SR *et al.* A National Cancer Institute Workshop on Microsatellite Instability for cancer detection and familial predisposition: development of international criteria for the determination of microsatellite instability in colorectal cancer. Cancer Res 1998; 58: 5248–57.

131. Perucho M. Correspondence re: C.R. Boland *et al*, A National Cancer Institute workshop on microsatellite instability for cancer detection and familial predisposition: development of international criteria for the determination of microsatellite instability in colorectal cancer. Cancer Res. 1998; 58: 5248–57. Cancer Res 1999; 59: 249–56.

132. Eshleman JR, Markowitz SD. Mismatch repair defects in human carcinogenesis. Hum Mol Genet (5 Spec. No.) 1996; 5 : 1489–94.

133. Fishel R, Lescoe MK, Rao MR *et al.* The human mutator gene homolog MSH2 and its association with hereditary nonpolyposis colon cancer [Published erratum appears in Cell 1994; 77: 167]. Cell 1993; 75: 1027–38.

134. Nicolaides NC, Papadopoulos N, Liu B *et al.* Mutations of two PMS homologues in hereditary nonpolyposis colon cancer. Nature 1994; 371: 75–80.

135. Nystrom-Lahti M, Parsons R, Sistonen P *et al.* Mismatch repair genes on chromosomes 2p and 3p account for a major share of hereditary nonpolyposis colorectal cancer families evaluable by linkage. Am J Hum Genet 1994; 55: 659–65.

136. Papadopoulos N, Nicolaides NC, Wei YF *et al.* Mutation of a mutL homolog in hereditary colon cancer. Science 1994; 263: 1625–9.

137. Liu B, Parsons R, Papadopoulos N *et al.* Analysis of mismatch repair genes in hereditary non-polyposis colorectal cancer patients. Nat Med 1996; 2: 169–74.

138. Nystrom-Lahti M, Wu Y, Moisio AL *et al.* DNA mismatch repair gene mutations in 55 kindreds with verified or putative hereditary non-polyposis colorectal cancer. Hum Mol Genet 1996; 5: 763–9.

139. Akiyama Y, Sato H, Yamada T *et al.* Germ-line mutation of the hMSH6/GTBP gene in an atypical hereditary nonpolyposis colorectal cancer kindred. Cancer Res 1997; 57: 3920–3.

140. Papadopoulos N, Lindblom A. Molecular basis of HNPCC: mutations of MMR genes. Hum Mutat 1997; 10: 89–99.

141. Lipkin SM, Wang V, Jacoby R *et al.* MLH3: a DNA mismatch repair gene associated with mammalian microsatellite instability. Nat Genet 2000; 24: 27–35.

142. Borresen AL, Lothe RA, Meling GI *et al.* Somatic mutations in the hMSH2 gene in microsatellite unstable colorectal carcinomas. Hum Mol Genet 1995; 4: 2065–72.

143. Moslein G, Tester DJ, Lindor NM *et al.* Microsatellite instability and mutation analysis of hMSH2 and hMLH1 in patients with sporadic, familial and hereditary colorectal cancer. Hum Mol Genet 1996; 5: 1245–52.

144. Cunningham JM, Christensen ER, Tester DJ *et al.* Hypermethylation of the hMLH1 promoter in colon cancer with microsatellite instability. Cancer Res 1998; 58: 3455–60.

145. Esteller M, Levine R, Baylin SB, Ellenson LH, Herman JG. MLH1 promoter hypermethylation is associated with the microsatellite instability phenotype in sporadic endometrial carcinomas. Oncogene 1998; 17: 2413–7.

146. Herman JG, Umar A, Polyak K *et al.* Incidence and functional consequences of hMLH1 promoter hypermethylation in colorectal carcinoma. Proc Natl Acad Sci USA 1998; 95: 6870–5.

147. Esteller M, Catasus L, Matias-Guiu X *et al.* hMLH1 promoter hypermethylation is an early event in human endometrial tumorigenesis. Am J Pathol 1999; 155: 1767–72.

148. Fleisher AS, Esteller M, Wang S *et al.* Hypermethylation of the hMLH1 gene promoter in human gastric cancers with microsatellite instability. Cancer Res 1999; 59: 1090–5.

149. Eads CA, Danenberg KD, Kawakami K, Saltz LB, Danenberg PV, Laird PW. CpG island hypermethylation in human colorectal tumors is not associated with DNA methyltransferase overexpression. Cancer Res 1999; 59: 2302–6.

150. Fleisher AS, Esteller M, Tamura G *et al.* Hypermethylation of the hMLH1 gene promoter is associated with microsatellite instability in early human gastric neoplasia. Oncogene 2001; 20: 329–35.

37 | Dysplasia in inflammatory bowel disease: clinical pathology and current surveillance methods

CATHERINE J. STREUTKER, RODGER C. HAGGITT AND ROBERT H. RIDDELL

Introduction

Inflammatory bowel disease (IBD) predisposes to the development of colorectal carcinomas. In ulcerative colitis (UC) the highest risk occurs in those patients with extensive colitis for more than 10 years. This risk is accentuated if the disease began at an early age [1–3], and appears to be less if the inflammation is confined to the left side of the colon [4]. Crohn's colitis, while initially thought to have a low risk [4] is now recognized to have a risk comparable to that of UC [4–6].

The management of the cancer risk in those patients with IBD can be problematic. Patients with severe symptoms are more likely to have a colectomy as a result of these symptoms, while those with minimal or no symptoms are actually at the highest risk as their colons are spared. As it is difficult to apply relative risks to the individual patient, the patient's age and general health are considerations when considering the relative morbidity and mortality of possible options. Fortunately, the advent of ileal pouch–anal anastomosis techniques has made prophylactic colectomy more attractive, particularly to the young, as an alternative to continent or non-continent ileostomies.

Periodic surveillance by colonoscopy with adequate biopsies of the epithelium to assess for dysplasia has also become utilized to aid in controlling the risk of carcinoma. The rationale for this method of surveillance derives from the hypothesis that cancer in UC evolves through a premalignant phase of dysplasia which can be detected on biopsy [7], and which identifies the patient who requires a colectomy for cancer prevention even if the colon is clinically asymptomatic. The results of long-term studies suggest that surveillance by biopsy may have an effect on reducing cancer risk and mortality [8–11], though since most patients with UC will not develop cancer, the cost-effectiveness is moderate [12].

This chapter will examine the morphologic criteria for dysplasia in idiopathic IBD, the biologic characteristics and significance of dysplasia, and summarize current management and surveillance strategies.

Definition and grading of dysplasia

Definition and gross features

Dysplasia is defined as an unequivocal neoplastic alteration of the colonic epithelium that remains confined within the gland in which it arose [13]. The gross appearance of dysplastic epithelium depends upon the stage of its development. Early lesions may not be visible grossly. With progression the dysplastic mucosa may appear granular, pebbly, velvety or shaggy (particularly if villous structures are present). A spectrum of plaques, nodules and excrescences that resemble adenomas may develop. Still later, overt polypoid, ulcerating and/or stricturing malignancies may be seen.

Dysplasia grading

The epithelium in IBD may show a wide spectrum of changes, both inflammatory and dysplastic. It may appear normal or close to normal, or there may be significant reactive changes present (Fig. 1). The term 'indefinite for dysplasia' is utilized for those cases in which there is marked atypicality of the epithelial cells but the degree of abnormality is insufficient to give a diagnosis of dysplasia (Fig. 2). This diagnosis is frequently given in the setting of marked acute inflammation, though as inflammatory changes become better recognized this subcategory is becoming uncommon. Dysplasia, as elsewhere in the gastrointestinal tract, shows a spectrum from slight to marked changes which are

Stephan R. Targan, Fergus Shanahan and Loren C. Karp (eds.), Inflammatory Bowel Disease: From Bench to Bedside, 2nd Edition, 719–729.
© 2003 *Kluwer Academic Publishers. Printed in Great Britain*

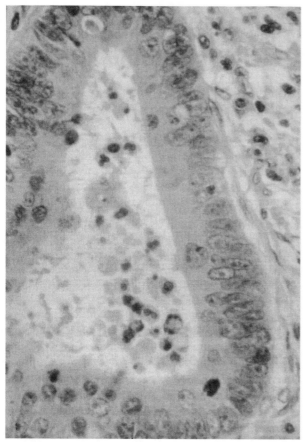

Figure 1. Reactive change in a patient with long-standing ulcerative colitis. There are neutrophils within the crypt lumen. The nuclei are enlarged, stratified and crowded and there is loss of goblet cell mucus (H&E, approximate original magnification × 250).

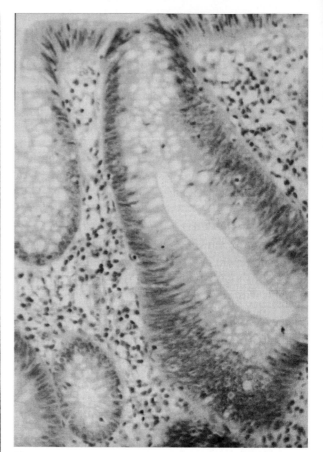

Figure 2. Mucosal biopsy histologically indefinite for dysplasia. The nuclei are enlarged, stratified and crowded, with more atypia than one would expect for reactive changes. However, there is maturation toward the surface of the crypt, which is more indicative of reactive than dysplastic change (H&E, approximate original magnification × 100).

separated into low-grade (LGD) and high-grade (HGD) dysplasia depending primarily on the degree of stratification of the nuclei.

Low-grade dysplasia

The crypt architecture tends to be preserved with only minimal, if any, distortion. Nuclear changes are similar to those seen in tubular adenomas: the nuclei are hyperchromatic and enlarged with nuclear crowding and overlapping. The nuclei lose their position at the base of the cell and start to stratify, though still restricted to the basal two-thirds of the cell. Mitotic figures may be present in the upper portion of the crypt (Fig. 3). Goblet cell mucin is usually moderately diminished but may be normal, increased or absent. Some of these cells may be 'dystrophic', in which the mucin droplet is present in the basal rather than the apical portion of the cell [14]. Paneth and endocrine cells may be present, occasionally in excessive numbers. These cells may also appear abnormal, with cytoplasmic granules in a perinuclear rather than the usual supranuclear and subnuclear locations, respectively [14]. Dysplastic changes generally involve the mucosal surface with extension down into the crypts; this may allow differentiation from reactive changes as these generally spare the mucosal surface. However, exceptions always exist, and specimens in which there is severe inflammation or poor orientation are difficult to interpret.

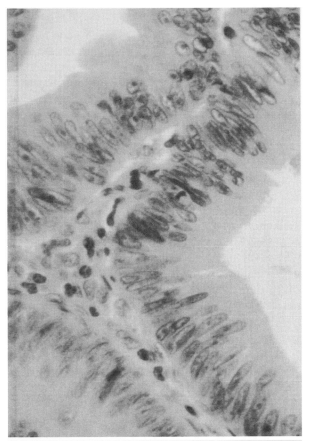

Figure 3. Mucosal biopsy containing low-grade dysplasia. Note the hyperchromatic, enlarged nuclei with stratification restricted to the lower portion of the cell (H&E, approximate original magnificationn × 100).

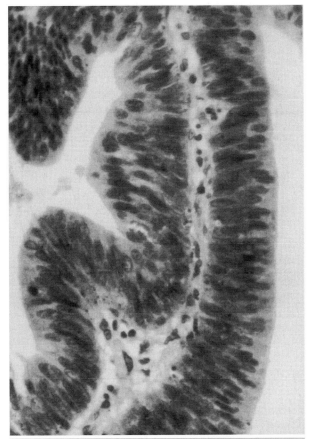

Figure 4. High-grade dysplasia. Note the markedly enlarged, hyperchromatic nuclei which show stratification up to the surface of the cell, as well as the absence of goblet cells (H&E, approximate original magnification × 100).

High-grade dysplasia

High-grade dysplasia encompasses all dysplastic epithelium with changes more marked than in LGD but the cells have not yet invaded into the lamina propria. This therefore includes cases previously called 'carcinoma-*in-situ*', since the treatment options are the same. In HGD, distortion of crypt architecture is usually present and may be marked: it comprises branching and lateral budding of crypts often yielding a complex architecture, intraglandular bridging of epithelium to form a cribriform pattern of 'back-to-back' glands, and frequently a villous surface contour. The villous surface contour may also be seen in non-dysplastic long-standing disease, and thus must be interpreted with consideration of other architectural and nuclear changes. In HGD the nuclear changes are also increased, with increased

variability in size, shape and chromaticity. Nuclear stratification reaches the top third of the cell, frequently to the crypt luminal surface. Nuclear polarity may be lost, so that the nucleus is no longer oriented perpendicular to the basement membrane (Fig. 4). Some variants characterized only by loss of nuclear polarity while remaining localized to the basal part of the cell can cause problems in interpretation. Goblet cell mucin may be diminished or absent, 'dystrophic' goblet cells may again be seen.

Indefinite for dysplasia

This category encompasses epithelial changes which are suspicious for dysplasia but features are also present that make an unequivocal determination impossible. Sometimes this occurs in the presence of marked acute inflammation where reactive changes mimic dysplasia. More frequently the nuclei are enlarged and hyperchromatic, but the changes are insufficient for a diagnosis of dysplasia. As this category can be subdivided into three subcategories (probably negative, probably positive and unknown) these are included in either of the latter, and are an indication for re-colonoscopy with multiple biopsies, often after therapy, to determine whether these changes persist or have resolved or are not detected. Some have advocated the elimination of the entire category due to concern over its application to clinical management [15]; we believe that it should be maintained due to the well-recognized difficulty in subjectively classifying certain cases.

Reliability of grading dysplasia

Inter-observer variability is recognized as a confounding factor in the diagnosis of dysplastic lesions. Among experienced gastrointestinal pathologists there is fairly good reproducibility and agreement when diagnosing 'negative for dysplasia' and HGD but there is less agreement in distinguishing LGD from indefinite lesions [7, 8, 13]. In recognition of the subjective nature of the histologic diagnosis of dysplasia, if the pathologist of record has any doubt about the diagnosis, or the clinician remains concerned about the accuracy of the diagnosis, confirmation of the diagnosis by a second, experienced pathologist should probably be obtained prior to colectomy [14, 15]. However, some would argue that even experienced gastrointestinal pathologists have difficulty in making the distinctions [16]. Observer variability in the diagnosis of dysplasia emphasizes the need for reliable, objective methods for its detection.

Differential diagnosis of dysplasia in IBD

Reactive and regenerative changes in actively inflamed epithelium can be difficult or impossible to distinguish from dysplasia; thus the development of the 'indefinite for dysplasia' category discussed above. Changes can include crowded, stratified, enlarged, hyperchromatic nuclei and abnormal mitotic figures, but the changes are usually most marked within the crypt and diminish toward the luminal surface. If the atypia involves the surface it is more suggestive of dysplasia. To recognize abnormal epithelium involving the surface, well-oriented biopsies are necessary. The nuclear–cytoplasmic (N/C) ratio is generally maintained in reactive cells while it is generally increased in dysplastic cells. Frequently the N/C ratio may even appear decreased in reactive cells, due to the presence of abundant eosinophilic cytoplasm. If active inflammation is present, and the patient is clinically symptomatic and not receiving optimum therapy, intensive medical therapy will sometimes suppress the inflammation. Post-treatment biopsies are frequently recommended, and may show a dramatic reduction in the intensity of inflammation and resolution of abnormalities that are reactive in nature, while dysplasia will be unaffected.

As a consequence of the ulcerating nature of IBD, epithelium may become displaced into the submucosa where it can be mistaken for invasive carcinoma [17]. If the misplaced epithelium is dysplastic it can be particularly difficult to differentiate from invasive carcinoma. Helpful criteria for recognizing misplaced epithelium include lamina propria surrounding the glands, absence of the typical desmoplastic stromal reaction of an invasive carcinoma, smooth contours of the glands rather than the sharply angulated appearance characteristic of most invasive carcinomas, and little or no cytologic atypism (unless the displaced epithelium is dysplastic).

Sporadic adenomas and dysplasia-associated lesion or mass (DALM)

Adenomas are, by definition, composed of dysplastic epithelium and thus are cytologically indistinguishable from dysplasia in UC/IBD. Dysplasia in UC can be difficult or impossible to differentiate from an adenoma, but typically it is distinctive because it originates and proliferates in the setting of pre-existing crypts and residual crypt architecture. In contrast, dysplastic epithelium in an adenoma forms glands or villi that proliferate to produce a mass. However, it should be noted that the dysplasia in IBD can also produce a mass. When a grossly visible dyplastic lesion is present within a background of dysplastic mucosa in UC, the lesion is termed a DALM (Fig. 5). The significance of these lesions is that there is a much higher frequency of associated carcinoma than in the 'flat' dysplasias [18]. Such lesions producing a mass, particularly on the first colonoscopy, are much more likely to be associated with an underlying invasive carcinoma than one detected on surveillance colonoscopy [19]. When dysplasia develops during follow-up of a patient with

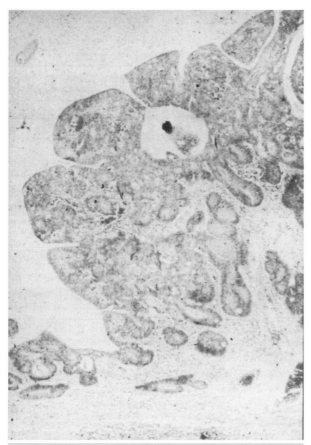

Figure 5. Dysplasia-associated lesions or mass (DALM). Note the dysplastic polypoid lesion with dysplastic changes also present in adjacent mucosa (H&E, approximate original magnification × 40).

previously negative biopsies, the dysplasia usually produces no endoscopically recognizable lesion.

In UC, if dysplasia arises as a mass or other endoscopically visible lesion, the relationship of the mass to the UC needs to be assessed. If the lesion is present in biopsy-proven normal mucosa proximal to the diseased portion of colon, the mass can be treated and followed up as any other adenomatous polyp [20–23]. If the mass has arisen in diseased colon the distinction of a DALM from an adenoma arising in a patient with UC can be difficult or impossible. Increasingly, if detected on surveillance endoscopy the algorithm used is based on whether the entire lesion can be removed endoscopically. If so, and if biopsies of the adjacent large bowel mucosa do not show dysplasia (thereby excluding this being the visible part of a more widespread area of dysplasia) and there are no other areas of dysplasia elsewhere in the affected large bowel, local excision of the

lesion appears to be a reasonable option which is not associated with an increased risk of associated or subsequent development of carcinoma [20]. In practice, 'true' dysplasias are invariably sessile or semisessile: a pedunculated lesion implies a sporadic adenoma arising within UC. An empirical approach to pedunculated adenomas is therefore to perform a colonoscopic polypectomy and to sample the mucosa in the stalk adjacent to the polyp and remote from it [9]. If there is no evidence of dysplasia outside the adenoma proper, nothing other than polypectomy is required.

Significance of dysplasia
Cancer risk in extensive ulcerative colitis

While there is a consensus that patients with UC have an increased risk of developing colorectal carcinoma, the precise magnitude of the risk has been controversial due to large variations between studies, as well as incorporated biases or methodologic errors such as referral bias, inclusion of patients who presented with cancer, and failure to adequately assess and control for disease extent and number of biopsies taken [12, 24–26]. That said, a meta-analysis performed by Eaden et al. [27] reports an overall prevalence of cancer in any patient with UC of 3.7%, which increases to 5.4% for those with pancolitis. Increased duration of disease has also been implicated as a risk factor for development of cancer: the meta-analysis demonstrated a cumulative probability of 2% at 10 years, 8% at 20 years and 18% at 30 years for any UC patient. The numbers for pancolitis were apparently similar, though the authors note this may be due to the small number of studies where this factor was reported as separate from all colitic patients. Geboes notes a relative risk of colorectal cancer of 14.8 for patients with pancolitis [28].

Cancer risk in left-sided ulcerative colitis

Cancer risk in left-sided (not extending proximal to the splenic flexure) UC is probably lower than in extensive disease, but higher than in the normal population [15]. Geboes lists a relative risk of 1.7 for patients with disease restricted to the rectum [28]. One study suggests that patients with left-sided disease will develop a risk of carcinoma approaching that of extensive disease if they are followed long enough [4].

Crohn's colitis

Patients with long-standing Crohn's disease (CD) of the colon are also at increased risk for developing dysplasia or carcinoma. This is now recognized to be comparable to the risk in UC [6, 29]. A study investigating the efficacy of surveillance colonoscopy in chronic CD detected dysplasia or cancer in 16% of patients who were followed since 1980 [29]. Dysplasia in CD is identical in appearance to that seen in UC.

Dysplasia/carcinoma sequence

There is a strong association between dysplasia and cancer, and the data support the hypothesis that dysplasia precedes carcinoma. However, many studies report patients who developed cancer in the absence of biopsies showing dysplasia. When colectomy has been performed because dysplasia alone was present in biopsies, 30–70% of patients have a clinically unsuspected carcinoma discovered in the resected colon [8, 9, 12, 19] (Table 1). Most such patients had the diagnosis of dysplasia made on their first colonoscopy, rather than during follow-up surveillance. The prevalence of carcinoma in colectomy specimens appears to be much lower when dysplasia is discovered on prospective follow-up biopsies, probably because the neoplastic process is being detected at an earlier stage in its development [9]. Both of these findings are consistent with the hypothesis that dysplasia is a precursor of carcinoma. However, some variants of carcinoma (signet-ring and endocrine carcinomas in particular) sometimes resemble their gastric counterparts by not having 'classical' dysplasia, but quite subtle variants not readily recognized or diagnosed in biopsies [30].

In non-IBD patients with adenomas, the progression from LGD to HGD to carcinoma is difficult to study, as it is uncommon to leave such lesions *in situ* for long-term follow-up. However, population studies evaluating the average ages at which these lesions are identified suggests that the time period is approximately 18 years [31]. In the study by Hoff *et al.*, polyps of less than 5 mm were followed for 2 years prior to resection: of the 35 adenomas evaluated, half grew from an average of 2.8 to 4.1 mm, 13 remained unchanged and five regressed from an average of 3.6 mm to 2.4 mm [32]. Similarly, in patients with IBD, the period of time for development of carcinoma from dysplasia is in the range of years. Rosenstock and colleagues followed six ulcerative colitis patients

Table 1. Post-surveillance colonoscopy diagnosis and probability of finding cancer*

Diagnosis	Probability of finding cancer	
	If colectomy done immediately	If colectomy done after some follow-up
DALM	43% (17/40)	Data not available
High-grade dysplasia	42% (10/24)	32% (15/47)
Low-grade dysplasia	19% (3/16)	8% (17/204)
Indefinite for dysplasia	Data not available	9% (9/95)
Negative for dysplasia	Data not available	2% (11/595)

*From Bernstein CN *et al.* Are we telling patients the truth about surveillance colonoscopy in ulcerative colitis? Lancet 1994; 343: 71–4

who had HGD but did not undergo colectomy an average of 4.7 years; none developed carcinoma during the follow-up interval [33].

There is a high prevalence of synchronous carcinoma in patients who had dysplasia on their initial biopsies [9]; this is probably related to more advanced progression along the pathway to neoplasia as compared to those who develop neoplasia while under surveillance. Gorfine *et al.* investigated patients who had colectomies for chronic UC: 13.1% had at lease one focus of dysplasia, and 6.4% had invasive carcinoma [34]. If dysplasia of any grade was present, there was a 36-fold increase in the likelihood of finding invasive carcinoma. Gorfine *et al.* conclude that dysplasia of any grade has a relatively high probability of coexisting with a carcinoma. The review by Bernstein *et al.* [19] indicates a 42% risk of finding a synchronous carcinoma when HGD is detected on biopsy, and 19% if LGD was detected on biopsy.

Interestingly, the investigation of molecular and genetic events in the development of carcinomas in IBD has indicated that, while the genetic changes that occur in the dysplasia-carcinoma sequence are basically similar in UC and non-UC patients, the changes occur at different times, in a different order. Many patients have widespread areas of aneuploidy throughout the colon well before histologically identifiable dysplasia is found [21], and this may predict the development of dysplasia. Investigation of non-neoplastic inflamed epithelium in colons removed from patients with UC showed an increased occurrence of microsatellite instability, particularly in those with severe inflammation [35]. Once dysplasia has developed, p53 mutations are found, though they seem to occur earlier in the sequence than in non-colitic dysplasias/carcinomas [36]. This is sometimes useful in that biopsies indefinite for dysplasia that have Ki-67 and p53 immunoreactivity that is diffuse and reaches the surface may well indicate patients who are at increased risk of developing dysplasia and carcinoma.

Surveillance strategy in IBD

General considerations

While surveillance programs remain a popular management strategy in UC, it must be remembered that some lethal cancers will develop despite a surveillance program. Furthermore, cost and compliance remain important factors, particularly among the young and poor. Thus, the benefits of surveillance programs remain controversial, particularly in light of estimates that about US$200 000 are spent in surveillance programs for every carcinoma found or prevented [12]. Estimating cost per year of life gained based on data from cohort studies has shown an incremental cost-effectiveness ration of $247 000 for yearly surveillance [37], comparable to that of cervical cancer screening every 3 years at $250 000.

Cancer surveillance may not be warranted in patients with the onset of colitis after the seventh decade of life because the increased risk of cancer will not then begin until the eighth decade, an age at which UC confers little or no additional risk above that in the general population.

Pancolitis

The available data do not permit a firm conclusion as to how frequently surveillance colonoscopy and biopsy should be performed. The surveillance interval is generally recommended to be 1–2 years [9–12, 18, 33, 38, 39]. Since the dysplasia–carcinoma sequence likely requires an extended period of time, every 2 years would seem appropriate after two consecutive annual colonoscopies at which no dysplasia was detected. The screening is generally recommended to begin 8 years after onset of pancolitis since occasionally patients will develop carcinoma before 10 years of disease [40].

Left-sided and Crohn's colitis

Again there were no firm data regarding the efficacy of surveillance programs in left-sided (distal to the splenic flexure) UC and Crohn's colitis. Since left-sided cancer may have a lesser risk of carcinoma, and it may develop later in its course, there may be a rational basis for a later initiation of surveillance. The American Cancer Society recommends colonoscopy with biopsy beginning 12–15 years after onset of disease [40]. In Crohn's colitis there are few data regarding screening and surveillance colonoscopy with biopsy. However Friedman *et al.* reported that, of 259 patients who underwent examinations at least every 24 months, 16% were found to have abnormal biopsies (10 indefinite, 23 LGD, four HGD and five cancers) [29]. The risk of dysplasia was increased with older age and increased symptoms. This suggests that patients with extensive and long-standing Crohn's colitis might also benefit from a screening program.

Colonoscopy and biopsy techniques

Colonoscopy performed as a surveillance procedure for dysplasia and carcinoma must be complete to the ileocecal valve, as even double-contrast barium enemas may fail to detect the flat lesions of dysplasia. If colonoscopy is not available, rigid or flexible sigmoidoscopy with biopsy is preferable to no follow-up at all, since about half of the carcinomas in UC will occur in the rectosigmoid. Multiple biopsies must be taken throughout the colon: it has been estimated that 33 biopsy specimens are needed to achieve a 90% confidence for detecting dysplasia [41]. A method that many have adopted is to take four-quadrant biopsies every 10 cm along the colon, and to place the biopsies from each segment into separately labeled bottles. This should translate into eight to ten bottles each containing four biopsies to be submitted to pathology. Utilizing 'jumbo' biopsy forceps increases the amount of tissue (to about 4 mm) and should not increase morbidity or mortality; it is thus highly recommended. Larger biopsies are easier to orient and increase the amount of mucosa sampled. Placing more than four biopsies in each bottle is not advisable – more than this will result in many of the biopsies being poorly oriented and uninterpretable [41].

Biopsy of obvious inflammatory polyps ('pseudopolyps') is to be avoided since they are less likely to contain dysplasia and are often difficult to interpret.

Any lesions greater than 1 cm, or those with abnormal color or configuration from the usual inflammatory polyp, should be extensively sampled or be removed completely [13]. If the lesion is suspected to be a DALM, additional biopsies of the mucosa around the stalk may be useful. Strictures in UC are suspicious of carcinoma and should be sampled extensively, since malignancy may be present in over one-third of cases [42]. Similarly, colonic strictures in Crohn's disease must be well sampled since a significant proportion (5–11%) may be malignant [43].

Management implications for dysplasia

General considerations

The Inflammatory Bowel Disease/Dysplasia Morphology Study group recommended colectomy for patients with HGD on biopsy, after confirmation of the diagnosis by an experienced gastrointestinal pathologist [13]. The group recommended short-interval follow-up for patients with biopsies that were indefinite for dysplasia and those with LGD. The algorithmic approach suggested by this group, as well as many approaches subsequently proposed by others, have limited clinical use since they can provide only a general outline, and individual factors such as the context of dysplasia (grossly apparent vs inapparent lesions, detected on initial vs follow-up examinations), patient factors (age, health status, psychological profile) as well as the availability of surgical options, particularly ileoanal pouch anastamosis, with good patient acceptance and relatively low morbidity and mortality. It is also becoming clear that even biopsies with LGD have a significant risk of synchronous carcinoma, and many are suggesting colectomy for these cases [19, 34].

Context of dysplasia

As discussed above, prospective studies imply that there is a fundamental difference in dysplasia detected on initial surveillance versus that detected during the course of a follow-up program [9]. Furthermore, it is likely that the dysplasia–carcinoma sequence requires years to evolve in most cases. Thus, when dysplasia is noted on the first examination, it cannot be determined where in the dysplasia–carcinoma sequence the lesion lies, and the patient is much more likely to have an invasive

carcinoma if colectomy is carried out. However, if prior biopsies were negative it is more likely that the process is being observed early in its natural history, and colectomy may be delayed if the patient is elderly or has other relative contraindications to surgery. Nevertheless, patients with LGD have demonstrated that they can produce neoplastic disease in their large bowel. As the purpose of the surveillance is to carry out colectomy in those patients at increased risk, in order to prevent the development of carcinoma, these patients clearly fall into that category. Further, if colectomy is not carried out, what is the next node in the management algorithm? Biopsies from even a short period of follow-up may result in HGD with its high risk of concomitant carcinoma and therefore risk of death from that disease. Because invasive carcinomas may only be found at colectomy, and may already be metastatic, a good case can be made for seriously considering procto-colectomy when LGD is initially detected. This is enhanced by the sampling problems of confirming that diagnosis on subsequent colonoscopy (the usual explanation for 'disappearing' dysplasia). Further, because the development of dysplasia may be modified by numerous factors, including the use of therapy, if dysplasia is becoming less frequent, then perhaps it should also be taken seriously when it occurs.

As stated previously, dysplasia that produces an endoscopically visible mass (DALM) has a significantly greater risk of being associated with a carcinoma than dysplasia that occurs in the absence of an endoscopically visible lesion. Again, this probably reflects the point in the dysplasia–carcinoma sequence at which one is observing the lesion; as dysplastic lesions age and grow, they tend to form masses. These masses then reflect temporally advanced dysplasia with a concurrent high risk of associated carcinoma, and if they cannot be excised locally, or are associated with dysplasia either adjacent or remotely, then colectomy should be very seriously considered.

Age and health factors

Age at onset of dysplasia is another factor that is important in determining potential therapy. Since the dysplasia–carcinoma sequence takes years to occur, if the dysplasia occurs later in life (seventh decade and beyond), one might consider continuing surveillance in patients with LGD, providing that it has developed during follow-up. Conversely, when

LGD develops in younger individuals (<40 years), one might wish to proceed with ileoanal-pouch anastomosis. The rationale for this recommendation is that functional results of ileoanal–pouch anastomosis are optimal in the young, the likelihood of living to one's life expectancy without intercurrent carcinoma is increased and the costs and inconvenience of a lifetime of surveillance may equal or exceed those of colectomy with ileoanal anastomosis. Another factor that should be considered is that some studies indicate that young age of onset of UC is an important risk factor for the subsequent development of carcinoma, particularly for children [27].

The severity of symptoms of the colitis, the overall health status of the patients, and their ability to tolerate the colectomy or care for and psychologically tolerate a possible ileostomy are other factors that must be considered. Significantly symptomatic patients may benefit from an early colectomy regardless of whether or not LGD was found, particularly if they are young, whereas surveillance may be most prudent in minimally asymptomatic, elderly patients.

Surgical options

Surgical options for chronic UC consist of colectomy with ileorectostomy, proctocolectomy with Brooke ileostomy, continent ileostomy of Kock, or ileal pouch–anal anastomosis [44–46]. The advantages of colectomy with ileorectostomy are that the surgery is technically simple, is associated with minimal morbidity and mortality when done electively, preserves bladder and sexual functions, and provides satisfactory anorectal function. However, because the diseased rectum is left in place, recurrent symptomatic disease and/or dysplasia/carcinoma may occur [45, 47]. As a surgical option for dysplasia/cancer, this procedure is perhaps best reserved for patients in whom the cancer is advanced and expected survival short, or for the elderly or debilitated for whom the lower morbidity of this procedure has advantages. Periodic surveillance with biopsies of the rectal stump is also an option.

Total proctocolectomy has the advantage of removing the entire diseased colon, thereby removing the risk of colorectal carcinoma. The necessity of wearing an external appliance with a Brooke ileostomy led to the development of 'continent' Kock ileostomies and subsequently the ileal pouch–anal anastomosis. In the latter two procedures an ileal reservoir is formed and attached to the abdominal skin (Kock procedure) or the dentate line after rectal mucosectomy (ileal pouch–anal anastomosis).

There is increasing enthusiasm for the ileal pouch–anal anastomosis, particularly for younger patients [48], with high patient satisfaction and quality of life among experienced surgeons [27, 49]. However, before the procedure is done it can be suggested that the patient's history and previous biopsies be reviewed with the intent of ensuring that the disease present is not CD. Performance of this surgery in a patient with CD will not only strongly increase the risk of disease recurrence at the anastomosis, but if there is significant disease then the pouch must be taken down with the subsequent loss of a significant length of small bowel. That said, some patients with CD do well with these pouches [50].

Unfortunately, the long-term risk of subsequent dysplasia and neoplasia in the pouch mucosa, while small, is present [51–53]. Pouchitis, a frequent (7–45%) long-term complication of ileal pouches, has a strong association with an original diagnosis of UC and is recognized by suggestive symptoms (bloody diarrhea, abdominal pain), mucosal inflammation on endoscopy and acute and chronic inflammation histologically. The histologic appearance of the pouch mucosa may closely resemble that of the colon and its mucin histochemical profile may also change to that of the colon (colonic metaplasia); these characteristics, combined with its strong association with UC, suggest that the pathogenesis of pouchitis, while still obscure, may be similar to that of UC [54–56. Increasing degrees of pouchitis and/or mucosal atrophy may pose greater risks for the development of dysplasia [52, 53].

Furthermore, there has been well documented occurrence of colonic metaplasia and carcinoma in ileostomy stomas in both UC [57–59] and CD [60] patients. Overall, however, the actual long-term risk of cancer in pouches and ileostomies is very small. Nonetheless, additional follow-up of this group of patients will be required. Although long-term surveillance of the ileal reservoir in post-proctocolectomy UC patients has been advocated [52], objective data regarding its need, efficacy and cost-effectiveness are not currently available.

38 | Hepatobiliary disorders

SUE CULLEN AND ROGER CHAPMAN

Hepatobiliary complications of inflammatory bowel diseases

The hepatobiliary system and the alimentary tract are closely linked embryologically, physiologically, biochemically and anatomically with all mesenteric venous drainage ascending via the portal vein into the liver. It is not surprising, therefore, that the liver is especially vulnerable to the development of complications of many different gastrointestinal diseases, particularly inflammatory bowel disease (IBD).

The first association between colonic ulceration and liver disease was made in 1874 by Thomas, who described a young man who died of a 'much enlarged, fatty liver in the presence of ulceration of the colon' [1]. The association was confirmed by Lister in 1899, who reported a patient with ulcerative colitis (UC) and secondary diffuse hepatitis [2]. Over the next 100 years it has become well established that there is a close relationship between IBD and various hepatobiliary disorders. These disorders are listed in Table 1.

In the past 20 years a different concept of hepatobiliary disorder in IBD has emerged. It is now apparent that the major hepatobiliary diseases seen in association with both UC and Crohn's disease (CD) – namely pericholangitis, primary sclerosing cholangitis (PSC), cirrhosis, cholangiocarcinoma, and most cases of autoimmune hepatitis – represent different aspects of the same spectrum of hepatobiliary disease.

Prevalence of liver disease

The prevalence of liver disease in patients with UC and CD has varied widely in different series. The discrepancy between the series may be largely due to differences in the number of patients included with severe, active, or extensive IBD, and also in the method used to investigate liver dysfunction.

Table 1. Hepatobiliary disorders associated with inflammatory bowel disease

	Associated with Ulcerative colitis	Associated with Crohn's disease
A *Primary sclerosing cholangitis (PSC)*		
Large duct PSC	+	+
Small duct PSC ('pericholangitis')	+	(+)
Cirrhosis	+	+
Hepatoma	+	+
Cholangiocarcinoma	+	(+)
B *Miscellaneous disorders*		
Fatty liver	+	+
Granulomas		+
Amyloidosis		+
Hepatic abscess		+
Gallstones		+
Autoimmune hepatitis	+	
Primary biliary cirrhosis	(+)	
Budd–Chiari sydrome	(+)	(+)

+, definite association; (+), possible association

Abnormal liver function tests are found in over half of patients with IBD requiring surgery, and are due to a number of factors such as malnutrition, sepsis, and blood transfusions with the subsequent risk of viral infection. However, significant liver disease is much less common. The true prevalence of hepatobiliary abnormality is difficult to determine, as it would involve obtaining liver histology and cholangiography on an unselected group of patients with IBD. Most series, therefore, have relied upon detecting persistent abnormalities on serum biochemical testing before proceeding to hepatic biopsy or endoscopic retrograde cholangiography. Technological advances such as magnetic resonance cholangiography and spectroscopy may allow more accurate assessments of the prevalence of liver abnormality to be made.

Stephan R. Targan, Fergus Shanahan and Loren C. Karp (eds.), Inflammatory Bowel Disease: From Bench to Bedside, 2nd Edition, 731–745.
© 2003 *Kluwer Academic Publishers. Printed in Great Britain*

In an early study from Oxford, 5–6% of 300 unselected adult patients with UC had significant histological abnormalities on hepatic histology compared with 10% of 100 unselected patients with CD; none of these patients underwent cholangiography [3, 4]. A group of 336 Norwegian patients with UC and persistently abnormal liver function tests were investigated using cholangiography [5]. The study found that more than 14% of patients had some form of hepatobiliary disease and 5% of all patients had PSC although most were asymptomatic (Table 2). Similar results were obtained in 1500 Swedish patients with UC [6]. In this thorough study, endoscopic cholangiography was obtained in 65 of 72 patients with elevated values of serum alkaline phosphatase. PSC was diagnosed in 3.7% of the UC group. The prevalence was 5.5% in patients with extensive colitis and only 0.5% in patients with distal disease [6]. This figure may be an underestimate, as a study from the Mayo Clinic has shown that standard liver function tests may be normal despite the presence of PSC on cholangiography [7].

PSC is also associated with CD but has only been reported in patients with extensive colonic involvement. A study from Norway has suggested that PSC is as common in patients with colonic CD as it is in UC [8]. Studies to date have suggested a prevalence of 1.3–13% of PSC among Crohn's patients [8–10].

The prevalence of hepatobiliary abnormalities with normal liver function tests in patients with UC has been investigated in a study from Sweden [11]. Liver biopsies were assessed from 74 patients with UC and normal liver function tests. Fifty percent had a completely normal liver biopsy. The biopsies of three patients with total colitis displayed concentric periductular fibrosis and the rest showed minimal portal inflammation or fatty filtration. The patients were then followed for a mean of 18 years. None of the three patients with concentric fibrosis developed abnormal liver function tests, although cholangiography was not performed. Two other patients developed liver disease; cirrhosis in one and autoimmune chronic hepatitis and cholangiocarcinoma in the other.

In summary, approximately 5% of adult patients with IBD will have significant hepatobiliary disease. Although the number of patients with hepatobiliary abnormality is approximately the same for UC and CD, severe significant liver disease is more commonly seen in patients with UC and when it occurs in CD it is usually associated with extensive colonic involvement.

Table 2. Prevalence of primary sclerosing cholangitis in patients with ulcerative colitis

Country of origin (ref.)	No. of patients with UC	Percentage with PSC
Oxford, UK [3]	681	2.9
Oslo, Norway [5]	336	5
Stockholm, Sweden [6]	1500	3.7 (5.5 in total colitis)

Primary sclerosing cholangitis

PSC is a chronic cholestatic liver disease characterized by an obliterative inflammatory stricturing fibrosis which usually involves the whole biliary tree [9, 12] (Fig. 1). The changes may sometimes be localized to either the extrahepatic or intrahepatic bile ducts, and the degree of involvement varies considerably from patient to patient.

Relationship of primary sclerosing cholangitis with IBD

Association with ulcerative colitis

Approximately 70% of northern European patients with PSC have coexisting UC, and PSC is the most common form of chronic liver disease found in UC [9, 12] (Table 3). Studies from southern Europe, however, have found only 36–44% of patients with PSC have underlying UC, although not all patients in these studies underwent total colonoscopy and colonic biopsies [13, 14]. Data from Japan suggest that the relationship is even weaker, with only 20% of PSC patients having a diagnosis of UC [15]. Some authorities believe that all patients with PSC will develop IBD at some point. Many studies from different parts of the world have reviewed the clinical features of patients with UC and PSC. The findings from all studies have been remarkably consistent. Paradoxically, the colitis is usually total but symptomatically mild, often with no rectal bleeding, and is often characterized by prolonged remissions [16]. Interestingly, patients with UC and PSC have a male predominance, with a male:female ratio of 2:1 which is in contrast to the slightly female predominance of UC in isolation [17].

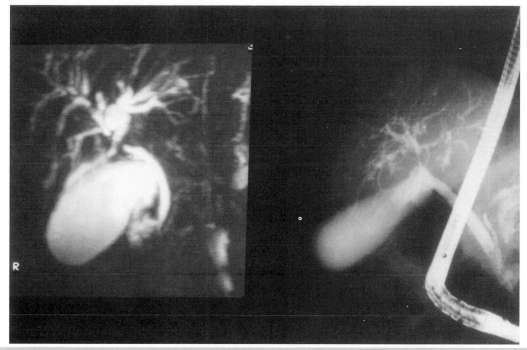

Figure 1. Cholangiogram from patient with ulcerative colitis and abnormal cholestatic liver function tests showing stricturing and dilation of extrahepatic and intrahepatic bile ducts.

Smoking

Cigarette smoking has been recognized as a protective factor against the development of UC. Two studies have suggested that cigarette smoking may also additionally protect against the development of PSC. Moreover, this protective effect was more marked in patients with PSC than UC and was seen in patients with and without IBD [18, 19, 20]. The mechanism of protection in both disorders remains unknown.

Onset

Although the symptoms of UC usually develop before those of sclerosing cholangitis, in some patients the onset of PSC may precede the symptoms of colitis by up to 4 years. Although large-scale studies have not been performed, there is some evidence that the prevalence of liver abnormality may be higher in children than adults with colitis. Abnormal liver function tests were detected in 60% of 34 children with UC; abnormalities were most commonly seen in total colitis. Cholangiography was performed in only two patients, one of whom had sclerosing cholangitis [21].

Table 3. Prevalence of inflammatory bowel disease in patients with primary sclerosing cholangitis (PSC)

Institution (country of origin) disease; ref.	No. of patients with PSC	Percentage with IBD
Royal Free Hospital (UK) [10]	29	72
Mayo Clinic (USA) [9]	50	70
Huddinge (Sweden)	305	72
King's College London (UK, children)	13	77
Okolicsanyi (Italy) [14]	82	54
Escorsell (Spain [13]	43	47

Outcome

The outcome of the hepatobiliary disease is completely unrelated to the activity, severity, or clinical course of the colitis. This is borne out by the fact that colectomy makes no difference to the clinical progression or to the mortality of patients with PSC. Indeed, liver disease may develop some years after a total colectomy has been performed [22]. Patients with combined UC and PSC may have a worse prognosis from liver disease than patients with PSC alone [17]. Involvement of the extrahepatic bile ducts alone is more frequently seen in patients who do not have IBD [17].

Biliary and colorectal cancer in ulcerative colitis and PSC

The association between UC and colorectal carcinoma has been recognized since the 1920s [23]. In 1995 Broomé *et al.* suggested that there was an increased risk of colorectal neoplasia in patients with concomitant PSC [24] (see Fig. 2). This hypothesis has been extensively tested since that date, with conflicting datasets published in recent years. Most experts currently agree that PSC is an independent risk factor for developing colorectal carcinoma. The possible mechanisms for the increased susceptibility to neoplasia are not clear, but genetic predisposition, alterations in the bile salt pool due to cholestasis, and folate deficiency are all possibilities [25]. Yearly colonoscopy is recommended in patients with UC and PSC.

Three recent studies have all shown that PSC patients consistently develop a more proximal colorectal carcinoma than patients with UC alone [26–28]. This observation may be explained by the higher exposure of the right side of the colon to the carcinogenic properties of the secondary bile acids produced in cholestasis, although this hypothesis remains unproven. The increased risk of carcinoma of the bile ducts, including gallbladder carcinoma, in patients with UC is also well established and now appears to occur almost exclusively in the context of pre-existing PSC. Furthermore, one study has suggested that cholangiocarcinoma develops significantly more often in patients with colonic dysplasia or carcinoma, thus suggesting that these patients may constitute a high-risk subgroup requiring increased colonic and biliary surveillance [29]. However, further prospective studies are needed to confirm these findings.

Orthotopic liver transplantation is the only effective treatment for PSC. The presence of IBD does not affect the outcome, but is associated with a higher rate of severe acute graft rejection [30, 31]. Surprisingly, there is some evidence that the clinical course of IBD worsens post-transplant despite the immuno-

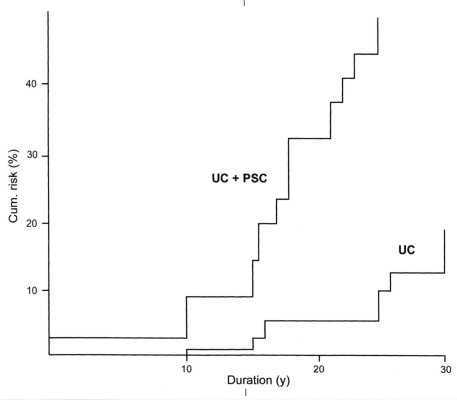

Figure 2. The cumulative risk of developing colonic or biliary dysplasia in 40 patients with primary sclerosing cholangitis (PSC) and ulcerative colitis (UC) compared with 80 matched controls with UC alone. (Reproduced with permission from ref. 23)

suppression given to protect the graft from rejection. A series published by the Royal Free Hospital found an increase in the clinical activity of the associated colitis in eight of 16 patients transplanted for PSC [31]. Similar data have been published from Birmingham, with nine of 26 (35%) of patients noticing a worsening of their symptoms of IBD [30]. In contrast, Gavaler *et al.* and Shaked *et al.* found no worsening of IBD symptoms post-transplant in 23 and 24 patients respectively [32, 33]. These conflicting data may in part be explained by the differences in immunosuppressive regimens used post-transplantation. The Royal Free and Birmingham centers usually withdraw steroids early, and maintain immunosuppression with cyclosporine or tacrolimus with or without azathioprine. The Gavaler and Shaked reports are from units where steroids are used as maintenance immunosuppression.

The risk of colon cancer in PSC increases after transplantation, occurring most commonly in the early post-transplant period, and is probably associated with high-level immunosuppression accelerating the growth of malignant cells. Colonoscopy with extensive mucosal biopsies is therefore recommended prior to transplantation, and annually thereafter in this particularly high-risk group [34, 35].

Pouchitis

Patients with UC treated by colectomy with an ileal reservoir (pouch) are sometimes affected by a non-specific inflammation of the pouch (pouchitis). This complication is much more common in patients with PSC and UC (64% of patients affected) than in those with UC alone (32% of patients affected) [36], and is the major complication of this operation. Prior to the development of pouch operations the Brooke ileostomy was the most commonly performed operation for UC. In patients with coexistent PSC, however, peristomal varices occur in approximately 25% of cases, and bleeding from these varices can be difficult to manage [37]. Although the intraoperative and postoperative complication rate and mortality is comparable in the two operations, pouchitis tends to present a less difficult management problem than recurrent peristomal variceal bleeds; therefore ileal pouch–anal anastomosis is usually the operation of choice in these patients.

Association with Crohn's disease

PSC is associated with CD although the prevalence is lower than for UC and the prevalence of bile-duct carcinoma is less in CD. The explanation for these apparent differences in prevalence between the two IBD is unclear, but may be related to the less frequent occurrence of total colonic involvement in patients with CD.

Epidemiology

The prevalence of PSC is unknown. As previously stated, there is a 2.4–7.5% prevalence of PSC in patients with UC. The prevalence of PSC in the United States has been estimated to be two to seven cases per 100 000 population, based on a prevalence of UC of 40–225 cases per 100 000. This estimate has been confirmed by the results from Olsson *et al.* [6], who noted the prevalence of UC and PSC to be 171 and 6.3 cases per 100 000 population respectively. The most recent data from Norway found a prevalence of 8.5 cases of PSC per 100 000 population [38]. These results, however, probably underestimate the actual prevalence of PSC, as the disease can occur in patients with normal serum levels of alkaline phosphatase, and 20–30% of patients with PSC have no associated IBD. PSC is more common than previously suspected, and may have a frequency similar to primary biliary cirrhosis.

Aetiology

The cause of PSC is unknown, but any proposed etiologic mechanism must incorporate the close association with UC. A number of hypotheses have been proposed to explain the association between colonic disease and biliary tract inflammation and fibrosis (Table 4). Recent studies have suggested that genetic and immunologic factors are important in

Table 4. Possible causes of primary sclerosing cholangitis

Portal bacteremia
Abnormal bile acids
Absorbed colonic toxins
Viral infections
Copper toxicity
Immunologic mechanisms
Genetic predisposition
Ischemic arteriolar injury

the pathogenesis of PSC. Three sets of siblings from three families have been described with PSC and UC [39–41]. Furthermore the frequency of HLA-B8, DR3 and DR52A is much higher in PSC patients than in controls [40–42]. More recently HLA-DR52A, which is closely associated with the HLA-B8 DR3 haplotype by linkage disequilibrium, has been shown to be the most closely associated HLA allele in PSC, as the HLA-B8 and DR3 haplotype is associated with a number of autoimmune diseases such as autoimmune chronic active hepatitis, myasthenia gravis and thyrotoxicosis [43]. Although the prevalence of HLA-B8 and DR3 is not increased in patients with UC, a patient with UC who is unfortunate enough to possess the HLA-B8 and DR3 haplotype, has a 10-fold increase in the relative risk of developing PSC.

There is some debate about which are the most important HLA associations. Studies from Scandanavia have suggested that DRB1*0301 and DRB1*1301 are the primary susceptibility alleles. More recent work has identified very strong associations with the tumor necrosis factor-α (TNF-α) promotor (TNF*2) allele and MICA*008 allele [44–47].

Non-MHC genes are also likely to contribute to the susceptibility to and progression of PSC. Unpublished data from Sweden have suggested an association with polymorphisms in genes encoding cytotoxic lymphocyte antigen-4 (CTLA-4 chromosone 2q32) and preliminary studies from Oxford have implicated a polymorphism in the matrix metalloproteinase 3 [48]. Both these findings, however, await confirmation.

The possible importance of immunologic factors has been emphasized by the number of recent reports which have shown humoral and cellular abnormalities in PSC.

Perinuclear antineutrophil cytoplasmic antibodies (ANCA) have been detected in the sera of 26–85% of patients with PSC with or without UC and up to 68% with UC only [49–51]. Current data suggest that the ANCA reactive antigens are similar, and may be indicative of a common immunopathologic mechanism. As for UC no correlation exists between disease activity and ANCA in PSC. Unfortunately the antigen(s) which is specific to mature neutrophils has not been isolated, although one group have recently suggested that a nuclear envelope protein may be the target antigen [52]. It remains unclear whether ANCA have pathogenic diagnostic or prognostic significance, or merely represent an epiphenomenon.

Current evidence would suggest that PSC is an immunologically mediated disease which requires exposure to bacterial products in the portal venous blood to trigger its expression. Vierling *et al.* hypothesized that bacteria might gain access to the portal venous blood in the setting of acute or chronic colitis. Hepatic macrophages would then secrete interleukins and TNF-α into the peribiliary space of the portal tracts stimulating secretion of chemokines and cytokines from the biliary epithelial cells, promoting regurgitation of bile into the peribiliary space and interfering with cholehepatic circulation. Neutrophils, monocytes, macrophages, T cells and fibroblasts would be attracted to the area and, together with platelet-derived growth factor (PDGF), could promote enzymatic digestion of extracellular matrix, and collagen synthesis resulting in peribiliary fibrosis and progressive inflammation and biliary obstruction [53]. This hypothesis does not, however, explain the pancreatic duct abnormality observed in 10–50% of PSC patients.

Clinical features

PSC is mainly a disease of young males, with a male:female ratio of 2:1. The majority of patients present between the ages of 25 and 40 years, although the disease has been diagnosed at any age between 1 and 90 years! The clinical presentation of PSC is variable but commonly includes fatigue, intermittent jaundice, weight loss, right upper quadrant abdominal pain and pruritus [9, 13]. Despite the name of the disease, only a minority of patients suffer attacks of acute cholangitis, and these usually follow reconstructive biliary surgery or some form of endoscopic interventional therapy.

Some patients with PSC may present with an established cirrhosis and portal hypertension without any previous symptoms of cholangitis or cholestasis. These patients may be diagnosed and treated as cryptogenic cirrhosis for many years before the diagnosis is established. Physical examination is abnormal in about half the symptomatic patients at presentation. Common abnormalities include hepatosplenomegaly and jaundice, although jaundice often appears only late in the course of the disease. The stigmata of liver disease – including spider naevi, palmar erythema and clubbing – are not usually found. An increasing number of asymptomatic patients with PSC are being diagnosed in whom physical examination is normal. The diagnosis is usually made incidentally when a persistently raised serum alkaline phosphatase is discovered in a patient with UC [6].

Laboratory investigations

Serum biochemical tests usually indicate cholestasis. However, the levels of alkaline phosphatase and bilirubin may vary widely in an individual patient during the course of the disease; increasing, for example, during periods of acute cholangitis and falling after appropriate therapy. Sometimes the levels may fluctuate for no apparent reason. Modest elevations in serum transaminases are usually found, while hypoalbuminemia and clotting abnormalities are found only at a late stage [9, 12].

The diagnostic role of antineutrophil cytoplasmic antibodies (ANCA) in PSC has been discussed earlier. Low titers of serum antinuclear and smooth-muscle antibodies have been found in patients with PSC but they have no diagnostic significance; serum mitochondrial antibody is invariably absent [9]. Increased serum IgM concentrations are seen in about half of symptomatic patients, and the levels of IgM are similar to those observed in patients with primary biliary cirrhosis. Elevation of IgG is found in about one-third of adult patients tested and 60–80% of children with PSC.

Radiographic features

Endoscopic cholangiography is the best method of demonstrating the biliary system in patients with sclerosing cholangitis. Although in skilled hands the bile ducts can be visualized by percutaneous trans-hepatic cholangiography, this technique is difficult in sclerosing cholangitis and has a higher morbidity rate. The cholangiographic appearances are diagnostic and consist of multiple stricturing and dilation (beading) of the intrahepatic and extrahepatic bile ducts [9, 12] (Fig. 1).

Occasionally involvement may be limited to the intrahepatic ducts alone, or more rarely in patients with concurrent UC only the extrahepatic bile ducts may be abnormal. Small diverticuli along the common bile duct are diagnostic, and found in about 25% of patients [54]. Magnetic resonance cholangio-pancreatography (MRCP) provides a non-invasive method of imaging the biliary tree and characteristic appearances of PSC on MRCP are being defined. Recent studies have reported 85–88% sensitivities and 92–97% specificities for the detection of PSC using MRCP [55]. The technique is still being assessed, but will probably become the diagnostic method of choice for PSC in the future.

Pathological features

Extrahepatic bile ducts appear macroscopically as thickened cords, although the overall diameter is not usually increased. In cross-section the lumen is narrow and the wall may be up to eight times the usual thickness. The inflammation and dense concentric fibrosis usually affect the submucosa and outer layers of the bile ducts, leaving the mucosa largely unaffected.

The histologic appearances of the liver biopsy are not usually diagnostic, although some form of biliary disease can usually be identified, indicating the need for cholangiography. The classical histologic feature of PSC, *viz.* 'onion-skin' concentric fibrosis, is seen in about one-third of patients (Figure 3).

Natural history

In the majority of patients PSC is a progressive disease. The median time of survival from the time of diagnosis of PSC is approximately 12 years [9, 13] in symptomatic patients. However, 75% of patients with asymptomatic disease are alive after 15 years of follow-up. The majority of patients die in hepatic failure following deepening cholestatic jaundice. However, approximately 10–20% of patients with long-standing PSC develop bile duct carcinoma, which often follows a very aggressive course [12, 56]. Up to 21% of patients will have an incidental biliary carcinoma found at the time of transplantation [34]. Mean survival after the diagnosis of cholangiocarcinoma is 9 months. Prognostic models have been developed to try to predict the clinical course of the hepatobiliary disease and the development of cholangiocarcinoma [57–60]. However, no model has been shown to be of any use in the individual patient, although most studies have shown that an elevated serum bilirubin level at presentation is associated with a poor prognosis. Further models are being developed to facilitate the timing of liver transplantation, and to evaluate the usefulness of monitoring the effect of experimental therapy on disease progression.

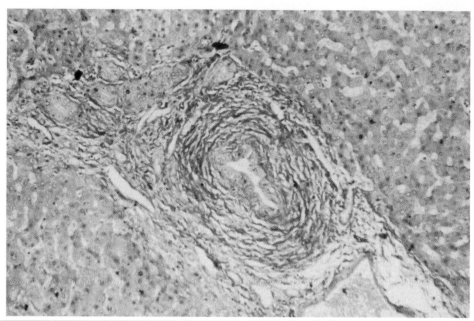

Figure 3. Bile duct surrounded by layers of concentric 'onion-skin' fibrosis.

Treatment

There is no curative treatment for PSC, but a plethora of medical, endoscopic and surgical approaches have been advocated. The treatment of PSC can be divided into the management of cholestasis, the management of the complications, and lastly, specific treatments of the disease process.

Management of cholestasis

Symptomatic patients are frequently troubled by pruritus. This is best managed initially by cholestyramine, and the dose should be increased until relief of pruritus is obtained. Both rifampicin and naltrexone are also sometimes effective. In addition, fat-soluble vitamin replacement is necessary for the jaundiced patient and this should be replaced by monthly intramuscular injections. Metabolic bone disease (usually osteoporosis) is a frequent complication of advanced PSC. No proven effective treatment is available for the prevention or management of osteopenia, although bisphosphates with calcium and vitamin D supplements should be considered in patients with osteoporosis, and in patients with advanced cholestasis.

Management of complications

Broad-spectrum antibiotics such as ciprofloxacin should be given for acute attacks of cholangitis but they have no proven prophylactic value and should not be used routinely on a long-term basis except in patients with recurrent cholangitis. If cholangiography shows well-defined obstruction to the main extrahepatic bile ducts, mechanical relief must be considered. In many patients the best therapeutic approach is by introducing a prosthesis (stent) through the obstruction. This may be placed non-operatively by the percutaneous transhepatic route or at endoscopic retrograde cholangiopancreatography (ERCP). Balloon dilation of the strictures prior to stenting may be useful in those few patients with well-defined localized strictures, and can lead to a striking improvement in symptoms and serum biochemistry [61]. The development of small biliary stones and sludge can lead to sudden clinical or biochemical deterioration. In these patients endoscopic sphincterotomy with extraction of the biliary debris is beneficial. Some authors have advocated nasobiliary drainage, but no long-term controlled results have been reported.

Patients with PSC and chronic UC treated by total colectomy and ileostomy may develop peristomal varices which can bleed profusely [22]. No effective measures are available once they have developed, although local measures such as injection of sclerosants have been tried.

Specific treatment

Medical treatment

Medical treatment of PSC has included uncontrolled trials of corticosteroids, immunosuppressive drugs, cholecystogogues and antibiotics, either alone or in combination. The results have been universally disappointing, although assessment of treatment in this uncommon disease is difficult because the clinical course fluctuates, survival is variable and some patients may remain asymptomatic for long periods of time.

The role of corticosteroid therapy in PSC is unclear. There have been no controlled trials of steroid therapy, but many patients with sclerosing cholangitis, particularly those who also have UC, will have received corticosteroids. Corticosteroids have been used both topically and systemically in small and generally uncontrolled trials in sclerosing cholangitis. A controlled trial of nasobiliary lavage with corticosteroids or placebo did not produce any significant benefit [62].

Good results with oral prednisolone have been reported in pilot studies. However, no benefit was seen in patients treated with prednisolone and colchicine for 2 years at the Mayo Clinic [63]. Controlled trials with bone-sparing agents such as bisphosphonates would be needed before this treatment could be widely recommended, in view of the dangers of bone disease being accentuated by steroid therapy.

A number of immunosuppressive agents have been tried, either alone or in combination, including penicillamine, methotrexate and cyclosporine. No benefit has been demonstrated.

Treatment with ursodeoxycholic acid is being assessed in clinical trials. A study from the Mayo Clinic has shown that ursodeoxycholic acid in standard doses (10–15 mg/kg per day) produces an improvement in biochemistry but has no effect on symptoms, histology or survival [64]. However, a recent pilot study has demonstrated that higher daily doses of ursodeoxycholic acid (20–25 mg/kg) may be efficacious [65].

Orthotopic liver transplantation

This is the only option available in young patients with PSC and advanced liver disease. Decisions regarding the optimum timing for transplantation are, however, made difficult by the variable clinical course of PSC and the potential risk of cholangiocarcinoma. Indications for transplantation are summarized in Table 5 [34].

Table 5. Indications for liver transplantation in PSC [27]

Accepted indications for transplantation
Cirrhosis complicated by:
Intractable ascites
Recurrent cholangitis
Variceal hemorrhage not controlled by banding or sclerotherapy
Muscle wasting
Recurrent bacterial peritonitis
Encephalopathy

Consideration for transplantation
Non-cirrhotic patients with intractable itching or fatigue
Biliary dysplasia (debatable)

Survival rates for patients transplanted for PSC without evidence of cholangiocarcinoma are excellent, with most series publishing 5-year survival rates of 85–90%. Recent data from the Mayo Clinic have demonstrated that post-transplant survival rates are clearly related to the pre-transplant Child-Pugh stage [66]. Survival rates in Child-Pugh A over 1, 2 and 5 years were: 98.1%, 97.0% and 91.0%: Child-Pugh B: 89.1%, 81.0%, and 55% and in Child-Pugh C: 73.0%, 53.0% and 16.0%, respectively. For this reason patients with PSC should be referred for transplantation earlier than other patients with chronic liver disease. Where cholangiocarcinoma is found incidentally in the explanted liver with no spread to regional lymph nodes the prognosis is comparable to patients with no evidence of cholangiocarcinoma [67]. Clinically apparent cholangiocarcinoma is, however, a contraindication to transplantation as the tumor rapidly recurs post-transplantation with immunosuppression [67].

PSC recurs in the liver graft in around 20% of cases [68]. Post-transplantation PSC appears have a survival rate similar to patients without evidence of recurrence. Several patients have required re-transplantation for advanced recurrent disease [69].

Small-duct primary sclerosing cholangitis 'pericholangitis'

Pericholangitis is a histological diagnostic term that has been used to describe inflammatory reactions in the portal zones of the liver which are characterized by periductular inflammation and fibrosis. For many years the term 'pericholangitis' was synonymous with involvement of the liver in IBD [70, 71]. Some patients with pericholangitis have been shown to progress to cirrhosis of the liver and cholangio-carcinoma [72]. However, it has become clear that the majority of patients with histologic pericholangitis and persistently abnormal liver function tests will have cholangiographic appearances diagnostic of PSC at ERCP [73, 74]. A minority of patients with UC will have persistently abnormal liver function tests, together with histologic appearances such as concentric fibrosis, but have normal bile ducts at cholangiography. The term 'small-duct primary sclerosing cholangitis' has been proposed to replace the term 'pericholangitis' in this group of patients as the evidence suggests that these conditions are all part of the same disease spectrum [75]. Wee and Ludwig have described two patients who progressed from small-duct PSC to develop extrahepatic biliary involvement diagnostic of sclerosing cholangitis [75]. It is clear that patients with small-duct PSC have a more favorable outlook than those with 'classical' disease in terms of risk for developing liver cirrhosis and cholangiocarcinoma [76, 77].

A number of other portal tract lesions such as chronic periportal inflammation and/or increased cellularity of portal tracts have also been described as 'pericholangitis' in patients with UC [70, 71].

In view of the confusing use of the term pericholangitis, which has been applied to a heterogeneous mixture of hepatobiliary disorders by different authors, it has been proposed that the term and concept of pericholangitis should be abandoned [78].

Autoimmune hepatitis

Autoimmune hepatitis has been reported to occur in association with UC [79]. However, interface hepatitis (piecemeal necrosis) on liver histology can accompany the classic bile-duct changes of PSC on cholangiography [12] and it seems likely that the majority of patients with autoimmune hepatitis and IBD will have either large- or small-duct PSC. The diagnosis of autoimmune hepatitis should not be made in patients with IBD unless cholangiography is normal. The diagnostic difficulties are compounded by the presence of circulating serum autoantibodies such as antinuclear antibodies, smooth muscle antibodies, antineutrophil cytoplasmic antibodies, and elevated serum immunoglobulins in some patients with PSC [80]. Moreover, both autoimmune hepatitis and PSC are associated with an increased prevalence of the tissue antigens HLA-B8 and HLA-DR3 [32] and

overlap syndromes exist [81]. It is unclear from current evidence whether the prevalence of autoimmune hepatitis without underlying sclerosing cholangitis is increased in patients with IBD.

Cirrhosis

The incidence of cirrhosis associated with IBD has varied in different series between 1% and 5% [82–85]. Most patients in these reports are classified as having biliary cirrhosis and, since patients with PSC can present with portal hypertension and established cirrhosis with no preceding symptoms, it seems likely that the majority of these patients will have underlying end-stage PSC. However, not all patients with cirrhosis and IBD will have PSC, and it is possible that some cases may be due to chronic hepatitis C infection [86] associated with previous blood transfusions. Patients with cirrhosis may present with the typical symptoms of liver failure including jaundice, ascites, and variceal hemorrhage. Although the variceal bleeding usually occurs from veins in the esophagus, patients with concomitant IBD who have undergone total proctocolectomy may bleed from peristomal varices some 6–13 years after formation of the ileostomy stoma [22].

Cholangiocarcinoma

Cholangiocarcinoma in UC usually occurs in the context of pre-existing PSC and is therefore associated with long-standing total colitis. A large study from the Cleveland Clinic has reported a prevalence rate of 0.5% [87]. Bile duct carcinoma has been reported in association with CD but it occurs much more rarely [88, 89].

The clinical presentation of bile duct cancer is usually that of a progressive cholestatic jaundice. Diagnosis of cholangiocarcinoma in the context of PSC can be extremely difficult. Cholangiography usually reveals a particularly narrow bile duct stricture. Brush cytology obtained endoscopically may be useful in confirming malignancy but suffers from low sensitivity. Computerized tomography (CT) scanning showing intrahepatic bile duct dilation is suggestive but not diagnostic of malignant change. Positron emission tomography (PET) scanning has been used with some success in the early diagnosis of small cholangiocarcinomas, and may become a useful tool in differentiating benign and malignant strictures [90].

The tumor usually pursues a progressive course and the prognosis is very poor, with a median survival of 9 months [91]. Liver transplantation for isolated cholangiocarcinoma occurring in PSC as previously discussed, has been disappointing, with rapid recurrence of tumor [92].

There has been considerable interest in developing a laboratory test to detect early cholangiocarcinoma in patients with PSC. A combination of the serum tumor markers CEA and CA 19-9 was thought to be promising, but appears to lack specificity and sensitivity in detecting small tumors [93]. There is currently no evidence that this test identifies patients with localized cholangiocarcinoma or biliary dysplasia who would benefit from surgery [94].

New techniques are currently being evaluated for the detection and characterization of biliary dysplasia. If vulnerable dysplastic tissue can be reliably identified on liver biopsy specimens, liver transplantation should be possible to prevent the subsequent development of neoplastic change. Unfortunately the current cytobrush specimen usually taken from suspicious areas at ERCP is usually inadequate for definitive diagnosis of dysplasia, and much less for distinguishing which subjects with dysplasia are most likely to progress quickly. Serial collection of material from the suspicious area and genetic analysis may in the future allow the likelihood of progression to cholangiocarcinoma to be predicted [95].

Hepatocellular carcinoma

Two case reports have described the development of fibrolamellar hepatocellular cancer in male patients with UC and PSC. Neither patient was cirrhotic [96, 97]. In the single patient who received a transplant the tumor recurred in the donor liver [96]. In common with most causes of chronic liver disease, patients with PSC and established cirrhosis have an increased risk of developing primary liver cell cancer [98].

Fatty change

Fatty liver or steatosis is the most common type of hepatobiliary lesion found in patients who have IBD. It has been recorded as occurring in 45% of patients with UC who undergo colectomy [99] and in 40% of patients with CD who undergo similar surgery [100]. The presence of fatty liver is related to the general state of health of these patients and the severity of the underlying colitis rather than any other specific factor. This is reflected by the fact that, in an unselected series, fatty liver was found in only 6.3% and 4% of patients with UC and CD, respectively [3, 4]. Moreover, the incidence of fatty change in patients with UC at autopsy is similar to that of other debilitated patients. The pathogenesis of fatty liver in IBD is unknown. It is probably multifactorial, secondary to causes such as poor nutrition, drugs, bacterial and chemical toxins, and unsuspected alcohol abuse. The steatosis is usually of the macrovesicular type and all types of distribution, including diffuse, periportal and centrilobular, have been described in patients with IBD.

There are no symptoms associated with fatty liver, although on abdominal examination hepatomegaly may be detected. Treatment of the underlying bowel disorder and improvement in the general health of the patient will normally result in a resolution of the fatty change. There is no evidence that the lesion progresses to chronic liver disease. In view of improvements in the management of IBD the incidence of fatty change has probably fallen.

Gallstones

Patients with CD of the small bowel have an increased incidence of gallstones. The reported incidence in patients with Crohn's ileitis, ileal resection, or intestinal bypass ranges from 13% to 34% [101–105]. However, the incidence of gallstones in patients with UC and those with CD confined to the colon is about 5%, and does not differ from that of the general population. Total colectomy with ileoanal anastomosis does not predispose to the formation of cholesterol gallstones [105]. The increased rate of formation of gallstones in patients with inflammation or absence of the terminal ileum is due to a reduction in bile-salt absorption, leading to depletion of the bile-salt pool. As a result the concentration of biliary bile salts falls, and there is a relative increase in the concentration of biliary cholesterol. Thus, bile may become supersaturated with cholesterol, which in turn increases cholesterol precipitation in the gallbladder and predisposes to the formation of cholesterol gallstones. There may be additional factors predisposing to gallstones in these patients. One study has demonstrated impaired gallbladder contractability, most marked in patients who have undergone bowel resection or have both large and small bowel disease [106].

Amyloidosis

Hepatic amyloidosis is a rare complication, occurring in less than 1% of patients with IBD; it is much more commonly associated with CD than UC. The development of amyloid can occur in association with CD involving either the small or large bowel.

The amyloid deposition in the liver is found in the media of portal blood vessels and in the sinusoidal wall, and eventually leads to atrophy and disappearance of hepatocytes. In addition to IBD, most patients who develop amyloidosis have either extra-intestinal foci of suppuration or arthropathy. In addition most CD patients who develop amyloid have chronically active disease. Aggressive anti-inflammatory treatment of the intestinal lesions probably reduces the chance of developing systemic amyloid. More effective recent treatment probably accounts for the reduced prevalence of amyloid. Although regression of amyloidosis has been reported after colectomy, in the majority of patients the prognosis is poor [107].

Granulomas

Granulomas are occasionally seen in the liver biopsy specimens of patients with CD, some of whom may show a moderate elevation of serum alkaline phosphatase [108]. The granulomas can be present in portal tracts as well as in the parenchyma. The presence of hepatic granulomas in patients with CD often reflects granulomas in the bowel [109]. There have been a few isolated reports of hepatic granulomas occurring in association with UC but the relationship remains unproven. Granulomas are found in 3–4% of liver biopsies from patients with PSC [109].

Liver abscess

Intra-abdominal abscess is a frequent complication of CD. However, the development of hepatic abscess in association with IBD is very uncommon. The abscesses are often multiple and are associated with a high mortality [110]. Streptococci, especially *Streptococcus milleri*, are the most frequent organisms isolated from the abscesses [111].

Primary biliary cirrhosis

Thirteen patients have been described with concomitant UC and primary biliary cirrhosis [112]. Prevalence of primary biliary cirrhosis in UC appears to be significantly higher than in the general population and there may be a true immunologic link between the two diseases.

Budd–Chiari syndrome

At least five patients with active UC have now been reported who have developed hepatic vein thrombosis and the clinical symptoms and signs of Budd–Chiari syndrome. Four of the five had no known risk factors for venous thrombosis [113–115]. The most recent patient reported was found to have positive anti-cardiolipin antibodies [116]. There has also been one report of Budd–Chiari syndrome in association with CD [117].

Drug-induced hepatitis

There have been a few case reports of drug-induced hepatitis in patients with IBD with mesalazine, sulfasalazine and azathioprine all having been implicated [118–121]. In practical terms, however, drug toxicity is a rare cause of hepatic injury in the context of IBD.

References

1. Thomas CH. Ulceration of the colon with a much enlarged fatty liver. Trans Pathol Soc Phil 1873; 4: 87–8.
2. Lister JD. A specimen of diffuse ulcerative colitis with secondary diffuse hepatitis. Trans Path Soc Lond 1988; 50: 130–5.
3. Perret AD, Higgins G, Johnston HH, Massarella G, Truelove SC, Wright R. The liver in ulcerative colitis. Q Med 1971; 40: 211–38.
4. Perret AD, Higgins G, Johnston HH, Massarella G, Truelove SC, Wright R. The liver in Crohn's disease. Q Med 1971; 40: 187–209.
5. Schrumpf E, Fausa O, Kolmannskog F, Elgjo K, Ritland S, Gjome E. Sclerosing cholangitis in ulcerative colitis. A follow-up study. Scand Gastroenterol 1982; 17: 33–9.
6. Olsson R, Danielson A, Jarnerot G, Lindstrome, Loof L, Rolny P. Prevalence of primary sclerosing cholangitis in patients with ulcerative colitis. Gastroenterology 1991; 100: 1319–23.
7. Balasubramaniam K, Wiesner RH, LaRusso NF. Primary sclerosing cholangitis with normal serum levels of alkaline phosphatase. Gastroenterology 1988; 95: 1395–8.
8. Rasmussen HH, Fallingborg JF, Mortensen PB, Vyberg M, Tage-Jensen U, Rasmussen SN. Hepatobiliary dysfunction

and primary sclerosing cholangitis in patients with Crohn's disease. Scand J Gastroenterol 1997; 32: 604–10.

9. Tobias R, Wright J, Kottler R. Primary sclerosing cholangitis associated with inflammatory bowel disease in Cape Town, 1975–1981. S Afr Med J 1983; 63: 229–35.

10. Wiesner RH, LaRusso NF. Clinicopathologic features of the syndrome of primary sclerosing cholangitis. Gastroenterology 1980; 79: 200–6.

11. Broome V, Glaumann H, Hultcrantz R. Liver histology and follow-up of 68 patients with ulcerative colitis and normal liver function tests. Gut 1990; 31: 468–72.

12. Chapman RW, Arborgh BA, Rhodes JM et al. Primary sclerosing cholangitis – a review of its clinical features, cholangiography and hepatic histology. Gut 1980; 21: 870–7.

13. Escorsell A, Pares A, Rodes J, Soli-Herruzo J, Miras M, de la Morena E. Epidemiology of primary sclerosing cholangitis in Spain. J Hepatol 1994; 21: 787–91.

14. Okolicsanyi L, Fabris L, Viaggi S, Carulli N, Podda M, Ricci G. Primary Italian multicentre study. The Italian PSC Study Group. Eur J Gastroenterol Hepatol 1996; 8: 685–91.

15. Takikawa H. Recent status of primary sclerosing cholangitis in Japan. J Hepatol Bil Panc Surg 1999, 6. 352–5.

16. Lundgrist K, Broome U. Differences in colonic disease activity in patients with primary sclerosing cholangitis. Dis Colon Rectum 1997; 40: 1–6.

17. Rabinovitz M, Gavalier JS, Schade RR, Dindzans VJ, Chien M-C, VanThiel DH. Does primary sclerosing cholangitis occurring in association with inflammatory bowel disease differ from that occurring in the absence of inflammatory bowel disease. Hepatology 1991; 11: 7–11.

18. Loftus EvJr, Sandborn WJ, Tremaine WJ et al. Primary sclerosing cholangitis is associated with non-smoking: a case–control study. Gastroenterology 1996; 110: 1496–502.

19. Van Erpecium KJ, Smits SJ, Van-de-Meeberg PC et al. Risk of primary sclerosing cholangitis is associated with non-smoking behaviour. Gastroenterology 1996; 110: 1503–6.

20. Mitchell SA, Thyssen M, Orchard TR, Jewell DP, Fleming KA, Chapman RW. Cigarette smoking, appendectomy, and tonsillectomy as risk factors for the development of primary sclerosing cholangitis: a case control study. Gut 2002; 51: 1–6.

21. Nemeth A, Ejderhamn J, Glaumann H, Strandvik B. Liver damage in juvenile inflammatory bowel disease. Liver 1990; 10: 239–48.

22. Wiesner RH, La Russo NF, Dozois RR, Beaver SJ. Peristomal varices after proctocolectomy in patients with primary sclerosing cholangitis. Gastroenterology 1986; 90: 316–22.

23. Bargen JA. Chronic ulcerative colitis associated with malignant change. Arch Surg 1928; 17: 561–76

24. Broome U, Lofberg R, Veress B, Eriksson LS. Primary sclerosing cholangitis: evidence for increased neoplastic potential. Hepatology 1995; 22: 1404–8.

25. Jayaram H, Satsangi J, Chapman RWG. Increased colorectal neoplasia in chronic ulcerative colitis complicated by primary sclerosing cholangitis: fact or fiction? Gut 2001; 48: 430–4.

26. Marchesa P, Lashner BA, Lavery IC et al. The risk of cancer and dysplasia among ulcerative colitis patients with primary sclerosing cholangitis. Am J Gastroenterol 1997; 92: 1285–8.

27. Shetty K, Rybicki L Bzezinski A, Carey WD, Lashner BA. The risk for cancer or dysplasia in ulcerative colitis patients with primary sclerosing cholangitis. Am J Gastroenterol 1999; 94: 1643–9.

28. Lindberg B, Broomé U, Persson B. Proximal colorectal dysplasia/cancer in ulcerative colitis. The impact of primary sclerosing cholangitis and sulfasalazine: results from a 20-year surveillance study. Dis Colon Rectum 2001; 44: 77–85.

29. Broome U, Lofberg R, Veress B, Eriksson LS. Primary sclerosing cholangitis and ulcerative colitis: evidence for increased neoplastic potential. Hepatology 1995; 22: 1404–8.

30. Miki C, Harrison JD, Gunson BK, Buckels JA, McMaster P, Mayer AD. Inflammatory bowel disease in primary sclerosing cholangitis: an analysis of patients undergoing liver transplantation. Br J Surg 1995; 82: 1114–17.

31. Papatheodoridis GV, Hamilton M, Rolles K et al. Liver transplantation and inflammatory bowel disease. J Hepatol 1998; 28: 1070–6.

32. Gavaler JS, Delemos B, Belle SH et al. Ulcerative colitis disease activity as subjectively assessed by patient-completed questionnaires following orthotopic liver transplantation for sclerosing cholangitis. Dig Dis Sci 1991; 36: 321–8.

33. Shaked A, Colonna JO, Goldstein L et al. The inter-relation between sclerosing cholangitis and ulcerative colitis in patients undergoing liver transplantation. Ann Surg 1992; 215: 598–603.

34. Gow PJ, Chapman RW. Liver transplantation for primary sclerosing cholangitis. Liver 2000; 20: 97–103.

35. Narumi S, Roberts JP, Emond JC, Lake J, Ascher NL. Liver transplantation for sclerosing cholangitis. Hepatology 1995; 22: 451–7.

36. Penna C, Duzois R, Tremaine W et al. Pouchitis after ileal pouch–anal anastomosis for ulcerative colitis occurs with increased frequency in patients with associated primary sclerosing cholangitis. Gut 1996; 38: 234–9.

37. Pemberton JH. The role of proctocolectomy in patients with primary sclerosing cholangitis and inflammatory bowel disease. 2000 Clinical Research Single Topic Conference. Primary Sclerosing Cholangitis: Controversies and Consensus. AASLD.

38. Boberg KM, Aadland E, Jahnsen J, Raknerud N, Stiris M, Bell H. Incidence and prevalence of primary biliary cirrhosis, primary sclerosing cholangitis and autoimmune hepatitis in a Norwegian population. Scand J Gastroenterol 1998; 33: 99–103.

39. Quigley EMM, La Russo NF, Ludwig J, MacSween RNM, Birnie GG, Watkinson G. Familial occurrence of primary sclerosing cholangitis and ulcerative colitis. Gastroenterology 1983; 85: 1160–5.

40. Chapman RW, Varghese Z, Gaul R, Patel G, Kokinon N, Sherlock S. Association of primary sclerosing cholangitis with HLA-B8. Gut 1983; 24: 38–41.

41. Schrumpf E, Fausa O, Forre O, Doblong JH, Ritland S, Thorsby E. HLA antigens and immunoregulatory T cells in ulcerative colitis associated with hepatobiliary disease. Scand J Gastroenterol 1982; 17: 187–91.

42. Donaldson PT, Farrant JM, Wilkinson MK, Hayllar K, Portmann BC, Williams R. Dual association of HLA DR2 and DR3 with primary sclerosing cholangitis. Hepatology 1991; 13: 129–33.

43. Olerup O, Olsson R, Hultcrantz R, Broomé U. HLA-DR and HLA-DQ are not markers for rapid disease progression in primary sclerosing cholangitis. Gastroenterology 1995; 108: 870–8.

44. Mitchell SA, Grove J, Spurkland A et al. Association of the tumour necrosis factor alpha-308 but not the interleukin 10-627 promoter polymorphism with genetic susceptibility to primary sclerosing cholangitis. Gut 2001;49: 288–94.

45. Bernal W, Moloney M, Underhill J, Donaldson PT. Association of tumor necrosis factor polymorphism with primary sclerosing cholangitis. J Hepatol 1999; 30: 237–41.

46. Wiencke K, Spurkland A, Schrumpf E, Boberg KM. Primary sclerosing cholangitis is associated to an extended B80DR3 haplotype including particular MICA and MICB alleles. Hepatology 2001; 34: 625–30.

47. Norris S, Kondeatis, Collins R et al. Mapping MHC-encoded susceptibility and resistance in primary sclerosing cholangitis: the role of MICA polymorphism. Gastroenterology 2001; 120: 1475–82.

48. Satsangi J, Chapman RW, Haldar N et al. A functional polymorphism of the stromelysin gene (MMP-3) influences susceptibility to primary sclerosing cholangitis. Gastroenterology 2001; 121: 124–30.

49. Duerr RH, Targan SR, Landers CJ, LaRusso NF, Lindsey KL, Wiesner RH. Neutrophil cytoplasmic antibodies: a link between primary sclerosing cholangitis and ulcerative colitis. Gastroenterology 1991; 100: 1381–5.

50. Lo SK, Fleming KA, Chapman RW. Prevalence of antineutrophil antibody in primary sclerosing cholangitis and ulcerative colitis using an alkaline phosphatase technique. Gut 1992; 33: 1370–5.

51. Lo SK, Fleming KA, Chapman RW. A two year follow-up study of antineutrophil antibody in primary sclerosing cholangitis. J Hepatol 1994; 21: 974–8.

52. Terjung B, Spengler U, Sauerbruch T, Worman HJ. 'Atypical p-ANCA' in IBD and hepatobiliary disorders react with a 50-kilodalton nuclear envelope protein of neutrophils and myeloid cell lines. Gastroenterology 2000; 119: 310–22.

53. Vierling JM. Immunologic and non-immunologic factors in the etiopathogenesis of sclerosing cholangitis. 2000 Clinical Research Single Topic Conference. Primary Sclerosing Cholangitis: Controversies and Consensus. AASLD.

54. Wells IP, Wheeler PG, Laws JW, Williams R. A new appearance of the comon bile duct in sclerosing cholangitis. Br J Radiol 1980; 53: 502–4.

55. Fulcher AS, Turner MA, Franklin KJ et al. Primary sclerosing cholangitis: evaluation with MR cholangiography – a case control study. Radiology 2000; 215: 71–80.

56. Broome U, Olsson R, Loof L et al. Natural history and prognostic factors in 305 Swedish patients with primary sclerosing cholangitis. Gut 1996; 38: 610–15.

57. Wiesner RH, Grambsch PM, Dickson ER et al. Primary sclerosing cholangitis; natural history, prognostic factors and survival analysis. Hepatology 1989; 10: 430–6

58. Farrant JM, Hayllar KM, Wilkinson ML et al. Natural history and prognostic variables in primary sclerosing cholangitis. Gastroenterology 1991; 100: 1710–17.

59. Dickson ER, Murtaugh PA, Wiesner RH et al. Primary sclerosing cholangitis: refinement and validation of survival models. Gastroenterology 1992; 103: 1893–901.

60. Kim WR, Poterucha JJ, Wiesner RH et al. The relative role of the Child-Pugh classification and the Mayo natural history model in the assessment of survival in patients with primary sclerosing cholangitis. Hepatology 1999; 29: 1643–8.

61. May GR, Bender CE, LaRusson NF, Wiesner RH. Non operative dilatation of dominant strictures in primary sclerosing cholangitis. Am J Radiol 1985; 145: 1061–4.

62. Allison MC, Burroughs AK, Noone P, Summerfield JA. Biliary lavage with corticosteroids in primary sclerosing cholangitis. J Hepatol 1986; 3: 118–22.

63. Lindor KD, Wiesner RH, Colwell LJ, Steiner BL, Beaver S, LaRusso NF. The combination of prednisolone and colchicine in patients with primary sclerosing cholangitis. Am J Gastroenterol 1991; 85: 57–61.

64. Lindor KD. Ursodiol for primary sclerosing cholangitis. N Engl J Med 1997; 336: 691–5.

65. Mitchell SA, Bansi DS, Hunt N, Von Bergmann K, Fleming KA, Chapman RW. A preliminary trial of high-dose ursodeoxycholic acid in primary sclerosing cholangitis. Gastroenterology 2001; 121: 900–7.

66. Shetty K, Rybicki L, Carey WD. The Child-Pugh classification as a prognostic indicator for survival in primary sclerosing cholangitis. Hepatology 1997; 25: 1049–53.

67. Goss JA, Shackleton CR, Farmer DG et al. Orthotopic liver transplantation for primary sclerosing cholangitis. A 12-year single centre experience. Ann Surg 1997; 225: 472–81.

68. Graziadei IW, Wiesner RH, Batts KP et al. Recurrence of primary sclerosing cholangitis following liver transplantation. Hepatology 1999; 29: 1050–6.

69. Ahrendt SA, Pitt HA. Surgical treatment for primary sclerosing cholangitis. J Hepatobil Panc Surg 1999; 6: 366–72.

70. Mistilis SP. Pericholangitis and ulcerative colitis: (pathology, aetiology and pathogenesis). Ann Intern Med 1965; 63: 1–16.

71. Mistilis SP, Skyring AP, Goulston SJM. Pericholangitis & ulcerative colitis: II. Clinical aspects. Ann Intern Med 1965; 63: 17–26.

72. Boden RE, Rankin JG, Goulston SJ, Morrow W.vThe liver in ulcerative colitis: the significance of raised serum alkaline phsophatase levels. Lancet 1959; 2: 245–8.

73. Blackstone MO, Nemchausky BA. Cholangiographic abnormalities in ulcerative colitis associated pericholangitis which resemble sclerosing cholangitis. Dig Dis Sci 1978; 23: 579–85.

74. Shepherd HA, Selby WS, Chapman RW et al. Ulcerative colitis and liver dysfunction. Q Med 1983; 52: 503–13.

75. Wee A, Ludwig J. Pericholangitis in chronic ulcerative colitis: primary sclerosing cholangitis of the small ducts? Ann Intern Med 1985; 102: 581–7.

76. Broome U, Glaumann H, Lindstom E et al. Natural history and outcome in 32 Swedish patients with small duct primary sclerosing cholangitis (PSC). J Hepatol 2002; 36: 586–9.

77. Bjornsson E, Cullen S, Fleming K et al. Patients with small duct primary sclerosing cholangitis have a favourable long term prognosis. Gut 2002 (in press).

78. Desmet VJ, Geboes K. Liver lesions in inflammatory bowel disorders. J Pathol 1987; 151: 247–55.

79. Olsson R, Hulten L. Concurrence of ulcerative colitis and chronic active hepatitis. Clinical courses and results of colectomy. Scand J Gastroenterol 1975; 10: 331–5.

80. Hashimoto E, Lindor KD, Homburger HA et al. Immunohistochemical characterization of hepatic lymphocytes in primary biliary cirrhosis in comparison with primary sclerosing cholangitis and autoimmune hepatitis. Mayo Clin Proc 1993; 68: 1049–55.

81. Gotike F, Lohse AW, Dienes HP et al. Evidence for an overlap syndrome of autoimmune hepatitis and primary sclerosing cholangitis. J Hepatol 1996; 24: 699–705.

82. Tumen HJ, Moaghan JF, Jobb E. Hepatic cirrhosis as a complication of chronic ulcerative colitis. Ann Intern Med 1947; 26: 542–53.

83. Holdsworth CD, Hall EW, Dawson AM. Ulcerative colitis in chronic liver disease. Q Med 1965; 34: 211–26

84. Lupinetti M, Mehigan D, Cameron JL. Hepato-biliary complications of ulcerative colitis. Am Surg 1980; 139: 113–17.

85. Schrumpf E, Elgjo K, Fausa O, Gjone F, Kolmannskog F, Ritland S. Sclerosing cholangitis in ulcerative colitis. Scand Gastroenterol1980; 15: 689–97.

86. Broome U, Glaumann H, Hellers G, Nilsson B, Sorstadt J, Hultcrantz R. Liver disease in ulcerative colitis: an epidimiologcal and follow-up study in the county of Stockholm. Gut 1994; 35: 84–9.

87. Mir-Madjlessi SH, Farmer RG, Sivak MV. Bile duct carcinoma in patients with ulcerative colitis. Dig Dis Sci 1987; 32: 145–54.

88. Berman MD, Falchuk KR, Trey C. Carcinoma of the biliary tree complicating Crohn's disease. Dig Dis Sci 1980; 25: 795–7.

89. Choi PM, Nugent FW, Zelig MP, Munson JL, Schoetz DJ Jr. Cholangiocarcinoma and Crohn's disease. Dig Dis Sci 1994; 39: 667–70.
90. Keiding S, Hansen SB, Rasmussen HH *et al.* Detection of cholangiocarcinoma in primary sclerosing cholangitis by positron emission tomography. Hepatology 1998; 28: 700–6.
91. Rosen CB, Nagorney DM, Wiesner RH, Coffey RJ, LaRusso NF. Cholangiocarcinoma complicating primary sclerosing cholangitis. Ann Surg 1991; 213: 21–5.
92. Stieber AL, Marino IR, Iwatsuki S, Starzl TE. Cholangiocarcinoma in sclerosing cholangitis: the role of liver transplantation. Int Surg 1989; 74: 1–3.
93. Ramage JK, Donaghy A, Farrant JM, Iorns R, Williams R. Serum tumour markers for the diagnosis of cholangiocarcinoma in primary sclerosing cholangitis. Gastroenterology 1995; 108: 865–9.
94. Harrison PM. Prevention of bile duct cancer in primary sclerosing cholangitis. Ann Oncol 1999; 10: 208–11.
95. Finklestein S. Cholangiocarcinoma associated with primary sclerosing cholangitis. 2000 Clinical Research Single Topic Conference. Primary Sclerosing Cholangitis: Controversies and Consensus. AASLD.
96. Klompmaker IJ, DeBruign KM, Gouw AS, Bams JL, Sloof MJH. Recurrence of hepatocellular carcinoma after liver transplantation. Br Med J 1988; 296: 1445.
97. Snook JA, Kelly P, Chapman RW, Jewell DP. Fibrolamellar hepatocellular carcinoma complicating ulcerative colitis with primary sclerosing cholangitis. Gut 1989; 30: 243–5.
98. Harnois DM, Goves GJ, Ludwig J, Steers JL, LaRusso NF, Wiesner RH. Are patients with cirrhotic stage primary sclerosing cholangitis at risk for development of hepatocellular cancer? J Hepatol 1997; 27: 512–16.
99. Eade MN. Liver disease in ulcerative colitis. I. Analysis of operative liver biopsy in 138 consecutive patients having colectomy. Ann Intern Med 1970; 72: 457–87.
100. Eade MN, Cooke WT, Brooke BN, Thompson H. Liver disease in Crohn's colitis. A study of 21 consecutive patients having colectomy. Ann Intern Med 1970; 74: 518–28.
101. Cohen S, Kaplan M, Glottlieb L, Patterson L. Liver disease and gallstones in regional enteritis. Gastroenterology 1971; 60: 243–5.
102. Marks JW. Gallstone prevalence of biliary lipid composition in inflammatory bowel disease. Am Dig Dis 1977; 22: 1097–100.
103. Baker EJ, Merritt CRB, Sullivan MA *et al.* Gallstones in inflammatory bowel disease. Am Dig Dis 1974; 19: 109–12.
104. Kangas E, Lehmusto P, Matikainen M. Gallstones in Crohn's disease. Hepatogastroenterology 1990; 37: 83–4.
105. Galatola G, Fracchia M, Gazrawi RP. Effect of colectomy with ileal and anal anastamosis on the biliary lipids. Eur J Clin Invest 1995; 25: 534–8.
106. Murray FE, McNicholas M, Stack W, O'Donoghue DP. Impaired fatty meal stimulated gall bladder contractivity in patients with Crohn's disease. Clin Sci 1993; 83: 689–93.
107. Fausa O, Nygaard K, Elgjo K. Amyloidosis and Crohn's disease. Scand J Gastroenterol 1977; 12: 657–62.
108. Mayer HL, Hughes RW, Jarrett HF, Mosenthal A. Granulomatous hepatitis associated with regional enteritis. Gastroenterology 1967; 53: 301–5.
109. Ludwig J, Colina F, Poterucha JJ. Granulomas in primary sclerosing cholangitis. Liver 1995; 15: 307–12.
110. Greenstein AJ, Schar DB, Lowenthal D, Goldofsky E, Aufses AH. Pyogenic liver abscess in Crohn's disease. Q J Med 1955; 56: 505–18.
111. Mir-Madjlessi SH, McHenry MC, Farmer RG. Liver abscess in Crohn's disease. Gastroenterology 1986; 91: 987–93.
112. Koulentaki M, Koutroubakis IE, Petinaki E *et al.* Ulcerative colitis associated with primary biliary cirrhosis. Dig Dis Sci 1999; 44: 1953–6.
113. Brinson RR, Curtis WD, Schuman BM, Mills LR. Recovery from hepatic vein thrombosis (Budd-Chiari styndrome) complicating ulcerative colitis. Dig Dis Sci 1988; 33: 1615–20.
114. Chesner IM, Muller S, Newman J. Ulcerative colitis complicated by Budd-Chiari syndrome. Gut 1986; 27: 1096–100.
115. Kraut K, Berman JH, Gunasekaran TS *et al.* Hepatic vein thrombosis (Budd-Chiari syndrome) in an adolescent with ulcerative colitis. J Pediatr Gastroenterol Nutr 1997; 25: 417–20.
116. Praderio L, Dagna L, Longhi P, Rubin G, Sabbadini MG. Budd-Chiari syndrome in a patient with ulcerative colitis: association with anticardiolipin antibodies. J Clin Gastroenterol 2000; 30: 203–4.
117. Maccini DM, Berg JC, Bell GA. Budd-Chiari and Crohn's disease. An unreported association. Dig Dis Sci 1989; 34: 1615–20.
118. Braun M, Fraser GM, Kunin M, Salamon F, Kaspa RT. Mesalamine-induced granulomatous hepatitis. Am J Gastroenterol 1999; 94: 1973–4.
119. Delentre P, Berson A, Marcellin P, Degott C, Biour M, Pessayre D. Mesalazine (5-aminosalicylic acid) induced chronic hepatitis. Gut 1999; 44: 886–8.
120. Besnard M, Debray D, Durand P, Cezard JP, Navarro J. Sulfasalazine-induced fulminant hepatitis in pediatric Crohn's disease: report of two cases. J Pediatr Gastroenterol Nutr 1998; 26: 119–20.
121. Romagnuolo J, Sadowski DC, Lalor E, Jewell L, Thomson AB. Cholestatic hepatocellular injury with azathioprine: a case report and review of the mechanisms of hepatotoxicity. Can J Gastroenterol 1998; 12: 479–83.

39 | Articular and ocular complications of inflammatory bowel disease

TIMOTHY R. ORCHARD AND DEREK P. JEWELL

Introduction

Articular and ocular complications of inflammatory bowel disease (IBD) are relatively common, and were recognized as far back as the 19th century. Despite causing a significant morbidity in IBD patients they have not been widely studied and their pathogenesis remains unclear. Recent studies have produced a clearer classification, and this in turn has led to new pathogenetic insights.

Arthritis

Historical considerations and classification

Peripheral arthritis

Hale White described postmortem abnormalities in the joints of patients with ulcerative colitis (UC) in 1895, and Bargen described arthritis in association with UC in the 1920s. Initially this was thought to be coincident rheumatoid arthritis, but in 1958 Bywaters and Ansell published a paper demonstrating that the arthritis was inflammatory with a lymphocytic infiltration of the synovium, but that it was not erosive or deforming and produced a negative rheumatoid factor [1].

Two large studies in the 1960s examined peripheral arthritis in UC: a retrospective study of 675 patients from Oxford demonstrated a polyarthritis [2], whereas a prospective study of 269 patients from Leeds showed a large joint arthritis in 11.5% of patients [3]. Subsequent studies in Crohn's disease (CD) found a similar distribution of disease [4]. However, many studies did not differentiate between arthritis and arthralgia. This is potentially a very important distinction, as was demonstrated by a study from Israel [5]: this compared arthritis and arthralgia in a group of 54 CD patients with age- and sex-matched controls. Forty-four percent of the CD patients complained of arthralgia, but 46% of

controls also had joint pains. When objective evidence of joint inflammation was sought 7.4% of CD patients had arthritis, compared to none of the controls. Thus arthralgia is a common problem in both CD patients and healthy controls, but inclusion of patients with arthralgia in studies of arthritis may considerably distort the results.

Recently a large study from Oxford studied arthritis in 976 UC patients and 483 CD patients, studying only those with objective evidence of articular inflammation [6]. This found two distinct forms of peripheral arthritis associated with IBD, both seronegative, with differing patterns of joint involvement and natural histories.

1. Type 1 (pauciarticular) affects less than five joints including a weightbearing joint and is asymmetrical. The swelling is acute and self-limiting and associated with relapse of the IBD in the majority of cases. It lasts for a maximum of 10 weeks, although, like reactive arthritis (ReA), 10–20% will develop persistent problems. There is a strong association with other extraintestinal features such as erythema nodosum and uveitis.

2. Type 2 (polyarticular) affects five or more joints, and affects a wide range of joints but particularly the metacarpophalangeal (MCP) joints. It may cause persistent problems with a median duration of 3 years. It is associated with uveitis, but not erythema nodosum.

The onset of arthritis may occur at any time during the course of the IBD or before it becomes clinically manifest. It is not related to disease extent in UC but in CD it is possibly more common in colonic disease. In both types of arthropathy there is little or no joint destruction and patients are seronegative.

Stephan R. Targan, Fergus Shanahan and Loren C. Karp (eds.), *Inflammatory Bowel Disease: From Bench to Bedside, 2nd Edition*, 747–756.
© 2003 *Kluwer Academic Publishers. Printed in Great Britain*

In the Oxford series of 1459 patients the prevalence of type 1 was 3.6% in UC and 6.0% in CD and for type 2 was 2.5% in UC and 4.0% in CD. These figures are slightly lower than in some other studies, which may reflect the strict entry criteria and the retrospective nature of the study. In total between 5% and 10% of UC patients develop peripheral arthritis and 15–20% of CD patients. This study demonstrates that careful clinical characterization of patients may lead to the detection of new clinical entities. This in turn may lead to new pathogenic insights.

Axial arthritis

In some ways the association of axial arthritis with IBD is clearer than peripheral arthritis. Both ankylosing spondylitis and isolated sacroiliitis are known to be associated with IBD, but there remain a number of questions unanswered.

Ankylosing spondylitis (AS) is a seronegative inflammatory arthropathy affecting the vertebral column, characterized by sacroiliitis and progressive ankylosis (fusion) of the vertebral facet joints. This progressive fusion leads to a characteristic 'question mark' posture and may lead to respiratory embarrassment secondary to poor chest expansion and upper lobe pulmonary fibrosis. It is associated with peripheral arthritis in about 30% of cases. Its prevalence in the general population is between 0.25% and 1%, with a male:female ratio of 3:1 [7, 8]. The prevalence of AS in IBD is 1–6% [9, 10], varying according to the study population, and the proportion of female patients is higher than in idiopathic AS, accounting for up to 50% of patients in some series. Otherwise the clinical features are identical to idiopathic AS and it runs a course independent of the IBD.

Whilst AS, with sacroiliitis, back pain, restriction of movement and respiratory embarrassment, is progressive over a number of years, isolated sacroiliitis, without these features, has also been described in IBD. Its prevalence is largely dependent upon the means of diagnosis, and it is often asymptomatic.

Radiographic surveys suggest a prevalence of up to 18% [10], but more recent studies have suggested a higher prevalence. Diagnosis on radiographic grounds alone is hampered by a large degree of inter-observer and intra-observer error [11]. Computerized tomographic (CT) imaging studies have detected sacroiliitis in 32% of patients with IBD [12] and studies using radioisotope scintigraphy have found uptake abnormalities in up to 52% of patients with CD and 42% with UC [13]. However, the significance of these findings is not clear, and long-term follow-up studies to demonstrate progression to AS have not been undertaken. It may be that in the majority of patients this is a non-progressive condition.

Pathogenesis

Spondyloarthropathies

Before considering the IBD-associated arthropathies it is worth considering the spondyloarthropathies, with which they are often classified. AS is the model for this group of rheumatological conditions. It includes reactive arthritis (post enteric and urogenital), psoriatic arthritis and IBD-associated arthritis [14]. They are all seronegative inflammatory arthritides, and they share important clinical and pathogenic features. These include the presence of inflammatory low back pain, an increased prevalence of AS, an association with erythema nodosum and uveitis, and (with the exception of IBD peripheral arthritis) an association with HLA-B27. This association was first recognized in AS, where it is strongest, with 94% of patients possessing HLA-B27 in a recent study, compared to 10% of the general population [15]. The association is weaker, but still significant, in the peripheral arthritides: In reactive arthritis approximately 70% of patients possess HLA-B27, although the prevalence varies widely between studies [16]. In the peripheral arthritides it appears that it is those patients who are HLA-B27-positive who develop the long-term complications of disease – namely sacroiliitis, acute uveitis or recurrent arthritis [17, 18].

Behçet's disease is sometimes included in the spondyloarthropathy group, but its inclusion remains controversial [19]. The reported prevalence of HLA-B27 is only modestly increased, and the association with sacroiliitis is weak. However, there is an increase in mucocutaneous complications such as erythema nodosum and uveitis (although this is characteristically posterior, in contrast to uveitis in spondyloarthropathy which is anterior).

IBD arthritis

IBD arthritis is likely to be caused by the interaction of genetic and environmental factors.

Genetic factors

Axial arthritis

As mentioned above, AS associated with IBD appears clinically to be identical to idiopathic AS, and it runs a course independent of the IBD. Some authors have suggested that it is generally milder than idiopathic AS, but ascertainment bias is a problem in these studies, and currently there is no consensus on this point.

The HLA- B27 association of IBD AS is different, being considerably weaker: 50–80% of IBD AS patients possess HLA-B27 [20–22] compared to 94% of idiopathic AS patients [15]. The pathogenic significance of this difference is unclear, but some possibilities are discussed later.

The genetic associations of isolated sacroiliitis are less clear. This is partly because it is not clear what proportion of patients with sacroiliitis have early progressive disease (and will ultimately develop AS), and what proportion have true isolated sacroiliitis. Large follow-up studies are required to address this question.

The only study of sacroiliitis performed so far is a small study in 136 patients with CD, which studied patients with symptomatic back pain [23]. This demonstrated that 29% of these patients had evidence of sacroiliitis, including 7% who had AS. Those patients with sacroiliitis in the absence of AS were less likely to be HLA-B27-positive. However, a full clinical assessment was not undertaken to differentiate inflammatory from mechanical back pain, and the study did not examine patients with asymptomatic sacroiliitis.

Thus it is probable that patients with isolated sacroiliitis do not have an increased prevalence of HLA-B27, and that HLA-B27 is a marker of progressive axial disease rather than sacroiliitis *per se*, but clearly long-term follow-up studies are required.

Peripheral arthritis

Most studies of the peripheral arthritis of IBD have been small and have not made any distinction between different patterns of disease. Possibly as a result of this they failed to find any association between HLA-B27 and arthritis.

In a recent study of the immunogenetics of IBD arthritis, patients were subdivided according to the clinical classification described above. By doing this, distinct HLA associations were discovered [24]. These are shown in Table 1.

Table 1. HLA associations of peripheral arthropathy in IBD (percentages)

HLA type	Type 1 arthropathy (n = 30)	Type 2 arthropathy (n = 30)	Controls (n = 603)
HLA-B27	27*	3	7+
HLA-B35	33**	7	15++
HLA-B44	13	63***	31+++
HLA-DR103	40****	0	3++++

Type 1 vs controls: + $p = 0.001$, RR = 4.0; ++ $p = 0.01$, RR2.2; ++++ $p < 0.0001$, RR = 12.1.

Type 2 vs controls: +++ $p_c = 0.01$, RR = 2.1.

Type 1 vs type 2: *$p = 0.03$, RR = 8.0; **$p = 0.02$, RR = 5.0; ***$p = 0.0001$, RR = 4.8; ****$p = 0.0001$, RR = incalculable.

Type 1 (the large joint arthritis) is associated with HLA-B27, but type 2 has a distinct association, with HLA-B44. The association of type 1 with HLA-B27 is, perhaps, unsurprising, as type 1 peripheral arthritis (PeA) is clinically very similar to ReA, in which approximately 70% of patients are HLA-B27-positive. In addition in type 1 there was a very strong association with the rare HLA class II allele HLA-DR103 (DRB1*0103). This association is also seen in postenteric ReA. Interestingly in ReA the HLA-B27 association is twice as strong as in type 1 IBD PeA, whereas the HLA-DR103 association is twice as strong in type 1 IBD PeA.

The pathogenic significance of these associations (and any functional significance) is difficult to gauge, and the associations described may simply represent linkage disequilibrium with pathogenic genes located close by. This possibility is well illustrated by type 2 PeA. In this condition there is a strong association with HLA-B44, but there is a stronger association with the nearby gene MICA (MHC class I chain-like gene A). MICA codes for a non-classical HLA molecule which is known to be expressed on the gastrointestinal epithelium, and is up-regulated under conditions of cellular stress. It interacts with $\gamma\delta$ T cells, but does not appear to require exogenous antigen for this interaction. Its role appears then, to be in regulating the immune response, and so is a good candidate for involvement in immune-mediated inflammation. Ninety-nine percent (44/45) of patients studied with type 2 PeA possessed the MICA*008 allele compared to 72% of IBD controls and 73% of healthy controls ($p = 0.001$).

The associations described above provide good evidence that genes in the MHC region of chromosome 6 play an important role in both axial and peripheral arthritis associated with IBD. However, the exact nature of this role remains unclear.

Environmental factors

There is little known about the environmental factors involved in the pathogenesis of arthritis in IBD, but some clues can be gained from studying similar conditions in humans and animal models.

It has been suggested that idiopathic AS is associated with antibodies to *Klebsiella* species [25], and that an abnormal immune response involving HLA-B27 is of pathogenetic importance. In AS associated with IBD the association with HLA-B27 is less marked, and this might suggest that in the presence of an inflamed gut, with increased permeability, more antigen may be presented, allowing other HLA-B alleles to act pathogenically. However, in IBD no associations between AS and bacteria have been demonstrated and in idiopathic AS the evidence in favor of *Klebsiella* as opposed to other gut flora is unconvincing.

In contrast, the association between postdysenteric ReA and bacterial infection is well established. Gram-negative enterobacteria such as *Salmonella, Escherichia coli, Yersinia, Klebsiella* and *Campylobacter* are all associated with arthritis, and bacterial antigens may be isolated from the affected joints. These conditions are clinically very similar to type 1 PeA seen in IBD, and so it seems likely that presentation of bacterial antigen may be important in the initiation of type 1 IBD arthritis. This is plausible given the association between type 1 arthritis and active disease. In these circumstances the gut is inflamed, and therefore more permeable; a similar situation to acute bacterial enterocolitis. Proliferative T cell responses to the relevant bacteria have been demonstrated from the synovial fluid of patients with ReA, but interestingly most of these appear to be HLA-DR restricted rather than HLA-B restricted [26–28]. This suggests that the HLA class II alleles may be more important than HLA-B27 in the peripheral arthritides associated with enteropathy.

Further information regarding the role of bacteria in initiating arthritis in the presence of gut inflammation has been gained from the study of the HLA-B27 transgenic animal models. Whilst the rat and mouse models differ in some respects they provide useful working models. These animals spontaneously develop a colitis and arthritis when reared under normal conditions [29, 30]. However, if reared in a germfree environment, the gut and joint inflammation is abrogated [30]. Furthermore Rath and colleagues have demonstrated that different bacteria induce gut and joint inflammation with differing efficiency, with *Bacteroides vulgatus* and a cocktail of bacteria isolated from CD patients being the most efficient, whilst *E. coli* is ineffective [29, 31].

Thus it appears likely that bacteria are important in the pathogenesis of the type 1 PeA of IBD and possibly IBD-associated AS, but the mechanisms by which they interact with the immune system are unclear.

The exact site within the gut where this interaction occurs is also a matter for debate, and in this area animal models may also provide some useful information: Rath et al. have demonstrated in the HLA-B27 transgenic rat that diversion of the fecal stream away from the cecum abrogates distant inflammation, whilst leaving the colitis unaffected [32]. They have postulated a role for bacterial overgrowth in the cecum in the pathogenesis of extracolonic inflammation. In humans the cecum is relatively much smaller than in the rat, and so these data cannot be extrapolated directly. However, in a study of 434 patients with CD it has been shown that there is a significant decrease in the incidence of new joint complications after resection of the ileocecal region – from one complication for every 89 years of follow-up to one complication every 701 years of follow-up [33]. This is illustrated as Kaplan–Meier survival curves in Fig. 1. This is highly significant, even when correcting for the time spent in remission from CD after surgery. Although this study provides circumstantial evidence that the ileocecal region may be important in the development of arthritis in IBD it does not help determine whether it is stasis proximal to the ileocecal valve or cecal bacteria that are of importance. Neither is it clear whether it is the interaction of bacteria with up-regulated HLA class II molecules in the ileum or with newly induced class II molecules in the colon (or another mechanism) that is important.

Taking the genetic and environmental data together it is possible to hypothesize concerning the mechanisms involved in the arthritides associated with IBD. Classical type 1 peripheral arthritis of IBD occurs in genetically susceptible individuals, and may be caused by the interaction between gut bacteria and HLA class II molecules in the context of

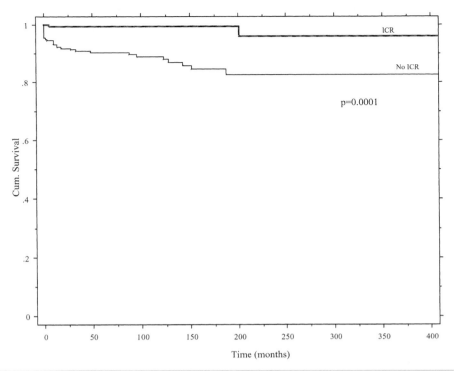

Figure 1. Kaplan–Meier curves of survival free of joint complications in Crohn's disease patients who had never undergone surgery and patients after ileocecal resection (ICR).

an actively inflamed, and therefore abnormally permeable, gut. Whether this interaction is proximal or distal to the ileocecal valve is unclear, and further work is required.

In contrast, the axial complications, such as AS, seem more likely to be mediated by typical or atypical interactions between HLA class I molecules and the immune system, although intestinal inflammation may make the conditions more favorable for the development of axial inflammation. This would be consistent with the observation that the HLA-B27 association in IBD is weaker than in idiopathic AS, suggesting that the presence of intestinal inflammation may allow the development of joint disease even in patients without the usual genetic predisposition.

The pathogenetic mechanisms in type 2 peripheral arthritis are less clear, and although there is a strong HLA class I association this may be secondary to linkage disequilibrium with other genes in the region such as the non-classical class I gene MICA.

All the hypotheses described above remain largely speculative, and there are others, including the suggestion that arthritis and other extraintestinal manifestations are an autoimmune reaction to self antigens such as isoforms of tropomyosin found in the gut, eye and joint [34]. However, these do not account for the HLA associations found, and the evidence has not yet been widely replicated.

Clinical features

Diagnosis

Axial disease

Symptomatic disease

Low back pain is a common complaint in both IBD and the general population. In IBD it may represent inflammatory arthritis of the sacroiliac joints (sacroiliitis) or progressive AS. It has been suggested that the course of AS associated with IBD is less severe than idiopathic AS, but this is not universally accepted. In a patient presenting with back pain it is therefore important to distinguish between mechanical low back pain and the inflammatory back pain associated with sacroiliitis and AS.

The clinical features of inflammatory low back pain are an insidious onset over months, morning stiffness and exacerbation of pain by rest and pain radiating into the buttocks (rather than central back pain). It tends to occur in patients under 40 years of age. Mechanical back pain may be of sudden onset, is often central and is better after rest, occurring generally in older patients. Plain radiographs of the sacroiliac joints are the conventional means of diagnosis, but X-ray changes occur only after several months and magnetic resonance imaging scanning (with or without gadolinium enhancement) is more sensitive and avoids the necessity of a radiation dose.

If radiologic evidence of sacroiliitis is found then a further assessment should be made to detect evidence of progressive axial disease. This should include the modified Schober test of lumbar flexion, lateral lumbar flexion and chest expansion.

The most useful blood test in diagnosis is HLA-B27 status, although in IBD a negative HLA-B27 status does not preclude the diagnosis of AS, and patients with low back pain or decreased spinal mobility in the presence of sacroiliitis should be treated as having AS .

Asymptomatic disease

Up to 20% of IBD patients may have asymptomatic sacroiliitis detectable by plain radiology, and it may be diagnosed on the basis of routine abdominal X-rays. In many cases there is no history of inflammatory back pain even on direct questioning. If sacroiliitis is diagnosed a clinical assessment of spinal mobility should be undertaken along with HLA-B27 status. If there is evidence of decreased spinal mobility patients should be treated as having early AS.

Peripheral arthritis (PeA)

As mentioned above, there are two distinct forms of PeA, and in addition arthralgia may occur. This is often in conjunction with reducing doses of corticosteroids or the commencement of immunosuppressants such as azathioprine. These normally settle with time and rarely require specific treatment.

Both forms of arthritis are rheumatoid factor-negative and are not generally erosive or deforming. If there is evidence of erosive disease then further investigation by a rheumatologist is required.

Diagnosis of IBD PeA is largely based upon clinical grounds, but other joint disease should be excluded.

For type 1 arthritis the differential diagnosis includes gout and pseudogout, septic arthritis and arthritis following genitourinary infections such as *Chlamydia* and gonorrhea. These causes should be actively sought, particularly where there is no apparent relation to activity of the bowel disease, and serum urate and calcium should be checked routinely. Joint aspiration and examination should be performed in cases where there is any doubt. For type 2 arthritis a rheumatoid factor and autoantibody screen should be performed to exclude seropositive rheumatic disease. Arthritis associated with IBD is very rarely erosive or deforming and is not associated with other manifestations of rheumatoid arthritis such as subcutaneous nodules. X-rays of the most severely affected joints should therefore be performed if symptoms are persistent, to exclude erosive disease.

Management of IBD arthritis

General points

The management of arthritis in IBD depends upon the nature and duration of the arthritis, as discussed below. The aims of treatment are to alleviate symptoms and preserve joint function for the future, particularly in axial disease. Because of the relatively small number of patients involved no controlled trials of treatment have been conducted and most treatment modalities rely on general principles.

Physical treatments (rest, range of movement exercises and physiotherapy) are important components of management and should not be ignored. These may be enhanced by simple measures such as splinting affected joints and the use of assistive devices such as a walking stick.

Analgesia is a key element in management, and is a potentially difficult area, as many analgesics have undesirable effects on the gut. A stepped approach to the prescription of analgesics should be used, starting with simple analgesia such as paracetamol, progressing to stronger analgesics as required. Analgesics containing opioids may cause problematic constipation, particularly in patients with resistant distal colitis.

Non-steroidal anti-inflammatory drugs (NSAIDs) should be avoided if at all possible. They may cause enterocolitis in their own right and may trigger or exacerbate relapse of pre-existing IBD. This may be associated with significant lower gastrointestinal bleeding. They should not be used at all in patients with active disease, and in these situations other therapies should be used. The recent advent of cyclo-oxygenase2 (COX-2) specific NSAIDs has raised the prospect of fewer unwanted gastro-intestinal problems, particularly in the stomach. However, experiments in animals have demonstrated that the enterocolitis of NSAIDs is not mediated by the cyclo-oxygenase pathway, and that the role of the COX isoforms in inflammation may be quite complex. It is therefore likely that COX-2 specific NSAIDs may not improve the tolerability of these drugs in IBD patients, and they should still be avoided.

Axial disease

Patients with AS should be managed in conjunction with a rheumatologist. Physical therapies are of particular importance and all patients should take regular exercise to maintain the mobility of the spine. This may include swimming and spinal exercises with regular physiotherapy if necessary. These forms of exercise should also be recommended to patients with sacroiliitis associated with any form of low back pain or decreased spinal mobility. For patients with severely reduced spinal mobility or severe low back pain injection of steroid into the sacroiliac joints may help, particularly in association with a period of intensive inpatient physiotherapy. The period of relief from sacroiliac injection alone may be brief.

Drug treatments

Simple analgesics should be used if possible. NSAIDs are the drugs of choice in idiopathic AS, and if there is active spinal disease in the absence of active IBD then it is reasonable to use NSAIDs. However, they should be stopped if the IBD flares up. Sulfasalazine can be used for both the IBD and joint symptoms, but it is most effective in patients with associated peripheral joint problems. Other 5-aminosalicylic (5-ASA) drugs are not as effective, as it is thought to be the sulfapyridine component that confers the articular effects rather than the 5-ASA.

If oral steroids are required for active disease then they will also have a beneficial effect on the spinal disease. However long-term steroid therapy for spinal disease alone should be avoided. This may be achieved by using methotrexate, which may be effective in both gut and spinal disease.

In severe progressive disease unresponsive to the measures outlined above radiotherapy remains a last resort; however, the increased risk of hematologic malignancy associated with this form of treatment means it is rarely used.

The most important part in the successful management of patients with AS and IBD is good communication between patient, gastroenterologist and rheumatologist to maximize the effectiveness of the available therapeutic options.

Isolated sacroiliitis should be treated symptomatically with simple analgesia, and regular exercise should be encouraged. However, further treatment should not be required in the absence of decreased spinal mobility or severe pain.

Peripheral joint disease

Type 1 arthritis

This is usually self-limiting, so treatment is largely symptomatic.

Resting the joint is important, and use of a walking stick or splint to take pressure off the joint may lead to a significant improvement. Range of movement exercises should be performed to minimize any periarticular muscle atrophy and to prevent contractures. In severe cases formal physiotherapy may be required to improve function.

Analgesia should be with simple analgesia, and, as type 1 arthritis is usually associated with active bowel disease, NSAIDs should not be used. A good, but relatively seldom used, therapy is intra-articular injection of steroid. This may provide very effective symptom relief and may remove the requirement for other treatments. If oral steroids are used to treat the active bowel disease then these will normally treat the arthritis effectively. If not, an empirical change of 5-ASA drug to sulfasalazine may give good symptom relief. If sulfasalazine fails then low doses of oral steroid specifically for the joint disease may be effective, but this should not be prolonged for more than a few weeks.

Long-term treatment is not usually required, although maintenance with sulfasalazine as the 5-ASA of choice may be appropriate, particularly in patients at risk of recurrent disease such as those who are HLA-DR103-positive. In the minority of patients with persistent problems the treatment options are those of type 2 arthritis (see below).

Type 2 arthritis

These patients generally have persistent problems and may require long-term treatment. Again, as the disease is usually non-erosive and non-deforming symptomatic relief is the major aim.

Again, splinting of affected joints and rest are important components of management, but the persistent and polyarthritic nature of this condition makes this harder to achieve than in type 1 arthritis.

Simple analgesia should be tried initially. NSAIDs should be considered only in patients with quiescent disease unresponsive to simple or combination analgesia, but if there is any evidence of an increase in the activity of the bowel disease NSAIDs should be stopped.

For patients with persisting problems sulfasalazine, or low-dose prednisolone, may be used. However, prolonged courses of oral steroids should be avoided. In patients with active bowel disease it may be appropriate to use methotrexate as the first-line immunosuppressant rather than azathioprine, in order to treat both gut and joints.

Patients who show evidence of erosive joint disease, a positive rheumatoid factor, or who do not respond to the measures outlined above, should be managed jointly with a rheumatologist.

New therapies for IBD arthritis

The major possible new therapy for IBD-associated arthritis is the use of infliximab. This is a monoclonal antibody to the proinflammatory cytokine Tumor necrosis factor alpha. This drug is licensed for use in resistant CD and rheumatoid arthritis, where it has been demonstrated to be effective in improving symptoms and decreasing inflammation. Small open-label trials in spondyloarthropathy have demonstrated that it is again effective in reducing inflammation and symptoms [35, 36]. In IBD-associated arthritis the published experience is limited to case reports but, unsurprisingly here also a reduction in inflamed joints and inflammatory markers has been reported [37]. Thus infliximab may well be an alternative treatment in patients with severe resistant joint disease associated with IBD. As in other rheumatic diseases this may be combined with other immunosuppressants such as methotrexate [38]. However, further studies are required to confirm its efficacy and the best treatment regimens.

Ocular manifestations of IBD

Epidemiology and clinical features

Ocular inflammation in IBD was first documented by Crohn in 1925. If left untreated it is potentially a cause of blindness; however, prompt treatment with topical steroids can minimize this risk.

The prevalence of ocular inflammation varies widely between studies – from 2% to 13% depending on the population and methodology. Various forms have been described including iritis, episcleritis, scleritis and anterior uveitis. In our retrospective study of 1459 patients (976 UC and 483 CD patients) 3% of UC and 5% of CD patients had eye complications. The commonest were iritis (60%), episcleritis (30%) and uveitis (10%). However, in the vast majority of cases the inflammation caused no lasting ocular damage [39].

The female:male ratio was 2.9:1, the eye complications were present at or before diagnosis in 19% of cases, and in 72% of cases the eye complications were associated with active IBD. Thirty percent of patients went on to have recurrent episodes of ocular inflammation.

In common with other studies patients who suffered eye complications were more likely to suffer other mucocutaneous complications, notably arthritis and erythema nodosum.

Pathogenesis

The clinical observation that ocular inflammation occurs more commonly in those patients with other extraintestinal manifestations has led to several hypotheses to explain it.

The first suggested that the eye, the joints, the skin and the liver expressed a particular isoform of tropomyosin, to which an autoimmune reaction was generated [40]. However, although this antigen was found in the target organs it was not found in the components that became inflamed. Thus it was expressed in chondrocytes but not synovium, and in ciliary muscles but not the iris. In addition this hypothesis fails to explain why in some patients ocular inflammation may occur as a single manifestation and in others as part of a complex of extraintestinal manifestations (EIM).

This phenomenon of the EIM being distinct but overlapping clinical entities may be explained by a genetic-based hypothesis. This suggests that the presence of the different EIM is determined by different genes located in the same region. Linkage disequilibrium between these genes would mean that the genes for different manifestations are inherited together more frequently than would be expected by chance, leading to the clinical clustering of the EIM. Given the HLA associations described above we have studied the HLA-B and DR regions in 52 patients with ocular complications of IBD. This study found that there are associations between ocular complications and HLAB27 (40% vs 9% in

IBD controls, $p < 0.0001$), HLA-B58 (12% vs 1%, $p = 0.002$) and HLA-DR103 (20% vs 8%, $p = 0.001$). These associations appear independent of the HLA-B27 and DR103 associations seen in arthritis [41]. This suggests strongly that there are genes in the HLA region of chromosome 6 which determine the different EIM and that linkage disequilibrium between these genes may account for the clinical observation of distinct but overlapping clinical syndromes.

Management of ocular manifestations

For a proper diagnosis to be made the patient should undergo a full ophthalmologic assessment including slit-lamp examination. Treatment normally consists of topical steroid treatment initially frequently (hourly) but reducing subsequently, although a course of treatment lasting 6–8 weeks in total is usual. A cycloplegic agent such as atropine is often added to prevent the formation of posterior synechiae. Occasionally oral steroids may be required for acute anterior uveitis, and often in scleritis. Oral or topical NSAIDs may be useful in anterior scleritis, but have no role in anterior uveitis. Their use carries the risks to the IBD described above.

Thus patients with acute ocular inflammation should have a rapid assessment by an ophthalmologist, who should guide their treatment, which normally consists of topical or oral corticosteroid therapy. Failure to treat the inflammation effectively may lead to long term complications or even blindness, although these situations are rare.

References

1. Bywaters E, Ansell B. Arthritis associated with ulcerative colitis: a clinical and pathological study. Ann Rheum Dis 1958; 17: 169–83.
2. Edwards F, Truelove S. The course and prognosis of ulcerative colitis. III. Complications. Gut 1964; 5: 1–15.
3. Wright V, Watkinson G. The arthritis of ulcerative colitis. Br Med J 1965; 2: 670–5.
4. Greenstein A, Janowitz H, Sachar D. Extra-intestinal complications of Crohn's disease and ulcerative colitis. Medicine 1976; 55: 401–12.
5. Stein H, Volpin G, Shapira D, Suir E, Stevenberg A, Eidelman S. Musculoskeletal manifestations of Crohn's disease. Bull Hosp Jt Dis 1993; 53: 17–20.
6. Orchard TR, Wordsworth BP, Jewell DP. Peripheral arthropathies in inflammatory bowel disease: their articular distribution and natural history. Gut 1998; 42: 387–91.
7. van der Linden S, van der Heijde DM. Clinical and epidemiologic aspects of ankylosing spondylitis and spondyloarthropathies. Curr Opin Rheumatol 1996; 8: 269–74.
8. Calin A. Ankylosing spondylitis. In: Maddison PJ, Isenberg DA, Woo P, Glass DN, eds. Oxford Textbook of Rheumatology. Oxford: Oxford University Press, 1998: 1058–70.
9. Dekker-Saeys B, Meuwissen S, VandenBerg-Loonen E, De Haas W, Agenant D, Tytgat G. Prevalence of peripheral arthritis, sacroiliitis and ankylosing spondylitis in patients suffering from inflammatory bowel disease. Ann Rheum Dis 1978; 37: 33–5.
10. Wright V, Watkinson G. Sacroiliitis and ulcerative colitis. Br Med J 1965; 2: 675–80.
11. Hollingsworth P, Cheah P, Dawkins R, Owen E, Calin A, Wood P. Observer variation in grading sacroiliac radiographs in HLA-B27 positive individuals. J Rheumatol 1983; 10: 247–54.
12. McEniff N, Eustace S, McCarthy C, O'Malley M, Morain C, Hamilton S. Asymptomatic sacroiliitis in inflammatory bowel disease. Assessment by computed tomography. Clin Imaging 1995; 19: 258–62.
13. Agnew JE, Pocock DG, Jewell DP. Sacroiliac joint uptake ratios in inflammatory bowel disease: relationship to back pain and to activity of bowel disease. Br J Radiol 1982; 55: 821.
14. Dougados M, Linden S, Juhlin R et al. The European Spondyloarthropathy Study Group preliminary criteria for the classification of spondyloarthropathy. Arthritis Rheum 1991; 34: 1218–27.
15. Brown MA, Pile KD, Kennedy LG et al. HLA class I associations of ankylosing spondylitis in the white population in the United Kingdom. Ann Rheum Dis 1996; 55: 268–70.
16. Leirisalo-Repo M, Suoranta H. Ten year follow-up study of patients with Yersinia arthritis. Arthritis Rheum 1988; 31: 533–7.
17. Calin A, Fries JF. An 'experimental' epidemic of Reiter's syndrome revisited. Follow-up evidence on genetic and environmental factors. Ann Intern Med 1976; 84: 564–6.
18. Thomson GT, DeRubeis DA, Hodge MA, Rajanayagam C, Inman RD. Post-Salmonella reactive arthritis: late clinical sequelae in a point source cohort. Am J Med 1995; 98: 13–21.
19. Olivieri I, Salvarani C, Cantini F. Is Behçet's disease part of the spondyloarthritis complex? [Editorial]. J Rheumatol 1997; 24: 1870–2.
20. Dekker-Saeys B, Meuwissen S, Berg-Loonen EVD et al. Clinical characteristics and results of histocompatibility typing (HLA B27) in 50 patients with both ankylosing spondylitis and inflammatory bowel disease. Ann Rheum Dis 1978; 37: 36–41.
21. Brewerton D, Caffery M, Nicholls A, Walters D, James D. HL-A27 and arthropathies associated with ulcerative colitis and psoriasis. Lancet 1974; 1: 956–8.
22. Mallas EG, Mackintosh P, Asquith P, Cooke WT. Histocompatibility antigens in inflammatory bowel disease. Their clinical significance and their association with arthropathy with special reference to HLA-B27 (W27). Gut 1976; 17: 906–10.
23. Steer S, Jones H, Hibbert J, Gibson T, Sanderson J. CT defined sacroiliitis and HLA-B27 in Crohn's disease. Gut 1999; 44(Suppl 1.): A41.
24. Orchard TR, Thiyagaraja S, Welsh KI, Wordsworth BP, Hill Gaston JS, Jewell DP. Clinical phenotype is related to HLA genotype in the peripheral arthropathies of inflammatory bowel disease. Gastroenterology 2000; 118: 274–8.
25. Ebringer A. Ankylosing spondylitis is caused by Klebsiella. Evidence from immunogenetic, microbiologic, and serologic studies. Rheum Dis Clin N Am 1992; 18: 105–21.
26. Gaston J, Life P, Granfors K et al. Synovial T lymphocyte recognition of organisms that trigger reactive arthritis. Clin Exp Immunol 1989; 76: 348–53.

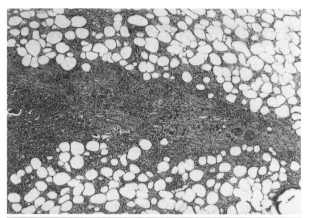

Figure 1. Predominantly septal panniculitis with secondary involvement of surrounding fat lobules, typical of erythema nodosum.

with CD, perianal fissures and fistulas were found in 36% of patients [9]. Only 25% of those patients with small bowel disease alone had perianal involvement, whereas more than 40% of patients with colonic disease exhibited perianal disease [9]. The perianal fissures and fistulas of IBD are typically multiple and involve the anus circumferentially. Abscesses, undermined ulcers, and skin tags or 'pseudo' skin tags formed by edematous skin are often noted on the perineum. The edema can be so severe as to produce lymphedema [10]. Histologic examination of the perianal inflammatory lesions characteristically shows transmural inflammation with lymphoid aggregates and non-caseating sarcoidal-type granulomas typical of CD. In one series of 29 biopsies, granulomas were identified in 25 [11]. The clinical and histologic findings may help distinguish CD from UC, as perianal disease is rare in UC. Perifistular and peristomal disease is less helpful diagnostically; since once a colostomy has been performed or cutaneous fistulas have developed, the diagnosis of CD is secured.

Oral Crohn's disease

Examination of the oral cavity allows clinicians to readily observe two of the classic morphologic features of CD: ulceration and cobblestoning. The ulcers are often tiny, herpetiform, occasionally linear, and may resemble ordinary aphthae. They can, of course, become large, undermining and indolent. When linear ulcers or tissues connect and the intervening mucosa is edematous, a 'cobblestone' appearance develops [10].

The oral manifestations of CD tend to vary by location within the mouth. The buccal mucosa appears to be the most common site of cobblestoning, while the gingival and alveolar mucosae often exhibit tiny nodular growths [12]. Linear ulcers are more common in sulci [12]; the lips may become swollen, hardened, or ulcerated, especially at the angles of the mouth [13]. Because of the granulomatous histology the lip changes have been called cheilitis glandularis [14]. It is unclear from previous studies how often granulomatous inflammation of the lip is associated with CD as compared to being associated with Melkerson–Rosenthal syndrome or being idiopathic. Finally, there may even be inflammation and ulceration of the epiglottis and larynx [10].

While nodules or ulcers with granulomatous histology strongly implicate CD, the role of aphthous ulcers is less clear. Some studies [12] have suggested that they are a non-specific finding, while others [10] suggest that they may be the most frequent oral lesions seen in CD. Aphthae, oral lesions, and oral ulcerations have been estimated to occur in between 4% and 20% of CD patients [15, 16]. In the UCEDS study only five of 569 patients (1%) had aphthae at the beginning of the study, but another 23 (4%) developed them during the study even on systemic therapy [17]. These figures are not incompatible with the presence of aphthae in the general population. Although aphthae in CD have not been studied in depth histologically, they do not appear to be granulomatous.

Despite these caveats the presence of apthhae can suggest the diagnosis of CD [16]. If a biopsy shows a granulomatous histology, CD should be the major consideration in the microscopic differential diagnosis. Recurrent aphthae may be the first manifestation of CD; thus a history of their presence may prove useful in the work-up of patients with chronic diarrhea and/or abdominal pain.

Metastatic Crohn's disease

Metastatic CD refers to nodules, plaques, or ulcerated lesions that demonstrate a granulomatous histology identical to that of the IBD, and that are located in the skin and subcutaneous tissue at sites distant from the gastrointestinal lesions of CD. Metastatic cutaneous CD is rare; studies [18] have emphasized a flexural distribution, and have shown that metastatic CD may be non-ulcerative and may even mimic erythema nodosum [19, 20].

Metastatic CD can be viewed as still another 'great imitator' both clinically and histologically. Cases have been initially diagnosed as factitial dermatitis, intertrigo, severe acne, hidradenitis suppurativa, chronic cellulitis, or erythema nodosum among many other entities [10]. Metastatic CD does not seem to appear in the absence of gastrointestinal CD. Histologically, most patients present with typical sarcoidal granulomas, raising the microscopic differential diagnosis of infection, sarcoid, and a foreign-body reaction. Rarely, cases of metastatic CD may differ histologically. Two patients with erythema nodosum-like lesions showed granulomatous perivasculitis [10].

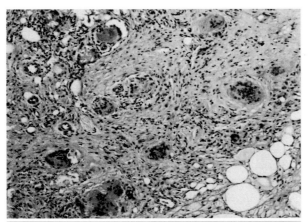

Figure 2. Close-up view of the septal inflammatory process includes characteristic multinucleated giant cells and small non-caseating granulomata.

Reactive cutaneous lesions of IBD

Erythema nodosum (EN) typically presents as tender red nodules on the anterior aspect of the lower legs that gradually resolve in several weeks. EN has been reported in 1–10% of patients with UC, however, a more reasonable figure is around 4% [21], and it appears to be more common in female patients. It may occur before the diagnosis of IBD or in conjunction with a clinical flare-up of the disease, and it may occur in unusual locations and in chronic forms [2]. Ulceration is common and concomitant arthropathy is often noted. Significant skin involvement may be accompanied by fever and malaise [21].

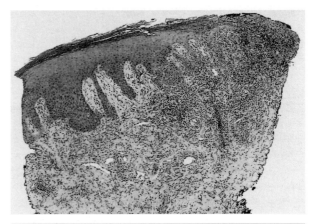

Figure 3. Focal ulceration of the epidermis with underlying predominantly neutrophilic infiltrate, characteristic of pyoderma gangrenosum and other neutrophilic dermatoses.

EN does not appear to be a good marker for CD. In large series of patients with EN, very few have CD [2]. Furthermore, all nodose lesions on the extremities of CD patients are not erythema nodosum. Histologically, in addition to the septal panniculitis of EN, one may see polyarteritis or granulomatous inflammation. Thus, in a CD patient with EN-like lesions clinically, a biopsy of sufficient depth and size to evaluate the subcutaneous fat as well as the dermis is a necessity.

EN is believed to represent the expression of a hyperimmune response and may be seen in association with various disease entities and as a reaction to various drugs (Figs 1 and 2). The possibility of a drug reaction should be considered in all patients with EN, especially those being treated with sulfa derivatives. It is interesting to note that studies have suggested that EN may be the most common extracolonic manifestation of UC in children [1] and that usually the lesions heal without scarring.

Pyoderma gangrenosum

Pyoderma gangrenosum (PG) usually begins with small papules, plaques, or hemorrhagic blisters that rapidly enlarge and ulcerate with violaceous undermined edges. The lesions may occur anywhere on the skin, but most frequently are located on the lower extremities. Patients may give a history of preceding trauma to the area. Lesions are sterile and are characterized by a dense dermal infiltrate of neutrophils (Figs 3 and 4). PG has been noted in approxi-

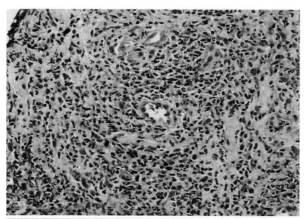

Figure 4. Close-up reveals a predominantly neutrophilic dermatosis surrounding reactive blood vessels without evidence of vasculitis. These histologic findings are typical of any of the various neutrophilic dermatoses, including pyoderma gangrenosum.

mately 5% of patients with UC and is roughly three times more common in UC than in CD [22]. However, one series found a higher incidence of PG in CD – it occurred in 8% of these patients [23]. Approximately 50% of patients with PG have underlying UC [23, 24]. This makes UC by far the most common identifiable underlying cause. The course of IBD-associated PG tends to parallel that of the underlying gastrointestinal disease [6, 25] and may even begin years before the onset of bowel symptoms [26].

The pathogenesis of PG, as well as the basis of its standing association with UC, remain obscure. Evidence favors an altered immune response and most investigators believe that the pathogenesis of the skin disorder and its association with UC are both based on immunologic mechanisms. Confusion persists in the fact that the immune defects reported vary greatly from patient to patient, and no one common defect has as yet become apparent. No consistent genetic markers have been identified in various groups of patients studied [21].

The treatment of PG, as with EN, is first directed at the underlying disease but, in contrast to the latter, PG may not respond nearly as rapidly during remissions of UC. In fact, PG has been reported occurring years after apparent cure of UC [21].

Vesiculopustular eruption

A vesiculopustular eruption that can be localized or generalized has been described in some patients with UC [27]. The lesions consist of grouped erythematous vesiculopustules (3–5 mm in size) that sequentially crust and heal, resulting in postinflammatory hyperpigmentation. Some authors consider this entity to be a *forme fruste* of PG; cases have been reported in which most lesions of a vesiculopustular eruption have resolved while a few lesions developed into typical PG [28, 29]. Histologic examination reveals intraepidermal neutrophilic abscesses with mixed inflammatory dermal infiltrates [27].

Pyoderma vegetans

Pyoderma vegetans has been described in several patients with UC [21, 30]. It initially appears mainly in intertriginous areas with vegetating plaques and vesiculopustules that resolve with postinflammatory hyperpigmentation. Mucosal involvement may also occur (pyostomatitis vegetans), Histologically, the principal features include pseudoepitheliomatous hyperplasia and intraepidermal abscesses that contain neutrophils and eosinophils. Pyoderma vegetans may also represent a *forme fruste* of PG (Fig. 3) [21].

Cutaneous vasculitis and polyarteritis nodosa

Cutaneous vasculitis is a rare cutaneous manifestation of IBD [31]. Both leukocytoclastic vasculitis and cutaneous polyarteritis nodosa have been reported. Vasculitis is more commonly associated with UC whereas polyarteritis nodosa has been documented only in association with CD [2].

Necrotizing (leukocytoclastic) vasculitis generally presents as palpable purpura, ulcerations, and, rarely, gangrene [2]. The usual sites of involvement are the legs and anal areas. Mixed cryoglobulinemia may sometimes be demonstrated in these patients. Histologic examination reveals fibrin thrombi and/or fibrinoid necrosis of blood vessel walls with associated leukocytoclasia and extravasated erythrocytes.

Cutaneous polyarteritis nodosa is characterized by tender or painful erythematous nodules which often ulcerate. They are commonly located on the legs but may affect other areas of the body. The lesions can be clinically mistaken for EN, metastatic CD or PG. The biopsy specimen exhibits a necrotizing leukocytoclastic panarteritis that may show granulomatous features and often a variable infiltrate of eosinophils. Associated features of cutaneous polyarteritis nodosa include livedo reticularis, peripheral neuropathy, arthralgias, and myalgias; severe systemic involvement does not occur. Cutaneous polyarteritis nodosa usually runs a benign but chronic course that is usually unrelated to the activity of the bowel disease [31, 32]. Cutaneous polyarteritis nodosa usually presents after the diagnosis of CD has been established, but may occur before the diagnosis of IBD [31–34]. Circulating immune complexes have been demonstrated and may contribute to the pathogenesis [33, 34].

Epidermolysis bullosa acquisita (EBA)

There appears to be a greater than chance association between EBA and IBD, particularly CD. EBA is an acquired blistering disorder that occurs mainly on the knees, elbows, hands, and feet. It is mediated by antibody deposition and immune activation at the dermo-epidermal junction [34–36]. When it occurs in relation to CD it usually begins many years after the onset of the bowel disease – it may be best considered a long-term complication of CD.

Other associations

Reactive eruptions such as erythema multiforme and urticaria may occur in patients with IBD [24]. These may be due in part to a response to the disease or its treatment. An increased incidence of thromboembolic events, clubbing, psoriasis, and vitiligo has also been noted in patients with IBD [24, 37, 38]. Palmar erythema has been associated with CD [10]. A case report of acne fulminans has suggested an association with CD [39]. The association of psoriasis and vitiligo with IBD may be related to HLA linkage rather than a true cause-and-effect relation [24]. Secondary amyloidosis may rarely develop in the setting of chronic inflammatory disorders including CD and UC [2].

Conclusion

It is important to become acquainted with the various cutaneous manifestations of IBD because some of them may serve as sentinels of the disease

Table 2. Skin conditions more common in Crohn's disease than ulcerative colitis

Fissures and fistulas
Oral Crohn's disease
Metastatic Crohn's disease
Cutaneous polyarteritis nodosa
Epidermolysis bullosa acquisita
Vitiligo
Acne fulminans
Palmar erythema

Table 3. Skin conditions more common in ulcerative colitis than Crohn's disease

Erythema nodosum
Pyoderma gangrenosum (by most reports)
Vesiculopustular eruption
Pyoderma vegetans
Leukocytoclastic vasculitis

Table 4. Cutaneous manifestations which may precede the development of IBD

Perianal disease
Aphthous ulcers
Pyoderma gangrenosum
Erythema nodosum
Cutaneous polyarteritis nodosa

and may actually help to clarify a diagnosis. Approximately one-quarter of all Crohn's patients will present initially with perianal disease [10], and oral changes may precede intestinal symptoms. The skin conditions which have been reported to precede the development of IBD are listed in Table 4. Moreover, skin disease may help to clarify a diagnosis and aid in the distinction between CD and UC, still a challenging clinical and histopathologic differential diagnosis. Some cutaneous changes are far more common in CD than in UC and vice-versa (Tables 2 and 3). When a patient presents with perioral disease or granulomatous skin disease at multiple sites or the oral cavity, the intestinal disease will invariably be CD. Conversely, the presence of a vesiculopustular eruption, pyoderma vegetans, or even a leukocytoclastic vasculitis favors a diagnosis of UC.

The pathogenesis of the cutaneous aspects of IBD probably reflects the immunologic basis of the intestinal disease. The presence of skin changes suggests that the same factors which elicit and propagate the gut disease are capable of stimulating an abnormal immune response in the skin. Whether or not these responses are the result of crossreacting antigens or the deposition of circulating immune complexes remains unclear. It remains to be seen whether the immunologic/microbiologic advances which promise to unlock the secrets of the etiologies of CD and UC in the near future will similarly shed light on the pathogenesis of the many and varied cutaneous changes which may herald and accompany these diseases

References

1. Samitz MH, Greenberg MS. Skin lesions in association with ulcerative colitis. Gastroenterology 1951; 19: 476–9.
2. Gregory B, Ho VC. Cutaneous manifestations of gastro-intestinal disease. Part II. J Am Acad Dermatol 1992; 26: 371–83.
3. Greenstein AJ, Janowitz HD, Sachar DB. The extra-intestinal complications of Crohn's disease and ulcerative colitis: a study of 700 patients. Medicine 1976; 55: 401–12.
4. Bianchi CA. Cutaneous manifestations of the malabsorption syndrome. Med Cutan Ibero Lat Am 1984; 12: 277–85.
5. Delahoussaye AR. Cutaneous manifestations of nutritional diseases. Dermatol Clin 1989; 7: 559–70.
6. Basler RSW, Dubin HV. Ulcerative colitis and the skin. Arch Dermatol 1976; 112: 531–4.
7. Tremaine WJ. Treatment of erythema nodosum, aphthous stomatitis, and pyoderma gangrenosum in patients with IBD. Inflam Bowel Dis 1998; 4: 68–9.
8. Habif TP. Clinical Dermatology: A Color Guide To Diagnosis and Therapy, 3rd edn. St Louis: Mosby, 1998.
9. Rankin GB, Watts HD, Melnyck CS et al. National Cooperative Crohn's Disease Study: extraintestinal manifestations and perianal complications. Gastroenterology 1979; 77: 914–20.
10. Burgdorf W. Cutaneous manifestations of Crohn's disease. Am Acad Dermatol 1981; 5: 689–95.
11. Lockhart-Mummery HE, Morson BC. Crohn's disease of the large intestine. Gut 1964; 5: 493–509.
12. Bernstein ML, McDonald JS. Oral lesions in Crohn's disease: report of two cases and update of the literature. Oral Surg 1978; 46: 234–45.
13. Issa MA. Crohn's disease of the mouth. Br Dent J 1971; 130: 247–8.
14. Kolokotronis A, Antoniades D, Trigonidis G, Papanagiotou P. Granulomatous cheilitis: a study of six cases. Oral Dis 1997; 3: 188–92.
15. Basu MK, Asquith P, Thompson RA, Cooke WT. Oral manifestations of Crohn's disease. Gut 1975; 16: 249–54.
16. Kraft SC. Crohn's disease of the mouth. Ann Intern Med 1975; 83: 570–1.
17. Rankin GB, Watts HD, Melnyk CS, Kelley ML Jr. National Cooperative Crohn's Disease Study: extraintestinal manifestations and perianal complications. Gastroenterology 1979; 77: 914–20.
18. Shum DT, Guenther L. Metastatic Crohn's disease: case report and review of the literature. Arch Dermatol 1990; 126: 645–8.
19. Parks AG, Morson BC, Pegum JS. Crohn's disease with cutaneous involvement. Proc R Soc Med 1965; 58: 241–2.
20. Witkowski JA, Parish LC, Lewis JE. Crohn's disease – non-caseating granulomas on the legs. Acta Derm Venereol (Stockh) 1977; 57: 181–3.
21. Basler RSW, Ulcerative colitis and the skin. Med Clin N Am 1980; 64: 941–54.
22. Loeffel ED, Koya D. Cutaneous manifestations of gastrointestinal disease. Cutis 1978; 21: 852–61.
23. Paller AS. Cutaneous changes associated with inflammatory bowel disease. Pediatr Dermatol 1986; 3: 439–45.
24. Samitz MH. Dermatologic manifestations of gastrointestinal disease. In: Berk EJ, ed. Gastroenterology. Philadelphia: WB Saunders, 1985: 285–315.
25. Edwards FC, Truelove SC. The course and prognosis of ulcerative colitis. Gut 1964; 5: 1–15.
26. Powell FC, Perry HO. Pyoderma gangrenosum in childhood. Arch Dermatol 1984; 120: 757–61.
27. Fenske NA, Gern JE, Pierce D et al. Vesiculopustular eruption of ulcerative colitis. Arch Dermatol 1983; 119: 664–9.
28. Callen JP, Woo TY. Vesiculopustular eruption in a patient with ulcerative colitis. Arch Dermatol 1985; 121: 399–404.
29. O'Loughlin S, Perry HO. A diffuse pustular eruption associated with ulcerative colitis. Arch Dermatol 1978; 114: 1961–4.
30. Johnson ML, Wilson HTH. Skin lesions in ulcerative colitis. Gut 1969; 10: 255–63.
31. Kahn EI, Daum F, Aiges HW et al. Cutaneous polyarteritis nodosa associated with Crohn's disease. Dis Colon Rectum 1980; 23: 258–62.
32. Chalvardjian A, Nethercott JR. Cutaneous granulomatous vasculitis associated with Crohn's disease. Cutis 1982; 30: 645–55.
33. Goslen JB, Graham W, Lazarus GS. Cutaneous polyarteritis nodosa: report of a case associated with Crohn's disease. Arch Dermatol 1983; 119: 326–9.
34. Solley GO, Winkelmann RK, Rovelstad RA. Correlation between regional enteritis and cutaneous polyarteritis nodosa: two cases and review of the literature. Gastroenterology 1975; 69: 235–9.
35. Pegum JS, Wright JT. Epidermolysis bullosa acquisita and Crohn's disease. Proc R Soc Med 1973; 66: 234.
36. Livden JK, Nilsen R, Thunold S et al. Epidermolysis bullosa acquisita and Crohn's disease. Acta Derm Venereol (Stockh.) 1978; 58: 241–4.
37. Ray TL, Levine JB, Weiss W et al. Epidermolysis bullosa acquisita and inflammatory bowel disease. J Am Acad Dermatol 1982; 6: 242–52.
38. McPoland PR, Moss RL. Cutaneous Crohn's disease and progressive vitiligo. J Am Acad Dermatol 1988; 19: 421–5.
39. McAuley D, Miller RA. Acne fulminans associated with inflammatory bowel disease: report of a case. Arch Dermatol 1985; 121: 91–3.

41 | Fertility and pregnancy in inflammatory bowel disease

WILLIAM CONNELL

Introduction

Most patients with inflammatory bowel disease (IBD) experience concerns regarding fertility and pregnancy at some point of their reproductive life. These may relate to uncertainties concerning the future ability to have children, the wisdom and timing of pregnancy in IBD, the impact of disease on fetal development and delivery, and the safety of drug usage during this time. Anxiety regarding such issues is not always expressed, especially when the prospect of pregnancy is not a matter of immediate relevance. Nevertheless, many pregnancies are unexpected, and it is important for the clinician to prepare patients for such a possibility by introducing a general discussion of the topic soon after disease diagnosis. More specific details can then be provided to those who are actually pregnant or planning parenthood in the near future.

In the past, attention has focused on the relevance of these issues among women with IBD. However, there is an increasing recognition that the disorder and its treatment may also impact on male fertility and the wellbeing of babies born to men with the condition.

Genetic counseling

Although no prenatal test for IBD is currently available, genetic counseling is still appropriate for couples contemplating pregnancy in which one or both partners have IBD. Generally, this involves a discussion of the estimated risk to an offspring developing IBD as well as providing a perspective of the risk by highlighting background rates of malformation, miscarriage and perinatal death that apply in all pregnancies. Several studies have shown IBD tends to run in families, and a positive family history is reported to occur in 8–25% [1]. A higher frequency of IBD occurs among relatives of patients with Crohn's disease (CD) rather than ulcerative colitis (UC), and among relatives of patients who are Jewish [2]. Where one parent has CD the empiric risk of a child developing CD or IBD is estimated to be 7.4%, and 10.5% respectively [1]. There is preliminary evidence suggesting the transmission of susceptibility to CD in offspring may be higher if the affected parent with IBD is the mother [3]. If both parents have IBD the lifetime risk to children is quite high [4].

Because of a reluctance to use any medication during pregnancy, the indications for therapy and potential impact on fetal development are best discussed prior to conception. The effects of medication include those related to their use during pregnancy and lactation, as well as those exerted on men and women receiving therapy prior to, and at the time of, conception. Women with active disease who are unwilling to accept any possible risk of medical treatment may be best advised to consider surgical therapeutic alternatives or, in special circumstances, arrange egg storage. The need for folic acid supplements, which are routinely recommended before conception to reduce the risk of neural tube defects, should be emphasized to women using sulfasalazine.

Fertility

Although experience from the 1950s and 1960s suggested fertility rates were lower among women with UC [5], contemporary evidence shows this is not the case, at least in those with an intact colon [6–8]. Two large uncontrolled studies from the UK showed that 70–81% of women with UC under the age of 45 conceived normally, depending on the rate of voluntary birth control [7, 8]. The consistent finding in both studies was a 7–9% involuntary infertility rate, a figure that compares favorably with that occurring in

Stephan R. Targan, Fergus Shanahan and Loren C. Karp (eds.), Inflammatory Bowel Disease: From Bench to Bedside, 2nd Edition, 763–771.
© 2003 Kluwer Academic Publishers. Printed in Great Britain

the general population. In contrast, fecundity (the biological ability to conceive) appears to be substantially reduced in women with UC who have undergone restorative proctocolectomy, probably due to the development of pelvic adhesions [6].

Evidence shows fertility rates are decreased in females with CD. Early series suggested 32–53% of women with CD were infertile, especially those with Crohn's colitis [9, 10]. More recent surveys from Oxford and northeast Scotland recorded an involuntary infertility rate of 12–14% [8, 11]. An extensive case-controlled study from five different European countries showed a significant reduction in the proportion of women with CD who became pregnant and a reduced number of offspring in this group [12].

There are several factors which may explain why women with CD have fewer pregnancies. Among these, the most important appears to be a personal preference to avoid pregnancy [13]. In some cases women are discouraged from becoming pregnant by clinicians who focus excessively on the possible negative effects of drug therapy during this time [14]. Reduced sexual activity is more common among women with CD, especially in those with perianal inflammation, because of dyspareunia, abdominal pain, diarrhea and fear of incontinence [15].

It is well recognized that sulfasalazine may cause reversible infertility in men by reducing sperm motility and function [16]. This effect is usually transient, and not encountered with other 5-aminosalicylic agents. It has been presumed that this therapy accounts for the reduction in fertility observed among men with IBD. However, a study from the United Kingdom found that males with CD (but not UC) had fewer children, an effect that was independent of sulfasalazine usage [17]. The possible reasons for this finding are not explained, but a previous report has highlighted that long-term effects of disease activity or malnutrition may lead to oligospermia in some males with CD [18].

Neonatal outcome

According to the cumulative experience derived from several uncontrolled studies evaluating neonatal outcome in pregnant women with UC and CD, the chances of delivering a normal, full-term, live infant appear to be generally good [5–11, 19–25]. However, two case-controlled surveys have observed higher rates of neonatal complications among

women with IBD [26, 27]. A population-based study of women who had single births in Sweden during a 12-month period showed an increased rate of Cesarian section, prematurity and low-birthweight infants among IBD patients compared to healthy controls [26]. Details regarding underlying disease diagnosis and degree of disease activity were not reported in this study.

There is no evidence from either uncontrolled or case-controlled studies that neonatal complications are increased in UC [5–7, 19–24, 28]. In contrast, less favorable neonatal outcomes have been observed in CD [12–13, 28, 29]. A report from Denmark during a 10-year period showed a higher risk of prematurity and low-birthweight babies among women with CD compared to controls [29]. These findings support the findings of two earlier case-controlled studies in which an increased risk of prematurity was observed among patients with CD [12, 13].

There is considerable evidence linking disease activity, especially at the time of conception, to a higher frequency of fetal complications in IBD. In UC, women with quiescent disease at conception have higher rates of normal live births, and reduced rates of prematurity and spontaneous abortion compared to those with active disease at conception [22]. An increased rate of malformations has been described among medically treated women with active, but not inactive, UC [7].

In CD 80% of patients with quiescent disease at conception had a normal, uncomplicated live birth, compared to 50% of those with active disease [30]. Prematurity and spontaneous abortion are significantly increased in women with active disease at conception [25]. In women with active CD at conception, neonatal outcome is more favorable when inflammation improves during the remainder of pregnancy compared to when it is persistent [30].

Disease progress in pregnancy

In general the course of UC during pregnancy depends on the degree of intestinal inflammation at conception. According to the results of several uncontrolled studies evaluating pregnant patients with quiescent colitis at conception, approximately two-thirds remain in remission and one-third relapse. This proportion is similar to expected rates in the non-pregnant UC population. However, if colitis is active at conception, one-third improve, one-third remain persistently active and another third deteriorate. In other words, if UC is active at conception, two-thirds continue to have ongoing, persistent inflammation throughout pregnancy [5–7, 19–20, 22]. These symptoms can be particularly troublesome to control, thereby requiring vigorous medical therapy. Data from Israel raised the possibility that relapses were more common when pregnancy was unplanned [23].

Disease activity at conception also determines the course of CD during pregnancy. Uncontrolled studies of patients with quiescent CD at conception indicate that 75% remain in remission. In contrast, disease that is active at conception is likely to remain in this state, or actually deteriorate during pregnancy [9–11, 25]. Furthermore, the more severe the disease at conception, the more likely it is to remain active during pregnancy [30].

Whereas early studies suggested that post-partum flare-ups in CD were common [9, 10], recent data suggest this is not the case [8, 11, 25]. The reason for such a discrepancy is not known, but possibly relates to the past practice of elective withdrawal of sulfasalazine late in pregnancy due to concerns regarding the risk of neonatal kernicterus developing from sulfur-containing drugs [31]. In the light of further evidence showing this actual risk to be negligible, nowadays the drug is continued throughout this time [32].

The onset of UC in pregnancy or the puerperal period is not uncommon. In a study of 147 women with UC from Oxford, 8% experienced its onset during pregnancy and 4% post natally. Most cases were mild to moderate, and generally brought under control. Neonatal outcome was no different than if the disease preceded pregnancy [7]. The onset of CD appears relatively rare in pregnancy, possibly because of a natural reluctance to investigate pregnant women with pain and diarrhea. In the past the prognosis of such an event was thought to be poor [33], but data collected subsequently are more encouraging [8, 11, 25, 30].

Mode of delivery

For patients with quiescent colitis the risk of perineal sepsis following childbirth is low, and the mode of delivery is governed by obstetric indications [28]. It is unknown if patients with more active colitis are at higher risk of perineal complications. To avoid sphincter damage, Caeserian section has been advised for women with active, relapsing or fulmi-

nant disease, where the future prospect of ileoanal pelvic pouch surgery is high [34].

Information concerning the perianal consequences of vaginal delivery and episiotomy in patients with CD are conflicting. A highly selected survey of 117 female members of the Crohn's and Colitis Foundation of America who were free of perianal disease prior to pregnancy found 18% reported the development of complications in this region following vaginal delivery, most of which occurred within the first 2 months [35]. In contrast, a larger population study from Canada showed vaginal delivery rarely initiated the development of perianal disease in women without a previous history of this problem, and did not evoke a deterioration of symptoms in those with pre-existing inactive perianal disease. However, one-quarter of patients with active perianal disease at birth experienced an aggravation of their condition after vaginal delivery [36]. Accordingly, Ceserian section seems justified for women with active perianal CD, but not when perianal disease is absent or inactive prior to birth. It is important for obstetricians to exercise excellent care of the perineum if vaginal delivery is to be undertaken, and when episiotomy is required a mediolateral incision is preferable to reduce the risk of rectal tear [35].

Patients who have previously undergone total colectomy and iloestomy have an increased risk of stomal complications during pregnancy. Clinically, this may result in stomal dysfunction, prolapse, skin irritation, leakage, and sometimes intestinal obstruction [37]. Vaginal delivery may be undertaken in most of these patients without compromising maternal or neonatal outcome.

Patients who have previously undergone ileoanal pelvic pouch surgery for UC may experience an aggravation of stool frequency and incontinence during pregnancy. These effects are usually transient, and return to normal after delivery. Cesarian section is often recommended, though this practice is necessary only in patients with a scarred, non-compliant perineum, unless other obstetric reasons apply. For the majority of women with pelvic pouches, vaginal delivery and episotomy is well tolerated and rarely associated with the development of a rectal tear [38].

Investigations

Generally, investigations should be minimized during pregnancy and undertaken only when there is a very good clinical reason to do so. Provided it is done with exquisite care, flexible sigmoidoscopy and biopsy may be performed during pregnancy. In contrast, more extensive evaluation by colonoscopy should be reserved only for exceptional cases where its undertaking will influence management decisions; in which case fetal monitoring should be performed [39]. Investigations containing ionizing radiation should be avoided. Where necessary, ultrasound or magnetic resonance image scanning may be used to provide information regarding abscess formation or to assess bowel wall thickness. If obstruction or incipient toxic dilation is suspected, it is reasonable to perform a single plain abdominal X-ray. The risk of fetal toxicity from this investigation is extremely small, and outweighed by the consequences of these potentially serious maternal complications [40].

Surgery

The indications for surgery in IBD during pregnancy are similar to those in the non-pregnant state, namely severe hemorrhage, perforation, obstruction or severe disease unresponsive to medical therapy. The risks to mother and baby increase when surgical intervention is unduly delayed. Fetal morbidity is probably related more to the effects of underlying disease rather than the operation itself, since bowel surgery in pregnancy for reasons other than IBD has a relatively low risk to fetus. Although maternal mortality from emergency surgery for fulminant UC during pregnancy is declining, the risk of fetal death and social morbidity among parents thereafter is high [41].

Drug therapy

In view of the evidence associating a more favorable neonatal outcome with inactive maternal IBD, pharmacotherapy is often required to control disease activity before conception and to maintain remission or treat flare-ups during pregnancy. Although drugs may be associated with side-effects, the risk to the fetus is greater from uncontrolled disease inflammation [24]. The choice of agents depends on the severity of the disease, potential for side-effects, and the preference of the individual patient.

Clinical studies evaluating drug treatment in pregnant women with IBD are largely limited to 5-aminosalicylic acid drugs and corticosteroids.

Published data among IBD patients using other treatments in pregnancy are limited. Information regarding the safety of these drugs is mainly derived from the results of animal studies or clinical experience among patients with other conditions, such as organ transplantation or connective tissue disorders.

A summary of the effects of commonly used drugs for IBD during pregnancy and lacation is shown in Table I.

5-Aminosaliylic acid

Sulfasalazine and other 5-aminosalicylic formulations appear to be safe in pregnancy when used in recommended doses [42, 43]. The rates of spontaneous abortion, premature delivery, or congenital malformations for women with either UC or CD taking sulfasalazine are not increased [7, 11, 21, 22, 24]. A recent study showed that men with IBD who fathered a congenitally abnormal child were more likely to have used sulfasalazine [17]. Clinical series have demonstrated the overall safety in pregnancy of other 5-aminosalicylic formulations when used in low to moderate doses [43, 44]. A single case of renal insufficiency was reported in a newborn exposed to 4 g/day Pentasa during the mid-trimester [45]. Both sulfasalazine 5-aminosalicylic agents may be used during breast feeding, though isolated cases of transient acute diarrhea in the newborn have been reported [46, 47]. Concentrations of sulfasalazine and sulfapyridine in breast milk are insufficient to cause kernicterus [32].

Corticosteroids

Controlled and uncontrolled studies in patients with IBD, asthma and connective tissue disorders have shown no overall increase in the rate of any malformations nor fetal morbidity among babies exposed to steroids during pregnancy [21, 42, 48, 49]. Animal studies indicate an increased risk of oral cleft among offspring exposed to high doses of corticosteroids [50], and a report from the 1950s suggested this complication may also occur in humans [51]. A controlled study of 468 pregnant women treated with corticosteroids during pregnancy observed two cases of cleft palate in newborns, compared to 0.2 expected – numbers that were too small to be meaningful [52]. It can be presumed that any possible risk of cleft lip or palate from steroids is likely to be small, and one that must be weighed up

Table 1. Effects of drugs used for IBD in pregnancy and lacation

Drug	Pregnancy	Breast feeding
Sulfasalazine	Risk of miscarriage, prematurity or malformations not increased. Folate supplements recommended	Safe – reduce dose if neonatal jaundice is present
5-Aminosalicylic acid	Probably safe in doses < 3 g/day; higher doses may be nephrotoxic	Safe – occasional reports of reversible neonatal diarrhea
Corticosteroids	Probably safe – conflicting evidence regarding risk of oral cleft	Safe
Azathioprine	Malformations do not appear to be increased, but possible. Small risk of prematurity, low birthweight, fetal myelotoxicity, immunosuppression, transient chromosomal aberrations. Potential toxicity must be discussed with parents in advance and used only when clinically necessary	Not recommended due to risk of neonatal myelotoxicity or immunosuppression
6-Mercaptopurine	Teratogenic in animals at high doses. Human data sparse, but so far reassuring. Risks probably similar to azathioprine	Not recommended due to risk of neonatal myelotoxicity or immunosuppression
Methotrexate	Contraindicated due to risk of congenital abnormalities and abortion	Contraindicated
Cyclosporine	Possibly associated with prematurity and low birthweight	Not recommended
Metronidazole	Safe in short courses (< 10 days) but not recommended in high doses for prolonged periods	Not recommended
Ciprofloxacin	Defects in developing cartilage in animals. Short courses in human probably safe but not recommended for prolonged periods	Not recommended

against the drug's known beneficial effects in appropriate clinical circumstances. Women requiring prednisolone should not be discouraged from lactation [53]. There are no published data regarding the use of controlled-release budesonide preparations during pregnancy.

Azathioprine/6-mercaptopurine

Of all the various drug options to treat IBD, the safety of azathioprine and 6-mercaptopurine during pregnancy is the most controversial. Historically, pregnant women were cautioned against using these agents, due to early concerns about teratogenesis [54]. However, further data during the past two decades from patients with organ transplantation or connective tissue diseases have shown azathioprine to be generally well tolerated [55–58]. Occasional malformations have been reported, but the overall frequency is no different compared to observed rates in the general population, and no characteristic pattern of abnormality is evident [57, 58]. It is possible that the fetal immune system is transiently compromised from azathioprine exposure during the second and third trimesters, and this may result in growth retardation [59]. Cases of prematurity, neonatal myelotoxicity, thymic atrophy and transient chromosomal abnormalities have also been reported with azathioprine usage in pregnancy [58, 60]. Importantly, long-term follow-up effects among children who were exposed to the drug antenatally are lacking. One study in IBD observed no congenital abnormalities or subsequent health problems in 16 children born to mothers treated with azathioprine during pregnancy [61]. Provided the drug is used in recommended doses during pregnancy, the risks associated with azathioprine appear to be small. Because potential complications may be serious, its use should be reserved for refractory maternal disease only.

Little clinical information exists concerning 6-mercaptopurine usage in pregnancy, leading to uncertainty about its safety [49, 62]. In animals, 6-mercaptopurine is teratogenic and long-term effects have been described on germ cells of exposed offspring [63]. A study among patients with IBD observed rates of prematurity and significant congenital malformation to be 3% and 5% respectively [62]. Until more data are available the use of this drug in pregnancy will remain controversial.

Increasing attention has been drawn to the possible effects of azathioprine or 6-mercaptopurine on spermatogenesis. Among 13 children born to fathers receiving 6-mercaptopurine for IBD at conception, the rate of congenital malformations and spontaneous abortions was higher than in a control group of men who did not receive the drug [64]. In contrast, 58 of 60 babies born to male transplant recipients treated with azathioprine at conception were normal [65]. A recent study showed that semen quality was not affected by azathioprine, and in a small number of children born to fathers treated with azathioprine at conception, fetal outcome and post natal development were normal [66]. At present, there is insufficient evidence to discourage the use of either azathioprine or 6-mercaptopurine in men contemplating fatherhood.

Azathioprine is transferred to breast milk in small quantities, and lactating babies may be at slight risk of immunosuppression and myelotoxicity [67]. Its use is not generally recommended during breast-feeding, but a decision regarding this should take into account the benefits of breast milk, as well as the personal preference of the mother [58].

Cyclosporine

Occasionally, cyclosporine may be justified in pregnancy for patients with severe UC who would otherwise require emergency surgery. Two large series of transplant recipients receiving cyclosporine during pregnancy observed rates of congenital malformations that were similar to that expected in the general population [55, 68]. However, the drug has been associated with growth retardation and prematurity in patients with organ transplants [58].

Fetal and maternal outcomes were satisfactory according to a single case report when cyclosporine was administered during the second trimester for severe UC [69]. Due to concerns regarding possible nephrotoxicity or immunosuppression, cyclosporine has not been recommended during lactation. However, a recent report showed concentrations of the drug in breast milk to be low, and breast-fed babies did not develop any adverse effects [70].

Methotrexate

The elective use of methotrexate is contraindicated in pregnancy because of its embryotoxic and teratogenic effect [49]. The critical period of exposure is between 6 and 8 weeks of gestation, and the harmful effects on the fetus may be dose-related [71]. Its use in pregnancy can also be associated with fetal growth retardation, neonatal bone marrow suppression and possible chromosomal aberration [72]. Methotrexate may temporarily impair male fertility, and its effects can persist for several months after drug withdrawal. Accordingly, men and women are advised to discontinue methotrexate for several months before attempting conception [49]. Methotrexate is excreted into breast milk in small amounts, and is contraindicated during breast-feeding.

Antibiotics

Metronidazole and ciprofloxacin are increasingly used as primary therapy for CD. According to two large meta-analyses, treatment with metronidazole for less than 10 days during the first trimester was not associated with an increased risk of malformations [73, 74]. Moreover, this therapy does not seem to be associated with an increased frequency of stillbirths, growth retardation or prematurity [75]. Ciprofloxacin has been associated with the development of arthropathy in the offspring of animals exposed to the drug antenatally [76]. However, a prospective study in humans demonstrated no increased risk of malformations or musculoskeletal problems in 38 women receiving either ciprofloxacin or norfloxacin during the first trimester for urinary tract infection [77]. Nonetheless, there are no published data concerning the safety of either drug in IBD, especially when given at high doses for a prolonged period. Because the effects on breast-fed babies are uncertain, their use in lactation is not recommended.

Infliximab

There is little published information regarding the safety of infliximab on the developing fetus or breast-fed infant. Mutagenesis was not observed in preclinical studies with infliximab, and successful live births have occurred following its use in pregnancy [78]. However, the drug should not be used electively during pregnancy or lactation until more data are available.

Does pregnancy alter the natural history of IBD?

The future outcome of pregnancy in IBD cannot be predicted on the basis of what happened in a previous pregnancy [7]. However, it is possible that parity may improve the long-term outcome of IBD. A study of patients with CD showed the mean number of resections was lower and the interval between resections was longer in parous women than non-parous individuals [79]. A small study from Italy found rates of relapse from IBD to be reduced 3–4 years after delivery compared to the corresponding period prior to pregnancy [80].

Summary

Most women with IBD can expect an uneventful pregnancy. Evidence compiled over many years indicates the importance of controlling disease activity at the time of conception and during pregnancy to optimize the outcome for mother and baby. For this reason drug therapy is often required to treat flare-ups and maintain remission during this time. Where possible, women with IBD should plan a pregnancy to coincide with times when the disease is quiescent, and drug treatment minimal. In practice, however, many pregnancies are unexpected or occur in women with active disease that requires intensive medical therapy. Provided adequate information has been supplied in advance of conception, much of the apprehension that accompanies these events can be substantially reduced. Ongoing supervision by the clinician during pregnancy and the puerperium provides invaluable support, and enables maternal disease flare-ups to be identified and treated as expediently as possible.

References

1. Peeters M, Nevens H, Baert F *et al*. Familial aggregation in Crohn's disease: increased age-adjusted risk and concordance in clinical characteristics. Gastroenterology 1996; 111: 597–603.
2. Yang H, McElree C, Roth MP, Shanahan F, Targan SR, Rotter JI. Familial empirical risks for inflammatory bowel disease: differences between Jews and non-Jews. Gut 1993; 34: 517–24.
3. Akolkar PN, Gulwani-Akolkar B, Heresbach D *et al*. Differences in risk of Crohn's disease in offspring of mothers and fathers with inflammatory bowel disease. Am J Gastroenterol 1997; 92: 2241–4.
4. Bennett RA, Rubin PH, Present DH. Frequency of inflammatory bowel disease in offspring of couples both presenting with inflammatory bowel disease. Gastroenterology 1991; 100: 1638–43.
5. de Dombal FT, Watts JM, Watkinson G, Goligher JC. Ulcerative colitis and pregnancy. Lancet 1965; 2: 599–602.
6. Olsen KO, Juul S, Berndtsson I, Oresland T, Laurberg S. Ulcerative colitis: female fecundity before diagnosis, during disease and after surgery compared with a population sample. Gastroenterology 2002; 122: 15–19.
7. Willoughby CP, Truelove SC. Ulcerative colitis and pregnancy. Gut 1980; 21; 469–74.
8. Hudson M, Flett G, Sinclair TS, Brunt PW, Templeton A, Mowat NAG. Fertility and pregnancy in inflammatory bowel disease. Int J Gynecol Obstet 1997; 58: 229–37.
9. Fielding JF, Cooke WT. Pregnancy and Crohn's disease. Br Med J 1970; 2: 76–7.
10. De Dombal FT, Burton IL, Goligher JC. Crohn's disease and pregnancy. Br Med J 1972; 3: 550–3.
11. Khosla R, Willoughby CP, Jewell DP. Crohn's disease and pregnancy. Gut 1984; 25: 52–6.
12. Mayberry JF, Weterman IT. European survey of fertility and pregnancy in women with Crohn's disease: a case control study by European collaborative group. Gut 1986; 27: 821–5.
13. Baird DD, Narendranathan M, Sandler RS. Increased risk of preterm birth for women with inflammatory bowel disease. Gastroenterology 1990; 99: 987–94.
14. Korelitz BI. Inflammatory bowel disease and pregnancy. Gastroenterol Clin N Am 1998; 27: 213–24.
15. Moody GA, Probert CSJ, Srivastava EM, Rhodes J, Mayberry JF. Sexual dysfunction amongst women with Crohn's disease: a hidden problem. Digestion 1992; 52: 179–83.
16. O'Morain C, Smethurst P, Dore CJ, Levi AJ. Reversible male infertility due to sulphasalazine: studies in men and rats. Gut 1984; 25: 1078–84.
17. Moody GA, Probert C, Jayanthi V, Mayberry JF. The effects of chronic ill health and treatment with sulphasalazine on fertility amongst men and women with inflammatory bowel disease in Leicestershire. Int J Colorectal Dis 1997; 12: 220–4.
18. Farthing MJG, Dawson AM. Impaired semen quality in Crohn's disease – drugs, ill health or undernutrition? Scand J Gastroenterol, 1983; 18; 57–60.
19. MacDougall I. Ulcerative colitis and pregnancy. Lancet 1956; 2: 641–3.
20. McEwan HP. Ulcerative colitis in pregnancy. Proc R Soc Med. 1972; 65: 279–81.
21. Mogadam M, Dobbins WO, Korelitz BI, Ahmed SW. Pregnancy in inflammatory bowel disease: effect of sulfasalazine and corticosteroids on fetal outcome. Gastroenterology 1981; 80: 72–6.
22. Nielsen OH, Andreasson B, Bondesen S, Jarnum S. Pregnancy in ulcerative colitis. Scand J Gastroenterol 1983; 18: 735–42.

23. Levy N, Roisman I, Teodor I. Ulcerative colitis in pregnancy in Israel. Dis Colon Rectum, 1981; 24: 351–54.

24. Baiocco PJ, Korelitz BI. The influence of inflammatory bowel disease and its treatment on pregnancy and fetal outcome. J Clin Gastroenterol 1984; 6: 211–16.

25. Nielsen OH, Andreasson B, Bondesen S, Jacobsen O, Jarnum S. Pregnancy in Crohn's disease. Scand J Gastroenterol 1984; 19: 724–32.

26. Kornfeld D, Cnattingius S, Ekbom A. Pregnancy outcomes in women with inflammatory bowel disease – a population-based cohort study. Am J Obstet Gynecol 1997; 177: 942–6.

27. Fedorkow DM, Persaud D, Nimrod CA. Inflammatory bowel disease: a controlled study of late pregnancy outcome. Am J Obstet Gynecol 1989; 160: 998–1001.

28. Porter RJ, Stirrat GM. The effects of inflammatory bowel disease on pregnancy: a case-controlled retrospective analysis. Br J Obstet Gynaecol 1986; 93: 1124–31.

29. Fonager K, Sorensen HT, Olsen J, Dahlerup JF, Rasmussen SN. Pregnancy outcome for women with Crohn's disease: a follow-up study based on linkage between national registries. Am J Gastroenterol 1998; 93: 2426–30.

30. Woolfson K, Cohen Z, McLeod RS. Crohn's disease and pregnancy. Dis Colon Rectum 1990; 33: 869–73.

31. Silvermann WA, Andersen DH, Blanc WA, Crozier DN. A difference in mortality rate and incidence of kernicterus among infants allotted to two prophylactic antibacterial regimens. Pediatrics 1956; 18: 614–24.

32. Esbjorner E, Jarnerot G, Wranne L. Sulphasalazine and sulphapyridine serum levels in children to mothers treated with sulphasalazine during pregnancy and lactation. Acta Paediatr Scand 1987; 76: 137–42.

33. Jarnerot G Fertility, sterility, and pregnancy in chronic inflammatory bowel disease. Scand J Gastroenterol 1982; 17: 1–4.

34. Kelly MJ, Hunt TM, Wicks ACB, Mayne CJ. Fulminant ulcerative colitis and parturition: a need to alter current management? Br J Obstet Gynaecol 1994; 101: 166–7.

35. Brandt LJ, Estabrook SG, Reinus JF. Results of a survey to evaluate whether vaginal delivery and episiotomy lead to perineal involvement in women with Crohn's disease. Am J Gastroenterol 1995; 90: 1918–22.

36. Ilnyckyji A, Blanchard JF, Rawsthorne P, Bernstein CN. Perianal Crohn's disease and pregnancy; the role of the mode of delivery. Am J Gastroenterol 1999; 94: 3274–8.

37. Gopal KA, Amshel AL, Shonberg IL, Levinson BA, VanWert M, VanWert J. Ostomy and pregnancy. Dis Colon Rectum 1985: 28: 912–16.

38. Juhasz ES, Fozard B, Dozois RR, Ilstrup DM, Nelson H. Ileal pouch–anal anastomosis function following childbirth: an extended evaluation. Dis Colon Rectum 1995; 38: 159–65.

39. Cappell MS, Colon VJ, Sidhom OA. A study at 10 medical centers of the safety and efficacy of 48 flexible sigmoidoscopies and 8 colonoscopies during pregnancy with follow-up of fetal outcomes and with comparison to control groups. Dig Dis Sci 1996; 41: 2353–61.

40. Subhani JM, Hamiliton MI. Review article: the management of inflammatory bowel disease during pregnancy. Alimen Pharmacol Ther 1998; 12: 1039–53.

41. Anderson JB, Turner GM, Williamson RCN. Fulminant ulcerative colitis in late pregnancy and the puerperium. J R Soc Med, 1987; 80: 492–4.

42. Donaldson RM. Management of medical problems in pregnancy – inflammatory bowel disease. N Engl J Med 1985; 312: 1616–9.

43. Marteau P, Tennenbaum R, Elefant E, Lemann M, Cosnes J. Foetal outcome in women with inflammatory bowel disease treated during pregnancy with oral mesalazine microgranules. Alimen Pharmacol Ther 1998; 12: 1101–8.

44. Diav-Citrin O, Park YH, Veerasuntharam G *et al.* The safety of mesalamine in human pregnancy: a prospective controlled cohort study. Gastroenterology 1998; 114: 23–8.

45. Colombel J, Brabant G, Gubler MC *et al.* Renal insufficiency in infant: side-effect of prenatal exposure to mesalazine? Lancet 1994; 344: 620–1.

46. Branski D, Kerem E, Gross-Kieselstein E *et al.* Bloody diarrhea possible complication of sulfasalazine transferred through human breast milk. J Pediatr Gastroenterol Nutr 1986; 5: 316–17.

47. Nelis GF. Diarrhoea due to 5-aminosalicylic acid in breast milk. Lancet 1989; 1: 383.

48. Schatz M. Asthma treatment during pregnancy. What can be safely taken? Drug Safety 1997; 16: 342–50.

49. Bermas BL, Hill JA. Effects of immunosuppressive drugs during pregnancy. Arthritis Rheum 1995; 38: 1722–32.

50. Pinski L, DiGeorge AM. Cleft palate in the mouse: a teratogenic index of glucocorticoid potency. Science 1965; 147: 402–3.

51. Harris JWS, Ross IP. Cortisone therapy in early pregnancy: relation to cleft palate. Lancet 1956; 1: 1045–7.

52. Fraser FC, Sajoo A. Teratogenic potential of corticosteroids in humans. Teratology 1995; 5: 45–6.

53. Ost L, Wettrell G, Bjorkhem I *et al.* Prednisolone excretion into breast milk. J Pediatr 1985; 106: 1008–11.

54. Registration Committee of the European Dialysis and Transplant Association. Successful pregnancies in women treated by dialysis and kidney transplantation. Br J Obstet Gynaecol 1980; 87: 839–45.

55. Armenti VT, Ahlswede KM, Ahlswede BA *et al.* National transplantation pregnancy registry: outcomes of 154 pregnancies in cyclosporin-treated female kidney transplant recipients. Transplantation 1994; 57: 502–6.

56. Ramsay-Goldman R, Mientus JM, Kutzer JE *et al.* Pregnancy outcome in women with systemic lupus erythematosus treated with immunosuppressive drugs. J Rheum 1993; 20: 1152–7.

57. Ramsey-Goldman R, Schilling E. Immunosuppressive drug use during pregnancy. Rheum Dis Clin N Am 1997; 23: 149–67.

58. Armenti VT, Moritz MJ, Davison JM, Drug safety issues in pregnancy following transplantation and immunosuppression. Drug Safety 1998; 19: 219–32.

59. Little BB. Immunosuppressive therapy during gestation. Semin Perinatol 1997; 21: 143–8.

60. Leb DE, Weisskopf B, Kanovitz BS. Chromosome aberrations in the child of a kidney transplant recipient. Arch Inern Med 1971; 128: 441–4.

61. Alstead EM, Ritchie JK, Lennard-Jones JE *et al.* Safety of azathioprine in pregnancy in inflammatory bowel disease. Gastroenterology 1990; 99: 443–6.

62. Marion JF. Toxicity of 6-mercaptopurine/azathioprine in patients with inflammatory bowel disease. Inflam Bowel Dis 1998; 2: 116–7.

63. Reimers TJ, Sluss PM. 6-Mercaptopurine treatment of pregnant mice; effects on second and third generations. Science 1978; 201; 65–7.

64. Rajapaske RO, Korelitz BI, Zlatanic J, Baiocco PJ, Gleim GW. Outcome of pregnancies when fathers are treated with 6-mercaptopurine for inflammatory bowel disease. Am J Gastroenterol 2000; 95: 684–8.

65. Penn I. Parenthood following renal transplantation. Kidney Int 1980; 18: 221–33.

66. Dejaco C, Mittermaier C, Reinisch W *et al.* Azathioprine treatment and male fertility in inflammatory bowel disease. Gastroenterology 2001; 121: 1048–53.

67. Grekas DM, Vasiliou SS, Lazarides AN. Immunosuppressive therapy and breast-feeding after renal transplantation. Nephron 1984; 37: 68

68. Lamarque V, Leleu MF, Monka C *et al.* Analysis of 629 outcomes in transplant recipients treated with Sandimmun. Transplant Proc 1997; 29: 2480

69. Bertschinger P, Himmelmann A, Risti B, Follath F. Cyclosporine treatment of severe ulcerative colitis during pregnancy. Am J Gastroenterol 1995; 90: 330

70. Nyberg G, Haljamae U, Frisenette-Fich C, Wennergren M, Kjellmer I. Breast-feeding during treatment with cyclosporine. Transplantation 1998; 65; 253–5.

71. Feldkamp M, Carey JC. Clinical teratology counselling and consultation case report: low dose methotrexate exposure in the early weeks of pregnancy. Teratology 1993; 47: 533–9.

72. Connell W, Miller A. Treating inflammatory bowel disease during pregnancy. Risks and safety of drug therapy. Drug Safety 1999: 21: 311–23.

73. Burtin P, Taddio A, Ariburnu O *et al.* Safety of metronidazole in pregnancy: a meta-analysis. Am J Obstet Gynecol 1995; 172: 525–9.

74. Caro-Paton T, Carvajal A, de Diego IM *et al.* Is metronidazole teratogenic? A meta-analysis. Br J Clin Pharmacol 1997; 44: 179–82.

75. Dobias L, Cerna M, Rossner P *et al.* Genotoxicity and carcinogenicity of metronidazole. Mutat Res 1994; 317: 177–94.

76. Mayer DG. Overview of toxicological studies. Drugs 1987; 34 (Suppl. 1): 150–3.

77. Berkovitch M, Pastuszak A, Gazarian M *et al.* Safety of the new quinolones in pregnancy. Obstet Gynecol 1994; 84: 535–8.

78. Hommes DW, van de Heisteeg BH, van der Spek M, Bartelsman JFWM, van Deventer SJH. Infliximab treatment for Crohn's disease: one year experience in a Dutch academic hospital. Inflam Bowel Dis 2002; 8: 81–6.

79. Nwokolo CU, Tan WC, Andrews HA, Allan RN. Surgical resections in parous patients with distal ileal and colonic Crohn's disease. Gut 1994; 35: 220–3.

80. Castiglione F, Pignata S, Morace F *et al.* Effect of pregnancy on the clinical course of a cohort of women with inflammatory bowel disease. Ital J Gastroenterol 1996; 28: 199–204.

42 | Special considerations in the diagnosis and management of inflammatory bowel disease in the pediatric age group

ERNEST G. SEIDMAN AND ARLENE CAPLAN

Introduction

The diagnosis and management of inflammatory bowel disease (IBD) in children and adolescents is a challenge to patients and their families as well as to members of the health-care team. There are many similarities in terms of the clinical features and therapeutic options in IBD, irrespective of the patient's age. Thus, much of what has been included in other chapters pertains to IBD in the pediatric age group, and is not repeated here. However, IBD often occurs at a particularly vulnerable period of childhood and adolescence, with potentially adverse effects on growth, quality of life and psychosocial functioning. This chapter focuses on specific issues in pediatric IBD, dealing with those problems that are unique to children and adolescents, such as growth failure and pubertal delay. It also emphasizes certain clinical dilemmas that are particularly important in this age group, including an approach to dealing with diagnostic uncertainty in the child with recurrent abdominal pain, therapeutics and adherence issues, as well as psychosocial problems.

Epidemiologic aspects

Crohn's disease (CD) and ulcerative colitis (UC) are the most common chronic inflammatory disorders of children and adolescents in North America and most of Europe. An almost 7-fold increase in the incidence of CD was reported among a primarily Caucasian population in Olmsted County, Minnesota, between 1940 and 1993 [1]. Notably, an increasing proportion of new cases was diagnosed in individuals below age 20, reaching 17% by 1990 [1]. This has led to a decrease in the median age at diagnosis. Other data on the incidence of CD among children in Europe,

the United States and Canada support the evidence for an earlier age at diagnosis, rather than a true increase in disease incidence [2]. Another study revealed that the incidence of CD (7–12 per 100 000) and UC (5–6.9 per 100 000) among African-American children in the state of Georgia was similar to that observed in the age-matched population overall [3]. The data revealed that IBD is more prevalent among African-American children than previously thought. A recent prospective study in the British Isles yielded similar results, with an incidence of 5.2 cases of childhood IBD per 100 000 population [4]. UC was more frequent in children of Asian descent. In our IBD clinic the incidence of new cases of CD has increased 4-fold over the past two decades; that for UC does not appear to have changed over the same time period.

Distinctive clinical presentations

In general, the symptoms and signs of IBD are dependent upon the sites involved, their extent as well as severity, rather than the age of the patient [5, 6]. However, there are certain clinical presentations that are either unique or more common to the pediatric age group (Table 1). Notorious among these is growth failure, seen in up to half of patients at the time of diagnosis [5–7]. It is important to recognize that this mode of presentation, far more common in CD than UC, may occur in the absence of gastrointestinal complaints. Unfortunately, this may lead to a delay in diagnosis, often entailing one or more years until IBD is suspected. Affected patients usually have delayed puberty accompanying their poor growth. As discussed below, the management of such patients is a major challenge, in terms of

Stephan R. Targan, Fergus Shanahan and Loren C. Karp (eds.), *Inflammatory Bowel Disease: From Bench to Bedside, 2nd Edition*, 773–790.
© 2003 *Kluwer Academic Publishers. Printed in Great Britain*

Table 1. Particular clinical presentations of IBD in the pediatric age group

Unique	Common
Growth failure	Recurrent abdominal pain
Delayed sexual maturation/ puberty	Short stature
	Recurrent unexplained fever
	Arthralgias/arthritis
	Perianal disease
	Anorexia
	Recurrent aphthous mouth ulcers

improving growth as well as the psychosocial implications of short stature and pubertal delay.

Other 'atypical' clinical presentations which should make the physician suspicious of IBD in the pediatric age group are recurrent unexplained fever, arthralgias or arthritis, perianal disease (tags, fissures, abscesses and/or fistulas), aphthous mouth ulcers or perianal skin tags, and unexplained anorexia [5, 8].

Diagnostic approach to the child suspected of IBD

The differential diagnosis of CD and UC in the pediatric age group is summarized in Table 2. As in adults, the recognition and diagnosis of IBD is straightforward in children and adolescents when the clinical presentation is unambiguous. Thus, for example, a diagnosis of colitis (UC or CD) is strongly suspected in patients who present with typical symptoms, such as bloody diarrhea, urgency and abdominal discomfort. These clinical findings are then promptly confirmed by standard radiologic, endoscopic and histologic criteria, and an accurate diagnosis is promptly arrived at [5, 6, 9].

On the other hand, a diagnostic challenge arises in children who present with non-specific and indolent intestinal and extraintestinal symptoms that can be characteristic of both IBD and functional bowel disorders. In the face of such diagnostic uncertainty some clinicians may rely on invasive diagnostic testing, which entails at minimum a barium upper gastrointestinal series and small bowel follow-through (UGI and SBFT), as well as a complete colonoscopy with biopsies in order to confirm or exclude IBD.

In adults over the age of 50, performing a colonoscopy in the setting of a functional bowel disorder is perhaps justifiable on the basis of the merits of screening for colonic tumors. On the other hand, it is inappropriate to pursue these investigations among children in the setting where IBD is very unlikely. Generally speaking, children suspected of IBD have not experienced significant health problems prior to onset of their symptoms. Therefore, one should consider the emotional impact of intrusive testing in the patient who very likely has a functional bowel disorder. Given these clinical challenges, clinical investigators have searched for a marker or a combination of non-invasive tests that may enable clinicians to screen for IBD. The diagnostic approach to the child suspected of IBD should depend upon the level of doubt (Table 3).

Infectious causes of chronic diarrhea are usually sought in this setting (Table 2), requiring stool cultures and search for ova and parasites. In view of the fact that children are often exposed to antibiotic therapy, assay for *Clostridium difficile* toxin is frequently indicated. A complete blood count is usually obtained, with particular attention paid to the presence of a microcytic anemia and thrombocytosis, commonly seen in IBD. Hypoalbuminemia, often observed in the presence of a protein-losing enteropathy, is also frequent, but not specific for IBD. Elevated levels of circulating markers of acute-phase reactants, such as the erythrocyte sedimentation rate (ESR), C-reactive protein, and orosomucoid, are more common in active CD than in UC [10]. In addition to their lack of specificity for IBD, these tests may be all normal in up to one-third of patients [10–12]. The recently developed highly specific serologic tests can be useful adjunctive aids in discriminating IBD in its mild forms from functional bowel disorders [13–16]. Perinuclear anti-neutrophil cytoplasmic autoantibodies (pANCA) have been established as an autoimmune marker most characteristic of UC in the pediatric age group. On the other hand, antibodies to oligomannosidic epitopes of the yeast *Saccharomyces cerevisiae* (ASCA) have been shown to be a reliable marker of CD. Double positivity (both IgA and IgG) for ASCA was found to be 100% specific for pediatric CD [15]. The potential sensitivity of these markers as screening tests for IBD is maximized when the two assays are combined. Table 3 summarizes our approach to the child suspected of IBD, depending on the severity of symptoms and the level of clinical suspicion.

Table 2. Differential diagnosis of disorders resembling IBD in the pediatric age group

	CD	UC
Infectious etiologies		
Acute appendicitis	++	−
Mesenteric adenitis	++	−
Enteritis (*Yersinia* enterocolitica, enteropathogeneic *E. coli*,	++	+
Campylobacter jejuni, *Salmonella*, *Shigella*, *Entamoeba histolytica*,		
Giardia lamblia, *Dientamoeba fragilis*, *Mycobacterium*		
tuberculosis, etc.)		
Pseudomembraneous or antibiotic-associated colitis	++	+++
Vascular disorders		
Hemolytic uremic syndrome, Henoch Schoenlein Purpura, Behçet's	+	+++
disease, polyarteritis nodosum, systemic lupus erythematosus,		
ischemic bowel disease, dermatomyositis		
Immunodeficiency disorders (congenital acquired)	++	++
Iatrogenic		
Radiation, chemotherapy (typhlitis), graft-versus-host disease	+	+
Obstetric and gynecologic causes		
Ectopic pregnancy, ovarian cysts, tumors, endometriosis	+	+
Allergic		
Eosinophilic gastroenteropathies	+	+
Neuromuscular		
Hirschsprung's disease, pseudo-obstruction syndromes	+	++
Others		
Intussusception, Meckel diverticulum, tumors	+	++

Table 2. Differential diagnosis of disorders resembling IBD in the pediatric age group

Clinical index of suspicion high
Upper gastrointestinal and small bowel follow-through barium X-rays
Complete colonoscopy with multiple biopsies
Upper endoscopy (if clinically indicated)
Rule out microbial causes
Exclude immunodeficiency disorder
Exclude autoimmune enteropathy
Exclude allergic disorder

Clinical index of suspicion low
Verify normal physical examination
Verify normal growth parameters
Carry out limited investigations:
    CBC: hemoglobin, platelet count, ESR
    Serum albumin, iron, ferritin
    Serological assays: pANCA, ASCA
    Abdominal ultrasound + Doppler assessment of mucosal vessel density

Table 4. Commonly employed medications for IBD in the pediatric age group

Drug and dose	Potential side-effects
Aminosalicylates Sulfasalazine (40–60 mg/kg per day; t.i.d.); 5-ASA/ mesalamine/ olsalazine (40–70 mg/kg per day; b.i.d. or t.i.d.);	Headaches, nausea, hypersensitivity reactions (skin), pancreatitis, pericarditis, granulocytopenia, thrombocytopenia
Topical 5-ASA (enema, 2–4 g; or suppository; 0.5 to 1 g, both q 12–24 h)	Side-effects of topical applications are seldom encountered
Corticosteroids Prednisone (1–2 mg/kg max. 50 mg/day; q.a.m. or divided b.i.d.). Topical enemas (hydrocortisone; 50–100 mg q 12–24 h; or methylprednisolone, 10–40 mg in 30–60 ml NaCl 0.9%, q 12–24 h)	Acne, moon facies, striae, growth impairment, hypertension, aseptic necrosis or bone fractures, depression or other mood alterations, sleep disorder, osteopenia, myopathy
Budesonide (9 mg/day; q.a.m.)	Budesonide: less systemic side-effects
Antimetabolite therapy 6-Mercaptopurine (1.25–1.5 mg/kg per day).* Azathioprine (2.25–3 mg/kg per day)*	Idiosyncratic: pancreatitis, rash, fever. Leukopenia, hepatitis (associated with increased metabolite levels). Nausea
Methotrexate (15 mg/m^2 s.c.)	Nausea; teratogenicity; hepatotoxicity; myelosuppression; pulmonary toxicity; anorexia
Immunosuppressive therapy Cyclosporine A and tacrolimus (dose adjusted according to drug levels)	Nephrotoxicity, headaches, paresthesias, hirsutism, oral thrush. Diabetes
Biological therapy Anti-tumor necrosis factor alpha (infliximab, 5 mg/kg i.v.)	Serum sickness-like reactions. Lupus-like syndrome. Lymphomas?
Antibiotics Metronidazole (10–15 mg/kg per day). Ciprofloxacin (restricted to >16 years; 250–750 mg b.i.d., according to weight)	Long-term use: peripheral neuropathy. Bone pain; potential for altered bone health

*Dose adjusted according to TPMT genotype and metabolite levels

term remission while preventing steroid dependence or resistance for most cases [38].

Despite the established efficacy of AZA and 6-MP in controlled trials, dose-ranging studies have not been carried out. Over the past few years, however, pharmacogenetic advances have led to the development of new strategies in order to optimize and individualize therapy with AZA and 6-MP, maximizing efficacy, while minimizing toxicity [29, 38]. AZA is an inactive prodrug that undergoes a series of enzymatic reactions via competing pathways, leading to two major metabolites (Fig. 1). One route leads to the production of 6-thioguanine nucleotides (6-TG), shown to be the active metabolite [39]. However, excessive levels of 6-TG are potentially myelotoxic. In the competing pathway, thiopurine methyltransferase (TPMT) yields 6-methylmercaptopurine ribonucleotides. The latter metabolites appear to be therapeutically inactive but potentially hepatotoxic at high levels [29, 39, 40]. Co-dominantly inherited polymorphic alleles confer variable TPMT enzyme activity levels, with about 11% of individuals heterozygous and 0.3% homozygous for common TPMT mutations. Such individuals have intermediate and low/absent TPMT activity, respectively. Heterozygous patients with intermediate activity generate higher therapeutic 6-TG levels, but are at a greater risk for myelosuppression. The identification of a patient's TPMT genotype or phenotype can thus allow the physician to adjust the dose of the drug accordingly, avoiding early leukopenic events [41]. Patients with subtherapeutic 6-TG levels, due either to under-dosing, poor compliance or excessive TPMT activity are more likely to be refractory to therapy with these drugs [40]. Thus, AZA and 6-MP are generally well tolerated in pediatric IBD patients

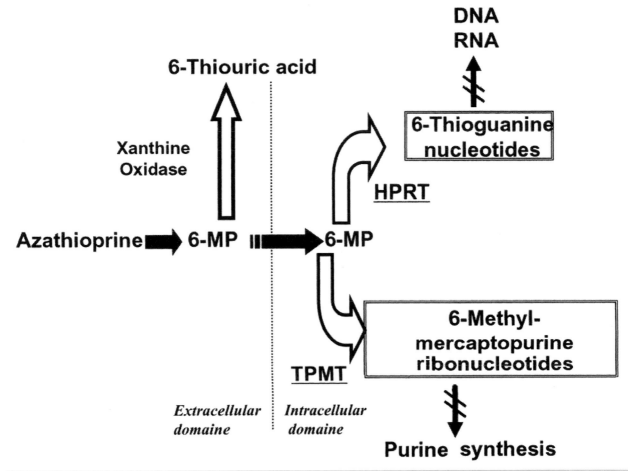

Figure 1. Pathways in the metabolism of azathioprine and 6-mercaptopurine. Oral azathioprine is rapidly converted to 6-MP by a non-enzymatic process. Initial 6-MP transformations occur along competing catabolic (xanthine oxidase; TPMT: thiopurine methyltransferase) and anabolic (HPRT: hypoxanthine phosphoribosyltransferase) enzymatic pathways. The latter intracellular enzyme (dashed line) transforms the drug into 6-thioguanine nucleotides, which have been shown to be the most important factor associated with treatment efficacy. TPMT converts the drug into 6-methyl-mercaptopurine ribonucleotides. Patients heterozygous for a mutant allele of TPMT will convert a higher proportion of the drug into 6-TG. This translates into a higher success rate, but with an increased risk of myelosuppression.

[42]. Measuring 6-MP metabolite levels and TPMT molecular analysis provide clinicians with useful tools for optimizing therapeutic response to 6-MP/ AZA, as well as for identifying individuals at increased risk for drug-induced toxicity [29, 38, 40].

Methotrexate is considered to be in the class of antimetabolite therapies, due to its antagonistic effect on folic acid metabolism [43]. Among adults, almost 40% of steroid-refractory chronically active CD patients have been found to respond to weekly injections of methotrexate (25 mg). No similar, controlled trials have been done in the pediatric age group. In pediatrics this therapy has generally been employed in moderate to severe CD, refractory to corticosteroids [44]. Weekly injections (15 mg/m^2 weekly subcutaneously) are effective in pediatric patients who had previously failed therapy with 6-MP. In one published open trial of 14 cases, nine showed symptomatic improvement after 4 weeks of therapy [45]. Hepatotoxicity is a major concern of long-term therapy. A recent study in children with juvenile rheumatoid arthritis showed that liver enzyme elevation more than 40% of the time was associated with an increased risk of fibrosis [46]. Obesity may add to the risk.

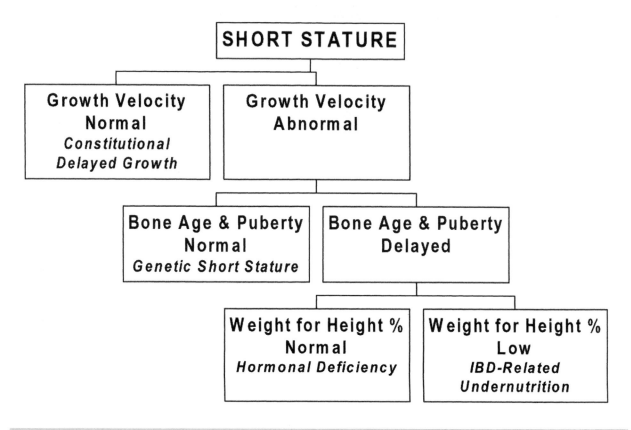

Figure 2. Assessment of the cause of short stature in pediatric IBD patients.

subject with cessation of linear growth over a period of 6 months or by a decrease exceeding one or more standard deviations in height percentile. An easy bedside rule of thumb is that growth velocity generally exceeds 4 cm per year in prepubertal boys and 3.5 cm in girls. Peak height velocity occurs before menarche in female adolescents. Therefore, it is important to recognize and treat malnutrition before it is too late to achieve any catch-up. For many adolescent patients with IBD, impaired growth leading to short stature and the accompanying delayed maturation of secondary sexual characteristics may be more troubling and debilitating than their underlying disease [5, 7]. Therapy for correcting growth failure is detailed below.

The proper management of short stature in the IBD child requires a precise evaluation of its cause, as summarized in Fig. 2. The clinician must ascertain whether the growth failure is due to inadequate intake of calories as a result of the IBD itself, or due to potential hormonal deficiency (growth hormone,

thyroxin or cortisol). In the former but not the latter scenario the weight for height percentile will almost invariably be abnormally low.

Therapy of active Crohn's disease

The potential role of nutritional therapy in children with IBD can be subdivided into two categories: either as primary therapy in order to induce remission in active CD or UC, or as adjunctive therapy to help maintain remission and to enhance growth [68, 69]. Although several randomized controlled trials have suggested that elemental and semi-elemental diets are as effective as steroids, meta-analyses have shown an overall statistical advantage for corticosteroids [70]. Nevertheless, nutrition is still a logical choice as primary therapy for active CD in selected cases, especially those children and adolescents with marked undernutrition and growth failure [68, 69]. Patients who tend to respond best (75% remission rate) are those with newly diagnosed CD involving the terminal ileum with or without the cecum or proximal colon [69]. Individuals with long-standing disease or extensive colitis generally respond less favorably (50% and 35%, respectively). Although steroids more often induce remission, their use is associated with a net loss of mineral bone density, negative nitrogen balance and with impaired linear growth [68]. On the other hand, nutritional therapy enhances growth, induces net anabolism with positive nitrogen balance, and improves bone health. Another clinical scenario favoring diet as primary therapy is for adolescents with CD who refuse a course of corticosteroids due to concerns for growth, cosmetic or other adverse effects [69].

Drawbacks to the use of nutrition as primary therapy for CD include the relatively high cost, the unpleasant taste and monotony of defined formula diets when employed as sole source of nutrition. The availability of flavor packets has improved the acceptance and oral tolerance of elemental and semi-elemental formulas. Whichever formula is selected, a major objective is to avoid parenteral nutrition, unless the enteral route has failed or is contraindicated. Defined formulas are as effective as, and certainly safer and less costly than, parenteral nutrition. In order to induce remission we generally administer a semi-elemental diet as sole source of nutrition (40–70 kcal/kg ideal body weight per day), for 4 consecutive weeks. The patients drink the formula during the day, along with clear fluids, as tolerated. The balance is administered nocturnally, by nasogastric tube or via a gastrostomy [9].

In addition to inducing remissions for active disease, nutritional therapy has been employed on an intermittent, cyclical manner (4 out of every 16 weeks) in order to sustain growth as well as to maintain remission off steroids [71, 72]. Patients who received intermittent semi-elemental diet had significantly fewer relapses and markedly improved growth velocity, compared to those treated with low-dose, alternate-day prednisone. In addition to improving symptoms, elemental diets reduce excessive intestinal permeability, reverse the protein-losing enteropathy and decrease intestinal and systemic markers of inflammation [73]. An alternative approach is to employ AZA or 6-MP, as detailed above. Novel defined formulas that include cytokines such as transforming growth factor-β or an enhanced content of antioxidants are currently under investigation, with promising preliminary results.

The mechanisms underlying the beneficial effects of nutritional therapy remain incompletely under-stood. Several theories have been postulated: removal of dietary antigens, elimination of pro-inflammatory nutrients such as omega-6 fatty acids and nucleotides, altered eicosanoid production, bowel gut hormones and flora, as well as diminished pancreatic, hepatobiliary and intestinal secretions [68]. Patients with active IBD have increased production of arachidonic acid metabolites derived from dietary sources of omega-6 fatty acids such as vegetable oils, leading to high levels of proinflammatory eicosanoids such as leukotriene B_4, a potent neutrophil chemoattractant [68]. Fish oils contain eicosapentaenoic acid, an unsaturated fatty acid that is metabolized through the cyclo-oxygenase pathway, leading to leukotriene B_5, 30 times less potent than its leukotriene B_4 counterpart. Studies using fish oil supplements have lent support to the potential role of dietary fatty acids in the pathogenesis as well as therapy of IBD [68]. One study using enteric-coated fish oil was highly effective in reducing relapses in CD, supporting this hypothesis [74]. Another novel approach to the use of neutriceuticals to alter the inflammatory process in IBD was to employ N-acetyl glucosamine (N-AG) to assist in tissue repair mechanisms. In a pilot study, treatment-resistant pediatric IBD patients were treated with N-AG orally or rectally [75]. There appeared to be some short-term benefit in several cases, including patients with strictures.

Approach to growth failure

The nutritional impact of IBD is particularly severe in the prepubertal patient. Many patients ingest an insufficient quantity of calories in order to meet their energy needs, as well as the metabolic costs of growth. Thus, growth failure is a common, serious complication that is unique to the pediatric age group, encountered in up to half of CD and about 10% of UC patients [7, 65, 66]. Normal growth is an important indicator of remission and an outcome parameter of therapeutic efficacy in pediatric IBD. However, despite 'appropriate medical therapy,' CD results in permanent short stature in 20–35% of adults who had the disease prior to their puberty [76]. There is a time limit for achieving potential 'catch-up' growth because of progressive bone maturation and eventual epiphyseal fusion. Weight gain can be achieved in weeks, whereas growth acceleration requires many months of sustained treatment. In order to be effective, therefore, therapy must be initiated well before bone maturation is

Table 7. Specific surgical indications in pediatric IBD

Crohn's disease	Ulcerative colitis
Intractable symptoms; failure of medical management	Prolonged steroid dependence, intolerance to immunosuppressive agents
Hemorrhage	Hemorrhage
Fulminant colitis with or without toxic megacolon	Fulminant colitis, with or without toxic megacolon
Suspected perforation or abscess	Suspected perforation
Obstruction of upper and/or lower gastrointestinal tract. Fistulas: enteroenteral, enterocutaneous, enterovesical, enterovaginal. Intractable perirectal disease	Chronically active, unremitting disease
Growth failure despite nutrition support	Growth failure despite nutrition support
High risk of dysplasia, carcinoma	High risk of dysplasia, carcinoma

character', especially when it comes to challenging parental authority and expressing anger or exhibiting aggression. However, it is unclear to what extent these changes are due to the illness as opposed to the effects of systemic corticotherapy.

The children may report feeling 'different inside' or having 'changed forever' as a result of their IBD. They frequently feel less in control of their emotions and behavior. Some experience bouts of crying, often without apparent reason. Many state that they have become more withdrawn and unsociable; others report that they no longer feel like enjoying themselves. They may consciously withdraw from recreational activities or social contact because they fear other children will find out that they have a disease and will treat them differently. Others withdraw simply because they feel unable to participate or enjoy themselves. The aversion of being questioned, feelings of embarrassment, or reluctance to be confronted with their disease often makes it difficult for children and adolescents with IBD to return to school after long absences due to their illness. These reactions of shame and embarrassment often contribute to depressive feelings of psychological isolation, fragility and instability.

Problems related to compliance with therapy are notorious in pediatric populations. For many children, 'forgetting' to take their medications is a way of psychologically denying their disease. For others it may be more conscious, and related to the lack of efficacy, or side-effects of the drug. In addition to the adverse effects of steroids on mood, cognition and behavior, psychological factors in children, parents or the family at large may also contribute to poor compliance and adherence to therapy. Nutritional therapy can also have important effects on psycho-

social functioning. During periods of treatment, patients endure prolonged periods of food-deprivation and experience frustration due to disruption of social and family activities. Special formula diets are particularly difficult for children who eat their meals at school. They are often already embarrassed about their disease. Thus, nutrition as primary therapy potentially exacerbates the child's feeling of being different due to the disease itself, and may contribute to his/her sense of alienation. There is the additional consideration that the feeding tube and pump apparatus makes the disease more visible, both to patients and to those around them. This can accentuate feelings of self-consciousness and heighten embarrassment in social situations. Some patients experience the insertion of a nasal gastric tube as intrusive or aggressive on the part of the medical team. The psychological meaning patients attribute to treatment procedures, as well as their emotional reactions (e.g. anxiety, fear, and depression), may be more influential than their physical response in determining treatment success. More data on the psychological effects of medical and nutritional therapies are needed to provide a better understanding of the factors affecting compliance with treatment and the relationship to the medical team. Further study in this area would increase understanding of these factors, allowing gastroenterologists to provide higher-quality care and improved treatment strategies for pediatric IBD.

Children with IBD have been reported to have a significantly impaired quality of life [82]. They fear everyday childhood activities and are concerned for their future employment. These children need sympathetic management, and efforts should be concentrated on improving their daily psychosocial functioning, enabling them to lead as normal a life as possible. This can best be achieved by medically controlling their disease activity, achieving normal growth and development through nutritional interventions, and providing psychosocial support to them and their family members.

Surgical considerations

As in adults, the surgical approach to the child with IBD must always bear in mind that unlike UC, CD is not a surgically curable disorder. Surgical interventions are thus reserved either for complications of CD, or for symptoms that cannot be managed medically (Table 7). In the latter situation intractability of symptoms generally infers a poor prognosis postoperatively, with clinical relapse within 1 year in 50% of cases [93]. On the other hand, young patients operated upon for ileal strictures or local abscesses have a far better prognosis, with a 50% recurrence rate after 5 years. As summarized in Table 7, other surgical indications include recurrent episodes of partial bowel obstruction, or an abscess that fails to respond to conservative measures. Entero-enteric fistulas are not necessarily an indication for surgery. Although an enterovesical fistula is not an absolute indication for surgery, most patients will require an operation eventually. Perianal CD also calls for a conservative approach. Abscesses should be drained and fistulas laid flat or treated with setons when possible. Although surgical resection has not been shown to influence the natural history of CD, it can lead to dramatic growth acceleration and attainment of normal adult height in some, but not all, cases [77, 78]. The type of intervention depends on the extent and severity of the disease [94].

The principal indications for surgery in UC [95] include intractable disease (64%), refractory growth failure (14%), toxic megacolon (6%), hemorrhage (4%), perforation (3%) and cancer prophylaxis (2%). Despite the relative success of CsA, tacrolimus and other immunosuppressive agents, it must be borne in mind that colectomy can be a lifesaving procedure in a child with fulminant colitis or toxic megacolon. CsA and tacrolimus are not only short-term solutions, they are associated with considerable morbidity as well as potential mortality, as reviewed above.

The increased risk of developing colon cancer among patients with onset of UC during childhood is well established [9]. Proctocolectomy has been the most commonly practiced and accepted operation. If rectal involvement is mild, some surgeons prefer to carry out a colectomy and ileoanal anastomosis in one stage. Meticulous supervision of the conserved rectum is mandatory, as it might be a site for later cancer. Successful ileoanal–endorectal anastomosis after total colectomy and a mucosal proctectomy is often achieved. The rectal mucosa is stripped from its muscular wall, and the ileal mucosa is sutured on. The creation of a neorectum with an ileal pouch affords decreased stool frequency. This is now the treatment of choice in the pediatric population. An important factor regarding continence is the level at which the ileoanal anastomosis is performed [95, 96]. Colon cancer may also occur in the case of Crohn's colitis [97]. The relative risk depends largely upon the extent, as well as the duration, of the colitis [98]. Screening is usually initiated after about 8 years of clinical presentation for cases of extensive colitis.

References

1. Loftus EV Jr, Silverstein MD, Sandborn WJ, Tremaine WJ, Harmsen WS, Zinsmeister AR. Crohn's disease in Olmsted County, Minnesota, 1940–1993: incidence, prevalence, and survival. Gastroenterology 1998; 114: 1161–8.
2. Logan RFA. Inflammatory bowel disease incidence: up, down or unchanged. Gut 1998; 42: 309–11.
3. Ogunbi SO, Ransom JA, Sullivan K, Schoen BT, Gold BD. Inflammatory bowel disease in African-American children living in Georgia. Pediatrics 1998; 138: 103–7.
4. Sawczenko A, Sandhu BK, Logan RF *et al.* Prospective survey of childhood inflammatory bowel disease in the British Isles. Lancet 2001; 357: 1093–4
5. Seidman E. Inflammatory bowel diseases. In: Roy C, Silverman A, Alagille D, eds. Pediatric Clinical Gastroenterology, 4th edn. St Louis: CV Mosby, 1995: 417–93.
6. Marx G, Seidman EG. Inflammatory bowel diseases. In: C Lifschitz, ed. Pediatric Gastroenterology and Nutrition in Clinical Practice. New York: Marcel Decker, 2002: 651–82.
7. Seidman EG. Growth and nutritional problems in pediatric IBD. In: Bayless TM, Hanauer SB, eds. Advanced Therapy of Inflammatory Bowel Disease, 2nd edn. Hamilton, Ontario: BC Decker, 2002 (In press).
8. Pittock S, Drumm B, Fleming P *et al.* The oral cavity in Crohn's disease. J Pediatr 2001; 138: 767–71.
9. Seidman EG. Role of endoscopy in pediatric inflammatory bowel disease. Gastrointest Endosc Clin N Am 2001; 11: 641–57.
10. Murch SH, Walker-Smith J, Beattie RM. Indications for investigation of chronic gastrointestinal symptoms. Arch Dis Child 1995; 73: 354–5.
11. Holmquist L, Ahren C, Feallstreom SP. Relationship between results of laboratory tests and inflammatory activity assessed by colonoscopy in children and adolescents with UC and Crohn's colitis. J Pediatr Gastroenterol Nutr 1989; 9: 187–93.
12. Dubinsky MC, Seidman EG. Diagnostic markers of inflammatory bowel disease. Curr Opin Gastroenterol 2000; 16: 337–42.

94. Davies G, Evans CM, Shand WS, Walker-Smith JA. Surgery for Crohn's disease in childhood: influence of site of disease and operative procedure on outcome. Br J Surg 1990; 77: 891–4.

95. Telander RL. Surgical management of inflammatory bowel disease in children: In: Telander R, ed. Problems in General Surgery: Surgical Treatment of Inflammatory Bowel Disease. Philadelphia, JB Lippincott, 1993.

96. Martin LW, LeCoultre C, Schubert WK. Total colectomy and mucosal proctectomy with preservation of continence. Ann Surg 1977; 186: 477–80.

97. Tiszlavicz L, Kapin M, Varkonyi A, Lorincz A, Bartyik K, Varkonyi T. Adenocarcinoma of the colon developing on the basis of Crohn's disease in childhood. Eur J Pediatr 2001; 160: 168–72

98. Gillen CD, Walmsley RS, Prior P *et al*. Ulcerative colitis and Crohn's disease: a comparison of the colorectal cancer risk in extensive colitis. Gut 1994; 35: 1590–2.

43 | Microscopic colitis: collagenous and lymphocytic colitis

DIARMUID O'DONOGHUE AND KIERAN SHEAHAN

Introduction

Microscopic colitis is now an accepted member of the inflammatory bowel disease family. Recognition came slowly following Lindstrom's classical description of collagenous colitis in 1976 [1]. Read *et al.* first used the term microscopic colitis to describe a diffuse increase in inflammatory cells in colorectal biopsies from patients with chronic diarrhea [2]. Numerous reports have followed as the critical importance of obtaining colonic biopsies from patients with diarrhea, despite normal-looking mucosa, has been appreciated. The term 'lymphocytic colitis' was employed to distinguish patients who, like those with collagenous colitis, presented with watery diarrhea and a normal colonoscopy, had an expansion of intraepithelial lymphocytes but no increase in the subepithelial collagen layer [3]. Microscopic colitis is now the accepted terminology encompassing collagenous and lymphocytic colitis. Whether these are two separate conditions, or represent ends of a spectrum of a single disease, is a moot point.

Incidence and prevalence

As many cases of microscopic colitis are probably undiagnosed it is difficult to assess incidence or prevalence figures. Bohr and colleagues in Sweden, in a retrospective study of pathology material and case records, estimated the prevalence of collagenous colitis to be 15.7 per 100 000 inhabitants with an annual incidence of 1.8 [4]. A recent study from Spain records an incidence figure of 1.8/100 000 for collagenous colitis and 3.1 for the lymphocytic variety [5]. In this study microscopic colitis was identified in 9.5% of patients with watery diarrhea and a normal-looking mucosa. Females dominate in all large series; more so in collagenous than lymphocytic colitis [4–6]. Likewise all studies show a peak at diagnosis in the late 50s and early 60s age groups. Thus, microscopic colitis is now the first disease to consider in the older woman presenting with chronic watery diarrhea.

Etiologic theories and associations

The etiology of microscopic colitis is unknown; indeed lymphocytic infiltration and collagen formation may be the histologic end-points of a variety of insults. The female predominance, especially of collagenous colitis, lends credence to an autoimmune theory, and many diseases with a putative immune basis are associated with these conditions. Celiac disease, thyroid disorders, rheumatoid arthritis and diabetes are just some of the more common conditions greatly overrepresented in patients with microscopic colitis [7–11]. However, apart from a non-significant increase in antinuclear factor, autoantibodies are not increased in patients with collagenous colitis [12]. A higher than expected occurrence of microscopic colitis within families suggests a genetic predisposition for this disease [13].

The relationship between celiac disease and microscopic colitis is, perhaps, the most intriguing. All major reports on microscopic colitis have highlighted an unexpectedly high concurrence of the two disorders. Bohr's study from Sweden records celiac disease in 8% of 163 patients with collagenous colitis [4]. Although initially associated with collagenous colitis, it is now recognized to occur with both histologic varieties [14–16]. Gluten does not appear to be the offending substance, as many cases of microscopic colitis come to light when the diarrhea of celiac disease fails to resolve on a gluten-free diet despite good histologic recovery of the small bowel pathology [17]. The close relationship between these conditions has led to the investigation of the small bowel in a number of studies which, although based

Stephan R. Targan, Fergus Shanahan and Loren C. Karp (eds.), Inflammatory Bowel Disease: From Bench to Bedside, 2nd Edition, 791–798.
© 2003 *Kluwer Academic Publishers. Printed in Great Britain*

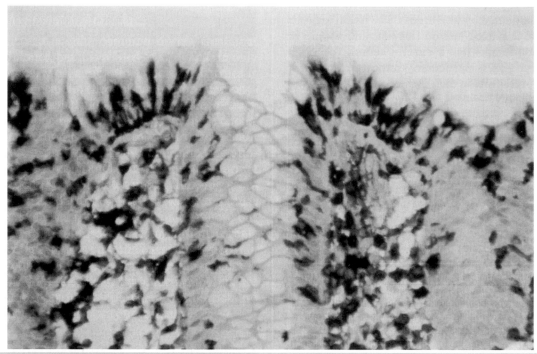

Figure 2. Common leukocyte antigen (CLA) immunostaining confirming the diagnosis of lymphocytic colitis (× 400).

mean number of surface IELs in lymphocytic colitis is 40 (range 20–60) [36]. Others who have performed quantitative studies showed a mean of 24.6 [3] and 37 lymphocytes per 100 surface epithelial cells [34]. Our study has used quantitative immunohistochemistry and therefore may be the more accurate. We also find that a confirmatory immunohistochemical stain for common leukocyte antigen (CLA) is useful on many occasions (Fig. 2).

Focal intraepithelial lymphocytosis only (involvement of some but not all biopsies) is insufficient for diagnosis, and has been addressed in a few studies. Focal lymphocytic and collagenous colitis have been described as preceding Crohn's disease in one report [37]. Other features, however, including focal involvement of biopsies, abnormal colonoscopic findings, presence of numerous neutrophils and a foreign-body-type granuloma between the collagen fibers, helped to distinguish these cases in retrospect. In our experience differentiation from Crohn's disease is rarely a problem if strict histologic diagnostic criteria are applied and correlated with clinical and endoscopic findings. In addition, it is always difficult to entirely exclude so-called 'Brainerd' or epidemic diarrhea, which is most likely infectious in etiology [34, 38].

Using a cut-off of 15 lymphocytes per 100 surface colonocytes, Wang and colleagues have suggested abandoning the name lymphocytic colitis and replacing it with the term colonic epithelial lymphocytosis [15]. In this study 28 of 40 patients fitted the classical description of lymphocytic colitis but the remaining 12 were atypical, fulfilling the histologic but not the clinical or endoscopic criteria. These patients represented a heterogeneous group of disorders including idiopathic constipation, Crohn's disease and infectious colitis. A recent commentary suggests that the term 'colonic epithelial lymphocytosis' be reserved for these atypical cases which do not satisfy all the criteria for classic lymphocytic colitis [39].

Collagenous colitis

All of the features of lymphocytic colitis outlined above are seen in collagenous colitis but the number of IELs tends to be lower [36, 39]. The *sine qua non* for the diagnosis of collagenous colitis is a thickened subepithelial collagen layer. There has been considerable controversy with regard to the exact thickness necessary to make the diagnosis. The upper limit of normal is stated to be 7 μm. A rule of thumb states that > 10 μm raises the possibility, while > 15 estab-

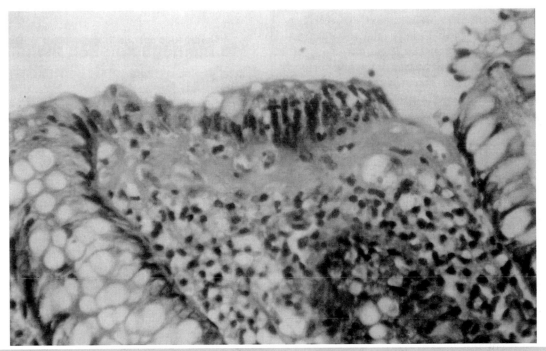

Figure 3. Lacy infiltration of superficial lamina propria by collagen (Masson-Trichrome × 400).

lishes a diagnosis in the proper setting. More importantly, in our experience, is the pattern of injury; in particular, the lacy infiltration of the superficial capillaries of the lamina propria is characteristic and in doubtful cases can clinch the diagnosis (Fig. 3). This has previously been highlighted by Lazenby *et al.* who state that no absolute or minimum quantitative measure of subepithelial collagen should be used for the diagnosis [40]. The collagen accumulation is usually diffuse but can be patchy in up to 20% of cases. Prominent eosinophils are an occasional feature. Pericryptal myofibroblasts are also prominent. We have seen one case of collagenous colitis with pseudomembranes [41]. and other groups have also reported this finding [42, 43].

Pathogenesis

It now seems clear that collagenous colitis is due to an aberrant activation of intestinal subepithelial myofibroblasts (ISEMF) [44]. It appears that the normal type IV collagen of the basement membrane is unaltered in the disease. A recent study has shown that pericryptal myofibroblasts normally secrete small amounts of types I, III and VI collagen around the deep parts of the crypts. In the upper part of the crypts, and in the subepithelial location, increased amounts of type VI collagen and the matrix glycoprotein tenascin are produced. It is tenascin and type VI collagen which accumulate and comprise the majority of the subepithelial band. It has been suggested by this group that decreased synthesis of matrix metalloproteinases (MMP) may be responsible for the abnormal collagen accumulation, i.e. that the delicate balance between collagen production and resorption is disturbed [45]. This finding has been confirmed by Gunther and colleagues, who demonstrated reduced MMP1 but also increased levels of the tissue inhibitor of matrix metalloproteinase 1 (TIMP1) in 12 cases [46]. They also confirmed the accumulation of tenascin, while also showing an absence of undulin. This tenascin/undulin dichotomy is a feature of a rapidly remodeling extracellular matrix as compared with the high undulin/low tenascin content in long-standing scar tissue. This may explain why these deposits can be removed within periods of a few months upon fecal stream diversion [26]. Controversy persists, however, with a recent report stating that type III collagen is predominant in the condition [47]. It is interesting to note that other forms of colonic fibrosis (e.g. Crohn's strictures) are composed predominantly of collagen types I, III and V [48]. Finally, elegant electron microscopy work has shown deficient fibroblast cell processes, focally deficient basal lamina and surface epithelial cells resting directly on a thickened collagen layer in this condition [49].

Immune mechanisms have been proposed as being important in microscopic colitis. The abnormalities detected have been similar in both conditions. These include an accumulation of CD4 positive-cells in the lamina propria and abnormal expression of class II MHC molecules on colonic epithelial cells. The increased surface IEL are predominantly CD8-positive, T cell receptor (TCR)αβ phenotype [50]. No increase in TCRγδ cells was identified. A number of groups are beginning to find differences in the colonic intraepithelial lymphocytosis seen in celiac disease. In particular, the majority of IEL in the colon in refractory sprue are CD8-negative [51]. This requires further study, but it is interesting that a recent report suggests that a loss of IEL CD8 expression correlated with refractory sprue and often heralded a cryptic intestinal lymphoma [52].

Pathophysiology

The mechanism of the diarrhea seen in microscopic colitis has been evaluated in a small number of patients, with conflicting results. Giardiello and colleagues reported net fluid secretion, as distinct from the expected absorption, in the small bowel and colon of one subject and net jejunal secretion and reduced colonic absorption in a second patient. The induction of water and electrolyte secretion by the dihydroxy bile acids is a likely source of the diarrhea in those patients with bile salt malabsorption [8]. In contrast, a recent study has demonstrated reduced colonic water absorption in all six patients evaluated. These abnormalities were shown to be due to reduced active and passive sodium and chloride absorption and to reduced CL/HCO^3 exchange [23]. The pathophysiology of the diarrhea appears to correlate with lamina propria cellularity and not the thickness of the collagen layer, suggesting that the inflammatory reaction is the important component in the causation of the diarrhea [53]. Elevated levels of prostaglandin E_2 have been postulated as a circulating secretagogue in a single case study [54]. A recent and elegant study from Burgel and colleagues strongly supports the view that, in the collagenous variety of the disease, reduced sodium and

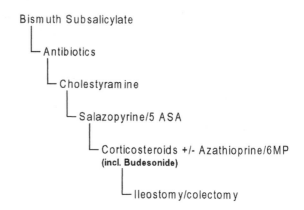

Figure 4. Therapeutic options in microscopic colitis.

chloride absorption along with active chloride secretion are the main components of the diarrhea. The subepithelial collageous band is felt to act as a diffusion barrier while down-regulation of tight junction molecules may contribute to a 'leak flux mechanism' [55].

Treatment

Microscopic colitis usually follows a benign course [6, 56, 57] and treatment options must keep this in mind. It is our experience that most patients, by the time of diagnosis, have already tried simple remedies such as antidiarrheal agents and need more effective therapy. Treatment is empirical, as with many diseases of unknown cause, but recent reports now allow for a more structured approach. Fine and Lee's study of the effectiveness of bismuth subsalicylate makes this the first drug to consider [27]. In this report 11 of 13 patients responded to the drug given orally for 8 weeks. This was mirrored by histopathologic improvement, including resolution of the thickened subepithelial collagen in the six patients who displayed this feature prior to therapy. The treatment was well tolerated and nine of the group remained in remission with a follow-up of 7–28 months. Options thereafter are outlined in Fig. 4. The case for antibiotics is less certain and based on retrospective analysis [7, 57]. Nevertheless, the hope of avoiding long-term medication makes this approach attractive. Metronidazole is the most frequently used antimicrobial. Ung *et al.*'s report of symptom resolution in 21 of 27 patients given a bile salt-binding agent would make this the third line of treatment [21]. These drugs are not always well tolerated, and this may limit their effectiveness. Thereafter the choice of treatment is based on little more than case reports and personal experience. Thirty-seven of 108 patients treated in a Swedish study benefited from salazopyrine while 45 individuals could not tolerate the medication [7]. Corticosteroids are effective but unacceptably high dosage is often required and relapse is common on reduction or withdrawal. This is far from ideal in a population that is predominantly female and postmenopausal. This has led Pardi and colleagues to use azathioprine in patients with steroid-dependent disease [58]. Budesonide, a locally acting corticosteroid with low systemic activity, may alleviate concerns regarding steroid toxicity and has recently been shown to be effective in collagenous colitis [59]. Surgery is occasionally required for severe disease [31] but a diversion ileostomy might be a better option and would have the benefit of allowing time for other therapies to act.

Acknowledgements

The authors wish to acknowledge the immense contribution made by Dr Darren Treanor to the scientific background and preparation of this chapter.

References

1. Lindstrom CG. 'Collagenous colitis' with watery diarrhoea – a new entity? Pathol Eur 1976; 11: 87–9.
2. Read NW, Krejs GJ, Read MG, Santa Ana CA, Morawski SG, Fordtran JS. Chronic diarrhea of unknown origin. Gastroenterology 1980; 78: 264–71.
3. Lazenby AJ, Yardley JH, Giardiello FM, Jessurun J, Bayless TM. Lymphocytic ('microscopic') colitis: a comparative histopathologic study with particular reference to collagenous colitis. Hum Pathol 1989; 20: 18–28.
4. Bohr J, Tysk C, Eriksson S, Jarnerot G. Collagenous colitis in Orebro, Sweden, an epidemiological study 1984–1993. Gut 1995; 37: 394–7.
5. Fernandez-Banares F, Salas A, Forne M, Esteve M, Espinos J, Viver JM. Incidence of collagenous and lymphocytic colitis: a 5-year population-based study. Am J Gastroenterol 1999; 94: 418–23.
6. Baert F, Wouters K, D'Haens G et al. Lymphocytic colitis: a distinct clinical entity? A clinicopathological confrontation of lymphocytic and collagenous colitis. Gut 1999; 45: 375–81.
7. Bohr J, Tysk C, Eriksson S, Abrahamsson H, Jarnerot G. Collagenous colitis: a retrospective study of clinical presentation and treatment in 163 patients. Gut 1996; 39: 846–51.
8. Giardiello FM, Bayless TM, Jessurun J, Hamilton SR, Yardley JH. Collagenous colitis: physiologic and histopathologic studies in seven patients. Ann Intern Med 1987; 106: 46–9.
9. Jessurun J, Yardley JH, Giardiello FM, Hamilton SR, Bayless TM. Chronic colitis with thickening of the subepithelial collagen layer (collagenous colitis): histopathologic findings in 15 patients. Hum Pathol 1987; 18: 839–48.
10. Soulier C, Baron D, Saraux A, Robert FX, Le Goff P. Four new cases of collagenous colitis with joint symptoms. Rev Rhum Engl Ed 1996; 63: 593–9.
11. van Tilburg AJ, Lam HG, Seldenrijk CA et al. Familial occurrence of collagenous colitis. A report of two families. J Clin Gastroenterol 1990; 12: 279–85.
12. Bohr J, Tysk C, Yang P, Danielsson D, Jarnerot G. Autoantibodies and immunoglobulins in collagenous colitis. Gut 1996; 39: 73–6.
13. Jarncrot G, Hertervig E, Granno C et al. Familial occurrence of microscopic colitis: a report on five families. Scand J Gastroenterol 2001; 36: 959–62.
14. DuBois RN, Lazenby AJ, Yardley JH, Hendrix TR, Bayless TM, Giardiello FM. Lymphocytic enterocolitis in patients with 'refractory sprue'. J Am Med Assoc 1989; 262: 935–7.
15. Wang N, Dumot JA, Achkar E, Easley KA, Petras RE, Goldblum JR. Colonic epithelial lymphocytosis without a thickened subepithelial collagen table: a clinicopathologic study of 40 cases supporting a heterogeneous entity. Am J Surg Pathol 1999; 23: 1068–74.
16. Wolber R, Owen D, Freeman H. Colonic lymphocytosis in patients with celiac sprue. Hum Pathol 1990; 21: 1092–6.
17. Fine KD, Meyer RL, Lee EL. The prevalence and causes of chronic diarrhoea in patients with celiac sprue treated with a gluten-free diet [Published erratum appears in Gastroenterology 1998; 114: 424–5]. Gastroenterology 1997; 112: 1830–8.
18. Fine KD, Do K, Schulte K et al. High prevalence of celiac sprue-like genes and enteropathy in patients with the microscopic colitis syndrome. Am J Gastroenterol 2000; 95: 1974–82.
19. Moayyedi P, O'Mahony S, Jackson P, Lynch DA, Dixon MF, Axon AT. Small intestine in lymphocytic and collagenous colitis: mucosal morphology, permeability, and secretory immunity to gliadin. J Clin Pathol 1997; 50: 527–9.
20. Marteau P, Lavergne-Slove A, Lemann M et al. Primary ileal villous atrophy is often associated with microscopic colitis. Gut 1997; 41: 561–4.
21. Ung KA, Gillberg R, Kilander A, Abrahamsson H. Role of bile acids and bile acid binding agents in patients with collagenous colitis. Gut 2000; 46: 170–5.
22. Veress B, Lofberg R, Bergman L. Microscopic colitis syndrome. Gut 1995; 36: 880–6.
23. Bo-Linn GW, Vendrell DD, Lee E, Fordtran JS. An evaluation of the significance of microscopic colitis in patients with chronic diarrhoea. J Clin Invest 1985; 75: 1559–69.
24. Riddell RH, Tanaka M, Mazzoleni G. Non-steroidal anti-inflammatory drugs as a possible cause of collagenous colitis: a case–control study. Gut 1992; 33: 683–6.
25. Andersen T, Andersen JR, Tvede M, Franzmann MB. Collagenous colitis: are bacterial cytotoxins responsible? Am J Gastroenterol 1993; 88: 375–7.
26. Jarnerot G, Tysk C, Bohr J, Eriksson S. Collagenous colitis and fecal stream diversion. Gastroenterology 1995; 109: 449–55.
27. Fine KD, Lee EL. Efficacy of open-label bismuth subsalicylate for the treatment of microscopic colitis. Gastroenterology 1998; 114: 29–36.

28. Carpenter HA, Tremaine WJ, Batts KP, Czaja AJ. Sequential histologic evaluations in collagenous colitis. Correlations with disease behavior and sampling strategy. Dig Dis Sci 1992; 37: 1903–9.

29. Thaysen EH, Pedersen L. Idiopathic bile acid catharsis. Gut 1976; 17: 965–70.

30. Arlow FL, Dekovich AA, Priest RJ, Beher WT. Bile acid-mediated postcholecystectomy diarrhoea. Arch Intern Med 1987; 147: 1327–9.

31. Bowling TE, Price AB, al Adnani M, Fairclough PD, Menzies-Gow N, Silk DB. Interchange between collagenous and lymphocytic colitis in severe disease with autoimmune associations requiring colectomy: a case report. Gut 1996; 38: 788–91.

32. Sylwestrowicz T, Kelly JK, Hwang WS, Shaffer EA. Collagenous colitis and microscopic colitis: the watery diarrhoea–colitis syndrome. Am J Gastroenterol 1989; 84: 763–8.

33. Teglbjaerg PS, Thaysen EH, Jensen HH. Development of collagenous colitis in sequential biopsy specimens. Gastroenterology 1984; 87: 703–9.

34. Bryant DA, Mintz ED, Puhr ND, Griffin PM, Petras RE. Colonic epithelial lymphocytosis associated with an epidemic of chronic diarrhoea. Am J Surg Pathol 1996; 20: 1102–9.

35. Goldman H, Antonioli DA. Mucosal biopsy of the rectum, colon, and distal ileum. Hum Pathol 1982; 13: 981–1012.

36. Treanor DT, Morgan S, O'Donoghue DP, Sheahan K. Microscopic colitis: a detailed clinicopathological study. Gut 2000; 46: A8 (Abstract).

37. Goldstein NS, Gyorfi T. Focal lymphocytic colitis and collagenous colitis: patterns of Crohn's colitis? Am J Surg Pathol 1999; 23: 1075–81.

38. Osterholm MT, MacDonald KL, White KE et al. An outbreak of a newly recognised chronic diarrhoea syndrome associated with raw milk consumption. J Am Med Assoc 1986; 256: 484–90.

39. Lamps LW, Lazenby AJ. Colonic epithelial lymphocytosis and lymphocytic colitis: descriptive histopathology versus distinct clinicopathologic entities. Adv Anat Pathol 2000; 7: 210–13.

40. Lazenby AJ, Yardley JH, Giardiello FM, Bayless TM. Pitfalls in the diagnosis of collagenous colitis: experience with 75 cases from a registry of collagenous colitis at the Johns Hopkins Hospital. Hum Pathol 1990; 21: 905–10.

41. Treanor DT, Gibbons DG, O'Donoghue DP, Sheahan K. Pseudomembranes in collagenous colitis. Histopathology 2001; 38: 83–4.

42. Giardiello FM, Hansen FC, Lazenby AJ et al. Collagenous colitis in setting of nonsteroidal antiinflammatory drugs and antibiotics. Dig Dis Sci 1990; 35: 257–60.

43. Reyes V, Bronner M, Haggitt R. Pseudomembranes and collagenous colitis. Am J Clin Pathol 1999; 112: A542 (Abstract).

44. Powell DW, Mifflin RC, Valentich JD, Crowe SE, Saada JI, West AB. Myofibroblasts. II. Intestinal subepithelial myofibroblasts. Am J Physiol 1999; 277: C183–201.

45. Aigner T, Neureiter D, Muller S, Kuspert G, Belke J, Kirchner T. Extracellular matrix composition and gene expression in collagenous colitis. Gastroenterology 1997; 113: 136–43.

46. Gunther U, Schuppan D, Bauer M, Matthes H, Stallmach A, Schmitt-Graff A et al. Fibrogenesis and fibrolysis in collagenous colitis. Patterns of procollagen types I and IV, matrix-metalloproteinase-1 and -13, and TIMP-1 gene expression. Am J Pathol 1999; 155: 493–503.

47. Lamps LW, Bonsib SM, Mitros FA. Collagenous colitis: not your basic basement membrane abnormality. Mod Pathol 2000; 13: A83 (Abstract).

48. Graham MF, Diegelmann RF, Elson COS et al. Collagen content and types in the intestinal strictures of Crohn's disease. Gastroenterology 1988; 94: 257–65.

49. Hwang WS, Kelly JK, Shaffer EA, Hershfield NB. Collagenous colitis: a disease of pericryptal fibroblast sheath? J Pathol 1986; 149: 33–40.

50. Mosnier JF, Larvol L, Barge J et al. Lymphocytic and collagenous colitis: an immunohistochemical study. Am J Gastroenterol 1996; 91: 709–13.

51. Fine KD, Lee EL, Meyer RL. Colonic histopathology in untreated celiac sprue or refractory sprue: is it lymphocytic colitis or colonic lymphocytosis? Hum Pathol 1998; 29: 1433–40.

52. Cellier C, Delabesse E, Helmer C et al. Refractory sprue, coeliac disease, and enteropathy-associated T-cell lymphoma. Lancet 2000; 356: 203–8.

53. Lee E, Schiller LR, Vendrell D, Santa Ana CA, Fordtran JS. Subepithelial collagen table thickness in colon specimens from patients with microscopic colitis and collagenous colitis. Gastroenterology 1992; 103: 1790–6.

54. Rask-Madsen J, Grove O, Hansen MG, Bukhave K, Scient C, Henrik-Nielsen R. Colonic transport of water and electrolytes in a patient with secretory diarrhoea due to collagenous colitis. Dig Dis Sci 1983; 28: 1141–6.

55. Burgel N, Bojarski C, Mankertz J, Zeitz M, Fromm M, Jorg D. Mechanisms of diarrhea in collagenous colitis. Gastroenterology 2002; 123: 433–43.

56. Bonderup OK, Folkersen BH, Gjersoe P, Teglbjaerg PS. Collagenous colitis: a long-term follow-up study. Eur J Gastroenterol Hepatol 1999; 11: 493–5.

57. Mullhaupt B, Guller U, Anabitarte M, Guller R, Fried M. Lymphocytic colitis: clinical presentation and long term course. Gut 1998; 43: 629–33.

58. Pardi DS, Loftus EV, Tremaine W, Sandborn WJ. Treatment of refractory microscopic colitis with azathioprine and 6-mercaptopurine. Gastroenterology 2001; 120: 1483–4.

59. Miehlke S, Heymer P, Bethke B et al. Budesonide treatment for collagenous colitis: a randomized, double-blind, placebo-controlled, multicenter trial. Gastroenterology 2002; 123: 978–84.

44 | Colon ischemia

SETH E. PERSKY AND LAWRENCE J. BRANDT

Introduction

Colon ischemia (CI) is the most common form of gastrointestinal ischemia, accounting for more than 50% of all cases of such ischemic injuries [1]. Although colonic gangrene has been recognized for more than 100 years it was not until the 1950s and 1960s that milder forms of CI were described [2]. Today we recognize six patterns of CI: reversible colopathy, transient colitis, chronic ulcerating colitis, gangrene, stricture, and fulminant universal colitis. While CI most often is idiopathic, some episodes can be linked to proven etiologies. CI commonly is misdiagnosed as inflammatory bowel disease (IBD); however, clinicians must be able to differentiate these two causes of colitis, as their management and prognosis differ markedly. This chapter will discuss current knowledge of the etiologies, pathogenesis, presentations, and management of CI.

Incidence/etiology

Although CI is the most common form of gastrointestinal ischemia it remains largely under-diagnosed. Stated to be the cause of 1 in 2000 hospitalizations [3], its exact incidence remains unknown, since a large number of cases go undetected; they are either subclinical in nature, mild and resolve spontaneously before patients present to a physician, or are misdiagnosed as infectious colitis or IBD [4]. While the incidence of IBD classically has been described as having a bimodal age distribution, most cases in the second peak actually are cases of CI rather than of new onset IBD [4, 5]. In one series [4], after reviewing the clinical, radiographic and pathologic findings of patients who developed new-onset colitis after age 50, 75% of these cases were classified as definite CI, whereas only 15% of these cases were classified as definite ulcerative or Crohn's colitis. In the remaining 10% of cases a definitive diagnosis could not be established. Therefore, when encountering a patient over the age of 50 with new-onset colitis, CI is the most likely cause, and new-onset IBD should be considered only after carefully excluding CI.

CI affects both sexes equally, and unlike IBD, which predominantly affects young patients, 90% of sporadic cases of CI occur in patients over age 60. Affected patients often have atherosclerotic vascular disease, although there is no close correlation between the severity of such changes and the occurrence of CI. There are several recent small case series [6–8] that report a lesser proportion of cases in the elderly, with up to 34% of cases of CI occurring in patients below the age of 50 [7]. It is this subset of patients who are often misdiagnosed with IBD. Unlike IBD, however, the vast majority of patients with CI improve spontaneously, i.e. with no or conservative therapy, whereas patients with IBD usually improve only after receiving definitive therapy with aminosalicylates or corticosteroids.

The proven etiologies of CI in the older population differ markedly from those in younger patients (Table 1). Most commonly, however, no etiology is found and it is believed that CI develops as a result of spontaneous episodes of local 'nonocclusive' ischemia, in association with small vessel atherosclerotic disease. Angiograms in affected patients rarely correlate with clinical disease, and only show age-related changes such as narrowing and tortuosity of the inferior mesenteric artery and its branches [56]. Less commonly, systemic alterations in blood flow, such as hypoperfusion from underlying cardiovascular disease, sepsis, hypovolemia, or inferior mesenteric artery (IMA) thrombosis, lead to CI. Constipation and straining during bowel movements also have a deleterious, albeit transient, effect on colonic blood flow, and therefore may render the colon susceptible to ischemic injury.

There are two special clinical problems which have a significant association with CI. First, up to 10% of patients undergoing elective abdominal aortic sur-

Stephan R. Targan, Fergus Shanahan and Loren C. Karp (eds.), Inflammatory Bowel Disease: From Bench to Bedside, 2nd Edition, 799–810.

Table 1. Characteristics of colon ischemia in young vs. older subjects*

	Younger patients	Elderly patients
Identifiable causes	(Approximately 40% of patients) Coagulopathies Vasculitis Infections Long-distance running Medications: Oral contraceptives, pseudoephedrine, danazol, sumatriptan, psychotropic agents, cocaine, alosetron	(Approximately 10% of patients) Aortic surgery Cardiac failure/dysrhythmias Arterial embolus/thrombosis Shock Medications: digoxin, psychotropic agents, flutamide, hormone replacement therapy
Idiopathic etiology associations	Approximately 60% of cases	Approximately 90% of cases Distal obstructing lesions ($\sim$5%): carcinoma, volvulus, constipation, fecal impaction; colonic stricture; diverticulitis
Course	May be recurrent. Progression to chronic CI (i.e. chronic ulcerating colitis, stricture) unstudied	Single episode. Progression to chronic CI (i.e. chronic ulcerating colitis, stricture) uncommon
Location	Right side Rectum	Splenic flexure Sigmoid colon
Differential diagnosis	IBD; infection	Infection; carcinoma; IBD less likely

*The presentation and clinical course is usually identical in both younger and older patients; this table merely emphasizes differences that *may* occasionally be seen.

gery develop CI. This is related to hypotension, intraoperative trauma to the colon, IMA loss during aneurysmectomy, or prolonged cross-clamp time. In the setting of emergent aortic surgery for repair of a ruptured abdominal aortic aneurysm, CI develops in up to 60% of cases. By assessing colonic perfusion intraoperatively with laser Doppler flowmetry [57, 58] and photoplethysmography [59], several investigators have been able to predict the development of postoperative CI. The intramural pH of the sigmoid colon before and after cross-clamping the aorta, as determined by tonometry, has also been used to predict postoperative CI [60]. Routine intraoperative reimplantation of the IMA to prevent postoperative CI has been advocated by one group [61], but is not routinely performed.

The second clinical problem associated with an increased risk of CI is colon obstruction. Approximately 20% of older patients with CI have a distal and potentially obstructing lesion, such as carcinoma, stricture, fecal impaction, diverticulitis, or volvulus. CI probably develops from distension of the colon proximal to the obstructing lesion, which leads to increased intraluminal pressure and decreased mucosal blood flow. Less commonly such lesions are within a segment of ischemic colon and, rarely, distal to it.

The causes of CI in younger persons are markedly different from those in elderly patients. Often these causes may not be immediately apparent to the clinician, and making a diagnosis of CI instead of new-onset IBD may be especially challenging. A well-described but rare cause of CI in young patients is mesenteric vasculitis. Such vasculitides include polyarteritis nodosa [31, 32], Takayasu's arteritis, or Buerger's disease [30], as well as systemic autoimmune disease, such as systemic lupus erythematosus (SLE) [27, 28] or Sjögren's syndrome [62]. Hypercoagulable states, such as protein S or C deficiency, antithrombin III deficiency, or activated protein C resistance (APCR, factor 5 Leiden) may also lead to CI in young patients. The anticoagulant actions of the protein C system are important in maintaining microvasculature patency [63]. Heterozygosity for APCR is present in approximately 5% of the general population, with affected individuals having an eight-fold risk of venous thrombotic disease [25]. For the rare individual with the homo-

Table 2. Causes of colon ischemia

Non-Iatrogenic causes	Iatrogenic causes
Non-occlusive ischemia	Surgical
Cardiac failure or dysrhythmias	Aneurysmectomy
Shock	Aortoiliac reconstruction
Obstructing colon carcinoma	Gynecologic operations
Volvulus	Exchange transfusion
Strangulated hernia	Colonic bypass
Arterial embolus	Lumbar aortography
Inferior mesenteric artery thrombosis	Colectomy with IMA ligation
Cholesterol emboli [9, 10]	Colonoscopy and barium enema [35, 36]
Phlebosclerosis [11, 12]	
Pancreatitis [13, 14]	Medications
Amyloid [10, 15–17]	Digitalis
Idiopathic dysautonomia [18]	Estrogens [25, 37, 38]
Allergy [19, 20]	Danazol [39]
Trauma	Progestins [40]
Ruptured ectopic preganancy	Gold compounds
Long-distance running [21]	Psychotropic drugs [41]
Pit viper toxin [22]	Pseudoephedrine [42]
Pheochromocytoma [23]	Sumatriptan [43]
Kawasaki's disease [24]	Cocaine [44]
Hematologic disorders	Immunosuppressive agents [45]
Protein C and S deficiencies	NSAID [46]
Sickle cell disease	Imipramine [47]
Antithrombin III deficiency	Methamphetamines [48, 49]
Activated protein C resistance [25]	Vasopressin [50]
Prothrombin 20210A mutations [26]	Ergot [51]
Vasculitis	Oral hyperosmotic saline laxatives [52]
Systemic lupus erythematosus [27–29]	Interferon Alpha [53]
Rheumatoid arthritis	Glycerin enema [54]
Thromboangitis obliterans [30]	Flutamide [55]
Periarteritis nodosa (hepatitis B) [31–32]	Alosetron
Takaysu's arteritis	
Infections	
Escherichia coli 0157:H7 [33, 34]	
Angiostrongylus costaricensis	
Cytomegalovirus	
Hepatitis B (polyarteritis nodosa) [31, 32]	

zygous defect for APCR the risk of thrombosis increases 50–100-fold. Recently, a young woman with APCR was reported to develop ischemic colitis [25]; she was also taking oral contraceptives, another risk factor for ischemic colitis. Lastly, another hypercoagulable state is linked to genetic mutations in the prothrombin 20210 A allele, and bowel ischemia has recently been described in patients with this mutation [26]. In that report one of the two cases had CI.

There are a host of medications which may cause CI (see Table 2). Use of these medications may lead to ischemic injury via mesenteric vasoconstriction or thrombosis. The most commonly implicated medica-

tions have been oral contraceptive agents; in one study [37], 59% of younger individuals with reversible CI used these preparations. As mentioned above, patients with underlying hypercoagulable states who use oral contraceptive agents may be at a particularly increased risk for CI. Several other medications have recently been described in case reports to cause CI, including: sumatriptan [43], interferon-alpha [53], pseudoephedrine [42], non-steroidal anti-inflammatory agents [46], vasopressin [50], Danazol [39], imipramine [47], psychotropic agents [41], and digitalis. Several illicit drugs may also lead to CI, including cocaine [44] and methamphetamine [48, 49].

Anatomy of colonic vasculature and pathogenesis of colon ischemia

Blood is supplied to the colon by the superior mesenteric artery (SMA), and the inferior mesenteric artery (IMA), which respectively carry blood to the proximal and distal parts of the colon. The SMA gives off the middle colic artery and then branches into: (a) the right colic artery, which supplies the distal ascending colon, hepatic flexure, and proximal half of the transverse colon; and (b) the ileocolic artery, which supplies the terminal ileum, cecum, and proximal ascending colon. The IMA, which is smaller than the SMA, branches into: (a) the left colic artery, which supplies the distal half of the transverse colon and the descending colon; (b) multiple sigmoid arteries, which supply the sigmoid colon; and (c) the superior rectal artery, which supplies the rectum. The distal rectum is also supplied by the middle and inferior rectal arteries, which are branches of the internal iliac artery. Additionally, there are extensive collateral arteries between the SMA and the IMA, limiting the propensity of the colon to ischemic injury. These collateral vessels include: (a) the marginal artery of Drummond, which is close to and parallels the wall of the intestine; (b) the central anastomotic artery, which is larger and more centrally placed; and (c) the arc of Riolan at the base of the mesentery. If either the SMA or IMA is occluded, a large collateral vessel, termed the 'meandering artery', may develop, representing a dilated central anastomotic artery or arc of Riolan. Resting blood flow to the colon is relatively low (8–44 ml/min per 100 g tissue) in comparison to other parts of the gastrointestinal tract [64], and colonic blood flow is even more diminished during functional motor activity of the colon, e.g. bowel movements, making the colon uniquely susceptible to ischemia.

There are certain areas of the colon where collateral flow between the SMA and the IMA is crucial to maintain colonic integrity; these are the areas especially prone to ischemic injury. The most important of these 'watershed' areas is the splenic flexure, or Griffith's point, which has the highest propensity for CI, especially in individuals in whom the marginal artery of Drummond is diminutive or absent. The rectosigmoid junction, or the point of Sudeck, is another so-called watershed region. This region is dependent on anastomotic branches of the IMA and

the internal iliac artery, and CI may develop if these anastomotic branches are limited.

CI results from local hypoperfusion, with or without reperfusion injury. During hypoperfusion the involved colonic segment is deprived of important nutrients and oxygen; during extensive periods of hypoperfusion tissue hypoxia leads directly to cell death, with damage progressing outward from the mucosa to the serosa [65]. It has been shown that high levels of renin and angiotensin, which are elevated during periods of systemic hypotension, may exacerbate splanchnic vasospasm, leading to further colonic hypoperfusion and ischemia [66].

During relatively short periods of hypoperfusion, however, most of ischemic damage results from subsequent reperfusion injury. In one study [67], the injury observed after 3 h of hypoperfusion and 1 h of reperfusion was more severe than that observed after 4 h of isolated hypoperfusion. There are extensive data showing that, during reperfusion, there is mucosal neutrophil accumulation, with release of reactive oxygen metabolites by activated neutrophils as part of the inflammatory process [64]. In an equine model of CI [68], one group of horses was subjected to 6 h of hypoperfusion, and another group to 3 h of hypoperfusion followed by 3 h of reperfusion. Concentrations of neutrophils within the mucosa were significantly higher during reperfusion as compared with the corresponding times in the group subjected to prolonged hypoperfusion. The reactive oxygen metabolites released from activated neutrophils are derived from molecular oxygen, and mediate both mucosal damage and disruption of microvascular integrity. Reactive oxygen metabolites cause peroxidation of lipids, thereby disrupting cell membranes and destroying cell compartmentation, resulting in cell lysis. Reactive oxygen metabolites also alter nucleotide function, and damage cellular proteins and enzymes. These effects ultimately lead to impaired cellular function or necrosis.

Several reactive oxygen metabolites are released during reperfusion injury (Table 3). First, the univalent reduction of oxygen produces the superoxide anion radical, O_2^-. The cellular toxicity associated with superoxide is usually attributed to its role as a precursor to more reactive oxygen species, such as hydrogen peroxide (H_2O_2) and the hydroxyl radical ($\cdot OH$), which is formed via the Haber–Weiss reaction ($O_2^- + H_2O_2$). The Haber–Weiss reaction is accelerated by the presence of transition metals, such as iron, which are present in high concentrations in intestinal mucosa. Hypochlorous acid (HOCl) is

Table 3. Xanthine oxidase pathway for induction of ischemia

In Non-Ischemic Tissue:

$$\text{Hypoxanthine} + H_2O + NAD^+ \xrightarrow{\text{XDH}} \text{Xanthine} + NADH + H^+$$

During Tissue Ischemia:

$$\text{Hypoxanthine} + H_2O + 2O_2 \xrightarrow{\text{XO}} \text{Xanthine} + \boxed{O_2^- + H_2O_2}$$

$$\text{Xanthine} + 2O_2 + H_2O \xrightarrow{\text{XO}} \text{Uric Acid} + \boxed{O_2^- + H_2O_2}$$

$$\boxed{O_2^- + H_2O_2} \to \mathbf{H_2O_2}, \cdot OH$$

Reactive Oxygen Metabolite Production:

$$\text{Univalent reduction of oxygen} \longrightarrow O_2^-$$

$$O_2^- \xrightarrow{\text{divalent reduction or dismutation}} H_2O_2 \quad \text{(Hydrogen Peroxide Radical)}$$

$$O_2^- + H_2O_2 \xrightarrow{\text{Haber-Weiss Reaction}} \cdot OH \quad \text{(Hydroxyl Radical)}$$

another potent oxidizing agent formed from the reaction of H_2O_2 with Cl^- and H^+ when activated neutrophils secrete the enzyme myeloperoxidase (MPO). In animal models of reperfusion injury, treatment with antioxidants, such as superoxide dismutase (SOD), catalase, and dimethyl sulfoxide (DMSO), as well as with iron chelators, such as desferoxamine, has been shown to attenuate reperfusion injury by suppressing the formation of these reactive oxygen metabolites [8, 69, 70]; such agents have not been tested clinically in CI.

In addition to their direct cytotoxic effects, reactive oxygen metabolites also initiate the production and release of leukocyte chemoattractants, such as leukotriene B_4 and platelet-activating factor (PAF), which increase polymorphonuclear leukocyte migration, leading to further oxidant production [71, 72]. Activated neutrophils also release a variety of enzymes, such as collagenase and elastase, that can directly injure mucosa and the microvasculature.

Reactive oxygen metabolites are also formed by the oxidant-producing enzyme, xanthine oxidase (XO). In ischemic tissue XO has the ability to generate O_2^- and H_2O_2 during the oxidation of xanthine and hypoxanthine. Normally, i.e. in non-ischemic tissue, XO does not produce reactive oxygen metabolites, as it uses NAD^+ instead of O_2 as an electron-acceptor. During tissue ischemia, however, due to a proteolytic conversion in the enzyme, XO uses O_2 as an electron-acceptor, generating reactive oxygen metabolites. The XO inhibitor, allopurinol, has been shown to attenuate both the epithelial cell necrosis and the increased microvascular permeability observed after reperfusion of the rat small intestine [73], but this agent has not been tested in the clinical setting.

Clinical presentation

The clinical presentation of CI varies with the underlying cause, extent of vascular obstruction, and presence or absence of comorbity. The spectrum of CI is wide (Table 4), and includes reversible colopathy, transient colitis, chronic ulcerating colitis, gangrene, stricture, and fulminant universal colitis. Most patients with CI present with the acute onset of mild, crampy, left lower quadrant pain, followed by the urge to defecate. These symptoms are followed over the next 24 h by the passage of bright red or maroon blood mixed with diarrheal stool. In one study of 47 patients, 87% had abdominal pain, 68% had diarrhea, and 38% had nausea and vomiting [74]. Gastrointestinal blood loss is not of hemodynamic significance. If there is hemodynamic instability, or if significant blood loss requiring transfusion occurs, other diagnoses should be considered. Approximately 10% have only subclincal disease and present later with constipation or obstruction secondary to stricture formation. The elderly may also present with altered levels of consciousness. Prior to the onset of symptoms the vast majority of patients with CI feel well. CI, however, may also develop shortly after a major cardiac event, such as a myocardial infarction or new-onset atrial fibrillation, or during hemodialysis-associated hypotension; these patients have higher mortality than do patients without these precipitating factors. In several reports [7, 75], approximately 30% of CI cases occurred immediately following such episodes of systemic hypotension. Unfortunately, even with classic presentations, the diagnosis is often overlooked. In one series [7], CI

Table 4. Types and approximate incidences of colon ischemia

Type	Incidence (%)
Reversible colonopathy	30–40
Transient colitis	15–20
Chronic ulcerating colitis	20–25
Stricture	10–15
Gangrene	15–20
Fulminant universal colitis	< 5

was initially considered only in 17% of patients ultimately diagnosed with CI.

Physical examination usually reveals mild to moderate tenderness over the involved segment of bowel. Low-grade fever is present in a minority of patients. In more severe cases patients may also have abdominal distension from an ileus. Approximately 15–20% of patients present with peritoneal signs from colonic perforation. The vast majority of patients, however, look well at presentation. Laboratory analysis may show a mild leukocytosis, which may parallel the extent of injury. The hematocrit is usually at the patient's baseline since blood loss is minimal, and hemoconcentration from fluid losses is not severe.

Any segment of the colon may be affected by ischemia' however, the 'watershed' areas of the sigmoid colon and splenic flexure are most commonly involved (Fig. 1). In the largest series to date, ischemia isolated to the right colon was seen in 8% of patients, ischemia isolated to the rectum in 6%, and segmental ischemia proximal to the splenic flexure was seen in 12%.

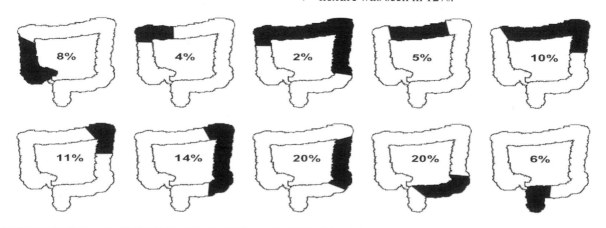

Figure 1. Ischemia of the colon: patterns of involvement in 250 cases.

Specific etiologies tend to involve specific areas of the colon. Systemic low flow states usually produce CI of the ascending colon as a result of vasoconstriction within the distribution of the SMA. Spontaneous non-occlusive ischemic injury usually involves the watershed areas of the left colon. Colon ischemia after abdominal aortic surgery typically involves the descending colon, due to operative IMA injury. Ischemia isolated to the rectum accounts for only 3–6% of all cases of CI [1, 76], and is seen in patients with aorto-iliac atherosclerotic disease; in up to half of these cases ischemia is preceded by a superimposed hemodynamic event, leading to systemic hypotension. In this situation severe atherosclerotic disease combined with hypotension compromises the collateral blood supply to the rectum. The length of affected bowel also varies with the cause of ischemia. Atheromatous emboli involve short segments, whereas non-occlusive injuries involve longer portions of colon.

The diagnosis of CI depends on prompt clinical suspicion, followed by appropriate laboratory, roentgenographic, and colonoscopic studies. Using these studies other causes of colitis (e.g. infections, IBD), can be excluded, as can other diagnoses that are often considered, such as diverticulitis and colon carcinoma. A thorough stool analysis for potential causes of infectious colitis should be performed. Stool should be cultured for common pathogens, such as *Salmonella*, *Shigella*, and *Campylobacter*, as well as for *E. coli* O157:H7. In one study [34], immunohistologic staining for *E. coli* O157:H7 was performed in a retrospective manner on archived colonic biopsy specimens from 24 patients with various colitides. Biopsies from 27.3% of patients initially diagnosed with CI were found to stain positively for *E. coli* O157:H7 antigens, thereby implicating an infectious etiology for some cases of CI previously considered to be idiopathic in origin. If there is concomitant hemolysis or renal failure, thereby increasing the clinical suspicion for this infection, immunohistochemical staining may be performed on biopsy specimens if stool cultures for *E. coli* O157:H7 were not obtained at the time of presentation.

Radiologic evaluation is performed commonly in the initial assessment of patients with CI. Whereas these examinations provide information regarding location and severity of disease, they are neither sufficiently sensitive nor specific in most situations to diagnose CI definitively. Plain films of the abdomen are important initially, and findings suggestive of CI may be identified in 30% of patients [77]; colonic thumbprinting, which represents submucosal hemorrhage and edema, may be seen; an ileus or colonic pseudo-obstruction may be present, and toxic megacolon has been described [78]. In severe cases pneumatosis coli, intraperitoneal air, or both, may be seen. In addition to the above findings, computerized tomography scanning may reveal segmental colonic thickening with narrowing of the colonic lumen, and may demonstrate mild to moderate amounts of free intraperitoneal fluid; portal venous gas may also be seen in advanced cases. Rarely, patients with CI may have intrahepatic abscess formation [79]. Unfortunately, none of these findings is specific for CI. Recently, scintigraphic imaging with technectium-99m was reported to localize a segment of CI [80]. Nuclear imaging with indium-111 has also been described in the literature 6[81, 82]. These tests, however, are expensive, lack specificity, and are not routinely used to diagnose CI.

If CI is suspected, and the patient has no signs of peritonitis, colonoscopy or the combination of sigmoidoscopy and a gentle barium enema should be performed within 48 h of the onset of symptoms. Evaluation should be performed early, because submucosal hemorrhages are resorbed and mucosal abnormalities may improve quickly. Barium enema was the first method used to diagnose CI, and has a reported sensitivity of 60–80% [83, 84]. Thumbprinting, segmental longitudinal ulcers, and mucosal abnormalities are delineated well by barium enema. Barium enema is also a useful technique for the evaluation of strictures, which may develop after an acute episode of CI. Colonoscopy, however, provides a better assessment of mucosal abnormalities than does barium enema [84], is the procedure of choice in the acute and chronic setting, and is safe if performed carefully [84]. Colonoscopic evaluation may demonstrate submucosal hemorrhagic nodules, which are the equivalent of radiologic thumbprinting. Such nodules are blue or red; however, black nodules may also be seen, and indicate colonic gangrene. Colonic ulcerations exhibit a spectrum ranging from small aphthae to large, wide, parallel longitudinal ulcers, known as 'bearclaw' ulcers. In the mildest form of CI, i.e. reversible colopathy, submucosal hemorrhages are resorbed quickly, and mucosal ulceration is not seen on colonoscopy. In cases of transient colitis the mucosa covering submucosal hemorrhages breaks down, blood is exuded into the lumen, and erythema, edema, ulceration, and mucosal friability are seen on colonoscopy. Mural spasm and luminal narrowing may also be present. Occasionally, pseudomembranes are observed, mimicking *Clostridium difficile* colitis. If the inflammatory response to ischemia is vigorous there may be a heaping-up of the mucosa and submucosa, which may mimic a stricturing or polypoid neoplasm.

Morphologic changes after an ischemic insult vary with the duration and severity of the injury. Repeat colonoscopy or barium enema 1 week after the initial study should reflect evolution of the injury, either by demonstrating normalization of the colonic mucosa or replacement of submucosal hemorrhagic nodules with a transient segmental ulcerative colitis. Over time, in cases of more severe injury, granulation tissue replaces the mucosa and submucosa. Persistence of submucosal nodules on follow-up examination should suggest another diagnosis, such as carcinoma, lymphoma, IBD, or amyloidosis. Although colonoscopy can only survey the mucosal aspect of the colon, future studies with endoscopic ultrasound may help assist with diagnosis, and perhaps help predict prognosis by evaluating the entire thickness of the colonic wall [85].

Colonoscopy also affords the clinician an opportunity to biopsy affected as well as normal-appearing mucosa. In the early stages of CI the biopsies are usually non-specific. As in other forms of acute colitis, cryptitis, crypt abscesses, and an acute inflammatory infiltrate may be present, and usually do not help in differential diagnosis. Additionally there may be fibrin thrombi in submucosal capillaries, submucosal hemorrhage, vascular congestion, loss of normal crypt architecture, an absence of surface epithelial cells, and mucin depletion. Although the use of biopsies in the diagnosis of CI is limited because of the superficial and often non-specific nature of the small specimens, findings that are diagnostic of CI on histologic analysis are mucosal gangrene and the presence of ghost cells. Biopsy is also important to exclude other entities, such as IBD. In the presence of pseudomembranes, histologic evidence of hyalinization of the lamina propria, presence of atrophic-appearing microcrypts, full-thickness mucosal necrosis, and lamina propria hemorrhage are more suggestive of CI than of *C. difficile* colitis [86].

During colonoscopy or barium enema, it is important to avoid overdistension of the colon, because colonic blood flow is diminished at intraluminal pressures greater than 30 mmHg. Additionally, at this pressure, blood is shunted from the mucosa to the serosa, exacerbating ischemic injury. In a dog model [87] a 22–72% decrease in colonic blood flow persisted even after release of distension. Insufflation of carbon dioxide rather than room air during colonoscopy may reduce this potential complication of overdistension, as carbon dioxide increases colonic blood flow during colonic distension, and it is rapidly absorbed from the intestine, thus decreasing post-procedure colonic distension [88]. Another key to limiting complications during colonoscopy in patients with CI is to limit intubation to only the affected region, and not continue proximal to affected bowel because of the risk of perforation. If clinically indicated, the segment of the colon proximal to the ischemic segment should be surveyed only after the acute episode of ischemia has resolved.

Angiography is rarely of any benefit in the evaluation of CI, because colonic blood flow has usually returned to normal by the time patients become symptomatic and, as mentioned earlier, anatomic abnormalities in the mesenteric circulation rarely explain the cause for CI. Therefore, angiography should not be used routinely in the evaluation of patients with CI. If, however, the clinical presentation is more consistent with acute mesenteric ischemia (e.g. the patient has severe abdominal pain), angiography plays an important role in the differential diagnosis. In a minority of patients with isolated right-sided colon ischemia, angiography may play a role in documenting and treating SMA disease, since such patients may be at risk for concomitant or subsequent small bowel ischemia. If the clinical presentation is confusing, and it is unclear whether the patient has CI or acute mesenteric ischemia, an alternative approach to differentiate the two is by administering an 'air' enema. Air can be instilled by a hand bulb or during sigmoidoscopy, and is followed by fluoroscopy. Submucosal hemorrhage and edema are seen as relative radiodensities against the column of air. If thumbprinting is isolated to the right colon, angiography is warranted to confirm SMA disease; defects confined to the left colon do not warrant angiographic evaluation.

Therapy and prognosis

Once the diagnosis of CI is confirmed, initial management is largely supportive (Fig. 2). Any drug potentially implicated in the ischemic episode should be discontinued, and the patient's cardiac status should be optimized. Marked colonic distension, if present, should be treated with rectal tube decom-

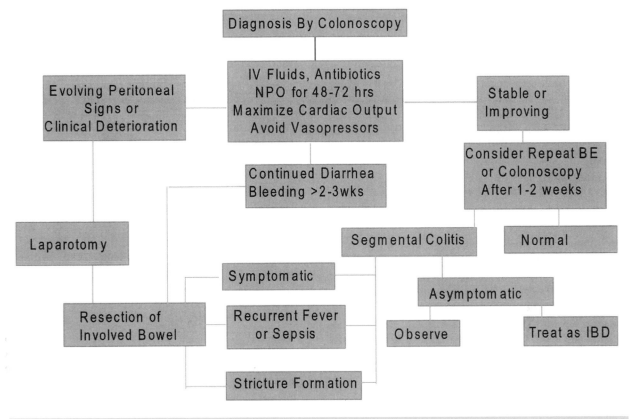

Figure 2. Algorithm for management of colon ischemia.

pression. Vasopressors should be avoided. The patient should be placed on bowel rest, and given intravenous fluids. Broad-spectrum antibiotics should be administered to cover anaerobic bowel flora, as several animal studies have demonstrated that the concentration of luminal anaerobic bacteria increases after ischemic injury to the bowel [89–91], largely due to their proliferation in an ischemia-induced hypoxic environment. Additionally, ischemic injury disrupts the mucosal barrier, allowing for bacterial translocation and portal bacteremia. Metronidazole has been shown to prolong survival in rats subjected to mesenteric ischemia [91], and its use is recommended in patients with CI. In only two patients short-chain fatty acid enemas have been reported to speed healing in CI [92]. A large-scale, randomized trial is needed to validate the efficacy of this therapy. Infusions of splanchnic vasodilators, such as papaverine or prostaglandin E_1, have been shown to increase colonic blood flow in experimental models of CI [93], but are not used clinically in the management of CI, since blood flow has returned to normal by the onset of symptoms, and vasodilators do not improve outcome.

Unfortunately it is impossible to predict the outcome of an ischemic insult from the initial clinical, radiologic, and colonoscopic findings. Patients who initially look well may deteriorate quickly, despite the results of initial studies. With conservative or even no medical therapy, however, patients with reversible colopathy or transient ischemic colitis will have a complete clinical and endoscopic recovery. Fortunately these patients encompass approximately 60–70% of all cases of CI. Symptoms improve over 3–4 days, and complete endoscopic regression of colitis ensues over 4–6 weeks. Only 5% of patients with complete healing will have a subsequent recurrence of CI. Complete endoscopic regression of colitis may take up to 6 months, but during this time patients are often asymptomatic. These patients may require repeat colonoscopic examination to document healing or development of a stricture or chronic colitis.

Continued symptoms or protein-losing colopathy for more than 2–3 weeks is worrisome and is best treated by resection of the involved segment of colon. The extent of the resection should be guided by the distribution of disease as revealed by preoperative studies, rather than by the appearance of the serosal surface of the colon at the time of operation, because if the injury is not transmural, mucosal injury may be extensive despite a normal-appearing serosa.

Approximately 15% of patients with CI will develop full-thickness colonic gangrene during their initial presentation. These patients require resection of the involved colonic segment. Several alarm symptoms and signs that warrant prompt surgical intervention include severe pain or bleeding, persistent or increasing fevers, presence of rebound, involuntary guarding, or distension on abdominal examination. After segmental resection, symptoms improve and prognosis is excellent if perforation did not occur. If perforation is present at the time of surgery the patient's overall prognosis depends on his or her underlying age and comorbid status, as well as the timing of surgery and the ability to control concomitant sepsis.

One recent study identified two factors which may be predictive of a more severe colitis; an increased need for surgical resection and a higher mortality rate [94]. These factors were: chronic renal failure requiring hemodialysis, and ischemia involving the right colon. In that study up to 82% of hemodialysis patients with CI developed isolated right-sided ischemia [94], likely attributed to repeated episodes of systemic hypotension in the hemodialysis sessions. As mentioned earlier, isolated right colonic involvement may indicate compromised SMA blood flow, warranting early angiography and surgical exploration due to the increased risk of more severe disease.

Approximately 20% of patients with CI will develop a chronic ulcerating ischemic colitis, manifest by continued symptoms of abdominal pain, diarrhea, fevers, or hematochezia. They may also have a protein-losing colopathy with resultant hypoalbuminemia. Differentiation from Crohn's colitis may be difficult on follow-up barium enema or colonoscopy; in both of these entities chronic ulceration, erythema, friable mucosa, edema and blunted vasculature may be seen. Mucosal nodularity may also be present in both conditions, and pseudopolyposis has been described as a consequence of chronic ulcerating colitis [95]. However, patients with a non-healing segment of chronic ulcerating ischemic colitis do not respond to corticosteroid therapy or other traditional therapies for IBD. Additionally, repeat biopsies from areas of chronic ulcerating ischemic colitis may show glandular dropout with associated ghost cells, as well as an increased deposition of mucosal and submucosal fibrous tissue. These biopsy findings are quite different from those seen in IBD, in which branching of glands and granulomata are commonly seen. Patients with symptomatic chronic ulcerating ischemic colitis may benefit from a segmental resection; after resection, recurrence is rare.

Lastly, approximately 10% of patients develop a stricture after an acute episode of colon ischemia. Strictures develop as a consequence of damage to the muscularis propria and its replacement with fibrous tissue. These patients may not present during the acute episode of ischemia, but develop constipation or colonic obstruction weeks to months later. Patients with ischemic strictures can be observed if asymptomatic, since some strictures will regress in 12–24 months with no specific therapy. Symptoms from strictures, such as worsening constipation, usually do not respond to laxative therapy. While gentle use of bulk laxatives may dilate strictures, they may be hazardous if used in a zealous fashion. Endoscopic dilation may be attempted if the stricture is short, although there are no data on the efficacy of this approach. Most symptomatic strictures should be surgically resected.

Summary

CI is the most common cause of mesenteric ischemia, and encompasses a wide clinical spectrum from mild, reversible disease to life-threatening colonic gangrene. While most commonly seen in elderly patients, younger patients are also at risk, especially if an underlying risk factor such as vasculitis, hypercoagulability, or certain medication use such as oral contraceptives, pseudoephedrine, cocaine, or ergot, is present. Colonoscopic evaluation is critical in the evaluation of patients with CI, although it must be kept in mind that CI may mimic or be mimicked by other entities, such as IBD or carcinoma. Conservative management usually leads to a full clinical recovery, although several subsets of patients may require segmental resection. Clinicians should always consider CI in the differential diagnosis of acute colitis, especially in elderly patients.

References

1. Brandt LJ, Boley SJ. Colonic ischemia. Surg Clin N Am 1992; 72: 203–29.

2. Boley SJ, Schwartz S, Lash J *et al.* Reversible vascular occlusion of the colon. Surg Gynecol Obstet 1963; 121: 789.

3. Cappell MS. Intestinal (mesenteric) vasculopathy II. Ischemic colitis and chronic mesenteric ischemia. Gastroenterol Clin N Am 1998; 27: 827–60.

4. Brandt LJ, Boley SJ, Goldberg L *et al.* Colitis in the elderly. Am J Gastroenterol 1981; 76: 239–45.

5. Wright HG. Ulcerating colitis in the elderly: epidemiological and clinical study of an in-patient hospital population. Thesis, New Haven, Yale University, 1970.

6. Habu Y, Tahashi Y, Kiyota K. Reevaluation of clinical features of ischemic colitis: analysis of 68 consecutive cases diagnosed by early colonoscopy. Scand J Gastroenterol 1996; 31: 881–6.

7. Arnott ID, Ghosh S, Ferguson A. The spectrum of ischemic colitis. Eur J Gastroenterol Hepatol 1999; 11: 295–303.

8. Dalsing M, Grosfeld J, Shiffler M *et al.* Superoxide dismutase: a cellular protective enzyme in bowel ischemia. J Surg Res 1983; 34: 589–96.

9. Jaeger HJ, Mathias KD, Gissler HM *et al.* Rectum and sigmoid colon necrosis due to cholesterol embolization after implantation of an aortic stent-graft. J Vasc Interv Radiol 1999; 10: 751–5.

10. Bayne SR, Donovan DL, Henthorne WA. A rare complication in elective repair of an abdominal aortic aneurysm: multiple transmural colonic infarcts secondary to atheroemboli. Ann Vasc Surg 1994; 8: 290–5.

11. Arimura Y, Kondoh Y, Kurokawa S. Chronic ischemic colonic lesion caused by phlebosclerosis with calcification. Am J Gastroenterol 1998; 93: 2290–2.

12. Maruyama Y, Watanabe F, Kanaoka S. A case of phlebosclerotic ischemic colitis: a distinct entity. Endoscopy 1997; 29: 334.

13. Srivastava DN, Gulati MS, Tandon RK. Colonic infection in acute pancreatitis: an unusual cause of gastrointestinal hemorrhage. Am J Gastroenterol 1998; 93: 1186–7.

14. Yamagiwa I, Obata K, Hatanaka Y *et al.* Ischemic colitis complicating severe acute pancreatitis in a child. J Pediatr Gastroenterol Nutr 1993; 16: 208–11.

15. Kyzer S, Korzets A, Zevin D *et al.* Ischemic colitis complicating AA amyloidosis and familial Mediterranean fever. Isr J Med Sci 1993; 29: 212–14.

16. Trinh TD, Jones B, Fishman EK. Amyloidosis of the colon presenting as ischemic colitis: a case report and review of the literature. Gastrointest Radiol 1991; 16: 133–6.

17. Perarnau JM, Raabe JJ, Courrier A *et al.* A rare etiology of ischemic colitis – amyloid colitis. Endoscopy 1982; 14: 107–9.

18. Woodward JM, Sanders DS, Keighley MR *et al.* Ischaemic enterocolitis complicating idiopathic dysautonomia. Gut 1998; 43: 285–7.

19. Sacca JD. Acute ischemic colitis due to milk allergy. Ann Allergy 1971; 29: 268–9.

20. Ohrui T, Sekizawa K, Seki H *et al.* Ischemic colitis during an asthma attack. J Allergy Clin Immunol 1998; 102: 692–3.

21. Lucas W, Schroy PC. Reversible ischemic colitis in a high endurance athlete. Am J Gastroenterol 1998; 93: 2231–4.

22. Iwakiri R, Fujimoto K, Hirano M *et al.* Snake-strike induced ischemic colitis with colonic stricture complicated by disseminated intravascular coagulation. South Med J 1995; 88: 1084-5.

23. Sohn CI, Kim JJ, Lim YH. A Case Of Ischemic colitis associated with pheochromocytoma. Am J Gastroenterol 1998; 93: 124–6.

24. Fan St, Law WY, Wong KK. Ischemic colitis in Kawasaki disease. J Pediatr Surg 1986; 21: 964–5.

25. Mann DE, Kessel ER, Mullins DL *et al.* Ischemic colitis and acquired resistance to activated protein C in a woman using oral contraceptives. Am J Gastroenterol 1998; 93: 1960–2.

26. Balian A, Veyradier A, Naveau S. Prothrombin 20210G/A mutation in two patients with mesenteric ischemia. Dig Dis Sci 1999; 44: 1910–13.

27. Korkut M, Erhan Y, Osmanoglu H *et al.* A case of severe ischemic colitis caused by systemic lupus erythematosus. J Pak Med Assoc 1995; 45: 271–2.

28. Reissman P, Weiss EG, Teoh TA. Gangrenous ischemic colitis of the rectum: a rare complication of systemic lupus erythematosus. Am J Gastroenterol 1994; 89: 2234–6.

29. Papa MZ, Shiloni E, McDonald HD. Total colonic necrosis: a catastrophic complication of systemic lupus erythematosus. Dis Colon Rectum 1986; 29: 576–8.

30. Guay A, Janower ML, Bain RW. A case of Buerger's disease causing ischemic colitis with perforation in a young male. Am J Med Sci 1976; 271: 239–40.

31. Okada M, Konishi F, Sakuma K *et al.* Perforation of the sigmoid colon with ischemic change due to polyarteritis nodosa. J Gastroenterol 1999; 34: 400–4.

32. Ruiz-Irastorza G, Egurbide MV, Aguirre C. Polyarteritis nodosa presenting as ischemic colitis. Br J Rheumatol 1996; 35: 1333–4.

33. Dalal BI, Krishnan C, Laschuk B *et al.* Sporadic hemorrhagic colitis associated with *Escherichia coli*, Type O157:H7: unusual presentation mimicking ischemic colitis. Can J Surg 1987; 30: 247–8.

34. Su D, Brandt LJ, Sigal SH. The immunohistological diagnosis of *E. coli* O157:H7 Colitis: possible association with colonic ischemia. Am J Gastroenterol 1998; 93: 1055–9.

35. Cremers MI, Olivera AP, Freitas J. Ischemic colitis as a complication of colonoscopy. Endoscopy 1998; 30: S54.

36. Champman AH, El-Hasani S. Colon Ischaemia secondary to Barolith obstruction. Br J Radiol 1998; 71: 983–4.

37. Deana DG, Dean PJ. Reversible ischemic colitis in young women. Association with oral contraceptive use. Am J Surg Pathol 1995; 19: 454–62.

38. Gurbaz AK, Gurbuz B, Salas L *et al.* Premarin induced ischemic colitis. J Clin Gastroenterol 1994; 19: 108–11.

39. Miyata T, Tamechika Y, Torisu M. Ischemic colitis in a 33 year old woman on danazol treatment for endometriosis. Am J Gastroenterol 1988; 83: 1420–3.

40. Gelfand MD. Ischemic colitis associated with a depot synthetic progestogen. Am J Dig Dis 1972; 17: 275–7.

41. Patel YJ, Scherl ND, Elias S *et al.* Ischemic colitis associated with psychotropic drugs. Dig Dis Sci 1992; 37: 1148–9.

42. Dowd J, Bailey D, Moussa K *et al.* Ischemic colitis associated with pseudoephedrine use: four cases. Am J Gastroenterol 1999; 94: 2430–4.

43. Knudsen JF, Friedman B, Chen M. Ischemic colitis and sumatriptan use. Arch Intern Med 1998; 158: 1946–8.

44. Papi C, Candia S, Masci P *et al.* Acute ischemic colitis following intravenous cocaine use. Ital J Gastroenterol Hepatol 1999; 31: 305–7.

45. Gomella LG, Gehrken GA, Hagihara PF *et al.* Ischemic colitis and immunosuppression. An experimental model. Dis Colon Rectum 1986; 29. 99–101.

46. Carratu R, Parisi P, Agozzino A. Segmental ischemic colitis associated with nonsteroidal anti-inflammatory drugs. J Clin Gastroenterol 1993; 16: 31–4.

47. Basse P, Rordam P. Ischemic colitis complicating imipramine overdose and alcohol ingestion. Case report. Eur J Surg 1992; 158: 187–8.

48. Dirkx CA, Gerscovich EO. Sonographic findings in methamphetamine induced ischemic colitis. J Clin Ultrasound. 1998; 26: 479–82.

49. Johnson TD, Berenson MM. Methamphetamine induced ischemic colitis. J Clin Gastroenterol 1991; 13: 687–9.

50. Lambert M, De Peyer R, Muller AF. Reversible Iichemic colitis after intravenous vasopressin therapy. J Am Med Assoc 1982; 247: 666–7.

51. Stillman AE, Weinberg M, Mast WC *et al.* Ischemic bowel disease attributable to ergot. Gastroenterology 1977; 72: 1336–7.

52. Oh JK, Meiselman M, Lataif LE Jr. Ischemic colitis caused by oral hyperosmotic saline laxatives. Gastrointest Endosc 1997; 45: 319–22.

53. Tada H, Saitoh S, Nakagawa Y *et al.* Ischemic colitis during interferon alpha treatment for chronic active hepatitis C. J Gastroenterol 1996; 31: 582–4.

54. Chang RY, Tsai CH, Chou YS, Wu TC. Nonocclusive ischemic colitis following glycerin enema in a patient with coronary artery disease. A case report. Angiology 1995; 46: 747–52.

55. Barouk J, Doubremelle M, Faroux R. Ischemic colitis after taking flutamide. Gastroenterol Clin Biol 1998; 22: 841.

56. Binns JC, Isaacson P. Age related changes in the colonic blood supply: their relevance to ischemic colitis. Gut 1978; 19.:384.

57. Redaelli CA, Schilling MK, Carrel TP. Intraoperative assessment of intestinal viability by laser Doppler flowmetry for surgery of ruptured abdominal aortic aneurysms. World J Surg 1998; 22: 283–9.

58. Sakakibara Y, Jikuya T, Saito EM *et al.* Does laser Doppler flowmetry aid the prevention of ischemic colitis in abdominal aortic aneurysm surgery? Thorac Cardiovasc Surg 1997; 45: 32–4.

59. Garcia-Granero E, Alos R, Uribe N *et al.* Intraoperative photoplethysmographic diagnosis of ischemic colitis. Am J Surg 1997; 63: 765–8.

60. Schiedler MG, Cutler BS, Fiddian-Green RG. Sigmoid intramural pH for prediction of ischemic colitis during aortic surgery: a comparison with risk factors and inferior mesenteric artery stump pressure. Arch Surg 1987; 122: 881–6.

61. Seeger JM, Coe DA, Kaelin LD *et al.* Routine reimplantation of patent inferior mesenteric arteries limits colon infarction after aortic reconstruction. J Vasc Surg 1992; 15: 635–41.

62. Lie T. Isolated necrotizing and granulomatous vasculitis causing ischemic bowel disease in primary Sjögren's syndrome. J Rheumatol 1995; 22: 2375–7.

63. Esmon CT. The roles of protein C and thrombomodulin in the regulation of blood coagulation. J Biol Chem 1989; 264: 4743–6.

64. Thomson A, Hemphill D, Jeejeebhoy KN. Oxidative stress and antioxidants in intestinal disease. Dig Dis 1998; 16: 152–8.

65. Zimmerman BJ, Granger DN. Reperfusion injury. Surg Clin N Am 1992; 72: 65–83.

66. Bailey RW, Bulkley GB. Pathogenesis of nonocclusive ischemic volitis. Ann Surg 1986; 203: 590–8.

67. Parks DA, Granger DN. Contributions of ischemia and reperfusion to mucosal lesion formation. Am J Physiol 1986; 250: G749.

68. Moore RM, Bertone AL, Bailey MQ. Neutrophil accumulation in the large colon of horses during low-flow ischemia and reperfusion. Am J Vet Res 1994; 55: 1454–63.

69. Lehmann CH, Luther B, Holzapfel A *et al.* Perioperative vascular flushing perfusion in acute mesenteric artery occlusion. Eur J Vasc Endovasc Surg. 1995; 10: 265–71.

70. Zimmerman BJ, Granger DN. Reperfusion injury. Surg Clin N Am 1992; 72: 65–83.

71. Zimmerman BJ, Grisham MB, Granger DN. Role of oxidants in ischemia/reperfusion induced granulocyte infiltration. Am J Physiol 1990; 258: G185.

72. Mangino MJ, Anderson CB, Murphy MK *et al.* Mucosal arachidonate metabolism and intestinal ischemia–reperfusion injury. Am J Physiol 1989; 257: G299.

73. Granger DN, McCord JM, Parks DA *et al.* Xanthine oxidase inhibitors attenuate ischemia-induced vascular permeability changes in the cat intestine. Gastroenterology 1986; 90: 80.

74. Longo WE, Ballantyne GH, Gusberg RJ. Ischemic colitis: patterns and prognosis. Dis Colon Rectum 1992; 35: 726–30.

75. Guttormson NL, Bubrick MP. Mortality from ischemic colitis. Dis Colon Rectum 1989; 26: 469–72.

76. Bharucha AE, Tremaine WJ, Johnson CD, Batts KP. Ischemic proctosigmoiditis. Am J Gastroenterol 1996; 91: 2305–9.

77. Wolf EL, Sprayregen S, Bakal CW. Radiology in intestinal ischemia: plain film, contrast, and other imaging studies. Surg Clin N Am 1992; 72: 107–24.

78. Markoglou C, Avgerinos A, Mitrakou M. Toxic megacolon secondary to acute ischemic colitis. Hepatogastroenterology 1993; 40: 188–90.

79. Balthazar EJ, Yen BC, Gordoen RB. Ischemic colitis: CT evaluation of 54 cases. Radiology 1999; 211: 381–8.

80. Hyun H, Pai E, Blend MJ. Ischemic colitis: Tc-99m HMPAO leukocyte scintigraphy and correlative imaging. Clin Nucl Med 1998; 23: 165–7.

81. Bell D, Jackson J, Connaughton JJ. Indium-111 neutrophil imaging in ischemic colitis. J Nucl Med 1986; 27: 1782.

82. Vijayakumar V, Bekerman C, Blend MJ. Preoperative prediction of extent and severity of ischemic colitis by imaging with In-111 labeled leukocytes. Clin Nucl Med 1991; 16: 98.

83. Iida M, Matsui T, Fuchigami T. Ischemic colitis. Serial changes in double contrast barium enema examinations. Radiology 1986; 159: 337–41.

84. Scowcroft CW, Sanowski RA, Kozarek RA. Colonoscopy in ischemic colitis. Gastroenterol Endosc 1981; 27: 156–61.

85. Shimizu S, Tada M, Kawai K. Endoscopic ultrasonography in inflammatory bowel diseases. Gastroenterol Endosc Clin N Am 1995; 5: 851–9.

86. Dignan CR, Greenson JK. Can ischemic colitis be differentiated from C. *difficile* colitis in biopsy specimens? Am J Surg Pathol 1997; 21: 706–10.

87. Tunick PA, Treiber WF, Martin BA *et al.* Pathophysiological effects of bowel distention on intestinal blood flow. II. Curr Top Surg Res 1970; 2: 59–69.

88. Brandt LJ, Boley SJ, Sammartano R. Carbon dioxide and room air insufflation of the colon. Gastrointest Endosc 1986; 32: 324–9.

89. Bennion RS, Wilson SE, Williams RA. Early portal anaerobic bacteremia in mesenteric ischemia. Arch Surg 1984; 119:151–5.

90. Redan JA, Rush BF, Lysz TW *et al.* Organ distribution of gut-derived bacteria caused by bowel manipulation or ischemia. Am J Surg 1990; 159: 85–9.

91. Plonka AJ, Schentag JJ, Messinger S. Effects of enteral and intravenous antimicrobial treatment on survival following intestinal ischemia in rats. J Surg Res 1989; 46: 216–20.

92. Mortensen FV, Hessov I, Rasmussen A. Ischemic colitis treated with short chain fatty acids: report of two cases. J Gastroenterol 1996; 31: 302–3.

93. Nakai M, Uchida H, Hanaoka T. Beneficial effects of prostaglandin E_1 on ischemic colitis following surgery on the abdominal aorta. Jpn J Surg 1998; 28: 1146–53.

94. Flobert C, Cellier C, Berger A *et al.* Right colonic involvement is associated with severe forms of ischemic colitis and occurs frequently in patients with chronic renal failure requiring hemodialysis. Am J Gastroenterol 2000; 95: 195–8.

95. Levine DS, Surawicz CM, Spencer GD. Inflammatory polyposis two years after ischemic colon injury. Dig Dis Sci 1986; 31: 1159–67.

45 | Diversion colitis

KONRAD H. SOERGEL

Introduction

Diversion colitis is an inflammatory bowel disease (IBD) that has attracted considerable clinical and scientific interest during the past 15 years. Indeed, the histologic features of this entity were recognized only 28 years ago [1] and in that time it has acquired several names, including bypass colitis, exclusion colitis, and disuse colitis. Since its first clinical description in 1981 [2], a number of case reports and series have been published [2–30]. Certain observations have sparked the current curiosity:

1. It is the only model of non-infectious 'experimental' colitis in humans, with the possible exception of radiation colitis. It occurs in 50–100% of cases following exclusion of the distal colorectum and is predictably reversible by surgical reanastomosis [2, 17, 18, 21].

2. It is caused by diversion of the fecal stream, most likely by deprivation of short-chain fatty acids (SCFA) [13], the preferred metabolic substrate of the colonic epithelium [31–33].

3. This 'nutritional deficiency' leads to an inflammatory process similar to that of other colitides [34–36].

4. The disease has recently been reproduced in laboratory animals [37].

Thus, diversion colitis presents an ideal opportunity to study the pathophysiology of an IBD in humans: its occurrence after surgical bypass of normal colon is frequent, characteristics of inflammation may be studied as they develop, and successful treatment by either surgical or medical means can be monitored.

Table 1. Possible etiologic mechanisms of diversion colitis [13]

Luminal short-chain fatty acid deficiency
Deficient short-chain fatty acid metabolism by colonocytes
Pathogenic microorganisms – direct invasion or toxin elaboration
Stasis – bacterial overgrowth (similar to bypass enteritis)
Bile acid deficiency

Pathophysiology/colonic SCFA metabolism

While the clinical setting in which diversion colitis develops is well established, little is known regarding the etiologic mechanism. The sequence of events following surgical bypass that culminates in inflammation and clinical symptoms remains poorly understood. Several theories have been proposed (Table 1). Among these, only the virtual absence of SCFA from the lumen of the bypassed segment is supported by substantial evidence. Thus, no pathogenic microorganisms or toxins have been discovered in the contents of the inflamed segments [13, 26, 38]. Quantitative bacteriologic studies revealed a decrease in anaerobic bacteria by two log units with frequent absence of *Eubacteria* and *Bifidobacteria* strains as compared to normal feces [38]. A stasis colitis, similar to the bypass enteritis observed after jejunoileal bypass for obesity, is unlikely since saline irrigations are ineffective in diversion colitis [13]. Luminal 'casts' composed of cell detritus and mucus glycoproteins are also rare occurrences in this disease [30]. There are no data to support or refute the theory of luminal bile salt deficiency. However, colitis is not a feature of biliary obstruction. Excess bile acids rather than deficiency, in the colon, cause secretion and mild cellular injury. Decreased ability of the colonic epithelium to metabolize SCFA is contradicted by several observations: the near-

Stephan R. Targan, Fergus Shanahan and Loren C. Karp (eds.), Inflammatory Bowel Disease: From Bench to Bedside, 2nd Edition, 811–821.
© 2003 *Kluwer Academic Publishers. Printed in Great Britain*

absence of these acids in the contents of diverted segments [13] and the healing of mucosal inflammation when they are supplied by irrigation or by surgical reanastomosis.

The concentration of SCFA (acetate + propionate + n-butyrate) in the sparse, mucoid contents of rectosigmoid segments affected by diversion colitis is only < 5 mmol/L, compared to 100–200 mmol/L in normal stool [39–41]. This reduction is caused by the exclusion of contents from the proximal colon where the bulk of anaerobic carbohydrate fermentation occurs, by the reduced number of anaerobic bacteria [38] and by the absence of fermentable exogenous carbohydrate. The reduced bacterial flora of these inflamed bowel segments is incapable of fermenting glucose at a rate sufficient to cause a rise in breath H_2 concentration [13]. The following observations support the SCFA deficiency hypothesis of diversion colitis:

1. SCFA, especially n-butyrate, are the preferred metabolic substrate of the colonic epithelium [31, 32, 42]. SCFA are abundantly produced by anaerobic fermentation and are rapidly absorbed in the human ileum and colon by a combination of a distinct anion exchange transport system and non-ionic diffusion [39–41, 43–49].

2. The preference for SCFA as the source of metabolic fuel increases aborally along the colon [32, 42]. Thus, from cecum to rectum an increasing percentage of metabolic need is derived from SCFA. Diversions involving proximal colonic segments are less likely to develop colitis [36], and the surgical creation of neobladders from the proximal or transverse colon does not result in inflammation [50].

3. Blood concentrations of SCFA (except acetate) are negligible, so they must enter the colonocyte from the colonic lumen.

4. Deprivation of luminal contents following surgical diversion results in colitis only in the diverted segment [36].

5. Treatment of the colitis with SCFA irrigations decreases the inflammation [13].

6. Metabolic inhibition of colonocyte SCFA metabolism produces experimental colitis in animals [51, 52].

7. The crypt cell production rate is decreased after surgical diversion [53–55] and irrigation with an SCFA solution restores the cell proliferation rate to normal [56].

8. Decreased colonic SCFA concentrations during therapy with broad-spectrum antibiotics have been implicated in the pathogenesis of *Clostridium difficile*-negative antibiotic-associated diarrhea [57].

9. All three major SCFA (n-butyrate, propionate, acetate) potently inhibit colonic secretion induced by cholera toxin and *E-coli* heat-stable enterotoxin [58].

Luminal deficiency of SCFA caused by surgical diversion of the fecal stream results in a state of energy deficiency. Presumably, this leads to a 'weakened' epithelium when the colonocyte is unable to satisfy its metabolic requirements with alternate substrates such as glucose, ketone bodies, and glutamine [32, 42]. Increased epithelial permeability develops, allowing bacterial translocation resulting in a local inflammatory response. The transition from weakened epithelium to inflammation is poorly understood, but it may resemble so-called starvation colitis [33]. While SCFA deficiency is the key to the development of diversion colitis, nutritional deprivation may not be the only explanation. As Table 2 demonstrates, these acids have several additional effects on colonic function, any of which may contribute to maintaining the functional and morphologic integrity of the colonic epithelium.

Table 2. Physiologic functions of colonic short-chain fatty acids

Preferred metabolic fuel for colonocytes [31, 32, 42]
Enhance Na, Cl, and water absorption [48, 79]
Acid–base balance: HCO_3 secretion [45, 46]
Regulation of motility [62]
Mucosal growth [53, 70, 80, 81]
Increase cell differentiation [53, 54]
Carbohydrate caloric salvage [40, 44, 48]
Bacteriostatic properties
Increase colonic blood flow [56, 79]
Increase colonic oxygen consumption [79]

The sparse, predominantly anaerobic bacterial flora may play a contributory role. Compared to controls, patients with diversion colitis have an increased number of rectal nitrate-reducing bacteria which may have pathogenic potential via enhanced production of NO [59].

Clinical presentation

The incidence of diversion colitis is difficult to assess, for several reasons. Some reports include patients with pre-existing inflammation of the rectosigmoid, while in others only symptomatic patients were examined. No longitudinal studies are available, although the disease has been found as early as 1 month after the surgical diversion procedure [30]. Based on endoscopic criteria the prevalence varies between 40–50% [7, 10, 11, 30, 38, 55] to 70% [5], 80% [26], and 90–100% [2, 4, 9, 17–19]. Histologic examination of mucosal biopsies revealed inflammatory changes in 68% [12], 83% [30], and 100% [7] of cases. The true incidence of diversion colitis will probably approach 100% when patients are examined sequentially and when clinicians and pathologists become more familiar with this entity.

The most common symptom is an increase in the frequency and amount of mucoid discharge from the anus or the mucus fistula. Bleeding, usually painless [25], may be noticed, ranging from blood-tinged discharge to significant blood loss [4], which may require resection of the diverted segment [23]. Pain in the pelvic area, the left lower quadrant, or the rectum is another rare complaint. The pain may be dull or cramping and is occasionally associated with the presence of mucoliths in the lumen [10, 30]. One patient represented with copious mucoid discharge of 400 ml/day; histologic study, however, revealed no inflammation but the presence of goblet cell hyperplasia [3]. Other reported complaints include low-grade fever, anal irritation by the mucoid discharge, and anal fissure. The reported frequency of any symptom attributable to diversion colitis varies between zero [5, 20, 22, 60], 10–20% [6, 9, 61], 28–33% [26, 62], and 50% [7, 9, 11]. Furthermore, there is no correlation between the severity of inflammation and the presence and degree of symptoms [7].

Asymptomatic cases tend to be recognized in one of three settings: (a) endoscopic re-evaluation following a bypass operation for IBD when either new inflammation or, less likely, worsening of pre-existing disease is found [15–17]; (b) routine examination

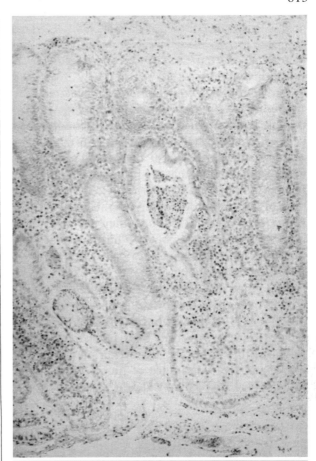

Figure 1. Severe diversion colitis. Histology resembles ulcerative colitis with mucosal surface exudate, crypt distortion, crypt abscesses, and a mixed inflammation infiltrate in the lamina propria. Note marked mucosal edema (H&E, original magnification × 50). (Courtesy of Richard A. Komorowski, MD, Milwaukee, WI.)

prior to planned surgical restitution of colorectal continuity; (c) a prospective search for diversion colitis [5]. These asymptomatic patients may exhibit the entire spectrum from chronic inflammation, apparent only on histologic study, to severe inflammation easily recognized during endoscopy. Late stricture formation and areas of stenosis [6] may obviate plans for surgical reanastomosis.

Histopathology

The histologic spectrum of diversion colitis has been summarized [7, 14, 21]. The disease is largely limited to the mucosa, although fibrosis of the lamina propria [17] progressing to thickening of the muscularis propria [1, 63] may develop over time. The morphologic appearance varies with the severity of the disease and its duration. Many of its features (Table 3) overlap with those of idiopathic and infectious colitides.

Active diversion colitis mimics idiopathic ulcerative colitis (UC) in many respects (Fig. 1). The picture is dominated by marked mucosal edema, surface exudate, mucin depletion, a mixed inflammatory infiltrate, and crypt abscesses. The degree of edema, and the fact that the histologic changes may be non-uniform [2, 17], differ from the usual appearance of UC. Aphthous lesions are rarely identified in tissue sections [7], although they are commonly described by the endoscopist. While mucin granulomas have been presented, true mucosal granulomas have been reported only once [21], and their presence should raise the question of Crohn's colitis [64]. Villous changes of the surface epithelium have been described [14]. Subacute or healing diversion colitis (Fig. 2) is characterized by a persistent chronic inflammatory infiltrate, distortion of the colonic crypt, and the appearance of numerous lymphoid follicles [4, 12] which may appear as small polypoid

Table 3. Histologic findings in diversion colitis [1, 7, 12, 14, 21, 23, 63]

Common
- Mucosal edema
- Mucin depletion
- Reactive crypt epithelium
- Lymphocytic infiltrate
- Lymphoid follicles
- Crypt abscesses
- Crypt distortion and atrophy
- Neutrophilic infiltrate
- Mucosal ulceration
- Surface exudate

Rare
- Increased mucin production
- Goblet cell hyperplasia
- Mucin granulomas
- Villous surface changes
- Pseudomembranes
- Aphthous lesions

Never
- True granulomas

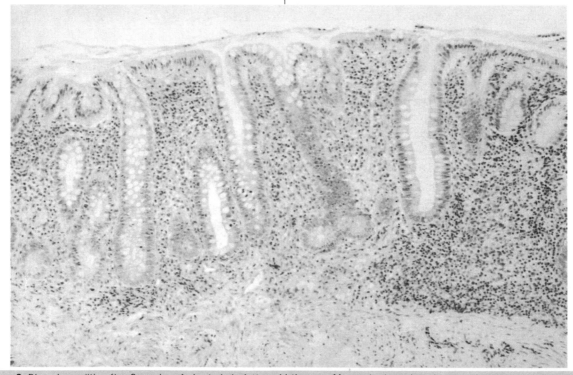

Figure 2. Diversion colitis after 2 weeks of short-chain fatty acid therapy. Mucosal edema has decreased and acute inflammatory infiltrate and exudate are diminished; crypts are shortened, irregular, non-parallel, and bifid with a chronic inflammatory infiltrate still present in the lamina propria (H&E, original magnification × 50). (Courtesy of Richard A. Komorowski, MD, Milwaukee, WI.)

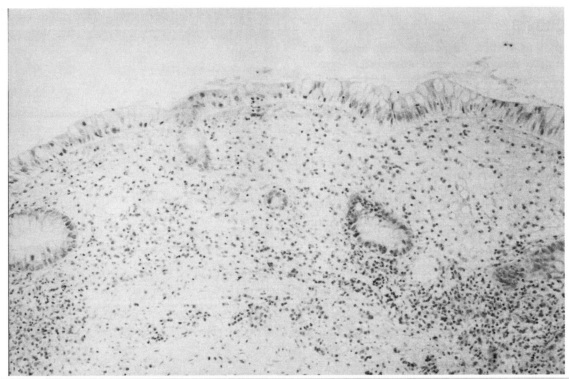

Figure 3. Long-standing diversion colitis on maintenance therapy with short-chain fatty acid irrigations. There is marked crypt atrophy with persisting mild chronic inflammation (H&E, original magnification × 7C). (Courtesy of Richard A. Komorowski, MD, Milwaukee, WI.)

excrescences on gross inspection. Lymphoid follicular hyperplasia within the lamina propria, featuring a high percentage of germinal centers, is nearly universal in diversion colitis. This is not a specific finding, however, as it may also be present in chronic UC and in lymphoid follicular proctitis [63]. The chronic inactive stage (Fig. 3) presents with a striking reduction in the number and depth of the colonic crypts [53], mild chronic inflammation, and persistence of the nodular lymphoid hyperplasia. The appearance is that of atrophy involving the mucosa [22], but not the muscularis propria and myenteric plexus [65].

The clinically important distinction of diversion colitis from other types of colonic inflammation can rarely be made on the basis of a single set of mucosal biopsies. A histologic appearance compatible with this diagnosis during the active phase of the disease, followed by resolution of mucosal edema, superficial ulcerations, and neutrophilic infiltration with therapy, strongly supports the diagnosis. The two effective therapeutic modalities consist of SCFA irriga-

tions (Figs. 1 and 2) and of surgical reanastomosis. By contrast, the response of distal UC to topical SCFA therapy is less predictable and less complete [66–68]. According to some reports, patients with Crohn's disease (CD) showing acute inflammation in their excluded rectosigmoid appear to suffer from diversion colitis rather than reactivation of their underlying disease [13, 15–17, 35]. By contrast, chronic radiation proctitis may respond clinically and histologically to topical SCFA therapy [69] but the distinction between diversion and radiation proctitis is clinically non-problematic.

In summary, there is an evolving concept of the pathology of diversion colitis involving a continuum of minimal non-specific inflammation progressing to acute inflammation, then chronic inflammatory changes, eventually resulting in fibrosis and mucosal atrophy. This continuum exhibits wide variability with regard to time of onset following diversion, the severity of inflammation, and the rate of evolution.

Diagnosis

In a patient with a surgical colonic bypass and preoperative documentation of normal rectosigmoid mucosa the diagnosis of diversion colitis is straightforward. The inflammation should involve the entire diverted segment, albeit non-uniformly, both in the longitudinal and circumferential axes [7]. The distal rectum tends to be most severely affected [30] while the blind end of Hartmann's pouch, or the area near a mucus fistula, may only show edema with loss of vascularity. Furthermore, the colonic segment in continuity with fecal stream should be free of inflammation. Marked erythema, edema, friability, granularity, and erosions covered by exudate are found in the acute stage (Fig. 4). Moderately active or healing disease is indicated by mild edema, erythema, and irregularly shaped erosions (Fig. 5). The inactive or healing stage can be recognized by edema, reduced vascular markings, and gradual narrowing of the lumen [6, 7] (Fig. 6). Diffuse mucosal modularity caused by aggregates of enlarged lymph follicles has been observed [2, 17], and masses of inspissated cell detritus and mucus may be present [30]. Contrast radiographs confirm the findings of mucosal modularity [18, 70] and diffuse luminal narrowing [6, 22]. An indium^{111}-labeled leukocyte scan was positive in a single patient [71]. Fistulas and abscess formation have not been reported as complications of diversion colitis.

The major problem in differential diagnosis is idiopathic IBD. Patients with CD frequently undergo colonic bypass procedures and the surgeon is reluctant to re-establish anatomic continuity in the presence of active inflammation in the bypassed segment. There exist several observations to suggest that reanastomosis may safely proceed in this situation [35].

1. CD activity generally requires the presence of intestinal or colonic contents [72] and it subsides after these contents have been diverted.

2. A total of nine patients [16, 17, 19] (also personal observations) experienced healing of the inflammation after the bypassed segment had been reconnected to the fecal stream.

3. Ten patients with CD were treated with instillation of an SCFA solution and all responded within 6 weeks [15 (also personal observations). Although topical SCFA therapy of Crohn's colitis has not yet been investigated, there is little reason to expect that it would be effective.

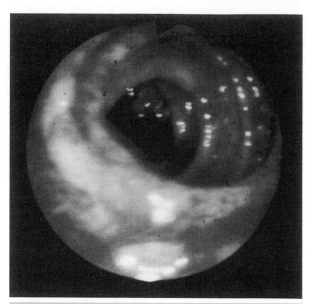

Figure 4. Severe diversion colitis. Marked friability with spontaneous bleeding, exudate, and superficial ulceration dominate the endoscopic appearance.

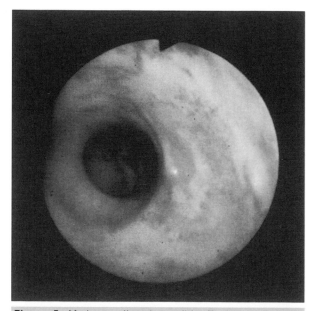

Figure 5. Moderate diversion colitis. Typical endoscopic findings include edema with loss of vascular markings, granularity and irregular areas of exudation, and superficial ulceration.

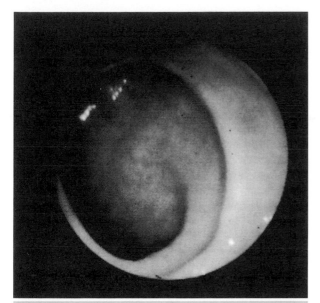

Figure 6. Diversion colitis after 4 weeks of short-chain fatty acid irrigation. Friability and ulceration have disappeared and vascular markings are noticeable, although mucosal edema remains (same patient as in Fig. 4).

Only an occasional patient with UC will undergo colectomy with plans for a later ileorectal anastomosis. Persistent inflammation of the isolated rectum usually represents diversion colitis rather than UC, particularly if lymphoid follicular hyperplasia and surface exudates are present on histologic examination [73]. A therapeutic trial with instillations of neutral isotonic SCFA solution cannot distinguish between diversion colitis and persistent distal idiopathic UC because some patients with ulcerative proctosigmoiditis will improve [66–68]. The differential diagnosis should also include antibiotic-associated colitis; while this is a theoretical possibility, it has not yet been reported. Finally, there may be mild focal 'colitis' associated with diverticulitis in the bypassed colon, but this entity does not involve the entire excluded segment [10].

Treatment

Indications

Decisions regarding the management of diversion colitis arise in different clinical settings: First there is the patient with endoscopic and histologic findings compatible with diversion colitis and documented absence of mucosal disease prior to the surgical diversion procedure. The surgeon should proceed with a planned reanastomosis without the need for preoperative medical therapy. Diversion colitis disappeared completely in all patients after colonic continuity had been re-established [2, 10, 16, 18, 21, 30, 55]. Second is the patient with symptomatic diversion colitis where reanastomosis or resection of the bypassed segment is contraindicated and which represents an indication for medical treatment. Third there are patients with asymptomatic diversion colitis who are not candidates for reanastomosis. The decision for medical treatment rests on the question of whether progressive stenosis and the uncertain risk of neoplasia developing in the diverted segment (see 'Prognosis') justify chronic topical therapy. No recommendations can be given at this time because there are no observations on the efficacy of medical therapy in preventing these complications. Fourth is the patient with an inflamed segment and pre-existing IBD. Here a diagnosis of diversion colitis will favor a planned reanastomosis while active CD or UC would militate against it. As discussed earlier, patients with known CD had a uniformly favorable outcome after continuity of the fecal stream had been re-established. In addition, three such patients were treated by the authors with SCFA irrigations; the inflammation subsided and did not reappear after surgical reanastomosis. One may conclude, tentatively, that an inflamed diverted colorectal segment in a patient with CD represents diversion colitis. While the same reasoning may also apply to UC, a favorable response to topical SCFA therapy does not distinguish between ulcerative and diversion colitis, as discussed earlier.

Miscellaneous therapy

The experience with medications known to be effective in other IBD is largely anecdotal. Two patients with diversion colitis responded to 5-aminosalicylate enemas (Rowasa) [60, 74], while one did not [24]; one other failed to improve with Azulfidine suppositories [17]. Treatment with corticosteroid enemas caused improvement in six patients [2, 4, 11, 60], while six other patients did not respond [17, 23, 24].

Topical SCFA therapy

The rationale for this therapy is to supply a mixture of the three SCFA predominant in stool water by slow instillation into the diverted segment, either per rectum or through a mucus fistula. The composition

Table 4. Short-chain fatty acid solution for treatment of diversion colitis [13]*

Acetic acid 7.206 g
Propionic acid 4.448 g
n-Butyric acid 7.049 g

Add 500–600 ml of deionized water; titrate with 1 N NaOH to pH7.0. Add NaCl, 2.500 g.
Add water to total volume of 2.0 L. Osmolality: 285–290 mOsm/kg.
Composition: acetate, 60 mmol/L; propionate, 30 mmol/L; n-butyrate, 40 mmol/L; Na, 152 mEq/L.

May be kept in a screw-topped plastic container. Stable for 3 months, if refrigerated.

*This solution is not commercially available. Its use has not been reviewed by the US Food and Drug Administration.

of the solution used by the author is shown in Table 4. Sixty milliliters is instilled twice daily with a syringe, either through a soft enema tip or an inflated Foley catheter. The patient remains supine for at least 30 min in order to avoid premature leakage. The initial four patients so treated experienced resolution of symptoms, normalization of endoscopic appearance, and disappearance of histologic evidence of acute inflammation [13]. Improvement generally is noted at 2 weeks, but complete healing requires a treatment period of 4–6 weeks. The authors have since treated six additional patients with identical favorable results [75]. Two children with diversion colitis also responded [12]. After healing has been achieved, relapse will occur within 1–4 weeks if treatment is discontinued. Remission can be maintained by reducing the frequency of the instillations progressively to one daily for 1–2 months, then to three instillations/week. Instillations of the patient's own colostomy effluent into the diverted segment have been suggested [29]. This would avoid the need and cost of preparing the malodorous SCFA solution in the pharmacy or research laboratory, but this logical idea has not yet been tested. No improvement was reported in a placebo-controlled study of diversion colitis, but the duration of observation was only 2 weeks, which may have been too little [8]. Negative results with SCFA enemas were obtained in a 3-week crossover trial of patients with underlying IBD [76], as well as in a 12-week study in which 14 of 21 patients had IBD [77]. By contrast, in a 12-week study of seven patients with CD and an excluded distal colorectum, marked improvement was noted beginning at 2 weeks of treatment [15]. In summary, the effect of topical SCFA therapy on diversion colitis continues to be debated. It appears, however, that most patients receiving this therapy for at least 4 weeks, without underlying IBD and without the use of a solution preservative [76] will respond favorably.

Prognosis

The prognosis of diversion colitis is good, although prospective evaluations of patient groups over long periods of time are not available. Progressive luminal narrowing and stricture formation have been observed repeatedly [1, 6] and may begin as early as 9 months following the diversion procedure [30]. Surgical reanastomosis is not advisable in the presence of a narrowed or strictured rectosigmoid segment. There are no data to document whether maintenance treatment with SCFA or corticosteroid irrigations will stop the progression to a distal 'microcolon,' although this may be expected to occur.

There is no evidence of an increased risk of neoplasia in the disused segment. On theoretical grounds the decreased epithelial proliferation rate in diversion colitis [53–55] supports this view, but the differentiating effect of SCFA, especially n-butyrate, on various cell lines [53, 54] raises some concern in this regard. In one series of 45 patients with a Hartmann's pouch, polyps were found in four and carcinoma in seven patients. However, these patients all had pre-existing conditions that placed them at increased risk for colorectal neoplasia [11]. Patients with ureterosigmoidostomies and an intact fecal stream are at high risk of developing carcinoma of the sigmoid, but this complication has not been described in patients who underwent isolation of colonic segments for the creation of neobladders [50, 78]. Certainly, patients who underwent colonic resection for carcinoma with colostomy and a rectal Hartmann's pouch may develop metachronous carcinomas [9, 10] and should therefore undergo regular endoscopic surveillance regardless of the presence of diversion colitis.

Concern has been expressed regarding bacterial invasion of the 'weakened' epithelium in the diverted segment, especially in patients with central venous catheters who are prone to septicemia [26].

In summary, the only definite risk of long-term diversion colitis is progressive narrowing of the involved segment, which may preclude planned surgical reanastomosis.

Future directions

Research in diversion colitis will continue to focus on the pathophysiology of this disease and its treatment. There is considerable interest in the overlap between idiopathic UC and diversion colitis, since both conditions share many histologic features as well as a favorable response to topical SCFA therapy [67]. Scientific inquiry into this disease is complicated by the limited number of surgical diversions performed at any one medical center. An animal model of this disease has recently been described [37], but has not yet been evaluated as to its applicability to humans. Specific areas of promising research directions include the following questions:

1. What events are involved in the apparent link between metabolic starvation of the colonic epithelium and the subsequent initiation of immune/inflammatory responses?

2. Are diverted segments at increased risk of malignant transformation?

3. How do SCFA irrigations reverse diversion colitis – direct replacement of a critical, obligate substrate, merely a nutritional adjuvant to help heal inflamed tissue, or local vasodilatory effects?

4. Do diversion colitis and idiopathic UC share pathophysiologic mechanisms? Why are SCFA irrigations effective in both diseases, although to a lesser extent in UC?

References

1. Morson BC, Dawson IMP. Gastrointestinal Pathology, 1st edn. London: Blackwell, 1972: 485.
2. Glotzer DJ, Glick ME, Goldman H. Proctitis and colitis following diversion of the fecal stream. Gastroenterology 1981; 80: 438–41.
3. Bories C, Miazza B, Galian A et al. Idiopathic chronic watery diarrhea from excluded rectosigmoid with goblet cell hyperplasia cured by restoration of large bowel continuity. Dig Dis Sci 1986; 31: 769–72.
4. Bosshardt RT, Abel NIE. Proctitis following fecal diversion. Dis Colon Rectum 1984; 27: 605–7.
5. Ferguson CM, Siegel RJ. A prospective evaluation of diversion colitis. Am Surg 1991; 57: 46–9.
6. Flesh P. Wurbs D, Krueger P. Die Diversionskolitis. Dtsch Med Wochenschr 1986; 111: 1566–9.
7. Geraghty JM, Talbot IC. Diversion colitis: histological features in the colon and rectum after defunctioning colostomy. Gut 1991; 32: 1020–3.
8. Guillemot F, Colombel F, Neut C et al. Treatment of diversion colitis by short-chain fatty acids: prospective and double-blind study. Dis Colon Rectum 1991; 34: 861–3.
9. Haas PA, Haas GP. A critical evaluation of the Hartmann's procedure. Am Surg 1988; 54: 330–85.
10. Haas PA, Fox TA Jr, Szilagy EJ. Endoscopic examination of the colon and rectum distal to a colostomy. Am J Gastroenterol 1990; 85: 850–4.
11. Haas PA, Fox TA Jr. The fate of the forgotten rectal pouch after Hartmann's procedure without reconstruction. Am J Surg 1990; 159: 106–11.
12. Haque S, West AB, Nioyer NIS. Correlation of clinical and pathologic features in pediatric patients with diversion colitis. Gastroenterology 1991; 100: A215 [Abstract].
13. Harig JM, Soergel KH, Komorowski RA et al. Treatment of diversion colitis with short-chain fatty acid irrigation. N Engl J Med 1989; 320: 23–8.
14. Komorowski RA. Histologic spectrum of diversion colitis. Am J Surg Pathol 1990; 14: 548–54.
15. Körber J, Soudah B, Schmidt FW. Effects of short-chain fatty acids irrigation on excluded inflamed segments of the colon in Crohn's disease. Gastroenterology 1992; 102: A648 [Abstract].
16. Korelitz BI, Cheskin LJ, Sohn N et al. Proctitis after fecal diversion in Crohn's disease and its elimination with reanastomosis: implications for surgical management. Report of four cases. Gastroenterology 1984; 87: 710–13.
17. Korelitz BI, Cheskin LJ, Sohn N et al. The fate of the rectal segment after diversion of the fecal stream in Crohn's disease: its implications for surgical management. J Clin Gastroenterol 1985; 7: 37–43.
18. Lechner CL, Frank W, Jantsch H et al. Lymphoid follicular hyperplasia in excluded colonic segments: a radiologic sign of diversion colitis. Radiology 1990; 17: 135–6.
19. Löhr HF, Mayet WJ, Singe CC et al. Diversionskolitis bei Morbus Crohn. Z Gastroenterol 1989; 27: 221–4.
20. Lusk LB, Reichen J, Levine JS. Aphthous ulceration in diversion colitis: clinical implications. Gastroenterology 1984; 87: 1171–3.
21. Ma CK, Gottlieb C, Haas PA. Diversion colitis: a clinicopathologic study of 21 cases. Hum Pathol 1990; 21: 429–36.
22. Mingazzini PL, Guiliana A, Caporale A et al. Defunctioned colon: clinical, endoscopical, radiological, and histopathological observations. Ital J Gastroenterol 1987; 19: 329–33.
23. Murray FE, O'Brien MJ, Birkett DH et al. Diversion colitis: pathologic findings in a resected sigmoid colon and rectum. Gastroenterology 1981; 93: 2404–8.
24. Nobels F, Colemont L. Van Nioer E. A case of diversion colitis. Acta Clin Belg 1989; 44: 202–4.
25. Ona FV, Boger JN. Rectal bleeding due to diversion colitis. Am J Gastroenterol 1985; 80: 40–1.
26. Ordein JJ, Di Lorenzo C, Flores A et al. Diversion colitis in children with severe gastrointestinal motility disorders. Am J Gastroenterol 1992; 87: 88–90.
27. Orkin VA, Telander RL. The effect of intra-abdominal resection or fecal diversion on perianal disease in pediatric Crohn's disease. J Pediatr Surg 1985; 20: 343–7.
28. Roe AM. The effects of diversion colitis in the Defunctioned anorectum. Gastroenterology 1991; 100: A244 [Abstract].
29. Spector P. Diversion colitis [Letter]. J. Clin Gastroenterol 1990; 12: 480.
30. Winte VJ, Creiner L, Schubert GE. Kolitis im funktionslosen Rektosigmoid nach Anlegen eines endstandigen Anus practernaturalis. Z Gastroenterol 1983; 21: 27–33.

46 | Pseudomembranous colitis and *Clostridium difficile* infection

RICHARD J. FARRELL, LORRAINE KYNE AND CIARÁN P. KELLY

Introduction

Clostridium difficile was first identified in 1935 as a commensal organsim in the fecal flora of healthy nconatcs [1]. Thc organism was given its name because it grew very slowly in culture and was difficult to isolate. Although it produced cytotoxins, and was pathogenic for guinea-pigs and rabbits, the organism was considered part of the normal neonatal gut flora that disappeared after weaning. *C. difficile* remained a laboratory curiosity until 1978, when Bartlett and colleagues [2] identified it as the source of a cytotoxin found in the stool of patients with antibiotic-associated pseudomembranous colitis. Since that time the incidence of *C. difficile* infection has increased dramatically and the organism is now recognized as the most frequent cause of nosocomial infectious diarrhea in developed countries [3–5]. Incidence rates of nosocomial infection range from 0.1 to 30 per 1000 hospital admissions in non-epidemic settings [6–11]. Over 30% of high-risk patients, such as those admitted to acute-care general medical medical wards and receiving antibiotics, may be colonized with *C. difficile* [12, 13]. In community populations the reported prevalence of *C. difficile*-associated diarrhea ranges from 8 to 12 per 100 000 person-years [14, 15].

As shown in Fig. 1, the sequence of events leading to *C. difficile* diarrhea and colitis in susceptible individuals comprises disturbance of the normal colonic microflora, exposure to and colonization by *C. difficile*, toxin production and toxin-mediated intestinal injury and inflammation. Depending on host factors, especially the immune response to *C. difficile* toxins, the outcome of colonization is either asymptomatic carriage or a spectrum of disease ranging from mild diarrhea to life-threatening pseudomembranous colitis.

During the two decades since its identification as a pathogen our understanding of the epidemiology,

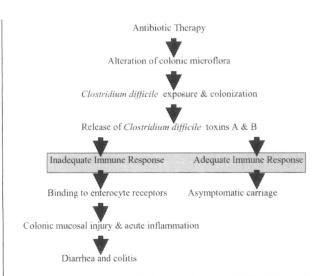

Figure 1. Pathogenesis of *C. difficile* diarrhea and colitis.

pathogenesis and management of disease caused by *C. difficile* has increased dramatically. Yet despite this increased knowledge there has been no substantial decline in the frequency of hospital-acquired *C. difficile* diarrhea and colitis.

Clostridium difficile

Clostridium difficile is a Gram-positive, obligate anaerobic rod that grows best in selective media containing cycloserine and cefoxitin and enriched with fructose and egg yolk [16]. This selective medium can detect as few as 2000 organisms in a stool sample. Individual strains of *C. difficile*, identified by agglutinating antisera [17], or DNA fingerprinting [18], may differ with regard to virulence [19]. Hospital outbreaks have been attributed to toxin-producing epidemic strains [20]. The organism forms spores, allowing it to survive in harsh environments and withstand antibiotic therapy.

Stephan R. Targan, Fergus Shanahan and Loren C. Karp (eds.), Inflammatory Bowel Disease: From Bench to Bedside, 2nd Edition, 823–844.

Pathogenesis

C. difficile diarrhea is a toxin-mediated disease. Pathogenic strains of *C. difficile* produce two potent protein exotoxins, toxin A and toxin B. These toxins are encoded by two distinct genes in close proximity on the bacterial genome [21–23]. They are structurally similar and show 49% homology at the amino acid level [22].These high molecular weight proteins are believed to bind receptors on the luminal aspect of the colonic epithelium and are then transported into the cytoplasm. However, specific cell surface receptors for toxin A or toxin B have not yet been characterized. In rabbit ileum the brush-border ectoenzyme, sucrase-isomaltose, binds *C. difficile* toxin A and functions as a cell surface receptor [24]. Since this enzyme is not present in human colonic mucosa, other membrane surface glycoproteins presumably serve as toxin receptors. Both toxins potently activate cell signaling molecules including NF-κB and MAP kinases in human monocytes, leading to the production and release of proinflammatory cytokines including IL-1β, TNF-α, and IL-8. These proinflammatory effects appear to precede toxin internalization and may be mediated by cell surface receptor binding [24, 25].

The aminoterminal regions of both toxins carry a series of repeated protein sequences that are believed to mediate toxin binding to the host cell membrane, while the carboxyterminal regions of both toxins possess similar glucosyltransferase activity. Once internalized, both toxins inactivate Rho proteins, a family of small GTP-binding proteins. The critical enzymatic action is the glycosylation of a specific, conserved threonine amino acid on Rho [26, 27]. The Rho protein targets of toxins A and B are rhoA, rac and cdc42, key cell signaling molecules that direct gene expression and are essential to maintain the actin cytoskeleton. Consequently, toxin-mediated Rho inactivation results in depolymerization of actin filaments, disruption of the cytoskeleton, cell rounding and cell death [24, 28]. In contrast to cholera toxin or *E. coli* heat-stable toxin, *C. difficile* toxins have no effects on intracellular levels of cyclic AMP or GMP. However, a number of other bacterial toxins target Rho proteins in a similar manner [29]. For example the cytotoxins from *C. sordellii* and *C. novyi* add a glucose to Rho and toxins from *Bacillus cereus* and *Staphylococcus aureus* also modify Rho family proteins. Thus it appears that *C. difficile* toxins and other structurally unrelated bacterial cytotoxins modify host cell structure and function by attacking Rho family proteins that are vital for maintenance of normal cell architecture and function.

Toxin A is an inflammatory enterotoxin that induces fluid secretion, increased mucosal permeability and marked enteritis and colitis when injected into the intestinal lumen of animals [24]. Toxin A also possesses weak cytotoxic activity against cultured cells [30, 31]. Although toxin B is an extremely potent cytotoxin, it has no enterotoxic activity in animal intestine *in vivo* [28, 30, 32, 33]. This led to the widely held belief that toxin B did not participate in the pathogenesis of *C. difficile* diarrhea and colitis in humans. However, recent evidence appears to contradict this hypothesis and suggests that toxin B may indeed be pathogenic in humans. First, toxin A and toxin B both cause injury and electrophysiological changes in human colonic strips *in vitro*. Toxin B is 10 times more potent than toxin A in inducing these changes [34]. Second, there have been reports of the isolation of toxin A-negative/toxin B-positive strains of *C. difficile* from patients with antibiotic-associated diarrhea and colitis [19, 35–38]. Toxin A-negative/ toxin B-positive strains accounted for 3% of clinical isolates referred for typing to the Public Health Laboratory Service Anaerobic Reference Unit in England and Wales [19].

Both toxins of *C. difficile* bind to and damage human colonic epithelial cells [34]. *C. difficile* toxins produce colonic injury as a result of damage to the enterocyte cytoskeleton and disruption of tight junction function [34, 39]. The toxins also cause a severe inflammatory reaction in the lamina propria with the formation of microulcerations of the colonic epithelium that are covered by an inflammatory pseudomembrane. A characteristic of *C. difficile* infection is the intense acute neutrophilic inflammation seen in pseudomembranous colitis patients and in animal models of the disease. In contrast to cholera toxin, which stimulates massive intestinal fluid secretion without a significant inflammatory response, *C. difficile* toxin A stimulates fluid secretion accompanied by considerable mucosal edema, inflammatory cell infiltration and necrosis.

Interactions between neuropeptides and inflammatory mediators released from inflammatory cells of the intestinal lamina propria and from epithelial cells are also critical initiators of the toxin A-induced inflammatory process (Fig. 2). Pothoulakis and colleagues reported the release of the neuropeptides substance P (SP) and calcitonin gene-related peptide (CGRP) from sensory nerves, and degranulation of mast cells within 15 min of luminal application of

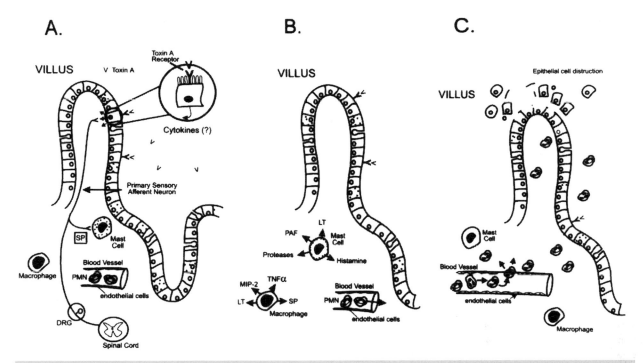

Figure 2. Pathogenesis of inflammatory diarrhea caused by *C. difficile* toxin A. **A**: Toxin A binds to its brush-border receptor(s) on intestinal epithelial cells, causing release of cytokines from these cells which diffuse into the lamina propria and activate primary sensory afferent neurons whose cell bodies are present in the dorsal root ganglia (DRG). Activation of primary sensory neurons causes early release of substance P (SP) which stimulates mucosal mast cells and other resident immune cells, such as macrophages. **B**: Significant mucosal mast cell degranulation occurs early after toxin A administration, releasing several proinflammatory mediators, such as histamine, platelet-activating factor (PAF), leukotriene C4 (LT), and proteases (rat mast cell protease II). Activated intestinal lamina propria macrophages also release potent inflammatory mediators, such as macrophage inflammatory protein-2 (MIP-2), LT, tumor necrosis factor-α (TNF-α), and SP. These mediators directly stimulate fluid secretion from epithelial cells and also up-regulate expression of adhesion molecules on endothelial cells and polymorphonuclear neutrophils (PMN). **C**: PMN subsequently enter into the intestinal mucosa and release more proinflammatory mediators, which act on epithelial cells, causing acute destruction and necrosis of villus enterocytes 2–3 h after toxin A exposure. Toxin A can also directly damage enterocytes by inactivating rho proteins and by damaging the enterocyte cytoskeleton. (Adapted from ref. 40, with permission of the publisher.)

toxin A in animal intestine [41]. This is followed by release of TNF-α from macrophages and up-regulation of adhesion molecules on endothelial cells, allowing neutrophil attachment and invasion. Pretreatment of rabbits with a monoclonal antibody directed against the neutrophil adhesion molecules CD18 prevented neutrophil infiltration and substantially reduced toxin A-induced secretion and mucosal injury [42]. The importance of sensory neuropeptides in *C. difficile* diarrhea is also demonstrated by a report that prevention of SP and CGRP release from sensory neurons by administration of specific SP or CGRP antagonists substantially inhibits toxin-A-mediated diarrhea and inflammation [43]. Moreover, mice genetically deficient in the NK-1 (SP)

receptor are largely protected from the secretory and inflammatory changes induced by toxin A, and mast cell-deficient mice have markedly diminished responses to the toxin [44].

Recent work also suggests that the proinflammatory chemokine macrophage inflammatory protein-2 (MIP-2) plays a pivotal role in mediating the early interaction between sensory nerves and mast cells and macrophages of the intestinal lamina propria following luminal exposure to toxin A. Intestinal epithelial cells release MIP-2 within 15 min of exposure to toxin A, well before the onset of fluid secretion or inflammation [45]. Moreover, an antibody to MIP-2 substantially inhibited intestinal secretion and inflammation in this model, support-

Table 1. Antimicrobial agents that predispose to *C. difficile* diarrhea and colitis

Frequently	Infrequently	Rarely or never
Ampicillin and amoxicillin	Tetracyclines	Parenteral aminoglycosides
Cephalosporins	Sulfonamides	Metronidazole
Clindamycin	Macrolides (including erythromycin)	Bacitracin
	Chloramphenicol	Vancomycin
	Trimethoprim	
	Quinolones	

Adapted from ref. 46, with permission of the publisher.

ing the view that release of this chemokine is critical for pathogenesis. These results suggest that inflammatory mediators such as MIP-2 and IL-1β released from enterocytes in response to toxin A activate sensory nerves in the subjacent lamina propria. Sensory nerves then release proinflammatory neuropeptides such as SP and CGRP, which in turn stimulate inflammatory cells leading to release of proinflammatory cytokines such as TNF-α and leukotrienes that elicit neutrophil recruitment via activation of adhesion molecules on vascular endothelial cells.

Predisposing factors

As shown in Table 1 almost all antibiotics have been associated with *C. difficile* diarrhea and colitis, including metronidazole and vancomycin [46–49] However, the precise risks associated with individual agents are difficult to establish [3, 50, 51]. While the duration of antibiotic therapy, the number of different antibiotics used, and the route of administration significantly influence the risk of *C. difficile* diarrhea [51–53]. pseudomembranous colitis associated with a single preoperative antibiotic dose has been reported [54]. A recent meta-analysis demonstrated that the 'big three' classes of antibiotics predisposing to *C. difficile* diarrhea are clindamycin, cephalosporins, and ampicillin/amoxicillin [51]. While early work focused attention on the prominent role of clindamycin as an inducing agent, subsequent studies have shown that cephalosporins are the most common agents implicated in *C. difficile* diarrhea, especially in nosocomially acquired cases [55]. Ampicillin, amoxicillin, or amoxicillin-clavulanate (Augmentin) are also common causes, especially in outpatients. Less commonly implicated antibiotics include penicillins other than ampicillin/amoxicillin,

macrolides (erythromycin, clarithromycin, and azithromycin), tetracyclines, sulfonamides, trimethoprim, chloramphenicol, and quinolones. Antibiotics that are rarely or never associated with *C. difficile* infection include parenteral aminoglycosides, vancomycin, bacitracin, nitrofurantoin, or antimicrobial agents whose activity is restricted to fungi, mycobacteria, parasites, or viruses. Antineoplastic agents that possess antibacterial properties, principally methotrexate, have occasionally been implicated. Presumably these agents induce a sufficient disturbance of the intestinal microflora to allow colonization with *C. difficile* [56].

Immunity and host defense factors

The first line of defense again *C. difficile* infection is the normal bowel microflora that inhibits growth of this pathogen *in vitro* and *in vivo* [57]. Indeed, normal adults not exposed to antibiotics are rarely infected with *C. difficile*. While *C. difficile* is frequently cultured from the stools of healthy neonates it is seldom part of the normal colonic microflora in healthy children above age 2, or in adults. Colonization by *C. difficile* follows alteration of the endogenous microflora by antibiotics, or cancer chemotherapy agents. The protective effect of the normal stable intestinal flora is frequently referred to as 'colonization resistance'. Disruption of this barrier by antibiotics and subsequent infection with *C. difficile* was originally demonstrated in animal models [58–60]. *C. difficile* can colonize the intestine of 'germ-free' mice. Wilson *et al.* demonstrated that inoculation of these animals with fecal flora from normal mice led to the disappearance of *C. difficile*, confirming the importance of the normal flora in preventing colonization [60]. The phenomenon of 'colonization resistance' has also been demonstrated *in vitro* where the growth of *C. difficile* is inhibited by emulsions of feces from healthy adults but not by sterile extracts [61]. The specific organism or group of organisms of the normal adult microflora that exclude *C. difficile* is not entirely clear, but anaerobic species including *Bacteroides* may be especially important. For example, treatment with lyophilized *Bacteroides* species can inhibit the growth of *C. difficile* in the stool of patients with chronic recurrent infection [62]. Healthy neonates and infants have poor 'colonization resistance' because they have not yet developed a stable complex colonic microflora [57, 63]. Colonization rates with *C. difficile* of 25–80% have been reported in infants and children up to the age of 2 years; however, despite the presence of toxin, they rarely develop *C. difficile*-associated diarrhea [3, 64]. Immaturity of their enterocytes with absence of toxin receptor expression is a possible mechanism for this clinical phenomenon [65]. Although cats, dogs, horses, and donkeys are colonized by *C. difficile*, there is no evidence that animals serve as reservoirs for colonization of humans [21].

The humoral immune system provides a second line of defense against C. *difficile*. Immunization of laboratory animals against toxin A protects against a subsequent challenge with *C. difficile* [66, 67]. Infant hamsters who drink milk from mothers immunized against toxins A and B are also protected [66]. The fact that only one-third of *C. difficile* carriers develop diarrhea [68] suggests that the host's ability to produce antitoxin antibodies may play a similar role in humans in modifying disease expression. Serum antibodies against *C. difficile* toxins are present in the majority of the adult population [71]. Secretory IgA antitoxin is present in colonic secretions and can inhibit binding of toxin A to its specific brush-border receptor, providing a possible mechanism of immune protection [72]. High levels of serum and intestinal antitoxin antibodies may be associated with mild colitis or asymptomatic carriage of *C. difficile* [69, 70, 73]. Conversely, a deficient antibody response may predispose to severe, prolonged, or recurrent *C. difficile* colitis [74–76].

In a recent prospective study of nosocomial C. *difficile* infection 41% of 47 patients who acquired *C. difficile* remained asymptomatic [13]. At the time of colonization, serum levels of IgG antibody against toxin A were three times higher in asymptomatic carriers compared to patients who developed *C. difficile* diarrhea (Fig. 3). Multivariable analyses indicated that patients with a low serum level of IgG antitoxin A were 48 times more likely to develop *C.*

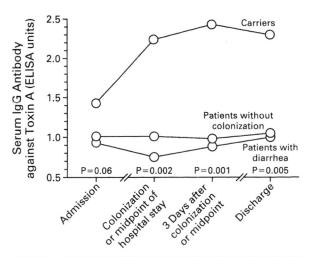

Figure 3. Serum IgG antibody levels against toxin A in asymptomatic carriers and patients with *C. difficile* diarrhea during hospitalization. The median levels of IgG antibody against toxin A are shown for 28 patients in whom *Clostridium difficile* diarrhea developed, 19 asymptomatic carriers, and 187 patients without colonization at the time of hospitalization, at the time of colonization by *C. difficile*, 3 days after colonization, and at discharge. The median interval between admission and colonization was 3 days (range 3–33), and the median interval between the third day after colonization and discharge was 12 days (range 2–56). Serum levels of IgG antibody against toxin A were three times higher in asymptomatic carriers compared to patients who developed *C. difficile* diarrhea. The *p*-values refer to the comparison among the three groups (by the Kruskal–Wallis test). (Reproduced from ref. 13, with permission of the publisher.)

difficile diarrhea compared to patients who had high antibody levels ($p < 0.001$). Although no protective association was found for serum IgG antitoxin B levels, these were significantly correlated with IgG levels against toxin A in the asymptomatic carriers. While we await controlled trials, open-label studies have demonstrated the efficacy of passive immunotherapy using pooled human immune globulin (containing antitoxin A IgG antibody) in patients with recurrent or refractory *C. difficile* diarrhea [77, 78].

A third protective factor is gastric acid, which reduces the number of viable spores [79]. Normal intestinal peristalsis is also important as a defense mechanism by eliminating *C. difficile* and its toxins. Conversely, antidiarrheal medications that reduce intestinal peristaltic activity may delay clearance of the organism and its toxins, and worsen the duration or intensity of illness.

Epidemiology

C. difficile infection occurs primarily in hospitalized patients, causing approximately 250 000–500 000 cases of diarrhea and colitis per year in the United States [12, 80], compared to only 20 000 cases per year in outpatients [14]. Carriage of *C. difficile* is rare in healthy adults not taking antibiotics; intestinal carriage rates of 0% to 3%, have been reported in American and European populations [81–83]. It remains unclear whether carriage is a temporary or permanent state [19]. In contrast, the incidence of *C. difficile* carriage is unusually high following admission to hospital and treatment with antibiotics. In one study, 7% of patients admitted to an acute-care hospital had positive stool cultures for *C. difficile* and another 21% became colonized with *C. difficile* during their hospital stay [12]. At the time of discharge, 82% of hospital carriers were still excreting *C. difficile* in their stools [12], accounting for the high rate of infection in nursing homes and chronic-care facilities. More recent hospital studies have reported similar *C. difficile* carriage rates [10, 13].

C. difficile survives in the hospital environment as antibiotic-resistant spores that are ingested by patients. Infected patients, environmental surfaces, inanimate objects, and the hands of health-care workers are all potential sources of *C. difficile* in the hospital setting [84]. In one study, patients sharing a room with a *C. difficile* carrying room-mate acquired *C. difficile* more rapidly than patients who were in single rooms or with room-mates who were culture-negative (mean time to acquisition 3.2 days compared to 18.9 days respectively) [12]. The same group of investigators also cultured *C. difficile* from the hands of 59% of hospital personnel caring for patients with positive *C. difficile* cultures as well as from bedrails, commodes, toilets, floors, scales, call-buttons, windowsills, dust-mops, and in the rooms where these patients were nursed [12]. Thus, cross-infection may occur by patient-to-patient spread or through environmental contamination [12, 80, 85–87]. The spread of infection can be interrupted by careful hand washing after examining patients and by the use of disposable gloves [88].

Although asymptomatic carriers rarely go on to develop *C. difficile*-associated diarrhea [68], they can contaminate the hospital environment and serve as a reservoir of infection. McFarland *et al.* demonstrated that 29% of cultures taken from rooms of asymptomatic carriers were positive for *C. difficile*, whereas only 8% of cultures from rooms of culture-negative patients were positive [12]. Asymptomatic carriers have also been implicated as the source of strains of *C. difficile* that caused *C. difficile*-associated diarrhea in other hospital inpatients [89]. In antibiotic-treated animals the infective dose of toxigenic *C. difficile* may be as low as two organisms [81]. If human susceptibility is similar, control of *C. difficile* infection in hospitals will continue to be a major challenge, as the organism is excreted in high numbers in liquid feces (up to 10^9 organisms/g) [85, 90]. Furthermore, *C. difficile* can be cultured in a hospital room 40 days after discharge of an infected patient [73], and it is likely that spores of *C. difficile* may persist for many months in hospital wards, as they are particularly resistant to oxygen, desiccation, and to many disinfectants [85].

While antibiotic exposure is the most important risk factor for *C. difficile* infection, other risk factors include increasing age (after infancy), and severity of underlying disease. In England and Wales 75% of all reports of *C. difficile* to the Public Health Laboratory Service Communicable Disease Surveillance Centre between 1992 and 1996, occurred in patients over 64 years of age [91]. Studies in the US have also demonstrated that increasing age is an independent risk factor for *C. difficile* diarrhea [79, 92]. Independent of age, sicker patients are also more likely to acquire *C. difficile* [13]. In a recent study of antibiotic recipients, patients with severe underlying disease at the time of hospital admission were 8 times more likely to develop *C. difficile* infection compared to patients who were less severely ill [13].

An increased incidence of *C. difficile* infection in oncology and HIV patients appears to be related to specific risk factors among these groups of patients. Low intensity of chemotherapy, reflecting a lower frequency of neutropenia, lack of parenteral vancomycin use and hospitalization within the previous 2 months were independently predictive of *C. difficile* colitis in hospitalized oncology patients [9]). A $CD4^+$ cell count less than 50/mm^3, in addition to clindamycin and penicillin, use were independent factors significantly associated with *C. difficile* colitis among HIV-infected patients [94].

Other reported risk factors for *C. difficile* infection include the presence of a nasogastric tube, non-surgical gastrointestinal procedures, acid antisecretory medications, intensive-care unit stay, and duration of hospital stay [51]. The strengths of the associations of these risk factors with *C. difficile* vary from study to study. Because these factors are often markers of disease severity and/or older age, their association with *C. difficile* may lose its significance after controlling for these confounding variables [13, 79, 92].

Pathology

When the human colon is exposed to *C. difficile* toxins, loss of actin filaments leads to cell rounding and shedding of cells from the basement membrane into the lumen, leaving a shallow ulcer on the mucosal surface. Serum proteins, mucus, and inflammatory cells flow outward from the ulcer, creating the characteristic colonic pseudomembrane. The spewing forth of the inflammatory exudate from the mucosal microulceration produces the typical 'volcano' or 'summit' lesion of *C. difficile* colitis (Fig. 4). On gross or sigmoidoscopic inspection of the colonic or rectal mucosa, pseudomembranes appear as yellow or off-white raised plaques 0.2–2.0 cm in diameter scattered over a fairly normal-appearing intervening mucosa. Edema and hyperemia of the full thickness of the bowel wall are common, and this is reflected by the typical radiographic appearance of 'thumbprinting', or massive wall thickening on computerized tomography scanning of patients with pseudomembranous colitis.

The patchy distribution of the pseudomembranes is probably related to a toxin dose–response effect. For example, when human colonic mucosal strips *in vitro* were exposed to different concentrations of toxin B, cellular damage was very patchy at low concentrations but, as the toxin concentration was raised, the area of damage increased until it was nearly confluent [34]. Similarly, some patients with early pseudomembranous colitis have only scattered lesions on the colonic mucosa, while others exhibit a confluent pseudomembrane covering the entire mucosa.

The pathologic features of pseudomembranous colitis (PMC) have been classified into three distinct types [95]: in type 1 PMC, the mildest form, the major inflammatory changes are confined in the superficial epithelium and immediately subjacent lamina propria. Typical pseudomembranes and summit lesions are present, and crypt abscesses are occasionally noted. Type 2 PMC is characterized by more severe disruption of glands and marked mucin secretion, and more intensive inflammation of basal lamina. Type 3 PMC is characterized by severe, intense necrosis of the full thickness of the mucosa with a confluent pseudomembrane. In practice,

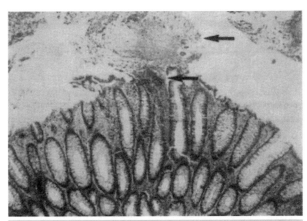

Figure 4. Endoscopic-biopsy specimen from a patient with pseudomembranous colitis and a 'summit' or 'volcano' lesion (hematoxylin and eosin, × 55). Focal ulceration of the colonic mucosa (lower arrow) is evident, with exudation of a pseudomembrane (upper arrow) made up of inflammatory cells, fibrin, and necrotic debris. The adjoining mucosa is intact. (Reproduced from ref. 3, with permission of the publisher.)

colonic histology is often normal in mild cases and may reveal only type 1 changes in the majority of cases, while the classical type 3 pseudomembranous colonic changes are seen in only a minority of patients.

Clinical features

Infection with *C. difficile* can produce a wide spectrum of clinical manifestations ranging from the asymptomatic carrier state in infants and adults to fulminant colitis with megacolon or perforation.

Asymptomatic carrier state

Asymptomatic carriage of *C. difficile* is common in hospitalized patients. Several large epidemiologic studies have demonstrated that 10–16% of patients in hospital may be carriers of the organism [12, 13, 96]. Despite the fact that over 50% of *C. difficile* isolates from these patients are toxigenic, they do not appear to be at an increased risk of developing symptomatic disease [6, 27]. The basis for this variability in response is not entirely clear but, as mentioned above, the host immune response appears to be more important than bacterial virulence factors. Other important host response factors may include toxin receptor density and the presence or absence of the normal barrier flora.

Antibiotic-associated diarrhea

Mild diarrhea is quite common during treatment with antibiotics, but it is related to *C. difficile* in only 20% of cases. Most antibiotic-associated diarrhea is related to an osmotic effect of unabsorbed carbohydrate [97]. In normal individuals unabsorbed dietary carbohydrate delivered to the large intestine undergoes fermentation by the microflora to short-chain fatty acids, hydrogen, methane, and other metabolites. However, during antibiotic therapy this normal fermentation process is interrupted, allowing accumulation of carbohydrates that bind water and cause diarrhea. Diarrhea is watery, containing mucus but not blood. Sigmoidoscopic examination reveals normal colonic mucosa or mild edema or hyperemia of the rectum. Obvious colitis or pseudomembrane formation does not occur. Systemic symptoms are absent and diarrhea stops when antibiotics are discontinued in the majority of patients.

C. difficile diarrhea without pseudomembrane formation

This is the most common clinical manifestation of *C. difficile* infection. The incubation period for diarrhea after colonization is not known, but is likely to be less than a week, with a median time of onset of approximately 2 days [10, 12, 13, 80]. *C. difficile* diarrhea is a more serious illness than simple antibiotic-associated diarrhea. *C. difficile* diarrhea is typically watery and foul-smelling [96]. Mucus or occult blood may be present but visible blood is rare [98]. Some patients may present with fever, leukocytosis, and crampy abdominal pain [96]. Extraintestinal manifestations of *C. difficile* infection such as septic arthritis, bacteremia or splenic abscess may occur, but are extremely rare [99–102], while asymmetrical arthropathy affecting large, weight-bearing joints is more common [103]. Fecal leukocytes may be present in the stools but are not a reliable indicator of *C. difficile* colitis, as they were absent in 72% of toxin-positive stools in one study [104]. Sigmoidoscopy may reveal a non-specific diffuse or patchy erythematous colitis without pseudomembranes.

Pseudomembranous colitis (PMC)

This entity is the classic manifestation of full blown *C. difficile* colitis and is accompanied by similar, but often more severe, symptoms than observed in *C. difficile* diarrhea. Sigmoidoscopic examination

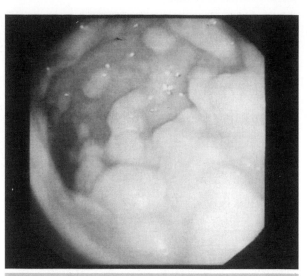

Figure 5. Colonoscopy view of pseudomembranous colitis resulting from refractory *C. difficile* infection. In the lower part of the figure coalescing pseudomembranes are visible (raised, adherent yellow plaques on the colonic mucosa that vary in size from 2 to 20 mm). In the upper part of the figure there is non-specific erythema of the colonic mucosa, with isolated pseudomembranes visible.

reveals the classic pseudomembranes, raised yellow plaques ranging from 2 to 20 mm in diameter scattered over the colorectal mucosa (Fig. 5). In severely ill patients, white blood cell counts of 20 000 or greater and hypoalbuminemia of 3.0 g/dl or lower may be observed. Most patients with PMC have involvement of the rectosigmoid area, but as many as one-third of patients have pseudomembranes limited to the more proximal colon [105]. There have been a few reported cases of pseudomembrane formation involving the small intestine [106]. A number of these were in postsurgical patients and included involvement of a defunctionalized limb of a jejunal–ileal bypass [107], an ileal conduit [108], or an end-ileostomy. Although abdominal CT scan in patients with PMC is not highly specific, it may reveal mucosal edema, thumbprinting, pancolitis, pericolonic inflammation, and pronounced thickening of the colonic wall that may involve the entire colon, collections of fluid in the lower abdomen or pelvis as well as the characteristic 'accordion sign' of contrast trapped among the thickened folds [109–111] (Fig. 6). A neutrocytic ascites with a low serum-to-ascites albumin gradient may occur in patients with hypoalbuminemia [112, 113]. Ascites may even be the presenting manifestation of PMC. A recent

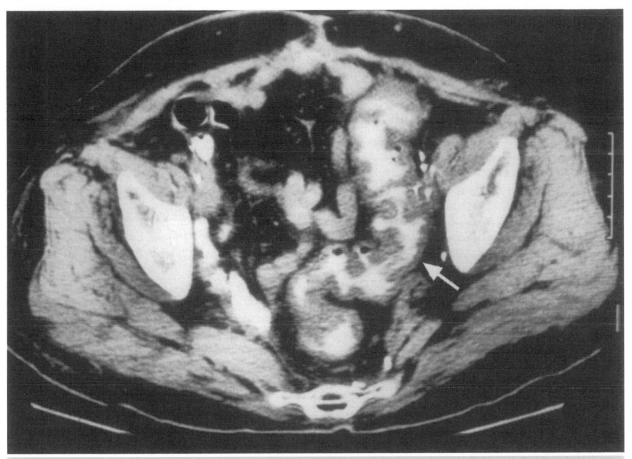

Figure 6. Computerized tomograph of the abdomen in *C. difficile* colitis. There is marked thickening of the colonic wall in the sigmoid colon (arrow). The accordion pattern is evident, produced by a series of broad edematous colonic haustral folds. (Reproduced from ref. 111, with permission of the publisher.)

radiologic review of typical sonographic appearances of common colonic diseases reported ascites in 64% of patients with PMC, compared to 24% of patients with diverticulitis, cancer, inflammatory or ischemic bowel disease [114].

Fulminant colitis

Fulminant colitis in *C. difficile* infection occurs in approximately 3% of patients but accounts for most of the serious complications including perforation, prolonged ileus, megacolon, and death [115]. Patients with fulminant colitis may complain of severe abdominal pain, diarrhea, and distension. Some patients exhibit high fever, rigors, dehydration, and marked leukocytosis. Diarrhea is usually prominent, but may be minimal in patients who

develop an ileus resulting in the pooling of secretions in the dilated, atonic colon. Hypoalbuminemia may also occur because of a severe protein-losing enteropathy. An abdominal radiograph may reveal a dilated colon (> 7 cm in its greatest diameter), consistent with toxic megacolon. Patients with megacolon may also have dilated small intestine on plain abdominal radiographs with air-fluid levels mimicking an intestinal obstruction or ischemia (pseudo-obstruction) [64]. In some patients fulminant *C. difficile* infection may present with signs and symptoms of bowel perforation. Typically, these patients have abdominal rigidity, involuntary guarding, rebound tenderness, and reduced bowel sounds. Abdominal radiographs may reveal the presence of free abdominal air.

C. difficile infection in patients with chronic inflammatory bowel disease

Infection with *C. difficile* may complicate the course of ulcerative colitis or Crohn's disease [116, 117]. Patients with inflammatory bowel disease (IBD) are often exposed to antibiotics and are frequently hospitalized, placing them at increased risk. Patients infected with *C. difficile* may develop diarrhea, abdominal pain, and low-grade fever mimicking a flare of their IBD. The diagnosis is established by identification of *C. difficile* toxin in a stool sample. Pseudomembrane formation is rare in this setting, probably because the colon is already involved by IBD. *C. difficile* diarrhea and colitis responds promptly to appropriate therapy with metronidazole or vancomycin. Some patients have developed *C. difficile* at the onset of their first attack of IBD, a situation that can lead to considerable diagnostic confusion. Infection with *C. difficile* in patients with ulcerative colitis or Crohn's disease requires prompt diagnosis and management, since failure to diagnose the infection may lead to inappropriate treatment with corticosteroids or immunosuppressive agents.

Diagnosis

The diagnosis of *C. difficile* diarrhea or colitis is based on a history of recent or current antibiotic therapy, development of diarrhea, or other evidence of acute colitis and demonstration of infection by toxigenic *C. difficile*, usually by detection of toxin A or toxin B in a stool sample [3, 118].

The diagnosis of *C. difficile* diarrhea should be suspected in any patient with diarrhea who has received antibiotics within the previous 2 months and/or whose diarrhea began 72 h or more after hospitalization [118]. Recent studies have shown that up to 40% of patients with *C. difficile* diarrhea at tertiary referral centers are symptomatic on admission to hospital [12, 13, 119]. Therefore, it is also prudent to consider the diagnosis in patients who present to hospital with antibiotic-associated diarrhea, especially if there is a history of recent discharge or transfer from another hospital or nursing home.

Testing of non-diarrheal stools for *C. difficile* by culture or toxin assay is not recommended because many patients in hospital may be asymptomatic carriers of the organism [12, 13, 98]. Treatment of asymptomatic carriers is not recommended, as it may prolong the carrier state [120]. For the same reason, 'test-of-cure' of *C. difficile* in asymptomatic patients with recent episodes of *C. difficile* diarrhea is not indicated. The duration of stool carriage of this organism following an episode of *C. difficile* diarrhea is unclear, but may persist for at least 3–6 weeks [121].

Fecal specimens

If *C. difficile* diarrhea is suspected, a freshly taken fecal sample should be submitted immediately to the laboratory in a clean watertight container, to test for the presence of toxigenic *C. difficile* (usually by the detection of fecal toxin A or toxin B). Anaerobic culture or the use of transport media do not enhance recovery of the organism or its toxin, and therefore are not recommended [84]. Storage at ambient temperatures leads to possible denaturation of fecal toxin [19]. Therefore, samples should be tested immediately for toxin or refrigerated or frozen for future testing. As *C. difficile* readily forms spores, culture of the organism from stools should be largely unaffected by ambient storage.

Laboratory tests for C. difficile

A variety of laboratory tests are available for the diagnosis of *C. difficile*-associated diarrhea (Table 2). Enzyme immunoassays to detect toxin antigens in the stool are increasingly used in clinical practice. These tests have the advantages of being relatively inexpensive, quick, and highly specific. However, their sensitivity is not ideal, leading to frequent false-negative results. The tissue culture cytotoxicity assay is more sensitive, leading to greater diagnostic accuracy, but it is also more costly and time-consuming.

Tissue culture cytotoxicity assay

The 'gold standard' diagnostic test to identify *C. difficile* toxins in the stool of patients with antibiotic-associated diarrhea is the tissue culture cytotoxicity assay [122–124]. By inactivating Rho proteins (see above) toxins A and B effect a disintegration of the actin cytoskeleton of mammalian cells leading to cell rounding. A suspension of diarrheal stool in phosphate-buffered saline is centrifuged and filtered. The filtrate is then inoculated on to a monolayer of cultured cells (usually fibroblasts or Chinese hamster ovary (CHO) cells). The monolayer is examined after overnight incubation and again at 48 h for cell

Table 2. Stool tests for diagnosis of *C. difficile* infection

Test	Detects	Advantages	Disadvantages
Cytotoxin assay	Toxin B	'Gold standard'; highly sensitive and specific	Requires tissue culture facility; takes 24–48 h
Enzyme immunoassay	Toxin A or B	Fast (2–6 h); easy to perform; high specificity	Not as sensitive as the cytotoxin assay
Latex agglutination assay	Bacterial enzyme-glutamate dehydrogenase	Fast; inexpensive; easy to perform	Poor sensitivity and specificity
Culture	Toxigenic and non-toxigenic *C. difficile*	Sensitive; allows strain typing in epidemics	Requires aerobic culture; not specific for toxin-producing bacteria; takes 2–5 days
Polymerase chain reaction	Toxin A or B genes in isolates or directly in feces	High sensitivity and specificity	Requires expertise in molecular diagnostic techniques

Adapted from ref. 111, with permission of the publisher.

rounding [19]. The specificity of the test result is established by preincubating the sample with specific neutralizing antitoxin antibody [118].

The advantages of the cytotoxicity assay include its high sensitivity (67–100%) and specificity (85–100%), if performed correctly [84]. However, the sensitivity of the test may be reduced by inactivation of toxins during transport and storage, by the age and type of cell line used, and by the dilution titer of the stool sample [19, 125–127]. Therefore a negative cytotoxicity test does not completely rule out *C. difficile* as the cause of diarrhea. A positive stool cytotoxin test in a patient with antibiotic-associated diarrhea indicates that it is highly likely that *C. difficile* is the cause of diarrhea. The main disadvantages of the cytotoxicity assay are that it is relatively expensive; it requires a cell culture facility; and it is slow, requiring incubation of the fecal filtrate for 24–48 h.

Enzyme-linked immunoassay tests for toxin A or toxins A and B

There are several commercially available enzyme immunoassays (EIA) for the detection of toxin A or toxins A and B of *C. difficile* in stool specimens [122–124, 128, 129]. Most of the tests that are used in clinical practice are designed to detect toxin A by using a monoclonal antibody that reacts with an epitope located on the aminoterminal region of the toxin A molecule. The advantages of these tests are that they are easier to perform than the cytotoxicity test, they are relatively inexpensive, results may be available within 2–6 h, and they have high specificity (75–100%) [84]. Their main disadvantage is that they are less sensitive than the cytotoxicity test (63–99%) [84]. In addition, if stool samples are tested for toxin A only, *C. difficile* diarrhea due to a toxin A-negative/toxin B-positive strain will not be diagnosed [35]. For this reason commercial kits that detect both toxins A and B have a slight advantage over those that detect toxin A alone [129].

Latex agglutination assay

The latex agglutination test was designed to detect toxin A in the stool, but instead recognizes glutamate dehydrogenase, another bacterial protein present in nontoxigenic strains of *C. difficile* and other non-pathogenic clostridia [130–132]. Thus the test is nonspecific and is also not sufficiently sensitive (48–59%) for the diagnosis of *C. difficile* diarrhea [3].

C. difficile culture

The stool culture test for *C. difficile* is sensitive (89–100%) but is not specific for toxin-producing strains of *C. difficile* [3, 84]. *In-vitro* testing for toxin production by isolates cultured from toxin-negative stools may improve specificity, but this is not a routine laboratory procedure and is costly and time-consuming. An advantage of stool culture of *C. difficile* is that it permits strain typing of individual isolates. The latter facilitates recognition of outbreaks of nosocomial infection.

Polymerase chain reaction for detection of toxin A or toxin B

Polymerase chain reaction (PCR), with the use of specific primers based on the gene sequences of toxins A and B, has been used to detect toxigenic C. difficile in clinical isolates [133–135]. Although this is a highly sensitive (100%) and specific (97–100%) test, it is laborious and requires initial culture of C. difficile. PCR methods for the detection of toxin genes directly in feces have been developed recently [136–140]. Using a nested PCR assay for the detection of toxin B in fecal specimens Alonso et al. reported 99% concordance with the cytotoxicity assay and sensitivity, and specificity of 96.3% and 100%, respectively [141]. Application of PCR methods in the clinical laboratory will require expertise in molecular diagnostic techniques and may not prove to be any more rapid or less expensive than stool cytotoxicity assay.

Endoscopic diagnosis of *C. difficile* diarrhea and colitis

Sigmoidoscopy or colonoscopy are not indicated for most patients with C. difficile diarrhea [3, 118]. Endosocopy is helpful, however, in special situations, such as when the diagnosis is in doubt or the clinical situation demands rapid diagnosis. In these situations limited flexible sigmoidoscopy or colonoscopy may be performed at the bedside. In severe PMC, because of the risk of perforation, only minimal amounts of air should be introduced. The presence of pseudomembranes in the rectum or sigmoid colon is sufficient to make a presumptive diagnosis of C. difficile colitis. It is important to note that the results of endoscopic examination may be normal in patients with mild diarrhea, or may demonstrate nonspecific colitis in moderate cases. The finding of rectal pseudomembranes in a patient with antibiotic-associated diarrhea is virtually pathognomonic for C. difficile colitis. Some patients without any diagnostic features in the rectosigmoid will have pseudomembranes in the more proximal areas of the colon [105]. Other endoscopic findings include erythema, edema, friability, and nonspecific colitis with small ulcerations or erosions.

Treatment

Management of mild to moderately severe *C. difficile* diarrhea and colitis

The first step in the management of C. difficile diarrhea and colitis is to discontinue the precipitating antibiotic(s) if possible [3, 118]. Diarrhea will resolve in approximately 15–25% of patients without specific anti-C. difficile therapy [8, 142]. However, conservative management alone may not be indicated in patients who are severely ill, or who have multiple medical problems, as it is difficult to predict who will improve spontaneously and who will have ongoing diarrhea. If it is not possible to discontinue the precipitating antibiotic, because of other active infections, the patient's antibiotic regimen should be altered to make use of agents less likely to exacerbate C. difficile diarrhea, for example, parental aminoglycosides, trimethoprim, and quinolones [143].

Anti-peristaltic agents such as diphenoxylate plus atropine (Lomotil), loperamide (Imodium) or narcotic analgesics should be avoided because they may delay clearance of toxin from the colon and thereby exacerbate toxin-induced colonic injury or precipitate ileus and toxic dilation [118, 144–147].

Specific therapy to eradicate C. difficile should be used in patients with initially severe symptoms and in patients whose symptoms persist despite discontinuation of antibiotic treatment. Currently, the most widely accepted antimicrobials for the treatment of C. difficile diarrhea are metronidazole (250–500 mg four times a day for 10 days) and vancomycin (125 mg to 500 mg four times a day for 10 days). Bacitracin, teicoplanin, fusidic acid, and colestipol have also been used to treat this condition, but have few if any advantages over conventional antimicrobials. In a recent systematic review of the efficacy of different treatments of C. difficile intestinal disease, none of these agents showed clear therapeutic superiority in terms of response rates [147]. The advantages and disadvantages of specific therapeutic agents are discussed briefly below.

Metronidazole

Metronidazole is now the drug of first choice in the treatment of C. difficile diarrhea and colitis [118]. It is inexpensive ($0.50 per 250 mg tablet) and is highly effective for the treatment of this condition. A number of clinical studies have demonstrated that metronidazole therapy results in the resolution of diarrhea and colitis in the vast majority of patients treated (98% overall) [8, 148]. In a prospective randomized clinical trial, metronidazole (250 mg four times a day for 10 days) was found to be as effective as vancomycin (500 mg four times daily for 10 days) in terms of response and relapse rates for the treatment of *C. difficile* diarrhea [142].

Metronidazole, unlike vancomycin, is well absorbed when administered orally. Fecal concentrations are low or absent in healthy individuals or asymptomatic carriers of *C. difficile*, but higher concentrations are observed in patients with *C. difficile* colitis. In patients with diarrhea, metronidazole may be secreted through an inflamed intestinal mucosa or decreased intestinal transit times may result in decreased absorption [149, 150]. Intravenous metronidazole (500 mg four times per day) may be used if patients cannot tolerate oral medication because it is excreted into bile and can accumulate in bactericidal levels in the inflamed colon [149].

Systemic side-effects may occur with the oral use of metronidazole [151]. However, this antibiotic is remarkably well tolerated. In one institution, in a 10-year period, over 600 patients received metronidazole for the treatment of *C. difficile* diarrhea; only 1% of those treated experienced significant side-effects [8]. Adverse effects include nausea and vomiting, a metallic taste, peripheral neuropathy (with prolonged therapy) and a disulfiram-like reaction with alcohol. Metronidazole may potentiate the anticoagulant effects of warfarin, resulting in prolongation of the prothromin time. Its use in pregnant and nursing women is cautioned because of the unknown effect of metronidazole on fetal organogenesis, and reports of tumorgenictiy in rodents. Its safety in children has not been documented. Although the majority of *C. difficile* isolates are sensitive to metronidazole, occasional resistant isolates have been reported, as have occasional cases of *C. difficile* diarrhea induced by metronidazole [45, 118, 152, 153].

Vancomycin

Vancomycin has been successfully used for the treatment of *C. difficile* colitis since 1978 [154]. Its pharmacokinetic properties make vancomycin an ideal agent for the treatment of *C. difficile* diarrhea [3]. When given orally it is neither absorbed nor metabolized, and is excreted virtually unchanged, in high concentrations, in the feces. A number of controlled trials have confirmed the efficacy of vancomycin in the treatment of *C. difficile* colitis [142, 154–156]. Symptomatic improvement is usually evident within 72 h of initiating therapy, and complete resolution of diarrhea and colitis occurs in the majority of patients (96% overall) by the end of a 10-day treatment course [148]. In one observational study of 122 patients treated with vancomycin at one institution the response rate, drug intolerance rate, and relapse rate were 99%, 1%, and 10% respectively [8].

Fekety *et al.* demonstrated that vancomycin at a dose of 125 mg four times a day is as effective as vancomycin 500 mg four times a day [157]. The lower dose is recommended for patients with mild to moderate colitis but the higher dose is recommended if the patient is critically ill, or has impending ileus, colonic dilation, or fulminant PMC. Vancomycin may be administered by mouth, nasogastric tube, or enema [8, 118]. It should not be given intravenously as effective luminal concentrations of the agent cannot be obtained via this route [158, 159]. Systemic side-effects associated with the use of oral vancomycin are rare.

Despite the many advantages of therapy with vancomycin, it is now considered a second-line agent for the treatment of *C. difficile*. There are two main factors discouraging the use of oral vancomycin; first, it is expensive (a 10-day course may cost up to $800) and second, its use may encourage the spread of vancomycin resistance amongst nosocomial bacteria [160]. Oral vancomycin therapy should be reserved for patients who are intolerant of or fail to respond to metronidazole, have severe PMC, are pregnant, or are under the age of 10 years [118]. Table 3 compares metronidazole and vancomycin therapy of *C. difficile* diarrhea.

Other antibacterial agents

Bacitracin (25 000 U four times daily for 7–10 days) has been studied in several clinical trials and is less effective than metronidazole or vancomycin for the treatment of *C. difficile* diarrhea [148, 155, 162–164]. The overall response rate is only about 80% and the relapse rate (> 30%) appears to be higher than with conventional therapy. In randomized therapeutic trials teicoplanin, 100 mg twice a day for 10 days, has been shown to be as effective as vancomycin for the treatment of *C difficile* diarrhea [165, 166]. It also appears to be associated with a lower relapse rate (approximately 7%) [166]. However, teicoplainin is relatively expensive and, like bacitracin, it is not readily available for oral administration in the United States. The efficacy of fusidic acid for the treatment of *C. difficile* diarrhea has been tested in a

Table 3. Metronidazole and vancomycin for treatment of *C. difficile* diarrhea

	Metronidazole	Vancomycin
Dose	250–500 mg	125–500 mg
Frequency	t.i.d. or q.i.d.	t.i.d. or q.i.d.
Duration	10–14 days	10–14 days
Route	Oral or intravenous	Oral
Response rate	>96%	>96%
Cost (10-day oral course)	$20	$800
Disadvantages	Systemic side-effects; rare resistant strains of *C. difficile*	Encourages growth of nosocomial vancomycin-resistant bacteria

t.i.d., three times a day; q.i.d., four times a day.

Adapted from ref. 161, with permission of the publisher.

limited number of patients [166, 167]. Once again, it is less effective than metronidazole or vancomycin and is associated with a relapse rate of approximately 28% [166]. Treatment with the ion exchange resin, colestipol (10 g four times daily) is associated with a very low response rate (36%) and is not recommended as primary therapy for *C. difficile* diarrhea [156].

Management of severe pseudomembranous colitis

As with mild to moderate cases of *C. difficile* diarrhea, the first step in the management of severe PMC is to discontinue precipitating antibiotics if possible, and start therapy with metronidazole or vancomycin. Although there are no published data indicating that vancomycin is superior to metronidazole for the treatment of severe *C. difficile* colitis, vancomycin is recommended as a first-line agent if the patient is critically ill [118]. This recommendation is based on clinical observations that such patients appear to respond more rapidly to vancomycin than to metronidazole. Intravenous metronidazole should be given if oral medication is not tolerated. Intravenous vancomycin is not recommended, for the reasons mentioned above. For patients with ileus, vancomycin (500 mg every 6 h) may be administered via a nasogastric tube, with intermittent clamping [8]. For critically ill patients a combination of antibiotics administered by various routes may be indicated. In one series six of eight patients with severe ileus were successfully treated using a combination of vancomycin administered by nasograstric tube, intravenous metronidazole, and vancomycin-retention

enemas (500 mg of vancomycin in 100 cc of normal saline administered every 6 h via a no. 18 Foley catheter inserted into the rectum); patients treated with this regimen responded within 5–17 days [8]. Intracecal infusion of vancomycin has been reported, but is not recommended because of the risks associated with placement of a narrow-bore tube over a guidewire at colonoscopy in patients with severe active colitis [168].

Passive immunization with immunoglobulin products has been shown to be effective for patients with severe colitis, who do not respond to therapy with metronidazole or vancomycin [69, 70]. Patients with severe or prolonged *C. difficile* diarrhea have low serum and fecal concentrations of antibody against *C. difficile* toxins [73, 75–77, 120]. Intravenous infusion of normal pooled human immunoglobulin (IVIG) increases serum IgG antitoxin levels and has been used successfully to treat a small number of patients with severe *C. difficile* colitis [77, 78]. A vaccine, based on formalin-inactivated *C. difficile* toxins, has recently been developed and tested in human subjects [169]. The *C. difficile* toxoid vaccine may be used to stimulate antitoxin antibody responses in healthy volunteers and thereby produce a hyperimmune IVIG against *C. difficile* to treat patients with severe or recurrent *C. difficile* diarrhea and colitis.

The presence of extreme leukocytosis (>30 000), fever, hypotension, and metabolic acidosis despite medical therapy are danger signs in fulminant colitis, and may indicate the need for emergency laparotomy and colectomy in patients with impending or actual perforation [170, 171]. However, surgical intervention in this setting is also associated with a high mortality rate, making the decision to operate difficult. Ramaswamy and colleagues determined that the following factors predicted increased mortality in severe *C. difficile* colitis: a low serum albumin on admission to hospital (<2.5 g/dl); a fall in albumin greater than 1.1 g/dl at the onset of symptoms; exposure to more than 3 antibiotics; and persistent toxin in the stools 7 days or longer after therapy [172]. If surgery is required, the operation of choice is a subtotal colectomy and ileostomy [110, 171, 173]. In a review of the literature between 1976 and 1994, Grundfest-Broniatowski *et al.* found that subtotal colectomy and ileostomy was associated with a failure rate of 24% [174]. In comparison, nontherapeutic laparotomy, diverting stomas, and segmental resections were associated with failure rates of 77%, 75%, and 40%, respectively [174].

Management of recurrent *C. difficile* diarrhea

Approximately 15–20% of patients treated successfully for *C. difficile* diarrhea will have recurrence of diarrhea in association with a positive stool test for *C. difficile* toxin [3, 118]. Recurrence is manifested by the reappearance of diarrhea and other symptoms, usually within 1–2 weeks of stopping treatment with metronidazole or vancomycin. Symptomatic recurrence is rarely due to treatment failure or antimicrobial resistance to metronidazole or vancomycin. It may result from germination of *C. difficile* spores persisting in the colon despite treatment. Recent evidence now suggests that recurrence most likely results from reinfection with the same or a different strain of *C. difficile* from the environment [175, 176]. Using DNA fingerprinting, Wilcox *et al.* demonstrated that 56% of clinical recurrences of *C. difficile* diarrhea were due to infection with a different strain of *C. difficile* [177]. It is worth emphasizing that therapy with metronidazole or vancomycin perpetuates disruption of the colonic microflora and therefore predisposes to reinfection with *C. difficile*. An impaired host immune response to *C. difficile* toxins may also increase the risk of recurrent *C. difficile* diarrhea [3, 70].

Regardless of the mechanism of recurrence, treatment of this form of disease can be problematic. Approaches to management include conservative therapy or treatment with specific anti-*C. difficile* antibiotics, the use of anion-binding resins, therapy with micro-organisms (probiotics), and immunoglobulin therapy. The basic principles of management involve: (a) treatment of *C. difficile* diarrhea, and (b) reduction of the susceptibility of the individual to *C. difficile* reinfection and/or *C. difficile* toxin-mediated colonic injury.

Conservative therapy

As with initial episodes of *C. difficile* diarrhea, conservative management of recurrent diarrhea may be preferable to re-treatment with metronidazole or vancomycin. While diarrhea usually responds to these agents, they do little to eradicate *C. difficile* spores within the colon or in the environment. They also perpetuate the disturbance of the normal intestinal flora and the associated loss of 'colonization resistance' [118]. In clinical practice, however, it is often impossible to withhold antibiotic therapy, as many patients with recurrent disease are elderly and infirm and are not able to tolerate diarrhea [178]. Even in healthier patients persisting or worsening diarrhea caused by recurrent *C. difficile* infection are clear indications for active treatment.

Re-treatment with specific anti-*C. difficile* antibiotics

The most common therapy for recurrent *C. difficile* diarrhea is a second course of the same antibiotic used to treat the initial episode [118]. In one large observational study in the United States, 92% of patients with recurrent *C. difficile* diarrhea responded successfully to a single repeated course of therapy, usually with metronidazole or vancomycin [8]. In this study multiple recurrences were uncommon (8%); however, other investigators have found that patients with a history of recurrence have a high risk of further episodes of *C. difficile* diarrhea after antibiotic therapy is discontinued [179, 180]. In a 1994 study, patients with at least two previous relapses had a subsequent relapse rate of 65% after standard therapy with metronidazole or vancomycin [179]. Fortunately there is no evidence to suggest that sequential episodes become progressively more severe or complicated [180].

A variety of treatment schedules have been suggested for patients with multiple recurrences of *C. difficile* diarrhea (Table 4). One approach is to give a prolonged course of vancomycin (or metronidazole) using a decreasing dosage schedule followed by pulse therapy [181]. The unproven rationale for this treatment course is that pulse therapy with antibiotics allows *C. difficile* spores to vegetate on the off days and then be killed when the antibiotics are taken again [181]. A combination of vancomycin 125 mg four times a day and rifampicin 600 mg twice a day for 7 days was used successfully in a study of seven patients with relapsing disease [182]. However, this

Table 4. Approach to management of recurrent *C. difficile* colitis

First relapse
Confirm diagnosis
Symptomatic treatment if symptoms are mild
10–14-day course of metronidazole or vancomycin

Second relapse
Confirm diagnosis
Vancomycin* taper
      125 mg q6h for 7 days
      125 mg q12h for 7 days
      125 mg q.d. for 7 days
      125 mg q.o.d. for 7 days
      125 mg every 3 days for 7 days

Further relapse
Vancomycin in tapering dose as above plus cholestyramine 4 g b.i.d.
     or
Vancomycin 125 mg q.i.d. and rifampicin 600 mg b.i.d. for 7 days
     or
Therapy with micro-organisms, e.g. *Saccharomyces boulardii* in
  combination with metronidazole or vancomycin
     or
Intravenous immunoglobulin

*Metronidazole may be substituted for vancomycin, although there are no published data regarding its efficacy in this treatment regimen.

q6h, every 6 h; q.d., every day; q.o.d., every other day; b.i.d., twice daily; q.i.d., four times daily.

Adapted from ref. 111, with permission of the publisher.

Table 5. Practice guidelines for prevention of *C. difficile* diarrhea

1. Limit the use of antimicrobial drugs
2. Wash hands between contact with all patients
3. Use enteric (stool) isolation precautions for patients with *C. difficile* diarrhea
4. Wear gloves when contacting patients with *C. difficile* diarrhea or their environment
5. Disinfect objects contaminated with *C. difficile* with sodium hypochlorite, alkaline glutaraldehyde, or ethylene oxide
6. Educate the medical, nursing, and other appropriate staff members regarding the disease and its epidemiology

Adapted from ref. 118, with permisssion of the publisher.

study was uncontrolled and there is no evidence that this combination of antibiotics has any unique activity against *C. difficile* [118].

Anion-binding resins

Cholestyramine (4 g three or four times daily for 1–2 weeks), an anion-exchange resin, binds *C. difficile* toxins and may be used in conjunction with antibiotics to treat frequent relapsers [183]. Because cholestyramine may bind vancomycin as well as toxins, it should be taken at least 2–3 h apart from the vancomycin [184].

Biotherapy

Biotherapy (therapy with micro-organisms or 'probiotics') is an attractive approach to the management of recurrent *C. difficile* diarrhea because it aims to restore the 'colonization resistance' of a normal colonic flora. Several agents and routes of administration have been evaluated, including a mixture of colonic bacteria in saline administered as a rectal infusion, fresh feces administered as a rectal enema, *Lactobacillus GG* given as a concentrate in skim milk, oral administration of non-toxigenic *C. difficile*, brewer's or baker's yeast (*Saccharomyces cerevisiae*) taken by mouth and *Saccharomyces boulardii* given in capsule form [60, 179, 185–189]. Unfortunately many of these studies have been small, open-labeled and uncontrolled.

S. boulardii is a non-pathogenic yeast that has been reported to reduce the incidence of antibiotic-associated diarrhea [190]. A randomized, double-blind, placebo-controlled trial involving 124 patients examined the efficacy of *S. boulardii* (500 mg twice a day for 4 weeks) in combination with metronidazole or vancomycin in patients with *C. difficile* diarrhea [179]. *S. boulardii* significantly reduced recurrences compared with placebo in patients with multiple episodes of *C. difficile* diarrhea (recurrence rate 35% versus 65%, $p = 0.04$), but not in those with an initial episode of *C. difficile* diarrhea (recurrence rate 19% versus 24%; $p = 0.86$) [179]. The preparation of *S. boulardii* used in this trial is not currently approved for use in the US, but is available in other countries.

Immunoglobulin therapy

As mentioned earlier, there is now substantial evidence that the immune response to *C. difficile* toxins plays a major role in determining host susceptibility to disease [13, 69, 70]. Several investigators have found that serum antibody levels against *C. difficile* toxins are low in patients with recurrent *C. difficile* diarrhea [75–77, 191]. In a study of six children with relapsing *C. difficile* colitis, Leung *et al.* found that these children had low serum levels of IgG antibody against toxin A [77]. Treatment with normal pooled intravenous gamma globulin, that contains IgG antitoxin A, was associated with a marked increase in serum antitoxin antibody levels and resolution of recurrent *C. difficile* diarrhea [77]. Although this approach to the management of recurrent *C. difficile* diarrhea is promising, further controlled studies are required before gamma globulin can be recommended as a standard therapy for this condition.

Prevention

Published practice guidelines for the prevention of *C. difficile* diarrhea emphasize restriction of antimicrobial use (Table 5) [84, 118]. Although limitation or restriction of antibiotics known to be associated with *C. difficile* diarrhea (such as clindamycin or broad-spectrum cephalosporins) may be difficult to implement, observational studies demonstrate that this approach may be beneficial in preventing *C. difficile* diarrhea [20, 50, 192–195]. Other recommendations include handwashing between contact with patients, the use of gloves for the handling of body substances of patients with *C. difficile* diarrhea, and the use of enteric isolation precautions [84, 118]. Although there is a paucity of data regarding the efficacy of different cleaning agents and disinfectants for *C. difficile*, the American College of Gastroenterology recommends that instruments and contaminated surfaces in rooms of patients with *C. difficile* diarrhea should be disinfected using alkaline glutaraldehyde, sodium hypochlorite, or ethylene oxide [118]. The Society for Healthcare Epidemiology of America guidelines include a recommendation that electronic thermometers should be replaced with disposable thermometers if rates of *C. difficile* diarrhea are high [84]. This recommendation is supported by the results of two studies, one of which employed a randomized crossover design, in which replacement of electronic rectal with disposal thermometers was associated with a decreased incidence of *C. difficile* diarrhea [196, 197].

A recommendation that is likely to have a substantial impact on the spread of *C. difficile* infection emphasized by Fekety *et al.* is that medical, nursing, and other hospital staff members receive education on *C. difficile* diarrhea and its epidemiology [118]. Aggressive infection control policies which involve multiple disciplines are often necessary to control nosocomial infection with *C. difficile* [198]. Patient education regarding the mode of transmission of *C. difficile* is also likely to be important, but may be difficult in the patient population who are commonly affected, i.e. the old and infirm [198].

Future approaches to the control of nosocomial *C. difficile* infection may involve active or passive immunization of at-risk individuals [69, 70]. Increasing individual and herd immunity to *C. difficile* and its toxins may provide the best means of preventing this troublesome iatrogenic disease [199].

Acknowledgements

J. Thomas LaMont and Joanne K. Linevsky. This work was supported by grants from the National Institutes of Health (K23 DK02848-01 to Dr Farrell; and AG16956 to Drs Kyne and Kelly).

References

1.   Hall IC, O'Toole E. Intestinal flora in new-born infants: with a description of a new pathogenic anaerobe, *Bacillus difficilis*. Am J Dis Child 1935; 49: 390–402.
2.   Bartlett JG, Chang TW, Gurwith M, Gorbach SL, Onderdonk AD. Antibiotic-associated pseudomembranous colitis due to toxin-producing clostridia. N Engl J Med 1978; 298: 531–4.
3.   Kelly CP, Pothoulakis C, LaMont JT. *Clostridium difficile* colitis. N Engl J Med 1994; 330: 257–62.
4.   Guerrant RL, Hughes JM, Lima NL, Crane J. Diarrhea in developed and developing countries: magnitude, special settings, and etiologies. Rev Infect Dis 1990; 12(Suppl. 1): S41–50.
5.   McFarland LV. Epidemiology of infectious and iatrogenic nosocomial diarrhea in a cohort of general medicine patients. Am J Infect Control 1995; 23: 295–305.
6.   Samore MH. Epidemiology of nosocomial *Clostridium difficile* diarrhea. J Hosp Infect 1999; 43(Suppl.): S183–90.
7.   Alfa MJ, Du T, Beda G. Survey of incidence of *Clostridium difficile* infection in Canadian hospitals and diagnostic approaches. J Clin Microbiol 1998; 36: 2076–80.
8.   Olson MM, Shanholtzer CJ, Lee Jr JT, Gerding DN. Ten years of prospective *Clostridium difficile*-associated disease surveillance and treatment at the Minneapolis VA Medical Center, 1982–1991. Infect Control Hosp Epidemiol 1994; 15: 371–81.
9.   Lai KK, Melvin ZS, Menard MJ, Kotilainen HR, Baker S. *Clostridium difficile*-associated diarrhea: epidemiology, risk factors, and infection control. Infect Control Hosp Epidemiol 1997; 18: 628–32.
10. Samore MH, DeGirolami PC, Tlucko A, Lichtenberg DA, Melvin ZA, Karchmer AW. *Clostridium difficile* colonization and diarrhea at a tertiary care hospital. Clin Infect Dis 1994; 18: 181–7.
11. Struelens MJ, Maas A, Nonhoff C *et al.* Control of nosocomial transmission of *Clostridium difficile* based on sporadic case surveillance. Am J Med 1991; 91: 138S–44S.
12. McFarland LV, Mulligan ME, Kwok RY, Stamm WE. Nosocomial acquisition of *Clostridium difficile* infection. N Engl J Med 1989; 320: 204–10.
13. Kyne L, Warny M, Qamar A, Kelly CP. Asymptomatic carriage of *Clostridium difficile* and serum levels of IgG antibody against toxin A. N Engl J Med 2000; 342: 390–7.

14. Hirschhorn LR, Trnka Y, Onderdonk A, Lee ML, Platt R. Epidemiology of community-acquired *Clostridium difficile*-associated diarrhea. J Infect Dis 1994; 169: 127–33.

15. Levy DG, Stergachis A, McFarland LV *et al*. Antibiotics and *Clostridium difficile* diarrhea in the ambulatory care setting. Clin Ther 2000; 22: 91–102.

16. George WL, Sutter VL, Citron D, Finegold SM. Selective and differential medium for isolation of *Clostridium difficile*. J Clin Microbiol 1979; 9: 214–19.

17. Delmee M, Homel M, Wauters G. Serogrouping of *Clostridium difficile* strains by slide agglutination. J Clin Microbiol. 1985; 21: 323–7.

18. Kuijper EJ, Oudbier JH, Stuifbergen WN, Jansz A, Zanen HC. Application of whole-cell DNA restriction endonuclease profiles to the epidemiology of *Clostridium difficile*-induced diarrhea. J Clin Microbiol 1987; 25: 751–3.

19. Brazier JS. The epidemiology and typing of *Clostridium difficile*. J Antimicrob Chemother 1998; 41(Suppl. C): 47–57.

20. Johnson S, Samore MH, Farrow FA *et al*. Epidemics of diarrhea caused by a clindamycin-resistant strain of *Clostridium difficile* in four hospitals. N Engl J Med 1999; 341: 1645–51.

21. Dove CH, Wang SZ, Price SB *et al*. Molecular characterization of the *Clostridium difficile* toxin A gene. Infect Immun 1990; 58: 480–8.

22. von Eichel-Streiber C, Laufenberg-Feldmann R, Sartingen S, Schulze J, Sauerborn M. Cloning of *Clostridium difficile* toxin B gene and demonstration of high N-terminal homology between toxin A and B. Med Microbiol Immun 1990; 179: 271–9.

23. Barroso LA, Wang SZ, Phelps CJ, Johnson JL, Wilkins TD. Nucleotide sequence of *Clostridium difficile* toxin B gene. Nucleic Acids Res 1990;18:4004.

24. Pothoulakis C. Pathogenesis of *Clostridium difficile*-associated diarrhoea. Eur J Gastroenterol Hepatol 1996; 8: 1041–7.

25. Warny M, Keates AC, Keates S *et al*. p38 MAP kinase activation by *Clostridium difficile* toxin A mediates monocyte necrosis, IL-8 production, and enteritis. J Clin Invest 2000; 105: 1147–56.

26. Just I, Selzer J, Wilm M, von Eichel-Streiber C, Mann M, Aktories K. Glucosylation of Rho proteins by *Clostridium difficile* toxin B. Nature 1995; 375:500–3.

27. Just I, Wilm M, Selzer J, Rex G, von Eichel-Streiber C, Mann M, Aktories K. The enterotoxin from *Clostridium difficile* (ToxA) monoglucosylates the Rho proteins. J Biol Chem 1995; 270:13932–6.

28. Pothoulakis C, Barone LM, Ely R *et al*. Purification and properties of *Clostridium difficile* cytotoxin B. J Biol Chem 1986; 261: 1316–21.

29. Von Eichel-Streiber C, Boquet P, Souerborn M, Thalestam M. Large clostridial cytotoxins – a family of glycosyltransferases modifying small GTP-binding proteins. Trends Microbiol 1996; 4: 375–82.

30. Sullivan NM, Pellett S, Wilkins TD. Purification and characterization of toxins A and B of *Clostridium difficile*. Infect Immun 1982; 35: 1032–40.

31 Triadafilopoulos,G, Pothoulakis C, O'Brien MJ, LaMont JT. Differential effects of *Clostridium difficile* toxins A and B on rabbit ileum. Gastroenterology 1987; 93: 273–9.

32. Lyerly,DM, Saum KE, MacDonald DK, Wilkins TD. Effects of *Clostridium difficile* toxins given intragastrically to animals. Infect Immun 1985; 47: 349–52.

33. Mitchell TJ, Ketley JM, Haslam SC *et al*. Effect of toxin A and B of *Clostridium difficile* on rabbit ileum and colon. Gut 1986; 27: 78–85.

34. Riegler M, Sedivy R, Pothoulakis C *et al*. *Clostridium difficile* toxin B is more potent than toxin A in damaging human colonic epithelium in vitro. J Clin Invest 1995; 95: 2004–11.

35. Limaye AP, Turgeon DK, Cookson BT, Fritsche TR. Pseudomembranous colitis caused by a toxin A(–) B(+) strain of *Clostridium difficile*. J Clin Microbiol 2000; 38: 1696–7.

36. Kato H, Kato N, Watanabe K *et al*. Identification of toxin A-negative, toxin B-positive *Clostridium difficile* by PCR. J Clin Microbiol 1998; 36: 2178–82.

37. Kato H, Kato N, Katow S, Maegawa T, Nakamura H, Lyerly DM. Deletions in the repeating sequences of the toxin A gene of toxin A-negative, toxin B-positive *Clostridium difficile* strains. FEMS Microbiol Lett 1999; 175: 197–203.

38. Lyerly DM, Barroso LA, Wilkins TD, Depitre C, Corthier G. Characterization of a toxin A-negative, toxin B-positive strain of *Clostridium difficile*. Infect Immun 1992; 60: 4633–9.

39. Hecht G, Koutsouris A, Pothoulakis C, LaMont JT, Madara JL. *Clostridium difficile* toxin B disrupts the barrier function of T84 monolayers. Gastroenterology 1992; 102: 416–23.

40. Pothoulakis C, Castagliuolo I, LaMont JT. Neurons and mast cells modulate secretory and inflammatory responses to enterotoxins. News Physiol Sci 1998; 13: 58–63.

41. Pothoulakis C, Castagliuolo I, Leeman SE *et al*. Substance P receptor expression in intestinal epithelium in *Clostridium difficile* toxin A enteritis in rats. Am J Physiol 1998; 275: G68–75.

42. Kelly CP, Becker S, Linevsky JK *et al*. Neutrophil recruitment in *Clostridium difficile* toxin A enteritis in the rabbit. J Clin Invest 1994; 93: 1257–65.

43. Keates AC, Castagliuolo I, Qiu B, Nikulasson S, Sengupta A, Pothoulakis C. CGRP upregulation in dorsal root ganglia and ileal mucosa during *Clostridium difficile* toxin A-induced enteritis. Am J Physiol 1998; 274: G196–202.

44. Wershil BK, Castagliuolo I, Pothoulakis C. Diect evidence of mast cell involvement in *Clostridium difficile* toxin A-induced enteritis in mice. Gastroenterology 1998; 114: 956–64.

45. Castagliuolo I, Keates AC, Wang CC *et al*. *Clostridium difficile* toxin A stimulates macrophage-inflammatory protein-2 production in rat intestinal epithelial cells. J Immunol 1998; 160: 6039–45.

46. Kelly CP, LaMont JT. Treatment of *Clostridium difficile* diarrhea and colitis. In: Wolfe MM, ed. Gastrointestinal Pharmacotherapy. Philadelphia: WB Saunders, 1993: 199–212.

47. Saginur,R, Hawley CR, Bartlett JG. Colitis associated with metronidazole therapy. J Infect Dis 1980; 141: 772–4.

48. Thomson G, Clark AH, Hare K, Spilg WG. Pseudomembranous colitis after treatment with metronidazole. Br Med J 1981; 282: 864–5.

49. Hecht JR, Olinger EJ. *Clostridium difficile* colitis secondary to intravenous vancomycin. Dig Dis Sci 1989; 34: 148–9.

50. Gorbach SL. Antibiotics and *Clostridium difficile*. N Engl J Med 1999; 341: 1690–1.

51. Bignardi GE. Risk factors for *Clostridium difficile* infection. J Hosp Infect 1998; 40: 1–15.

52. Ambrose N. The effects of single doses of antibiotics on faecal flora with a reference to their mode of excretion. J Drug Dev 1989; 1: 233–41.

53. Nord CE, Edlund C. Impact of antimicrobial agents on human intestinal microflora. J Chemother 1990; 2: 218–37.

54. Freiman JP, Graham DJ, Green L. Pseudomembranous colitis associated with single-dose cephalosporin prophylaxis. J Am Med Assoc 1989; 262: 902.

55. Golledge CL, McKenzie T, Riley TV. Extended spectrum cephalosporins and *Clostridium difficile*. J Antimicrob Chemother 1989; 23: 929–31.

56. Anand A, Glatt AE *Clostridium difficile* infection associated with antineoplastic chemotherapy: a review. Clin Infect Dis 1993; 17: 109.

57. Borriello SP. The influence of the normal flora on *Clostridium difficile* colonisation of the gut. Ann Med 1990; 22: 61–7.

58. Wilson KH, Silva J, Fekety FR. Suppression of *Clostridium difficile* by normal hamster cecal flora and prevention of antibiotic-associated cecitis. Infect Immun 1981; 34: 626–8.

59. Onderdonk AB, Cisneros RL, Bartlett JG. *Clostridium difficile* in gnotobiotic mice. Infect Immun 1980; 28: 277–82.

60. Wilson KH, Freter R. Interaction of *Clostridium difficile* and Escherichia coli with microfloras in continuous-flow cultures and gnotobiotic mice. Infect Immun 1986; 54: 354–8.

61. Borriello SP, Barclay FE. An in-vitro model of colonisation resistance to *Clostridium difficile* infection. J Med Microbiol 1986; 21: 299–309.

62. Tvede M, Rask-Madsen J. Bacteriotherapy for chronic relapsing *Clostridium difficile* diarrhea in six patients. Lancet 1989; 1: 1156–60.

63. Larson HE, Barclay FE, Honour P, Hill ID. Epidemiology of *Clostridium difficile* in infants. J Infect Dis 1982; 146: 727–33.

64. Kelly CP, LaMont JT. *Clostridium difficile* infection. Annu Rev Med 1998; 49: 375–90.

65. Eglow R, Pothoulakis C, Itzkowitz S *et al*. Diminished *Clostridium difficile* toxin A sensitivity in newborn rabbit ileum is associated with decreased toxin A receptor. J Clin Invest 1992; 90: 822–9.

66. Kim KH, Iaconis JP, Rolfe RD. Immunization of adult hamsters against *Clostridium difficile*-associated ileocecitis and transfer of protection to infant hamsters. Infect Immun 1987; 55: 2984–92.

67. Libby JM, Jortner BS, Wilkins TD. Effects of the two toxins of *Clostridium difficile* in antibiotic-associated cecitis in hamsters. Infect Immun 1982; 36: 822–9.

68. Shim JK, Johnson S, Samore MH, Bliss DZ, Gerding DN. Primary symptomless colonisation by *Clostridium difficile* and decreased risk of subsequent diarrhoea. Lancet 1998; 351: 633–6.

69. Kelly CP. Immune response to *Clostridium difficile* infection. Eur J Gastroenterol Hepatol 1996;8: 1048–53.

70. Kyne L, Kelly CP. Prospects for a vaccine for *Clostridium difficile*. BioDrugs 1998; 10: 173–81.

71. Viscidi R, Laughon BE, Yolken R *et al*. Serum antibody response to toxins A and B of *Clostridium difficile*. J Infect Dis 1983; 148: 93–100.

72. Kelly CP, Pothoulakis C, Orellana J, LaMont JT. Human colonic aspirates containing immunoglobulin A antibody to *Clostridium difficile* toxin A inhibit toxin A-receptor binding. Gastroenterology 1992; 102: 35–40.

73. Mulligan ME, Miller SD, McFarland LV, Fung HC, Kwok RY. Elevated levels of serum immunoglobulins in asymptomatic carriers of *Clostridium difficile*. Clin Infect Dis 1993; 16: S239–44.

74. Aronsson B, Granstrom M, Mollby R, Nord CE. Enzyme-linked immunosorbent assay (ELISA) for antibodies to *Clostridium difficile* toxins in patients with pseudomembranous colitis and antibiotic-associated diarrhoea. J Immun Methods 1983; 60: 341–50.

75. Aronsson B, Granstrom M, Mollby R, Nord CE. Serum antibody response to *Clostridium difficile* toxins in patients with *Clostridium difficile* diarrhoea. Infection 1985; 13: 97–101.

76. Warny M, Vaerman JP, Avesani V, Delmee M. Human antibody response to *Clostridium difficile* toxin A in relation to clinical course of infection. Infect Immun 1994; 62: 384–9.

77. Leung DY, Kelly CP, Boguniewicz M, Pothoulakis C, LaMont JT, Flores A. Treatment with intravenously administered gamma globulin of chronic relapsing colitis induced by *Clostridium difficile* toxin. J Pediatr 1991; 118: 633–7.

78. Salcedo J, Keates S, Pothoulakis C, Castagliuolo I, LaMont JT, Kelly CP. Intravenous immunoglobulin therapy for severe *Clostridium difficile* colitis. Gut 1997; 41: 366–70.

79. McFarland LV, Surawicz CM, Stamm WE. Risk factors for *Clostridium difficile* carriage and *C. difficile*-associated diarrhea in a cohort of hospitalized patients. J Infect Dis 1990; 162: 678–84.

80. Johnson S, Clabots CR, Linn FV, Olson MM, Peterson LR, Gerding DN. Nosocomial *Clostridium difficile* colonisation and disease. Lancet 1990; 336: 97–100.

81. Larson HE, Price AB, Honour P, Borriello SP. *Clostridium difficile* and the aetiology of pseudomembranous colitis. Lancet 1978; 1: 1063–6.

82. Viscidi R, Willey S, Bartlett JG. Isolation rates and toxigenic potential of *Clostridium difficile* isolates from various patient populations. Gastroenterology 1981; 81: 5–9.

83. Aronsson B, Molby R, Nord CE. Antimicrobial agents and *Clostridium difficile* in acute disease: epidemiological data from Sweden, 1980–1982. J Infect Dis 1985; 151: 476–81.

84. Gerding DN, Johnson S, Peterson LR, Mulligan ME, Silva Jr J. *Clostridium difficile*-associated diarrhea and colitis. Infect Control Hosp Epidemiol 1995; 16: 459–77.

85. Fekety R, Kim KH, Brown D, Batts DH, Cudmore M, Silva Jr J. Epidemiology of antibiotic-associated colitis; isolation of *Clostridium difficile* from the hospital environment. Am J Med 1981; 70: 906–8.

86. Kim KH, Fekety R, Batts DH *et al*. Isolation of *Clostridium difficile* from the environment and contacts of patients with antibiotic-associated colitis. J Infect Dis 1981; 143: 42–50.

87. Nolan NP, Kelly CP, Humphreys JF *et al*. An epidemic of pseudomembranous colitis: importance of person to person spread. Gut 1987; 28: 1467–73.

88. Johnson S, Gerding DN, Olson MM *et al*. Prospective, controlled study of vinyl glove use to interrupt *Clostridium difficile* nosocomial transmission. Am J Med 1990; 88:137–40.

89. Clabots CR, Johnson S, Olson MM, Peterson LR, Gerding DN. Acquisition of *Clostridium difficile* by hospitalized patients: evidence for colonized new admissions as a source of infection. J Infect Dis 1992; 166: 561–7.

90. Hoffman, P. *Clostridium difficile* in hospitals. Curr Opin Infect Dis 1994; 7: 471–4.

91. Djuretic T, Wall PG, Brazier JS. *Clostridium difficile*: an update on its epidemiology and role in hospital outbreaks in England and Wales. J Hosp Infect 1999; 41: 213–8.

92. Brown E, Talbot GH, Axelrod P, Provencher M, Hoegg C. Risk factors for *Clostridium difficile* toxin-associated diarrhea. Infect Control Hosp Epidemiol 1990; 11: 283–90.

93. Hornbuckle K, Chak A, Lazarus HM *et al*. Determination and validation of a predictive model for *Clostridium difficile* diarrhea in hospitalized oncology patients. Ann Oncol 1998; 9: 307–11.

94. Barbut F, Meynard JL, Guiget M *et al*. *Clostridium difficile*-associated diarrhea in HIV-infected patients: epidemiology and risk factors. J Acquir Immun Defic Syndr Hum Retrovirol 1997; 16:176–81.

95. Price AB, Davies DR. Pseudomembranous colitis. J Clin Pathol 1977; 30: 1–12.

96. Gerding DN, Olson MM, Peterson LR *et al*.*Clostridium difficile*-associated diarrhea and colitis in adults. A prospec-

tive case-controlled epidemiologic study. Arch Intern Med 1986; 146: 95–100.

97. Rao SS, Edwards CA, Austen CJ, Bruce C, Reed NW. Impaired colonic fermentation of carbohydrates after ampicillin Gastroenterology 1988; 94: 928–32.

98. Spencer RC. Clinical impact and associated costs of *Clostridium difficile*-associated disease. J Antimicrob Chemother 1998; 41(Suppl. C): 5–12.

99. Wolf LE, Gorbach SL, Granowitz EV. Extraintestinal *Clostridium difficile*: 10 years' experience at a tertiary-care hospital. Mayo Clin Proc 1998; 73: 943–7.

100. Pron B, Merckx J, Touzet P *et al.* Chronic septic arthritis and osteomyelitis in a prosthetic knee joint due to *Clostridium difficile*. Eur J Clin Microbiol Infect Dis 1995; 14: 599–601.

101. Feldman RJ, Kallich M, Weinstein MP. Bacteremia due to *Clostridium difficile*: case report and review of extraintestinal *C. difficile* infections. Clin Infect Dis 1995; 20: 1560–2.

102. Studemeister AE, Beilke MA, Kirmani N. Splenic abscess due to *Clostridium difficile* and *Pseudomonas paucimobilis*. Am J Gastroenterol 1987; 82: 389–90.

103. Cope A, Anderson J, Wilkins E. *Clostridium difficile* toxin-induced reactive arthritis in a patient with chronic Reiter's syndrome. Eur J Clin Microbiol Infect Dis 1992;11: 40–3.

104. Marx CE, Morris A, Wilson ML, Reller LB. Fecal leukocytes in stool specimens submitted for *Clostridium difficile* toxin assay. Diagn Microbiol Infect Dis 1993; 16: 313–15.

105. Tedesco FJ, Corless JK, Brownstein RE. Rectal sparing in antibiotic-associated pseudomembranous colitis: a prospective study. Gastroenterology 1982; 83: 1259–60.

106. Tsutaoka B, Hansen J, Johnson D, Holodniy M. Antibiotic-associated pseudomembranous enteritis due to *Clostridium difficile*. Clin Infect Dis 1994; 18: 982–84.

107. Kralovich KA, Sacsner J, Karmy-Jones RA, Eggenberger JC. Pseudomembranous colitis with associated fulminant ileitis in the defunctionalized limb of a jejunal-ileal bypass: case report. Dis Colon Rectum 1997; 40: 622–4.

108. Shortland JR, Spencer RC, Williams JL. Pseudomembranous colitis associated with changes in an ileal conduit. J Clin Pathol 1983; 36: 1184–7.

109. Fishman E, Kavuru M, Jones B *et al.* CT of pseudomembranous colitis: radiologic, clinical, and pathologic correlation. Radiology 1991; 180: 157–61.

110. Cleary RK. *Clostridium difficile*-associated diarrhea and colitis: clinical manifestations, diagnosis, and treatment. Dis Colon Rectum 1998; 41: 1435–49.

111. Linevsky JK, Kelly CP. *Clostridium difficile* colitis. In: JT Lamont, editor. Gastrointestinal Infections: Diagnosis and Management. New York: Marcel Dekker; 1997: 293–325.

112. Zuckerman E, Kanel G, Ha C, Kahn J, Gottesman BS, Korula J. Low albumin gradient ascites complicating severe pseudomembranous colitis. Gastroenterology 1997; 112: 991–4.

113. Jafri SF, Marshall JB. Ascites associated with antibiotic-associated pseudomembranous colitis. South Med J 1996; 89: 1014–17.

114. Truong M, Atri M, Bret PM *et al.* Sonographic appearances of benign and malignant conditions of the colon. Am J Roentgenol 1998; 170: 1451–5.

115. Rubin MS, Bodenstein LE, Kent KC. Severe *Clostridium difficile* colitis. Dis Colon Rectum 1995; 38: 350–4.

116. Bolton RP, Sherriff RJ, Read AE. *Clostridium difficile* associated diarrhea: a role in inflammatory bowel disease? Lancet 1980; 1: 383–4.

117. LaMont JT, Trnka YM. Therapeutic implications of *Clostridium difficile* toxin during relapse of chronic inflammatory bowel disease. Lancet 1980; 1: 381–3.

118. Fekety R. Guidelines for the diagnosis and management of *Clostridium difficile*-associated diarrhea and colitis. Amer-

ican College of Gastroenterology, Practice Parameters Committee. Am J Gastroenterol 1997; 92: 739–50.

119. Kyne L, Merry C, O'Connell B, Keane C, O'Neill D. Community-acquired *Clostridium difficile* infection. J Infect 1998; 36: 287–8.

120. Johnson S. Gerding DN, Janoff EN. Systemic and mucosal antibody responses to toxin A in patients infected with *Clostridium difficile*. J Infect Dis 1992; 166: 1287–94.

121. Issack MI, Elliott TS. *Clostridium difficile* carriage after infection. Lancet 1990; 335: 610–11.

122. Barbut F, Kajzer C, Planas N, Petit JC. Comparison of three enzyme immunoassays, a cytotoxicity assay, and toxigenic culture for diagnosis of *Clostridium difficile*-associated diarrhea. J Clin Microbiol 1993; 31: 963–7.

123. Merz CS, Kramer C, Forman M *et al.* Comparison of four commercially available rapid enzyme immunoassays with cytotoxin assay for detection of *Clostridium difficile* toxin(s) from stool specimens. J Clin Microbiol 1994; 32: 1142–7.

124. Whittier S, Shapiro DS, Kelly WF *et al.* Evaluation of four commercially available enzyme immunoassays for laboratory diagnosis of *Clostridium difficile*-associated diseases. J Clin Microbiol 1993; 31: 1632–5.

125. Peterson LR, Kelly PJ. The role of the clinical microbiology laboratory in the management of *Clostridium difficile*-associated diarrhea. Infect Dis Clin N Am 1993; 7: 277–93.

126. Walker RC, Ruane PJ, Rosenblatt JE *et al.* Comparison of culture, cytotoxicity assays, and enzyme-linked immunosorbent assay for toxin A and toxin B in the diagnosis of *Clostridium difficile*-related enteric disease. Diagn Microbiol Infect Dis 1986; 5: 61–9.

127. Tichota-Lee J, Jaqua-Stewart MJ, Benfield D, Simmons JL, Jaqua RA. Effect of age on the sensitivity of cell cultures to *Clostridium difficile* toxin. Diagn Microbiol Infect Dis 1987; 8: 203–14.

128. Doern GV, Coughlin RT, Wu L. Laboratory diagnosis of *Clostridium difficile*-associated gastrointestinal disease: comparison of a monoclonal antibody enzyme immunoassay for toxins A and B with a monoclonal antibody enzyme immunoassay for toxin A only and two cytotoxicity assays. J Clin Microbiol 1992; 30: 2042–6.

129. Lyerly DM, Neville LM, Evans DT *et al.* Multicenter evaluation of the *Clostridium difficile* TOX A/B TEST. J Clin Microbiol 1998; 36: 184–90.

130. De Girolami PC, Hanff PA, Eichelberger K *et al.* Multicenter evaluation of a new enzyme immunoassay for detection of *Clostridium difficile* enterotoxin A. J Clin Microbiol 1992; 30: 1085–8.

131. DiPersio JR, Varga FJ, Conwell DL, Kraft JA, Kozak KJ, Willis DH. Development of a rapid enzyme immunoassay for *Clostridium difficile* toxin A and its use in the diagnosis of *C. difficile*-associated disease. J Clin Microbiol 1991; 29: 2724–30.

132. Lyerly DM, Barroso LA, Wilkins TD. Identification of the latex test-reactive protein of *Clostridium difficile* as glutamate dehydrogenase. J Clin Microbiol 1991; 29: 2639–42.

133. Wren B, Clayton C, Tabaqchali S. Rapid identification of toxigenic *Clostridium difficile* by polymerase chain reaction. Lancet 1990; 335: 423.

134. Kato N, Ou CY, Kato H *et al.* Identification of toxigenic *Clostridium difficile* by the polymerase chain reaction. J Clin Microbiol 1991; 29: 33–7.

135. Alonso R, Pelaez T, Cercenado E, Rodriquez-Creixems M, Bouza E. Rapid detection of toxigenic *Clostridium difficile* strains by a nested PCR of the toxin B gene. Clin Microbiol Infect 1997; 3: 145–7.

136. Green GA, Riot B, Monteil H. Evaluation of an oligonucleotide probe and an immunological test for direct detection of toxigenic *Clostridium difficile* in stool samples. Eur J Clin Microbiol Infect Dis 1994; 13: 576–81.

137. Gumerlock PH, Tang YJ, Meyers FJ, Silva Jr J. Use of the polymerase chain reaction for the specific and direct detection of *Clostridium difficile* in human feces. Rev Infect Dis 1991; 13: 1053–60.

138. Boondeekhun HS, Gurtler V, Odd ML, Wilson VA, Mayall BC. Detection of *Clostridium difficile* enterotoxin gene in clinical specimens by the polymerase chain reaction. J Med Microbiol 1993; 38: 384–7.

139. Kato N, Ou CY, Kato H *et al*. Detection of toxigenic *Clostridium difficile* in stool specimens by the polymerase chain reaction. J Infect Dis 1993; 167: 455–8.

140. Gumerlock PH, Tang YJ, Weiss JB, Silva Jr J. Specific detection of toxigenic strains of *Clostridium difficile* in stool specimens. J Clin Microbiol 1993; 31: 507–11.

141. Alonso R, Munoz C, Gros S, Garcia de Viedma D, Pelaez T, Bouza E. Rapid detection of toxigenic *Clostridium difficile* from stool samples by a nested PCR of toxin B gene. J Hosp Infect 1999; 41: 145–9.

142. Teasley DG, Gerding DN, Olson MM *et al*. Prospective randomised trial of metronidazole versus vancomycin for *Clostridium difficile*-associated diarrhoea and colitis. Lancet 1983; 2: 1043–6.

143. Spencer RC. The role of antimicrobial agents in the aetiology of *Clostridium difficile*-associated disease. J Antimicrob Chemother 1998; 41(Suppl C.): 21–7.

144. Novak E. Lee JG, Seckman CE, Phillips JP, DiSanto AR. Unfavorable effect of atropine-diphenoxylate (Lomotil) therapy in lincomycin-caused diarrhea. J Am Med Assoc 1976; 235: 1451–4.

145. Walley T, Milson D. Loperamide related toxic megacolon in *Clostridium difficile* colitis. Postgrad Med J 1990; 66: 582.

146. Burke GW, Wilson ME, Mehrez IO. Absence of diarrhea in toxic megacolon complicating *Clostridium difficile* pseudomembranous colitis. Am J Gastroenterol 1988; 83: 304–7.

147. Zimmerman MJ, Bak A, Sutherland LR. Review article: treatment of *Clostridium difficile* infection. Aliment Pharmacol Ther 1997; 11: 1003–12.

148. Peterson LR. Antimicrobial agents. In: Rambaud JC, Ducluzeau R, eds. *Clostridium difficile*-associated Intestinal Diseases. Paris: Springer-Verlag, 1990: 115–27.

149. Bolton RP, Culshaw MA. Faecal metronidazole concentrations during oral and intravenous therapy for antibiotic associated colitis due to *Clostridium difficile*. Gut 1986; 27: 1169–72.

150. Ings RM, McFadzean JA, Ormerod WE. The fate of metronidazole and its implications in chemotherapy. Xenobiotica 1975; 5: 223–35.

151. Bartlett JG. Antimicrobial agents implicated in *Clostridium difficile* toxin-associated diarrhea of colitis. Johns Hopkins Med J 1981; 149: 6–9.

152. Bingley PJ, Harding GM. *Clostridium difficile* colitis following treatment with metronidazole and vancomycin. Postgrad Med J 1987; 63: 993–4.

153. Thomson G, Clark AH, Hare K, Spilg WG. Pseudomembranous colitis after treatment with metronidazole. Br Med J (Clin Res Ed) 1981; 282: 864–5.

154. Keighley MR, Burdon DW, Arabi Y *et al*. Randomised controlled trial of vancomycin for pseudomembranous colitis and postoperative diarrhoea. Br Med J 1978; 2: 1667–9.

155. Young GP, Ward PB, Bayley N *et al*. Antibiotic-associated colitis due to *Clostridium difficile*: double-blind comparison of vancomycin with bacitracin. Gastroenterology 1985; 89: 1038–45.

156. Mogg GA, Arabi Y, Youngs D, Johnson M, Bentley S, Burdon DW. Therapeutic trials of antibiotic associated colitis. Scand J Infect Dis Suppl 1980; 22: 41–5.

157. Fekety R, Silva J, Kauffman C, Buggy B, Deery HG. Treatment of antibiotic-associated *Clostridium difficile* coli-

158. tis with oral vancomycin: comparison of two dosage regimens. Am J Med 1989; 86: 15–19.

158. Kleinfeld DI, Sharpe RJ, Donta ST. Parenteral therapy for antibiotic-associated pseudomembranous colitis. J Infect Dis 1988; 157: 389.

159. Oliva SL, Guglielmo BJ, Jacobs R, Pons VG. Failure of intravenous vancomycin and intravenous metronidazole to prevent or treat antibiotic-associated pseudomembranous colitis. J Infect Dis 1989; 159: 1154–5.

160. Recommendations for preventing the spread of vancomycin resistance: recommendations of the Hospital Infection Control Practices Advisory Committee (HICPAC). Am J Infect Control 1995; 23: 87–94.

161. Kelly CP, LaMont JT. Treatment of *Clostridium difficile* diarrhea and colitis. In: Wolfe MM, editor. Therapy of Digestive Disorders. Philadelphia: WB Saunders, 2000: 513–22.

162. Dudley MN, McLaughlin JC, Carrington G, Frick J, Nightingale CH, Quintiliani R. Oral bacitracin vs vancomycin therapy for *Clostridium difficile*-induced diarrhea. A randomized double-blind trial. Arch Intern Med 1986; 146: 1101–4.

163. Chang TW, Gorbach SL, Bartlett JG, Saginur R. Bacitracin treatment of antibiotic-associated colitis and diarrhea caused by *Clostridium difficile* toxin. Gastroenterology 1980; 78: 1584–6.

164. Tedesco FJ. Bacitracin therapy in antibiotic-associated pseudomembranous colitis. Dig Dis Sci 1980; 25: 783–4.

165. de Lalla F, Nicolin R, Rinaldi E *et al*. Prospective study of oral teicoplanin versus oral vancomycin for therapy of pseudomembranous colitis and *Clostridium difficile*-associated diarrhea. Antimicrob Agents Chemother 1992; 36: 2192–6.

166. Wenisch C, Parschalk B, Hasenhundl M, Hirschl AM, Graninger W. Comparison of vancomycin, teicoplanin, metronidazole, and fusidic acid for the treatment of *Clostridium difficile*-associated diarrhea. Clin Infect Dis 1996; 22: 813–18.

167. Cronberg S, Castor B, Thoren A. Fusidic acid for the treatment of antibiotic-associated colitis induced by *Clostridium difficile*. Infection 1984; 12: 276–9.

168. Pasic M, Jost R, Carrel T, Von Segesser L, Turina M. Intracolonic vancomycin for pseudomembranous colitis. N Engl J Med 1993; 329: 583.

169. Giannasca PJ, Zhang ZX, Lei WD *et al*. Serum antitoxin antibodies mediate systemic and mucosal protection from *Clostridium difficile* disease in hamsters. Infect Immun 1999; 67: 527–38.

170. Morris LL, Villalba MR, Glover JL. Management of pseudomembranous colitis. Am Surg 1994; 60: 548–52.

171. Bradbury AW, Barrett S. Surgical aspects of *Clostridium difficile* colitis. Br J Surg 1997; 84: 150–9.

172. Ramaswamy R, Grover H, Corpuz M, Daniels P, Pitchumoni CS. Prognostic criteria in *Clostridium difficile* colitis. Am J Gastroenterol 1996; 91: 460–4.

173. Morris JB, Zollinger Jr. RM, Stellato TA. Role of surgery in antibiotic-induced pseudomembranous enterocolitis. Am J Surg 1990; 160: 535–9.

174. Grundfest-Broniatowski S, Quader M, Alexander F, Walsh RM, Lavery I, Milsom J. *Clostridium difficile* colitis in the critically ill. Dis Colon Rectum 1996; 39: 619–23.

175. Fekety R, Shah AB. Diagnosis and treatment of *Clostridium difficile* colitis. J Am Med Assoc 1993; 269: 71–5.

176. Wilcox MH. Treatment of *Clostridium difficile* infection. J Antimicrob Chemother 1998; 41(Suppl C.): 41–6.

177. Wilcox MH, Fawley WN, Settle CD, Davidson A. Recurrence of symptoms in *Clostridium difficile* infection – relapse or reinfection? J Hosp Infect 1998; 38: 93–100.

178. McFarland LV, Surawicz CM, Rubin M, Fekety R, Elmer GW, Greenberg RN. Recurrent *Clostridium difficile* disease: epidemiology and clinical characteristics. Infect Control Hosp Epidemiol 1999; 20: 43–50.

179. McFarland LV, Surawicz CM, Greenberg RN *et al*. A randomized placebo-controlled trial of *Saccharomyces boulardii* in combination with standard antibiotics for *Clostridium difficile* disease. J Am Med Assoc 1994; 271: 1913–18.

180. Fekerty R, McFarland LV, Surawicz CM, Greenberg RN, Elmer GW, Mulligan ME. Recurrent *Clostridium difficile* diarrhea: characteristics of and risk factors for patients enrolled in a prospective, randomized, double-blinded trial. Clin Infect Dis 1997; 24: 324–33.

181. Tedesco FJ, Gordon D, Fortson WC. Approach to patients with multiple relapses of antibiotic-associated pseudomembranous colitis. Am J Gastroenterol 1985; 80: 867–8.

182. Buggy BP, Fekety R, Silva Jr J. Therapy of relapsing *Clostridium difficile*-associated diarrhea and colitis with the combination of vancomycin and rifampin. J Clin Gastroenterol 1987; 9: 155–9.

183. Tedesco FJ. Treatment of recurrent antibiotic-associated pseudomembranous colitis. Am J Gastroenterol 1982; 77: 220–21.

184. Taylor NS, Bartlett JG. Binding of *Clostridium difficile* cytotoxin and vancomycin by anion-exchange resins. J Infect Dis 1980; 141: 92–7.

185. Gorbach SL, Chang TW, Goldin B. Successful treatment of relapsing *Clostridium difficile* colitis with *Lactobacillus* GG. Lancet 1987; 2: 1519.

186. Seal D, Borriello SP, Barclay F, Welch A, Piper M, Bonnycastle M. Treatment of relapsing *Clostridium difficile* diarrhoea by administration of a non-toxigenic strain. Eur J Clin Microbiol 1987; 6: 51–3.

187. Schellenberg D, Bonington A, Champion CM, Lancaster R, Webb S, Main J. Treatment of *Clostridium difficile* diarrhoea with brewer's yeast. Lancet 1994; 343: 171–2.

188. Chia JKS, Chan SM, Goldsein H. Baker's yeast as adjunctive therapy for relapses of *Clostridium difficile* diarrhea. Clin Infect Dis 1995; 20: 1581.

189. Surawicz CM., McFarland LV, Elmer G, Chinn J. Treatment of recurrent *Clostridium difficile* colitis with vancomycin and *Saccharomyces boulardii*. Am J Gastroenterol 1989; 84: 1285–7.

190. Surawicz CM, Elmer GW, Speelman P, McFarland LV, Chinn J, van Belle G. Prevention of antibiotic-associated diarrhea by *Saccharomyces boulardii*: a prospective study. Gastroenterology 1989; 96: 981–8.

191. Bacon 3rd AE, Fekety R. Immunoglobulin G directed against toxins A and B of *Clostridium difficile* in the general population and patients with antibiotic-associated diarrhea. Diagn Microbiol Infect Dis 1994; 18: 205–9.

192. McNulty C, Logan M, Donald IP *et al*. Successful control of *Clostridium difficile* infection in an elderly care unit through use of a restrictive antibiotic policy. J Antimicrob Chemother 1997; 40: 707–11.

193. Climo MW, Israel DS, Wong ES, Williams D, Coudron P, Markowitz SM. Hospital-wide restriction of clindamycin: effect on the incidence of *Clostridium difficile*-associated diarrhea and cost. Ann Intern Med 1998; 128: 989–95.

194. Pear SM, Williamson TH, Bettin KM, Gerding DN, Galgiani JN. Decrease in nosocomial *Clostridium difficile*-associated diarrhea by restricting clindamycin use. Ann Intern Med 1994; 120: 272–7.

195. Settle CD, Wilcox MH, Fawley WN, Corrado OJ, Hawkey PM. Prospective study of the risk of *Clostridium difficile* diarrhea in elderly patients following treatment with cefotaxime or piperacillin-tazobactam. Aliment Pharmacol Ther 1998; 12: 1217–23.

196. Brooks SE, Veal RO, Kramer O, Dore L, Schupf N, Adachi M. Reduction in the incidence of *Clostridium difficile*-associated diarrhea in an acute care hospital and a skilled nursing facility following replacement of electronic thermometers with single-use disposables. Infect Control Hosp Epidemiol 1992; 13: 98–103.

197. Jernigan JA, Siegman-Igra Y, Guerrant RC, Farr BM. A randomized crossover study of disposable thermometers for prevention of *Clostridium difficile* and other nosocomial infections. Infect Control Hosp Epidemiol 1998; 19: 494–9.

198. Worsley MA. Infection control and prevention of *Clostridium difficile* infection. J Antimicrob Chemother 1998; 41(Suppl C.): 59–66.

199. Starr JM, Rogers TR, Impallomeni M. Hospital-acquired *Clostridium difficile* diarrhea and herd immunity. Lancet 1997; 349: 426–8.

47 | Infectious colitis

Michael J.G. Farthing

Introduction

Many infections of the gastrointestinal tract are transient, self-limiting illnesses, and thus are generally not confused with chronic non-specific inflammatory bowel disease (IBD). However, others, particularly those due to invasive enteropathogens which cause an ileocolitis, may mimic ulcerative colitis or Crohn's disease. It is thus essential to distinguish rapidly between these conditions since inappropriate use of corticosteroids or immunosuppressive drugs may adversely affect outcome. Similarly, delay in administering an appropriate antibiotic for a colonic infection may increase morbidity, including the likelihood of developing complications. In the past, misdiagnosis of amoebiasis for example, has occurred with inappropriate use of corticosteroids which in some cases has resulted in colectomy and litigation. Some self-limiting colonic infections will resolve despite administration of steroids and mesalazine, but it is clearly inappropriate to commit an individual to lifelong maintenance therapy when further problems would not be expected following a single attack of infective colitis. Thus, precision regarding prognosis demands an accurate initial diagnosis of the etiology of an attack of colitis.

Clinicians in the developing world, where the micro-organisms responsible for infectious colitis are endemic, are accustomed to routinely searching for an infectious cause for colitis before making a diagnosis of non-specific IBD. In the industrialized world for several decades the reverse situation has existed, with IBD always being the most likely diagnosis. However, in recent years there has been a steady increase in reports of intestinal infection to agencies responsible for the surveillance of infectious diseases in the United Kingdom and USA. In the UK there has been a steady increase in reports of Salmonella spp. and Campylobacter jejuni infections (Fig. 1) and a number of important outbreaks of enterohemorrhagic E. coli (EHEC) infection with a reported mortality of 1–2% and a relatively high incidence of serious complications such as the hemolytic–uremic syndrome. The continued increase in foreign travel has further contributed to the importance of infectious colitis in individuals living in the industrialized world [1], as has the increasing use of broad-spectrum antibiotics and the well-recognized association of antibiotic-related diarrhea and pseudomembraneous colitis due to infection with Clostridium difficile.

Thus, despite the widespread implementation of public health measures to prevent transmission of intestinal enteropathogens in the industrialized world, intestinal infectious disease remains a significant problem which can be attributed to a number of factors including transmission of enteropathogens through food. Thus, clinicians must exercise increased vigilance in patients with diarrhea, particularly bloody diarrhea, and ensure that an appropriate search is made for an infective agent before a final diagnosis of non-specific IBD is made.

Epidemiology

The enteric pathogens responsible for infectious colitis are distributed worldwide both in industrialized and resource-poor countries [2,3]. However, the relative prevalence varies between different geographic locations; amebiasis, for example, is found most commonly in the Indian subcontinent, sub-Saharan Africa and Latin America, particularly Mexico, although it is an endemic infection of low prevalence in many countries in the northern hemisphere including North America and the United Kingdom. Salmonella spp. and Campylobacter jejuni are important foodborne pathogens which, during the last two decades, have been reported with increasing frequency in the United Kingdom. Many chicken flocks in the UK are contaminated with these human pathogens such that up to 70% of chicken carcasses in UK supermarkets may be contaminated.

Stephan R. Targan, Fergus Shanahan and Loren C. Karp (eds.), Inflammatory Bowel Disease: From Bench to Bedside, 2nd Edition, 845–861.
© 2003 Kluwer Academic Publishers. Printed in Great Britain

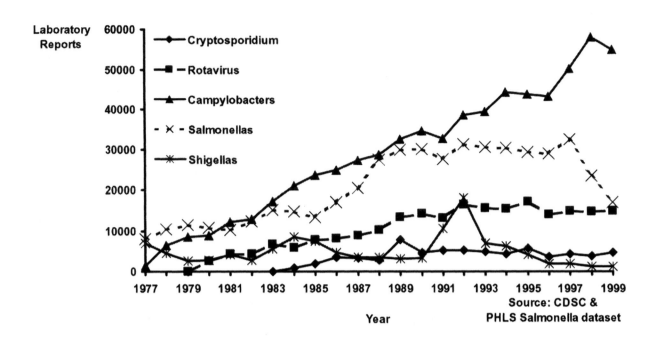

Figure 1. Reports of enteropathogens to the Public Health Laboratory Service 1977–1999.

A recent survey of general practice confirmed the high prevalence of intestinal infections in the United Kingdom [4] and concluded that many infections are not reported either to general practitioners or to communicable disease surveillance agencies.

Humans continue to be important reservoirs of the organisms responsible for infective colitis; some infections such as shigellosis and amebiasis are restricted to humans. Other infections such as those due to *Salmonella* spp. and *Campylobacter* spp. are zoonoses, since animal reservoirs have been shown to be increasingly important for the rising incidence of these infections in humans.

Transmission is nearly always by the fecal–oral route. Water may become contaminated either directly by human contact or indirectly by inadequate separation of domestic water supplies and sewage systems. In addition to the risks associated with contaminated drinking water, infectious colitis may also be acquired by swimming in contaminated swimming pools, freshwater lakes and seawater [5, 6]. Well-documented outbreaks of shigellosis and EHEC infection have been described following recreational swimming in a freshwater lake in Ore-

gon [7]. Intensive food production methods have increased the risk of contaminating poultry carcasses (*Salmonella* spp. and *Campylobacter jejuni*), beef (EHEC) and pork (*Yersinia enterocolitica*) [8]. Although contaminating organisms will be destroyed by adequate cooking, bacteria may survive on the hands of a food preparer and then be transferred to uncooked salads, fruit or vegetables by direct contact. EHEC on fresh beef has been transferred to cold cooked meats in a butcher's shop, leading to a local outbreak of EHEC infection as a result of ingestion of the contaminated, cold precooked meat. EHEC has also been responsible for outbreaks following ingestion of hamburger meat, presumably as a result of inadequate cooking [8].

Person-to-person transmission also occurs between children in schools and day-care centers and during sexual contact. Direct spread of infection between humans is particularly common with infections such as shigellosis in which only 10–100 organisms are required to initiate clinical infection.

There are a number of particular risk factors and epidemiologic settings that increase the risks of acquiring infectious colitis (Table 1). Infants, young

Table 1. Risk factors for infectious colitis

Risk factors	Groups at risk
Age	Infants and young children; the elderly
Non-immune host defense – gastric acid	The elderly; hypo- and achlorhydria; recipients of acid-inhibitory drugs
Immunodeficiency	Congenital immunodeficiency; HIV/AIDS; cancer and cancer chemotherapy; undernutrition
Increased exposure to enteropathogens	Travelers; contaminated food and water
Antibiotics	Especially the elderly and cancer patients

children and the elderly are at increased risk of acquiring intestinal infection partly because of relative impairment of host immune defense mechanisms but also, in the case of young children, due to increased exposure during the weaning period. Breast-fed infants however, are relatively protected during the first few months of life. Innate host defense, particularly gastric acid, presents an important barrier to invading enteropathogens. Acid secretion decreases in the presence of gastric atrophy (as a result of *Helicobacter pylori* infection or pernicious anemia) or during ingestion of acid-inhibitory drugs such as the H_2 receptor-antagonists and proton-pump inhibitors [9, 10]. There is now compelling evidence that the risks of acquiring *Salmonella* and *Campylobacter* infections are increased by these acid-inhibitory drugs.

About 30% of travelers from industrialized countries to resource-poor parts of the world will experience an attack of traveler's diarrhea almost always due to intestinal infection. Although enterotoxigenic *E. coli* is the most common cause of acute watery diarrhea in travelers, invasive enteropathogens such as *Salmonella* spp., *Shigella* spp., *Campylobacter jejuni* and *Entamoeba histolytica* all occur in travelers and can produce infectious colitis. Travelers to the developing world have increased exposure to these enteropathogens not only by ingestion of contaminated food and beverages [11–13] but also through recreational activities such as water sports.

It is now well established that immunocompromised individuals, particularly those with HIV infection, are at increased risk of infectious colitis, particularly that due to cytomegalovirus (CMV) infection. *Entamoeba histolytica* is also often isolated from homosexual men but invasive amebiasis is uncommon since infection is usually with the non-pathogenic *Entamoeba dispar*. However, the classic invasive enteropathogens such as *Salmonella* and

Shigella spp. are commonly isolated from HIV-infected individuals.

The widespread use of broad-spectrum antibiotics, both in the community and in hospitalized patients, has been another contributory factor to the increase in intestinal infection, particularly that due to *Clostridium difficile* (see Chapter 46). There is increasing evidence that *C. difficile* infection accounts for only a proportion of antibiotic-associated diarrhea and it is likely that other clostridia are also involved.

Etiology of infectious colitis

A broad spectrum of viruses, bacteria, protozoa and helminths are known to produce infectious colitis (Table 2). Many of these organisms, particularly the bacterial enteropathogens, are found worldwide, whereas others clearly have major geographic restrictions. Gastrointestinal infection with *Mycobacterium tuberculosis* has predominated in the developing world, although is now increasingly common in some parts of Europe and North America following the arrival of immigrants from parts of Asia and particularly the Indian subcontinent [14]. The enteropathogenic protozoa *Entamoeba histolytica* and *Balantidium coli* are again predominantly pathogens of the tropics and subtropics, although cases of intestinal amebiasis are not uncommon in the northern hemisphere and are not all necessarily acquired as a result of foreign travel. Infection with *B. coli* is limited almost exclusively to communities who have a close coexistence with pigs, for example as the inhabitants of Papua New Guinea.

Intestinal schistosomiasis and trichuriasis are again diseases of the tropics and subtropics and schistosomiasis occurs only in areas that are inhabited by the freshwater snail which is its specific intermediate host. However, acute schistosomiasis

Table 2. Enteropathogens responsible for infectious colitis
Viruses
Cytomegalovirus
Bacteria
Enteroinvasive *E. coli*, enterhemorrhagic *E. coli*, *Shigella* spp., *Salmonella* spp., *Campylobacter* spp., *Yersinia enterocolitica*, *Clostridium difficile*, *Mycobacterium tuberculosis*, Aeromonas hydrophila, Plesiomonas shigelloides
Protozoa
Entamoeba histolytica, *Balantidium coli*
Helminths
Schistosoma spp., *Trichuris trichiura*

is recognized to occur in travelers to these endemic areas when it usually presents as the acute infection syndrome, Katayama fever.

CMV infection is limited almost exclusively to the immunocompromised, particularly those with HIV infection, and *Clostridium difficile*-related pseudomembranous colitis is almost always associated with treatment with broad-spectrum antibiotics.

Pathogenesis

The microbial enteropathogens that are responsible for infectious colitis produce their effects on the host by a diverse series of mechanisms [15, 16]. Some organisms such as *Entamoeba histolytica* are able to destroy host epithelial cells merely by attaching to the apical membrane of the colonocyte; others such as enterohemorrhagic *E. coli* attach and then disrupt the apical membrane of the epithelial cell and then subsequently enter the mucosa through specialized M cells which overlay lymphoid cell collections in the intestine. Other organisms rely predominantly on the production of cytolethal substances such as cytotoxins; this is perhaps best exemplified by *Clostridium difficile*. However, the best-recognized mechanism for destruction of the colonic epithelium and associated inflammation is that of invasion, a mechanism utilized by many of the classic bacterial enteropathogens such as *Shigella* spp., *Salmonella enteritidis* and *Camplyobacter jejuni*. Finally, acute and chronic inflammatory responses in the mucosa and submucosa may be stimulated by the presence of micro-organisms such as *M. tuberculosis* or the ova of *Schistosoma* spp., or the direct presence of a helminth such as *Trichuris trichiura*. The latter is also able to induce local anaphylaxis.

Pathogenetic processes in infectious colitis

Contact-dependent cytolysis

Although *Entamoeba histolytica* is often considered to be an invasive enteropathogen this is not strictly true. *E. histolytica* produces its cytolethal effects through cell–cell contact. Initial engagement depends on a surface membrane-associated galactose-binding lectin which mediates adherence to the host epithelial cell [17] followed by release of a variety of hydrolytic enzymes and pore-forming proteins. Considerable attention has been directed toward the pore-forming protein, amoebapore which is released and inserted into the host cell membrane, producing high-conductance ion channels leading to a rapid increase in intracellular calcium and cell death [18]. *E. histolytica* also synthesizes a number of other potentially cytolytic proteins including hemolysins, proteolytic enzymes including a cathepsin B proteinase, an acidic proteinase and a collagenase. These proteinases appear to be involved in disruption of the extracellular matrix, which enables the trophozoites to penetrate into the deeper layers of the mucosa and submucosa. Amebic cytolytic activity is dependent on a number of parasite factors including microfilament function, calcium and a calcium-dependent phospholipase A.

Adherence and effacement

Enterohemorrhagic *E. coli*, like enteropathogenic *E. coli*, contain a series of genes known collectively as the locus of enterocyte effacement (LEE) which encode proteins which produce the attaching and effacing lesions [19, 20]. This lesion is characterized by localized effacement of microvilli, intimate attachment of the bacillus to the host cell membrane and formation of a pedestal-like structure in the host cell which contains cytoskeletal proteins including polymerized actin, α-actinin, ezrin and myosin. The LEE encodes for a type III secretion system which produces a number of secreted proteins which mediate these processes. Initial attachment is now thought to be mediated by EspA, which is present on small filamentous projections of the organisms [20]. The bundle-forming pillus, previously thought to be involved in mediating non-intimate attachment, is now probably mainly involved in allowing EHEC organisms to adhere together. EspA filaments are then thought to stimulate release and entry of the translocated intimin receptor (previously known as host protein 90) which then becomes the receptor for intimin, an EHEC attachment protein also encoded by the LEE. Following intimate attachment, EspB and EspD are then also translocated and are considered to be important for the polymerization of actin and other cytoskeletal rearrangements which lead to the formation of the pedestal lesion.

Although EHEC are not classic invasive enteropathogens they do penetrate the mucosa, probably through M cells, where they proliferate and release Shiga toxins. These are potent cytolethal toxins which act locally in the gut by inhibiting protein synthesis; they are also released into the systemic circulation and are probably responsible for one of the most devastating complications of this infection, namely the hemolytic–uremic syndrome.

Cytotoxin-induced colitis

Although many organisms responsible for infectious colitis liberate cytolethal substances as part of the pathogenesis of infection, a few enteropathogens, particularly *Clostridium difficile*, rely almost exclusively on cytotoxin production to cause disease. *C. difficile*, which is a non-invasive spore-forming anerobic bacillus, releases two potent toxins: toxin A (308 kDa) which is a potent 'enterotoxin' and toxin B (270 kDa) which is an extremely potent cytotoxin but is devoid of enterotoxic activity in rabbit ileum [21, 22]. However, toxin A also possesses cytotoxic and hemagglutinating activity and is a potent neutrophil chemoattractant. Both toxins are lethal when administered parenterally to animals. The genes for these toxins have been cloned and sequenced, and are located on the bacterial chromosome. Although toxin A is generally referred to as an enterotoxin, it does not produce intestinal secretion by the classic pathways of *E. coli* LT and ST and cholera toxin. Toxin A primarily elicits an inflammatory response with an inflammatory infiltrate in the lamina propria and increased concentrations of PGE_2 and LTB_4 accompanied by fluid secretion. In addition, there is increased intestinal permeability, which appears to be related to disaggregation of the actin-containing filaments in the peri-junctional actinomyosin ring. There is increasing evidence to suggest that it is the presence of neutrophils and neutrophil products that mediates these changes. Toxin B also elicits fluid secretion and increases permeability, and releases PGE_2 into the intestinal lumen although its precise role in pathogenesis is less well characterized. There is, however, evidence that the effects of toxins A and B are synergistic. Specific receptors for toxin A have been identified in some mammalian microvillus membranes. The receptor is a glycoconjugate with a

trisaccharide, galactose-$\alpha 1 \rightarrow 3$ galactose-$\beta 1 \rightarrow 4$N-acetylglucosamine, which contains the binding site [23]. Like the Shiga toxin receptor, toxin A receptor is not present in mammalian neonates, and this probably explains the absence of disease in human infants infected with *C. difficile*. Both toxins utilize the same intracellular signal transduction system since they act as enzymes to catalyze the glucosylation of rho, which is a family of proteins which are small GTPases and are essential for maintenance of the actin cytoskeleton [24–27]. The glucosylation of rho causes disaggregation of actin filaments, cell rounding and cell death.

Invasion of the epithelium

The mechanisms by which invasive organisms such as *Salmonella*, *Shigella* and enteroinvasive *E. coli* enter the host epithelial cell depend on their ability to trigger a signaling cascade which leads to a cytokeletal rearrangement that permits entry of the organism into the cell in an endocytotic vesicle. Following contact of the organism with the host surface membrane there is localized membrane ruffling, rearrangement of actin filaments and capping of host surface proteins [28].

Salmonella invasion is rapid, with internalization of bacteria in vacuoles within minutes and associated with calcium influx and activation of the inositol phosphate transduction pathways [29]. Regulation of the cytoskeletal rearrangement appears to be under the control of CD42, one of the *ras*-related superfamilies of small GTPases [30]. *Salmonella* has a chromosomal pathogenicity island SP-1 containing several invasion operons including *inv/spa* which are homologous with invasion genes of other invasive bacteria [31].

Shigella invades by a similar mechanism again involving actin-polymerization, but in this case dependent on the small GTPase rho [32]. Invasion is mediated by three surface effector proteins, IpaB, IpaC and IpaD, which trigger the host endocytotic process followed by release of shigellae from the vacuole, mediated by IpaB [33]. These invasion mechanisms exemplify the stealth of enteropathogenic bacteria in using their own surface or secreted proteins to subvert host cell structures to advance the colonization process [34, 35].

Once shigella has entered the epithelial cell it is then able to use the contractile protein actin to propel it through the cell and to penetrate and invade other cells in the epithelium. It is also able to release shiga toxin which causes irreversible inhibition of protein synthesis by a highly specific action on the 60s mammalian ribosomal subunit.

Most invasive enteropathogens stimulate the host epithelial cell to produce a variety of chemokines, notably IL-8 [36, 37]. These are potent chemoattractants which promote a rapid influx of neutrophils into the lamina propria. This is an appropriate host response to limit the progress of an infecting microorganism, but the presence of large numbers of neutrophils enhances the inflammatory cascade and ultimately increases tissue damage and the secretory response within the epithelium. Inhibition of neutrophil influx by administration of antibody to the cell adhesion molecule CD18 reduces the mucosal inflammatory response and structural damage and also diminishes fluid and electrolyte secretion by epithelial cells [38].

Inflammatory responses to mucosal enteropathogens

In addition to the acute and chronic intestinal inflammatory responses that are associated with invasive enteropathogens, chronic inflammation is the major pathway for pathogenesis of *Schistosoma* spp. and *Mycobacterium tuberculosis* infection. The adult worms of *Schistosoma* spp. reside in the tributaries of the portal vein, and the female worm releases a continuous supply of ova which are disseminated through the portal venous system to a number of sites including the liver (*S. mansoni*), the bladder (*S. haematobium*) and the intestine (*S. mansoni*, *S. haematobium* and *S. japonicum*). The ova release a number of antigens which produce a chronic inflammatory response including granuloma formation. Chronic inflammation can lead to epithelial destruction and hemorrhage, with healing by fibrosis sometimes complicated by stricture formation. Similarly, *M. tuberculosis* bacilli in the intestinal wall induce a chronic inflammatory response, again with granuloma formation, although in this case the granulomata are caseating. Chronic inflammation can produce ulceration and stricture formation.

The colonic helminth, *Trichuris trichiura*, directly invades the intestinal mucosa with its thin anterior end buried usually in the proximal colon. However, in heavy infections worms may be found from the terminal ileum to the rectum. Mucosal inflammation usually only occurs at the site of attachment of the worm, and may consist of breaches in the epithelium, subepithelial hemorrhages and infiltration with eosinophils, lymphocytes and plasma cells. A local immediate hypersensitivity reaction in the colonic mucosa may be involved in the pathogenesis of the so-called trichuris dysentery syndrome.

Clinical features

The distinction between infectious colitis and non-specific IBD (ulcerative colitis and Crohn's colitis) can present major difficulties to the clinician. Although infectious colitis usually has an abrupt onset, often associated with fever and cramping abdominal pain, these features are not always present and are not exclusive to intestinal infection. Infectious colitis can have a more indolent course typified by the gradual onset of symptoms in amebic colitis which may occur over many days or weeks. A history of foreign travel may be helpful, although in one series 15% of patients returning from abroad with persistent diarrhea were presenting for the first time with non-specific IBD [39]. Similarly, a history of diarrhea that followed a meal in which food or water could be a potential vehicle for infection, particularly if other family or friends had similar symptoms, might suggest an infective origin for the symptoms. Finally, infectious colitis is usually self-limiting and will often resolve without any specific interventions. However, when symptoms persist beyond 7–10 days clinical evaluation alone is usually inadequate to make a firm diagnosis and thus further investigation is usually required.

Bacterial colitis

Salmonella spp.

Non-typhoidal salmonellosis is a common cause of food poisoning usually occurring 12–48 h after eating contaminated food. Nausea, vomiting and headache occur early in the illness, usually followed by fever, cramping abdominal pain and watery diarrhea. In moderate to severe infections a dysenteric form of the illness can develop with small frequent mucoid, bloody stools, severe cramping abdominal pain and tenesmus. Recovery usually occurs in 2–14 days. Some types of *Salmonella*, such as *S. dublin*, are highly invasive and produce a typhoid fever-like illness. These invasive organisms can produce focal infections including mycotic aneurysms, septic arthritis (0.2–2.5%) and osteomyelitis. Occasionally *Salmonella* infection can cause cholecystitis and cholangitis, meningitis and splenic abscess.

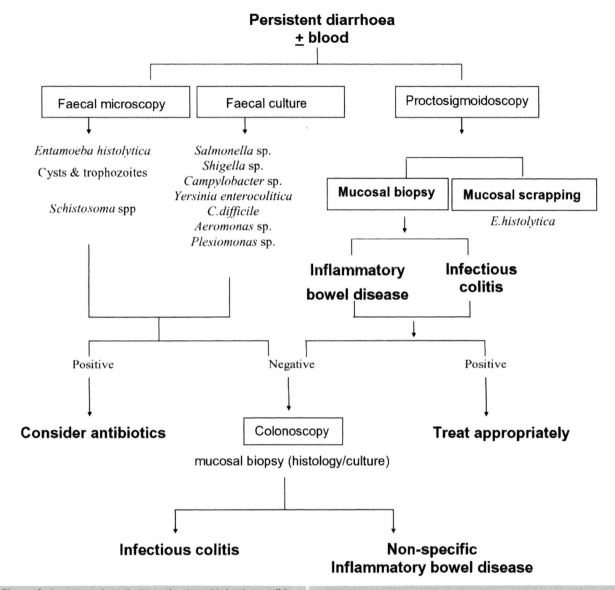

Figure 2. An approach to the investigation of infectious colitis.

Shigella spp. and enteroinvasive *E. coli*

Shigellosis gradually evolves through an incubation period of 1–4 days which is then followed by fever, headache and anorexia. These constitutional symptoms are followed by watery diarrhea which then declines but is generally followed by small-volume, mucoid bloody stools almost invariably accompanied by moderate to severe lower abdominal cramping pain and tenesmus. *Shigella* infections are often accompanied by extraintestinal manifestations in children including seizures, the hemolytic–uremic syndrome and thrombotic thrombocytopenic purpura. Focal infections are uncommon. Enteroinvasive *E. coli* has a similar presentation to shigellosis as these organisms can be regarded as non-shiga toxin-producing shigella. The complications due to shiga toxin (namely, seizures and hemolytic–uremic syndrome) are thus not associated with EIEC infection.

Enterohemorrhagic *E. coli*

The incubation period is usually 3–9 days, although it may be more prolonged in children. A typical presentation is of bloody diarrhea, blood usually appearing in the stool early in the illness. This is usually accompanied by lower abdominal pain and tenderness, abdominal distension, and in children rectal prolapse. As EHEC produces shiga toxin, seizures and hemolytic–uremic syndrome thus occur as in shigellosis, the latter being responsible for many of the deaths associated with this infection [8]. The majority of infections resolve in 7–21 days but mortality continues to be 3–5%.

Campylobacter jejuni

The incubation period is 2–3 days which is followed by a prodrome of headache, myalgia and fever. Diarrhea and severe cramping lower abdominal pain then supervene. Nausea, vomiting, anorexia and overt rectal bleeding occur in about 50% of patients. The illness usually resolves within 7–21 days. The severity of the abdominal pain may suggest the presence of an acute surgical abdomen such as appendicitis. *Campylobacter* infection may be complicated by reactive arthritis or a full Reiter's syndrome (arthritis, urethritis and conjunctivitis) particularly in patients who are HLA-B27-positive. *Campylobacter* infections are also complicated by the Guillain–Barré syndrome, which usually occurs 1–3 weeks after the intestinal infection [40]. The Guillain–Barré syndrome which follows *Campylobacter* enteritis is predominantly a motor syndrome with a relatively poor outcome because of residual motor deficit.

Yersinia enterocolitica

Infection usually produces watery diarrhea but in up to 25% of patients bloody diarrhea, fever and abdominal pain may be major symptoms. There is often a marked terminal ileitis with enlargement of local mesenteric lymph nodes, which in some situations results in a presentation similarly to acute appendicitis. *Yersinia* is also characterized by extra-enteric manifestations including erythema nodosum and erythema multiforme-like skin rashes. Reactive arthritis and Reiter's syndrome also occur, and like *Campylobacter* infection, this is more common in individuals who are HLA-B27-positive.

A serious complication of *Yersinia enterocolitica* infection is septicemia, which is particularly prevalent in individuals with iron overload, such as hemochromatosis, and those with chronic hemolytic anemias such as thalassemia.

Aeromonas and Plesiomonas spp. infections

Although the pathogenicity of these organisms has been controversial, there is compelling evidence that these organisms can produce infectious colitis which is indistinguishable from ulcerative colitis.

Mycobacterium tuberculosis infection

The presentation of ileocecal and colorectal tuberculosis is usually slowly progressive and may produce a variety of symptoms including chronic diarrhea with or without blood, abdominal pain and a tender abdominal mass in the right iliac fossa, and symptoms suggestive of subacute small bowel obstruction [14]. In addition, there are usually nonspecific symptoms including fever, general malaise and weight loss. Anorectal symptoms may be those of ulceration, anal fissure, perianal or ischiorectal abscess and fistula.

Viral colitis

Cytomegalovirus colitis occurs predominantly in immunocompromised individuals with HIV infection, although it is well recognized to occur in the immunocompetent. CMV usually presents as an acute colitis with abdominal pain and diarrhea with or without blood. Pain is often a predominant symptom and at least 50% of patients have a fever. The symptoms of infection usually persist for several weeks and, in the immunocompromised, usually do not resolve until antiviral treatment is administered. When infection is segmental in the colon the presentation may be accompanied by an abdominal mass, and when severe there is a substantial risk of perforation.

Protozoal colitis

Entamoeba histolytica

Infection with *E. histolytica* ranges from an asymptomatic carrier state to acute colitis which may be fulminant and complicated by perforation. The onset of amebic colitis is usually insidious with abdominal discomfort, loose stools often initially without blood or mucus. When fulminant, however, symptoms may be abrupt in onset and progress rapidly. Constitutional symptoms are often mild. Fulminant amebic colitis is usually the result of extensive colonic ulceration and may be indistinguishable from fulminant ulcerative colitis. There may be the clinical picture of toxic megacolon with abdominal distension and tenderness, high fever and tachycardia. Complications include severe hemorrhage and perforation, and may progress to amebic liver abscess.

Balantidium coli

The clinical features of this infection resemble amebic colitis. Again an asymptomatic carrier state can exist, although infection may present as acute colitis which can be fulminant. In the acute form of the disease, diarrhea with blood and mucus usually begins abruptly and is often associated with nausea, abdominal discomfort and marked weight loss. Again colonic dilation and perforation with peritonitis can occur with this infection. Occasionally balantidial appendicitis occurs.

Helminthic colitis

Schistosoma spp.

Acute schistosomiasis may be evident clinically 4–6 weeks after infection, and is characterized by fever, cutaneous and respiratory allergic manifestations, enlargement of the liver and spleen, lymphadenopathy and peripheral eosinophilia. This early clinical syndrome is sometimes known as Katayama fever. Intestinal schistosomiasis may present clinically months or years after infection. The major symptoms are of colitis with diarrhea which may contain blood, and these are often associated with non-specific abdominal pain. There may also be constitutional symptoms including tiredness, anorexia and weight loss. Symptoms may be particularly severe in *S. mansoni* infection, which is known to be associated with multiple inflammatory colonic polyps. These can result in severe blood and protein loss from the colon. *S. japonicum* also produces colitis, and with long-standing disease there is an increased risk of developing colorectal cancer. *S. haematobium* is particularly associated with disease in the distal colon and rectum. Inflammatory masses may also occur in the colon; these bilharziomas can masquerade as a colorectal neoplasm.

Trichuris trichiura

Light infections which involve only the proximal colon are often asymptomatic. However, heavy infections may result in the trichuris-dysentery syndrome which is characterized by frequent low-volume stools with blood and mucus. The predominant symptoms may be blood and mucus alone without significant diarrhea. There may be accompanying abdominal pain, tenesmus and rectal prolapse with constitutional symptoms including anorexia and weight loss. Anemia and finger clubbing are also associated with severe infection, and in children there may be impairment of growth and development.

There are some organisms that typically produce an isolated infectious proctitis (Table 4).

Diagnosis

Although the majority of episodes of acute infective diarrhea resolve without the need for making a specific diagnosis of the etiologic agent responsible, persistent diarrhea, particularly when associated with blood, always requires further investigation. Precision in diagnosis is important to ensure that antibiotics are made available for those infections in which there is a proven role for antimicrobial chemotherapy in reducing the duration and severity of disease, and also to distinguish infective colitis from non-specific IBD. This is particularly important in severely ill patients when delay in starting appropriate treatment might significantly alter the outcome. Confident exclusion of an infective etiology is rarely achieved in less than 24–48 h and, although imprecise, clinical assessment is important for guiding management during this early phase of the illness.

History

Identification of potential risk factors for intestinal infection may be acquired from the clinical history (see Table 1). Even patients with established IBD are at risk of acquiring intestinal infection; thus an infective etiology should be considered in all patients with IBD who are apparently in relapse.

Examination

General physical examination rarely distinguishes between infection and non-specific IBD unless there are obvious perianal stigmata of Crohn's disease, other signs suggestive of HIV infection (Kaposi's sarcoma, hairy leukoplakia or oral candidiasis) or typical extraintestinal manifestations of IBD, such as erythema nodosum, aphthous ulceration, pyoderma

Table 3. Endoscopic appearances of the rectum in infectious colitis and proctitis

Endoscopic appearances	Clinical diagnosis
'Colitis' but may be normal	Salmonellosis, shigellosis, campylobacteriosis, yersiniosis, tuberculosis, *Clostridium difficile* infection, amebiasis
Deep ulcers	Amebiasis, tuberculosis, syphilis
Pseudomembrane	*Clostridium difficile* infection
Vesicles	Herpes simplex virus
Beads of pus	Gonorrhea

Table 4. Infective proctitis

Bacteria	*Chlamydia trachomatis* non-LGV, *Chlamydia trachomatis* LGV, *Neisseria gonorrhoeae*, *Treponema pallidum*, *Mycobacterium tuberculosis*
Viruses	Herpes simplex virus, cytomegalovirus
Helminths	*Schistosoma* spp.

LGV, lymphogranuloma venereum.

gangrenosum and arthralgia. However, as stated previously, joint symptoms may accompany infection due to certain invasive enteropathogens, and may form part of a Reiter's syndrome.

Abdominal examination rarely distinguishes acute infectious colitis from non-specific IBD. Any form of severe colitis can give rise to abdominal tenderness, distension and in some cases reduced bowel sounds due to ileus. Rigid sigmoidsocopy should form part of the initial clinical assessment and may confirm the presence of a colitis. Although some forms of infective proctitis do have specific features which might favor a diagnosis of infection (Table 3) ulceration in the rectum can occur in infection and in non-specific IBD; pseudomembrane may be a feature of ischemic colitis as well as *C. difficile* infection. In addition, the endoscopic appearances in the rectum may be normal in many forms of infective colitis, which may be limited to the right colon (Table 3).

Routine blood tests

Similarly, routine laboratory investigations are rarely informative. In acute infectious colitis there may be anemia, a raised neutrophil count and evidence of an inflammatory process with a raised ESR, C-reactive protein and platelet count. However, these abnormalities also occur in colitis due to ulcerative colitis and Crohn's disease.

Thus, clinical assessment, while being important for assessing the severity of a colitis, is rarely sufficient to distinguish infection from non-specific inflammation. A variety of other diagnostic procedures are therefore acquired (Figure 2).

Microbiology

Microscopy

Microbiological examination of feces or rectal swab is the standard approach to identify an enteropathogen responsible for an infectious colitis. Light microscopic examination of three sequential fecal specimens continues to be important for the identification of protozoa such as *Entamoeba histolytica* and *Balantidium coli*. It is essential to examine fresh specimens as the fragile trophozoites of *E. histolytica* begin to lose their motility at room temperature and rapidly disintegrate; *E. histolytica* cysts are more robust and survive storage. *E. coli* is a large motile ciliate and can sometimes be seen with a hand lens. Fecal microscopy is also of potential value in identifying the ova of *Schistosoma* spp., and a skilled parasitologist can identify the various subspecies by ova morphology.

Culture

Stool culture will usually isolate the classic invasive enteropathogens providing appropriate culture conditions are employed. One of the major disadvantages of fecal culture is the inevitable delay before culture information is available to the clinician. It is unusual for a bacterial enteropathogen to be identified in less than 24–48 h, and for the slower-growing organism such as *Yersinia enterocolitica* and *Campylobacter jejuni*, information may not be forthcoming for 3–5 days. DNA-based technology, usually directed toward specific virulence factors of these enteropathogens, offers the opportunity to make a rapid, highly specific diagnosis. These techniques are widely used in research laboratories to investigate the role of potential virulence factors in pathogenesis, and will ultimately be incorporated into clinical practice. There continue to be difficulties in developing tests that will work on crude fecal extracts, but this technology had been satisfactorily used on tissue and other body fluids, particularly for the identification of *M. tuberculosis*.

Blood culture should be performed in ill patients with fever and other systemic symptoms. Invasive organisms that produce an enteric fever-like illness, including *Salmonella* spp., *Campylobacter jejuni* and *Yersinia entercolitica*, can be detected by this approach.

Serology

Serology is generally disappointing as a method of diagnosis for the majority of intestinal infections. However, in amebic colitis serology will be positive in 80–90% of patients, and is an important screening test alongside fecal microscopy if amebiasis is an important diagnostic candidate. Serology is also useful in detection of *Yersinia enterocolitica* infection although results are not usually positive for at least 10–14 days after the onset of the illness; thus the results may become available only as the diarrhea resolves. ELISAs are now available for the diagnosis of strongyloidiasis and schistosomiasis and should be regarded as first-line screening tests for these infections. These tests are particularly useful in travelers returning from endemic areas, but are of less value in the indigenous population once an infection has been diagnosed and treated, since antibodies may persist for months or even years after the initial infection.

Serotyping continues to be available for a number of bacterial enteropathogens including *Salmonella* spp., *Campylobacter jejuni* and enterohemorrhagic *E. coli*, and are still of value in identifying the source of outbreaks and monitoring their extent.

Abdominal imaging

A variety of imaging techniques are available, and may be useful both in establishing a primary diagnosis and in the assessment of the severity and extent of the disease.

Ileocolonoscopy

If rigid sigmoidoscopy reveals the presence of colitis in the rectum, then it is usually unnecessary to pursue this further with a more extensive examination of the colon and distal ileum. A rectal biopsy should, however, be taken for microscopic examination. If the rectum is normal then it is usually appropriate to examine the proximal colon endoscopically. However, the endoscopic differentiation between acute infectious colitis and other forms of colitis is difficult. Appearances of *Shigella*, *Salmonella* and *Campylobacter* infections are macroscopically indistinguishable from non-specific IBD. These infections may produce a predominantly right-sided colitis that macroscopically resembles ulcerative colitis; this finding should raise the index of suspicion for infection. Ileocaecal and rectal tuberculosis may produce identical endosopic appearances to Crohn's disease. However, an experienced endoscopist may be able to identify the typical amebic ulcers, which are shallow lesions with undermined edges often covered with a yellow exudate. The intervening mucosa appears normal, which distinguishes it from ulcerative colitis and other invasive bacterial infections of the colon. However, the diagnosis must be confirmed by microscopic examination of ulcer slough for trophozoites.

The presence of pseudomembranes in the colon (which appear as pale, white/yellow excrescences on the epithelium which when removed, leave an area of spontaneous bleeding separated by areas of normal mucosa) are generally indicative of *C. difficile* infection although pseudomembrane is not specific for this condition and may occur in ischemia.

Colonic and ileal strictures should be examined endoscopically so that multiple biopsies can be obtained for histology and microbiology. Strictures are classic features of intestinal tuberculosis and schistosomiasis. Multiple colonic polyps are well recognized to occur in severe colonic schistosomiasis usually due to infection with *S. mansoni*. Endoscopic polypectomy has been advocated when polyp formation is extensive and associated with hypoalbuminemia. Larger mass lesions should also be examined endoscopically, and biopsies to exclude neoplasia but benign inflammatory masses are well recognized in amebiasis (amebomata) and schistosomiasis (bilharziomas).

Endoscopic examination of the terminal ileum might reveal strictures (tuberculosis) or discreet ulceration (yersiniosis). Biopsies should be taken for microbiological culture and histology.

Endoscopic examination of the colon may also reveal the colonic helminth, *Trichuris trichiura*, where multiple worms can be seen to be adherent to the colonic mucosa. Multiple colonic biopsies should always be taken, as in some instances it may be possible to directly detect the presence of an enteropathogen in tissue (*M. tuberculosis, E. histolytica, Schistosoma* spp. and CMV).

Plain abdominal radiograph

A supine plain abdominal radiograph can be invaluable in assessing the severity and extent of infectious colitis. A gas-filled colon devoid of feces is consistent with total colitis; loss of haustration and colonic dilation is indicative of severe inflammation. The examination is also useful for detecting free air in the abdominal cavity, a sign of colonic perforation.

Transabdominal ultrasound

An ultrasound scan may reveal bowel wall thickening in invasive ileocolitis and enlarged lymph nodes in yersiniosis and abdominal tuberculosis. The examination may also be invaluable in detecting complications of intestinal infections such as amebic liver abscess, and in confirming the presence of hepatosplenomegaly and portal hypertension in schistosomiasis.

Histology

The histologic appearances of colonic mucosa in the later stages of infection with invasive enteropathogens such as *Salmonella* spp., *Shigella* spp. and *Campylobacter jejuni* are often indistinguishable from those of non-specific IBD. However, if biopsies are taken within the first 24–72 h, features which might suggest infectious colitis include mucosal edema, straightening of the glands, an acute inflammatory infiltrate including polymorphonuculear leukocytes which can sometimes be seen penetrating the epithelium [41, 42]. In *C. difficile* infection an acute inflammatory infiltrate is also apparent, combined with the typical 'erupting volcano' lesion which is the histologic counterpart of pseudomembrane. Colonic and ileal biopsies in tuberculosis may reveal caseating granulomata and occasionally acid-fast bacilli can be detected by light microscopy although, when tuberculosis is suspected, biopsies should always be sent for microbiologic culture. Other organisms which can be identified in mucosal biopsy include the trophozoites of *E. histolytica* and the 'owl's eye' inclusion bodies indicative of CMV infection. Ova of *Schistosoma* spp. can also be detected in mucosal biopsies, and it may be possible to differentiate one species from another on the basis of egg morphology.

Treatment

The treatment of infectious colitis may be considered at two levels, namely: (a) general supportive and symptomatic therapy and (b) specific antimicrobial chemotherapy aimed to alter the natural history of infection and reduce duration and severity of the illness.

General supportive therapy

Although infectious colitis is usually not associated with major fluid and electrolyte losses, many infections such as *Salmonella* spp. and *Shigella* spp. begin with acute watery diarrhea which can lead to deficits in fluid and electrolyte balance. These should be replaced by oral rehydration therapy with a glucose–electrolyte solution. This is particularly important in infants and young children, and in the elderly, who have a low tolerance for dealing with these losses, although otherwise healthy adults can usually replace fluid and electrolytes informally by increasing oral fluid intake by taking salty soups (sodium), fruit juices (potassium) and a source of complex carbohydrate such as rice, bread or pasta [43, 44].

Although antidiarrheal agents such as loperamide and diphenoxylate/atropine combination are frequently used to reduce bowel frequency in acute watery diarrhea [45–48], their use in dysentery is generally not encouraged. These drugs act predominantly by decreasing intestinal motility, and there is concern that in dysentery these agents may prolong colonization with the enteropathogen and possibly also increase the risk of colonic dilation. However, the evidence that these adverse effects are directly related to the use of these agents is poorly established, and a more recent study suggests that loperamide is safe in bacillary dysentery.

Table 5. Efficacy of antimicrobial chemotherapy in bacterial and protozoal colitis

	Bacterial colitis	Protozoal colitis
Proven efficacy	Dysenteric shigellosis; severe salmonellosis (dysentery, fever); C. difficile diarrhea; *Yersinia* septicemia; *Campylobacter* dysentery/sepsis	*Entamoeba histolytica, Balantidium coli*
Possible efficacy	EIEH; *Campylobacter* enteritis	
Doubtful efficacy	*Salmonella* enterocolitis; *Yersinia* enteritis (uncomplicated); EHEC	
Hazardous	? EHEC	

EPEC, enteropathogenic *E. coli;* EIEC, enteroinvasive *E. coli;* EHEC, enterohaemorrhagic *E. coli.*

Antimicrobial chemotherapy

The micro-organisms responsible for infectious colitis can be categorized as to whether antibiotics have been shown to be *definitely effective* in treating the infection, conditions in which these agents are *possibly effective* and finally conditions in which antimicrobial agents are *probably not effective* or possibly even *hazardous* (Table 5). However, there is evidence which clearly shows that antibiotics can reduce the severity and duration of some forms of infectious colitis, particularly in severe invasive bacterial infections and in colitis due to colonic protozoa and CMV.

Antibiotics are indicated for the treatment of dysenteric shigellosis [49–54], *C. difficile* associated diarrhea [55–58], amebiasis [59] and balantidiasis [60] (Table 6). Antibiotics are also of value in *Yersinia* septicemia and when there are associated bone and joint infections [61, 62] but their value in milder forms of *Yersinia* enteritis has not been established, probably because the antibiotic has been administered late in the natural history of infection [63]. The role of antibiotic therapy in *Campylobacter* infection remains controversial [64, 65]. There is good evidence that the natural history of the illness is not altered if treatment is begun more than 4 days after the onset of symptoms. One randomized controlled trial has shown that treatment with erythromycin early in the infection significantly reduces the duration of the illness in children [66], although a second study has failed to confirm these findings [67].

A role for antibiotics in the treatment of enteroinvasive *E. coli* infection has not been established, although in severe cases with evidence of systemic involvement it would be reasonable to treat along the same lines as those recommended for dysenteric shigellosis. There is a major controversy as to whether antibiotics should be used in EHEC infection, although the balance of evidence at present is that antibiotics, particularly when given after infection is well established, do not significantly improve the outcome [68]. In addition, there is increasing evidence that administration of antibiotics at this stage can promote the development of the hemolytic–uremic syndrome [69, 70]. This is presumed to relate to the massive lysis of organisms and release of shiga toxin and endotoxin. Current evidence therefore suggests that antimicrobial chemotherapy should not be used in children with proven EHEC infection. Antiviral agents such as ganciclovir and foscarnet are effective in CMV colitis but prolonged courses may be required in the immunocompromised [71–73].

Intestinal tuberculosis should be treated according to the current recommendations of the British Thoracic Society using isoniazid (330 mg) and rifampicin (450–600 mg) should be given for 6 months, with pyrazinamide (20–30 mg/kg daily, maximum 3 g daily) included for the first 2 months [74]. A fourth drug such as ethambutol or streptomycin should be added initially if drug resistance is suspected, particularly in patients who may have imported the disease from a developing country.

Antimicrobial chemotherapy is also indicated for protozoal [59, 60] and helminth infections in the colon (Table 6). Infectious proctitis of bacterial, viral [71, 73, 75, 76] and helminth origin is also responsive to antibiotic therapy (Table 7).

Non-specific colitis and intestinal infection

There is continuing controversy as to whether intestinal infection can act as a trigger for relapse in patients with ulcerative colitis and Crohn's colitis. There are a number of case reports in the literature demonstrating close temporal relationships between

Table 6. Antimicrobial chemotherapy for infectious colitis

	Drug of choice	Alternative(s)
Viruses		
Cytomegalovirus	Ganciclovir 5 mg/kg per 12 h, 14–21 days [71, 72]	Foscarnet 60 mg/kg per 8 h [73], 14–21 days; maintenance therapy may be required
Bacteria		
Shigella spp.*	TMP-SMX two tabs twice daily, 5 days [49] [3]Ciprofloxacin 500 mg twice daily, 5 days [50]	Short-term quinolone [52–54] [1]Cefixime 400 mg daily, 5–7 days; nalidixic acid 1g four times daily, 5–7 days
Salmonella spp.**	[2,3]Ciprofloxacin 500 mg twice daily, 10–14 days	TMP-SMX, ampicillin, amoxycillin
C. jejuni***	Erythromycin 250–500 mg four times daily, 7 days [64–67]	[3,4]Ciprofloxacin 500 mg twice daily, 5–7 days Azithromycin 500 mg daily, 3 days
Y. enterocolitica	[3]Ciprofloxacin 500 mg twice daily, 7–10 days [61, 62]	Tetracycline 250 mg four times daily, 7–10 days [61, 62]
C. difficile	Metronidazole 400 mg three times daily, 7–10 days [55]	Vancomycin 125 mg four times daily, 7–10 days [55–57]; fusidic acid, teicoplanin [58]
EIEC	? as Shigella spp	
EHEC	None	
Aeromonas hydrophila	Ciprofloxacin 500 mg twice daily, 7–10 days	TMP-SMX two tabs twice daily, 7–10 days
Plesiomonas shigelloides	Ciprofloxacin 500 mg twice daily, 7–10 days	TMP-SMX two tabs twice daily, 7–10 days
Protozoa		
E. histolytica	Metronidazole 750 mg three times daily, 5 days [59] Diloxanide furoate 500 mg three times daily, 10 days [59]	Paromomycin 25–35 mg/kg three times daily, 7–10 days [59]
Balantidium coli	Metronidazole 400 mg three times daily 10 days [59, 60]	Tetracycline 500 mg four times, daily 10 days [59, 60]
Helminths		
Schistosoma spp.	Praziquantel 40[5]–60[6] mg/kg per day	
Trichuris trichiura	Albendazole 400 mg single dose	Mebendazole 100 mg twice daily, 3 days

[1] And other third-generation cephalosporins.

[2] Usually only for bacteremia.

[3] And other fluoroquinolones such as ofloxacin, norfloxacin, fleroxacin and cinoxacin.

[4] Increasing resistance to quinolones being recognized.

[5] Schistosoma mansoni, Schistosoma haematobium.

[6] Schistosoma japonicum

EIEC; enteroinvasive E. coli, EHEC; enterohemorrhagic E. coli TMP-SMX; trimethoprim-sulphamethoxazole.

*Multiple resistance to tetracycline, TMP-SMX, ampicillin and chloramphenicol in South America, Greece, Spain and Thailand.
**Chronic carrier state, norfloxacin 400 mg twice daily, 28 days.
***May only shorten duration of illness when given early.

Table 7. Treatment of infectious proctitis

Drug of Choice	Alternative(s)	
Bacteria		
Chlamydia trachomatis		
Non-LGV	Doxycycline 100 mg twice daily for 7 days	Erythromycin 500 mg four times daily
LGV	Doxycycline 100 mg twice daily for 3 weeks or more	TMP-SMX two tabs twice daily
Neisseria gonorrhoeae	*Ceftriaxone 250 mg i.m.	Oral cefixime, ciprofloxacin or ofloxacin
Treponema pallidum	Benzathine penicillin G 2.4 million units, single oral dose	Procaine penicillin 600 000–900 000 units i.m. for 10 days; doxycycline 100 mg twice daily orally for 15 days
Mycobacterium tuberculosis	See text	
Viruses		
Herpes simplex virus	Acyclovir 5 mg/kg i.v. 8-hourly for 7–10 days [75]	Forscarnet 40–60 mg/kg i.v. 8-hourly for 2–3 weeks [76]
Cytomegalovirus	See Table 6	
Helminths		
Schistosoma spp.	See Table 6	

*Plus doxycyline 100 mg twice daily, orally for 7 days.

the onset of an attack of colitis and the detection of the presence of an enteropathogen in the stool. Several pathogens have attracted particular attention, including *Clostridium difficile* [77, 78] *Campylobacter* spp. [79, 80] *Aeromonas* spp. [81, 82] and CMV infection. There is no question that these and other infections can occur in association with established non-specific IBD and may be isolated during an apparent relapse, but it is not clear as to whether they are of etiologic importance in precipitating IBD in a previously healthy individual.

There are limited prospective studies of sufficient power to answer this question. One study examined 64 patients during their first attack of ulcerative colitis and 30 others during a relapse of known disease, and found no evidence that bacterial enteropathogens were important triggers in either group [83]. Another study searched for enteropathogens in 64 patients with a relapse of known IBD [80]. *C. difficile* was isolated in six patients, *Campylobacter jejuni* in one patient and *Salmonella typhimurium* in one patient. It was considered that these infrequent isolations indicated that intestinal infection played only a minor role in exacerbations of IBD. However, these studies confirm that the two conditions can coexist, and that an etiologic agent should be excluded in patients presenting for the first time with possible IBD. Many clinicians would routinely test for infection in patients with known IBD on the basis that intestinal infections are common even in industrialized countries, and that it is virtually impossible to distinguish clinically between a simple relapse of IBD and a relapse associated with a co-infection.

Intestinal infection associated with a relapse of IBD should be treated in the same way as recommended for infection in an otherwise healthy individual. In such patients with a relapse of non-specific colitis it is usually wise to treat both the infection and the IBD particularly when the patient is moderately or severely affected. In mild disease it may be possible to treat only the infection while closely monitoring the activity of the colitis.

References

1. Handszuh H, Waters SR. Travel and tourism patterns. In: DuPont HL, Steffen R, eds. Textbook of Travel Medicine and Health. Hamilton: Decker, 1997.
2. Farthing MJG, DuPont HL, Guandalini S *et al.* Treatment and prevention of travellers' diarrhoea. Gastroenterol Int 1992; 5: 162–75.
3. DuPont HL, Ericsson CD. Prevention and treatment of traveler's diarrhea. N Engl J Med 1993; 328: 1821–7.
4. Wheeler JG, Sethi D, Cowden JM *et al.* Study of infectious intestinal disease in England: rates in the community, presenting to general practice, and reported to national surveillance. Br Med J 1999; 318: 1046–50.

5. Balarajan R, Raleigh VS, Yuen P *et al.* Health risks associated with bathing in seawater. Br Med J 1991; 303: 1445–5.

6. Walker A. Swimming – the hazards of taking a dip. Br Med J 1992; 304: 242–5.

7. Keene WE, McAnulty JM, Hoesly FC *et al.* A swimming-associated outbreak of hemorrhagic colitis caused by *Escherichia coli* O157: H7 and *Shigella sonnei.* N Engl J Med 1994; 331: 579–84.

8. Boyce TG, Swerdlow DL, Griffin PM. *Escherichia coli* O157: H7 and the hemolytic–uremic syndrome. N Engl J Med 1995; 333: 364–8.

9. Neal KR, Brij SO, Slack RCB *et al.* Recent treatment with H2 antagonists and antibiotics for gastric surgery as risk factors for *Salmonella* infection. Br Med J 1994; 308: 176.

10. Neal KR, Scott HM, Slack RCB. Omeprazole as a risk factor for *Campylobacter* gastroenteritis: case control study. Br Med J 1996; 312: 414–15.

11. Kozicki M, Steffen R, Schar M. 'Boil it, cook it, peel it, or forget it': does this rule prevent travellers' diarrhoea? Int J Epidemiol 1985; 14: 169–72.

12. Bandres JC, Mathewson JJ, DuPont HL. Heat susceptibility of bacterial enteropathogens. Arch Intern Med 1988; 148: 2261–3.

13. Sheath NK, Wisniewski TR, Franson TR. Survival of enteric pathogens in common beverages. An *in vitro* study. Am J Gastroenterol 1988; 83: 658–60.

14. Farthing MJG. Mycobacterial disease of the gut. In: Phillips RKS, Northover JMA, eds. Modern Coloproctology. London: Edward Arnold, 1992: 174–89.

15. Strauss EJ, Falkow S. Microbial pathogenesis: genomics and beyond. Science 1997; 276: 707–12.

16. Finley BB, Falkow S. Common themes in microbial pathogenicity revisited. Microbiol Med Biol Rev 1997; 61: 136–69

17. Mann BJ, Vedvick T, Torian B, Petri WA. Cloning of the 170 kDa subunit of the galactose-specific adherence lectin of *Entamoeba histolytica.* Proc Natl Acad Sci USA 1991; 88: 3248–52.

18. Leippe M, Ebel S, Schoenberger OL, Horstmann RD, Muller-Eberhard HJ. Pore-forming peptide of pathogenic *Entamoeba histolytica.* Proc Natl Acad Sci USA 1991; 88: 7659–63.

19. Kenny B, DeVinney R, Stein M *et al.* Enteropathogenic *E. coli* (EPEC) transfers its receptor for intimate adherence into mammalian cells. Cell 1997; 91; 511–20.

20. Knutton S, Rosenshine I, Pallen MJ *et al.* A novel EspA-associated surface organelle of enteropathogenic *Escherichia coli* involved in protein translocation into epithelial cells. EMBO J 1998; 17: 2166–76.

21. Triadafilopoulos G, Pothoulakis C, O'Brien M, LaMont JT. Differential effects of *Clostridium difficile* toxins A and B on rabbit ileum. Gastroenterology 1987; 93: 273–9.

22. Triadafilopoulos G, Pothoulakis C, Weiss R, Giampaolo C, LaMont JT. Comparative study of *Clostridium difficile* A and cholera toxin in rabbit ileum. Gastroenterology 1989; 97: 1186–92.

23. Krivan HC, Clark GF, Smith DF, Wilkins TD. Cell surface binding site for *Clostridium difficile* enterotoxin: evidence for a glycoconjugate containing the sequence 1-3-Galβ1-4GlcNAc. Infect Immun 1986; 53: 573–81.

24. Just I, Fritz G, Akatories K *et al. Clostridium difficile* toxin B acts on the GTP-binding protein Rho. J Biol Chem 1994; 269: 10706–12.

25. Just I, Selzer J, von Eichel-Streiber C, Aktories K. The low molecular mass GTP-binding protein Rho is affected by toxin A from *Clostridium difficile.* J Clin Invest 1995; 95: 1026–31.

26. Just I, Selzer J, Wilm M, von Eichel-Streiber C, Mann M, Aktories K. Glucosylation of Rho proteins by *Clostridium difficile* toxin B. Nature 1995; 375: 500–3.

27. Just I, Wilm M, Selzer J *et al.* The enterotoxin from *Clostridium difficile* (ToxA) monoglucosylates the Rho proteins. J Biol Chem 1995; 270: 13932–6.

28. Francis CL, Ryan TA, Jones BD, Smith SJ, Falkow S. Ruffles induced by *Salmonella* and other stimuli direct macropinocytosis of bacteria. Nature 1993; 364: 639–42.

29. Ruschkowski S, Rosenshine I, Finlay BB. *Salmonella typhimurium* induces an inositol phosphate flux in infected epithelial cells. FEMS Microbiol Lett 1992; 74: 121–6.

30. Chen LM, Hobbie S, Galan JE. Requirement of CDC42 for *Salmonella*-induced cytoskeletal and nuclear responses. Science 1996; 274: 2115–18.

31. Galan JE. Molecular genetics bases of *Salmonella* entry into host cells. Mol Microbiol 1996; 20: 263–71.

32. Adam T, Giry M, Bowuet P, Sansonetti P. Rho-dependent membrane folding causes *Shigella* entry into epithelial cells. EMBO J 1996; 15 3315–21.

33. Menard R, Prevost MC, Gounon P, Sansonetti P, Dehio C. The secreted Ipa complex of *Shigella flexneri* promotes entry into mammalian cells. Proc Natl Acad Sci USA 1996; 93: 1254–8.

34. Cossart P. Subversion of the mammalian cell cytoskeleton by invasive bacteria. J Clin Invest 1997; 99: 2307–11.

35. Finlay BB, Cossart P. Exploitation of mammalian cell function by bacterial pathogens. Science 1997; 276: 718–25.

36. Eckmann L, Kagnoff MF, Fierer J. Epithelial cells secrete the chemokine interleukin-8 in response to bacterial entry. Infect Immun 1993; 61: 4569–74.

37. Yang S-K, Eckmann L, Panja A, Kagnoff MF. Differential and regulated expression of C-X-C, C-C and C chemokines by human colon epithelial cells. Gastroenterology 1997; 113: 1214–23.

38. Elliott EJ, Zhi Li, Bell C, Stiel D *et al.* A monoclonal antibody against the CD18 adhesion molecule inhibits colonic structural and ion transport abnormalities caused by enterohemorrhagic *E. coli* O157: H7 in rabbits. Gastroenterology 1994; 106: 1554–61.

39. Harries AD, Myers B, Cook GC. Inflammatory bowel disease: a common cause of bloody diarrhoea in visitors to the tropics. Br Med J 1985; 291: 1686–7.

40. Rees JH, Soudain SE, Gregson NA *et al. Campylobacter jejuni* infection and Guillain-Barré syndrome. N Engl J Med 1995; 333: 1374–9.

41. Allison MC, Hamilton-Dutoit SJ, Dhillon AP, Pounder RE. The value of rectal biopsy in distinguishing self-limited colitis from early inflammatory bowel disease. Q J Med 1987; 65: 985–95.

42. Nostrant TT, Kumar NB, Appelman HD. Histopathology differentiates acute self-limited colitis from ulcerative colitis. Gastroenterology 1987; 92: 318–28.

43. Farthing MJG. History and rationale of oral rehydration and recent development in formulating an optimal solution. Drugs 1988; 36(Suppl. 4): 80–90.

44. Farthing MJG. Dehydration and rehydration in children. In: Arnaud MJ, ed. Hydration Throughout Life. Paris: John Libbey Eurotext 1998: 159–73.

45. Kaplan MA, Prior MJ, McKonly KI, DuPont HL, Temple AR, Nelson EB. A multicentre randomized controlled trial of a liquid loperamide product versus placebo in the treatment of acute diarrhea in children. Clin Pediatr 1999; 38: 579–91.

46. Owens JR, Broadhead R, Hendrickse RG, Jaswal OP, Gangal RN. Loperamide in the treatment of acute gastroenteritis in early childhood. Report of a two centre, double-blind, controlled clinical trial. Ann Trop Paediatr 1981; 1: 135–41.

47. Bergstrom T, Alestig K, Thoren K, Trollfors B. Symptomatic treatment of acute infectious diarrhoea: loperamide versus placebo in a double-blind trial. J Infect 1986; 12: 35–8.

48. Bowie MD, Hill ID, Mann MD. Loperamide for treatment of acute diarrhoea in infants and young children. A double-blind placebo-controlled trial. S Afr Med J 1995; 85: 885–7.

49. Tauxe RV, Puhr ND, Wells JG, Hargrett-Bean N, Blake PA. Antimicrobial resistance of *Shigella* isolates in the USA: the importance of international travelers. J Infect Dis 1990; 162: 1107–11.

50. Bennish ML, Salam MA, Haider R, Barza M. Therapy for shigellosis. II. Randomized, double-blind comparison of ciprofloxacin and ampicillin. J Infect Dis 1990; 162: 711–16.

51. Khan WA, Seas C, Dhar U, Salam MA, Bennish ML. Treatment of shigellosis: V. comparison of azithromycin and ciprofloxacin. A double-blind, randomized, controlled trial. Ann Intern Med 1997; 126: 697–703.

52. Bassily S, Hyams KG, el-Masry NA *et al.* Short-course norfloxacin and trimethoprim-sulfamethoxazole treatment of shigellosis and salmonellosis in Egypt. Am J Trop Med Hyg 1994; 51: 219–23.

53. Gotuzzo E, Oberhelman RA, Maguina C *et al.* Comparison of single-dose treatment with norfloxacin and standard 5-day treatment with trimethoprim-sulfamethoxazole for acute shigellosis in adults. Antimicrob Agents Chemother 1989; 33: 1101–4.

54. Bennish ML, Salam MA, Khan WA, Khan AM. Treatment of shigellosis. III. Comparison of one or two-dose ciprofloxacin with standard 5 day therapy. A randomized, blinded trial. Ann Intern Med 1992; 117: 727–34.

55. Teasley DG, Gerding DN, Olson MM *et al.* Prospective randomised trial of metronidazole versus vancomycin for *Clostridium difficile*-associated diarrhoea and colitis. Lancet 1983; 2: 1043–6.

56. Wilcox MH, Howe R. Diarrhoea caused by *Clostridium difficile*: response time for treatment with metronidazole and vancomycin. J Antimicrob Chemother 1995; 35: 673–9.

57. Young GP, Ward PB, Bayley N *et al.* Antibiotic-associated colitis due to *Clostridium difficile*: double blind comparison of vancomycin with bacitracin. Gastroenterology 1985; 89: 1038–45.

58. Wenisch C, Parschalk B, Hasenhundl M, Hirschl AM, Graninger W. Comparison of vancomycin, teicoplanin, metronidazole and fusidic acid for the treatment of *Clostridium difficile*-associated diarrhea. Clin Infect Dis 1996; 22: 813–18.

59. Kelly MP, Farthing MJG. Infections of the gastrointestinal tract. In: O'Grady F, Lambert HP, Finch RG, Greenwood D, eds. Antibiotic and Chemotherapy, 7th edn. London: Churchill Livingstone, 1997: 708–20.

60. Garcia-Laverde A, de Bonilla L. Clinical trials with metronidazole in human balantidiasis. Am J Trop Med Hyg 1975; 24: 781–3.

61. Gayraud M, Scavizzi MR, Mollaret HJH, Guillevin L, Hornstein MJ. Antibiotic treatment of *Yersinia enterocolitica* septicemia: a retrospective review of 43 cases. Clin Infect Dis 1993; 17: 405–10.

62. Crowe M, Ashford K, Ispahani P. Clinical features and antibiotic treatment of septic arthritis and osteomyelitis due to *Yersinia enterocolitica*. J Med Microbiol 1996; 45: 302–9.

63. Pai CH, Gillis F, Tuomanen E, Marks MI. Placebo-controlled double-blind evaluation of trimethoprim-sulfamethoxazole treatment for *Yersinia enterocolitica* gastroenteritis. J Pediatr 1984; 104: 308–11.

64. Anders BJ, Lauer BA, Paisley JW, Reller LB. Double-blind placebo controlled trial of erythromycin for treatment of *Campylobacter* enteritis. Lancet 1982; 1: 131–2.

65. Mandal BK, Ellis ME, Dunbar EM, Whale K. Double-blind placebo-controlled trial of erythromycin in the treatment of clinical *Campylobacter* infection. J Antimicrob Chemother 1984; 13: 619–23.

66. Salazar-Lindo E, Sack RB, Chea-Woo E *et al.* Early treatment with erythromycin of *Campylobacter jejuni*-associated dysentery in children. J Pediatr 1986; 109: 355–60.

67. Williams MD, Schorling JB, Barrett LJ *et al.* Early treatment of *Campylobacter jejuni* enteritis. Antimicrob Agents Chemother 1989; 33: 248–50.

68. Proulx F, Turgeon JPJ, Delage G, Lafleur L, Chicoine L. Randomized, controlled trial of antibiotic therapy for *Escherichia coli* O157: H7 enteritis. J Pediatr 1992; 121: 299–303.

69. Carter AO, Borczyk AA, Carlson JA *et al.* A severe outbreak of *Escherichia coli* O157-H7-associated hemorrhagic colitis in a nursing home. N Engl J Med 1987; 317: 1496–500.

70. Wong CS, Jelacic S, Habeeb RL, Watkins SL, Tarr PI. The risk of the hemolytic–uremeic syndrome after antibiotic treatment of *Escherichia coli* O157: H7 infections. N Engl J Med 2000; 342: 1930–6.

71. Dieterich DT, Kotler DP, Busch DF *et al.* Ganciclovir treatment of cytomegalovirus colitis in AIDS: a randomized, double-blind, placebo-controlled multicenter study. J Infect Dis 1993; 167: 278–82.

72. Nelson MR, Connolly GM, Hawkins DA, Gazzard BG. Foscarnet in the treatment of cytomegalovirus infection of the esophagus and colon in patients with the acquired immune deficiency syndrome. Am J Gastroenterol 1991; 86: 876–81.

73. Salzberger B, Stoehr A, Jablonowski H *et al.* Foscarnet 5 versus 7 days a week treatment for severe gastrointestinal CMV disease in HIV-infected patients. Infection 1996; 24: 121–4.

74. Joint Tuberculosis Committee of the British Thoracic Society. Chemotherapy and management of tuberculosis in the United Kingdom: recommendations 1998. Thorax 1998; 54: 536–48.

75. Genereau T, Lortholary O, Bouchaud O *et al.* Herpes simplex eosophagitis in patients with AIDS: report of 34 cases. Clin Infect Dis 1996; 22: 926–31.

76. Safrin S, Crumpacker C, Chatis P *et al.* controlled trial comparing foscarnet with vidarabine for acyclovir-resistant mucocutaneous herpes simplex in the acquired immunodeficiency syndrome. N Engl J Med 1991; 325: 551–5.

77. Lee DK, Cooper BT, Barbezat GO. *Clostridium difficile* toxin in chronic idiopathic colitis. NZ Med J 1986; 99: 620–2.

78. Kochar R, Ayyagari A, Goenka MK, Dhali GK, Aggarwal R, Mehta SK. Role of infectious agents in exacerbations of ulcerative colitis in India. A study of *Clostridium difficile*. J Clin Gastroenterol 1993; 16: 26–30.

79. Farmer RG. Infectious causes of diarrhea in the differential diagnosis of inflammatory bowel disease. Med Clin N Am 1990; 74: 29–38.

80. Weber P, Koch M, Heizmann WR, Scheurlen M, Jenss H, Hartmann F. Microbic superinfection in relapse of inflammatory bowel disease. J Clin Gastroenterol 1992; 14: 302–8.

81. Doman DB, Golding MI, Goldberg HJ, Doyle RB. *Aeromonas hydrophila* colitis presenting as medically refractory inflammatory bowel disease. Am J Gastroenterol 1989; 84: 83–5.

82. Willoughby JM, Rahman AF, Gregory MM. Chronic colitis after *Aeromonas* infection. Gut 1989; 30: 686–90.

83. Brown WJ, Hudson MJ, Patrick S *et al.* Search for microbial pathogens in patients with ulcerative colitis. Digestion 1992; 53: 121–8.

48 | Human immunodeficiency virus and inflammatory bowel disease

CHARLES MEL WILCOX

Introduction

We have now completed the second decade of the acquired immunodeficiency syndrome (AIDS) that first came to attention in 1981 [1]. The early years of the epidemic were devoted to describing the vast spectrum of, and defining optimum treatments for, the complications of AIDS. Over the past 10 years, there has been intense investigation into the virology of the human immunodeficiency virus (HIV) and, consequently, rapid progress in our understanding of the pathogenesis of this devastating worldwide infectious disease. These efforts have culminated in the development of highly active antiretroviral therapies, termed HAART, which have profoundly changed the paradigms for management of HIV-related complications including those involving the gastrointestinal tract [2, 3]. Because of the widespread availability of these drugs and access to care [4] the fall in AIDS-related morbidity and mortality has been most pronounced in the developed world, whereas in contrast, and for the foreseeable future, complications related to HIV-associated immunodeficiency will continue unabated in developing countries [1, 5].

Before the development of HAART, gastrointestinal disorders occurred almost uniformly in patients with AIDS. Problems referable to the colon, usually diarrhea, were observed in 50% or more of patients at some point during the course of HIV and AIDS [5]. Although opportunistic infections and neoplasms comprise the majority of the colonic disorders in these patients, a number of cases of inflammatory bowel disease (IBD), both Crohn's disease (CD) and ulcerative colitis (UC), have been described [6–22]. In addition, an idiopathic inflammatory disease of the colon, apparently distinct from IBD, has also been recognized [23, 24]. Given the potential for confusion clinically, endoscopically, and pathologically between opportunistic infections of the colon and IBD, an appreciation of the clinical presentation, differential diagnosis, and management of IBD in HIV-infected patients is important. In this chapter the relationship of HIV infection and IBD will be explored, focusing on the pathogenesis of IBD and what lessons we can learn from coexistent HIV infection; the chapter will review the clinical presentation and relationship to immunodeficiency of the reported patients with HIV infection; outline the differential diagnosis of IBD in the setting of HIV; and review management. Finally, criteria will be proposed for the diagnosis of idiopathic IBD in the setting of HIV infection.

Pathogenesis of IBD in relation to HIV Infection

Since the key element in the pathogenesis of IBD is the inflammatory cascade which includes T cells, and HIV disease is characterized by the destruction of CD4 T lymphocytes leading to immunodeficiency, it follows that the prevalence and natural history of IBD may be altered in patients with HIV infection. Thus, the reported cases of coexistent HIV and IBD may provide insight into the pathogenesis of IBD.

It is well recognized that T cells play an important role in the expansion and perpetuation of the inflammatory response in IBD [25]. When presented with specific antigens the T cell population expands, and these cells then interact with B cells, resulting in an expansion of antigen-specific B cells. Activated T cells recruit and activate macrophages and neutrophils, which in turn produce cytokines amplifying and further perpetuating the inflammatory response. CD4 T cells, the pivotal cell destroyed in HIV infection, play an important role in the pathogenesis of IBD. This has been directly demonstrated in multiple experimental models of IBD. Such studies have demonstrated that certain CD4 T cell subsets

Stephan R. Targan, Fergus Shanahan and Loren C. Karp (eds.), *Inflammatory Bowel Disease: From Bench to Bedside, 2nd Edition*, 863–873.
© 2003 *Kluwer Academic Publishers. Printed in Great Britain*

exist that can cause colitis, and other subsets exist that prevent it. Two of the major CD4 T cell subsets are T-helper 1 and T-helper 2. The Th1 subset produces IL-2 and interferon gamma (IFN-γ)and mediates cell-mediated immunity. The Th2 subset produces IL-4, IL-5, IL-6, and IL-10, and mediates antibody production. Based on the profile of measured cytokine production, CD appears to be most associated with Th1 lymphocytes while UC may be more associated with Th2 lymphocytes, although this is much less clear.

Regulatory CD4 T cell subsets also exist. A CD4$^+$ T cell subset denoted Th3 produces large amounts of active transforming growth factor β1 (TGF-β$_1$), a cytokine with broad inhibitory effects on lymphocytes. The T-regulatory 1 (Tr1) CD4$^+$ T cell produces large amounts of IL-10, another inhibitory cytokine, along with some TGF-β$_1$. It is likely that more regulatory CD4$^+$ T cell subsets will be identified in the future.

Several studies have examined T cell subsets in bowel tissue from HIV-infected patients. Generally, T lymphocyte subsets in the gut reflect the concentration in the systemic circulation. HIV-infected patients with advanced immunodeficiency have markedly reduced numbers of CD4 cells both in the circulation and small bowel, with a corresponding increase in CD8 cells [26, 27]. Likewise, quantitation of CD4 and CD8 cells in colonic biopsy samples from AIDS patients shows a similar pattern. Thus, the systemic CD4/CD4 T cell ratio and the absolute values of each subset reflect what can be found in the gut.

There is little information regarding cytokine production in bowel tissue from HIV-infected patients, especially those with more severe degrees of immunodeficiency. Snijders *et al*. [28] biopsied the jejunum of HIV-infected patients with diarrhea, some of whom had small intestinal pathogens, HIV-infected patients without diarrhea, and HIV-seronegative controls. No significant differences were detected in cytokine levels among the groups with low levels uniformly detected. In contrast, McGowan *et al*. [29] found a significant increase in inflammatory cytokines, IL-1β and IFN-γ in HIV-infected patients compared to controls, but lower levels of IL-10 in colonic biopsies. Proinflammatory cytokines have also been detected in rectal mucosa of AIDS patients with peak expression of TNF-α and IL-1β in late-stage patients compared to patients with earlier-stage disease [30]. In contrast, one study [31] suggested defective function of colonic mono-nuclear cells in AIDS patients as reflected by a reduction in TNF-α secretion. The relationship of cytokine production to HIV-infected mucosal inflammatory cells is unclear. Overall, the number of HIV-infected cells identified in the lamina propria has been consistently low [32, 33].

If CD4 cells are important in the pathogenesis of IBD, then animal models of IBD with perturbations of CD4 T cell subsets would provide an ideal assessment of their role. Loss of CD4 T cells does improve disease activity in animal models. However, selective knockout of subpopulation has yet to be performed.

It follows from the above that the relationship between HIV infection and IBD is likely to be complex. Assuming that the CD4 T cell depletion occurs in all CD4 T cell subsets, including those that both mediate and prevent IBD, the net effect on the course of IBD will depend on which subset is more affected. For example, if the Th1 subset were to be disproportionaltely depleted in a patient with CD, the activity of the IBD might improve. Conversely, if the regulatory CD4 T cell subset were to be disproportionately depleted, IBD activity might worsen. Indeed, both improvement and worsening of IBD activity has been reported in patients with IBD who also develop HIV.

Review of reported cases of IBD and HIV infection

Although there have been a number of reported cases of coexistent HIV infection and IBD, given the millions of patients with HIV infection worldwide, coupled with the predominance of IBD in young patients – those most afflicted by HIV – one might anticipate many more reported cases. Two studies have provided estimates of the prevalence of coexistent HIV and IBD [10, 11]. In a retrospective study [10], hospital discharge records for a 4-year period were reviewed, and only three patients with IBD of 1839 patients with a discharge diagnosis of HIV/AIDS were identified. Four additional patients were identified by phone survey of clinicians in related outpatient clinics. Since both IBD and HIV infections are primarily treated in the outpatient setting, these results are likely to be an underestimate. In the study of Sharpstone *et al*. [11], HIV clinic records were cross-referenced with pharmacy records for 5-ASA compounds and rectal steroid preparations. Eight patients were identified, yielding a mean incidence of 41/100 000 and a prevalence of

364/100 000. These numbers are high compared to recent US studies [34] and may reflect the small sample size.

A number of important considerations must be kept in mind when reviewing the case series of IBD in HIV-infected patients. First, the time-course of IBD and HIV infection should be well documented. The majority of the reported cases consist of patients with IBD who later became HIV-infected, or both disorders were diagnosed together. Importantly, the acquisition of HIV infection can rarely be precisely timed; thus, a long lag time between infection and the diagnosis of IBD is likely in most patients, which means there could be considerable overlap in the duration of the two diseases. Second, the stage of HIV-related immunodeficiency in relationship to the timing of the diagnosis of IBD must be characterized. Most reported cases of *de-novo* IBD have been in HIV-infected patients with only modest immune dysfunction. The marker for staging immune dysfunction most frequently used, and for which there is compelling evidence, is the CD4 lymphocyte count [35, 36]. It is well established that significant immune dysfunction, as reflected clinically by the occurrence of opportunistic disorders, does not occur until the CD4 count falls below 200/μl, and most opportunistic infections involving the gastrointestinal tract do not manifest until the CD4 count falls below 100/μl [3, 5, 35]. Thus, reports of HIV-infected patients with CD4 counts less than 100/μl with active IBD may provide better insight into any relationship between HIV-associated immunodeficiency and IBD. Third, it is important to reflect on any differences as compared to non-HIV-infected patients in the manifestations and outcome of IBD, such as location and extent of disease, presence of extraintestinal complications, and response to therapy, both medical and surgical. Fourth, it is critical that a thorough histopathologic examination of colonic and/or small bowel biopsies be performed to exclude opportunistic disorders which may masquerade as IBD. Since a number of opportunistic infections, most notably cytomegalovirus (CMV), may mimic IBD, the diagnosis of IBD may be difficult to establish conclusively. Also, the characteristic histologic findings of IBD should be specifically documented, including crypt distortion, chronic inflammation, etc. This potential confusion is further perpetuated by the absence of specific criteria for the diagnosis of IBD in the setting of AIDS.

Crohn's disease

To date there have been eight reports of CD [6–14] totalling 12 HIV-infected patients (Table 1). Consistent with the epidemiology of AIDS, the majority of the patients were male homosexuals ranging in age from 14 to 48 years. Five of the 12 patients presented with CD after well-established HIV infection. Of the other seven patients with CD, the timing of HIV infection could be accurately determined in only two [13] (contaminated blood products) and, as noted above, it is likely that in many cases there was overlap of the two diseases. The descriptions of the radiographic and endoscopic findings were typical for CD. The diagnosis of CD was made by the findings on pathologic specimens, usually post-surgical, and non-caseating granulomas were reported as present in less than half the cases either on endoscopic biopsy or in the surgical specimen. Histologic examination was generally extensive to exclude other diseases. However, long-term follow-up of the HIV-infected patients who subsequently

Table 1. Reported cases of Crohn's disease in HIV-infected patients

Reference	Year	No. of patients	Sequence	CD4 count	Location
6	1984	1	AIDS →Crohn's	230*	Colon, terminal ileum
7	1988	1	Crohn's →HIV	410	Colon
8	1994	1	HIV →Crohn's	480	Colon, terminal ileum
9	1996	1	Crohn's →HIV	270*	Colon, terminal ileum
10	1996	1	HIV →Crohn's	210	NA
12	1997	1	HIV →Crohn's	100	Colon, terminal ileum
11	1996	2	Crohn's →HIV	336, 442	Colon, small bowel/rectum
13	1998	4	Crohn's →HIV	320, 50*, 162, 34*	Colon, terminal ileum

*CD4 count determined years after initial diagnosis of CD.

developed CD, which would add further security to the diagnosis, was rarely performed, including colonoscopic re-examination.

The gastrointestinal tract involvement with CD appeared similar to what might be anticipated with most patients having both colon and terminal ileal disease and with no apparent site predilection. Fistulous disease was reported in one patient [12] and extraintestinal manifestations were not described in any patient. To our knowledge there are no cases in which perianal disease was the sole manifestation.

One reported patient [14] had documented UC for 14 years and subsequently, at the time of recurrent symptoms, had colonoscopy as well as barium enema that was most suggestive of CD; granulomas were not seen on colon biopsy, and extensive histologic examination to exclude opportunistic disorders was not reported. Testing for HIV was not available at the time of publication (1986), but the helper-suppressor T cell ratio was very low, suggesting severe immunodeficiency. Whether this patient truly had UC or an overlap syndrome is unknown.

One of the most important features of these cases is the course of HIV-related immunodeficiency in relationship to the timing of IBD. Of the five HIV-infected patients who later developed CD, the CD4 lymphocyte counts at the time CD was first documented were 100/µl, 210/µl, 230/µl, 336/µl, and 480/µl. Only one of these patients had a history of opportunistic infections, and HIV testing was not available at the time of publication [6]. One additional reported patient with apparently advanced immunodeficiency, as reflected by the presence of opportunistic infections, had a low helper suppressor T cell ratio (0.25, normal 2.5) although the CD4 count was not reported [14]. As noted above, given these CD4 counts, only one of these three patients had substantial immunodeficiency, and this leaves open the possibility that severe immunodeficiency could be protective against the development of CD. Since some reports [14] preceded the recognition of AIDS-related diseases which mimic CD, it is perhaps possible that some of these cases could represent a missed opportunistic infection. The relationship of the response to therapy, as well as natural history with regard to stage of HIV infection, will be discussed below.

Ulcerative colitis

To date there have been nine reports [10, 11, 14, 15, 17–22] of UC totaling 17 HIV-infected patients (Table 2). In four of these patients UC and HIV were diagnosed simultaneously. The CD4 count at diagnosis was 500/µl or greater in six patients tested, and greater than 200/µl in 13 (87%). Histologic criteria for diagnosis followed objective criteria in one [10], were not described in another [15] while the histology was reported as 'nonspecific' in one [18] or demonstrated acute inflammation and crypt abscess

Table 2. Reported cases of UC in HIV-infected patients

Reference	Year	No. of patients	Sequence	CD4 count	Extent
10	96	2	HIV→UC	680, 700	Proctitis, NA
		2	UC→HIV	530, 130	NA, right colon
11	96	6	HIV →UC	460	NA
			HIV →UC	270	
			UC →HIV	256	
			HIV →UC	462	
			HIV →UC	228	
			HIV →UC	283	
14	86	1	UC→AIDS	NA	NA
15	90	1	UC/HIV	500	Transverse colon
18	91	1	UC/HIV	546	Pancolonic
19	92	1	HIV →UC	170	T colon
20	96	1	HIV →UC	NA	Pancolonic
21	97	1	HIV/ UC	450	Pancolonic
22	99	1	HIV/ UC	930	Transverse colon

NA = not available.

in the others. A missing element in most reports is a description of the characteristic histologic changes of chronicity which should be apparent at the time of diagnosis [37]. Of the patients undergoing colonoscopy the disease was limited to the rectum [10], reached the transverse colon [19] and right colon [10] in one patient each and was pancolonic in the other patient. Fulminant colitis requiring surgery was reported in four patients [11, 17, 22]. One patient developed significant articular symptoms (sacroiliitis, arthritis) and later uveitus with flares of disease [21]. When described, the endoscopic appearance of the colon was typical for UC. As mentioned above for CD, the rigor with which other potential causes of colitis were excluded varied, extensive histologic examination was not always performed to exclude infection or evidence of chronicity documented, and long-term follow-up to best assess diagnostic accuracy was not always reported.

Differential diagnosis

Given the apparent infrequency of IBD in AIDS, when confronted with an AIDS patient with suspected IBD the patient is more likely to have an AIDS-related disorder than idiopathic IBD. In contrast, when immunodeficiency is not advanced (CD4 count > 200/μl), gastrointestinal complaints are more likely non-HIV-related. Thus, recognition of the opportunistic disorders which may mimic IBD and their relationship to the stage of immunodeficiency is critical. Furthermore, when correctly diagnosed, the majority of these AIDS-related disorders are amenable to therapy.

When evaluating any HIV-infected patient with gastrointestinal symptoms the level of immunodeficiency must first be staged by the CD4 lymphocyte count. Numerous studies have consistently shown that opportunistic disorders rarely manifest above a CD4 count of 200/μl with most occurring at levels less than 100/μl [35]. Recent evidence also suggests that HIV viral load provides additional prognostic information for disease progression, including the development of opportunistic disorders [38]. Two common gastrointestinal pathogens that occur in the setting of advanced immunodeficiency are cytomegalovirus (CMV) and *Mycobacterium avium* complex (MAC) which commonly involve the colon and small bowel, respectively, and which may mimic IBD [39–44]. In addition, some processes may cause pathologic changes of chronicity that may suggest underlying IBD (unpublished observations). The many reported cases of opportunistic infections which mimicked IBD clinically, radiologically, endoscopically, and/or histologically in this setting emphasize the importance of a high index of suspicion for these diseases, as well as appropriate endoscopic tissue sampling and histologic processing.

Another point to consider when discussing the differential diagnosis of IBD in the setting of HIV infection is that patients with IBD may develop opportunistic infections characteristic of AIDS caused by treatment-related immunodeficiency. The best example of this is CMV colitis complicating high-dose prednisone therapy. In this scenario one may be concerned that the patient has underlying HIV infection and CMV colitis rather than IBD complicated by CMV colitis. Likewise, apparent exacerbation of IBD in HIV-infected patients can reflect intercurrent CMV infection [11].

The most important disease in the differential diagnosis of IBD, especially UC, is CMV colitis. Patients with CMV colitis almost uniformly present with a CD4 count less than 100/μl [39, 45]. In one study [39] the median CD4 count was 15/μl. CMV colitis can also be the index presentation of HIV infection. The most common manifestations of CMV colitis are crampy lower abdominal pain, chronic watery diarrhea which may be bloody, and proctitis symptoms, particularly when distal disease is prominent. Weight loss is also frequent and may be profound, while fever is uncommon. The similarity of these symptoms compared with IBD is readily apparent.

Endoscopically there are also many similarities of CMV colitis and IBD. In a study characterizing the endoscopic appearance of CMV colitis in 56 AIDS patients, Wilcox *et al.* [39] showed that the most common endoscopic manifestation was subepithelial hemorrhage, which was often confluent. Disease was located throughout the colon in 74%, but was limited proximal to the rectosigmoid colon in only 13%. Well-circumscribed ulcerations typical for CD were observed in six patients, while a pancolitis characteristic of UC was noted in three patients. Pseudopolyps have not been reported as a manifestation of CMV colitis. These findings demonstrate that the endoscopic appearance of CMV colitis may be suggestive of either UC or CD.

To best diagnose CMV colitis, multiple biopsies (at least six) of abnormal-appearing tissue should be obtained with close inspection of the characterisitc viral cytopathic effect of CMV. Immunohisto-chemical staining for CMV antigens may further assist in the diagnosis. Although not recommended routinely, viral culture of tissue biopsies may rarely be helpful. It should be noted that, in general, CMV colitis in AIDS is associated with numerous viral inclusions in the biopsies. Therefore, if the the viral cytopathic effect is rare (only one or two positively staining cells with numerous biopsies), one should consider another diagnosis; this should be considered as CMV 'infection' rather than true 'disease' [46].

Other colonic infections in AIDS which have been reported to mimic IBD include *Isospora* [47], and histoplasmosis [48]. Although commonly reported as a cause of colonic disease, herpes simplex virus (HSV) is actually a very rare cause of colonic infection in AIDS. Usually herpes simplex virus of the colon presents with limited anorectal disease. A number of other opportunistic diseases could theoretically mimic IBD also, but no specific reports detailing these associations in HIV-infected patients have been published (Table 3).

Terminal ileal disease suggesting CD may result from either CMV or MAC infection. In a report of terminal ileitis and AIDS [44], small bowel follow-through showed nodularity and ulceration of the terminal ileum characteristic of CD. However, histopathologic examination of the resected ileum demonstrated numerous acid-fast bacilli diagnostic of MAC.

Several cases of colonic Kaposi's sarcoma (KS) mimicking UC have been reported [16, 17]. However, in these AIDS patients KS was not identified on the initial evaluation, but rather on follow-up colonoscopy. In one case [17], IBD was treated aggressively with corticosteroid therapy for 3 months prior to the identification of KS; thus, colonic KS found on subsequent colonoscopy could represent a recognized complication of steroid (immunosuppressive) therapy. The other patient [16] was treated with hydrocortisone enemas prior to the diagnosis of colonic KS. The lesions of KS are characterized endoscopically as circumscribed hemorrhagic lesions of variable size, and it is well recognized that deep biopsies are required to identify the characteristic histologic findings as the tumor generally resides in the submucosa.

As HIV-infected patients are growing older, age-related colonic diseases which may mimic IBD must also be considered. Focal inflammation in the setting of diverticulosis (diverticular colitis) is being increas-

Table 3. Differential diagnosis of IBD in HIV-infected patients

Infection
    Bacterial colitis
    Cytomegalovirus
    Mycobactrium avium complex
    Mycobacterium tuberculosis
    Amebiasis
    Isospora belli
    Histoplasmosis

Non-Infectious
    Ischemia
    Drug-induced colitis
    Peridiverticulitis

Neoplasm
    Kaposi's sarcoma

ingly recognized [49]. Ischemic colitis typically presents with a segmental colitis which may mimic CD or CMV colitis; however, the histologic features of ischemia are usually apparent. Colonic neoplasms may occur in HIV-infected patients including adenocarcinoma, and colonic lymphomas may appear indistinguishable endoscopically from adenocarcinoma. Also, mass lesions have been reported with CMV colitis due to an exuberant inflammatory response, further highlighting the importance of adequate tissue sampling [5].

We and others have described HIV-infected patients with colorectal symptoms in whom focal areas of colitis and/or ulcers have been identified and which have remained idiopathic despite an extensive histologic examination for infections and neoplasms [23, 24]. These patients typically present with ulcers which can be large, and histologic examination of multiple biopsies shows granulation tissue; rarely crypt distortion was present which could mimic IBD. These ulcerative lesions are similar to the well-recognized idiopathic ulcer of the esophagus [50].

Hing *et al.* [24] reported on six HIV-infected patients with a chronic colitis presenting as a chronic diarrhea ranging from three to more than 10 stools per day. The CD4 counts at diagnosis ranged from 256 to 449/µl. Stool studies were negative and colonoscopy showed a diffuse colitis consisting of ulceration, hemorrhage, and erosions, and in one patient mild erythema. Histologically, crypt architecture was preserved with a mixed inflammatory cell population of plasma cells, lymphocytes and neutrophils. Crypt abscess, crypt destruction, and granulomas were absent and CMV and HSV were adequately excluded. Four patients entered remission 6–27 months following the diagnosis, although steroids and sulfasalazine were provided. Zidovudine (AZT) was given to five patients. This report suggests that a mild inflammatory disease of the colon distinct from UC can occur in these patients. The role of anti-inflamatory therapy or HIV-directed treatment (HAART) for this entity is unclear.

An increase in inflammatory cells of the distal colon [51] as well as small bowel [52, 53] has also been documented in HIV-infected patients. The mechanism(s) for this increase in inflammatory cells of these patients also remains unexplained.

Treatment

Because of the small number of reported cases of active IBD and HIV infection, the optimal treatment for both UC and CD in these patients is unknown. In addition, the recognized variability in response to medical therapy in IBD combined with the absence of controlled trials in this setting, makes it difficult to determine if the response to standard therapy for IBD in HIV-infected patients is altered either favorably or unfavorably.

Crohn's disease

For those patients with CD in whom therapy was described and follow-up reported, the clinical response does not appear different from non-HIV-infected patients. Three reports document the clinical response to standard therapy for CD. Corticosteroids with or without aminosalicylates were usually given, and the initial dose of prednisone was ≥ 40 mg per day. Of the three patients with active CD, all responded promptly to instituted therapy, achieving a clinical remission. One patient was treated with antibiotics and hydrocortisone suppositories. One of these patients had multiple relapses [9], all of which were treated successfully with prednisone and aminosalicylates. No long-term data are available describing the efficacy of maintenance therapy with aminosalicylates, and routine endoscopic follow-up after therapy has not been reported.

Surgical therapy has also been undertaken for CD in these HIV-infected patients. Bernstein *et al.* [8] reported one patient who required surgical resection for small bowel obstruction at the time of initial diagnosis. Postoperatively the patient did well, and 6-month follow-up found no recurrence. Other patients have required colectomy for toxic megacolon, some of whom had colonic infections complicating IBD [11, 17, 22].

Ulcerative colitis

Of the reported patients with active UC and HIV, treatment was effective in the majority, at least at the initial presentation, often resulting in clinical remission. One patient [11] was treated with prednisone chronically, but after HIV seroconversion, his clinical course appeared to moderate. However, the medication regimens during this later time were not specifically defined (see below). One patient [18] had experienced several recurrences of disease, all of which responded to therapy; however, one episode later in the course of HIV infection was poorly responsive to high-dose corticosteroid therapy, ultimately requiring 1 month hospitalization. His CD4 count during this severe flare fluctuated between 260/μl and 520/μl. Toxic megacolon refractory to standard therapy required surgery in a patient with minimal immune dysfunction [17]. None of the above-reported patients received additional immunosuppressive therapies such as azathioprine. Like the patients with CD, endoscopic follow-up with biopsies was not routinely performed to best document remission.

There appear to be few therapy-related side-effects from the use of standard treatment for IBD in HIV-infected patients. One of the main treatment concerns is the use of an immunosuppressive drug, such as prednisone, in patients who are already immunosuppressed. Of the 10 reported IBD patients who received prednisone in doses of 40 mg or greater, usually in combination with aminosalicylates, side-effects were reported in three. One patient with a history of UC was found to be HIV-infected during an exacerbation [14]. Following 40 mg of prednisone and sulfasalazine only a slight improvement in symptoms was noted. A CD4 count was not reported, although the T cell helper suppressor ratio was low (0.19). After receiving prednisone and sulfasalazine for approximately $2\frac{1}{2}$ months, he developed diffuse cutaneous KS. The prednisone therapy was discontinued and his cutaneous lesions improved substantially. One additional patient developed widespread KS following 3 months of high-dose steroid therapy [17]. *Candida* esophagitis was reported in one additional patient [9]. It is tempting to speculate that corticosteroid-induced immunosuppression may have predisposed these HIV-infected patients to the development of cutaneous KS.

Prednisone has been used for a variety of indications in HIV-infected patients, even in those who are profoundly immunosuppressed, with little apparent toxicity [54]. Importantly, precipitation of other opportunistic infections or malignancies appears to be rare. The most common reported toxicity of prednisone in HIV-infected patients is oropharyngeal and esophageal candidiasis. Endocrinologic complications such as diabetes may occur with prednisone as in any other patient. Because of the effect on cytokine production, prednisone has been shown to decrease HIV RNA in blood, suggesting a potential saluatory effect [55]. In the patient with severe immune dysfunction and prior CMV infection, caution must be exercised when tapering prednisone, given the possibility of unmasking adrenal insufficiency from CMV adrenalitis.

The use of aminosalicylates should be encouraged as primary therapy as there are no specific contraindications to their use in HIV-infected patients. Although there are numerous drug interactions with the protease inhibitors and other antiretroviral agents, there are no reported interactions with the aminosalicylates. There are also no reports on the use of azathioprine for the treatment of refractory IBD in HIV-infected patients. Likewise, there are no studies on the use of remicade (infliximab) in this setting. The use of infliximab may be contraindicated, however, in patients with active infection, and HIV infection has been an exclusion criterion in trials of this agent.

Given the above we recommend that HIV-infected patients be treated similarly to any other IBD patient. The use of prednisone should not necessarily be discouraged; rather the patient should be monitored closely for complications. For those patients with more severe immunodeficiency and history of thrush, prophylaxis with Nystatin or oral azoles should be considered. For the patient with distal colonic disease, local therapy with enemas should be considered as first-line therapy.

Natural history

There have been tantalizing suggestions that, as HIV-related immunodeficiency progresses, remission of IBD may occur. Given that IBD is characterized by periods of remission and exacerbation, it is important, however, to place these reports in the proper perspective. James [7] reported a patient with longstanding CD disease who subsequently developed HIV infection. This patient had experienced typical Crohn's symptoms on an intermittent basis for the preceding 8 years. HIV testing was performed as a routine and was found to be positive; at that time the CD4 count was 410/μl. Following the diagnosis of HIV infection the patient experienced no further symptoms of disease for the ensuing 2 years of follow-up.

Pospai *et al.* [13] reported four patients with moderately active CD ranging in duration from 4 to 21 years who subsequently acquired HIV infection. In only one of these four cases, however, could the exact date of HIV acquisition be documented. In this patient in whom the timing of HIV could be precisely determined (HIV infection was linked to contaminated blood products), multiple exacerbations had occurred over the preceding 15 years, but the patient went into apparent remission after HIV infection. Interestingly, within 1 year of acquiring HIV infection this patient had a CD4 count, when first

Table 4. Suggested criteria for the diagnosis of IBD in HIV-infected patients

1. Since there is no gold standard for the diagnosis of IBD, a combination of clinical presentation, endoscopic findings, response to therapy and follow-up must be employed

2. Exclusion of colonic and intestinal pathogens is mandatory
   A. Stool studies for bacterial pathogens
   B. Stool studies for parasitic diseases
   C. Blood cultures for mycobacteria

3. Extensive histologic examination of multiple biopsy specimens is mandatory
   A. Cytomegalovirus immunohistochemical staining
   B. Stains for fungi, mycobacteria

4. Documentation of the characteristic histologic changes of IBD including crypt distortion and type of inflammatory cell infiltrate

5. Appropriate follow-up to document response to therapy; both endoscopic and histologic follow-up after therapy should be performed

measured, of 320/μl. In the other three cases the patients had experienced exacerbations for many years, but lasting remission was noted following the estimated time of HIV infection. The long symptom-free intervals in these three patients in whom the time of acquisition of HIV infection could not be documented and the minimal immunodeficiency, particularly early on in HIV infection, makes the relationship between remission and HIV-associated immunodeficiency highly speculative. Also, patients did not routinely undergo follow-up colonoscopic evaluation or other imaging studies to evaluate for disease activity.

Yoshida *et al.* [10] reported one patient with UC who subsequently developed HIV infection. Following the initial diagnosis (the CD4 count was 450/ml), the patient's symptoms appeared to decline over time coincident with the fall in the CD4 count. Six years after HIV seroconversion, at a time when the CD4 count was 20/μl, the patient underwent sigmoido-scopy and biopsy for an acute diarrhea, which demonstrated cryptosporidiosis but no active inflammatory bowel disease; the patient had not received any medical therapy for IBD during the preceding 14 months. Of six patients with IBD (four UC, two CD) followed by Sharpstone *et al.* [11], none developed a flare of disease when the CD4 count fell below 200/μl.

Conclusions

Given the long latency between HIV infection and development of symptoms referable to AIDS, coupled with the variability in the natural history of IBD, it may be impossible to conclude that the progressive immunodeficiency of AIDS results in remission of IBD. The complex nature of the inflammatory response in IBD would suggest that loss of CD4 cells alone may not be 'therapy' for IBD. In addition, the multitude of opportunistic infections, some of which may mimic IBD, as well as the potential for some disorders (CMV) to result in histologic changes of chronicity further complicates any apparent relationship between HIV-related immunosuppression and the course of IBD. Guidelines for the diagnosis of IBD in the setting of HIV are appropriate (Table 4).

More intriguing is the possibility that improvement in immune function may exacerbate IBD in HIV-infected patients. Some of the reported patients did receive AZT therapy without apparent effect on the IBD; however, single-agent therapy with this drug generally has little long-lasting effect on immune function. Now that effective combination antiretroviral therapy is available, we may see reports of exacerbations of IBD in HIV-infected patients who receive HAART. Nevertheless, similar caveats as pointed out for the reverse situation still hold; opportunistic infections must be carefully excluded and spontaneous remissions and exacerbations are always a consideration. Better objective markers for active IBD are required to truly determine whether IBD can be turned off or on by HIV-related immunodeficiency.

References

1. Fauci AS. The AIDS epidemic. N Engl J Med 1999; 341: 1046–11050.
2. El-Sadr WM, Burman WJ, Grant LB *et al.* Discontinuation of prophylaxis against *Mycobacterium avium* complex disease in HIV-infected patients who have a response to antiretroviral therapy. N Engl J Med 2000; 342: 1085–92.
3. Monkemuller KE, Call SA, Lazenby AJ, Wilcox CM. Declining prevalence of opportunistic gastrointestinal disease in the era of combination antiretroviral therapy. Am J Gastroenterol 2000; 95: 457–62.
4. Whitman S, Murphy J, Cohen M, Sherer R. Marked declines in human immunodeficiency virus-related mortality in Chicago in women, African Americans, Hispanics, young adults, and injection drugs users, from 1955 through 1997. Arch Intern Med 2000; 160: 365–9.
5. Monkemuller KE, Wilcox CM. Diagnosis and treatment of colonic disease in AIDS. Gastrointest Endocrinol Clin N Am 1998; 8: 889–911.
6. Dhar JM, Pidgeon ND, Burton AL. AIDS in a patient with Crohn's disease. Br Med J 1984; 288: 1802–3.
7. James SP. Remission of Crohn's disease after human immunodeficiency virus infection. Gastroenterology 1988; 95: 1667–9.
8. Bernstein BB, Gelb A, Tabanda-Lichauco R. Crohn's ileitis in a patient with longstanding HIV infection. Am J Gastroenterol 1994; 89: 937–9.
9. Christ AD, Sieber CC, Cathomas G, Gyr K. Concomitant active Crohn's disease in the acquired immunodeficiency syndrome. Scand J Gastroenterol 1996; 31: 733–5.
10. Yoshida EM, Chan NHL, Herrick RA *et al.* Human immunodeficiency virus infection, the acquired immunodeficiency syndrome, and inflammatory bowel disease. J Clin Gastroenterol 1996; 23: 24–8.
11. Sharpstone DR, Duggal A, Gazzard BG. Inflammatory bowel disease in individuals seropositive for the human immunodeficiency virus. Eur J Gastroenterol Hepatol 1996; 8: 575–8.
12. Lautenbach E, Lichtenstein GR. Human immunodeficiency virus infection and Crohn's disease: the role of the CD4 cell in inflammatory bowel disease. J Clin Gastroenterol 1997; 25: 456–9.
13. Pospai D, Rene E, Fiasse R *et al.* Crohn's disease stable remission after human immunodeficiency virus infection. Dig Dis Sci 1998; 43: 412–19.
14. Liebowitz D, McShane D. Nonspecific chronic inflammatory bowel disease and AIDS. J Clin Gastroenterol 1986; 8: 66–8.

15. Franke M, Kruis W, Heitz W. First manifestation of ulcerative colitis in a patient with HIV infection. Gastroenterology 1990; 98: 544–5.

16. Weber JN, Carmichael DJ, Bolyston A, Monro A, Whitear WP, Pinching AJ. Kaposi's sarcoma of the bowel – presenting as apparent ulcerative colitis. Gut 1985; 26: 295–300.

17. Biggs BA, Crowe SM, Lucas CR, Ralston M, Thompson IL, Hardy KJ. AIDS related Kaposi's sarcoma presenting as ulcerative colitis and complicated by toxic megacolon. Gut 1987; 28: 1302–6.

18. Bernstein CN, Snape WJ. Active idiopathic ulcerative colitis in a patient with ongoing HIV-related immunodepression. Am J Gastroenterol 1991; 86: 907–9.

19. Sturgess I, Greenfield SM, Teare J, O'Doherty MJ. Ulcerative colitis developing after amebic dysentery in a hemophiliac patient with AIDS. Gut 1992; 33: 408–10.

20. Wilcox CM, Schwartz DA, Cotsonis GA, Thompson WE III. Evaluation of chronic unexplained diarrhea in human immunodeficiency virus infection: determination of the best diagnostic approach. Gastroenterology 1996; 110: 30–7.

21. Louis E, Moutschen MP, De Marneffe P *et al.* Extensive ulcerative colitis and extraintestinal manifestations in a patient with HIV infection and significant CD4 T cell lymphopenia. Gastroenterol Clin Biol 1997; 21: 884–7.

22. Silver S, Wahl SM, Orkin BA, Orenstein JM. Changes in circulating levels of HIV, CD4, and tissue expression of HIV in a patient with recent-onset ulcerative colitis treated by surgery. J Human Virol 1999; 2: 52–7.

23. Wilcox CM, Schwartz DA. Idiopathic anorectal ulceration in patients with human immunodeficiency virus infection. Am J Gastroenterol 1994; 89: 599–604.

24. Hing MC, Holdshmide C, Mathijs JM, Cunningham AL, Cooper DA. Chronic colitis associated with human immunodeficiency virus infection. Med J Aust 1992; 156: 683–7.

25. Elson CO. Experimental models of intestinal inflammation: new insights into the mechanisms of mucosal homeostasis. In: Ogra PL, Mcstecky J, Lamm ME, Strober W, Bienenstock J, McGhee JR, eds. Mucosal Immunology, 2nd edn. San Diego, CA: Academic Press, 1999: 1007–24.

26. Rodgers VD, Fassett R, Kagnoff MF. Abnormalities in intestinal mucosal T cells in homosexual populations including those with the lymphadenopathy syndrome and acquired immunodeficiency syndrome. Gastroenterology 1986; 90: 552–8.

27. Ellakany S, Whiteside TL, Schade RR, Van Theil DH. Analysis of intestinal lymphocyte subpopulations in patients with acquired immunodeficiency syndrome (AIDS) and AIDS-related complex. Am J Clin Pathol 1987; 87: 356–64.

28. Snijders F, van Deveter SJH, Bartelsman JFW *et al.* Diarrhea in HIV-infected patients: no evidence of cytokine-mediated inflammation in jejunal mucosa. AIDS 1995; 9: 367–73.

29. McGowan I, Randford-Smith G, Jewell DP. Cytokine gene expression in HIV-infected intestinal mucosa. AIDS 1994; 8: 1569–75.

30. Reka S, Garro ML, Kotler DP. Variation in the expression of human immunodeficiency virus RNA and cytokine mRNA in rectal mucosa dining the progression in infection. Lymph Cyto Res 1994; 13: 391–8.

31. Steffen M, Reinecker HC, Petersen J *et al.* Differences in cytokine secretion by intestinal mononuclear cells, peripheral blood monocytes and alveolar macrophages from HIV-infected patients. Clin Exp Immunol 1993; 91: 30–6.

32. Jarry A, Cortez A, Rene E, Muzeau F, Brouse N. Infected cells and immune cells in the gastrointestinal tract of AIDS patients. An immunohistochemical study of 127 cases. Histopathology 1990; 16: 133–40.

33. Kotler DP, Reka S, Borcich A, Cronin WJ. Detection, localization, and quantitation of HIV-associated antigens in intestinal biopsies from patients with HIV. Am J Pathol 1991; 139: 823–30.

34. Loftus EVJR, Silverstein MD, Sandborn WJ, Tremaine WJ, Harmen WS, Zinmeister AR. Ulcerative colitis in Olmsted County Minnesota, 1940–1993: incidence, prevalence, and survival. Gut 2000: 46: 336–43.

35. Mocroft A, Youle M, Phillips AN *et al.* The incidence of AIDS-defining illnesses in 4883 patients with human immunodeficiency virus infection. Arch Intern Med 1998; 158: 491–7.

36. Ledergerber B, Egger M, Erard V *et al.* AIDS-related opportunistic illnesses occurring after initiation of potent antiretroviral therapy. J Am Med Assoc 1999; 282: 2220–6.

37. Carpenter HA, Talley NJ. The importance of clinicopathological correlation in the diagnosis of inflammatory conditions of the colon: histological patterns with clinical implications. Am J Gastroenterol 2000; 95: 878–96.

38. Hubert JB, Burgard M, Dussaix E *et al.* Natural history of serum HIV-1 RNA levels in 330 patients with a known date of infection. AIDS 2000; 14: 123–31.

39. Wilcox CM, Chalasani N, Lazenby A, Schwartz DA. Cytomegalovirus colitis in AIDS: an endoscopic and clinical study. Gastrointest Endosc 1998; 48: 39–43.

40. Roskell DE, Hyde GM, Campbell AP, Jewell DP, Gray W. HIV associated cytomegalovirus colitis as a mimic of inflammatory bowel disease. Gut 1995; 37: 148–50.

41. Caroline DF, Hilpret PL, Russin VL. CMV colitis mimicking Crohn's disease in a patient with acquired immune deficiency syndrome (AIDS). J Can Assoc Radiol 1997; 38: 227–8.

42. Kotler DP, Baer JW, Scholes JV. Isolated ileitis due to cytomegalovirus in a patient with AIDS. Gastrointest Endosc 1991; 37: 571–4.

43. Wajsman R, Cappell MS, Biempica L, Cho KC. Terminal ileitis associated with cytomegalovirus and the acquired immune deficiency syndrome. Am J Gastroenterol 1989; 84: 790–3.

44. Schneebaum CW, Novick DM, Chapon AB, Strutynsky N, Yancovitz SR, Freund S. Terminal ileitis associated with *Mycobacterium avium-intracellulare* infection in a homosexual man with acquired immune deficiency syndrome. Gastroenterology 1987; 92: 1127–32.

45. Dieterich DT, Rahmin M. Cytomegalovirus colitis in AIDS: presentation in 44 patients and a review of the literature. J Acquir Immune Def Syndr Hum Retrovirol 1991; 1: S29.

46. Beaugerie L, Cywiner-Golenzer C, Monfort L *et al.* Definition and diagnosis of cytomegalovirus colitis in patients infected by human immunodeficiency virus. J Acq Immun Defic Syn Hum Retrovirol 1997; 14: 423–9.

47. Alfandari S, Ajana F, Senneville E, Beuscart C, Chidiac C, Mouton Y. Hemorrhagic ulcerative colitis due to *Isospora belli* in AIDS. Int J STD AIDS. 1995; 6: 216.

48. Balthazar EJ, Megibow AJ, Barry M, Opulencia JF. Histoplasmosis of the colon in patient with AIDS: imaging findings in four cases. Am J Radiol 1993; 161: 585–7.

49. Imperiali G, Meucci G, Alvisi C *et al.* Segmental colitis associated with diverticula: a prospective study. Am J Gastroenterol 2000; 95: 1014–16.

50. Wilcox CM, Schwartz DA, Clark WS. Esophageal ulceration in human immunodeficiency virus infection: causes, response to therapy, and long-term outcome. Ann Intern Med 1995; 123: 143–9.

51. Clayton F, Reka S, Cronin WJ, Torlakovic E, Sigal SH, Kotler DP. Rectal mucosal pathology varies with human immunodeficiency virus antigen content and disease stage. Gastroenterology 1992; 103: 919–33.

52. Kotler DP, Reka S, Clayton F. Intestinal mucosa inflammation associated with human immunodeficiency virus infection. Dig Dis Sci 1993; 38: 1119–27.

53. Bjarnason I, Sharpstone DR, Francis N *et al.* Intestinal inflammation, ileal structure, and function in HIV. AIDS 1996; 10: 1385–91.

54. Castro M. Treatment and prophylaxis of *Pneumocystis carinii* pneumonia. Sem Respir Infect 1998; 13: 296–303.

55. Kilby JM, Tabereaux PB, Mulanovich V, Shaw GM, Bucy RP, Saag MS. Effects of tapering doses of oral prednisone on viral load among HIV-infected patients with unexplained weight loss. AIDS Res Human Retrovir 1997; 13: 1533–7.

49 | Bone metabolism and inflammatory bowel disease

MARIA T. ABREU

Introduction

A serious and silent complication of inflammatory bowel disease (IBD) is the development of osteoporosis [1–3]. Osteoporosis is a systemic skeletal disease characterized by low bone mass, microarchitectural deterioration of bone tissue and increased bone fragility and susceptibility to fracture [4]. Milder bone loss or osteopenia is defined as a bone mineral density (BMD) that is 1.0–2.49 standard deviations below a control population, and osteoporosis as BMD that is less than 2.5 standard deviations below a control population [5] (Table 1). Estimates of osteopenia in IBD range from 31% to 59% [6, 7] and osteoporosis from 5% to 41% [1, 8–11]. Bone loss is more prevalent in patients with Crohn's disease (CD) than those with ulcerative colitis (UC), and this may be related to the fact that childhood onset of CD does not allow children to reach peak bone mass [1]. In a prospective series of patients with IBD the rate of bone loss over a 19-month period was –3.1 for CD, –6.4 for UC (includes patients on steroids) and +2.0 for UC after an ileoanal anastomosis [12]. The reasons for development of osteopenia and osteoporosis are multiple and include steroid-induced bone loss [12–15], malabsorption of nutrients [16, 17], vitamin D deficiency [18], smoking [19], and inflammatory cytokines [9, 20] (Table 2).

Based on the high prevalence of osteopenia and osteoporosis in patients with IBD, a baseline evaluation of BMD is warranted, especially in patients with CD [21]. The diagnosis of osteopenia and osteoporosis is most often made by dual-energy X-ray absorptiometry (DEXA) of the lumbar spine, proximal femur, and forearm, but can be made using other techniques such as calcaneal ultrasound or quantitative computed tomography [22, 23]. In addition to DEXA scanning for BMD, other serum and urinary markers are available for assessment of bone turnover. In patients with IBD, measurement of urinary N-telopeptide crosslinked of Type 1 collagen, a marker of bone resorption, was the best predictor of spinal bone loss over a 2-year follow-up period compared with other markers, including bone alkaline phosphatase, osteocalcin, parathyroid hormone (PTH) and vitamin D levels [10, 24, 25].

Table 1. World Health Organization criteria for assessment of disease severity in patients at risk for osteoporosis

Diagnostic criteria*	Classification
$T = 0$ to -1 SD	Normal
$T = 1$ to -2 SD	Osteopenia
$T \leqslant -2.5$ SD	Osteoporosis
$T \leqslant -2.5$ SD + fragility fractures	Severe osteoporosis

*T scores refer to the number of standard deviations (SD) below or above the peak bone mass in a young adult reference population of the same sex.

Table 2. Factors leading to bone loss in patients with inflammatory bowel disease

1. Corticosteroids
2. Vitamin D/calcium deficiency
3. Inappropriately high 1,25(OH) vitamin D (granulomatous disease)
4. Malnutrition
5. Physical inactivity
6. Immunosuppressive drugs (cyclosporine, tacrolimus, methotrexate)
7. Cytokine-mediated changes in bone metabolism
8. Smoking
9. Hypogonadism

Corticosteroid-induced osteoporosis

The principal cause of secondary osteoporosis in patients with IBD is corticosteroid use [26]. The unfortunate sequelae of chronic corticosteroid use are fractures which occur in 30–50% of steroid users

Stephan R. Targan, Fergus Shanahan and Loren C. Karp (eds.), *Inflammatory Bowel Disease: From Bench to Bedside, 2nd Edition*, 875–883.
© 2003 *Kluwer Academic Publishers. Printed in Great Britain*

[4]. Corticosteroids have multiple effects on bone including direct inhibition of bone formation, impaired calcium absorption across the intestine and increased renal calcium excretion, all of which result in a negative calcium balance [27] (Fig. 1). As a result of calcium wasting, secondary hyperparathyroidism results and increases bone resorption. Corticosteroids induce a myopathy which reduces the bone-stimulating effects of muscle activity. In animal models corticosteroids have been shown to induce apoptosis of osteoblasts and osteocytes, thereby resulting in diminished bone formation [11]. More recently, corticosteroids have been shown to regulate bone metabolism through their effect on members of the TNF receptor family, the osteoprotegerins (Fig. 2). Osteoclasts express the RANK receptor [28]. Binding of osteoprotegerin ligand (OPGL) to RANK activates osteoclastic activity. This osteoclastic activity can be blocked by a soluble receptor osteoprotegerin (OPG) that binds OPGL. Corticosteroids decrease OPG expression by 90% and increase OPGL expression by 3-fold, resulting in increased osteoclastic activity [28]. Corticosteroids also cause a 3-fold increase in osteoclast numbers. Finally, corticosteroids inhibit adrenal production of androgens, contributing to bone loss.

The effect of corticosteroids on bone loss is most marked in the first 6–12 months of therapy; therefore even short courses of steroids (<6 months) will result in marked bone loss [4, 29–31]. Even within 1 week of high-dose steroid exposure, markers of bone resorption are increased [32]. Bone loss secondary to steroids is dependent on both the dose and the duration of steroid use, with doses greater than 7.5 mg/day associated with five times the risk of fractures [33–37]. In studies of chronic exposure to steroids, average steroid doses of as little as 5.6 mg/day resulted in BMD loss of 2%/year [32, 38, 39]. In a large cohort of patients in the United Kingdom the relative risk of vertebral fracture compared to a control population was 1.55 times higher with a standardized daily dose of steroids of 2.5 mg of prednisolone, and increased to 5.18 for standardized doses of 7.5 mg or greater [37]. Importantly, all fracture risks declined rapidly after cessation of steroids, suggesting that therapy should be given during the time of corticosteroid use. Budesonide is a new-generation steroid with less pituitary axis suppression because of extensive first-pass metabolism in the liver, and has been shown to be effective in the treatment of ileocolic CD [40, 41]. Studies of osteoporosis in patients using inhaled budesonide

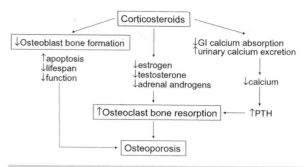

Figure 1. Pathophysiology of corticosteroid-induced osteoporosis: bone formation and resorption.

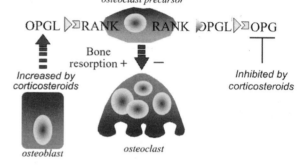

Figure 2. Osteoprotegerin ligand (OPGL) stimulates osteoclastogenesis. OPG is a soluble, inactivating receptor for OPGL. Local OPG:OPGL ratios control bone resorption rates. Corticosteroids decrease OPG expression by 90% and increase OPGL expression by 3-fold resulting in increased osteoclastica activity.

have demonstrated an inverse correlation between BMD and use of this steroid [42]. In patients with primary biliary cirrhosis, oral budesonide therapy resulted in worsening of their osteoporosis [43]. In patients with CD treated with budesonide for 10 weeks versus prednisolone (32 mg) for 3 weeks, and then tapered, there was decreased osteoblastic activity in the prednisolone-treated group but no changes in bone resorption markers during this time [44]. In short courses (less than 2 weeks), topical rectal steroids do not increase bone turnover in patients with IBD but long-term therapy with these agents will lead to bone loss [45]. These studies demonstrate that no steroid is completely safe with respect to bone loss.

With respect to steroid-induced bone loss, approximately 70% of IBD patients are treated with at least one course of steroids, and cumulative steroid use in IBD patients is inversely correlated with BMD [3, 8, 12]. A comparison of the prevalence of osteopenia in IBD patients revealed that osteopenia was present in 58% of patients treated with steroids compared with 28% not on steroids [15]. The annual rate of bone loss in IBD patients is 3–6%/year, and this rate is largely dependent on steroid use [2, 12, 26, 46, 47]. Patients with IBD who are treated with corticosteroids are at risk for the complications of osteoporosis, such as vertebral compression fractures and aseptic necrosis of the hip, and clinicians treating IBD should be proactive in preventing corticosteroid-induced osteoporosis and vigilant for the sequelae of corticosteroid use [48]. In spite of adequate therapy to prevent and treat osteoporosis, only 20% of patients on chronic corticosteroids (> 1 year) undergo some type of evaluation for bone loss, and only 30% of patients are treated for osteoporosis [49].

Additional causes of bone loss in IBD

In addition to bone loss secondary to treatment with steroids, patients with IBD, especially CD, have greater bone loss than expected for the amount of steroid exposure suggesting that other factors contribute to bone loss [50]. Symptoms of greater than 6 months duration prior to the diagnosis of IBD are significantly correlated with low BMD in the absence of disease-specific therapy [51]. Severe osteoporosis can be the presenting problem of children with CD [52]. At least part of the reason for bone loss in CD patients is low vitamin D levels leading to secondary hyperparathyroidism. Osteoporosis is most prominent in CD patients with previous surgical resections [24]. Vitamin D deficiency is related to malabsorption and correlates with previous surgical resections and lack of sun exposure [16, 17, 53]. Postmenopausal women with IBD are especially vulnerable to osteoporosis [2, 3, 54]. In addition to mechanisms leading to increased bone resorption in patients with IBD, histomorphometric analysis of iliac crest bone biopsies from patients with IBD revealed reduced bone formation [14]. For this reason, even in patients with current corticosteroid exposure or a history of corticosteroid use, a full evaluation should be performed to determine if more than one cause of bone loss exists (Fig. 3).

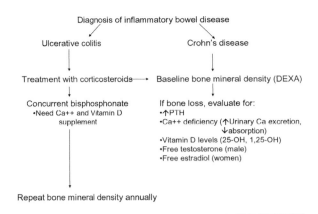

Figure 3. Maintenance of bone health in IBD.

Role of inflammatory cytokines in bone metabolism

In addition to known risk factors for bone loss, intestinal inflammation may have systemic consequences with respect to bone metabolism distinct from its effects on absorption of vitamins and nutrients. Patients with newly diagnosed CD may present with osteopenia or osteoporosis, suggesting that other factors may be contributing to increased bone turnover [51, 52]. In the 2,4,6-trinitrobenzenesulfonic acid (TNBS) rat model of colitis, colitic animals have significantly suppressed cancellous bone formation to 30% of that in control animals [55]. The inflammatory cytokines IL-1, IL-6 and TNF-α are elevated in the systemic circulation of patients with CD. *In vitro*, TNF-α causes osteoclastic bone resorption and inhibits bone collagen synthesis [6, 7, 56–58]. IL-1 and IL-6 also increase bone resorption through activation of osteoclast activity [59]. In addition to their effect on osteoclasts, TNF-α and IL-1β increase Fas-mediated apoptosis of osteoblasts [60]. TNF-α further propagates bone resorption by stimulating IL-6 secretion by osteoblasts [61]. TNF-α inhibits the action of 1,25(OH) vitamin D through activation of a nuclear inhibitor that antagonizes the effect of vitamin D [62]. Inhibition of TNF-α or IL-1 in ovariectomized mice prevents bone loss, suggesting that, in animal models, blockade of high TNF-α states is beneficial to the treatment of osteopenia and osteoporosis [63]. Recently a chimeric Fc fusion form of human OPG with enhanced biological activity was used to inhibit osteoclastic bone resorption in animals challenged with IL-1β, TNF-α, or 1,25(OH) vitamin D3 [64].

These data suggest that inflammatory cytokines mediate their osteoclastic effects through OPGL, and that blocking OPGL may be beneficial in osteoporosis in chronic inflammatory states.

Because of the role of proinflammatory cytokines in bone turnover, a study was performed in patients with IBD to identify genetic factors associated with increased bone loss [20]. The genetic markers assessed included IL-1 receptor antagonist, IL-6, heat-shock protein 70-2, and heat-shock protein 70-hom alleles. A specific IL-1 receptor antagonist allele (A2) and IL-6 allele (130 bp) were independently associated with increased bone loss, and the presence of both alleles led to significantly greater bone loss than either singly. Further studies will likely address the correlation of inflammatory cytokine production (phenotype) to actual bone turnover in patients with IBD.

Vitamin D metabolism in Crohn's disease: role in osteopenia and osteoporosis

One of the pathognomonic features of intestinal inflammation in CD is granuloma formation. As with other granulomatous diseases such as sarcoidosis [65], a subset of patients with CD have extrarenal 1-hydroxylase enzyme activity, leading to inappropriately high levels of the active 1,25-dihydroxylated form of vitamin D [66]. The consequence of increased $1,25(OH)_2$ vitamin D levels is increased bone resorption with hypercalcemia and hypercalciuria. In a prospectively identified series of patients, Kantorovich *et al.* have found that 31% of patients with CD have $1,25(OH)_2$ vitamin D levels that are above normal [67]. TNF-α may be one of the cytokines produced in the granulomatous milieu that contributes to 1-hydroxylase activation in macrophages and hyper-$1,25(OH)_2$ vitamin D. These CD patients are at increased risk for the development of osteopenia and osteoporosis. Strategies to reduce bone loss in these patients include treatment of the underlying IBD and, potentially, hydroxychloroquine which inhibits the conversion of 25-OH vitamin D to 1,25(OH) vitamin D [68].

Drug-induced bone loss

Although corticosteroids are a classic cause of drug-induced bone loss, other immunosuppressive therapies can also result in osteopenia and osteoporosis. In patients with rheumatoid arthritis methotrexate monotherapy is not associated with increased bone loss, but the combination of methotrexate and pre-

dnisone >5 mg/day led to greater bone loss than prednisone therapy alone [69, 70]. The calcineurin phosphatase inhibitors cyclosporine and tacrolimus both cause osteopenia and osteoporosis by increasing bone turnover which is reflected in high levels of osteocalcin [71, 72]. Renal transplantation patients given cyclosporine alone, however, did not have significant bone loss at the end of 18 months, whereas those treated with corticosteroids plus cyclosporine experienced the greatest losses, suggesting that corticosteroids are the worst offenders in this regard [73].

Treatment of corticosteroid-induced osteoporosis

As stated above, patients are at highest risk for hip and vertebral fractures while on corticosteroids, and the risk is directly proportional to the dose [37]. Although avoidance or discontinuation of corticosteroids is ideal, patients with moderate to severe IBD will likely require corticosteroids. Several strategies have been used to delay or partially reverse bone loss due to steroid use. Calcium and vitamin D supplementation has been shown to reduce bone loss in steroid-treated patients and should be started in all patients receiving corticosteroids [74–76]. Calcitonin has a modest effect on steroid-induced bone loss, delaying bone loss compared with placebo-treated patients [77–83]. The most effective drug therapy for osteoporosis is bisphosphonate therapy [84]. Bisphosphonates prevent dexamethasone-mediated apoptosis of cultured mouse osteoblasts and osteocytes, and prevent dexamethasone-mediated apoptosis of osteoblasts and osteocytes in prednisolone-treated mice [85]. A recent meta-analysis comparing the various options available for steroid-induced bone loss found that bisphosphonates are more effective with respect to preservation of bone density than vitamin D, fluoride or calcitonin [74] (Figs. 4 and 6). The change in lumbar spine BMD in patients treated with vitamin D was +1.96, calcitonin +2.11, compared with bisphosphonates which demonstrated +5.31 increases in BMD. Most of these studies have been performed in patients treated with corticosteroids for rheumatologic or pulmonary diseases, but the results are applicable to patients with IBD.

Two approaches have been used in clinical trials of bisphosphonates for corticosteroid-induced osteoporosis: (1) prevention and (2) treatment of existing bone loss. Studies of cyclical etidronate have consistently found a benefit in lumbar spine BMD when given to prevent steroid-induced bone loss [84, 86]. Similarly, studies with daily alendronate or risedronate for prevention of steroid-induced bone loss have demonstrated increases in BMD compared with losses in BMD in placebo-treated patients [87–89]. Data from prevention trials of risedronate performed in 228 patients (largely rheumatologic) demonstrated that risedronate 5 mg/day led to increased BMD at the lumbar spine (+0.59), femoral neck (0.75), and femoral trochanter (+1.42) compared with bone loss of –2.83, –3.06, and –3.06, respectively, in placebo-treated patients [88, 90]. Importantly, studies of bone loss 'prevention' have been done in patients exposed to corticosteroids for less than 3 months – a time when significant bone loss has already occurred. With respect to treatment of existing bone loss in patients taking steroids, the bisphosphonates etidronate, alendronate and risedronate are all effective in improving axial BMD [34, 91, 92]. In addition to the efficacy of bisphosphonates in increasing BMD in patients receiving corticosteroids, large randomized placebo-controlled trials have demonstrated a 70% reduction in the incidence of vertebral fractures in risedronate-treated (5 mg/day) patients compared with placebo-treated patients [88, 89]. Currently the only bisphosphonate that has an FDA indication for steroid-induced osteoporosis is risedronate.

Management of osteopenia and osteoporosis in patients with IBD

In spite of the great need to prevent and treat bone loss in patients with IBD, few clinical trials have been performed in this population of patients. Hormone replacement therapy has been used in postmenopausal women with CD or UC and results in increased bone mass, although few patients in this study were treated with steroids and this approach is for a very limited group of patients [54]. In corticosteroid-treated patients with IBD a randomized, placebo-controlled trial using calcium 1 g and vitamin D 250 units per day failed to confer a benefit in bone loss prevention at the end of 1 year [93]. Fluoride in combination with calcium and vitamin D was associated with small gains in BMD in CD patients with osteopenia previously treated with corticosteroids [94]. Vitamin D therapy by itself prevents ongoing bone loss in patients with CD but does not lead to increases in BMD [95]. Bisphosphonates have been

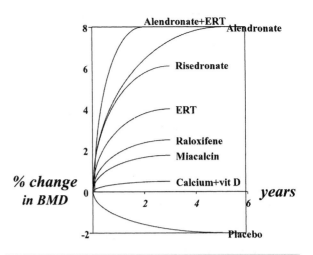

Figure 4. Relative effectiveness of antiresorptives in corticosteroid-induced osteoporosis. ERT is estrogen replacement therapy.

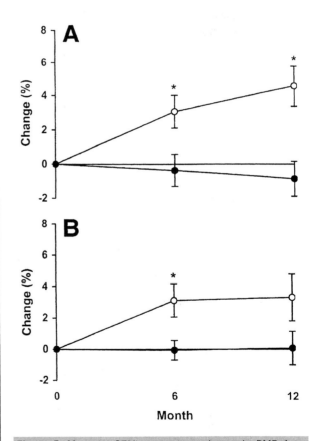

Figure 5. Mean (±SEM) percentage change in BMD from baseline to 12 months in the alendronate (open circle) and placebo (image) groups. **A**: Lumbar spine L2-L4; **B**: femoral neck. Data were analyzed on intention-to-treat basis. Asterisks indicate significant differences between treatment groups. From Haderslev *et al.* Gastroenterology 2000.

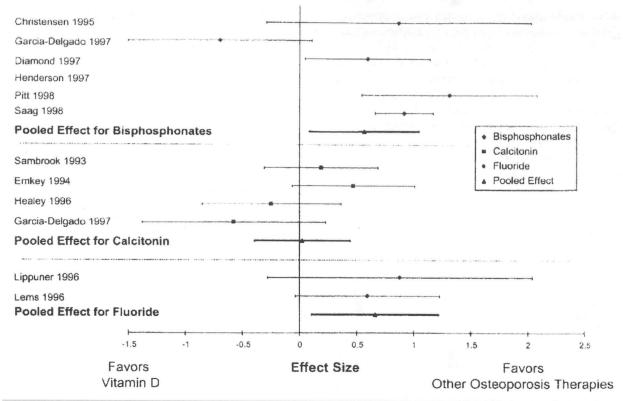

Figure 6. Meta-analysis comparing vitamin D for steroid-induced osteoporosis compared with bisphosphonate, fluoride or calcitonin therapy. Amin S *et al.* Arthritis Rheumat 1999; 42: 1740–51.

Table 3. Strategies to prevent and treat corticosteroid-induced osteoporosis

1. Minimize corticosteroid exposure
2. Initiate bisphosphonates concurrently with corticosteroids
3. Replace calcium and vitamin D (not sufficient as monotherapy)
4. Calcitonin (can be administered as nasal spray)
5. Hormone replacement therapy

used empirically in IBD patients. A large multicenter study examining the effect of alendronate on steroid-induced bone loss included some IBD patients (24 out of 477 patients) [87]. Thus far, one randomized controlled trial of bisphosphonates has been done in patients with CD and osteopenia defined as a bone mass T score of –1 at the hip or lumbar spine [96]. Patients were randomly assigned to receive placebo or alendronate 10 mg/day for 12 months. Patients were in remission at the time of the study and both groups had similar cumulative corticosteroid use, although current corticosteroid use was not permitted. At the conclusion of the study, patients

receiving alendronate had an increase of 4.6% in BMD whereas the control group experienced a decrease of 0.9% (Fig. 5). Although heartburn and dyspepsia occurred more frequently in the alendronate group, the overall rate of adverse events was low in both groups; specifically no increase in diarrhea was found in the alendronate group. Based on this study, as well as published studies demonstrating the efficacy of bisphosphonates for treatment of corticosteroid-induced osteoporosis, clinicians taking care of patients with IBD should prescribe bisphosphonates for their corticosteroid-treated patients and should obtain baseline bone densitometry studies on all their patients to determine if bone loss has already occurred, and treat appropriately (Fig. 3).

Patients with IBD may have multiple causes for bone loss and these should be addressed with specific therapies [5]. In addition to corticosteroid-induced osteoporosis, bisphosphonates are effective in bone loss secondary to cyclosporine [97]. All patients, including those taking bisphosphonates, should be concurrently receiving 1 g of elemental calcium and 400 units of vitamin D, as well as getting adequate sun exposure [75]. Patients with active IBD should receive appropriate therapy to control the intestinal inflammation, preferably not corticosteroids, in an effort to reduce inflammatory cytokine production, decrease extrarenal production of 1,25(OH) vitamin D and increase intestinal absorption of nutrients and vitamins. Hypogonadism should be treated specifically with hormone replacement therapy in men and women [98].

References

1. Adachi JD, Rostom A. Metabolic bone disease in adults with inflammatory bowel disease. Inflam Bowel Dis 1999; 5: 200–11.
2. Clements D, Motley RJ, Evans WD et al. Longitudinal study of cortical bone loss in patients with inflammatory bowel disease. Scand J Gastroenterol 1992; 27: 1055–60.
3. Motley RJ, Clements D, Evans WD et al. A four-year longitudinal study of bone loss in patients with inflammatory bowel disease. Bone Miner 1993; 23: 95–104.
4. Lukert BP, Raisz LG. Glucocorticoid-induced osteoporosis: pathogenesis and management. Ann Intern Med 1990; 112: 352–64.
5. Adachi JD, Olszynski WP, Hanley DA et al. Management of corticosteroid-induced osteoporosis. Semin Arthritis Rheum 2000; 29: 228–51.
6. Bertolini DR, Nedwin GE, Bringman TS, Smith DD, Mundy GR. Stimulation of bone resorption and inhibition of bone formation *in vitro* by human tumour necrosis factors. Nature 1986; 319: 516–18.
7. Lader CS, Flanagan AM. Prostaglandin E2, interleukin 1alpha, and tumor necrosis factor-alpha increase human osteoclast formation and bone resorption *in vitro*. Endocrinology 1998; 139: 3157–64.
8. Dinca M, Fries W, Luisetto G et al. Evolution of osteopenia in inflammatory bowel disease. Am J Gastroenterol 1999; 94: 1292–7.
9. Pollak RD, Karmeli F, Eliakim R, Ackerman Z, Tabb K, Rachmilewitz D. Femoral neck osteopenia in patients with inflammatory bowel disease. Am J Gastroenterol 1998; 93: 1483–90.
10. Schulte C, Dignass AU, Mann K, Goebell H. Reduced bone mineral density and unbalanced bone metabolism in patients with inflammatory bowel disease. Inflam Bowel Dis 1998; 4: 268–75.
11. Weinstein RS, Jilka RL, Parfitt AM, Manolagas SC. Inhibition of osteoblastogenesis and promotion of apoptosis of osteoblasts and osteocytes by glucocorticoids. Potential mechanisms of their deleterious effects on bone. J Clin Invest 1998; 102: 274–82.
12. Roux C, Abitbol V, Chaussade S et al. Bone loss in patients with inflammatory bowel disease: a prospective study. Osteoporosis Int 1995; 5: 156–60.
13. Compston JE, Judd D, Crawley EO et al. Osteoporosis in patients with inflammatory bowel disease. Gut 1987; 28: 410–15.
14. Croucher PI, Vedi S, Motley RJ, Garrahan NJ, Stanton MR, Compston JE. Reduced bone formation in patients with osteoporosis associated with inflammatory bowel disease. Osteoporosis Int 1993; 3: 236–41.
15. Abitbol V, Roux C, Chaussade S et al. Metabolic bone assessment in patients with inflammatory bowel disease. Gastroenterology 1995; 108: 417–22.
16. Compston JE, Horton LW, Laker MF et al. Bone disease after jejuno-ileal bypass for obesity. Lancet 1978; 2: 1–4.
17. Compston JE, Ayers AB, Horton LW, Tighe JR, Creamer B. Osteomalacia after small-intestinal resection. Lancet 1978; 1: 9–12.
18. Compston JE, Horton LW. Oral 25-hydroxyvitamin D3 in treatment of osteomalacia associated with ileal resection and cholestyramine therapy. Gastroenterology 1978; 74: 900–2.
19. Silvennoinen JA, Lehtola JK, Niemela SE. Smoking is a risk factor for osteoporosis in women with inflammatory bowel disease. Scand J Gastroenter 1996; 31: 367–71.
20. Schulte CM, Dignass AU, Goebell H, Roher HD, Schulte KM. Genetic factors determine extent of bone loss in inflammatory bowel disease. Gastroenterology 2000; 119: 909–920.
21. Compston JE. Detection of osteoporosis in patients with inflammatory bowel disease. Eur J Gastroenterol Hepatol 1997; 9: 931–3.
22. Cranney A, Welch V, Tugwell P et al. Responsiveness of endpoints in osteoporosis clinical trials – an update. J Rheumatol 1999; 26: 222–8.
23. Robinson RJ, Carr I, Iqbal SJ, al-Azzawi F, Abrams K, Mayberry JF. Screening for osteoporosis in Crohn's disease. A detailed evaluation of calcaneal ultrasound. Eur J Gastroenterol Hepatol 1998; 10: 137–40.
24. Dresner-Pollak R, Karmeli F, Eliakim R, Ackerman Z, Rachmilewitz D. Increased urinary N-telopeptide cross-linked type 1 collagen predicts bone loss in patients with inflammatory bowel disease. Am J Gastroenterol 2000; 95: 699–704.
25. Robinson RJ, Iqbal SJ, Abrams K, Al-Azzawi F, Mayberry JF. Increased bone resorption in patients with Crohn's disease. Aliment Pharmacol Ther 1998; 12: 699–705.
26. Silvennoinen JA, Karttunen TJ, Niemela SE, Manelius JJ, Lehtola JK. A controlled study of bone mineral density in patients with inflammatory bowel disease. Gut 1995; 37: 71–6.
27. Adachi JD. Corticosteroid-induced osteoporosis. Am J Med Sc 1997; 313: 41–9.
28. Hofbauer LC, Gori F, Riggs BL et al. Stimulation of osteoprotegerin ligand and inhibition of osteoprotegerin production by glucocorticoids in human osteoblastic lineage cells: potential paracrine mechanisms of glucocorticoid-induced osteoporosis. Endocrinology 1999; 140: 4382–9.
29. Saito JK, Davis JW, Wasnich RD, Ross PD. Users of low-dose glucocorticoids have increased bone loss rates: a longitudinal study. Calcif Tiss Int 1995; 57: 115–19.
30. Bornefalk E, Dahlen I, Michaelsson K, Ljunggren O, Ljunghall S. Age-dependent effect of oral glucocorticoids on markers of bone resorption in patients with acute asthma. Calcif Tissue Int 1998; 63: 9–13.
31. Adachi JD, Bensen WG, Bianchi F et al. Vitamin D and calcium in the prevention of corticosteroid induced osteoporosis: a 3 year followup. J Rheumatol 1996; 23: 995–1000.
32. Hodsman AB, Toogood JH, Jennings B. Differential effect of inhaled budesonide and oral prenisolone on serum osteocalcin. J Clin Endocrinol 1991; 72: 530–40.
33. Josse R, Adachi JD, Chines AA. Prevention of corticosteroid-induced osteoporosis with etidronate: one year follow-up with calcium only. Osteoporosis Int 1998; 8: 108.
34. Saag K, Emkey R, Cividino A. Effects of alendronate for two years on BMD and fractures in patients receiving glucocorticoids. Bone 1998; 23: S182.
35. Ruegsegger P, Medici TC, Anliker M. Corticosteroid-induced bone loss. A longitudinal study of alternate day

therapy in patients with bronchial asthma using quantitative computed tomography. Eur J Clin Pharmacol 1983; 25: 615–20.

36. Michel BA, Bloch DA, Fries JF. Predictors of fractures in early rheumatoid arthritis. J Rheumatol 1991; 18: 804–8.

37. van Staa TP, Leufkens HGM, Abenhaim L, Zhang B, Cooper C. Use of oral corticosteroids and risk of fractures. J Bone Miner Res 2000; 15: 993–1000.

38. LoCascio V, Bonucci E, Imbimbo B. Bone loss after glucocorticoid therapy. Calcif Tiss Int 1984; 36: 435–8.

39. Buckley LM, Leib ES, Cartularo KS. Calcium and vitamin D3 supplementation prevents bone loss in the spine secondary to low-dose corticosteroids in patients with rheumatoid arthritis. Ann Intern Med 1996; 125: 961–8.

40. Lowry PW, Sandborn WJ. A comparison of budesonide and mesalamine for active Crohn's disease. Gastroenterology 1999; 116: 1263.

41. Thomsen OO, Cortot A, Jewell D et al. A comparison of budesonide and mesalamine for active Crohn's disease. International Budesonide–Mesalamine Study Group. N Engl J Med 1998; 339: 370–4.

42. Wong CA, Walsh LJ, Smith CJ et al. Inhaled corticosteroid use and bone-mineral density in patients with asthma. Lancet 2000; 355: 1399–403.

43. Angulo P, Jorgensen RA, Keach JC, Dickson ER, Smith C, Lindor KD. Oral budesonide in the treatment of patients with primary biliary cirrhosis with a suboptimal response to ursodeoxycholic acid. Hepatology 2000; 31: 318–23.

44. D'Haens G, Verstraete A, Cheyns K, Aerden I, Bouillon R, Rutgeerts P. Bone turnover during short-term therapy with methylprednisolone or budesonide in Crohn's disease. Aliment Pharmacol Ther 1998; 12: 419–24.

45. Robinson RJ, Iqbal SJ, Wolfe R, Patel K, Abrams K, Mayberry JF. The effect of rectally administered steroids on bone turnover: a comparative study. Aliment Pharmacol Ther 1998; 12: 213–17.

46. Motley RJ, Crawley EO, Evans C, Rhodes J, Compston JE. Increased rate of spinal trabecular bone loss in patients with inflammatory bowel disease. Gut 1988; 29: 1332–6.

47. Bernstein CN, Seeger LL, Sayre JW, Anton PA, Artinian L, Shanahan F. Decreased bone density in inflammatory bowel disease is related to corticosteroid use and not disease diagnosis. J Bone Miner Res 1995; 10: 250–6.

48. Matsuda K, Watanabe T, Abo Y et al. Severe complications of ulcerative colitis after high-dose prednisolone and azathioprine treatment. J Gastroenterol 1999; 34: 390–4.

49. Hougardy DM, Peterson GM, Bleasel MD, Randall CT. Is enough attention being given to the adverse effects of corticosteroid therapy? J Clin Pharm Ther 2000; 25: 227–34.

50. Bjarnason I, Macpherson A, Mackintosh C, Buxton-Thomas M, Forgacs I, Moniz C. Reduced bone density in patients with inflammatory bowel disease. Gut 1997; 40: 228–33.

51. Schoon EJ, Blok BM, Geerling BJ, Russel MG, Stockbrugger RW, Brummer RJ. Bone mineral density in patients with recently diagnosed inflammatory bowel disease. Gastroenterology 1203; 119: 1203–8.

52. Thearle M, Horlick M, Bilezikian JP et al. Osteoporosis: an unusual presentation of childhood Crohn's disease. J Clin Endocrinol Metab 2000; 85: 2122–6.

53. Vogelsang H, Klamert M, Resch H, Ferenci P. Dietary vitamin D intake in patients with Crohn's disease. Wien Klin Wochenschr 1995; 107: 578–81.

54. Clements D, Compston JE, Evans WD, Rhodes J. Hormone replacement therapy prevents bone loss in patients with inflammatory bowel disease. Gut 1993; 34: 1543–6.

55. Lin CL, Moniz C, Chambers TJ, Chow JW. Colitis causes bone loss in rats through suppression of bone formation. Gastroenterology 1996; 111: 1263–71.

56. Giuliani N, Pedrazzoni M, Passeri G, Girasole G. Bisphosphonates inhibit IL-6 production by human osteoblast-like cells. Scand J Rheumatol 1998; 27: 38–41.

57. Thomson BM, Saklatvala J, Chambers TJ. Osteoblasts mediate interleukin 1 stimulation of bone resorption by rat osteoclasts. J Exp Med 1986; 164: 104–12.

58. Thomson BM, Mundy GR, Chambers TJ. Tumor necrosis factors alpha and beta induce osteoblastic cells to stimulate osteoclastic bone resorption. J Immunol 1987; 138: 775–9.

59. Manolagas SC, Bellido T, Jilka RL. Sex steroids, cytokines and the bone marrow: new concepts on the pathogenesis of osteoporosis. Ciba Found Symp 1995; 191: 187–96; discussion 197–202.

60. Tsuboi M, Kawakami A, Nakashima T et al. Tumor necrosis factor-alpha and interleukin-1beta increase the Fas-mediated apoptosis of human osteoblasts. J Lab Clin Med 1999; 134: 222–31.

61. Kurokouchi K, Kambe F, Yasukawa K et al. TNF-alpha increases expression of IL-6 and ICAM-1 genes through activation of NF-kappaB in osteoblast-like ROS17/2.8 cells. J Bone Miner Res 1998; 13: 1290–9.

62. Fernandez-Martin JL, Kurian S, Farmer P, Nanes MS. Tumor necrosis factor activates a nuclear inhibitor of vitamin D and retinoid-X receptors. Mol Cell Endocrinol 1998; 141: 65–72.

63. Votta BJ, Bertolini DR. Cytokine suppressive anti-inflammatory compounds inhibit bone resorption in vitro. Bone 1994; 15: 533–8.

64. Morony S, Capparelli C, Lee R et al. A chimeric form of osteoprotegerin inhibits hypercalcemia and bone resorption induced by IL-1beta, TNF-alpha, PTH, PTHrP, and 1, 25(OH)2D3. J Bone Miner Res 1999; 14: 1478–85.

65. Conron M, Young C, Beynon HL. Calcium metabolism in sarcoidosis and its clinical implications. Rheumatol (Oxf) 2000; 39: 707–13.

66. Bosch X. Hypercalcemia due to endogenous overproduction of 1,25-dihydroxyvitamin D in Crohn's disease. Gastroenterology 1998; 114: 1061–5.

67. Kantorovich V, Adams JS, Targan SR, Hassard PV, Vasiliauskas EA. Endogenous Overproduction of 1, 25-dihydroxyvitamin D in patients with Crohn's disease. American Society for Bone and Mineral Research Meeting 2000.

68. Barre PE, Gascon-Barre M, Meakins JL, Goltzman D. Hydroxychloroquine treatment of hypercalcemia in a patient with sarcoidosis undergoing hemodialysis. Am J Med 1987; 82: 1259–62.

69. Buckley LM, Leib ES, Cartularo KS, Vacek PM, Cooper SM. Effects of low dose methotrexate on the bone mineral density of patients with rheumatoid arthritis. J Rheumatol 1997; 24: 1489–94.

70. Bianchi ML, Cimaz R, Galbiati E, Corona F, Cherubini R, Bardare M. Bone mass change during methotrexate treatment in patients with juvenile rheumatoid arthritis. Osteoporosis Int 1999; 10: 20–5.

71. Epstein S, Shane E, Bilezikian JP. Organ transplantation and osteoporosis. Curr Opin Rheumatol 1995; 7: 255–61.

72. Inoue T, Kawamura I, Matsuo M et al. Lesser reduction in bone mineral density by the immunosuppressant, FK506, compared with cyclosporine in rats. Transplantation 2000; 70: 774–9.

73. Aroldi A, Tarantino A, Montagnino G, Cesana B, Cocucci C, Ponticelli C. Effects of three immunosuppressive regimens on vertebral bone density in renal transplant recipients: a prospective study. Transplantation 1997; 63: 380–6.

74. Amin S, LaValley MP, Simms RW, Felson DT. The role of vitamin D in corticosteroid-induced osteoporosis: a meta-analytic approach. Arthritis Rheum 1999; 42: 1740–51.

75. Anonymous. Recommendations for the prevention and treatment of glucocorticoid-induced osteoporosis. Ameri-

can College of Rheumatology Task Force on Osteoporosis Guidelines. Arthritis Rheum 1996; 39: 1791–801.

76. Homik J, Suarez-Almazor ME, Shea B, Cranney A, Wells G, Tugwell P. Calcium and vitamin D for corticosteroid-induced osteoporosis. Cochrane Database of Systematic Reviews [Computer file] 2000: CD000952.

77. Sambrook P, Birmingham J, Kelly P et al. Prevention of corticosteroid osteoporosis. A comparison of calcium, calcitriol, and calcitonin. N Engl J Med 1993; 328: 1747–52.

78. Healy JH, Paget S, Williams-Russo P. A randomized controlled trial of salmon calcitonin to prevent bone loss in corticosteroid treated temporal arteritis and polymyalgia rheumatica. Calcif Tissue Int 1996; 59: 73.

79. Adachi JD, Bensen WG, Bell MJ et al. Salmon calcitonin nasal spray in the prevention of corticosteroid-induced osteoporosis. Br J Rheumatol 1997; 36: 255–9.

80. Luengo M, Picado C, Del Rio L, Guanabens N, Montserrat JM, Setoain J. Treatment of steroid-induced osteopenia with calcitonin in corticosteroid-dependent asthma. A one-year follow-up study. Am Rev Respir Dis 1990; 142: 104–7.

81. Luengo M, Pons F, Martinez de Osaba MJ, Picado C. Prevention of further bone mass loss by nasal calcitonin in patients on long term glucocorticoid therapy for asthma: a two year follow up study. Thorax 1994; 49: 1099–102.

82. Ringe JD, Welzel D. Salmon calcitonin in the therapy of corticoid-induced osteoporosis. Eur J Clin Pharmacol 1987; 33: 35.

83. Kotaniemi A, Piirainen H, Paimela L et al. Is continuous intranasal salmon calcitonin effective in treating axial bone loss in patients with active rheumatoid arthritis receiving low dose glucocorticoid therapy? J Rheumatol 1996; 23: 1875–9.

84. Homik JE, Cranney A, Shea B et al. A metaanalysis on the use of bisphosphonates in corticosteroid induced osteoporosis. J Rheumatol 1999; 26: 1148–57.

85. Plotkin LI, Weinstein RS, Parfitt AM, Roberson PK, Manolagas SC, Bellido T. Prevention of osteocyte and osteoblast apoptosis by bisphosphonates and calcitonin. J Clin Invest 1999; 104: 1363–74.

86. Adachi JD, Bensen WG, Brown J et al. Intermittent etidronate therapy to prevent corticosteroid-induced osteoporosis. N Engl J Med 1997; 337: 382–7.

87. Saag KG, Emkey R, Schnitzer TJ et al. Alendronate for the prevention and treatment of glucocorticoid-induced osteoporosis. Glucocorticoid-Induced Osteoporosis Intervention Study Group. N Engl J Med 1998; 339: 292–9.

88. Reid D, Cohen S, Pack S, Chines A, Ethgen D. Risedronate reduces the incidence of vertebral fractures in patients on chronic corticosteroid therapy. Arthritis Rheum 1998; 41: S136.

89. Cohen S, Levy RM, Keller M et al. Risedronate therapy prevents corticosteroid-induced bone loss: a twelve-month, multicenter, randomized, double-blind, placebo-controlled, parallel-group study. Arthritis Rheum 1999; 42: 2309–18.

90. Reid D, Devogelaer JP, Hughes R et al. Risedronate is effective and well tolerated in treating corticosteroid-induced osteoporosis. American College of Rheumatology annual meeting 1998.

91. Reid D, Cohen S, Pack S. Risedronate is an effective and well-tolerated therapy in both the treatment and prevention of corticosteroid-induced osteoporosis. Bone 1998; 23: S402.

92. Adachi JD, Pack S, Chines AA. Intermittent etidronate and corticosteroid-induced osteoporosis. N Engl J Med 1997; 337: 1921.

93. Bernstein CN, Seeger LL, Anton PA et al. A randomized, placebo-controlled trial of calcium supplementation for decreased bone density in corticosteroid-using patients with inflammatory bowel disease: a pilot study. Aliment Pharmacol Ther 1996; 10: 777–86.

94. von Tirpitz C, Klaus J, Bruckel J et al. Increase of bone mineral density with sodium fluoride in patients with Crohn's disease. Eur J Gastroenterol Hepatol 2000; 12: 19–24.

95. Vogelsang H, Ferenci P, Resch H, Kiss A, Gangl A. Prevention of bone mineral loss in patients with Crohn's disease by long-term oral vitamin D supplementation. Eur J Gastroenterol Hepatol 1995; 7: 609–14.

96. Haderslav KV, Tjellesen H, Sorensen HA, Staun M. Alendronate increases lumbar spine bone mineral density in patients with Crohn's disease. Gastroenterology 2000; 119: 639–646.

97. Sass DA, Bowman AR, Yuan Z, Ma Y, Jee WS, Epstein S. Alendronate prevents cyclosporin A-induced osteopenia in the rat. Bone 1997; 21: 65–70.

98. Robinson RJ, Iqbal SJ, Al-Azzawi F, Abrams K, Mayberry JF. Sex hormone status and bone metabolism in men with Crohn's disease. Aliment Pharmacol Ther 1998; 12: 21–5.

Section III

BACK TO THE LABORATORY BENCH

50 | Epilogue: Bench to bedside and back to bench

STEPHAN R. TARGAN, LOREN C. KARP AND FERGUS SHANAHAN

Where we have been and where we are going

The preceding chapters combine to provide an excellent depiction of all facets of the study of IBD, from bench to bedside. The individual chapters are components of a coherent, albeit detailed, story of the local and systemic pathophysiology of intestinal inflammation, presented in association with a well-reasoned series of management strategies based on this knowledge. Research advances and current concepts of etiopathogenesis are described in the context of what is already known of the clinicopathologic features of these disorders. The book as a whole illustrates the effectiveness of a multilateral approach by basic scientists and clinician investigators in the field of IBD. The conclusions of the chapters were drawn purposefully to offer a glimpse of where the field is moving to stimulate research back at the bench.

The interplay of state-of-the-art technology and greater understanding of the pathophysiology in both human and animal disease has brought us far along our road, and has led to excellent translational research resulting in the development of better therapeutic options. Upon this model our efforts can be maximized, our scope expanded, and our progress expedited to take us the rest of the way. We know IBD comprises numerous discrete entities that can be stratified by a variety of subclinical and clinical markers that may well identify which patients are likely to respond to any particular therapeutic intervention. We also have made great progress toward defining the roles played by infectious agents in the etiology or pathogenesis of IBD. Evidence suggests that the elevated immune function, characteristic of these diseases, is in response to normal commensal bacteria rather than any specific pathogen. It is unlikely that the role of infectious agents correlates directly with the disease responses that are characteristic of IBD. More likely the process is indirect, requiring any number of combinations of genes, immune responses, and environmental triggers, to manifest as disease. Specific manipulation of bacterial expression and the corresponding immune response may be the basis of very effective therapies in the near future. Research over the past several years has changed the management of IBD. The effectiveness of therapeutic anti-tumor necrosis factor-α monoclonal antibodies (anti-TNF-α) in a portion of patients with Crohn's disease illustrates the unique immune mechanisms that underlie the intestinal inflammation in different subpopulations of patients.

The foundation of our *Bench to Bedside and Back to Bench* concept has been laid, and the planks of the foundation are described in detail by the chapters of this book. The final decades of the last century saw the Bench to Bedside portion of the equation evolve. New therapies based on laboratory science were developed, tested and some came to be used in clinical practice. At the very end of the last century only a few compounds were tested in humans with associated parallel basic science, or translational, investigations. Although such studies were few, the yield in terms of information was great.

Not long ago only a few animal models were available for the study of dysregulated intestinal inflammation. In the intervening years the number of models has grown to well over 30, mainly in the form of genetically engineered mouse strains. Analysis of these models has taught us that chronic colitis can be induced by diverse genetic abnormalities. However, the inflammatory patterns and their clinical expressions are also distinct, yielding new opportunities to link alterations in specific genetic loci with alterations of T cell responses, mucosal permeability, and *in-vivo* clinical patterns.

Another striking area of progress in IBD research that has traversed from the Bench to the Bedside and back again is related to the issue of a microbial pathogenesis of IBD. Despite more than 50 years of

Stephan R. Targan, Fergus Shanahan and Loren C. Karp (eds.), Inflammatory Bowel Disease: From Bench to Bedside, 2nd Edition, 887–891.
© 2003 *Kluwer Academic Publishers. Printed in Great Britain*

research a specific bacterial or viral organism has not been identified as a direct cause of IBD pathogenesis. Investigations in animals, however, identified a role for commensal bacteria in induction of dysregulated mucosal inflammation. Verification of bacterial involvement came with the finding that, despite the genetic or cellular manipulation in any given model, its attendant mucosal inflammation is lost in a pathogen-free environment.

We now know that there are two ways in which the mucosa responds to bacterial antigens. The antigen-specific T cell response is well characterized. A more complex relationship exists between bacterial structures such as lipopolysaccharides and peptido-glycans that have repetitive sequences that are recognized by cell receptors. The relationship is receiving a great amount of attention at the time of this writing. The most exciting of these receptors appear to be present on epithelial cells and macrophages and are known as toll-like receptors. First described in Drosophila, toll-like receptors engage bacterial structures and generate mucosal inflammation. Alterations in such receptor signaling may well play a key role in the inflammation of IBD. Bacterial antigens are likely to trigger certain T cell responses in the mucosa, and the balance of these responses is critical to regulating the intestinal immune response. T cell responses can be divided broadly into 'disease-inducing' and 'disease-preventing', depending upon the cytokines released. In the majority of animal models, the presence of effector cells secreting T helper-1 (Th1) cytokines (interferon-gamma, IFN-γ, TNF-α) is responsible for disease, and by this criterion these models are reflective of human Crohn's disease. One clear exception is the T cell receptor-alpha (TCR-α) 'knockout' mouse in which a unique subset of TCR-β dim/interleukin (IL)-4 producing cells is responsible for inflammation; this model may therefore be considered to be more similar to human ulcerative colitis. Two populations of disease-preventing or down-regulatory T cells have been described; Tr-1/IL-10 producing T cells and the T-helper-3 (Th3)/transforming growth factor-beta (TGF-β) producing T cells. Studies have demonstrated that these two T cell populations counterbalance the effector cells and protect against dysregulated inflammation. It is an imbalance between these effector and regulatory populations that presumably results in disease expression.

Renewed interest in commensal bacteria and their relationship to T cell responses in the mucosa has led to investigations demonstrating that the transfer of a specific subset of bacterial antigen-stimulated Th1 cells can induce colitis in animals. Furthermore, down-regulatory or T-regulatory-1 (Tr-1)/IL-10-producing cells, stimulated by the same bacterial antigens as the pathogenic Th1 cells, prevent expression of colitis when co-transferred with these antigen-specific Th1 cells. These bacterial antigen-triggered effector and regulatory cell populations clearly influence the interplay between clinical expression and mucosal inflammation. The diversity in expression of colitis, i.e. cecal involvement, rectal ulceration, specific ileal involvement, ulcerative lethal disease, is dependent upon any one or more genetic abnormalities. Furthermore, the same genetically altered animal can manifest a different expression of disease when raised in different housing facilities, suggesting an additional mechanism for the heterogeneity of these diseases. It is quite possible that genetic and microenvironmental heterogeneity in these animal models is similar to what is seen among patients with IBD. This paradigm is now the foundation of our understanding of pathogenic mechanisms in human disease.

The investigations in animal models of mucosal inflammation have proceeded in parallel with those in human IBD. Much progress has been made in identifying the genes associated with these inflammatory disorders. Genome-wide scanning and candidate gene approaches have revealed several disease-associated loci. One important implication of these studies is that IBD is an oligogenetic disease: genome-wide scans thus far have revealed at least four loci confirmed by independent groups, and an additional three others are suggested. Some of these chromosomes and loci are associated with Crohn's disease and/or ulcerative colitis individually, and others are associated with both. Marker antibodies and/or disease expression further refines the associations. Multiple studies in humans, as well as the animal studies summarized above, have demonstrated differing genetic associations with clinical phenotype as well as marker antibody expression. Allelic diversity at the susceptibility loci thus probably underlies the immunologic and clinical heterogeneity of IBD. The chromosome 16 locus was the first to be identified by a whole genome approach. The IBD1 gene (NOD2) has been identified by using a positional cloning strategy – linkage followed by linkage disequilibrium mapping. Three independent associations for Crohn's disease were discovered. Simultaneously, by a candidate gene approach, an independent group also demonstrated association between the NOD2 and Crohn's disease. Clearly, NOD2 is a susceptibility gene to Crohn's disease, as it increases an individual's risk for Crohn's disease, but it is neither sufficient nor necessary for the development of the disease.

Significant advances have already been made, based on the identification of NOD2 and its relationship to subtypes of Crohn's disease. Hugot *et al.* and Abreu *et al.* have recently published separate reports demonstrating that fibrosing Crohn's disease is associated with the dose effect of two mutations, and several other groups have further confirmed these findings, with results not yet published at the time of this writing. These studies indicate that ability to predict which patients will experience a more complicated course is in the immediate future. NOD2 will no doubt continue to shed light on the etiologic pathways of IBD and accelerate the discovery of additional susceptibility genes for IBD.

The identification of IBD-associated marker antibodies at the bench has made a great impact on patient care at the bedside, and in turn has stimulated further laboratory research. Since the discovery of perinuclear antineutrophil cytoplasmic antibodies (ANCA) more than 10 years ago, much has been learned about the significance of marker antibodies in the serum of patients with IBD. In addition to pANCA, interest has focused on antibodies to *Saccharomyces cerevisiae* (ASCA), which have been shown to differentiate between ulcerative colitis and Crohn's disease. Progress continues with these antibodies, and other bacterial antigens have been detected which identify strongly with disease-associated antibodies in IBD. These marker antibodies are important for their diagnostic utility and stratification of patients into distinct clinical phenotypes. These antibodies are associated not only with the different locations of disease, but also with aggressiveness of disease course and responses to treatment by specific manipulation of cytokines. It is of particular interest that some of the marker antibodies, such as pANCA, appear to be cross-reactive with commensal bacterial antigens. Therefore, the presence of marker antibodies provides a platform as a basis to study bacterial–host interactions as well as to define subsets of patients with Crohn's disease and ulcerative colitis. At the bench we shall now endeavor to define the relevance of these findings in animals to the diversity of human disease seen among patients with IBD. In addition we must determine which immune alterations and bacterial sensitivity in the different animal models are represented among the varied clinical expressions of disease seen in these disorders. From our findings in animal models, we assume that patterns of immune responses to environmental and bacterial antigens differ widely among groups of patients with Crohn's disease. Landers *et al.* have recently reported that expression of certain serologic markers clusters in certain patient subgroups. Even in groups of patients that have been classified as 'indeterminant', expression of certain markers remain consistent over time and suggest the clinical course that is ultimately taken, as has been shown by Joossens *et al.* Thus, what seemed futuristic only recently, clinically useful information derived from studying genes and their relationship to immunophysiologic responses will be obtainable in a much shorter time. It is therefore possible that certain antibiotics might be most effective in those patients who have the most robust responses to bacterial antigens. Likewise, the most robust responses to the broadest number of these antigens may define those patients who can best be treated by manipulation of the bacterial flora. If the antigens to which an individual is sensitive are among the anaerobic bacteria then metronidazole may be more effective. If these antigens are among the aerobic bacteria, then these patients may best be treated with ciprofloxacin. Finally, in patients who are immunoreactive to both aerobic and anaerobic populations, such patients may require a combination of both metronidazole and ciprofloxacin.

Although many inflammatory molecules are elevated in the mucosa of patients with IBD, their precise role in disease pathogenesis has never been determined. In animal models the success of treatment by manipulation of Th1 cytokines, e.g. antibodies to TNF-α, IFN-γ or IL-12, led to trials of anti-TNF-α for the treatment of Crohn's disease. Results of these trials showed for the first time that cytokine expression in the mucosa could alter disease course in the majority of patients with Crohn's disease. 'Back to Bench' research demonstrated down-regulation of Th1 cytokine-producing cells in the inflamed mucosa to the level of those in the uninflamed areas as one of the mechanisms responsible for the disease ameliorating effect. Unlike some animal models in which cecal bacterial antigens drive the dominant Th1 profile, no similar antigen trigger has been identified in human disease. A proportion of Crohn's disease patients can be treated by manipulation of the bacterial flora by either antibiotic therapy or a diversion of the fecal stream, which suggests diverse responses to bacterial antigens among the Crohn's disease population. In ulcerative colitis, patients with high levels of pANCA and serum IgG reactivity to the *E. coli* antigen, OmpC, are three times more likely to develop chronic pouchitis than patients without high levels of pANCA. These findings, taken together, highlight the potential importance of bacterial interactions in the induction or maintenance of inflammation. Overall, the diversity of clinical expression seen in IBD is very likely dependent upon a combination of genetic abnormalities and the presence of certain commensal bacteria.

The 21st century – the age of translationalism

With the rapidly growing body of knowledge, it behooves us to effect the most expeditious application of our findings to patient care and research in return. We must now determine which of the many discoveries made in animals are relevant to human disease. To do so requires a process by which ideas can be exchanged among investigators and work done simultaneously, crossing between animal models and *in-vitro* testing for human disease. Given what is already known about the heterogeneity of these disorders, this process is likely to be complex, and it is not yet possible to say how many combinations of genes and antigens are likely to result in some sort of chronic intestinal inflammation or extraintestinal disease. Nevertheless, these investigations are crucial to developing phenotypically defined disease groups.

Translational research will lead to some very exciting discoveries, based on the 'omics', genomics, proteinomics and phenomics. Genomic investigations of genes and their function are bringing about a revolution in our understanding of the molecular mechanisms of disease, including the complex interplay of genetic and environmental factors. Genomics is also stimulating the discovery of breakthrough pharmaceuticals by revealing hundreds of new biological targets for the development of drugs, and by giving scientists innovative ways to design new drugs, vaccines and diagnostics. Genomics-based therapeutics include 'traditional' small chemical drugs, protein drugs, and potentially gene therapy.

Proteinomics refers to the study of proteins expressed by genes and understanding the role of every human protein. By manipulation of these proteins the course of the disease process can be altered and potentially the expression of disease can be eliminated altogether.

Phenomics is the study of the result or sequelae of a gene's function, i.e. the disease manifestation. Phenomics is the ultimate point of tomorrow's drug discovery effort as it allows researchers to rapidly validate genes as potential targets for drug discovery and point them to the right individuals. At present, researchers use genomic 'knockout' animal models to determine the biological function of a gene, and then compare the function to that of humans. As diseases are related to subtle changes in protein activity, rather than to complete loss or gain in any one protein, researchers must produce varying changes in protein activity to determine a gene's relation to the specific disease process.

Through these efforts we can meet our challenge to refine patient subsets, not strictly from clinical points of view. There is a tendency among clinicians to 'lump' patients into groups based on certain clinical aspects of their disease; e.g. disease in the ileum. Nevertheless, not all patients with ileal disease are the same. Simultaneously we must refrain from 'splitting' so many subtypes so as not to lose sight of 'the forest for the trees.' To determine the phenotypes, the genetic and immunologic origins and clinical significance of the phenotypes requires a very certain type of investigator – the translationalist. We need to encourage a cadre of educated and creative translational investigators. Such individuals will have in-depth knowledge of disease pathogenesis combined with medical training and education in clinical investigation, and with these tools, they will bring about our expectations for the 21st century (Table 1).

Too many targets, too few patients

Estimates have placed the number of individuals affected with IBD at as high as two million. The actual pool of patients willing and able to participate in clinical trials is much, much smaller. A primary goal of the translationalists, then, must be the development of 'reagent-grade' patients. Well-defined populations will permit highly specific eligibility criteria for study participation. It is our challenge to accelerate our knowledge of these diseases without wasting our precious patient resources. In the 1990s we were successful in our efforts to capture the interest of the biotechnology and pharmaceutical industries to encourage them to focus on developing new and improved treatments for IBD. This success has strained our resources and there are now not

Table 1. IBD research in the 21st century

	Effort	Result
1.	Intercommunication of rodent and human genetic research findings	Identification of genetic mutations and interactions with relevance to human diseases
2.	Definition of IBD relevant bacterial antigens, i.e. commensal associated molecular patterns (CAMPs)	Definition of environmental triggers
3.	Prioritization of clinical trials via cooperation between academic institutions and the pharmaceutical industry	Rapid answers, targeted therapeutic efficacy
4.	Definition of 'reagent grade' patients	Customization of diagnosis and prognosis and therefore, therapeutic targets and treatment plans
5.	Crossbreeding of relevant rodent models to better approximate human IBD subtypes	Acceleration of the progress of 1–4

enough patients to do all of the trials necessary to bring a product to market. Thus, the responsibilities will fall upon this new generation of translationalists to prioritize the potential benefit of the compounds. We need to make highly informed, difficult decisions from among many promising options. Should the biopharm industry direct the emphasis of clinical testing or should translationalists influence which of the many targets are the best for medical intervention? It is our challenge to ensure that those with financial resources understand the clinical and pathophysiologic milieu in which their efforts are being devoted.

It is also important to coordinate the efforts in the academic laboratories with those of the biopharmaceutical industry. We would do well to determine which animal models are most relevant to human disease and ensure that these same models are those used by industry for their efficacy studies. There is already evidence that the molecules responsible for acute disease flares are different from those involved with chronic inflammation. Such findings need to be shared with industry so that therapeutic development can be targeted for such specific situations. A further need, which requires the coordination of academic and industry laboratories, is to apply novel

drug delivery systems to our models. For example, bacteria have been used to deliver IL-10 therapy in mouse models of colitis. Among the benefits of such cooperation are more limited immunomodulatory effects from treatments, and minimization of lengthy drug-administering infusions.

Given the current status of research in IBD, well-orchestrated cooperation between the basic and clinical sciences and academic and pharmaceutical industry research is likely to yield major advances in understanding of the disease and the development of treatments. The next edition of this textbook is sure to contain examples of the fruits of this cooperation and feature contributions from this new generation of well-trained translationalists. As we envision it, patient management in the 21st century would be far more efficient, with fewer discomforts for the patient, potentially altering the natural history of the disease. In a typical example a patient would present with diarrhea of 1 week's duration. A battery of non-invasive tests would be administered to characterize the immunogenetic phenotype of disease. A diagnosis and prognosis would be made, i.e. IBD#1, or IBD#2, etc. Finally, a specific, targeted therapeutic plan would be designed and implemented that would ameliorate the patient's disease.

Index

Stephan R. Targan, Fergus Shanahan and Loren C. Karp (eds.), Inflammatory Bowel Disease: From Bench to Bedside, 2nd Edition, 893–903.
© 2003 *Kluwer Academic Publishers. Printed in Great Britain*